CAM

WITHDRAWN FROM STOCK 21/05/24
RM

Cambridge Textbook of Effective Treatments in Psychiatry

This is a book of psychiatry at its most practical level. It aims to answer the sorts of questions psychiatrists ask on a daily basis. What treatments are available for the condition that I think this patient has? What is the relative value of each of these treatments? Are there any other treatments that I should be considering if a first approach has failed? Is there any value in combinations of treatment? And, can I be sure that the evidence and recommendations I read are free from bias?

The content is organised into three major parts. After an introductory section discussing the nature and classification of psychiatric disorders and the inherent problems of these diagnostic systems, the coverage moves on, in Part II, to review the major modalities of treatment and the priniciples involved. The core of the book is Part III, where treatments are discussed according to the diagnostic groupings. In almost all cases, the chapters have been written as partnerships, or group efforts, involving internationally recognised experts from North America and Europe, with synthesis of their recommendations.

All professionals in mental health want to give the best treatments for their patients. This book provides clinicians with the knowledge and guidance to achieve this aim.

Peter Tyrer is Professor of Community Psychiatry in the Department of Psychological Medicine, Imperial College, London, UK.

Kenneth R. Silk is Professor of Psychiatry and Director of the Personality Disorders Program in the Department of Psychiatry at the University of Michigan Medical School, Ann Arbor, USA.

Cambridge Textbook of Effective Treatments in Psychiatry

Peter Tyrer and Kenneth R. Silk

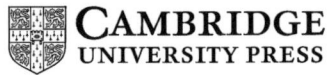

CAMBRIDGE UNIVERSITY PRESS
Cambridge, New York, Melbourne, Madrid, Cape Town, Singapore, São Paulo

Cambridge University Press
The Edinburgh Building, Cambridge CB2 8RU, UK

Published in the United States of America by Cambridge University Press, New York

www.cambridge.org
Information on this title: www.cambridge.org/9780521842280

First published 2008

Printed in the United Kingdom at the University Press, Cambridge

A catalogue record for this publication is available from the British Library

ISBN 978-0-521-84228-0 hardback

Cambridge University Press has no responsibility for the persistence or accuracy of URLs for external or third-party internet websites referred to in this publication, and does not guarantee that any content on such websites is, or will remain, accurate or appropriate.

Every effort has been made in preparing this publication to provide accurate and up-to-date information which is in accord with accepted standards and practice at the time of publication. Although case histories are drawn from actual cases, every effort has been made to disguise the identities of the individuals involved. Nevertheless, the authors, editors and publishers can make no warranties that the information contained herein is totally free from error, not least because clinical standards are constantly changing through research and regulation. The authors, editors and publishers therefore disclaim all liability for direct or consequential damages resulting from the use of material contained in this publication. Readers are strongly advised to pay careful attention to information provided by the manufacturer of any drugs or equipment that they plan to use.

Contents

Contributors

Kostas Agath
Westminster Substance Misuse Services
London, UK

Taryn M. Allen
Department of Psychiatry
Yale University School of Medicine,
USA

George W. Arana
Mental Health Service
RHJ VA Medical Center
Charleston
South Carolina, USA

David Baldwin
Clinical Neuroscience Division
University of Southampton
RSH Hospital
Southampton, UK

Yvonne Bannon
University of South Florida
College of Medicine
Department of Psychiatry and Behavioural Medicine
Tampa, FL, USA

James Barrett
Charing Cross Hospital
Gender Identity Clinic, Claybrook Centre
London, UK

Anthony Bateman
Halliwick Unit
St Ann's Hospital, St Ann's Road
London, UK

Shannon Bellefleur
University of Michigan
Addiction Psychiatry Training Program
Ann Arbor, MI, USA

Andrew Bennett
Weill Cornell Medical School
White Plains, NY, USA

Jeffrey A. Berman
Department of Psychiatry
Robert Wood Johnson Medical School
VA Health Care System
Lyons
New Jersey, NJ, USA

German E. Berrios
University of Cambridge
Addenbroke's Hospital
Cambridge, UK

Nancee Blum
University of Iowa
2880 JPP
Iowa City
Iowa, USA

Henrietta Bowden-Jones
Substance Misuse Services
Central North West London
Mental Health NHS Trust,
London, UK

Owen Bowden-Jones
Drug Treatment Centre
Chelsea and Westminster Hospital
London, UK

Cora Collette Breuner
Childrens' Hospital and Medical Center
Seattle
Washington, USA

Janet Brotchie
Lead Psychologist in Substance Misuse
Central and North West London Mental Health NHS Trust
London, UK

Kirk J. Brower
University of Michigan Addiction Research Center
Rachel Upjohn Building
Ann Arbor, MI, USA

Cara Brown
University of Toronto
Toronto, ON, Canada

Leslie L. Buckley
University Health Network
Toronto, ON, Canada

Alan J. Budney
Department of Psychiatry
University of Arkansas for Medical Sciences
Little Rock, AR, USA

Peter Bulow
Department of Psychiatry
Division of Brain Stimulation and Therapeutic Modulation
New York State Psychiatric Institute
NY, USA

Rose Calderon
Department of Child and Adolescent Psychiatry
University of Washington Medical School
Seattle, WA, USA

Rishi Caleyachetty
GKT Medical School
Guys Campus
London, UK

Laura Campbell-Sills
University of California
San Diego
La Jolla, CA, USA

Kathleen M. Carroll
Division of Substance Abuse
Yale University School of Medicine
New Haven, CT, USA

Edward Coffey
Department of Psychiatry
Henry Ford Health System
Detroit, MI, USA

Brent Collett
Department of Child and Adult Psychiatry
University of Washington Medical School
Seattle, WA, USA

David K. Conn
University of Toronto
Toronto, ON, Canada

Deirdre Conroy
University of Michigan Addiction Research Center
Department of Psychiatry and Addiction
Research Center
Ann Arbor, MI, USA

William H. Coryell
Department of Psychiatry
University of Iowa
Iowa City, IA, USA

Michelle Craske
Department of Psychology
University of California
Los Angeles, CA, USA

Mike Crawford
Department of Psychological Medicine
Imperial College London
Claybrook Centre
Charing Cross Campus
London, UK

Scott Crow
Department of Psychiatry
University of Minnesota Medical School
Minneapolis, MN, USA

Karim Dar
Gatehouse Alcohol Clinic
St Bernard's Hospital
Southall
Middx, UK

Ed. Day
Department of Psychiatry
Queen Elizabeth Psychiatric Hospital
Edgbaston
Birmingham, UK

Shoumitro Deb
Department of Psychiatry
University of Birmingham
Queen Elizabeth Psychiatric Hospital
Birmingham, UK

Michelle DeKlyen
Center for Research on Clinical Well-being
Princeton University
Princeton, NJ, USA

Angeles Diaz-Caneja
Wolverton Gardens Child and Family Consultation Service
London, UK

Christopher Dowrick
Department of Primary Care
University of Liverpool
Liverpool, UK

Melissa M. Dudas
New York College of Osteopathic Medicine
Norwalk, CT, USA

Caroline J. Easton
Division of Substance Abuse
Yale University School of Medicine
New Haven, CT, USA

Christopher Fairburn
Department of Psychiatry
Oxford University, Warneford Hospital
Oxford, UK

Peter Fonagy
University College London
Chief Executive
The Anna Freud Centre
Sub-Department of Clinical Health Psychology
University College London
London, UK

Laura Gage
Department of Psychiatry
University of Toronto
Toronto, ON, Canada

Elena Garralda
Imperial College London
Academic Unit of Child and Adolescent Psychiatry
St Mary's Campus
Norfolk Place
London, UK

John Geddes
Department of Psychiatry
University of Oxford
Warneford Hospital
Oxford, UK

Tony P. George
Department of Psychiatry
University of Toronto
Faculty of Medicine
Centre for Addiction and Mental Health (CAMH)
Toronto, ON, Canada

Rachel Gershenson
DePaul University
Chicago, IL, USA

Ian Goodyer
Cambridge University
Douglas House
Cambridge, UK

Jonathan Green
Academic Department of Child and
Adolescent Psychiatry
University of Manchester
Booth Hall Children's Hospital
Blackley, Manchester, UK

Sally Guthrie
The University of Michigan
College of Pharmacy
Ann Arbor, MI, USA

Alissa Haedt
Department of Psychology
University of Iowa
Iowa City, IA, USA

Katherine Halmi
New York Presbyterian Hospital
the Westchester Division
White Plains
NY, USA

Phil Harrison-Read
Department of Psychiatry
Royal Free Hospital
London, UK

Amy Henry
Division of Child and Adolescent Psychiatry
Department of Psychiatry and Behavioural Sciences
University of Washington School of Medicine
Seattle, WA, USA

Stefanie A. Hlastala
Department of Child and Adolescent Psychiatry
University of Washington School of Medicine
Seattle
WA, USA

Matthew Hodes
Imperial College London
St Mary's Campus
London, UK

Patricia Howlin
Department of Psychology
Institute of Psychiatry
King's College, London, UK

Philippa Hugo
Department of Psychiatry
St George's Medical School
Tooting
London, UK

Brian W. Jacobs
The Michael Rutter Centre
South London & Maudsley NHS Trust
London, UK

Anthony James
High Adolescent and Family Unit
Warneford Hospital
Oxford, UK

Peter B. Jones
Department of Psychiatry
Addenbrooke's Hospital
Cambridge, UK

Pamela K. Keel
Department of Psychology
University of Iowa
Iowa City, IA, USA

George A. Kenna
Center for Alcohol and Addiction Studies
Brown University
Providence, RI, USA

Adrienne J. Key
Department of Psychiatry
St George's Hospital Medical School
Tooting
London, UK

Michael King
Royal Free and University College Medial School
University College London
Royal Free Campus
London, UK

Thomas. R. Kosten
Department of Psychiatry
Baylor College of Medicine
Houston, TX, USA

Jonathan Krejci
Department of Psychiatry
Robert Wood Johnson Medical School
VA Health Care System
Lyons, NJ, USA

Manoj Kumar
Gatehouse Alcohol Clinic
St Bernard's Hospital
Southall
Middx, UK

Hower Kwon
Department of Child and Adolescent Psychiatry
University of Washington School of Medicine
Seattle, WA, USA

Krista L. Lanctôt
Department of Psychiatry
Sunnybrook Health Sciences Centre
Toronto, ON, Canada

Ariel J. Lang
Department of Psychiatry
University of California
San Diego, CA, USA

George Lewith
Complementary Medicine Research Unit, Mail Point OPH
Royal South Hants Hospital
Brintons Terrace
Southampton, UK

Sarah Hollingsworth Lisanby
Department of Psychiatry
Columbia University
Department of Biological Psychiatry
New York State Psychiatric Institute
NY, USA

Elizabeth McCauley
Department of Child and Adolescent Psychiatry
University of Washington Medical School
Seattle, WA, USA

Jon McClellan
Department of Child and Adolescent Psychiatry
University of Washington Medical School
Seattle, WA, USA

Daniel Maixner
University of Michigan
Dept of Psychiatry
Ann Arbor, MI, USA

Antonio Mantovani
Department of Psychiatry
Division of Brain Stimulation and Therapeutic Modulation
New York State Psychiatric Institute
NY, USA

Stephen R. Marder
West Los Angeles VA Healthcare Center
Los Angeles, CA, USA

Jane Marshall
Institute of Psychiatry
King's College London
London, UK

Randall D. Marshall
New York State Psychiatric Institute
NY, USA

Karen Milner
University of Michigan
Ann Arbor, MI, USA

Brent A. Moore
Department of Psychiatry
Yale University School of Medicine
Connecticut Mental Health Center
New Haven, CT, USA

Tara M. Neavins
Division of Substance Abuse
Yale University School of Medicine
Addiction and Substance Abuse Programs
New Haven, CT, USA

Sonya B. Norman
Department of Psychiatry
University of California
San Diego, CA, USA

David J. Nutt
Department of Psychopharmacology
University of Bristol
Psychopharmacology Unit
School of Medical Sciences
Bristol, UK

Erin L. O'Hea
Department of Psychology
La Salle University
Philadelphia, PA, USA

Heather Carmichael Olson
Division of Child Psychiatry
University of Washington School of Medicine
Seattle, WA, USA

Joel Paris
Institute of Community and Family Psychiatry
SMBD-Jewish General Hospital
Montreal, QC, Canada

Mark Parry
Bowman House
Reading Berkshire, UK

Kunal K. Patra
Department of Psychiatry
Henry Ford Health System
Detroit, MI, USA

Robert Patton
National Addiction Centre
London, UK

Bruce Pfohl
University of Iowa
Iowa City
IA, USA

Pauline S. Powers
University of South Florida
College of Medicine
Department of Psychiatry and Behavioural Medicine
Tampa, FL, USA

Mark Rapoport
University of Toronto
Sunnybrook Health Sciences Centre
Toronto, ON, Canada

Craig Ritchie
Department of Mental Health Sciences
Royal Free and University Medical School
Hampstead Campus
Hampstead
London, UK

Elizabeth A. R. Robinson
University of Michigan Addiction Research Center
Rachel Upjohn Building
Ann Arbor, MI, USA

Carol Rockhill
Department of Child and Adolescent Psychiatry
University of Washington School of Medicine
Seattle, WA, USA

Peter Roy-Byrne
Department of Psychiatry and Behavioural Sciences
University of Washington
Harborview Medical Center
Seattle, WA, USA

Steven B. Rudin
New York State Psychiatric Institute
New York, NY, USA

Kristi A. Sacco
Department of Psychiatry
Yale University School of Medicine
New Haven, CT, USA

Joel Sadavoy
University of Toronto
Mount Sinai Hospital
Toronto, Canada

Abhijeetha Salvaji
Doncaster Drug Team
Doncaster, UK

Elizabeth L. Sampson
Department of Mental Health Sciences
Royal Free and University College Medical School
London, UK

Paramala J. Santosh
Department of Psychological Medicine
Great Ormond Street Hospital for Children
London, UK

Kelly Schloredt
Childrens' Hospital and Regional Medical Centre
Seattle, WA, USA

Ulrike Schmidt
Institute of Psychiatry
De Crespigny Park
London, UK

Richard Schottenfeld
Yale University School of Medicine
Connecticut Mental Health Center
New Haven, CT, USA

Stephen Scott
Institute of Psychiatry
King's College, London, UK

Nicholas Seivewright
Substance Misuse Service
Fitzwilliam Centre
Sheffield, UK

Roz Shafran
Department of Psychiatry
Oxford University
Warneford Hospital
Oxford, UK

Michele Sie
Pharmacy
Mental Health
Charing Cross Hospital
London, UK

Kenneth R. Silk
Department of Psychiatry
University of Michigan Health System
Ann Arbor, MI, USA

Martine Simard
Laval University
Quebec City, QC, Canada

Mima Simic
Institute of Psychiatry
Department of Child and Adolescent Psychiatry
De Crespigny Park
London, UK

Helen Blair Simpson
New York State Psychiatric Institution
New York, NY, USA

Valerie J. Slaymaker
Hazelden Foundation
Center City, MN, USA

David Smelson
Department of Psychiatry
Robert Wood Johnson Medical School
VA Health Care System
Lyons, NJ, USA

Mehmet Sofuoglu
Department of Psychiatry
Yale University Medical School
VA Connecticut Healthcare System
Department of Psychiatry
West Haven, CT, USA

Matthew Speltz
Department of Child and Adolescent Psychiatry
University of Washington School of Medicine
Seattle, WA, USA

Arielle D. Stanford
Department of Psychiatry
Division of Brain Stimulation and Therapeutic Modulation
New York State Psychiatric Institute
New York, NY, USA

Murray B. Stein
University of California
San Diego
La Jolla, CA, USA

Ann Vander Stoep
Department of Psychiatry and Behavioural Sciences
University of Washington Medical School
Seattle, WA, USA

Michael Storck
Department of Child and Adolescent Psychiatry
University of Washington Medical School
Seattle, WA, USA

Stephen Strobbe
University of Michigan Addiction Research Center
Rachel Upjohn Building
Ann Arbor, MI, USA

Robert Swift
Center for Alcohol and Addiction Studies
Brown University Medical School
Providence, R1, USA

Michael A. Taylor
University of Michigan Medical Center
Psychiatry 9C, USA

Scott Temple
Penn State College of Medicine
Hershey Medical Center
Hershey, PA, USA

Janet Treasure
Department of Academic Psychiatry
Thomas Guy House
Guy's Campus
London, UK

Peter Tyrer
Imperial College London
Claybrook Centre
Charing Cross Campus
London, UK

Stephen Tyrer
University of Northumbria
Newcastle upon Tyne, UK

Robert van Reekum
Department of Psychiatry and Kunin-Lunenfeld
Applied Research Unit
Baycrest and Faculty of Medicine
University of Toronto
Toronto, ON, Canada

Ryan Vandrey
University of Vermont
VT, USA

Christopher K. Varley
Department of Child and Adolescent Psychiatry
University of Washington School of Medicine
Seattle, WA, USA

Jennifer A. Varley
Children's Hosptial and Regional Medical Center
Seattle, WA, USA

Pamela Walters
Camlet Lodge Regional Secure Unit
Chase Farm Hospital
The Ridgeway, Enfield
London, UK

Ming Wai Wan
University of Manchester
Manchester, UK

Sally L. Davidson Ward
Division of Pediatric Pulmonology
Children's Hospital
Los Angeles, USA

James Warner
Imperial College London
Claybrook Centre
Charing Cross Campus
London, UK

Wendy Weber
School of Naturopathic Medicine
Bastyr University, Kirkland
WA, USA

Andrea H. Weinberger
Department of Psychiatry
Yale University Medical School of Medicine
New Haven, CT, USA

Stacy Shaw Welch
Anxiety and Stress Reduction Center of Seattle/Evidence
Based Treatment Centers of Seattle
Seattle, WA, USA

Paul Wilkinson
Section of Developmental Psychiatry
Cambridge, UK

Nancy C. Winters
Department of Child and Adolescent Psychiatry
Oregon Health and Science University OP 02
Portland, OR, USA

Mary Zanarini
McLean Hospital
Belmont, MA, USA

Douglas M. Ziedonis
University of Massachusetts Memorial Medical Center
Worcester, MA, USA

Preface

All professionals in mental health want to give the best treatments for their patients, but how do we judge what is really best in a specific instance? The decisions about treatment are individual ones and yet the evidence in the literature is necessarily derived from groups, the larger the better. In editing this book we have tried to remember that, every time we make a treatment suggestion or recommendation, a busy clinician is tugging at our sleeve and asking 'how will this help me in treating my patient, who differs from others in having X, Y and Z?' We are both practising clinicians and are tuggers ourselves. We realise that evidence-based medicine (EBM), although it now trips easily off the tongue, is not nearly as straightforward as it may first appear. Real patients are seldom the same as those who are described in textbooks. Even at best, they only approximate to the sort of people who are described in good trials of evidence. We also have to remind ourselves that there must be hundreds of effective treatments that have not yet been shown to be effective, but this does not mean that clinicians should be deprived of their value because no one has done the hard work necessary to show that they are effective.

We are also fully aware that most of the evidence of efficacy comes from simple treatments such as drugs, which are much easier to evaluate than complex treatments, including most of the psychological therapies. The resources of the pharmaceutical companies are also quite naturally devoted to establishing good evidence as there is a strong commercial reason for doing so. As psychological therapies become more widely used and standardised, evaluation of these treatments may become methodologically less complicated, so we must be careful not to allege bias to one type of treatment only.

In planning and organizing this book we have had the practising clinician, the curious patient, and the disinterested researcher, all in mind. However, the needs of the practising clinician always take precedence here and we apologise to others for sometimes assuming that everyone looking at the text is in this role.

At the heart, we are hoping to answer five questions that we as clinicians ask ourselves when faced with the choice of treatment for a problem:

(1) What treatments are available for the condition that I think this patient has?

(2) What is the relative value of each of these treatments?

(3) Are there any other treatments that I should be considering now that my first approach has failed?

(4) Is there any value in combinations of treatment for this condition, and if so, which are likely to be most effective?

(5) Can I be reassured that the evidence and recommendations I read are free from bias?

Because there are so many treatments available in psychiatry, we have to group them by diagnosis and this explains the focus of the first section of this book, where the change in attitudes over the course of history is a salutary reminder of fashion in therapeutics. Because we, and indeed all independent thinkers, regard the diagnostic conditions in psychiatry as a weak approximation to the truth, and we make this clear, in advance of discussing individual treatments. Because diagnosis is inexact, most treatments have a wide spectrum across several disorders, and so we feel it important to discuss the main modalities of treatment and their principles. This is the subject of Part II. In Part III we discuss each treatment by diagnostic group, recognising that there is some significant overlap, both between diagnosis and between treatments at different stages of the lifespan.

As much as possible, we have tried to avoid duplication and have introduced relevant cross-referencing whenever we can. However, because of overlaps in diagnoses and in the treatments as well, we have tried to use cross-referencing judiciously. Otherwise, we could be cross-referencing every few pages, and the flow of the chapter and the text would suffer.

We recognise with appropriate humility that, despite the distinction and hard work of our section editors and contributors, much worthy evidence will be omitted in the following pages, and also acknowledge that many new pieces of important evidence could be added to this book by the time it is published. However, we feel that this volume, whatever its deficiencies, is the first attempt to bring together all treatments, both standard and complementary, into the evidence ring where they can compete openly with one another. There are often few head-to-head comparisons between all these treatments but we hope that their exposure, however brief, may help the practitioner in deciding on that critical set of decisions that will point the way to the solution of an individual problem.

We hope also that the reader will be reassured by our independence. We have not asked our authors to indicate their declarations of interest, because we, as the main editors, have examined every chapter and made modifications to ensure that the final conclusions are as independent as possible, even though we appreciate we are slaves to the data we have, not what we would like to see. Neither of the two editors has direct involvement in promoting any pharmacological or psychological treatment for personal gain, with the possible exception of nidotherapy, discussed in Chapter 44, for which PT is a product champion and which therefore should be read with allowances made for all the overstatements that accompany salesmanship.

We would like to thank all our contributors for staying with this project over the last 3½ years and bringing it forward to successful completion. We would also like to pay particular thanks to Richard Barling, who conceived this idea, to Richard Marley, who has kept us both on a delightfully long leash, and to Sandra O'Sullivan, who with the patience of a saint and the stamina of a marathon runner, has kept us both in order (no simple task indeed) right through to the end.

Peter Tyrer
Ken Silk
London, UK and Michigan, USA

Introduction

Classification of psychiatric disorders and their principal treatments

Peter Tyrer and Kenneth R. Silk

A kind of thought compulsion, a logical and aesthetic necessity, insists that we seek for well-defined, self-contained, clinical entities; but unfortunately our subjective need is no proof of the reality of which we desire. (Hoche, 1910)

Despite many proposed candidates, not one laboratory marker has been found to be specific in identifying any of the DSM-defined syndromes. Epidemiologic and clinical studies have shown extremely high rates of comorbidity among the disorders, undermining the hypothesis that the syndromes represent distinct etiologies. Furthermore, epidemiologic studies have shown a high degree of short-term diagnostic instability for many disorders. With regard to treatment, lack of treatment specificity is the rule rather than the exception. (Kupfer *et al.*, 2002, p. xvii)

Introduction

Why, you may well ask, has a book about treatment found it necessary to begin with a section on diagnosis? Since the introduction of DSM–III (American Psychiatric Association, 1980), diagnosis has seemed to become the 'holy grail' of psychiatry. Yet currently, diagnosis is in the doghouse, as the quotations above, spanning nearly a hundred years, illustrate. But, even though we despair at regular intervals, we continue to want a nice clean system that allows psychiatric patients to be pigeon-holed by clever clinicians who then have both an explanation of a disorder and its solution. For the hope has always been that if a specific diagnosis is made correctly, that the proper and best treatment will follow almost automatically.

If only psychiatry were that easy! If it was, then this book would not be necessary, for from the proper diagnosis would flow the essential treatment. But in psychiatry, and we would venture to say in most other specialties as well (though perhaps not so readily acknowledged by other practising physicians as in psychiatry), the diagnosis not only does not point directly towards treatment but can become a source of major conflict between clinicians and patients, and lead to allegations of the generation of stigma, labelling and other counter-productive arguments.

Then why do we persist with trying to refine and rework diagnoses and diagnostic manuals, and furthermore, why give it pride of place in this first chapter? In psychiatry, the path from correct diagnosis to correct explicit treatment is neither straight nor unambiguous and probably depends upon a number of different factors. The first factor might be the way diagnoses have evolved or developed in psychiatry, especially since, but not solely because of, the development of the editions of the DSM or the ICD that were advanced in the mid 1970s and became established as the DSM–III in 1980 (American Psychiatric Association, 1980) and the ICD–9 (World Health Organization, 1975, 1978) in 1975 with its clinical modification in 1978. Both of these then new iterations of prior diagnostic manuals profoundly changed the way psychiatrists approached diagnosis on both sides of the Atlantic. Rather than making a diagnosis based upon a number of different factors that included not only the 'chief' or presenting complaint, the specific symptoms that surrounded or accompanied the chief complaint, and the associated physiological and somatic concerns and complaints, while also considering the patient's capacity for empathy, the nature of his rapport or stance or 'posture' in relationship to the interviewing physician, the congruence of his affect with the content of his speech, and his ability to step back and view and comment on his own behaviour, the psychiatrist using the 'new' post 1980s approach basically needed to consider only the chief complaint with its accompanying symptoms, since together they were thought to be part of the package of the patient's overall psychophysiological, i.e. biologically determined, disorder. Empathy, relationship to the interviewer or to other people, capacity for insight, even motivation to change took on less

Cambridge Textbook of Effective Treatments in Psychiatry, ed. Peter Tyrer and Kenneth R. Silk. Published by Cambridge University Press.

significance, if any at all, as the new psychiatry, determined to look and feel like the rest of medicine, moved rapidly down the one diagnosis-one treatment road. If you got the diagnosis right, the choice of treatment would be, as they say, a 'no-brainer'.

This process can be compared with travelling on an expanding limited-access highway system where all you needed to know was what exit to take. Get on the correct road and take the correct exit and you would speedily be led to your desired destination. Get on the right diagnostic road and you will soon arrive at your destination, the right treatment. If the things that you needed at a specific exit were not that close by and to make things even clearer and more precise with less chance for error, more exits leading to more highways could be built (or more diagnostic entities created) so that you could arrive at your destination even more rapidly and efficiently. Of course, one of the problems with the interstate highway system, at least in the USA, is that, from the highway, all the roads look the same; and even when you get off the highway, the interchanges, with their almost standardized or perhaps operationalized conglomeration of fast food chains and service stations (symptoms and checklists), all, at least from some distance, look the same as well. You get little impression of the people who live and work in that particular area. But venture perhaps no more than a mile from the interstate, and you will find towns and cities and country roads that carry with them the specific distinction, flavour, and even peculiarity of the people and the geographical areas that you are passing through. Such a diversion from the interstate may not get you to your destination sooner, and it may not even appear initially to lend any valuable information to the journey. Yet it may convey a completely different and more complex sense experience and, in turn, appreciation of the trip that the shorter, faster, more direct route, the route the map searches on the computer produce when queried, places little or no value upon.

The second factor is related to other specific ideas about psychiatry, diagnosis and biology that developed throughout the 1970s. There evolved a number of ideas that took hold beginning in the late 1960s that were to change psychiatry and the diagnostic process profoundly. There developed the belief that we could, with enough expertise and diagnostic rigidity, isolate very specific diagnostic entities in psychiatry; and further that these specific entities were separate and distinct from other diagnostic entities. For example, there evolved the idea that depression, i.e. mood disorders, could clearly, in many cases, be distinguished from anxiety disorders. There was even a specific test developed, the dexamethasone suppression test (DST), that was purported to be able to distinguish

true melancholic depression from other entities. The title of that seminal paper in 1979, 'A specific laboratory test for the diagnosis of melancholia' conveys a good deal more about the wishes, not only of the authors, but of psychiatry in general, that there be specific laboratory tests that could help psychiatrists determine which patients had which diagnoses (Carroll *et al.*, 1981). If there was a biological or laboratory test that could help support that distinction, then psychiatry could have 'real' rather than imagined diagnoses (even though in most of medicine, there are actually very few diseases that have specific or pathognomonic tests that support their existence unequivocally). This is in no way to deny that the DST has gone on to become an important and useful measure of hypothalamic-pituitary-adrenal (HPA) activity and has led to many important areas of research and explorations into brain neurochemistry. And while the HPA axis is still thought to be overactive in some mood-disordered states, we now know that HPA overactivity may be a more general measure of an individual's reaction to stress and stressors rather than a specific laboratory test that reveals the presence of a specific mood disorder, or a mood disorder at all. What was originally proposed to be a specific laboratory test for a specific diagnostic entity turned out to be a laboratory test that cut across many of these so-called specific diagnostic groupings and appeared to be disordered across a number of conditions that all seemed to be linked together because of their relationship and reaction to stress. Stress certainly plays a role in many disorders, psychiatric as well as more purely medical.

Validity of psychiatric diagnoses

There has long been argument about the terms 'reliability', 'utility' and 'validity' of psychiatric diagnoses. Reliability, as a psychological construct, is the easiest of the three to resolve, as it is merely a measure of agreement between assessors of the same information. Thus for a diagnosis of a patient to be reliable, it is necessary for several people to see the same patient (preferable) or a set of proxy data (video recordings or transcripts) and show a level of agreement (measured by a standard measure of correlation) that is preferably above a level of 0.75 (Cicchetti & Sparrow, 1981). Confusion only arises when the lay interpretation of reliability is used (e.g. in a court of law counsel often asks if 'the evidence is reliable' when they really mean 'is the evidence valid', or can we really be confident that this evidence is a true record?). Validity is a much more difficult construct to achieve. Consider, for example, this quotation from two noted authorities on classification:

Table 1.1. Clinical Utility Total scores (CUTs) for some common psychiatric disorders

Diagnosis	Aetiology	Low comorbidity	Specificity of treatment	Natural history and course	CUT scores
Alzheimer's disease	−	+	+	+	3
Alcohol dependence syndrome	+	−	+	+	3
Generalized anxiety disorder	−	−	−	−	0
Adjustment disorder	+	+	−	−	2
Bipolar disorder	−	−	+	+	2
Schizophrenia	−	+	−	+	2
Dependent personality disorder	−	−	−	−	0
Bulimia nervosa	−	+	+	+	3
Social anxiety disorder	−	−	−	+	1
Obsessive-compulsive disorder	−	+	−	+	2

It is suggested that a score 0 or 1 renders the diagnosis suspect and ripe for reform.

We suggest, therefore, that a diagnostic category should be described as valid only if one of two conditions has been met. If the *defining characteristic* of the category is a syndrome, this syndrome must be demonstrated to be an entity, separated from neighboring syndromes and normality by a zone of rarity. Alternatively, if the category's defining characteristics are more fundamental – that is, if the category is defined by a physiological, anatomical, histological, chromosomal, or molecular abnormality – clear, qualitative differences must exist between these defining characteristics and those of other conditions with a similar syndrome. (Kendell & Jablensky, p. 7)

When current diagnostic practice is examined there can be only one, rather depressing, conclusion:

At present there is little evidence that most contemporary psychiatric diagnoses are valid, because they are still defined by syndromes that have not been demonstrated to have natural boundaries. This does not mean, though, that most psychiatric diagnoses are not useful concepts. In fact, many of them are invaluable. But, because utility often varies with the context, statements about utility must always be related to context, including who is using the diagnosis, in what circumstances, and for what purposes. (Kendell & Jablensky, p. 8)

Many, though not all, of the diagnostic concepts represented by the categories of disorder listed in contemporary nomenclatures such as DSM–IV and ICD–10 are extremely useful to practising clinicians, and most clinicians would be hard put to cope without them. Diagnostic categories provide invaluable information about the likelihood of future recovery, relapse, deterioration and social handicap; they guide decisions about treatment; and they provide a wealth of information about similar patients encountered in clinical populations or community surveys throughout the world. Diagnostic categories allow us to identify cohorts of like unwell people for whom we can collate their

frequency in the population, their demographic characteristics, family backgrounds and premorbid personalities, their symptom profiles and the evolution of those symptoms over time found in the results of clinical trials of different therapies. Research can then take place on the aetiology of the syndrome. This is all very useful and often provides invaluable information, whether or not the category in question is valid. Its usefulness depends mainly on two things: (1) the quantity and quality of the information in the literature (which depends on how long the category has been recognized and provided with adequate diagnostic criteria and how much competent research the category has generated) and (2) whether the implications of that information, particularly about aetiology, prognosis and treatment, are substantially different from the implications of analogous information about other related syndromes. But in recognizing the merits of usefulness, we must not go too far and imply validity to the diagnostic edifice we have constructed; it is a pragmatic solution, not a real one, and new data may quickly sweep it away.

We then might consider the following in attempting to rate or score the strength or clinical utility of a given diagnosis.

Aetiology

A good diagnosis indicates the cause, preferably silently rather than expressing it in the diagnostic description. Our suggested requirement for a positive score (see Table 1.1) is that the diagnosis indicates clearly which aetiological factors, up to a maximum of three, are involved. Few psychiatric diagnoses attain a satisfactory level at present of this factor. The aetiological factors can include genetic, social and environmental ones, and at least two of the main factors must be present in 90% of all cases. Conversely, the diagnosis cannot be made if these aetiological factors are absent.

Comorbidity

The original definition of comorbidity was 'the existence of two or more independent diseases in the same person at the same time' (Feinstein, 1970). In psychiatric classification this has been steadily eroded over the years so that now it is better defined as the presence of 'any distinct clinical entity that has existed or that may occur during the course of a patient who has the index disease under study' (Feinstein, 1970). Its absence indicates the 'zone of rarity that is considered to be essential for a valid diagnosis' (Kendell & Jablensky, 2003). Occasional comorbidity is to be expected even if a syndrome is clinically useful, but when it is extensive, it undermines the value of the diagnosis. We suggest that a lifetime comorbidity of 60% or more or a concurrent comorbidity of 40% or greater, the level required for extensive comorbidity among patients within a given diagnosis, raises serious questions as to the value of the diagnosis (and thus weighs against a positive score; see Table 1.1). The one exception is when the comorbid diagnosis is always secondary to the index one and can be claimed convincingly to be a consequence of its natural course.

Natural history and course

The natural history of most of the neuropsychiatric diagnoses is not known as therapeutic intervention is the rule and the interventions have, in most instances, modified that history (we hope in a positive direction). The study of the natural history of a given diagnosis might still be possible in lower middle income countries where treatment is in short supply. The course of any diagnosis, including its development over time in the presence of intervention (which may or may not be the same as the natural history), is now well recorded for most diagnoses. If we adopt a standard classification of the course of an illness (Frank et al., 1991), this would include recovery, remission with episodic relapse, remission with frequent relapse, unchanged clinical state, intermittent deterioration, continuous deterioration and death. A good diagnosis should predict its course and help it to be separated from other conditions. We suggest that for a diagnosis to be useful (to score positively – see Table 1.1) at least 50% of cases should be allocated to one of the main groups of outcome after 5 years. A heterogeneous course is not a good diagnostic criterion.

Specificity of treatment

For the practising clinician a good diagnosis is an ideal treatment selector. It plots a strategy of management better than any other single item of information. This idea of specificity of treatment also had an important role in introducing new diagnoses. For example, the introduction of 'panic disorder' to DSM–III was influenced heavily by Klein's suggestion (Klein & Fink, 1962; Klein, 1964) that imipramine showed 'pharmacological dissection' in treating panic disorder successfully but in failing to treat generalized anxiety disorder. The term 'psychological dissection' can also be used similarly for psychological interventions. Not all diagnoses yet have successful treatments but they still allow a management strategy to be set in place, even if it is an inactive one, when a good diagnosis is made. For a diagnosis to be useful (and achieve a high score on Table 1.1), we suggest that it should lead to a specific intervention plan (SIP) in at least 70% of cases. A SIP should contain no more than three elements of intervention to retain the definition of specificity, and these should not be shared by other diagnoses.

Comparison of Clinical Utility Total Scores (CUTs)

The comparison of clinical utility of some common diagnoses is illustrated in Table 1.1.

The current state of psychiatric diagnoses

The belief that psychiatry could define, isolate and separate specific diagnostic groupings appears to not have held up over time. Indeed we might argue that in many respects it has failed us in this task. The notion that one can clearly separate depression from anxiety might be possible in the most severe of instances of each of those states, but in general, there is a co-mingling of these states. Clinical experience would seem to suggest that the longer people remain depressed, the more that mantle of depression that they carry appears to be at least tinged with, if not layered throughout, with anxiety. Further, the more chronically anxious a person appears over time, the more depressed he also seems to become. In fact many patients with chronic states of mixed anxiety and depression often seem to drift into the large category that now bears the label of personality disorder.

Thus the specificity and separateness of current psychiatric diagnosis, upon which the current DSM and the ICD not only seemed to depend but also simultaneously helped to promote, appears to need some reworking. This does not mean that psychiatric diagnoses are non-existent, useless or unconnected to treatment; rather it says that much more study and work needs to be done in this area before any confident conclusions can be reached. By attempting to define precise and distinct diagnostic categories, the current diagnostic manuals have established certain well-defined areas for us to carve out and examine to see if the boundaries and points of distinction are correctly placed. Much important research and many significant biological and neuroanatomical discoveries would have been impossible if some genuine, categorical, data-based and empirically enhanced diagnostic system had not been created.

Creating diagnostic manuals is an iterative process, and we need to remain open to what it is that we actually see and experience clinically. From those observations there will come improvements in how we understand and utilize diagnoses. We need to remember that in general our patients do not read the DSM before they present to us (although given the ubiquity of the Internet, it does seem to be getting more common).

The idea of specificity of diagnosis was further driven by the rapid development of biological ideas into the practice of psychiatry. There were a number of forces that came together in the late 1960s and early 1970s to strengthen biological psychiatry and to promote the idea that there were biological underpinnings if not for all, for at least most, psychiatric disorders. As we proceed with the discussion, we want to emphasize that we believe that all feelings, thoughts, actions, cognitions and behaviours are rooted in and mediated by biological processes, lest the following discussion give the impression that we are 'anti-biological'. The success of medications developed and brought to market in the late 1950s and early 1960s conveyed new hope and offered a wide array of compounds for psychiatric practice. While the discovery of chlorpromazine opened the path towards much more precise pharmacological treatment of psychiatric illness, leaving the previous compounds with their weak non-specific sedating and mentally dulling effects way behind, the additional discovery of the antidepressants shortly thereafter heralded a way of thinking that was to revolutionize psychiatric practice.

Prior to the discovery of the antidepressants, the concept of depression, as put forth primarily by the psychoanalytic school, was based upon the idea that depression was anger turned against oneself, the result of a negative introject, because of a loss of an ambivalently felt loved object (person) (Jacobson, 1971). Unable to admit consciously or openly anything that could be considered negative or hostile towards the lost or departed figure, the depressed person turned those negative feelings against oneself and was thus able to preserve a positive memory or posture to the loved object. (One never, in some broad metaphorical sense, wants to say anything bad about the dead.) Then when Kuhn (1958) put forth the idea of a medication that was an antidepressant, psychiatrists of the day must have wondered how a medication, a biological intervention, could reverse the process of turning the negative aspects of one's ambivalence about a lost object away from the self, because such a cognitive process, at that time, was thought necessary to occur if depression was to be 'resolved' more than relieved. (To put these ideas into perspective, it can be pointed out that many people in psychiatry at that time believed that the success of electroconvulsive therapy [ECT] in depression was due to the fact that the ECT was a form of punishment that ultimately helped relieve the guilt the depressed patient felt about her anger towards the ambivalently loved but now lost object. The depressed person had now, through the pain and suffering of ECT, paid penance, as it were, to her guilt and now was able to recover and move forward!)

Max Hamilton (1960) was to redefine the assessment of depression and at the same time, perhaps unwittingly, shift psychiatry's attention, even more than perhaps the discovery of chlorpromazine and imipramine did, away from seeing things in psychodynamic or psychoanalytic terms and towards viewing psychiatric illness as a disease. These diseases had specific accompanying psychophysiological symptoms that were rooted in biology and formed a package that we would call a disorder. Hamilton's rating scale for depression (HRS-D; Hamilton, 1960) had nothing about introjects, ambivalence about lost objects, or turning anger against oneself, though it did have ratings for the mood state of depression, guilt and suicidality. But more importantly, by using the HRS-D, depression was to be defined primarily in physiological terms such as sleep, appetite, energy, sexual function and physical manifestations (or experiences) of anxiety. Further, these items within the HRS-D could be, in most instances, directly measured and scored. Different raters or clinicians could learn the scoring system and achieve reliability between them. Thus it was thought one could, with appropriate training and experience, be able to rate (and define) the degree of depression in one's patient and have it be related to the degree of depression in another patient of another therapist if both therapists had achieved a good level of reliability between them in the scoring of the HRS-D.

It was not an insignificant change when the categories that were identified as reactions (i.e. 'schizophrenic reactions') in DSM–I (American Psychiatric Association, 1952) became disorders (i.e. 'schizophrenic disorders') in

DSM–II (American Psychiatric Association, 1968). The idea of psychiatric illness was changing significantly. No longer were *reactions* thought to occur because the id overwhelmed the ego or because the defences failed to keep unwanted ideas out of the conscious mind or that mental conflicts (ambivalence) led directly to anxiety or somatic symptoms or conversion reactions. Rather, psychiatric *disorders* occurred because of biological irregularities or failures that were either predisposed and constitutionally determined or arose *de novo* because external events upset to a significant degree previous biological balances and/or compromises that the organism (individual) had attained.

The last 15–20 years have seen an explosion of biological research in psychiatry that now includes the most sophisticated aspects of pharmacological challenges, molecular biology, neuroimaging and genetic techniques. We have come much closer to understanding some of the biological processes that appear to be disordered in different disease states, but the precise relationship of those biological processes to the actual clinical symptoms and affects that the patients' experience still remains elusive. Further, there has been an explosion of new psychopharmacological compounds in the last 15 years that promise effectiveness equal to the older drugs (those discovered and brought to market in the late 1950s and through the 1960s) but whose side effects are purported to be much milder and more tolerable than those found among their predecessors.

But another explosion has occurred, an explosion that in many ways makes the organizing of this section on diagnosis somewhat challenging. That explosion has been the explosion in the number of specific psychiatric entities now in each of the diagnostic manuals, whether it is ICD–10 or DSM–IV. There are probably many reasons for the increase in diagnoses. One reason may be that the splitters currently rule the psychiatric nomenclature process. These are people who honestly believe that in breaking psychiatric diagnoses into smaller and smaller categories, we may find more precise (and hopefully more successful) treatments for each of the categories. Another reason may have to do with the issue of promotion of drug treatments. The more diseases that are available, the more pharmaceutical companies have the opportunity to show effectiveness of their compounds, and the more marketing mileage they may be able to gain in their attempts to promote the uniqueness (or the broad applicability) of their particular compound(s) when compared with those of their competitors. A further reason may be that the greater the number of narrowly defined diseases for which there can be developed evidence for specific treatments, then the more readily these diseases and disease states will be accepted as legitimate by

third party payers or by governmental agencies who want to know that their dollars or pounds or euros are being spent on the treatment of specific, well-defined entities rather than some global, somewhat nebulous concept of disease or unwellness rather than illness or disorder. Some more cynical observers note the exponential increase in diagnoses (and consequent increase in size of each new DSM volume) as a commercial matter, and regard the initials, DSM, as now standing for 'Diagnosis as a Source of Money' – for the American Psychiatric Association (Blashfield & Fuller, 1996).

Yet, while trying to reify these concepts of specific diseases and specific treatments, we found an opposite effect to that expected. Rather than finding that specific treatments worked only in specific diseases, we found the opposite, that specific treatments seem to work across a wide array of diseases. We turn once again back to the idea that in the 1970s there was the belief that in most instances depression or mood disorder was separate and distinct from anxiety disorder. One would have assumed from those studies in the 1970s that eventually we would find that the treatments, especially the biological treatment, for each of those large groups of disorders (or disorder categories) would be separate and distinct as well. But the opposite has happened. We now use the selective serotonin reuptake inhibitors (SSRIs) for a wide array of conditions that fall under the categories of both depression and anxiety. And further, the older tricyclic antidepressants (TCAs) that, as their name indicates and as Kuhn in 1958 so identified them, were thought to be specific for depression, are now used in a wide array of anxiety disorders as well. And the purported biological neurotransmitter activity is not the same between the TCAs and the SSRIs, for one is thought to interact primarily (though not exclusively) on the noradrenalin (norepinephrine) neurotransmitter system (TCAs) while the other is thought to interact primarily on the serotonin neurotransmitter system (SSRIs). This does not mean that these two neurotransmitters systems do not interact, perhaps very intimately and subtly, with one another. But the idea of one disease, one medication, or the idea of pharmacological specificity to accompany diagnostic specificity (described as pharmacologic(al) dissection by Klein, 1964), is being eroded as we learn more and more about various treatments and their tendency for their use to spread far beyond their original diagnostic targets.

Matching diagnosis, syndrome and treatment

Reflecting on these issues about diagnosis and specificity, we must arrive at some way to associate the current plethora of psychiatric diagnostic categories to provide a coherent and useful guide to treatment, if we are really going to live up to the title of this book. Our goal is, once again, to look at treatments in their broadest sense and to consider how each of them can be used to their maximum value. We do not want to be constricted too much by a diagnostic system that, while well intended, has turned out not to have fulfilled the promise of clarity and specificity all of us once hoped for. But we also do not want to give an unfair description of a treatment as effective when it is clearly ineffective if given for the wrong condition.

For this reason the evaluation of the general effectiveness of each of the main categories of treatment (and the more specific variations of treatment within the category) in psychiatry are presented in Part II. We leave the discussion of the specific value of each treatment to Part III, where we describe each treatment, sometimes in the context of a diagnosis and sometimes not, and summarize the evidence for each diagnosis in a concluding table for each chapter. Despite our criticisms of diagnosis, it is still the norm for clinicians, and indeed patients, to identify disorders and then to compare the treatments for these. Thus in practice we are pitting each treatment against all others in the relevant diagnostic group even when the diagnosis is of limited value. This is our best judgement as to how to approach the best way of testing effectiveness given all the limitations and gaps that we have in our knowledge base. Both practitioners and patients are keen on getting the best possible deal from the treatments available, and require their problems categorized in some way, so the competition is as much between treatments by diagnosis as by treatment in general. In choosing a treatment we also have to take into account other factors, particularly adverse effects, which may be complex to interpret as one person's poison may be another's elixir of life. Other relevant factors include comorbid medical illness, age and costs. Indeed, cost-effectiveness is rapidly becoming the watchword by which every treatment is being evaluated.

So we are left with a bit of a mishmash when it comes to fixing the current place of a treatment in psychiatry. Sometimes the treatment is so clear in its description that its diagnostic 'tag' appears to be unimportant; for others the treatment may be specifically linked to one diagnosis only. Thus in medicine penicillamine is used specifically to treat Wilson's disease (as this drug is a chelating agent that reduces the absorption of copper whose accumulation in the body becomes the manifestation of the disease). But a drug such as the benzodiazepine diazepam, despite being a sedative drug that reduces anxiety, can be used in many different ways because it is also an anticonvulsant as well as a muscle relaxant, so it can,

therefore, be used for a wide number of disorders. And if we turn to the symptom of anxiety, we find that it is such a prominent component of so many disorders, its main treatments can appear again and again and sometimes be in danger of duplication.

In deciding on which chapters should be confined to describing treatments only (Part II) and which to diagnoses and their treatments (Part III), we hope we have chosen correctly. Part II is concerned with the main modalities of treatment whereas Part III describes individual therapies, sometimes closely linked to standard diagnoses (e.g. panic disorder), and some by groupings that reflect experience in practice but which are not necessarily in DSM–IV and ICD–10 (e.g. the section of organic disorders). The choice of these has not necessarily been an easy process, and we and our editors for each of the diagnostic areas have not always met agreement in how we defined our sections. This lack of agreement again reflects the fact that while much has been accomplished in psychiatric diagnosis in the last 25–30 years, much still resides in the realm of opinion. Much more needs to be done in order to understand the relationship between what we frame as categories of psychiatric diagnosis and the treatment or treatments that for some of the patients within those categories appear to be effective.

Models of treatment for mental disorder

This subject is relevant when it comes to choice of treatment for any disorder. The selection of treatment will depend to some extent on the model each practitioner uses for mental disorders. These have been summarized as the disease, psychodynamic, cognitive-behavioural and social models (Tyrer & Steinberg, 2005), and they can be viewed as a hierarchy (Figure 1.1). Each of the models on its own is unsatisfactory but together they can be very useful. The disease model is the equivalent of the well-established medical model of common parlance and is well-suited to organic disorders as it is associated with demonstrable (physical) organic pathology, either gross or accessible by microscopic means. Once a disease is clearly present it allows four elements to be identified relatively clearly:

(1) The description of symptoms and main features of the disorder (the clinical syndrome matching the underlying pathology).
(2) Identification of the specific pathology (i.e. the structural or biological changes created by the illness).
(3) Study of the course (natural history) of the syndrome.
(4) Determination of its cause or causes.

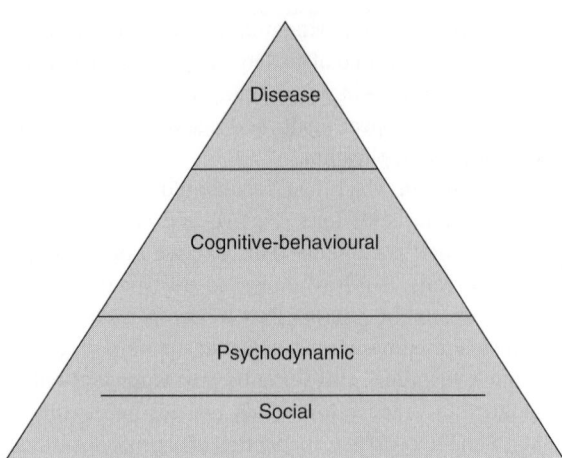

Fig. 1.1. The hierarchical model of mental disorders. Like all hierarchical models each level includes all disorders at that level and subsumes all those below (from Tyrer & Steinberg, 2005).

Although some disorders (e.g. Korsakoff's psychosis, Huntington's chorea) can satisfy all these requirements, most conditions encountered in psychiatry do not, and many do not get beyond the first element. The psychodynamic model does not even accept this element and maintains that the presentation of the complaint is a coded message that requires much further analysis (psychoanalysis) before a real understanding of the problem (or conflict) can be understood. The cognitive behavioural model blurs the distinctions between the disorders and examines the extent to which cognitive misinterpretations and distortions are present in the condition, so that, for example, in generalized anxiety disorder and obsessive–compulsive disorder the error may be in thinking, whereas in personality disorder the misinterpretation may be at the level of fundamental beliefs or schemas (Davidson, 2000; Tyrer & Davidson, 2000; Young et al., 2003). The social model abhors all diagnosis as stigmatic labelling, and that any advantages that they enjoy in terms of professional communication are more than offset by the depersonalization of diagnosis.

In practice most psychiatrists like to claim they are eclectic (i.e. they choose whichever model most fits the problem), but in the absence of clear guidelines this just looks like opportunism. However, by following diagnostic procedures and selecting treatment by diagnosis they are often accused by other practitioners and patients of following the 'medical model', a rather broader definition of the disease model described above. The proponents of alternative models are often dismissed or ignored but should not be. The simple fact is that a treatment that is

not perceived by either therapist or patient to be in the right 'frame of management' will rarely be effective in practice because it will not be followed. This is very important when considering the evidence base of different treatments. If a psychological treatment is marginally inferior to a drug treatment, but the patient and day-to-day therapists concerned are violently opposed to drug treatment, then it is desirable, one might say essential, for the psychological therapy to be chosen. It may not be the best treatment in an ideal world but pragmatic decisions are the best for such situations. Time and again in the ensuing pages the reader will come across treatments that are *likely from present evidence* to be very similar in efficacy (the reason for putting the words in italics is that so many treatments deriving from different models are seldom compared in randomized controlled trials). Under such circumstances the treatment that best fits the patient's perception of the correct treatment is probably the one that should be chosen.

Choosing treatments from diagnosis: the example of mood disorders

In setting forth the details of specific treatments in Part III, we have acknowledged the significance of diagnostic practice and have followed the standard order of classification in numbering our chapters. So we begin with the organic disorders, the true repository of the disease model, and move through substance disorders, to the schizophrenias, mood disorders and neurotic (yes, we do still use this word occasionally), anxiety and stress-related disorders to eating disorders and the rest, ending with child psychiatric disorders. Only intellectual disability is a little out of the standard order, with only Chapters 10 and 44 addressing specific treatments for this group, and unfortunately the evidence base here is very thin.

We do not have space to go through the relationship between treatments and every diagnostic group in this section as we would repeat ourselves, but it might be helpful if we concentrated on one group as an illustration. We have chosen the category of mood disorders for this exercise. We begin with a discussion, actually a form of text tabulation, of the ways the ICD and the DSM diagnose the mood disorders. We elucidate the categories and the subcategories, and we then try to point out the similarities and differences between the two systems. We then go on to discuss the various limitations to those diagnostic categories and subcategories, limitations and qualifications that will influence the practitioner and patient when deciding on effective treatments for this diagnostic group.

We could do this for each of the diagnostic categories, but that would, in essence, be another book in itself, and that book would be on the process of diagnosis rather than on the effectiveness of treatment, which is the focus of this text. We have chosen depression as an example because it is fairly ubiquitous, appears in many different forms and intensities or severities, and can be viewed in some people as arising endogenously from some internal dysregulated (we presume) source, and in other instances appears as a most human and natural reaction to loss, failure, pain, humiliation and disappointment.

The ICD–10 classification of mood disorders encompasses the major subcategories of manic episode, bipolar affective disorder, depressive episodes, recurrent depressive disorder, persistent mood disorder, other mood (affective) disorder, unspecified mood (affective) disorder. In a number of the major subcategories, the word 'mood' can be substituted with 'affective', which implies more of mood change or fluctuation and can include mood depression and elevation, and is not necessarily reserved for a 'negative' or 'depressed' state. Each of these major subcategories has further categories embedded or subsumed under them, but for purposes of economy, we will not list or review the categories labelled 'other' or 'unspecified', but we assume that in every instance such non-specified groupings are available to the diagnostician.

- **Manic episode** also includes mania with and without psychotic symptoms, and hypomania.
- **Bipolar affective disorder** includes a current episode of hypomania, episodes of mania with and without psychosis, a current episode of mild to moderate depression (with and without a somatic syndrome), severe depression with or without psychotic symptoms (and if psychotic symptoms are present, the psychotic symptoms can be classified as mood congruent or incongruent), a current mixed episode, or bipolar disorder currently in remission.
- **Depressive episodes** includes mild and moderate episodes (each with or without somatic syndrome), or a severe episode with or without psychosis (and if psychotic symptoms are present, the psychotic symptoms can be classified as mood congruent or incongruent).
- **Recurrent depressive disorder** includes recurrent episodes with the current episode being defined as mild or moderate (each with or without a somatic syndrome), or severe with or without psychosis (and if psychotic symptoms are present, are the psychotic symptoms mood congruent or incongruent), or a history of recurrent episodes now in remission.
- **Persistent mood disorders** include cyclothymia, and dysthymia.

The DSM–IV(TR) (TR stands for 'text-revised') category of mood disorders has two large subcategories, depressive disorders and bipolar disorders. For each of these categories, there are codings for subgroups, and the subgroupings have to do with severity (mild, moderate, severe with the severe category being divided into with or without psychotic features and the psychotic features being mood-congruent or incongruent), and remission (subcategories that would specify partial or complete remission).

- **Depressive disorders** include a single or recurrent depressive episode(s) and dysthymic disorder that can be further broken down into early or late onset dysthymia and whether there are any atypical features within the dysthymic disorder.
- **Bipolar disorders** include bipolar I disorder which then includes both single manic episode (with the opportunity to delineate whether the current and or the most recent episode is purely manic or mixed with depressive symptoms), bipolar II disorder (with the opportunity to delineate whether the current and or the most recent episode is purely hypomanic or mixed with depressive symptoms), cyclothymic disorder, and mood disorders secondary to either a general medical condition or substance-induced. In either of these two 'secondary' mood disorders, there are opportunities to describe the affective episode in terms of whether or not the episode has primarily depressive features including features so severe that they resemble a major depressive episode or manic features or features that are mixed. Included within the substance-induced mood disorder category is whether the affective features begin during the process of, including reaching the state of, intoxication or appear to begin during withdrawal.

But how are we to consider these multiple categories in a book on treatment? How do we define or cluster these various categories in order to make some sense as we proceed to discuss treatments, and to consider, in general, what treatments apply to these clusters that we determine.

Both the DSM and the ICD have probably brought a number of disparate, but consolidated through the common symptoms of either mood depression, mood elevation (mania or hypomania) or mood lability. They have also tried to classify or subclassify each of the mood presentations into the following:

- Is the disordered mood episodic or chronic?
- Is the episode or the disordered mood state mild, moderate or severe?
- If mild or moderate is there a preoccupation with bodily symptoms and function (though such a preoccupation might lead one to think about anxiety disorders as well)?

- If severe, is there a psychosis present, and if present, do the psychotic ideas coincide with the particular mood state that is being expressed (congruence)?
- Is there primarily one mood state being expressed (elation or depression) or is there a mixture of elation or depression currently, and historically has there been mixtures in the past, either within a given episode or across episodes?

Before we discuss the area of affective disorders in this text we will need to make inclusion and exclusion decisions because it appears that we will not be able to apply treatments coherently to the category of mood disorders that will make clinical sense since the category as defined by both DSM and ICD is so broad. Thus we will include under the category of mood disorders in this text the following: Any severe mood disorder whether psychotic or non-psychotic, mood-congruent on incongruent that involves mania, depression or a mixed affective state. The primary concept here is a mood disorder that is clearly severe and captures the old concept of endogenicity, i.e. being driven because of some internal state or process and is not really responsive or reactive to what is actually going on in the external world. This category will not include cyclothymic or dysthymic disorders (which seem to be very environmentally reactive), or bipolar II disorder as well unless the depressive episodes in the bipolar II disorder are at least in the moderate to severe range. Our category of mood disorders will not include mild depressive episodes, either single or multiple, although these are diagnostic categories in ICD-10 and can be regarded as appropriate ones as the features characteristic of depression (e.g. self-harm episodes) are present in mild depression and become more frequent with increasing severity (Kessing, 2004). Moderate depressive episodes are more difficult to quantify, and there is no system or operationalized criteria currently in use that defines the boundary between mild and moderate episodes, though there can probably be a better chance of reaching agreement as to where severe episodes begin, particularly if those episodes are marked by psychotic thinking. Without the psychosis, however, the boundary between moderate and severe is blurred as well. We will include moderate depression with a somatic syndrome only when the symptoms of that syndrome are primarily congruent with a depressive state or episode, but we will not include those patients whose somatic concerns fall more into what we would consider to be anxiety or other hypochondriacal symptoms. Secondary mood disorders, especially those secondary to a general medical condition, will be included if the clinical presentation coincides with our stated inclusion criteria for a mood disorder without the general medical condition, though more attention may need to be paid to drug–drug interactions or to the interplay between the general medical condition and certain somatic treatments.

We are not ignoring these other mood disorder classifications. Rather, we think that when considering treatments, especially effective treatments, the 'discarded' mood disorder categories are better regarded as neurotic or stress disorders under which we have subsumed anxiety disorders, or possibly even personality disorders. In doing this, we are not, through some form of subterfuge, trying to impose our own diagnostic schema. Rather, we think that in a book whose focus is primarily treatment effectiveness, that our classification revisions make sense from a treatment coherence/treatment review point of view. But obviously we will not be the final arbiters of the issue. What happens in practice decides that, and, whatever an individual may feel about the correct (or pure) classification of a clinical problem, in practice the ugly form of comorbidity is likely to present, and when one person has several diagnostic labels it is very difficult to know what treatment is acting on which disorder.

It then becomes a somewhat difficult task to determine the epidemiology of mood disorders if we are reclassifying the entire category. We will therefore present what is known about the epidemiology of the broader category as defined by the ICD and the DSM. Again, we are not trying to impose our view on the psychiatric world; rather we are trying to define categories that can lead to treatment coherence, and categories that will allow us to evaluate the effectiveness of the treatment for that category.

Certainly, as the prior discussion reveals, there is considerable overlap between mood disorders and other categories. Having a depressed mood is a ubiquitous phenomenon, and we might suggest that anyone who says that they have never experienced a depressed mood is either practising denial or suffers from alexithymia. We say that not in any way to try and resurrect the old idea that everyone is at least neurotic. In fact, we thoroughly oppose such smugness. Rather, we argue that depression is an omnipresent condition and can be triggered by many situations, and while some people may be more vulnerable or more ready to react to a wider array of different situations or disappointments with a feeling of depression, this does not mean that the depression reaches the level of a mood disorder. This again is the concept of depression we are striving to define for the purposes of this book. Certainly patients with chronic anxiety, stress, marital discord, family difficulties, job dissatisfaction, and in the recent throes of a loss through break up or death may experience depressive symptoms, often to a very significant degree. Further there appears to be a significant overlap or at least co-occurrence of depressive symptoms or episodes of depression in people who are classified as having personality disorders. And in almost all of these instances described above, if you ask the patient if she is depressed, she will most probably give endorsement to that mood state.

But differentiating these depressive reactions from mood disorders as defined in this book takes a certain amount of skill; but perhaps more than skill, it takes a certain amount of time and curiosity. It takes more than simply filling out a symptom checklist (driven or derived from the ICD or DSM) or determining a score on a rating scale. It involves understanding what the word depression means to the patient and where and how he learned to label that particular mood state in that particular way. It involves trying to understand how the patient has reacted to stressors and life events in the past, how incapacitated he was at those past times and how long it took to recoup and feel that the episode or the time of very difficult feeling had passed. It involves evaluating the patient's sense of hope, of the future, and of, at least on an intellectual level, the understanding that things will improve or that this current situation is temporary or that he realizes that he is looking and judging things too harshly at the current moment. And it involves the psychiatrist's experience of how the patient is behaving, relating, and grasping the present reality as well as the long-term perspective at the current time. Through this process of trying to exclude these many types of depressive reactions and states from our concept of mood disorder, we then can arrive, hopefully, at a reasonably explicit but certainly more narrow definition of mood disorders than the larger more sprawling category put forth by both the DSM and the ICD.

When we arrive at this definition or concept of mood disorders, it is most interesting to consider that each and every one of the classes of treatments we are reviewing in this book has been and is currently being applied in the treatment of people with mood disorders, and at least anecdotally, each is purported to have some success.

Thus, patients with mood disorders are very frequently prescribed psychopharmacological agents. Over the last decade and a half, the number of patients receiving such treatments for depression has increased while the 'bar' (i.e. the level of severity of depression in order to be considered for psychopharmacological intervention) has been lowered. As the definition of depression has expanded to include milder forms of depression (a 'type' of depressive reaction we are dissecting away from the category of mood disorders in this text), the number of people being medicated for depression and related disorders has expanded, even though the number of new drug discoveries has fallen (Shorter & Tyrer, 2003). There is a wide variety of medications, both older and newer, that are currently being used in the treatment of depression. Despite the ever-expanding number of antidepressants on the market, no antidepressant is viewed as more effective than any other (even though side effects may differ substantially). In fact, most antidepressants appear to be effective in somewhere between 50% and 70% of those who are prescribed them for depression. This does not mean that it is the same 30% who do not respond to any antidepressant. Any given antidepressant does not appear to work in at least 30% of those people for whom it is prescribed, though any given patient who fails to respond to one antidepressant, may respond to a different (same or different class) antidepressant (Sachs *et al.*, 2003).

Psychiatry's most prevalent somatic treatment, ECT, has been employed primarily for patients with mood disorders. It can be used not only for depression but for intractable or unresponsive mania as well. There are restrictions in some states as to when and how to use ECT, but nonetheless, it remains an effective, if not first line, treatment. Other somatic treatments that include transmagnetic stimulation (rTMS) and vagal nerve stimulation (VNS) are also gaining popularity as treatments for depression, particularly depression that appears to be non-responsive to pharmacological agents.

Mood disordered patients regularly utilize and undergo psychotherapy, and before the mid-to-late 1950s, psychotherapy, particularly psychodynamic and psychoanalytic psychotherapy (including classical psychoanalysis), was the primary and most popular form of treatment not only for depression but for almost all psychiatric illnesses. Psychotherapy remains a vital aspect of the treatment of people with depression, though attention has shifted away from the psychodynamic forms of treatment into more structured and less transference-based treatments. Interpersonal psychotherapy, which can be viewed as a modification of psychodynamic psychotherapy that focuses more on current relationships than on assumed attitudes about relationships as gleaned from the transference, has gained in popularity, along with many different variations of cognitive-behavioural therapy. In general, it is the cognitive aspects of cognitive-behavioural therapy, that have gained the most attention and utilization in mood disorders, and cognitive therapy can take place in individual and/or in group settings.

There has been evidence since Davenport's work in the 1970s (Davenport *et al.*, 1977) through Frank's work currently (Frank *et al.*, 2000), that educational and family therapy, or at least family members' awareness of the situations and events that can trigger mood disorder episodes or that can disrupt daily, and by extension psychophysiological, routines and rhythms, have an impact on the course of the disorder. Even though variations on educational interventions and family therapy for mood disorders (solely or as an adjunct to individual psychotherapy and/or pharmacotherapy) have been suggested for the last 25–30 years, their growth has been slow given the substantial increase in the number of people seeking help for depression.

The wide utilization of all of the above treatments often leads to a patient receiving treatment across at least two, if not more, of these modalities. We have chosen to label the treatment category where more than one type of treatment is being given to a patient as complex interventions. Certainly there are many efforts underway to try to appreciate the effectiveness of the combination of different treatments, most frequently some form of psychotherapy and pharmacotherapy, and the relative value of each alone versus both in combination.

And finally, depressed patients, especially those for whom the experience of depression has been a chronic one (perhaps separated from the question of severity), often seek out alternative therapies and self-help processes to assist them in overcoming the difficulty of living with a chronic mood disorder. This group often ignores the diagnostic practice behind depression altogether and goes for a natural remedy that is more in the spirit of the social model of psychiatry, along the lines of 'Do not listen to those people who want to medicalize your pain and suffering. Instead take a herbal remedy as the 'natural' method of healing and avoid the stigma of mental illness'. The 'success' of the herb St. John's wort (*Hypericum perforatum*) (see Chapter 7) has been one of the drivers for the recent surge in interest in alternative therapies for the treatment not only of depression but for many medical as well as psychiatric disorders. And even though the improvement in depression that this herbal treatment conveys is not at the top of the evidence tree, it is one that thousands of people prefer because it is an alternative to a system that so many abhor.

So we finish this account of the classification of mood disorders. It shows the problems of slavishly following a diagnosis that does very little to help in selecting a treatment and a great deal to support the brigade of obfuscation, and yet which is necessary to bring some order to the description of remedies that would have no anchor points if formal classification was abandoned.

The beginning starts here

We hope you are now ready to plunge into the web of evidence-based treatment in psychiatry with the right perspective, one which an Irish priest once implored his congregation to follow, 'the straight and narrow path between right and wrong'. Evidence is only a guide, but when there are so many false ones beckoning it is good to have one that is genuinely in the right territory.

There is an old comedy sketch that a comedian named Gabby Hayes used to perform. He plays an old weathered cowboy, covered with dust, wearing a large hat and leather chaps with a dirty beard that conceals his mouth. He is standing in the street when a bandit runs by him carrying a pistol and a bag of money. Shortly behind the fleeing robber comes the sheriff who stops in front of Hayes and asks him 'Which way did he go?' Hayes pauses for a moment, looking perplexed as he gazes in different directions while scratching his scraggly beard. But then he brightens and crosses his arms in front of his chest so that each hand points upward towards its opposite shoulder. Speaking through his beard in a voice so forceful that the part of the beard overhanging his mouth blows forward and back with each word, Hayes tells the sheriff 'He went that-a-away!'

We hope that we are somewhat better guides than our perplexing cowboy sending the posse off in all directions. But if we fail in helping you in your search for the elusive therapeutic booty, we can only apologize and congratulate you on the future success of your own efforts (which we will gladly reproduce in a future edition).

REFERENCES

American Psychiatric Association (1952). *Diagnostic and Statistical Manual, Mental Disorders*, 1st edn. Washington, DC: American Psychiatric Association.

American Psychiatric Association (1968). *Diagnostic and Statistical Manual of Mental Disorders*, 2nd edn. Washington, DC: American Psychiatric Association.

American Psychiatric Association (1980). *Diagnostic and Statistical Manual of Mental Disorders*, 3rd edn. Washington, DC: American Psychiatric Association.

Blashfield, R. K. & Fuller, A. K. (1996). Predicting the DSM-V. *Journal of Nervous and Mental Disease*, **184**, 4–7.

Carroll, B. J., Feinberg, M., Greden, J. F. *et al.* (1981). A specific laboratory test for the diagnosis of melancholia. Standardization, validation, and clinical utility. *Archives of General Psychiatry*, **38**, 15–22.

Cicchetti, D. V. & Sparrow, S. S. (1981). Developing criteria for the rating of specific items in a given inventory. *American Journal of Mental Deficiency*, **86**, 127–37.

Davenport, Y. B., Ebert, M. H., Adland, M. L. & Goodwin, F. K. (1977). Couples group therapy as an adjunct to lithium maintenance of the manic patient. *American Journal of Orthopsychiatry*, **47**, 495–502.

Davidson, K. (2000). *Cognitive Therapy for Personality Disorders: a Guide for Clinicians*. London: Butterworth-Heinemann.

Feinstein, A. R. (1970). The pre-therapeutic classification of co-morbidity in chronic disease. *Journal of Chronic Diseases*, **23**, 455–68.

Frank, E., Swartz, H. A. & Kupfer, D. J. (2000). Interpersonal and social rhythm therapy: managing the chaos of bipolar disorder. *Biological Psychiatry*, **48**, 593–604.

Frank, E., Prien, R. F., Jarrett, R. B. *et al.* (1991). Conceptualization and rationale for consensus definitions of terms in major depressive disorder – remission, recovery, relapse, and recurrence. *Archives of General Psychiatry*, **48**, 851–5.

Hamilton, M. (1960). A rating scale for depression. *Journal of Neurology, Neurosurgery and Psychiatry*, **23**, 56–62.

Hoche, A. (1910). Die Melancholiefrage. *Zeitschrift für die Gesellschaft für Nervenheilkunde und Psychiatrie*, **21**, 193–203.

Jacobson, E. (1971). *Depression: Comparative Studies of Normal, Neurotic, and Psychotic Conditions*. New York: International Universities Press.

Kendell, R. & Jablensky, A. (2003). Distinguishing between the validity and utility of psychiatric diagnoses. *American Journal of Psychiatry*, **160**, 4–12.

Kessing, L. V. (2004). Severity of depressive episodes according to ICD–10: prediction of risk of relapse and suicide. *British Journal of Psychiatry*, **184**, 153–6.

Klein, D. F. & Fink, M. (1962). Psychiatric reaction patterns to imipramine. *American Journal of Psychiatry*, **119**, 432–8.

Klein, D. F. (1964). Delineation of two drug-responsive anxiety syndromes. *Psychopharmacologia*, **5**, 397–408.

Kuhn, R. (1958). The treatment of depressive states with G22355 (imipramine hydrochloride). *American Journal of Psychiatry*, **115**, 459–64.

Kupfer, D., First, M. B. & Regier, D. E. (2002). Introduction. In *A Research Agenda for DSM-V*, pp. xv–xxiii. Washington, DC: American Psychiatric Association.

Sachs, G. S., Thase, M. E., Otto, M. W. *et al.* (2003). Rationale, design, and methods of the systematic treatment enhancement program for bipolar disorder (STEP-BD). *Biological Psychiatry*, **53**, 1028–42.

Shorter, E. & Tyrer, P. (2003). The separation of anxiety and depressive disorders: blind alley in psychopharmacology and the classification of disease. *British Medical Journal*, **327**, 158–60.

Tyrer, P. & Davidson, K. (2000). Cognitive therapy in personality disorders. In *Review of Psychiatry: personality disorders*, ed. G. O. Gabbard & J. Gunderson. Washington, DC: American Psychiatric Press.

Tyrer, P. & Steinberg, D. (2005). *Models for Mental Disorder: Conceptual Models in Psychiatry*, 4th edn. Chichester, UK: Wiley.

World Health Organization (1975). *International Classification of Diseases, 9th Revision, Clinical Modification*. Geneva: World Health Organization.

World Health Organization (1978). *International Classification of Diseases, 9th Revision, Clinical Modification*. Ann Arbor, MI: Commission on Professional and Hospital Activities.

Young, J. E., Klosko, J. S. & Weishaar, M. E. (2003). *Schema Therapy: A Practitioner's Guide*. New York: The Guilford Press.

The history of psychiatric therapies

German E. Berrios

Editor's note

Those who do not understand history are destined to repeat it, so Professor Berrios' reminder of the history of therapeutics is opportune. We often like to think of therapeutic discoveries being made in a logical sequence but so many of them are random. The famous Cambridge experimental psychologist, Frederick Bartlett, described a large part of our memory processes as 'effort after meaning', and this is illustrated excellently in this account. We are reminded that the meanings of words and our understanding of therapies almost has to be retranslated every hundred years. It is also chastening to find out how many of our treatments are discovered entirely by chance and on misplaced premises (read the section on ECT and psychosurgery and then look at Chapter 4II for the more recent arguments) and how long it took for ineffective treatments such as insulin coma therapy to be discredited. Readers of Orwell's *Animal Farm* will be interested to note that Cerletti and Bini's work on the introduction of ECT originated in observations with pigs, which is a logical sequence of sorts. The other illuminating aspect of this chapter is the way we have been almost seduced into the idea that all maladies have a cure, and that 'treatment resistance' formalizes the notion that out there is a successful treatment for every illness, and it just needs a clever therapist to find it. I hope we are not furthering this notion in publishing this book, which we admit is firmly in the tradition of selecting treatment as a 'scientific and mercantile transaction', even though we spare the reader the formal evaluation of cost-effectiveness in these pages.

Introduction

The understanding of the current notion of 'psychiatric treatment' depends on the coherence of concepts such

as mental disorder, effectiveness, evidence, probability, statistical significance, side effects, placebo, remission, resistance, chronicity, relapse, cure, etc. Since all such concepts are datable constructions, the study of psychiatric treatments requires an analysis of their history. Even the current distinction between biological, social and psychological treatments (which seems written in nature) is a distorted reflection of a classification of the sciences which only appeared during the eighteenth century. However, like the rest of the disciplines associated with psychiatry, history can only be as good as her methods.

Historiography

This chapter must therefore start with a brief analysis of the ways in which the history of psychiatric treatments can be (and has been) written in order to identify the most apposite historiography. *Apposite* here means rational, useful, predictive, aesthetically appealing, and adequately explanatory; *historiography* refers to techniques, rules and assumptions used to construct historical narratives (Lefevre, 1971; Kragh, 1987; Porter & Wear, 1987; Carbonell, 1991; Iggers, 1997). Historiographical awareness increases the probability (although it does not guarantee it) of writing good history.

Presentism

Many so-called histories of psychiatric treatment are no more than chronicles of progressive 'discoveries' (Laudan, 1977). This 'Whig approach' (Butterfield, 1931) is popular amongst clinicians who see history as a celebration of their achievements. Called also the 'whom to worship' (Young, 1966), 'who said it first' and 'latest is bestest' approach, this method makes use of categories such as discovery, genius, objectivity, evidence, science, serendipity, etc., and assumes that 'science' has monopoly over the truth. Such purview will also determine the type of 'historical' material to be used which almost exclusively will consist of 'peer-reviewed' papers reporting 'for the first time' successful 'new' treatments (Ruffat, 1996; Higby & Stroud, 1997). Since presentistic historians equate success with truthfulness, they will show little interest in unsuccessful treatments or in explaining success by means other than a correspondence with the 'truth'. They will also dismiss claims that old treatments have been successful because their success has not been assessed according to the latest statistical or methodological fashion. This leads to a dismissal of all such treatments as unscientific. It seems clear that when applied to the history of psychiatric therapies the Whig approach hampers understanding (Chast, 1995; Shorter, 1997). This is because it is blind to a nuanced analysis of the sociology or economy of 'success' (Vogel & Rosenberg, 1979; Bynum & Nutton, 1991; Porter, 1993; Porter & Teich, 1995; Braslow, 1997; Warner, 1997; Faure, 1999) and cannot handle the social phenomenon of post-hoc psychiatric diagnostic categories constructed around the prior 'discovery' of a 'miraculous' new treatment bullet (Cooper, 2005).

Historians of psychiatric treatments who believe in 'scientific progress' are happy to assume that mental disorders are concrete objects (natural kinds) (Laporte, 2004) whose very existence is independent from culture and language. This means that mental disorders are like rocks, dogs or orchids and exist in the world as autonomous entities. This ontological view underlies their 'naturalization', i.e. the reduction of mental disorders (without residuum) to genes, evolution, neurotransmitters, dysfunctions in neuropsychological pathways, etc. (Bennett & Hacker, 2003), and is also at the core of the linear, Whiggish historiography.

Periodicity and incommensurability

The history of psychiatric treatments can also be conceived of as the study of autonomous historical periods (called 'epistemes'), each having its own discourse, rules of meaning, and representations of life, society, person, mind, deviancy, disorder, ethics and social control (Berrios, 1994). Events and human actions can only be understood in terms of their episteme. No discourse, including that of 'science', can transcend its episteme and the concept of a theory-neutral 'description' of reality is considered as unintelligible. The collective representation of reality (Potter, 1996; Golinski, 1998) generated by each episteme depends upon the intertwined languages of

poetry, theology, science, ethics, politics, mythology, etc. Science cannot claim special privileges. Its current 'supremacy' is less due to its 'truth-obtaining power' than to its contribution to societal economy and stability. Because each historical period is self-contained, it cannot be understood (or judged) from the perspective of another historical period or from some absolute, external, 'objective' vantage point. Epistemes are thus incommensurate and incommensurable (Agazzi, 1985; Biagioli, 1990; Hoyningen-Huene, 1990; Chen, 1997).

This view originated in the late nineteenth century distinction between natural sciences (*Naturwissenschaften*) and human sciences (*Geisteswissenschaften*). Aimed at capturing meanings, experiences (*Erlebnisse*) and semantic Gestalts, the human sciences are based on hermeneutics (the discipline of interpretation). Schleiermacher, Droysen, Dilthey, Durkheim and Windelband developed this approach to the full (Grondin, 1991). Via Weber and Rickert (Oakes, 1988) this approach became well established in the social sciences of the twentieth century, and via Blondel and Bachelard it became applied to the natural sciences and eventually psychology and psychiatry. During a period in Paris, Thomas Kuhn learned of these ideas, and by the late 1950s he introduced a version of historical periodicity in the Anglo-Saxon world (Kuhn, 1962). Central to Kuhn's view is the claim that paradigms and their theories are incommensurable.

According to the *weak* programme of 'social constructionism', 'social factors' are only required at the moment in which scientific theories seek social acceptance. According to the '*strong* programme in the sociology of knowledge' (SSK), the very concept of 'evidence' is a social belief (Bloor, 1991) and hence social factors participate in the very legitimization of scientific theories.

This approach helps the historian to avoid anachronistic readings of the past, for example, the error of attributing to historical 'patients' and 'doctors' motivations and views that only belong to our present (Beier, 1987; Porter, 1985, 1995). This is because the understanding and concepts such as emotions, passions, sufferings, ailments, diseases, managing, helping, curing, etc. are different in each historical period (Graumann & Gergen, 1996; Danziger, 1997). For example, the current concept of 'emotion' was only constructed during the seventeenth century, and in terms of boundaries and experiential content is very different from 'passion', which is the word used to refer to 'orectic' mental functions before 1700 (Cogan, 1802; Levi, 1964; Brunschwig & Nussbaum, 1993; James, 1997; Despret, 1999; Dixon, 2003). From this it can be surmised that, say, the concept of melancholia had an entirely different experiential content in 1600 and in 2005 and hence 'treating' a person with melancholia in the former period has little to do with 'treating' one in our own day. The same differences can be predicated of the 'therapeutic attitude' itself when practised, say, in classic, medieval, modern and current times (Laín-Entralgo, 1970; Ackernecht, 1973; Porter, 1985; Beier, 1987; Bynum & Porter, 1987; Faure, 1999; Telesko, 2001; Nathan & Stengers, 2004).

This historiographical approach also throws a fresh light on the complex question of whether some earlier treatments may have actually worked (i.e. been efficacious). This question, asked by Rosenberg with special vigour (Rosenberg, 1997), concerns the meaning of 'efficacy', that is, should this elusive quality be defined from an absolute, objective, extra-epistemic perspective? And if so, should that perspective be that of the present? It has thus been claimed that bloodletting, the rotating chair, cold baths, moral treatment, insulin coma treatment, etc., have all worked well within their historical niche. Conventionally, such claims are explained away as: (1) inferentially false (e.g. due to observational bias); (2) true but trivial (e.g. due to spontaneous recovery, mis-diagnosis, placebo response); or (3) true and explicable in terms of modern science. Rarely, if ever, efficacy claims and the explanatory theory propounded *at the time* are accepted *simpliciter*.

Rosenberg's question is more acute in the field of psychiatric treatments because the definition of mental disorder remains prescriptive and underspecified, i.e. boundaries between disorders and normality depend on social criteria and systems of beliefs.

Psychiatric concepts related to treatments

'Treatment resistance' and 'treatment effectiveness'

The concept of 'treatment-resistance' is based on the assumptions that:
(1) some 'diseases' are susceptible to treatment;
(2) treatment-responsiveness is definable as the diminution or disappearance of symptoms for a reasonable (albeit unclear) period of time;
(3) improvement must be defined in terms of probability (e.g. 'statistical significance', 'power calculations', etc.);
(4) observed symptom-change should be attributed to the treatment in question if the assessment meets adequate methodological criteria;
(5) 'placebo response' is not an efficient 'explanation' and its contribution must be parcelled out statistically;

(6) a return of the illness (outside an indeterminate given time-period) should not count as evidence against the 'efficacy' of the treatment (to deal with this eventuality concepts of recrudescence or relapse have been constructed);
(7) 'psychiatric disorders' are structurally similar to medical disease and hence medical and psychiatric treatments should be evaluated by the same criteria;
(8) change in (certain) target symptoms constitutes evidence for treatment-response, even if the patient remains non-functional (to deal with this eventuality, the concept of partial response has been constructed);
(9) the mental symptoms that constitute the target 'disease' have similar value when it comes to assessing response to treatment;
(10) enough knowledge about the causes of the target disease is already available to define 'good' and 'appropriate' treatment; and,
(11) terms such as remission, relapse, recrudescence, chronicity, acuteness, etc. etc. reflect 'real events' in nature.

These assumptions reflect beliefs accumulated only since the nineteenth century. Before 1800, the concepts of treatment and cure were based upon a different theory of disease and upon different social expectations and hence cannot be compared with those which emerged after the early 1800s when the clinico-anatomical model of disease became predominant. Such epistemological breaks can to certain extent be found reflected in transcultural differences in the concepts of 'treatment' and 'cure'. For example, in some current (non-western) cultures such concepts are social rather than 'scientific' categories, that is, they are qualitative ways of looking at the result of the 'doctor-patient' interaction. In the 'developed' Western world, 'treatment' and 'cure' are embedded in 'medical acts' which are being increasingly re-defined as scientific and mercantile transactions ('health' has become a 'commodity', patients 'clients', clinicians 'purveyors of health'). This new approach demands that the medical act be measured and priced and rendered economically efficient. Like the selling of faulty goods, 'lack of response' to treatment is increasingly being considered as a violation of a putative trade descriptions act. Courts need 'operational criteria' to decide on whether a breach of trust has occurred, and these are being provided by the so-called treatment guidelines which bodies of experts are increasingly compiling. Non-response to treatment can only be called 'treatment-resistance' if the guidelines have been complied with, and this lets the therapist off the hook. In social and legal terms, the notion of 'treatment resistance' can thus be used as an alibi as it transfers the responsibility for the lack of response from the therapist to the disease or the patient.

The following definition is a good example of the above: 'the preferred outcome is *complete symptom remission*. In some cases one must accept a clinically significant *symptom reduction*. Depression may be difficult to treat because of the *nature of the condition itself; factors that interfere* with the proper delivery of optimal treatment (such as *poor adherence* or under-dosing); associated concurrent Axis I, II, or III disorders; or the lack of effective treatments. *If treatment is optimally delivered and an unsatisfactory outcome occurs, treatment resistance is said to be present.*'(my italics) (Rush *et al.*, 2003) Most of the assumptions listed above appear in this definition: the ideal of 'complete symptom-remission', the practical aim of 'symptom-reduction'; the blaming of the lack of response on 'the nature of the condition itself' and on 'factors that interfere' with the delivery of care; the mentioning of patient-related (negative) variables such as 'poor adherence'; and the tacit assumption that the model of depression or other disease used to diagnose the patient is the *true* one and could not possibly be the cause of the lack of response to treatment.

Chronicity and treatment resistance since the eighteenth century

Together with acute, sub-acute, response, remission, recovery, relapse, recurrence, etc. (Frank *et al.*, 1991), *chronicity* is a member (perhaps the oldest) of a 'family' of concepts constructed to qualify the nature of disease and its response to treatment. Hence, it is semantically dependent upon 'disease', 'treatment' and 'time'. Resistance, pseudo-resistance, refractoriness, etc., are recent members of the same family but on account of their negative (apophatic) definition they are epistemically weaker than the others.

Throughout history patients have either responded or failed to respond to treatment. Clinicians have attributed success to themselves and blamed failure to respond onto the patient, disease and other factors. 'Chronicity', in fact, is a good example of blaming the disease. Known since the time of Galen of Pergamum, the concept of 'chronic disease' was defined by him in terms of its 'longer' duration as compared with acute disease. Celsus introduced into the definition a *social* component: 'Swift or acute diseases may be cured spontaneously, with the aid sometimes of chance and sometimes of nature. And for this reason ignorant people often proudly avoid physicians and attribute these cures to new incantations or amulets or luck. . . . chronic or slow diseases, on the other hand, which are in

possession of the body by a previous crisis, can be helped only by the skilful physician. For neither nature or luck can effect a cure' (Caelius Aurelanius, 1950, p. 441).

Aretæus also blamed the disease or patient: 'of chronic diseases the pain is great, the period of wasting long, and the recovery uncertain; for either they are not dispelled at all, or the disease relapse upon any slight error; for neither have the patients the resolution to persevere to the end; or, if they do persevere, they commit blunders in a prolonged regime . . .' (Adams in Aretaeus, 1856, p. 293).

Interest in the concept of chronicity and chronic illness flared up during the late eighteenth and early nineteenth centuries (Buchner, 1753; Bordeu, 1775; Hounau, 1807; Dumas, 1812; Martinet, 1813). The entry on 'chronicity' in the *French Encyclopaedia* (written by M. le Chevalier de Jaucourt) started a trend: 'CHRONIQUE, adj. (*Médecine*) épithète qui se donne, & qui est consacrée aux maladies de longue durée. *Définition des maladies chroniques.* Les Médecins ayant divisés toutes les maladies, par rapport à la durée, en aiguës & en *chroniques*, nomment *maladies chroniques* toutes celles qui, douces ou violentes, accompagnées de fievre (sic) ou sans fievre, s'étendent au-delà de quarante jours.' (Diderot & D'Alembert, 1753, p. 388). De Jaucourt proposed three criteria: badly treated acute diseases can become chronic, inherent features that make some diseases chronic, and chronic is a disease lasting more than 40 days. This duration criterion was not taken up by the great writers on chronicity that followed him.

In the second edition of his great book on semiology, Landré-Beauvais developed a broader definition of chronicity. He also suggested that acute diseases could become chronic if age, constitution, physical state, climate and time of the year were unfavourable (Landré-Beauvais, 1813).

Chronicity and psychiatry

By the early nineteenth century it was still believed that madness was total and enduring and hence remissions were explained as 'lucid intervals' (madness always lurked in the background) (Berrios, 1996). During the 1810s, this metaphysical view of madness started to be challenged in the courts by the idea (of legal origin) that insanity could be 'partial'. After the 1850s, a second challenge to the totalistic view of madness arose from clinical observations made in the new mental asylums (Guillant *et al.*, 1964).

The medical concepts of acute and chronic disease arrived in psychiatry during this period. The latter caused little stir and was rapidly conflated with the old concept of total and enduring madness. 'Acute disease', on the other hand, found no counterpart amongst the various forms of madness as all were considered as enduring. By the 1850s, the conceptual panorama started to change as 'time' (as a dimension) became included into fashionable disciplines such as neurophysiology and the theory of evolution. For the first time, it became clear that chronic mental diseases could start as 'acute' disorders, and this created the need to explain the mechanisms of transition. Madness itself was seen as a 'process' occurring in time and space, and this led to the abandonment of the metaphysical claim of 'once mad always mad'. This temporalization of madness continued apace until 1863 when Kahlbaum suggested that madness could be defined in terms of course and the biological age at which it started (Kahlbaum, 1863).

In 1809, John Haslam suggested that the prediction of chronicity should be based on a distinction between a derangement and a decline of the intellect: 'the former may frequently be remedied; the latter admits of no assistance from our art'. He also cautioned that 'when the disorder has been induced from remote physical causes, the proportion of those who recover is considerably greater, than where it has arisen from causes of moral nature' (Haslam, 1809). A few years later, Pinel added criteria which are redolent of those listed by Aretæus: 'Forgetfulness, distraction or unclarity on the part of the clinician or natural indolence in the patient may keep the latter in bed beyond what is required by convalescence from an acute disease. A state of chronicity more or less dangerous may then issue out of the continuation of a weakening regime' (Pinel, 1813, p. 172). J. C. Heinroth echoed Haslam: 'All deviations of the psyche that are mixed with derangement of the intellect are less benign than those in which this derangement is absent; for this reason there is hope of recovery from this second species of insanity than from the first, especially if the disease has lasted for a long time...' The duration criterion is iterated soon afterwards: 'if the disease has persisted for more than a year, there is little hope of recovery' (Heinroth, 1975). In 1826, A. L. J. Bayle returned to the 'duration' criterion: 'the chronic meningitis which I have described is therefore an primary and particular disease, totally different from acute arachnoiditis and of its chronic form. The term chronic is useful to indicate that it goes on for a long time and is not related to its origin' (Bayle, 1826, p. 401).

By the second half of the nineteenth century the term 'chronic' starts to be used in psychiatry in a different fashion. This time it was attached to specific symptom clusters and disorders. As Lanteri-Laura has remarked, during this period chronicity became the hallmark of psychiatric illness and the world of institutional psychiatry was organized accordingly (Lanteri-Laura, 1997). Examples of this new usage can be found in the work of Kahlbaum (who influenced Kraepelin), Axenfeld and Magnan. Parallel to such changes is the establishment of the notion of 'degeneration' which provides another temporal foundation for the idea of chronicity: this time the latter is represented by the fact that successive generations of the same family are tainted by ever worsening mental disorders (Genil-Perrin, 1913).

Linking chronicity and treatment resistance

The twin concepts of 'treatment-response' and 'treatment-resistance' are meant to capture putative behavioural configurations occurring within a given period. Their study requires that the following be defined: (1) systems participating in the behavioural configurations; (2) what 'meaningful' change is or amounts to, (3) what measures of change are to be used, (4) the actors (doctor, patient and evaluator), and (5) contextual factors. These will generate a regional language with which to study the vicissitudes of treatment (both response and resistance).

For example, it is not always clear what of the *systems* participating in the therapeutic process is the primary target for assessment. To most it will be the disease or proxy variables representing the disease. However, this impersonal mode of evaluating response may not be sufficiently informative particularly when objectivity demands that the crucial variables be scores on a psychiatric instrument. Awareness of this problem, and of the relevance of ecological measures and qualitative assessments of psychosocial competence has led to the view that it is changes in the whole person that should be evaluated. This because persons are repositories of information relevant to treatment outcome which is not conventionally measured. Even more complex (and exact) methods of assessing treatment outcome should include the therapist (attitudes, beliefs, expectations) and the treatments themselves (posology, treatment patterns, side effects, social valence, cultural relevance and expectations, etc.).

Efforts to make treatment-resistance a 'scientific' concept have caused the neglect of contextual variables such as venue of treatment (in-patient, out-patient), time of the year, age, gender, social class, country, etc. Likewise there is little knowledge on whether or not the same definition of treatment-resistance should be used in medicine, psychiatry, clinical psychology, sociology, history, etc. This is because context modulates the way in which treatment is understood and works. In addition to obvious and measurable environmental variables, there are the cultural ones, that is, the way in which symbols, meanings and expectations will modulate the bioavailability of a treatment and its pharmacodynamic effects.

The rigidity and low heuristic yield of the concept of 'treatment-resistance' is due to the fact that it has been construed as the antonym of 'optimal outcome' (i.e. it is an apophatic notion). The latter, in turn, is currently defined nomothetically, that is, as the expected outcome to the correct application of certain treatment guidelines (Sachs & Rush, 2003). Within this narrow model, good outcomes to treatments not included in the guidelines must be considered as suspicious, and there is very little room for notions such as spontaneous recovery or the action of alternative remedial forces, the vis naturae medicatrix, and the placebo effect. As opposed to such a nomothetical definition, an idiographic definition (i.e. one which is developed in terms of each patient) could define 'optimal outcome' as a 'full return to premorbid levels of functioning' (Thase, 2003).

'Behavioural phenocopies'

The concept of 'behavioural phenocopy' is relevant to the issue of treatment and treatment failure and will be discussed briefly. It is used here as a generic name for behaviours and mental experiences that mimic or copy other behaviours and mental experiences (the 'originals'). The relationship between originals and their copies can best be described as one of phenomenological similarity, likeness or resemblance. Examples of behavioural phenocopies (of symptoms and diseases) are pain syndromes, fatigue, pseudoseizures, so-called 'dissociative' or 'conversion' symptoms (paralysis, dysphonia, paresthesiae, amnesia, etc.), depression-like pictures (e.g. organic depression), manic-like syndromes (e.g. secondary/organic mania), pseudo-dementia syndromes, obsessional-like symptoms (e.g. in HD/other dementias), psychotic symptoms, particularly in relation to neurological disease (e.g. hallucinations, delusion-like phenomena, misidentifications, etc.). Copies can act as confounders in diagnosis, prognosis, treatments, epidemiological and aetiological research and provide an explanatory mechanism for medically and psychiatrically unexplained symptoms. They can both overestimate or underestimate efficacy.

One problem with using 'original' and 'copy' is that their meaning is distorted by a false hierarchical relationship, namely, the belief that the copy is of less value than the original (as it might be between the original of Mona Lisa and one of its copies). This concrete situation is not transferable to descriptive psychopathology because both 'original' mental symptoms and what are called 'copies' are both constructs. The only reason why some are called the former and some the latter is an historical accident, namely that the 'original' was reported (published, noticed, etc.) first. Unfortunately, because 'originals' have been known for longer, they have received more social and scientific investment, have been enshrined earlier in official glossaries, etc., and hence have acquired a sort of groundless ontological primacy or autonomy. For example, the claim that pseudoseizures are 'copies' of some 'original' form of seizure (like some that can be seen in epilepsy) should only be understood as meaning that there is a surface resemblance between the two and not to that the pseudoseizure is (clinically or scientifically) less important than the original (Berrios & Marková, 2002).

Behavioural phenocopies are relevant to the diagnosis of 'treatment-resistance'. Because they are not the target disease (i.e. only look like it), they may not respond to the treatment created to deal with the target disease. In the absence of neurobiological markers, the clinician still relies on a description of surface resemblance and hence it is easy to get it wrong because it is likely that copies and originals present often together in clinical practice. Their relative proportion remains unknown for currently there is little awareness of their existence (except in some specific cases). It would seem clear now that the future development of more specific treatments for some psychiatric conditions will require that the incidence and prevalence, and differential diagnosis of copies are carefully studied.

The history of psychiatric treatments: from classical antiquity to the nineteenth century

There will be no space in this chapter to deal piecemeal with the way in which the treatment or management of madness and allied disorders changed from century to century. There will be just space to discuss general points and trends with the objective of raising historical awareness and showing how concepts such as patient, doctor, disease, complaint, treatment, cure, etc., are context-dependent.

Mental bothers derangements and their treatments

Psychiatric treatments can be defined as interventions aimed at modifying experiences and behaviours considered as undesirable. Because 'undesirability' is socially defined, psychiatric treatments are best described as socio-ethical acts. The manner in which such acts and their motivation were formed and have emerged from the cultures of the west remains little understood. This opaqueness has been made worse but the current fashion of presenting such acts as being purely 'scientific', 'evidence-based' and 'epistemologically independent' from all social factors. It is of course the case that everyone pays lip service to the sociology and ethics of medical treatments. A cursory examination, however, shows that social and ethical factors are not made to participate in the very definition of treatment acts but are considered as important to what can be called their organization and administration. In other words, a treatment is deemed 'effective' because its evaluation has met certain 'scientific criteria', that it, the truth of its effectiveness depends upon the statistical significance yielded by a set of randomized clinical trials and not by the fact that it is ethically or socially acceptable. Given the success of the current rhetoric of science, it is therefore unavoidable that earlier therapeutic acts will suffer when compared with current ones and be deemed non-scientific, capricious, backward, irrational, cruel or immoral. The historian must not fall into this trap. As mentioned in the first part of this chapter, historical evidence is accumulating that some earlier treatments have worked and this success should not be dismissed as placebo effect, bias or bad outcome assessments.

The rhetorical triumphalism of current drug trialists must be avoided as current treatments (and the statistical criteria used to evaluate them) will in due course become 'historical' and found equally wanting or false. Within each historical period, the historian finds that certain mental complaints, the treatments developed to deal with them, and the rules to evaluate their success are interdependent. The job of the historian is to throw light on what factors have determined such interdependences and to clarify the meaning of the claim that the latest methodology and rules of evaluation have to be 'better, superior, more exact, truer, etc.'.

For example, in classical times, the *'tekhne iatriké'* or *'ars medica'* dictated the objectives and boundaries of all therapeutic interventions. The *ars medica* itself reflected models of the world and of man upheld by the Greek and Roman cultures (Brock, 1929). Nowhere is this better illustrated than in 'The Art', one of the books of the Hippocratic Corpus. Written by a lay person (Protagoras and Hippias are the main authorial candidates), the text specifies that the *duty* and *right* of a physician, are, respectively, to *alleviate* suffering and *refuse* to treat incurable disorders. It also attacks the claims that patients get better spontaneously or through luck, that doctors select for treatment only those patients who they believe will get better, and that patients die in spite of treatment. This text is important for it suggests that by the fifth century BC the physician could already tell curable from incurable, and that he was already having difficulties in showing that his therapeutic intervention was a factor in the cure: '... no

patient who recovers without a physician can logically attribute the recovery to spontaneity. Indeed, under a close examination spontaneity disappears; for everything that occurs will be found to do so 'through something', and this 'through something' shows that spontaneity is a mere name, and has no reality. Medicine, however, because it acts 'through something', and because its results may be forecasted, has reality, as is manifest now and will be manifest for ever...' (Hippocrates, 1967, p. 201).

In Classical times ideas on treatment evolved in three stages: Hippocratic, Alexandrian-Roman and Galenic (Laín-Entralgo, 1978). The Hippocratic model revolved around the *vis medicatrix*, the healing power of nature. Following rather than fighting such power the physician could achieve his objectives of saving mankind, regaining of health, alleviating suffering and restoring the patient's decorum (Laín-Entralgo). In practice, the physician was enjoined to do no harm, to avoid trying the impossible (i.e. not to treat incurable diseases) and to treat the 'cause' of the disease ('cause' then meant something different from what it means now) (Wallace, 1972). Treatments had to be opportune, personalized, prudent, holistic, and aesthetically pleasing. There were three main modalities of treatment: the *pharmakón*, term which in Greek meant scapegoat, venom, and agent of nature (physiological); *dietetics*, which consisted in influencing health, encouraging life and attention to hygiene; and *'chirurgy'* which related to a cure by the use of the hands (*kheir*).

The Alexandrian-Roman physicians called into question the Hippocratic acceptance of the *vis medicatrix*, aspiring to a higher and more active role, namely, to become governors of nature. This they did by encouraging the development of surgery, particularly in areas such as gynaecology and ophthalmology, and the introduction of bloodletting (Médioni, 1992).

Galen, in turn, rationalized the concept of therapy by setting up canonical criteria which were to last well into the seventeenth century (Temkin, 1973). Although a believer in the *vis medicatrix*, Galen introduced the idea that knowledge of the structure and function of the bodily parts may empower the physician to enhance the healing powers of nature. To the four Aristotelian causes (formal, material, efficient & final) Galen added the concept of 'instrumental cause', (i.e. the antecedent conditions and physical dispositions leading to disease) and made it the foundation of his therapeutic approach. He believed that human health resulted from the equilibrium between blood, yellow bile, black bile, and phlegm. These four Hippocratic humours were, in turn, built up from combinations of the old Aristotelian qualities of hot, cold, wet, and dry (Garcia Ballester, 1972). Each disease resulted from a different type of humoural imbalance which was sited both in a specific organ and the body as a whole (Hankinson, 1998). His therapeutic approach was based on the definition and recognition of the 'instrumental causes': (a) patterns of humoural imbalance (the disease); (b) the organ affected, the temperament, biological constitution, dreams, age and gender of the patient; and (c) environmental factors (Siegel, 1973).

Because they were based on the dissection of animals, Galen's anatomical ideas survived for less time than his teleological physiology and other works which after being reintroduced in the West became the medical canon up to the Renaissance (Boudon, 2000). During the fifteenth century Galenic ideas on therapy reached their culmination in the famous correlational tables (*tacuinum sanitatis*) showing correspondences between profiles of humoural pathology and foodstuffs, plants, seasons, clothing, physical exercise, etc. For centuries, these tables were used as veritable therapeutic 'guidelines' (Telesko, 2001).

Galenism (Daremberg, no date) continued until challenged by Paracelsus who rejected the old theory of humours, renewed the materia medica by including alchemical minerals, and revived the old 'doctrine of signatures', namely, the view that the form, colour and other external features of plants predicted therapeutic indication and clinical efficacy (Virey, 1821; Chereau, 1881; Pachter, 1951). Most importantly, by proposing that treatments should be specific to diseases and not to 'clinical states', Paracelsus started the shift from symptomatic to aetiological therapy (Pagel, 1958). In general, these changes little affected the way in which madness was dealt with at the time.

Two views on the nature of disease and its treatment vied for supremacy during the seventeenth century (Boinet, no date). According to the iatromechanical view (Brown, 1970), treatments should address the mechanical alterations underlying disease (changes in fibres, tubules, nerves, etc.); according to the iatro chemical view, changes in chemical principles (including alchemic ones) caused diseases and their study and manipulation provided the rationale for all forms of therapy, including balneology (Coley, 1979). Iatromechanics was a development of the Cartesian mechanistic model of matter (Carter, 1983). Iatrochemistry was a continuation of Paracelsian therapeutic philosophy.

Thomas Willis, whose ideas on 'mental disorder' and its treatment are important to the history of psychiatric therapy (Conry, 1982), took a middle course. Whilst broadly adhering to the mechanistic approach, Willis resorted to non-mechanical concepts and occult qualities (Henry, 1986) to explain certain physiological changes. For example, he proposed that the change of 'blue' to 'red' blood

took place in the left ventricle aided by the presence of a ferment which digested foodstuff diluted in blue blood. In conceptual terms, this explanation was no different from Harvey's claim that blood was 'intrinsically' active (Frank, 1980). On account of his acceptance of the existence of occult principles in the workings of nature, it has been claimed that Willis was closer to Gassendi ('*qualitez occultes ou cachees*')(Bernier, 1674, p. 458) than to Descartes (Bynum, 1973).

Willis proposed treatments for melancholia, mania, phrensy, epilepsy, etc. Interpretation of his proposals is hampered by the fact that the current meaning of these terms has changed radically since Willis's times (Berrios, 1996). In all cases, success is claimed with bleeding, purgation and vomiting although the frequency of each treatment, the substances and methods with which it was achieved, and the aetiological model involved, were very much taken into account (Willis, 1685, pp. 370–494).

Rationale for the treatment of mental disorders, and the treatments themselves, vary little until the nineteenth century when major changes in the explanatory narratives of psychiatry underwent severe change (Bynum, 1964). This was brought about by the appearance of new ways of describing and interpreting the behavioural and subjective manifestations of mental disorder (semiology and descriptive psychopathology), by a new model of disease (anatomo-clinical model) that forced psychiatry to concentrate on the study of the brain as the seat of madness, and by the development of venues of care (e.g. large asylums) which encouraged the longitudinal and more or less consistent application of treatments (e.g. moral treatment) (Berrios & Freeman, 1991).

In addition to the traditional and newer treatments for insanity (e.g. the rotating chair) (Wade *et al.*, 2005), the nineteenth century saw the development of more social and psychological approaches. These were inspired by the reforming and humanitarian philosophy of the philanthropic movements (Gray, 1905; Jordan, 1959) whose main focus at the time was on poverty, slavery, penal reform, and prostitution. The care of the insane was also to benefit from such an important social movement. For example, in a classical report, Colombier and Doublet recommended that the insane, whether acute or chronic, must be offered special accommodation and 'treatment' (Colombier & Doublet, 1785). Echoes of this report can be heard in Daquin's oft-quoted 'La Philosophie de la Folie' (Daquin, 1792).

In regards to insanity, the therapeutic philosophy of the philanthropic movement (Curti, 1974) crystallized in what was then called 'moral treatment'. The term referred to a collection of attitudes, techniques and management approaches popular in Europe roughly between the end of the eighteenth century and the division of the nineteenth. Although 'moral' meant 'non-physical' or 'psychological' it was not free from 'moral' connotations (in the current sense of the term). On account of this, it was used to refer to a range of management practices which included hospitalization, isolation, entertainment, protection from stress and from the family, attempts to convince the individual of their wrong ideas and emotions, manipulation of emotions deemed to be upset in madness, active induction of anxiety and fear, and physical restraint (Séguin, 1846; Kraft, 1961; Ey, 1978; Postel, 1979; Baguenier-Desormeaux, 1983). By the middle of the nineteenth century, as alienists became more interventionist, aggressive forms of 'moral therapy' became popular. This can be shown in France by comparing the proposals of Colombier & Doublet (1785) with those by Amard (1807) at the beginning of the nineteenth century and with the content of the 1840s debate when Leuret openly discussed the failures of the intimidatory procedures of moral treatment and their combination with physical treatments (Leuret, 1838). Moral treatment followed a similar evolution in Germany and Great Britain (Scull, 1979; Digby, 1985; Suzuki, 1995).

The adoption by alienists of more aggressive forms of moral treatment is a reflection of their increasing professionalization and self-confidence and a response to the practical pressures brought about by asylums overcrowding, by the gradual erosion of the relationship between doctor and patient (as had developed in the small private madhouses of the eighteenth century) (Parry-Jones, 1972), and by changes in their beliefs about the mechanisms of madness (by the middle of the nineteenth century works began to appear providing a rationale for the way in which the manipulation of emotions and of physical activity (which were central to the concept of Moral Therapy) could help in medicine; Ribes, 1860). Moral treatments were also 'complemented' by physical methods such as water treatment, cold baths, and drugs. This means that it is very unlikely that 'moral treatment' can be considered as a precursor of psychotherapy (Carlson & Dain, 1960). Only at the turn of the century this melee was teased out into the categories we know and cherish now: physical, psychological, social and administrative treatments, and each was provided with explanatory narratives taken from allied sciences. For example, the physical treatments (whose mechanisms of action had until the 1860s been explained as mediated by 'psychological factors') began to be explained in terms of the language of the neurosciences; and psychological treatments were 'explained' in terms of the findings provided by clinical psychology and the nascent discipline of psychoanalysis. Thus, the

nineteenth century was not exception to the belief that in each historical period madness and allied behaviours are fitted into a different Procrustean bed. But it was also the century when for the first time books fully devoted to psychiatric treatments began to appear and when alienists accepted (perhaps for the last time) that their therapeutic endeavours were influenced by the social class, economic status, gender, ethnic origin, etc. of their charges.

Drugs, remedies and mental disorders

As discussed above, when writing on the history of drug treatments in psychiatry the historian must decide on whether or not to use a presentistic historiography. The latter demands that complex social choices and constructs be conceived of as 'discoveries' and be listed in a chronological line going from past to present (from worst to best). Such a decontextualizing approach negates the offering of a real historical explanation.

For three reasons this issue is relevant to the history of drug therapy in insanity. Firstly, up to the nineteenth century such drugs were part of the 300 or so items comprised in the materia medica of the West (and for that matter the East). In this regard, it has been claimed that 'a typical medicine chest of an 18th century physician was not very different from a 13th century physicians chest' (Riddle, 1992, p. 12). Secondly, for the last two millennia 'madness' was part of conventional nosology. Thirdly, the 'medical acts' whereby such drugs were administered to madmen were subsumed under the rest of general medical acts. It is thus difficult to talk about anything like a history of 'psychopharmacology' before the beginning of the nineteenth century.

Nineteenth century materia medica

Up to the division of the nineteenth century canonical texts of materia medica do not include sections on the treatment of madness (although some refer to 'brain diseases') (Petersen, 1877). This is the case of Barbier's great work where the 'appareil cérébral' is included as a rubric when he discussed the effects of classes of drugs on bodily systems (Barbier, 1824, p. 476). Milne-Edwards and Vavasseur also included a section on drugs with exciting effect specially on the 'nervous system' (1828, p. 341) but madness is not mentioned in that section. Examples can be multiplied. The situation changed by the second half of the century. Trousseau's 'Materia Medica', the standard textbook for generations of medical students, discussed in depth the use of drugs in alienism. For example, when dealing with Chloral detailed mention is made of

'Insomnia, agitation, delirium and insanity' in its indications (Trousseau & Pidoux, 1877, Vol. 2, pp. 350–351). The same is the case with the popular experimental therapeutics by Antoine de Störck who dealt with the effect of a number of drugs on madness, delusions, etc. (Störck, 1887).

The situation was different in regards to textbooks on alienism which from early in the nineteenth century carried chapters on treatment often including references to drugs. For example, Pinel discussed them in some detail although his conclusion was that drugs are only adjuvants of psychological (moral) and physical treatments. Since Pinel believed that the stomach and intestines contributed to the development of madness (e.g. mania), he averred that laxatives and purgatives helped manic patients; indeed, he reported the observation that spontaneous diarrhoeas could contribute to the remission of mania (Pinel, 1809, pp. 355–357). Little had changed by the second half of the century. In Griesinger, for example, drugs are included with other physical treatments such as cold baths, bleeding, cupping, blistering and cutaneous irritants. *Inter alia*, Griesinger discussed opium, digitalis, ether, chloroform, hydrocyanic acid, belladonna, emetics and purgatives (Griesinger, 1861).

The second half of the century was to witness the publication of works specially dedicated to the drug treatment of mental disorder. One of the earliest (organized in the manner of the old medical casuistries) was a book by a homeopathic physician, Hermeil, who grouped 164 cases of mental disorder under the active substance that had been administered, e.g. aconitum napellus (5), anancardium orientale (8), aurum (6), belladonna (24), calcarea carbonica (4), helleborus niger (4), hepar sulfurus calcarea (19),hyoscyamus (13), nux vomica (8), opium (7), pulsatilla (9), stramonium (10), sulphur (7), veratrum (14), etc. The clinical descriptions show the author's awareness of the ongoing nosological debates (Hermeil, 1856).

By the end of the century publications on psychiatric treatments had multiplied including both textbooks and monographs on specific therapies. Salient amongst these are the book by Luys which *inter alia* included chapters on out-patients (*aliénés en liberté*), high suicidal risk, psychosurgery and ethics thereof, incontinence, etc. (Luys, 1893). A major volume on the treatment of mental disorders, edited by Valentin Magnan, included chapters by Chaslin on acute and chronic delusional disorder and mental confusion; Mairet on General Paralysis of the Insane; Blin on mania and dementia; Ritti on melancholia; Sollier on mental handicap; and by Magnan himself on delusional disorders and intermittent madness. Each chapter had a standard format that included general clinical features,

treatments, general aspect of the therapy, etc. (Magnan, 1898). Equally important was the treatise by P. J. Kovalevsky (Professor of Psychiatry at Kharkov, now in Ukraine), one of few foreign psychiatric treatises to be translated into French. The book includes chapters on nutrition, clothing, ventilation, electrotherapy, hydrotherapy, kinesitherapy, drugs, psychological treatments, and asylum management. Kovalevsky (1890) introduced the chapter on drugs by stating that there seems to have been a diminution in the importance of drug therapies in the management of the insane and then listed comments upon each type: revulsive (bleeding, cupping, 'cooling of the head by ice', cold showers, blistering, purgatives, ergotization, use of calabarine (alkaloid found in the Calabar-bean), fortified alcohols and tonics, arsenic, quinine, arnica, digitalis, camphor, phosphates, potassium iodine, quick silver, opium, hyoscine, chloral hydrate, amyl nitrate, cocaine, and bromides.

Things were no different in Great Britain. Like Pinel at the beginning of the century, Hack Tuke recommends that the 'proximate cause of the attack of insanity' (that is, some organic disorder) is dealt with first: 'so long as a disordered liver disturbs the healthy action of the mind, so long as a disorder of the colon occasions melancholia . . . in short so long as any of the viscera are the seat of disease, and the physician disregards such disorder of the bodily organs, he clearly fails to fulfil the first indication of treatment . . .' (Tuke, 1892, p. 1290). Tuke also discusses drugs under the following headings: counter-irritation, depressants (bleeding, antimony, purgatives), tonics and stimulants (iron, arsenic, phosphorus quinine, strychnia), narcotics (opiates, hypodermic injections of morphia, hyoscyamus), sedatives (chloral, paraldehyde, bromides, sulphonal, cannabis), baths, electricity, and feeding.

German textbooks of psychiatry made similar points. Krafft-Ebing (1893), for example, sets out the two principles on which the treatment of madness should be based: understanding of the origin and nature of the physical changes underlying insanity and avoidance of all measures that may weaken the organism of the insane patient. The author recommends measures to 'reduce the fluxion of blood to the brain': depletion (bleeding), reduction of the activity of the heart via (digitalis), dilatation of peripheral vessels (baths, cascara, rhubarb), contraction of cerebral vessels (hydrotherapy, irritation of the skin, nicotine, hyoscyamus, nux vomica, etc.); and 'calming therapies' such as narcotics, hypnotics, tonics, diet, etc.

It would be fair to conclude then that up to the turn of the century a convergence of views on psychiatric therapeutics had been achieved in Europe. This continued into the early twentieth century when new treatments started to develop: some were specific, e.g. Salvarsan or hyperthermia for general paralysis of the insane; others general, e.g. psychopharmacology (the Oxford English Dictionary dates to 1920 the earliest usage of this term; Macht, 1920), insulin coma, electroconvulsive therapy and psychosurgery. As an example, the history of some of these approaches will now be discussed.

'Psychopharmacology'

In most current books on psychiatric treatments, the lion's share of space is dedicated to drugs and their effects on mental disorder. The shift in emphasis occurred during the early 1950s. For example, in the 1951 Meeting on 'Psychiatric Treatments' of the American Association for Research in Nervous and Mental Disease the lion's share of space in the proceedings is still occupied by the psychotherapies (Wortis *et al.*, 1953). A similar comment can be made about France (Claude & Rubenovitch, 1940; Cossa, 1945; Baruk, 1955).

Since the time when *Phantastica* was first published in 1924 (it compiled the effects of compounds from plants and synthetic chemicals on the mind, and gave rise to the discipline of ethno-botany; Lewin, 1998), knowledge on psychoactive substances seems to have accumulated fast to the point that by the late 1950s generic treatments such as amphetamines, barbiturates, chloral hydrate, and paraldehyde had been replaced by drugs which were being marketed for specific disorders. This specificity was made possible by the construction of concepts such as neurotransmitter, drug receptor and neurochemical localization, and by their statistical association with mental functions. Equally important to the predominance of psychotropic drugs has been the public relations work done on behalf of the ever growing pharmaceutical industry, ambivalence about the efficacy of psychological treatments, and the waning popularity of biological treatments such as ECT and psychosurgery. Although a minority are likely to remain hostile to drugs on account of their psychological views of mental disorder, they are considered by the Industry as numerically and economically unimportant. In this regard, it is sufficient for the economic success of psychopharmacology that the view that drugs are the treatment of choice for most mental ailments is accepted by a sizeable majority.

On account of their popularity, histories of psychopharmacology started to be written early (Gayral & Dauty, 1957; Gordon, 1958). Most of these works are little more than lists of discoveries (Lehmann & Ban, 1997; López-Muñoz & Álamo, 1998; Domino, 1999). Some authors, however, have valiantly studied the development of drugs as historical and social acts (Barcia, 1998), analysed issues pertaining to their historiography (Braslow, 1997, 2000), research ethics (Healy, 2002), efficacy, side effects, and long-term (as opposed to short-term) impact of disease (Moncrieff, 1999).

Of particular interest is the history of the methodology on the basis of which it is decided whether or not a drug works (Tröhler, 2000). Drug trial methodology and the statistical analyses which developed to make it 'significant' in the first half of the twentieth century (the idea that mathematics can be applied to quality and to the metier of the social sciences needed some time to develop; crucial to this process in England are works such as Edgeworth, 1881) are seen by many as part of the ineluctable progress of science. The view that probability may have epistemological value started to develop during the nineteenth century (Gigerenzer *et al.*, 1989). The style of thinking according to which the 'knowledge' generated by probability estimates is tantamount to 'evidence' is called 'statistical reasoning' (on the epistemological aspects of statistics, see Taper & Lele, 2004). It is currently believed that the latter offers adequate scientific and ethical purchase for social and political decision-making (Desrosières, 1998).

Declaring a drug efficacious on the basis of clinical experience alone is considered unscientific and the current summum bonum for such evaluations is the randomized controlled clinical trial (Matthews, 2000). Because of its 'impersonal, pure, and objective' nature, this methodology is regarded as the only path to truth and all efforts to conceptualize it as a 'social practice' are rejected (Marks, 1997). This damages all chances of studying its role in social, political and economic control (for example, in the demonization of alternative therapies). Drugs which 'pass the test' (however insignificant the statistical significance supporting them is) gain a magic status (licence) and the right to be administered to the public. However, the process of evaluating required by the licensing procedure remains largely in the hands of the pharmaceutical industry itself and this has led to concealment of data about side effects, and other serious infringements of objectivity (on this the work of Healy, 2004, is of great importance).

There is no space to write at length on the history of psychopharmacology nor is there any need to: in spite of 'major' claims made in favour of drug therapies they occupy just a small space on the broader canvas of history (for further information see many references listed above). Far more didactic from the ethical viewpoint is the history of treatments which in the recent past were supported by claims worryingly similar to those currently made in favour of psychopharmacology. Some of these will be discussed now.

Insulin coma therapy

At its zenith, insulin coma therapy was fully supported by medical theory (Geller, 1962) and the full paraphernalia of science (Rinkel & Himwich, 1959) and proved to be a popular (and some claimed successful) treatment for certain forms of insanity (Abély, 1939). Its history can be written in two ways: as that of a nonsensical treatment eventually rooted out by the power of the new statistical methodology of medicine (Cramond, 1987) or as a truly useful treatment which helped many patients, created a social revolution in the context of the asylum, and taught psychiatrists the value of therapeutic teams (James, 1992; Jones, 2000), and which was got rid of only when the space of treatment needed to be cleared up for the sale of neuroleptics (D'Aulney & Malineau, 1956). For example, much has been made of the Lancet papers (Bourne, 1953; Ackner et al., 1957) that are supposed to have sounded the knell of insulin coma therapy. The fact of the matter is that they did not. For example, in 1958, a meeting of experts (both clinicians and basic scientists) on insulin coma therapy was held at the New York Academy of Medicine to collate recent research and evaluate contradictory evidence, including the Lancet papers (an equally critical American paper was, however, not discussed nor was the author able to attend the New York meeting; David, 1954). The editors concluded that on the basis of the evidence presented that 'insulin therapy is not outmoded and is still essential in psychiatry' (Rinkel & Himwich, 1959, p. x). Indeed, the treatment continues well into the late 1960s in places where there was less pressure from the pharmaceutical industry to prescribe neuroleptics.

The basic facts on the origin, development and rationale of insulin coma therapy have been rehearsed many times before (Sakel, 1935; Braunmühl, 1938; James, 1992; Jones, 2000). In 1936, Dr Isabel Wilson was instructed by the Board of Control in England to study and report the new treatment. After visiting various psychiatric departments where the treatment was being implemented, including Sakel's in Vienna, and fully evaluating the literature, Dr Wilson produced an extraordinarily lucid report (Wilson, 1937). Her conclusions were:

(1) The results of Hypoglycaemic Shock Therapy as published in a number of countries indicate that the treatment is promising.
(2) The association between insulin treatment and clinical improvement is occasionally very striking.
(3) The degree of response to be expected cannot be clinically prophesied in any case or group of cases.
(4) Because of the difficulties of diagnosis and the variability in spontaneous course and in response to physical and psychological treatments which schizophrenia may show, published statistics on the effect of insulin therapy can only be regarded as tentative.
  (a) In groups of treated cases the percentage in whom remission or improvement can be definitely ascribed to insulin treatment, cannot be accurately deduced.
  (b) Longer and fuller experience will be needed before firm opinion can be reached on the influence of insulin treatment on the duration of remission or on the tendency to relapse.
(5) The method certainly merits ample clinical trial.
(6) The treatment is neither too dangerous nor too unpleasant to be used in a serious disorder.
(7) Many aspects of the action of insulin in the psychoses invite further study and research.

This report opened the doors to the introduction of the treatment in England and Wales and by the early 1950s great experience had been accumulated in at least 31 centres. These were overseen by the Board of Control and Dr Wilson acted as their consultant. Escaping Nazism many Continental doctors well trained in the technique came to England and they helped with the safe introduction of the procedure. From the start, one problem had been the lack of a standard protocol, for example, there were variations in both the depth of the coma (which admittedly was difficult objectively to ascertain) and its duration (it varied between 1 and 4 hours) and also in whether the treatment was administered alone or together with other treatments (Fleming, 1950). This meant that clinical results from the various centres were difficult to compare. It is not altogether clear why the treatment declined during the 1960s but historical evidence suggests that the reasons were other than negative outcome studies.

The convulsive therapies

The 'convulsive therapies' are procedures aimed at treating mental disorders by causing fits or seizures induced by either drugs (Metrazol, Fluorothyl) or an electrical current passed through the head. This section will deal only with the development of electroconvulsive therapy.

Originally, the convulsive therapies (i.e. by cardiazol) were based on the hypothesis that there was a negative correlation between schizophrenia and epilepsy (Meduna, 1938). Clinical observation (Krapf, 1928) suggested that having one disease protected from having the other; neuropathological evidence (Nyirö & Jablonsky, 1929) seemed to show that nerve fibres were thinner in schizophrenia than in epilepsy and that inducing artificial seizures in subjects with schizophrenia caused nerve hypertrophy and alleviation of the mental disorder (Meduna, 1934).

Three periods can be identified in the history of ECT. The first ends up in about 1945 and includes work on the neurophysiology of ECT, specific indications, and the control of side effects. The second period goes up to the late 1950s, and it includes the debate on unilateral and bilateral placing of electrodes. The third period reaches the present and comprises research into clinical indications, side effects, neurobiology and endocrinology, and 'seizure duration'. There is here space only to deal with the first period (for a full study of the history of ECT see Berrios, 1997).

The convulsive therapies find their origin in the work of Ladislas Joseph von Meduna.[1] At the 89th Meeting of the Swiss Psychiatric Association, Meduna argued that whilst there was no evidence for the view that insulin 'reversed the predominance of old over new fibres in the brain of schizophrenics': 'Between schizophrenia and epilepsy there exists a sort of biological antagonism which must be expressed in the pathological course of the two diseases ... I feel justified in asserting a priori that these courses are either mutually exclusive or they do, at least to a great degree, weaken each other in their mutual effects.' (Meduna, 1938, pp. 44–45).

The relationship between schizophrenia and epilepsy has a long history (Berrios, 1995). Up to the 1910s the view was popular that epilepsy and dementia praecox were associated (agonism hypothesis) but in the interbellum period the antagonism view had gained the upper hand. This 'biological antagonism hypothesis' received crucial support from the work of Glaus who in 6000 subjects with schizophrenia had found a prevalence of epilepsy as low as 0.13% and observed that in the eight patients in which both conditions were combined there was an *alternation* of the conditions (Glaus, 1931). By the late 1930s improved statistical analysis cast doubt on this finding. Esser (1938) reported that the prevalence of epilepsy in schizophrenia was, in fact, 1.5%; and Yde *et al.* (1941) went as far as saying that it was twice that of the general population.

[1] Von Meduna (1896–1964) was born in Hungary and completed his medical studies at the Royal Clinical School of Budapest in 1921. He started his academic career three years later as an assistant professor at the Neurological Institute in the same city and in 1927 became associate professor of psychiatry. In 1933 he was appointed consultant to the Leopold Field hospital. The Nazi threat led him to emigrate to the USA in 1939 where he continued his career at the University of Illinois. At the Neurological Institute he worked under the great Karl Schaffer on the distribution and type of neuroglia in the cortex of subjects with epilepsy and schizophrenia. He is credited with the development and implementation of cardiazol therapy. Later on he also developed the interesting clinical notion of 'oneirophrenia' (Meduna, 1950).

Von Meduna's early work

Following animal research which included injections of camphor in guinea pigs (Meduna, 1939), Meduna started treating patients on 23rd January 1934, and by the end of the year had treated 26. The response to cardiazol was of about 66% amongst acute and stuporous patients with schizophrenia. Meduna believed that cardiazol acted on the medulla oblongata, and that its convulsant effect was reached when 0.4–0.5 g given intravenously and diluted in a 10% solution. The convulsion usually occurred within 2 seconds of the injection and lasted anywhere between 30–80 seconds (Meduna, 1937). By the time he had emigrated to the USA, the antagonism hypothesis had been called into question. Meduna proposed instead that the shock worked at an endocrinological level re-establishing mental 'harmony' (Meduna, 1943). However, the Metrazol seizure was unreliable: it may not occur, or occur later and outside the intensive care period or last for too long; this encouraged the search for another stimulus that might provoke seizures.

The early use of an electric stimulus

In 1935, Ugo Cerletti, professor of Neuropathology and Psychiatry in Rome[2], sent one of his assistants to Meduna's department to learn the Metrazol technique. In the meantime, he had observed at a slaughter-house that electric shocks rendered animals comatose and that the amount of electricity correlated with the behavioural effects.[3] Together with Lucio Bini (said to have been crucial to the success of the research),[4] Ferdinando

[2] The son of an agricultural engineer, Ugo Cerletti was born at Conegliano Veneto, Italy, on 26th September 1877 and trained as a physician at Rome and Turin. He did his neuropsychiatric training in Paris under Pierre Marie and Ernest Dupré, and at Heidelberg and Munich under Kraepelin, Nissl, and Alzheimer. During the First World War, he is said to have invented a white camouflage for the Alpine troops, and also a delayed time fuse for the rifle. He became a professor in Rome in 1935, retired in 1948, and died on 25th July 1963 (Breathnach, 1990).

[3] Cerletti & Bini's (1938) *post-hoc* narrative must be considered as a *reconstruction* (in Lakatos's sense): When 'Cardiazol-induced convulsive therapy appeared in the scene, the authors thought *immediately* of using an electric current to achieve the same results' (p. 260).

[4] Lucio Bini was born on 18th September 1908, and when at age 30 he started his collaboration with Cerletti he had not yet trained as a psychiatrist. He was soon to do so and in the event was senior author of one of the leading Italian textbooks of psychiatry (Bini & Bazzi, 1954). He also wrote an important (and little known) monograph on dementia (Bini, 1948). At the time of his untimely death in 1964, he was a Clinic director at San Camillo Hospital in Rome.

There is some evidence that Cerletti tried to play down Bini's contribution. In 1950, for example, he stated that 'he was only a

Accornero[5] and Mario Felici,[6] Cerletti started exploring the usefulness of electricity as a seizure-inductor.

There is little point in repeating the oft-told story of this research, and of the first ECT in a human being (Passione, 2004). However, two historical issues are worth noticing. One concerns the discrepancies between the accounts given by Cerletti (1940, 1950, 1956; Impastato, 1960), who saw himself as the creator of the treatment, and those by Accornero and Kalinowsky who emphasized the contribution of other members of the team, particularly Bini. The crucial contribution by Bini seems to have been his realization that what killed about 50 per cent of dogs in Cerletti's preliminary experiments was the fact that electrodes were placed axially (head and rectum) and the current passed through their heart (Abrams, 1988). The other issue concerns the awareness shown by Cerletti and his team of the ethical implications of their experimental treatment. This is reflected in the painstaking research and animal trials undertaken before it was decided to go ahead with the first treatment in human beings. It also explains the fact that little is known about the *first* treatment which is said to have been carried out in secrecy. What is celebrated is the *second* treatment.

From the historical point of view, the survival and popularity of a treatment is as much a problem as its discovery. This is the case with ECT. By the early 1940s, it was known and used in the USA (Pulver, 1961), Britain (Fleming *et al.*, 1939), France (Lapipe & Rondepierre, 1941; Delmas-Marsalet, 1943), Germany (Braunmühl, 1947), and Spain (Gutiérrez *et al.*, 1990). Indeed, by 1945, a quick search identifies already more than 60 research papers on various aspects of the new treatment.

It is important to notice that although *ab initio* ECT was piggy-backed on other convulsive therapies, it soon developed a life of its own. By the early forties, as the biological antagonism between epilepsy and schizophrenia declined (Kennedy, 1940), the first clinical trials showed that ECT was more efficacious in the affective disorders. For example, Malzberg reported that 491 cases of dementia praecox did better on insulin treatment than ECT, and that 33% of

142 main-depressives, and 23% of 85 involutional patients responded better to ECT (Malzberg, 1943). Smith (1942) reported similar findings. The early 1940s can be described as a period during which researchers looked for new scientific basis for ECT, dealt with side effects, and extended the range of indications. For comparative purposes, these three points will be (briefly) discussed in relation to some European countries.

France

Claude & Rubenovitch (1940) believed that ECT was just a continuation of work done by the Frenchman Stéphane Leduc who 40 years earlier had sought to provoke sleep by means of low voltage, alternate currents (Leduc, 1902).

In 1941, and with the help of Dr Bargerton, a physiologist from the Paris Medical School, Lapipe & Rondepierre (1941) constructed a machine to deliver electric stimuli with durations of up to 10 seconds and energy of up to 1000 milliamps. To achieve good stimulus titration, they also carried out measurements of skull resistance. During the presentation of their work at the *Société Médico-Psychologique* (1941), Heuyer reported that 'he had been informed that the Siemens company from Germany had become interested in manufacturing a [similar] machine'; and Bour that stated that 'in England he had seen the treatment given to all manner of cases'. Gouriou pointed out that all animals treated by Leduc had, in fact, died, and that it might be safer to continue using cardiazol. Lapipe reassured those present that whilst Leduc had used a rectangular current of 100 cycles per second and with a duration of minutes, their machine delivered an alternate sinusoidal current for under a second.

The same year, two other clinical reviews in favour of the technique were published in France. Forel (1941) suggested that 'it was time for the new treatment to be evaluated and distinguished between aborted, incomplete and full seizures'. The latter were characterized by a tonic state with apnoea lasting between 40 to 60 seconds, followed by a clonic phase. Full seizures were accompanied by therapeutic success in about 65 per cent in patients with catatonia, melancholia and mania. However, the therapeutic gains needed to be consolidated by 'psychotherapy'. He also reported 'retrograde amnesia' in patients who were 'impressionable' or 'hypochondriacal'. Lamarche *et al.* (1941) administered ECT to 25 patients and concluded that it worked in all psychoses, could be combined with insulin coma, caused little anxiety, was cheap and could be repeated without causing harm. Furthermore, it was safe in the physically ill, agitated, and old.

---

technician' (Impastato, 1960) and Lothar Kalinowsky once confided that: 'Cerletti was very angry after the war that the method was called 'Cerletti-Bini', or even 'Bini-Cerletti'; he did his best to prevent Bini's academic advancement, and as a result, Bini never became a professor' (Abrams, 1988, p. 31). This damning view, expressed by someone who actually worked in Cerletti's clinic and knew those involved must be taken seriously.

[5] Ferdinando Accornero (1910–1985) was the third collaborator in the ECT project and was to write the most useful account of the events which surrounded the use of ECT in humans (Accornero, 1970).

[6] Much less is known on the fourth member of the team (Endler, 1988).

There was also a debate on the mechanisms of ECT. According to the so-called 'diencephalic theory' (Delay, 1950), ECT was a 'harmonizer' acting via modifications in the metabolism of mood. It followed that changes observed in non-affective symptoms such as delusions and hallucinations were secondary to a primary regulation of emotional function. According to a rival theory, developed from a Jacksonian perspective, symptoms resulted from 'partial dissolutions' and the convulsive therapies (including ECT) caused a total 'dissolution' of brain function. The ensuing 'reconstruction' returned psychological functioning to its normal level (Delmas-Marsalet, 1943).

Up to the middle 1940s, French psychiatrists remained divided as to the usefulness of ECT and a debate erupted at the *Société Médico-Psychologique* in 1945. Rondepierre, Guiraud and Minkowski defended ECT against the attack of Baruk (who was critical of its side effects), Delmas (who believed ECT had little efficacy but that failures were rearely reported), Sivadon (on the danger of spontaneous seizures), and Daumezón (on extreme variability of results). A paper showing that ECT was useful in the treatment of organic delirium appeared the same year (Delay & Maillard, 1945).

Germany

The work of Braunmühl, Weitbrecht, and Walter Ritter von Baeyer is important to map the acceptance of ECT in Germany, particularly during the post-war period which was one of special sensitivity in regards to all forms of biological treatments in psychiatry. Braunmühl was director of the Eglfing-Haar Hospital and professor at Munich and had been researching in convulsive therapy, particularly insulin coma, since before the war. In his book, he gave a detailed account of current variables, side effects, and both bilateral and unilateral placing of electrodes (Braunmühl, 1947, p. 148). Braunmühl recommended that Corberi's schema for electricity titration was used, i.e. one in which voltage (but not duration) was changed according to skull resistance; and also offered a classification and criteria to differentiate between abortive, incomplete and complete seizures. Lastly, he suggested a number of schedules for the administration ECT.

In his book on biological treatments for schizophrenia, Hans Jörg Weitbrecht (1949) dealt with ECT and discussed its rationale, particularly von Baeyer's view that ECT worked temporarily by 'abolishing pathological experiences' (*Erlebnisse*) and hence just postponed the onset of the disease. Weitbrecht argued that the delay hypothesis could not be understood in terms of what was known

about brain functioning and hence concluded that the basis of ECT were unknown (pp. 14–15).

Dedicated to all types of convulsive therapy, in the section on ECT Von Baeyer's book (1951) included an excellent survey of non-German literature. ECT caused a form of organic disorganization that postponed the development of the psychosis. Hence, the so-called *Blockmethode* (frequent treatments) could accelerate the process.

Great Britain

Electroconvulsive therapy found firm sponsors in Britain. G. W. T. H. Fleming, an influential figure in the *Royal Medico-Psychological Association* and F. Golla, director of the *Burden Neurological Institute*, wrote favourably about the new treatment and Grey Walter, gave it scientific respectability by exploring its electroencephalographic features.[7] All three went on to publish an influential article in the *Lancet*: 'it is not proposed to discuss here the therapeutic results of electroconvulsive therapy; it must stand or fall by the ultimate verdict on shock therapy in general. From the technical point of view there can be no doubt that the electrical method is greatly superior to any hitherto employed for the production of severe convulsions. For the operator, only a small amount of training is necessary' (Fleming *et al.*, 1939, p. 1354). After observing 75 shocks given to five subjects with schizophrenia they reported that 'no untoward results were observed … the claims of Cerletti and Bini are confirmed; the method is technically effective, simple, and safe and arouses no fear or hostility in the patients' (p. 1355).

A year later, at a meeting of the psychiatry section of the *Royal Society of Medicine*, Shipley & McGregor (1940) endorsed the treatment from the clinical point of view: ECT did not produced any of the side effects of cardiazol (fear, vomiting, confusion, thrombosis, patients did not struggle), was fully controllable, could be combined with cardiazol, was useful as a maintenance treatment, and in 200 treatments no fractures had been observed.

The following year Freudenberg (1941) published his review on the 'curability' of mental disease by ECT which he prefaced with an interesting analysis of the concept of 'curability' in schizophrenia. He then listed 'favourable' factors such as acute onset, short duration of illness, picnic or athletic constitution, and cyclothymia, and 'negative

[7] Fleming was at the time editor of the *Journal of Mental Science*; after a successful career at the Maudsley Hospital, Golla was appointed to the directorship of the *Burden Institute*. Grey Walter, a brilliant Cambridge neurophysiologist, had recently taken up a position in the same institution at Bristol.

factors' such as insidious onset, long duration of illness, dysplastic or leptosome constitution, schizothymia and 'process' symptoms. Freudenberg concluded that no factor by itself could predict outcome, that the affective psychoses responded better to shock therapy, and that insulin and the convulsive therapy (including ECT) should *complement* each other.

Even more influential was the paper by Hemphill & Walter (1941) reporting the treatment with ECT of over 200 in- and out-patients. It included indications for the right method of administration, a table to calculate the correlation between strength and duration of electrical stimulus (p. 261), an assessment of the factors governing seizure duration, and even the proposal that, in ideal conditions, seizure duration should be around 45 seconds (range 25–65 seconds). In regards to the relationship between efficacy and diagnosis, the authors concluded that: 'manic depressive and involutional melancholics respond best to treatment' (p. 274). This confirmed a report by Borgarello that ECT improved 50 per cent of 24 manic depressives but only 10 per cent of 56 schizophrenics (Borgarello, 1939); and another by Dawson (1939) that all convulsive therapies were efficacious in the affective psychoses.

Early British work on ECT is also characterized by pre-occupation with its clinical indications and side effects. J. C. Batt published his trial of ECT in a 100 depressive psychoses including manic depressives, 'menopausal, and senile affective psychoses' (Batt, 1943). The author concluded that although about 90 per cent of depressions 'reacted favourably to electrically induced convulsions . . . 13 per cent of all cases relapsed' (p. 294). He was, however, unable to identify a pattern of symptoms that might dis criminate between responders and non-responders.[8] More optimistically, Fitzgerald (1943) reported that the presence of premorbid 'melancholic trends' in the personality augured a good response to ECT.

Others sought to assess the efficacy of ECT by comparing matched samples with and without ECT. For example, Penrose & Marr (1943, p. 380) reported that 'fewer shock treated cases remained on the hospital books than are expected from considerations of the control sample'. Equally imaginative was the work of Moore who evaluated maintenance ECT in 45 cases suffering from a variety of psychoses: 'chronic psychotics whose behaviour

endangered their health, constituted a serious nursing problem, or whose mental state was one of misery were treated with electrically induced convulsions repeated at intervals, with the object of maintaining the improvement achieved after an initial course of treatment or of cutting short a particular phase of illness . . . all cases responded favourably except eleven of the schizophrenic group . . . in some cases treatment has been in progress for over two years . . . clinical observation shows no appreciable deterioration in personality or intelligence as a result of continued therapy' (Moore, 1943, p. 268).

In spite of early optimism that ECT caused only minor side effects, it soon became clear that fractures were a serious problem. For example, in 420 consecutive cases Samuel (1943) reported 12 fractures (2.8 per cent) (fractures of the spine 5, of the humerus 2, simple, of the right humerus 1, of femoral neck 5, and pelvis 1). Shorvon & Shorvon (1943) suggested that spinal anaesthesia might be superior than injections of curare, of concentrated magnesium sulphate solution or of beta-erythoidin hydrochloride. These authors reported that in cases with high risk for fractures the spinal injection of stovaine (which caused mild meningitic reactions) was justified. Lastly, work was done on stimulus duration and Finner (1954) showed that (given the same stimulus) women and older subjects have shorter seizures, and that duration shortens in the later shocks of a series.

It can be concluded that most of our current knowledge on the side effects and main indications of ECT was obtained in the period 1938–1958. It also became clear at that time that it was not easy to identify predictors of good response nor decide on which placing of electrodes was more advantageous (Braunmühl, 1947, p. 148). Although much work on mechanisms was carried out (Gordon, 1948 listed 27 biological and 23 psychological explanations) then as now little was known about how ECT works.

The origins of psychosurgery

Psychosurgery can be defined as a procedure that aims at alleviating mental disorder by directly causing more or less irreversible anatomical changes in 'normal' brain tissue by neurosurgical means. This definition is not free from ambiguity. For example, it does not help to decide whether operations to relieve CSF pressure or electrical stimulation by implanted devices which may lead to anatomical change should also count as psychosurgery. Likewise, it is unclear whether 'normal tissue' refers only to anatomy or should include physiology, neurochemistry and molecular biology. Further strain on the definition is caused by the fact that ideas governing the understanding

---

[8] Prediction of response greatly exercised British psychiatrists during the 1950s. See for example, findings by Roth that 'an atypical EEG is associated with a poor therapeutic response' (Roth, 1951, p. 278), and papers by Hobson (1953) and by Thorpe (1962) on the use of the Funkenstein Test, the sedation-threshold test, the amytal test, and psychological tests.

of mind and mental disorder have also changed since the nineteenth century.

Psychosurgery in Britain during the late nineteenth century

Late in 1889, T. C. Shaw[9] reported the case of a male patient suffering from general paralysis of the insane (GPI) whose madness had remitted after having had a piece of his temporo-parietal skull removed, his dura sectioned, and 'much yellow fluid' drained (Shaw, 1889). Shaw intimated that David Ferrier[10] had been consulted on 'performing an operation which might or might not be creditable to brain surgery' (p. 1091). Three months after surgery, and prior to his discharge, the patient had been declared 'no longer insane' by Clifford Allbutt.[11] Shaw suggested that the operation released the mechanical pressure compressing the brain. The correspondence column of the British Medical Journal was soon set alight. J. Adams (1889) suggested that it had been a spontaneous remission; G. Revington (1889) concurred and stated that three scientific and ethical criteria had not been met: (1) clear knowledge of the pathogenesis of the disease; (2) availability of technical and operatory means; and (3) a methodology to show that the improvement was due to the procedure. He called the increase fluid pressure hypothesis 'mechanical non-sense' and suggested that if fluid was to be important, it would be only in the

formation of oedema, and hence only slicing of the cortex (which had not been done) might have help.

Cripps, the surgeon who had carried out the operation, explained that the hypothesis had been conceived by extrapolation from the mechanism of glaucoma (Cripps, 1889, p. 1215). Batty Tuke[12] reported another operation leading to improvement and claimed the paternity of the increased CSF pressure hypothesis (Tuke, 1890). Percy Smith (1890) reported 'spontaneous remission' in four cases of GPI suggesting that Shaw's case belonged in this category; he also criticized Revington for having used the phrase 'mechanical non-sense'. Revington (1890) wrote again attacking Batty Tuke for not dealing with the spontaneous remission issue and criticized the increased pressure hypothesis. Invoking Clouston and Bevan Lewis he stated that mental symptoms resulted not from increased pressure but from degeneration of nervous tissue.

Shaw and Cripps performed a second operation, this time the case of a 29-year-old man with GPI whose left parietal eminence and underlying dura had been excised and his mental state (but not his motor symptoms) had improved to the point that he merited discharge. They also reported that after seven months of sustained improvement, their first patient had sadly developed epilepsy and died. They stated that the target of their operation were the mental and not the motor symptoms and defended the pressure hypothesis (Shaw & Cripps, 1890). Earlier the same year, the first American case, of a 32-year-old black patient, was reported (Wagner, 1890).

The 1891 Bournemouth meeting of the British Medical Association included a session on the surgical treatment of general paralysis of the insane (Anon., 1891). Shaw delivered a paper on the rationale of the operation which he based both on the release of pressure hypothesis and the new claim that it encouraged reactive vascularization and 'formation of new lymphatic vessels' thereby improving the drainage system and nutrition of the brain. He discussed criteria for deciding on the side of the operation, speculated on the mechanisms causing the increase in CSF pressure and reported a third case operated by Drs Barton and Gayton at the Brookwood Asylum (Shaw, 1891).

---

[9] Thomas Claye Shaw was born in Stockport in 1841, and died in Cheltenham in 1927. He trained at Kings's College London, where he was a gold medallist and did his psychiatry at the Colney Hatch Asylum. He then became physician superintendent of the Leavesden, a Metropolitan Asylum, and then of the Middlesex County Asylum at Banstead. He was a lecturer in Psychological Medicine at St Bartholomew's hospital, and soon acquired a reputation as a clear and outspoken lecturer. He was interested in the development of psychiatric units in general hospitals, in aftercare, and in alcoholism (Anon. 1927; Brown, 1955). A consultant at St Bartholomew's Hospital, Shaw supported its 'Reports' and was president of the Abernethian Society. He became a member of the Medico-Psychological Society in 1904 and in the same year published 'Ex-Cathedral Essays on Insanity', a collection of lectures and papers.

[10] A disciple of Alexander Bain (also a great Aberdonian), Sir David Ferrier was a believer in localizationism, and founder both of the Physiological Society and of the journal Brain. In 1889, he acceded to the chair of Neuropathology at King's College. Ferrier would not have been adverse to the rationale behind Claye Shaw's operation (Sherrington, 2004).

[11] Educated at Cambridge and St George's, Sir Thomas Clifford Allbutt spent a period in France with Trousseau and Duchenne. He was consulting physician at Leeds, Commissioner in Lunacy, and after 1892 Regius Professor of Physic at Cambridge. Since 1900 and until his death, he worked at Addenbrooke's hospital. He contributed to neurology, endocrinology and psychiatry (Rolleston, 2004).

[12] Sir John Batty Tuke (1835–1913) was born in Surrey and died in Edinburgh. He took his degree of the University of Edinburgh and after serving as an assistant physician at the Royal Edinburgh Asylum under Skae, he became medical superintendent of the Asylum for Fife & Kinross. He did neurobiological research under Rutherford, Goodsir and Stirling. Twice Morrison lecturer, in 1895 he became president the Royal College of Physicians of Edinburgh; he was also president of the British Neurological Society. He re-described 'miliary sclerosis' and published both in learned journals and in popular works such as Encyclopaedia Britannica.

During the discussion, Victor Horsley[13] congratulated Shaw and claimed no personal experience in this area. Charles Mercier[14] cautioned that the operation should not be done lightly, and if the main reason for it was to relieve pressure he asked why 'not just bore a small hole'. He stated that the claim that surgery could improve the grandiose delusions of GPI was tantamount to saying that a 'church ritual could be improved by taking few slates of the roof of the building'! McPherson, Herbert and Snow returned to the spontaneous remission hypothesis and Needham suggested that the patients might have been 'simulators who used the operation to abandon their symptoms'. Rather surprisingly, David Hack Tuke (Digby, 2004) defended Shaw, and Moritz Benedikt (1835–1920), who was attending the meeting as a foreign guest, stated that more empirical data were needed before theorizing.

A year later, Shaw undertook a 'general conceptual analysis' of insanity and concluded that the only way to test the increased pressure hypothesis was to operate upon an 'ordinary patient' whose insanity was not due to this mechanism. He then revealed that such a 'control' operation had in fact been carried out in a 28-year-old, impulsive and deluded subject refusing food and in danger of dying! Since his symptoms 'did not favour' a particular brain site, Mr Cripps had trephined on the middle line. After some initial hesitations, the patient had improved. Shaw concluded: 'that the operation will ever become more than an occasional one is doubtful; it takes much time, it requires special surgical skill, and the idea of it is formidable. At best, it seems only palliative, at any rate in its present development ...' (Shaw, 1892, p. 68). He was not to carry out, or at least report, another operation.

This notwithstanding, others followed. McPherson & Wallace from the Stirling Asylum reported short-term remission of mental symptoms occurring in three out of five cases; post-mortem in two patients showed no new lymphatic vessels and the authors concluded that Cripps's hypothesis was wrong. Perhaps the operation needed to be undertaken 'earlier' in the disease as in chronic patients was of 'no material benefit whatsoever' (McPherson & Wallace, 1892, p. 170). Sporadic cases continued to be reported in the UK but it is difficult to form an idea of how many operations were carried out. For example, Goodall (1893) published the case of a female patient from the Wakefield Asylum whose mental state improved although she had sustained cortical damage and later developed convulsions and bilateral musical hallucinations.

A final analysis of the effectiveness of the operation was made at the 1894 meeting of the Edinburgh Medico-Chirurgical Society (Anon., 1894). Batty Tuke claimed that most specialists had 'accepted his encephalic pressure hypothesis' and reported another seven cases been operated by J Duncan, in four of whom good results had been obtained (Tuke, 1891). Others did not agree. William Ireland stated that he did not believe that GPI could be treated by trepanning. Thomas Clouston[15] took a middle course, and referring to the English cases, stated that 'he did not believe that they were really cures although in hopeless cases the operation should still be tried'; he wondered whether in the successful cases the diagnosis of GPI had in fact been right; and called into question the increased pressure hypothesis.

The operation was tried and commented upon abroad (Rey, 1891; Blumer, 1892). Summarizing the British evidence, Guiseppe Seppilli stated that the number of reported cases 'was too small', that the increased pressure hypothesis was unlikely to be correct, and that further knowledge on the mechanisms involved in the production of symptoms was needed before more operations were carried out (Seppilli, 1891). Binet & Rebatel (1895) reported the case of an officer wounded in the head in 1870 who 20 years later had developed a melancholic depression; the surgeon Chandelux trephined his left fronto-parietal skull but nothing was found upon inspecting the brain; after a temporary aphasia, the patient

[13] Sir Victor Horsley was at the time a famous scientist. Trained under Bastian, Schäffer and Bevor, he first researched on the function of the thyroid gland and on rabies. At 29, Horsley become surgeon to the National Hospital at Queen Square, and soon after at the request of Gowers carried out a pioneering operation for a tumour of the spinal cord. At the Berlin Congress (where Burckhardt also presented his results) Horsley gave a paper reporting 44 neurosurgical operations (resulting in 10 deaths). A crusader for medical and educational reform, and an apostle of temperance, Horsley saw active duty during the Great War, and died in Mesopotamia of heat stroke. His views on Claye Shaw's operation remained positive (Paget, 2004). When reviewing the uses of trephining in insanity, Horsley accepted the need for the operation but called into question the lymphatic vessels hypothesis (Horsley, 1892).

[14] Of Huguenot descent, Charles Arthur Mercier (1852–1919) trained at the London Hospital and became superintendent of the small Bethel Hospital in Norwich before becoming assistant medical officer at the Leavensden Asylum. He lectured on nervous diseases at the Westminster Hospital and later at the Charing Cross. He was a prolific writer on insanity and also on its psychological and forensic aspects.

[15] Sir Thomas Smith Clouston was born in Orkney and trained at Aberdeen and Edinburgh. At this latter university, he came under the influence of Thomas Laycock which marked his views on neurosciences for life. He worked at the Royal Edinburgh Asylum first as an assistant to David Skae and then as its superintendent. His views on the taxonomy and clinical analysis of mental disease are contained in his famous 'Clinical Lectures' which went through many editions (Beveridge, 2004).

recovered his mental health. The same year, Semelaigne (1895)[16] published his masterly review on the uses of brain surgery in insanity. A believer in the organicity of all forms of insanity, he grouped all conditions together irrespective of whether they were associated with trauma, epilepsy or general paralysis. He concluded that surgical treatments should not be carried out until more data had been collected.

Burckhardt

Gottlieb Burckhardt carried out his solitary research at the Asylum of Préfargier. His work has only recently been given serious attention (Whittaker *et al.*, 1996). From the historical point of view, the fact that his operation did not catch on is less important than the fact that Burckhardt's rationale is similar to that inspiring the 1890s British experience, and what was to come in the mid 1930s.

Like Shaw, Burckhardt,[17] was a child of the second half of the nineteenth century who believed that all mental functions and disorders had physical basis and were related to specific brain sites. The nervous system comprised: (a) an input or afferent or sensory system, (b) a linking or connecting system (where information processing took place), and (c) an efferent, motor or output system. In terms of this model Burckhardt predicted that lesions in association areas might change behaviour: 'if excitation and impulsive behaviour are due to the fact

that from the sensory surfaces excitations abnormal in quality, quantity and intensity do arise, and do act on the motor surfaces, then an improvement could be obtained by creating an obstacle between the two surfaces. The extirpation of the motor or the sensory zone would expose us to the risk of grave functional disturbances and to technical difficulties. It would be more advantageous to practice the excision of a strip of cortex behind and on both sides of the motor zone creating thus a kind of ditch in the temporal lobe' (Burckhardt, 1891, p. 478).

Starting on 29th December 1888, Burckhardt operated on two females and four male patients (the first patient had four operations) (Berrios, 1997). The operations were carried out in a small room on the grounds of the Préfargier Clinic. Burckhardt had little surgical experience and used primitive instruments and technique. Five of his cases were suffering from *primäre Verrücktheit*[18] (a disorder that can be anachronistically re-diagnosed as schizophrenia). Patients were deluded, violent and with auditory hallucinations. Most of the patients developed serious side effects: for example, subject 6 died in status epilepticus 5 days after surgery (on post-mortem the destructive effects of the 'topectomy' were clearly visible). In three subjects, mental symptoms are said to have been 'partially improved'.

Burckhardt reported his findings at the Berlin Medical Congress of 1889, attended *inter alia* by Horsley, Erb, Schultze, Mendel, Magnan, Dagonet, and Kraepelin. Reports of this meeting appeared in a number of international journals, for example, Worcester (1891) presented a summary to his American colleagues emphasizing the side effects and the brevity of the follow-ups. Kraepelin was very critical: Burckhardt 'suggested that restless patients could be pacified by scratching away the cerebral cortex' (Kraepelin, 1893, p. 64). Writing for an Italian audience Sepelli stated that Burckhardt's localizationist views did not 'fit in well with the view held by most [experts] that the psychoses reflect a diffuse pathology of the cerebral cortex and [run counter to] the conception of the psyche as a unitary entity' (Sepelli, 1891, p. 371). Due to this theoretical weakness, Sepelli concluded, it would be unlikely that anyone might want to follow Burckhardt's example. Semelaigne also attacked Burckhardt's ideas and procedures and concluded that 'an absence of treatment was better than a bad treatment' (Semelaigne, 1895, p. 402). Lastly, in his book on 'The treatment of madness' Jules Luys commented upon the Berlin report and called into

[16] René Semelaigne (1855–1934) was director of the Saint-James hospital at Neuilly, up to 1921. A corresponding member of the Royal Medico-Psychological Association, he became an honorary member in 1911. A magnificent reviewer and compiler Semelaigne did not carry out much primary research. His work on the history of French psychiatry remains essential reading.

[17] Scion of a famous family, Gottlieb Burckhardt was born in Basle on 24th December 1836. He studied at Basel, Göttingen and Berlin, and graduated with a thesis on the epithelium of the urinary tract. After a period as a general practitioner in his hometown, in 1873 he became physician to the Waldau Psychiatric University Clinic of Berne where he worked under Schärer and became a regular reviewer for the *Korrespondenzblatt für Schweizer Ärtze*. Whilst at Waldau he published a book on the physiological diagnosis of nervous diseases and researched into the relationship between brain temperature and mental illness. In 1881, Eugen Bleuler became his assistant (Bach, 1907; Hagenbach, 1907; Müller, 1958).

    Between 1882 and 1896 Burckhardt was at the Préfargier Psychiatric Clinic, near the lake of Neuchâtel, and in 1888, he carried out his first 'topectomy'. After losing his wife and one of his sons he retired to Basle where he directed the Sonnhalde Clinic and died of pneumonia in 1907. Burckhardt remained a psychiatric outsider, is not listed as attending international meetings, and after his presentation of 1891 he does not seem to have written a major paper again. A great Swiss psychiatrist described him as a 'thoroughly sincere man' who seem to have shunned 'customary courtesies' (Forel, 1937, p. 207).

[18] This clinical category was re-introduced by Sander (1868) and made popular as *originäre Paranoia*, a hereditary delusional-hallucinatory psychosis starting around puberty, by Krafft Ebing (1893, pp. 408–13).

question the ethics of the operation stating that patients were too ill to give consent (Luys, 1893, pp. 271–281).

After the Berlin presentation, Burckhardt published a long report which included the six case histories, repeated mental state assessments, a full review of the clinical and experimental literature on brain localization, and some theoretical arguments (Burckhardt, 1891). He was never to write on the subject again. William Ireland summarized it thus: 'Dr Burckhardt has a firm faith in the view that the mind is made up of a number of faculties, holding their seats in distinct portions of the brain. Where excess or irregularity of function occurs he seeks to check it by ablation of a portion of the irritated centres. He defends himself from the criticisms which are sure to be directed against his bold treatment by showing the desperate character of the prognosis of the patients upon whom the operations were performed ...' (Ireland, 1891, pp. 617–18) and wondered 'whether any English physician would have the hardihood to imitate Burckhardt' (p. 614).

Five years after Burckhardt's death, a harsher criticism appeared. After summarizing his cases, Bechterew & Puuseppe (1912) added: 'We have quoted this data to show not only how groundless but also how dangerous these operations were. We are unable to explain how their author, holder of a degree in medicine, could bring himself to carried them out ...' (p. 85). In a talk given to the Medical Academy of Torino in 1937 Puuseppe returned to the point but went on to confess that in 1910 (Puuseppe, 1937) he (unsuccessfully) had, in fact, severed the 'association fibres' of the frontal and parietal lobes of one patient with manic-depressive psychosis and two with 'epileptic-equivalents'!

Apart from Puuseppe, no one else seemed to have repeated Burckhardt's operation. Psychoanalysis and the holistic approaches to brain localization as proposed by Goldstein, Monakow, Mourgue, and Lashley changed for a time early twentieth century views on mental disorder (Hécaen & Lanteri-Laura, 1977). However, by the early 1930s, the modular view had returned to provide Moniz with grounds to develop his ideas.

Moniz

The ideas that inspired Moniz's views on psychosurgery[19] were late nineteenth century localizationism and associationism. Even his therapeutic objective of targeting

[19] Antonio Caetano de Abreu Freire (a.k.a. Egas Moniz) was born in Avanca, Northern Portugal, on 27th November 1874 (Barahona Fernandez, 1956; Walker, 1970; Pereira & Pita, 2000). The name Egas Moniz belonged to a eleventh century Portuguese hero of the resistance against the Moors and it has been claimed that it was his godfather who gave him that name; it is more likely that Moniz

symptoms rather than diseases was typical for this period. However, his choice of the frontal lobes as target for the operation was a departure of conventional views and needs explanation. Piecing together the events leading to the 1935 operations is hampered by discrepancies between extant accounts. For example, Moniz's description in the 1936 book (written without posterity in mind) markedly differs from his elaborated apologia of 1948; and these two, in turn, differ from the official view.

According to the 'official view' (Tow, 1955), Moniz heard a presentation by Fulton & Jacobsen in the '1935 London Neurological Meeting' on the tranquillizing effects of frontal lobectomies in primates suffering from behavioural disorders. A form of 'neurotic behaviour' had been induced in these monkeys by training them to respond to opposed stimuli with opposing responses, and then presenting them with an ambiguous stimuli. The disruptive behaviour of the monkeys 'reminded' Moniz of the agitation of psychotic behaviour, and he wondered whether frontal lobectomies might work in such patients. When approached by Moniz with the idea, Fulton was rather 'startled' (Fulton, 1951). Upon returning to Lisbon, Moniz organized for 20 patients to receive the operation.

himself adopted such pen name during his political struggle against the monarchy.

Moniz graduated from the University of Coimbra in 1899. In 1902 he obtained his MD and left for France to train as a neurologist under Pitrés and Régis (Bordeaux), and Raymond, Pierre Marie, Babinski and Dejerine (Paris). He kept the pictures of Marie, Pitrés and Babinski close to him until his death (Anonymous, 1979). In 1911 (date of the initiation of the Republic), Moniz joined the University of Lisbon as a lecturer, and founded the Neurological Clinic of Santa Marta.

A distinguished political career followed and he served as Foreign Minister, Ambassador to Spain, and Portuguese signatory at the Treatise of Versailles. After 1920, his political fortune changed and this led him back to the neurosciences. His work on angiography culminated in 1927 with the publication of a famous paper on the use of sodium iodide as a contrasting medium and with a book on the same topic carrying an introduction by Babinski.

The third stage of his career is marked by his work on frontal leucotomy. Between the end of 1935 and early 1936 he was involved in organizing such operations for 20 patients from the Bombarda Asylum selected by its director, Professor Sobral Cid. Operated by Dr Almeida Lima, a neurosurgeon, the patients were baselined and followed-up by Dr H. J. Barahona Fernandez who trained under K. Kleist in Germany. In 1936, Moniz published a book on the subject and papers followed carrying an ever more embellished accounts. He retired in 1944, and in 1949 was awarded the Nobel Prize for Medicine and Physiology, the citation referring to 'his invention of a surgical treatment for mental illness and to his elaboration of the psychophysiological concepts that made it possible'. Aged 65, he was shot by a patient suffering from schizophrenia; partially recovered, he died on 18th December 1955.

Moniz's accounts from both 1936 and 1948 differ from the 'official view' and also from each other. The 1936 account shows Moniz's deep concern with the scientific and ethical warrants for the procedure and includes a lucid analysis of its scientific and ethical warrants: '[the operation] may jeopardize patients' lives, which have for us, physicians, the highest value' (Moniz, 1936, p. 5). With regards to the *origin* of his ideas Moniz stated that 'We had already told confidentially Dr Almeida Lima of our idea *more than two and a half years before*' (my italics) (p. 6). If true, this claim would date his thoughts on the operation to the year 1933, that is 2 years earlier than the London Meeting. In regards to his choice of the frontal lobes, it is of interest that in his 1936 book Moniz only mentioned as his sources Kleist, Claude, Choroscko, and Brickner's detailed report of a subject with amputated frontal lobes. He does not refer to Fulton and Jacobsen's experiments in any detail.

In his Birmingham lectures, Fulton noticed this absence of reference to his work with some relief: 'in the thoughtful prefatory chapters of Egas Moniz's monograph on lobotomy he indicates that for some years prior to 1935 he had entertained the thought of interrupting frontal lobe projections as a possible therapeutic weapon for dealing with some of the more severe psychoses. He cites the work of Henri Claude on the functions of the frontal lobe and also the observations of the late Clovis Vincent. He was likewise familiar with Richard Brickner's well-known case of a bilateral frontal lobe removal in man. Finally he directs attention to the report which I made with Jacobsen on the behavioural changes observed in chimpanzees following bilateral removal of the frontal areas. Although Moniz later stated that the results reported for the chimpanzee convinced him that the operation would be useful in man, one *should not forget that he had considered surgical interference long before hearing of our experimental results...*' (my italics) (Fulton, 1948, p. 62).

The role played by Fulton's work in Moniz's decision to go ahead with the operations requires more research. What is clear is that, after earlier hesitations, and once the procedure gained some ethical warrants, Fulton seems to have been more than happy to act as the intellectual 'patron' of American psychosurgeons, particularly of Watts (Valenstein, 1986; Pressman, 1988).

In 1948, Moniz returned to his earlier views that aberrant and fixed synaptic circuits may lead to mental disorder: 'sufferers from melancholia, for instance, are distressed by fixed and obsessive ideas ... and live in a permanent state of anxiety caused by a fixed idea which predominates over all their lives ... in difference to automatic actions, these morbid ideas are deeply rooted in the synaptic complex which regulates the functioning of consciousness, stimulating it

and keeping it in constant activity ... all these considerations led me to the following conclusion: *it is necessary to alter these synaptic adjustments and change the paths chosen by the impulses in their constant passage so as to modify the corresponding ideas and force thoughts along different paths...*' (my italics) (Moniz, 1948, p. 583).

In 1936, Moniz listed as theoretical bases for the operation the principles of 'substitution' (which he 'had been teaching for years') and of 'fixed connection'. According to the former, the brain was able functionally to adapt by replacing damaged areas (Moniz, 1936, p. 42); according to the latter, mental symptoms were caused by rogue brain circuits created by aberrant learning. It followed from this that their 'partial destruction' might lead to improvement (p. 46). This rationale is *different* from the explanation suggested by Fulton to account for the reduction in affective responses ('frustrational behaviour') shown by Becky (the chimpanzee) after bilateral excision of her frontal lobes (Fulton & Jacobsen, 1935; Jacobsen *et al.*, 1935). According to Fulton 'hypo-reactivity' resulted from damage to the anterior cingulate gyrus (area 24) leading to a loss of the animal's 'social conscience': 'monkeys lose some of the social fear and anxiety which normally governs their activity and thus lose the ability to accurately forecast the social repercussions of their own actions' (Fulton, 1948, p. 67). With regards to surgical technique there was also an important difference. Inspired by the well-known operation for trigeminal neuralgia, Moniz and Almeida Lima injected alcohol into the white matter of 10 of their cases; the Fulton & Jacobsen technique for excising tissue was used in the rest.

The 1936 book describes in detail the first 20 cases and reprints (verbatim) papers published by Moniz in *L'Encephale* and in *Lisboa Medica* (Moniz & Lima, 1936). Based on a naked eye assessment of his data, Moniz concluded that 35% cases showed great improvement, 35% mild improvement and 30% no change. He also attempted to determine outcome by symptom and by diagnoses but his sub-groups were too small, and he does not seem to have been aware of the statistical techniques available in his time. A statistical comparison of 'improvers' versus 'no-changers' shows that the operation gave better results in older patients ($P < 0.01$), female subjects ($P < 0.01$), and amongst those suffering from an affective psychosis ($P < 0.01$). Surgical technique and target symptom do not seem to have made any difference. (For an analysis of Moniz's cases see Berrios, 1991.)

The work of Freeman & Watts (1950) in the USA, and that of others in Europe and the rest of the world, provided the scientific warrant on the basis of which thousands of mentally ill patients were operated between the late 1930s and the 1950s. Analysis of the debates that the operation was to generate are beyond the scope of this chapter whose exclusive aim has been to contextualize Moniz's work against earlier psychosurgical attempts.

Discussion and conclusions

In Western culture, the history of treatments in psychiatry has resulted from the convergent evolution of disciplines and themes such as medicine, therapeutics, materia medica, natural history, theory of probability, the doctor-patient relationship, alienism, psychiatric nosology, deontology, and the politics of social control. Each has contributed themes and warrants and shaped questions such as: What is mental disorder? What does it meant to treat it? How and why should it be treated? These are the guiding questions for the historian of psychiatric therapeutics.

This chapter started by asking what was the best way to write a history of psychiatric treatments. It was concluded that since history seeks to understand people and events and render them accountable, the method of simply compiling linear chronologies of discoveries, priorities, geniuses, and serendipities would not generate any useful explanation. It was recommended that a social historiography be used, and one which considered each historical period as independent. This was based on the view that the act of treating was fundamentally a social interaction characterized by negotiations and exchanges; and 'treatments' were a commodity changing hands under the aegis of such interaction. Because concepts such as doctor, patient, treatment, etc. mean differently in each historical period, it is advisable to studied each according to its own rules, beliefs and laws (Keel, 2001). It follows that comparing periods (on whatever scale) is an empty exercise; this 'incommensurability' between periods renders the very concept of progress meaningless.

What behaviours are considered as problematic and in need to treatment also changes from period to period. History shows that there are no ailments *sub specie aeternitatis*. Each historical period not only dubs certain behaviours as 'diseased' but also decides which are 'treatment-worthy'. In the West, warrants for this have been successively provided by religion, the secular state, medicine and of late psychiatry. Psychiatry, in turn, has constructed such warrants in different ways. Like medicine earlier on, it used to found the treatment warrant on experiential authority (e.g. the views of a great alienist); now it bases it on science. This conceals two worrying changes. One concerns the shift from makers of warrants with a face, men who could be identified, personalized and

challenged (e.g. when two great authorities disagreed) to an impersonal, unidentifiable, source of warrants. The second change concerns the putting into place of a monopolistic system (science) which in the name of truth and objectivity does not allow the parallel operation of rival systems of explanation and renders itself self-perpetuating. The claim that science allows a democratic play of hypotheses does not deal with the accusation of monopolism for hypotheses are allowed only if they fit into the same system of thought and are subjected to the same evaluative process; in other words, conventional science does not allow the free existence of alternative systems of thought (for example naturist medicine; for a full history see Grasset, 1910) and of other ways (not the statistical one) of ascertaining the truth.

Within this monopolistic world, psychiatrists are allowed to believe that mental disorders exist (like stones or flowers) independently from the language used to describe them; that mental disorders dwell entirely in the brain, and that modifying the latter will do away with the former (Berrios & Marková, 2002). This is the view governing the understanding of all psychiatric treatments, including the 'psychological' which to some work because they also modify brain structures (as shown by neuroimaging).

Once the historian has decide on the best method to write the history of psychiatric treatments, he/she must develop a set of conceptual tools and in this chapter the concepts of treatment resistance, chronicity and behavioural phenocopies were chosen for analysis.

Then the general history of treatments was explored. To show how systems of thought interact with treatments the story was started in classic times and examples given between then and the nineteenth century. Lastly, some specific interventions were chosen as examples, that is, as illustrations of general principle, rule, or state of things.

The examples were chosen from the twentieth century as that is the period when the concept of specific treatment developed in earnest. Following a short account of psychopharmacology, insulin coma therapy, ECT and psychosurgery were dealt with in depth. These were chosen because they illustrate well the interaction between scientific and social variables which in other cases, particularly of treatments which are fashionable or predominant (like psychopharmacology) remains hidden as these treatments are presented as purely scientific.

REFERENCES

Abély, P. (1939). Le traitement actuel de la démence précoce et d'autres psychoses par l'insuline et le cardiazol. *Annales Médico-Psychologiques*, **97**, 555–66.

Abrams, R. (1988). Interview with Lothar Kalinowsky. *Convulsive Therapy*, **4**, 24–39.

Accornero, F. (1970) Testimonianza oculare sulla scoperta dell'electtroshock. *Pagina di Story della Medicina*, **14**, 38–52 [translated into English by Frank Sicuro and Giovanna Morena as: Accornero, F. (1988). An eyewitness account of the discovery of electroshock. *Convulsive Therapy*, **4**, 40–9].

Ackerknecht, E. H. (1973). *Therapeutics. From the Primitives to the 20th Century*. New York: Hafner Press.

Ackner, B., Harris, A. & Oldham, A. J. (1957). Insulin treatment of schizophrenia, a controlled study. *Lancet*, **i**, 607–11.

Adams, J. (1889). Is general paralysis of the insane a curable disease? *British Medical Journal*, **ii**, 1187.

Agazzi, E. (1985). Commensurability, incommensurability, and cumulativity in scientific knowledge. *Erkenntnis*, **22**, 51–77.

Amard, L. V. F. (1807). *Traité analytique de la folie et des moyens de la guérir*. Lyon: Ballanche.

Anonymous (1891). Surgical treatment of general paralysis of the insane. *British Medical Journal*, **ii**, 596.

Anonymous (1894). Edinburgh Medico-Chirurgical Society. Discussion on intracraneal surgery. *Lancet*, **i**, 607–9.

Anonymous (1927). Thomas Claye Shaw: Obituary. *Lancet*, **i**, 260.

Anonymous (1979). *Catalogue: 'Exposiao sobre a vida e obra de Egas Moniz'*. Bial, Porto: Faculdade de Medicine do Porto.

Aretaeus (1856). *The extant works of Aretaeus, The Cappadocian*, edited and translated by F Adams. London: Sydenham Society.

Bach, C. (1907). Nekrolog Dr. G Burckhardt. *Allgemeine Zeitschrift für Psychiatrie*, **64**, 529–34.

Baeyer, W. R. von (1951). *Die moderne psychiatrische Schockbehandlung*. Stuttgart: Georg Thieme.

Baguenier-Desormeaux, A. (1983). Étude sur le traitement moral et ses origines philosophiques. *Mémoire pour le C.E.S. de Psychiatrie*. Angers: Ronéot.

Barahona Fernandez, H. J. de (1956). Egas Moniz. In *Grosse Nervenärzte*, Vol. 1, ed. K. Kolle, pp. 187–8. Stuttgart: Thieme.

Barbier, J. B. G. (1824). *Traité Élémentaire de Matière Médicale*, 2nd edn, 3 Vols. Paris: Méquignon-Marvis.

Barcia, D. (ed.) (1998). *Historia de la psicofarmacología*. Madrid: You & Us.

Baruk, H. (1955). *Les Thérapeutiques Psychiatriques*. Paris: Presses Universitaires de France.

Batt, J. C. (1943). One hundred depressive psychoses treated with electrically induced convulsions. *Journal of Mental Science*, **89**, 289–96.

Bayle, A. L. (1826). *Traite des Maladies du Cerveau*. Paris: Gabon.

Bechterew, W. & Puuseppe, M. (1912). La chirurgie des Aliénés. *Archives de Neurologie*, **34**, 1–17, 69–89.

Beier, L. Mc. (1987). *Sufferers and Healers: the Experience of Illness in Seventeenth Century England*. London: Routledge.

Bennett, M. R. & Hacker, P. M. S. (2003). *Philosophical Foundations of Neuroscience*. Oxford: Blackwell.

Bernier, F. (1674). *Abregé de la Philosophie de Mr Gassendi*. Paris: Langlois.

Berrios, G. E. (1991). Psychosurgery in Britain and elsewhere. In *150 years of British Psychiatry*, ed. G. E. Berrios & Freeman H., pp. 180–96. London: Gaskell.

Berrios, G. E. (1994). Historiography of mental symptoms and diseases. *History of Psychiatry*, **5**, 175–90.

Berrios, G. E. (1996). *The History of Mental Symptoms*. Cambridge: Cambridge University Press.

Berrios, G. E. (1997). The origins of psychosurgery: Shaw, Burckhardt and Moniz. *History of Psychiatry*, **8**, 61–81.

Berrios, G. E. (1997). The scientific origins of electroconvulsive therapy. *History of Psychiatry*, **8**, 105–19.

Berrios, G. E. & Freeman, H. (ed.) (1991). *150 years of British Psychiatry 1841–1991*. London: Gaskell.

Berrios, G. E. & Marková, I. S. (2002). Biological psychiatry: conceptual issues. In *Biological Psychiatry*, ed. H. D'Haenen, J. A. den Boer & P. Willner, pp. 3–24. New York: John Wiley.

Beveridge, A. (2004). Clouston, Sir Thomas Smith (1840–1915). *Oxford Dictionary of National Biography*. Oxford: Oxford University Press.

Biagioli, M. (1990). The anthropology of incommensurability. *Studies in History and Philosophy of Science*, **21**, 183–209.

Binet & Rebatel (1895). Un cas d'affection mental guéri par la trépanation. *Lyon Medical*, 12th May 1895.

Bini, L. (1948). *Le Demenze Presenili*. Rome: Edizioni Italiane.

Bini, L. & Bazzi, T. (1954). *Trattato di Psichiatria*, 2 Vols. Milan: F. Vallardi.

Bloor, D. (1991). *Knowledge and Social Imagery*, 2nd edn. Chicago: The University of Chicago Press.

Blumer, A. (1892). The surgical treatment of insanity. *American Journal of Insanity*, **49**, 222.

Boinet, E. (no date). *Les Doctrines Médicales. Leur Évolution*. Paris: Flammarion.

Bordeu, A. (1775). *Recherches sur les maladies chroniques*. Paris.

Borgarello, G. (1939). Clinical results of one hundred cases of mental illness treated with electroshock. *Schizofrenie*, **9**, 131–6.

Boudon, V. (2000). Galien de Pergame. In *Dictionnaire des Philosophes Antiques*, Vol 3, ed. R. Goulet, pp. 440–66. Paris: CNRS Éditions.

Bourne, H. (1953). The insulin myth. *Lancet*, **II**, 964–8.

Braslow, J. T. (1997). *Mental Ills and Bodily Cures. Psychiatric Treatment in the First Half of the Twentieth Century*. Berkeley CA: University of California Press.

Braslow, J. T. (2000). Therapeutics and the history of psychiatry. *Bulletin for the History of Medicine*, **74**, 794–802

Braunmühl, A. von (1938). *Die Insulinshockbehandlung der Schizophrenie*. Berlin: Springer.

Braunmühl, A. von (1947). *Insulinshock und Heilkrampf in der Psychiatrie*. Stuttgart: Wissenschaftliche Verlagsgesellschaft.

Breathnach, C. S. (1990). Cerletti. *Irish Journal of Psychological Medicine*, **7**, 177.

Brock, A. J. (1929). *Greek Medicine*. London: J. M. Dent.

Brown, G. H. (1955). *Munk's Roll: Lives of the Fellows of the Royal College of Physicians of London 1826–1925*, Vol. IV. London: Royal College of Physicians.

Brown, T. (1970). The College of Physicians and the acceptance of iatromechanism in England 1665–1695. *Bulletin for the History of Medicine*, **44**, 12–30.

Brunschwig, J. & Nussbaum, M. C. (ed.) (1993). *Passions and Perceptions*. Cambridge: Cambridge University Press.

Buchner de, T. (1753). *De transitu morbi chronici in acutum, et acuti in chronicum*. Halle.

Burckhardt, G. (1891). Ueber rindenexcisionen, als beitrag zur operativen therapie der psychosen. *Allgemeine Zeitschrift für Psychiatrie*, **47**, 463–548.

Butterfield, H. (1931). *Whig Interpretation of History*. London: G. Bell and Sons.

Bynum, W. (1964). Rationales for therapy in British Psychiatry 1780–1835. *Medical History*, **18**, 317–34.

Bynum, W. F. (1973). The anatomical method, natural theology, and the functions of the brain. *Isis*, **64**, 444–68.

Bynum, W. F. & Porter, R. (ed.) (1987). *Medical Fringe and Medical Orthodoxy 1750–1850*. London: Croom-Helm.

Bynum, W. & Nutton, V. (ed.) (1991). *Essays in the History of Therapeutics*. Amsterdam, Atlanta: Clio Medica.

Caelius Aurelianus (1950). *On Acute Diseases*, edited and translated by I. E. Drabkin. Chicago: Chicago University Press.

Carbonell, C.-O. (1991). *L'Historiographie*. Paris: Presses Universitaires de France.

Carlson, E. T. & Dain, N. (1960). The psychotherapy that was moral treatment. *American Journal of Psychiatry*, **117**, 519–24.

Carter, R. B. (1983). *Descartes' Medical Philosophy*. Baltimore, MD: The Johns Hopkins University Press.

Cerletti, U. (1940). L'elettroshock. *Rivista Sperimentale di Freniatria*, **64**, 209–310

Cerletti, U. (1950). Old and new information about electroshock. *American Journal of Psychiatry*, **107**, 87–94.

Cerletti, U. (1956). Electroshock therapy. In *The Great Physiodynamic Therapies in Psychiatry*, ed. A. M. Sackler, M. D. Sackler, R. R. Sackler & F. Martinez-Ibañez, pp. 91–120. New York: Hoeber-Harper Book.

Chast, F. (1995). *Histoire contemporaine des medicaments*. Paris: La Découverte.

Chen, X. (1997). Thomas Kuhn's latest notion of incommensurability. *Journal for General Philosophy of Science*, **28**, 257–73.

Chereau, A. (1881). Signatures mystiques. In *Dictionnaire Encyclopédique des Sciences Médicales*, Vol. 90, ed. A. Dechambre, pp. 615–18.

Claude, H. & Rubenovitch, P. (1940). *Therapeutiques Biologiques des Affections Mentales*. Paris: Masson.

Cogan, T. (1802). *A Philosophical Treatise on the Passions*. London: S. Hazard.

Coley, N. G. (1979). 'Cures without care'. 'Chymical physicians' and mineral waters in seventeenth-century English medicine. *Medical History*, **23**, 191–214.

Colombier, J. & Doublet, F. (1785). *Instruction sur la maniére de gouverner les insensés*. Paris: L'Imprimerie Royale.

Conry, Y. (1982). Thomas Willis ou le Premier Discours Rationaliste en Pathologie Mentale. *L'information Psychiatrique*, **58**, 313–23.

Cooper, R. (2005). *Classifying Madness. A Philosophical Examination of the Diagnostic and Statistical Manual of Mental Disorders*. Berlin: Springer.

Cossa, P. (1945). *Thérapeutique neurologique et psychiatrique*. Paris: Masson.

Cramond, W. A. (1987). Lessons from the insulin history in psychiatry. *Australian and New Zealand Journal of Psychiatry*, **21**, 320–6.

Cripps, H. (1889). The surgical treatment of general paralysis. *British Medical Journal*, **ii**, 1215–16.

Curti, M. (1974). Philanthropy. In *The Dictionary of the History of Ideas: Studies of Selected Pivotal Ideas*, Vol. 3, ed. P. P. Wiener, pp. 486–93. New York: Charles Scribner's Sons.

D'Aulney, J. & Malineau, R. (1956). Depuis l'avènement de la chlorpromazine la cure de Sake est elle condamnée? *L'Encéphale*, **45**, 656–60.

Danziger, K. (1997). *Naming of the Mind*. London: Sage.

Daquin, J. (1792). *La Philosophie de la folie, ou Essai philosophique sur le traitement des personnes attaquées de folie*. Paris: Née de La Rochelle.

Daremberg, Ch. (no date). *Galien considéré comme philosophe*. Paris: De Fain.

David, H. P. (1954). A critique of psychiatric and psychological research on insulin treatment in schizophrenia. *American Journal of Psychiatry*, **100**, 774–6.

Dawson, W. S. (1939). Cardiazol convulsion therapy in the psychoses. *Medical Journal of Australia*, **26**, 497–501.

Delay, J. & Maillard, J. (1945). L'électrochoc dans les différentes formes cliniques de la confusion mentale. *Annales Médico-Psychologiques*, **103**, 474–8.

Delay, J. (1950). *Méthodes Biologiques en Clinique Psychiatrique*. Paris: Masson.

Delmas-Marsalet, P. (1943). *L'électrochoc thérapeutique et la dissolution-reconstruction*. Paris: J.B. Baillière.

Despret, V. (1999). *Ces emotions qui nous fabriquent*. Paris: Collection Les Empêcheurs de Penser en Rond.

Desrosières, A. (1998). *The Politics of Large Numbers. A History of Statistical Reasoning*. Translated by Camille Naish. Cambridge, MA: Harvard University Press.

Diderot, D. & D'Alembert, J. R. (1753). *Encyclopédie ou Dictionnaire raisonné des sciences, des arts et des métiers par une société de gens de lettres*. 3rd Vol. Paris: chez Briasson: David l'aîné: Le Breton: Durand.

Digby, A. (1985). Moral treatment at the Retreat, 1796–1846. In *Anatomy of Madness*, Vol. **II**.

Digby, A. (2004). Tuke, Daniel Hack (1827–1895). *Oxford Dictionary of National Biography*. Oxford: Oxford University Press.

Dixon, T. (2003). *From Passions to Emotions*. Cambridge: Cambridge University Press.

Domino, E. F. (1999). History of modern psychopharmacology: a personal view with an emphasis on antidepressants. *Psychosomatic Medicine*, **61**, 591–8.

Dumas, C. L. (1812). *Doctrine générale des maladies chroniques*. Paris.

Edgeworth, F. Y. (1881). *Mathematical Psychics: an Essay on the Application of Mathematics to the Moral Sciences.* London: Kegan Paul.

Endler, N. S. (1988). The origins of electroconvulsive therapy (ECT). *Convulsive Therapy*, **4**, 5–23.

Ey, H. (1978). La notion de 'maladie morale' et de 'traitement moral' dans la psychiatrie Française et Allemande du debut du XIXme Siècle. *Perspectives Psychiatriques*, **1**, 12–35.

Faure, O. (ed.) (1999). *Les Thérapeutiques: savoirs et usages.* Paris: Foundation Marcel Merieux.

Finner, R. W. (1954). Duration of convulsion in electric shock therapy. *Journal of Nervous and Mental Disease*, **111**, 530–7.

Fitzgerald, O. W. S. (1943). Experiences in the treatment of depressive states by electrically induced convulsions. *Journal of Mental Science*, **89**, 73–80.

Fleming, G. W. T. (1950). *Recent Progress in Psychiatry.* London: Churchill.

Fleming, G. W. T. H., Golla, F. L. & Walter, W. G. (1939). Electric-convulsion therapy of schizophrenia. *Lancet*, **II**, 1353–5.

Forel, A. (1937). *Out of my Life and Work*, translated by B. Miall. London: George Allen & Unwin.

Forel, O. L. (1941). L'Électroshoc en psychiatrie. *Annales Médico-Psychologiques*, **99**, 32–40.

Frank, E., Prien, R. F., Jarrett, R. B. *et al.* (1991). Conceptualization and rationale for consensus definitions of terms in major depressive disorder. Remission, recovery, relapse, and recurrence. *Archives of General Psychiatry*, **48**, 851–5.

Frank, R. G. (1980). *Harvey and the Oxford Physiologists. A Study of Scientific Ideas.* Berkeley: University of California Press.

Freeman, W. & Watts, J. (1950). *Psychosurgery; In Treatment of Mental Disorders and Intractable Pain.* Springfield, IL: Charles C. Thomas.

Freudenberg, R. (1941). On the curability of mental diseases by 'shock' treatment. *Journal of Mental Science*, **87**, 529–44.

Fulton, J. F. & Jacobsen, C. F. (1935). The functions of the frontal lobes: a comparative study in monkeys, chimpanzees and man. In *Proceedings of 2nd International Congress*, Neurology Abstracts.

Fulton, J. F. (1948). *Functional Localization in the Frontal Lobes and Cerebellum.* Oxford: Clarendon Press.

Fulton, J. F. (1951). *Frontal Lobotomy and Affective Behaviour. A Neurophysiological Analysis.* New York: W W Norton.

Garcia Ballester, L. (1972). *Alma y enfermedad en la obra de Galeno.* Valencia: Universidad de Valencia.

Gayral, L. & Dauty, R. (1957). *Nouvelles Chimiothérapies en Psychiatrie.* Paris: Masson.

Geller, M. R. (1962). *The Treatment of Psychiatric Disorders with Insulin 1936–1960. A Selected Annotated Bibliography.* Washington: United States Government Printing Office.

Genil-Perrin, G. (1913). *Histoire des origines et de l'évolution de l'idée de dégénérescence en médecine mentale.* Paris: A Leclerc.

Gigerenzer, G., Swijtink, Z., Porter, T. *et al.* (1989). *The Empire of Chance.* Cambridge: Cambridge University Press.

Golinski, J. (1998). *Making Natural Knowledge.* Cambridge: Cambridge University Press.

Goodall, E. (1893). Transient motor and sensory disturbance following upon trephining in a case of general paralysis of the Insane. *British Medical Journal*, **ii**, 117.

Gordon, H. L. (1948). Fifty shock therapy theories. *Military Surgeon*, **103**, 397–401.

Gordon, H. L. (ed.) (1958). *The New Chemotherapy in Mental Illness.* New York: Philosophical Library.

Grasset, H. (1910). *La médicine naturiste a travers les siècles.* Paris: Rousset.

Graumann, C. F. & Gergen, K. J. (ed.) (1996). *Historical Dimensions of Psychological Discourse.* Cambridge: Cambridge University Press.

Gray, B. (1905). *A History of English Philanthropy from the Dissolution of the Monasteries to the Taking of the First Census.* London: P.S. King and Son.

Griesinger, W. (1861). *Die Pathologie und Therapie der psychischen Krankheiten*, 2nd edn. Stuttgart: Krabbe.

Grondin, J. (1991). *Einführung in die philosophische Hermeneutik.* Darmstadt: Wissenschaftliche Buchgesellschaft.

Guillant, Le L., Bonnafé, L. & Mignot, H. (1964). *Problèmes posés par la chronicité sur le plan des institutions psychiatriques.* Paris: Masson.

Gutiérrez, M. T., Primo, F. & Gutiérrez, J. L. (1990). Apuntes para la historia del Hospital Psiquiátrico San Luis, de Palencia. *Informaciones Psiquiátricas*, **121**, 227–39.

Hagenbach, N. (1907). Dr. Gottlieb Burckhardt. *Korrespondenzblatt für Schweizer Arzte*, **37**, 257–60.

Hankinson, R. J. (1998). *Galen on Antecedent Causes.* Cambridge: Cambridge University Press.

Haslam, J. (1809). *Observations of Madness and Melancholy.* London: Callow.

Healy, D. (2002). *The Creation of Psychopharmacology.* Cambridge, MA: Harvard University Press.

Healy, D. (2004). *Let them eat Prozac.* New York: New York University Press.

Hécaen, H. & Lanteri-Laura, G. (1977). *Evolution des connaissances et des doctrines sur les localizations cérébrales.* Paris: Descleé de Brouwer.

Heinroth, J. C. (1975). *Textbook of Disturbances of Mental Life*, Vol. 1. Translated by J. Schmorak. Baltimore, MD: Johns Hopkins University Press.

Hemphill, R. E. & Walter, W. G. (1941). The treatment of mental disorders by electrically induced convulsions. *Journal of Mental Science*, **87**, 256–75.

Henry, J. (1986). Occult qualities and the experimental philosophy: active principles in pre-Newtonian Matter Theory. *History of Science*, **24**, 335–81.

Hermeil (1856). *Recherches sur le traitement de l'aliénation mentale.* Paris: Simon.

Higby, G. J. & Stroud, E. C. (ed.) (1997). *The Inside Story of Medicines. A Symposium.* Madison, WI: American Institute of the History of Pharmacy.

Hippocrates (1967). *The Art.* English Translation by W.H.S. Jones, Vol. 2, pp. 190–217. London: W. Heinemann.

Hobson, R. F. (1953). Prognostic factors in electro convulsive therapy. *Journal of Neurology, Neurosurgery and Psychiatry*, **16**, 275–81.

Horsley, V. (1892). Trephining. In *A Dictionary of Psychological Medicine*, Vol. 2, ed. D. H. Tuke, pp. 1324–7. London: Churchill.

Hounau, H. M. (1807). *Des principales sources des maladies chroniques*. Paris.

Hoyningen-Huene, P. (1990). Kuhn's conception of incommensurability. *Studies in History and Philosophy of Science*, **21**, 481–92.

Iggers, G. G. (1997). *Historiography in the Twentieth Century*. Hanover: Wesleyan University Press.

Impastato, D. J. (1960). The story of the first electroshock treatment. *American Journal of Psychiatry*, **116**, 1113–14.

Ireland, W. W. (1891). Operative treatment of insanity. *Journal of Mental Science*, **37**, 613–18.

Jacobsen, C. F., Wolfe, J. B. & Jackson, T. A. (1935). An experimental analysis of the functions of the frontal association areas in primates. *Journal of Nervous and Mental Disease*, **82**, 1–14.

James, F. E. (1992). Insulin treatment in psychiatry. *History of Psychiatry*, **3**, 221–35.

James, S. (1997). *Passion and Action*. Oxford: Oxford University Press.

Jones, K. (2000). Insulin coma therapy in schizophrenia. *Journal of the Royal Society of Medicine*, **93**, 147–9.

Jordan, W. (1959). *Philanthropy in England, 1480–1660: a Study of the Changing Patterns of English Social Aspirations*. London: G. Allen & Unwin.

Kahlbaum, K. (1863). *Die Gruppirung der psychischen Krankheiten und die Eintheilung der Seelenstrungen*. Danzig: A.W. Kafemann.

Keel, O. (2001). *L'Avènement de la medicine clinique moderne en Europe 1750–1815*. Montreal: Les Presses de L'Université de Montréal.

Kennedy, A. (1940). The treatment of mental disorders by induced convulsions. *Journal of Neurology and Psychiatry*, **3**, 49–82.

Kovalevsky, P. J. (1890). *Hygiène et traitement des maladies mentales et nerveuses*. Translated by W. de Holstein. Paris: Alcan.

Kraepelin, E. (1983). *Lebenserinnerungen*. Berlin: Springer.

Krafft-Ebing, R. von (1893). *Lehrbuch der Psychiatrie*, 5th edn. Stuttgart: Enke.

Kraft, I. (1961). Edouard Séguin and 19th century moral treatment of idiots. *Bulletin of the History of Medicine*, **35**, 393–418.

Kragh, H. (1987). *The Historiography of Science*. Cambridge: Cambridge University Press.

Krapf, E. (1928). Epilepsie und schizophrenie. *Archiv für Psychiatrie und Nervenkrankheiten*, **83**, 547–86.

Kuhn, T. (1962). *The Structure of Scientific Revolutions*. Chicago: Chicago University Press.

Laín-Entralgo, P. (1970). *The Therapy of the Word in Classical Antiquity*. Translated by L. J. Rather & J. M. Sharp. New Haven: Yale University Press.

Laín-Entralgo, P. (1978). *Historia de la Medicina*. Barcelona: Salvat.

Lamarche, A., Beaujeu, J. & Estienne, G. (1941). Le Traitement par l'électrochoc. *Annales Médico-Psychologiques*, **99**, 251–61.

Landré-Beauvais, A. J. (1813). *Séméiotique*. Paris: Brosson.

Lanteri-Laura, G. (1997). *La Chronicité en psychiatrie*. Paris: Collection de Les Empêcheurs de Penser en Rond, Synthélabo.

Lapipe, M. & Rondepierre, J. (1941). Essai d'un apparel français pour l'électroshoc. *Annales Médico-Psychologiques*, **99**, 87–95.

Laporte, J. (2004). *Natural Kinds and Conceptual Change*. Cambridge: Cambridge University Press.

Laudan, L. (1977). *Progress and its Problems towards a Theory of Scientific Growth*. Berkeley, CA: University of California Press.

Leduc, S. (1902). Production du sommel et de l'anesthésie générale par les courantes électriques. *Comptes Rendus de l'Académie des Sciences*, **135**, 878–9.

Lefevre, G. (1971). *La Naissance de l'historiographie moderne*. Paris: Flammarion.

Lehmann, H. E. & Ban, T. A. (1997). The history of the psychopharmacology of schizophrenia. *Canadian Journal of Psychiatry*, **42**, 152–62.

Leuret, F. (1838). *Du Traitement moral de la Folie*. Paris: Baillière.

Levi, A. (1964). *French Moralists. The Theory of the Passions 1585–1649*. Oxford: Clarendon Press.

Lewin, L. (1998). *Phantastica*. Rochester: Park Street Press.

López-Muñoz, F. & Álamo, C. (ed.) (1998). *Historia de la Neuropsicofarmacología*. Madrid: Eurobooks.

Luys, J. B. (1893). *Le Traitement de la Folie*. Paris: Rueff.

Macht, D. I. (1920). *Johns Hopkins Hospital, Bulletin*, **31**, 167.

Magnan, V. (ed.) (1898). Traitement des maladies mentales. In *Traité de Thérapeutique Appliqué*, ed. A. Robin. Paris: Rueff.

Malzberg, B. (1943). The outcome of electric shock therapy in the New York civil state hospitals. *Psychiatric Quarterly*, **17**, 154–63.

Marks, H. M. (1997). *The Progress of Experiment*. Cambridge: Cambridge University Press.

Martinet, J. F. (1813). *Traité des maladies chroniques*. Paris.

Matthews, J. N. S. (2000). *An Introduction to Randomized Controlled Clinical Trials*. London: Arnold.

McPherson, J. & Wallace, D. (1892). The surgical treatment of general paralysis of the insane. *British Medical Journal*, **ii**, 167–70.

Médioni, G. (1992). Dic griechische Medizin nach Hippokrates. In *Illustrierte Geschichte der Medizin*, Vol. 1, ed. R. Toellner, pp. 351–92. Erlangen: Müller.

Meduna, L. J. (1934). Über experimentelle Campherepilepsie. *Archiv für Psychiatrie und Nervenkrankheiten*, **102**, 333–9.

Meduna, L. J. (1937). *Die Konvulsionstherapie der Schizophrenie*. Halle: Carl Marhold.

Meduna, L. J. (1938). General discussion of the cardiazol therapy. *American Journal of Psychiatry*, **94** (Suppl.), 40–50.

Meduna, L. J. (1950). Genèse du traitement de la schizophrénie par le cardiazol. *Annales Médico-Psychologiques*, **97**, 546–54.

Meduna, L. J. (1943). Dysharmonism in psychosis and its correction by shock. *Journal of Nervous and Mental Disease*, **98**, 5–13.

Milne-Edwards, H. & Vavasseur, P. (1828). *Manuel de Matière Médicale*, 2nd edn. Paris: Compère Jeune.

Moncrieff, J. (1999). An investigation into the precendents of modern drug treatment in psychiatry. *History of Psychiatry*, 1999, **10**, 475–90.

Moniz, E. & Lima, A. (1936). Premiers essais de psycho-chirurgie. Technique et résultats. *Lisboa Medica*, **13**, 152–61.

Moniz, E. (1936). *Tentatives opératoires dans le traitement de certaines psychoses.* Paris: Masson.

Moniz, E. (1948). Mein weg zur leukotomie. *Deutsche Medizinische Wochenschrift,* **73**, 581–3.

Moore, N. P. (1943). The maintenance treatment of chronic psychotics by electrically induced convulsions. *Journal of Mental Science,* **89**, 257–69.

Müller, Ch. R. (1958). Gottlieb Burckhardt: Le Pére de la Topectomie. *Revue Médicale de la Suisse Romande,* **28**, 726–30.

Nathan, T. & Stengers, I. (2004). *Médicins et Sorciers.* Paris: Collection Les Empêcheurs de Penser en Rond.

Nyirö, J. & Jablonsky, A. (1929). Einige daten zur prognose der epilepsie, mit besonderer rücksicht auf die konstitution. *Psychiatrische Neurologische Wochenschrift,* **31**, 547–9.

Oakes, G. (1988). *Weber and Rickert. Concept Formation in the Cultural Sciences.* Cambridge, MA: MIT Press.

Pachter, H. M. (1951). *Paracelsus.* New York: Shuman.

Pagel, W. (1958). *Paracelsus: an Introduction to Philosophical Medicine in the Era of the Renaissance.* Basel: Karger.

Paget S. (2004). Horsley, Sir Victor Alexander Haden (1857–1916), rev. Overy, C. *Oxford Dictionary of National Biography.* Oxford: Oxford University Press.

Parry-Jones, W. (1972). *The Trade in Lunacy. A Study of Private Madhouses in England in the Eighteenth and Nineteenth Centuries.* London: Routledge & Kegan Paul.

Passione, R. (2004). Italian psychiatry in an international context: Ugo Cerletti and the case of electroshock. *History of Psychiatry,* **15**, 83–104.

Penrose, L. S. & Marr, W. B. (1943). Results of shock therapy evaluated by estimating chances of patients remaining in hospital without such treatment. *Journal of Mental Science,* **89**, 374–80.

Pereira, A. L. & Pita, J. R. (ed.) (2000). *Egas Moniz.* Coimbra: Minerva.

Petersen, J. (1877). *Haupmomente in der geschichtlichen Entwicklung der medicinischen Therapie.* Copenhagen: Höst.

Pinel, Ph. (1809). *Traité médico-philosophique sur l'alienation mentale,* 2nd edn. Paris: Brosson.

Pinel, Ph. (1813). Chronique. In *Dictionnaire des sciences médicales,* ed. Adelon *et al.* Paris: Panckoucke.

Porter, R. (ed.) (1985). *Patients and Practitioners. Lay Perceptions of Medicine in Pre-industrial Society.* Cambridge: Cambridge University Press.

Porter, R. (1993). *Disease, Medicine and Society in England 1550–1860,* 2nd edn. Cambridge: Cambridge University Press.

Porter, R. & Wear, A. (ed.) (1987) *Problems and Methods in the History of Medicine.* London: Croom Helm.

Porter, R. & Teich, M. (ed.) (1995). *Drugs and Narcotics in History.* Cambridge: Cambridge University Press.

Postel, J. (1979). Naissance et decadence du traitement moral pendant la première moitie du XIX Siècle. *L'Evolution Psychiatrique,* **44**, 585–616.

Potter, J. (1996). *Representing Reality.* London: Sage.

Pressman, J. D. (1988). Sufficient promise: John F. Fulton and the origins of psychosurgery. *Bulletin of the History of Medicine,* **62**, 1–29.

Pulver, S. E. (1961). The first electroconvulsive treatment given in the United States. *American Journal of Psychiatry,* **117**, 845–6.

Puuseppe, M. (1937). Alcune considerazioni sugli interventi chirurgici nelle malattie mentali. *Giornale Accademia Medica Torino,* **100**, 3–16.

Revington, G. (1889). Is general paralysis of the insane a curable disease? *British Medical Journal,* 1889, **ii**, 1187.

Revington, G. (1890). The surgical treatment of general paralysis of the insane. *British Medical Journal,* **i**, 749.

Rey, M. (1891). Trépan dans un cas de paralysie générale. *Archives de Neurologie,* **22**, 260.

Ribes, F. (1860). *Traité d'hygiène thérapeutique ou application des moyens de l'hygiène au traitement des maladies.* Paris: Ballière.

Riddle, J. M. (1992). The methodology of historical drug research. In *Quid pro quo: Studies in the History of Drugs,* Variorum Collected Studies Series CS367, pp. 1–19. Great Yarmouth.

Rinkel, M. & Himwich, H. E. (ed.) (1959). *Insulin Treatment in Psychiatry.* New York: Philosophical Library.

Rolleston, H. D (2004). Allbutt, Sir Thomas Clifford (1836–1925), rev. Alexander G. Bearn. *Oxford Dictionary of National Biography.* Oxford: Oxford University Press.

Rosenberg, C. E. (1997). The therapeutic revolution: medicine, meaning and social change in nineteenth century America. *Perspectives in Biology and Medicine,* **20**, 485–506.

Roth, M. (1951). Changes in the EEG under barbiturate anaesthesia produced by electro-convulsive treatment and their significance for the theory of ECT action. *Electroencephalography and Clinical Neurophysiology,* **3**, 261–80.

Ruffat, M. (1996). *175 ans d'industrie pharmaceutique française.* Paris: La Découverte.

Rush, A. J., Thase, M. E. & Dube, S. (2003). Research issues in the study of difficult-to-treat depression. *Biological Psychiatry,* **53**, 743–53.

Sachs, G. S. & Rush, A. J. (2003). Response, remission, and recovery in bipolar disorders: what are the realistic treatment goals? *Journal of Clinical Psychiatry,* **64** (Suppl. 6), 18–22.

Sakel, M. (1935). *Neue Behandlungsmethode der Schizophrenie.* Wien: Moritz Perles.

Samuel, E. (1943). Some complications arising during electrical convulsive therapy. *Journal of Mental Science,* **89**, 81–4.

Sander, W. (1868). Über eine spezielle Form der primären Verrücktheit. *Archiv für Psychiatrie und Nervenkrankheiten,* **1**, 387–419.

Scull, A. T. (1979). Moral treatment reconsidered: some sociological comments on an episode in the history of British psychiatry. *Psychological Medicine,* 9.

Séguin, É. (1846). *Traitement Moral, hygiéne et éducation des idiots et des autres enfants arriérés.* Paris: Baillière.

Semelaigne, R. (1895). Sur la chirurgie cérébrale dans les aliénations mentales. *Annales Médico-Psychologiques,* **1**, 394–420.

Seppilli, G. (1891). La cura chirurgica delle malattie mentali. *Rivista Sperimentale di Freniatria e di Medicina Legale,* **27**, 369–74.

Shaw, T. C. & Cripps, H. (1890). On the surgical treatment of general paralysis. *British Medical Journal,* **i**, 1364.

Shaw, T. C. (1889). The surgical treatment of insanity. *British Medical Journal*, **ii**, 1090–1.

Shaw, T. C. (1891). Surgical treatment of general paralysis of the Insane. *British Medical Journal*, **ii**, 581–3.

Shaw, T. C. (1892). Surgery and insanity. *Saint Bartholomew's Hospital Reports*, **28**, 55–68.

Sherrington, C. S. (2004). Ferrier, Sir David (1843–1928), rev. Michael Bevan. *Oxford Dictionary of National Biography*. Oxford: Oxford University Press.

Shipley, W. H. & McGregor, J. S. (1940). The clinical applications of electrically induced convulsions. *Proceedings of the Royal Society of Medicine*, **30**, 267–9.

Shorter, E. (1997). *A History of Psychiatry*. New York: Wiley.

Shorvon, H. J. & Shorvon, L. M. (1943). Spinal anaesthesia in electric convulsive therapy. *Journal of Mental Science*, **89**, 69–72.

Siegel, R. E. (1973). *Galen on Psychology, Psychopathology and Function and Diseases of the Nervous System*. Basel: Karger.

Smith, L. H. (1942). Electroshock treatment in the psychoses. *American Journal of Psychiatry*, **98**, 558–61.

Smith, P. (1890). The surgical treatment of general paralysis. *British Medical Journal*, **i**, 11–12.

Störck, A. de (1887). *Études de thérapeutique experimentale*. Translated by H. Piedvache. Paris: Baillière.

Suzuki, A. (1995). The politics and ideology of non-restraint. *Medical History*.

Taper, M. L. & Lele, S. R. (ed.) (2004). *The Nature of Statistical Evidence. Statistical, Philosophical and Empirical Considerations*. Chicago: The University of Chicago Press.

Telesko, W. (2001). *The Wisdom of Nature. The Healing Powers and Symbolisms of Plants and Animals in the Middle Ages*. Munich: Prestel.

Temkin, O. (1973). *Galenism*. Ithaca: Cornell University Press.

Thase, M. E. (2003). Evaluating antidepressant therapies: remission as the optimal outcome. *Journal of Clinical Psychiatry*, **64** (Suppl. 13), 18–25.

Thorpe, J. G. (1962). The current status of prognostic test indicators for electroconvulsive therapy. *Psychosomatic Medicine*, **24**, 554–68.

Tow, P. M. (1955). *Personality Changes following Frontal Leucotomy*. London: Oxford University Press.

Tröhler, U. (2000). *To Improve the Evidence of Medicine. The 18th century British Origins of a Critical Approach*. Edinburgh: Royal College of Physicians of Edinburgh Publications.

Trousseau, A. & Pidoux, H. (1877). *Traité de Thérapeutique et de Matière Médicale*, 9th edn, 2 Vols. Paris: Asselin.

Tuke, D. H. (1892). Therapeutics. In *A Dictionary of Psychological Medicine*, 2 Vols, ed. D. H. Tuke, pp. 1290–3. London: Churchill.

Tuke, J. B. (1890). The surgical treatment of intracranial fluid pressure. *British Medical Journal*, **i**, 8–11.

Tuke, J. B. (1891). A plea for the scientific study of insanity. *British Medical Journal*, **i**, 1161–6.

Valenstein, E. S. (1986). *Great and Desperate Cures. The Rise and Decline of Psychosurgery and other Radical Treatments of Mental Illness*. New York: Basic Books.

Virey (1821). Signature. In *Dictionaire des Sciences Médicales*, ed. Adelon *et al.* Vol. 51, pp. 262–7. Paris: C. L. F. Panckoucke.

Vogel, M. J. & Rosenberg, C. E. (ed.) (1979). *The Therapeutic Revolution: Essays on the Social History of American Medicine*. Pennsylvania: University of Pennsylvania Press.

Wade, N. J., Norrsell, U. & Presly, A. (2005). Cox's chair: 'a moral and a medical mean in the treatment of maniacs'. *History of Psychiatry*, **16**, 73–88.

Wagner, C. G. (1890). A case of trephining for general paralysis. *American Journal of Insanity*, **47**, 59–66.

Walker, A. E. (1970). Egas Moniz. In *The Founders of Neurology*, 2nd edn, ed. W. Haymaker & F. Schiller, pp. 489–92. Thomas, IL.

Wallace, W. A. (1972). *Causality and Scientific Explanation*, Vol. 1. Ann Arbor, MI: The University of Michigan Press.

Warner, J. H. (1997). *The Therapeutic Perspective. Medical Practice, Knowledge, and Identity in America 1820–1885*. Princeton: Princeton University Press.

Weitbrecht, H. J. (1949). *Studie zur psychopathologie krampfbehandelter Psychosen*. Stuttgart: Georg Thieme.

Whitaker, H. A., Stemmer, B. & Joanette, Y. (1996). A psychosurgical chapter in the history of cerebral localization: the six cases of Gottlieb Burckhardt. In *Classical Cases in Neuropsychology*, ed. C. Code, C.-W. Wallesch, Y. Joanette & A. Roch, pp. 275–304. Hove: Lawrence Erlbaum.

Willis, T. (1685). *The London Practice of Physick*. London: Basset.

Wilson, I. G. H. (1937). *A Study of Hypoglycaemic Shock in Schizophrenia*. London: His Majesty's Stationery Office.

Worcester, W. L. (1891). Surgery of the central nervous system (Account of the Berlin meeting). *American Journal of Insanity*, **47**, 410–13.

Wortis, S. B. *et al.* (ed.) (1953). *Psychiatric Treatment*. Baltimore: The Williams Wilkins Company.

Young, R. M. (1966). Scholarship and the history of the behavioural sciences. *History of Science*, **5**, 1–51.

Part II

Summary of treatment modalities in psychiatric disorders

3

A critical assessment of methods and processes used to develop psychiatric drug treatments

George W. Arana and David J. Nutt

Editor's note

While the double-blind, placebo-controlled randomized clinical trial (RCT) has become the gold standard, and while many of the data behind the determination of effectiveness of compounds or other treatments in this volume rely upon the RCT as the primary determinant of effectiveness, this chapter reminds us that the gold standard is probably made up of less pure gold than we would want to believe. The variables, assumptions and biases that are inherent in the RCT and in Cochrane reviews and other meta-analyses are described in this chapter. The goal of Arana and Nutt is not to make sceptics of us all. Rather it is to make us wiser consumers of the psychiatric, particularly the pharmacologic psychiatric, literature so that we may approach both the literature and our patients with better understanding as to how to appreciate their illnesses and the benefits and limitations of the agents we have at our disposal in providing treatment to them.

Introduction

This chapter seeks to describe in simple terms the models and methods used to identify, test and validate the efficacy and safety of drugs for use in psychiatric illnesses.

In the first section, we review the complexity inherent in an environment where three strong, related, yet independent vectors drive most of the discovery in new drug development: (1) the profit motive of large pharmaceutical firms; (2) the academic motive evident in university settings where much of the preclinical and clinical research is undertaken; and (3) the clinical motive that seeks to offer relief to patients. The authors ask the reader to focus on various aspects of clinical trials including the importance of study design, use of placebo, the impact of nosological reform on advances in clinical psychopharmacology, and the hidden pitfalls of clinical response in special populations of psychiatric disorders.

In the second section, we have chosen to demonstrate how a literature review might be conducted by presenting findings from a limited literature review on depression and the drugs commonly used to treat clinical depression in its various settings and presentations. This includes depression when it co-exists with other conditions such as in geriatric and medical populations, in dually diagnosed patients with depression and substance abuse, and in depression in patients with schizophrenia.

Models and methods used to test psychiatric drugs

General remarks

That chemical compounds can change behavior, cognition, emotions and level of consciousness, has been evident over the millennia. Over the past half century we have witnessed an unprecedented growth in the number and variety of compounds that have emerged for use in psychiatric diseases and their corollaries. Some compounds have come forward either via traditional pharmaceutical-technical routes while others have followed non-traditional venues. In today's highly competitive marketplace that seeks safe and effective psychiatric drugs, the traditional track usually includes the identification of specific chemical compounds that are studied in a variety of pre-clinical models. These drugs are brought to the clinical setting and tested for toxicity and subsequently for efficacy in various diagnostic categories. Few are ultimately found to be useful for psychiatric and behavioral presentations.

Cambridge Textbook of Effective Treatments in Psychiatry, ed. Peter Tyrer and Kenneth R. Silk. Published by Cambridge University Press.
© Cambridge University Press, 2008.

The gold standard: double-blind, placebo-controlled, randomized controlled trial

The standard of the "clinical psychopharmacologic trial" is the double-blind, placebo-controlled, randomized controlled trial (RCT) study of a putative effective agent. In this research model, specific inclusion criteria (accepted diagnostic criteria are applied to a population of study subjects) and exclusion criteria (possible confounds such as concomitant medical and neurological illnesses) are applied, the new agent (e.g. an antidepressant) is given to a randomly assigned sub-group of subjects while an identically prepared inert substance (placebo) is given to another sub-group of subjects, and certain outcome variables such as cardinal symptoms of depression are measured before, sometime during, but always, at the conclusion of, the trial which usually lasts for 6–12 weeks. Analysis of RCT data can be performed in several ways with regulators traditionally preferring the conservative intention-to-treat (ITT) analysis where all subjects entered into the treatment phase (all those randomized) are included. This means that the ratings of subjects who drop out early on (so who should have little chance of recovering) are incorporated in the final analysis, and are usually carried through each assessment point 'carrying' their last score before they dropped out. This tends to minimize the difference between active and placebo treatments especially for drug therapies that may be poorly tolerated initially and can then lead to a significant number of early dropouts.

The question may be raised as to why not use completer analysis instead of ITT? This is a complicated issue because many non-drug treatments are evaluated just on completers as this chapter will describe later. The main reason regulators dislike this approach is that it says less about the efficacy of a drug in the whole population than an ITT analysis since those staying in the trial until completion may have a peculiar positive response sensitivity to the drug or, more likely, a special resistance to adverse effects which would explain why they stay in treatment. In the area of mental health treatments, a trial in which less than 75% of those entered into active drug treatment complete the test period is often considered a "failed" trial. This approach is rather arbitrary as in other areas of psychiatric medicine much lower retention rates are acceptable. For example, in smoking cessation studies less than 10% of placebo-treated patients may complete a trial and so if 20% on the active drug-treated complete the trial, then this can be highly significant. Buproprion (Zyban) was licensed based on such data (Hughes et al., 2004).

Recently more sophisticated "mixed model" statistical analytical approaches have been explored as a means of optimizing the value of clinical trial data. These approaches are, in effect, a compromise between the extremes of ITT and completers because they allow some weight to be given to the time at which the drop-out occurred.

A novel approach to efficacy is now emerging from the insistence of the European Medicines Evaluation Agency that drugs that are seeking a license for enduring or life-long disorders (as many psychiatric ones are) must show evidence of enduring efficacy. In practical terms, this implies that the effects of the drug should last for at least 6 months. In other words, to obtain a license in Europe, companies now have to show that an antidepressant or anxiolytic continues to demonstrate efficacy for at least 6 months. There are several ways this evidence can be gathered. One is to extend the early proof-of-efficacy from the short term of a 4–8 week trial up to a length of 6 months. This is ethically challenging as some patients will stay on placebo for all this time. However, as they are under careful medical supervision, they can be withdrawn at any time and put into alternative (active) treatment.

The main alternative strategy is one in which a group of patients is treated in an open fashion and then randomized to either continuing on the drug or being switched to placebo. The frequency of relapse is monitored over the subsequent 6–12 month period. These are usually called relapse prevention trials though they do reveal long-term efficacy data as well.

The relapse prevention approach has two major benefits. The first is that it inevitably gives data on the nature and frequency of drug withdrawal symptoms. A good example is the claim that the SSRIs are like the benzodiazepines in causing dependence because they lead to recurrence of depression when they are withdrawn and so patients are forced to keep taking them to prevent this "withdrawal" from occurring. A comparison of the literature on the clinical effects of blind (a very important consideration here) withdrawal reactions from benzodiazepines (BZs) and SSRIs shows important differences. Only in BZ withdrawal does one see the acute recurrence of the underlying anxiety disorder in the period of drug withdrawal whereas with the SSRIs, recurrence of depression on discontinuation comes much later, frequently weeks or months after the drug is stopped. This suggests important differences in the nature of the therapeutic and withdrawal reactions to these two classes of drug. (For a more detailed discussion see Nutt, 2003.)

The other major benefit of these longer-term relapse prevention trials is that they demonstrate the continued value of drug treatment in any disorder where relapse is likely, such as in depression and schizophrenia. In both these disorders there is strong evidence that continued use of medication prevents relapse or recurrence of the disorder. In schizophrenia, extended drug therapy reduced relapse risk to a small fraction of that seen among those not on the drug. In depression, the effect of continued treatment may be even more profound as reported by Geddes *et al.* (2003) after examining data from 57 trials with nearly 6000 people. They found that the prophylactic action of antidepressants to prevent relapse in depression was one of the strongest treatment effects in the whole of medicine with a *P* value of < 0.00001.

In most major psychiatric illnesses such as anxiety, depression and schizophrenia, both the long-term placebo control or the placebo withdrawal approaches to proving long-term efficacy tend to show that there is progressive improvement in the active treatment arm from the end of the initial efficacy phase to the 6 or 12 month end point. These data are useful in giving further support for the ongoing value of the treatment agents in the specific disorders. For instance, although the placebo effect is usually of similar magnitude in depression and anxiety disorders, the effect in depression tends to wane more rapidly and profoundly which perhaps suggests a fundamentally different underlying mechanism of the placebo response in the two disorders.

The question of comparator drug studies is also worth considering. Whilst it is not an absolute requirement for the demonstration of efficacy of a new treatment, most new drugs are explored in at least one comparator study. Simple comparator trials (i.e. the new drug against an established one) were once the mainstay of evidence in the early days of regulation for licensing where, if the new drug showed no difference, i.e. was non-inferior when compared with the control drug, it was considered efficacious. Such trials are not acceptable today unless they also contain a placebo arm because it can be extremely difficult to adequately power such a study to reliably demonstrate significant differences between drugs. Hence, in this instance, the studies run the risk of a type II error, i.e. showing no difference when one does, in fact, exist. An ineffective drug could obtain a license in this way, and it seems likely that a number of older agents that were licensed using this method would not currently meet modern criteria for efficacy. The current practice is to use a proven drug in a trial of a new agent and placebo as a form of internal control (verum).

One spin-off from the use of comparator studies is that we now have better, and in some cases, the only data on the long-term response to various first-generation compounds. For instance, imipramine has many more placebo-controlled examples of efficacy in depression as a result of being a comparator to the SSRIs in numerous trials.

The SSRI fluoxetine has been extensively used as a comparator for the other SSRIs and other newer antidepressants and so has gathered an extensive database for both efficacy and safety. This database is much larger than could have been produced by any one company. Paradoxically the best data for the benzodiazepines in properly diagnosed DSM–III or DSM–IV generalized anxiety disorder comes from their use as comparators for new drugs, especially antidepressants, in the treatment of this disorder.

Use of placebos in psychopharmacologic trial

A placebo run-in phase is a technique used in clinical trials in which placebo responders are dropped from a study before they are randomly assigned to either the active or placebo treatment condition. Although this approach may favor the active treatment in clinical trials, a recent meta-analytic report of nearly 6800 subjects from 43 separate studies treated either with SSRIs or placebo comparing the effect size of randomized, placebo-controlled clinical trials in the treatment of depression found no difference in outcome between those studies with the placebo-run-in versus those studies without the placebo-run-in. The authors did find, however, that the practice of using placebo-run-in methodology did produce larger absolute effect sizes, and their recommendation is that future studies report both the use of the placebo-run-in method and the number of subjects dropped from the study due to early placebo response. Another possible confound recently reported from the analysis of a large data repository was that certain diagnostic entities tended to higher placebo response when treated with certain classes of drugs whereas other diagnostic groupings tended to poor responses both to active and placebo preparations. In this report, analysis of drug response rates from Brief Psychiatric Rating Scale (BPRS) profiles in over 2600 psychiatric patients suggested that depressive disorders with anxious and hostile features may have excessive placebo response rates, while withdrawn and disorganized thinking subjects may respond poorly to both active drug or placebo in trials of neuroleptic drugs (Overall & Rhoades, 1982). The use of placebo in the pediatric age group has come under increasing scrutiny over the past 20 years due to regulatory and ethical pressures. This group consensus process concluded that "in many but not all circumstances, inclusion of a placebo control is essential to meet the scientific goals of treatment outcome research" (p. 1046). Although they endorsed novel approaches to assuring full disclosure and adherence to ethical practice of scientific research, fundamentally they concluded that the "gold standard" in the determination of rational allopathic treatments were based in the double-blind, placebo-controlled, randomized, clinical trial (March *et al.*, 2004).

Another question raised by regulators, patient organizations and physicians is what is it that comprises a clinically meaningful placebo–drug difference? This question is often posed with the assumption that a small drug–placebo difference means that the drug is relatively ineffective. Some have suggested that because of the greater safety of placebo, they should be used as a therapeutic agent instead of the active drug. These are false assumptions for two reasons. The first is that such a difference is the full size of the "true" drug effect. As has been well discussed elsewhere (Guess *et al.*, 2002), the true drug effect is the total effect of the drug minus that which would have occurred if no treatment was given. As we know, the placebo arm of a clinical trial includes self- and doctor-rated assessments, meetings with other medical staff, clinic visits, and other interactions with the investigative team which would not occur if "no treatment" had been the option.

Second, the effect of placebo is not that of no drug because in double-blind trials both patients and doctor feel that patients on placebo may be on active treatment, and many will assume that they are. This therefore contrasts with the clinical situation where if a doctor were to prescribe a placebo it would be single blind so the doctor's expectations would be different and therapeutic benefit would likely be much less than in the clinical trial.

An important further consideration is that the use of the placebo-controlled trial is to establish that a drug is efficacious, so that regulatory authorities are then given the confidence to license it. Such trials are necessarily on small, relatively select populations that are usually free of co-morbid disorders, often of middle age, and mostly without other medical problems or taking other drugs. Only once a drug is licensed can its true clinical utility or effectiveness be established, and thus information is usually gathered in larger, phase 4 studies, in a wider range of patients.

Re-inventing psychiatric nosology: the linchpin of modern psychopharmacology

There is no question that over the past half century, the nature of psychiatric practice and concomitantly, the methods and techniques used in psychiatric research, have changed dramatically. With the advent in the 1960s and early 70s of more descriptive, atheoretical, methods for clinical psychiatric diagnosis that were outlined in the DSM–III, psychiatric research and nosology began to use a descriptively based rather than a theoretically based model for diagnosis as had been employed in DSM–II. The authors of the DSM–III took their lead from the Robins, Woodruff, & Guze's Criteria for Psychiatric Diagnosis which emanated from the Washington University psychiatric research group in St. Louis, Missouri (Feighner *et al.*, 1972). This distinction is best demonstrated by DSM–III's description of a diagnostic entity, "depressive disorder," in which no etiologic assumptions are made, followed by a set of criteria that included historical, temporal, symptomatic and descriptive elements. Conversely, DSM–II identified a diagnostic entity, "depressive neurosis," which, in the use of the term "neurosis," implied an etiology founded in a psychodynamic model of disease and symptom formation. Although DSM–III was similar to DSM–II in that there were criteria that included historical, temporal, symptomatic, and descriptive elements for depression, it was DSM–III's putative atheoretical position that set it apart from former nosological systems. This allowed for a descriptive approach to the various behavioral, cognitive and affective syndromes managed and treated by psychiatrists and mental health professionals without the 'etiological loading' that had been apparent over the prior 50–100 years of psychiatric diagnostics and treatment. Corresponding to this more atheoretical position in describing and categorizing mental illnesses, interventions, treatments and disease management approaches began to look at symptom and quality of life outcomes from a more atheoretical position as well.

Interpretation of the psychopharmacology literature

An atheoretical nosology may ideally serve not to bias investigators but to focus them on signs and symptoms of disease. But those who use this atheoretical system of diagnostics to test efficacy of new treatments certainly are at liberty to make assumptions about the etiology of disease and the importance of any given experimental finding. For example, when a chemical compound with known receptor-binding affinity for NMDA receptors in preclinical laboratory studies is used to treat poor memory, the investigators will speculate heartily about the importance of NMDA receptors in modulating cognition and memory in the mammalian brain, while hypothesizing about events in very complex brain neuro-circuitry. Thus although an atheoretical construct such as DSM–III may have aided in the investigator's case selection process, the investigator may make assumptions about the etiology of memory impairment as residing in NMDA receptor systems. Thus despite the atheoretical approach of the DSM, one must remain thoughtful in reviewing literature to be sure one reads the "Methods" and "Results" sections carefully and understand what compound was tested, the population tested, the selection methods used and a myriad of other details of the actual study and not confuse the remarks in the "Introduction" and in the "Discussion" as the actual *finding* of the study. It is safe to say that the neurobiological hypotheses, ideas and ruminations found in the countless "Introductions" and "Discussions" in the psychopharmacological literature are at best speculative, at worst, highly presumptive. Claims by authors or editors about any neurobiological specificity regarding the mechanism of action of a given compound needs to be carefully considered and in most cases, framed as speculative, and must be considered by the critical reader as just that, an idea by the authors of how a compound may have exerted its effect. In only a few cases has it proved possible to demonstrate categorically that the pharmacological mechanism of action of a drug is the means by which its therapeutic effect is manifest. One good example is the use of tryptophan depletion to reduce the levels of 5-HT in the brain, which has been shown to undermine the therapeutic benefit of the SSRIs in depression and some anxiety disorders (see Bell *et al.*, 2005).

Some argue that there is a clear emphasis, if not a semi-religious quality, to the importance and significance placed on studies that use the statistical principle of the null-hypothesis and the mathematics used to prove or disprove that null hypothesis. The majority of biological scientific findings depend heavily on measures and correlations that are given in terms of statistical probabilities, not absolutes. A statistical accuracy level that for all practical purposes might seem absolute is actually only an approximation of a theoretical truth, and not the actual truth.

Comments on meta-analyses of large databases

When large databases are mined for essentials of drug efficacy and toxicity in the treatment of psychiatric conditions, several major findings are quickly evident. First, the striking heterogeneity of study designs, populations, settings, duration, diagnostic methodology, symptom assessment, statistical approaches and methods used, conclusions reached, and finally, the accuracy, reliability and validity of the entire study process, makes meta-analyses difficult at best, treacherous at worst. The common denominator for these meta-analyses is that they were obtained from the pharmacological and psychiatric literature. The publications generally used are the peer-reviewed journals in which several experts in the field have looked critically at the methodological elements mentioned above. This, in

and of itself, is a sizeable assumption, yet without this element of assumable homogeneity, meta-analyses would be meaningless. Therefore, it is important for the reader to know that, although a certain grouping of reports will "make the cut" and be included in the final analyses, there are major assumptions being utilized here attesting to the soundness of numerous factors in the clinical research that could be confounds were they to be faulty.

Peer-review mechanisms for grant funding in psychopharmacologic research, whether they be national institutes, private foundations, or Veterans Administration or Department of Defense, to name but a few funding sources, generally approve and fund a proposed clinical study based on various factors. Among these the most important are the credentials of the principal investigator, the study design and the statistical analysis proposed, the resources available at the study site, and the feasibility that the investigator/s will complete the proposed intervention on time in the number of subjects proposed. Whether a 3–5-year study is completed as designed, adheres to the parameters outlined in the grant application, and whether a granting agency scrutinizes these issues on an ongoing, continual basis, is variable. Often the peers on the review boards will rotate on and off over a period of years, changing the nature and the emphasis of the critical review for both the initial applications and for the non-competitive renewals that often are performed annually in a rather perfunctory fashion, certainly not as critically as the initial assessment of the principal investigators and their proposed science. Therefore, in the studies funded by these agencies, performed by these investigators, and reported in the literature, the quality control for adherence to the proposed protocol and consistent application of the study tools over the course of the study, is assumed, and is fully in the hands of the principal investigator. Therefore, the intense scrutiny applied on the front end of funding peer-reviewed studies is not applied throughout the course of the research, and unless there is a record of continuous funding with continuous review of a body of data and knowledge generated by a group of investigators, peer-review up front does not always yield the high degree of critical-mindedness that might be necessary through the course of the study or at the conclusion of a research project.

A fundamental assumption of reviewing large numbers of published studies is that over larger populations, across 5–10-years periods of time, the results will "wash out" false positive or false negative findings and true positive and true negative findings will result. Yet how to assure that "true" reports are generated in sufficient numbers to ultimately balance the false reports, remains elusive. Our statistical colleagues teach us that there is comfort in numbers; 10 000 similarly diagnosed patients studied with similarly designed parameters taken from the same literature will yield a "truer" picture of outcomes than 100 like patients.

The pharmaceutical-industrial-complex

The impact of the "pharmaceutical-industrial-complex" (PIC) on the development and clinical study of potential compounds that may be of benefit for psychiatric illnesses can not be underestimated. Pharmaceutical firms often screen thousands of chemical compounds annually for possible use in psychiatric and behavioral syndromes. After testing in pre-clinical paradigms that assess possible effects in the mammalian brain, these drugs are run through behavioral models that more clearly further identify those compounds that may have promise in the clinical arena. Initial testing in normal adult humans continues to assess toxicity of the drugs, and finally, those agents that are minimally toxic with promise for treatment of a known psychiatric illness, are tried in the target disorder. This process can cost many hundreds of dollars and delays a compound "getting to market" by years. This impacts the drug's "patent-life" which is the only window of time that the pharmaceutical firm can profit from its sale, the revenue from which off-setting the development cost and maybe even generating profits.

The profit motive so inherent in the PIC naturally needs to be balanced by the great benefit these large corporations have brought to the treatment and management of human illness. Nevertheless, in light of controversy raised regarding Vioxx and the litigious climate presently surrounding Merck, we must maintain a cautious attitude about the presence and absence of critical data and information brought forward by these profitable giants. Recently, a critical eye has been cast on pharmaceutical industry-sponsored trials concluding that their comparative psychotropic drug trials may need more careful review because there were apparent design and reporting modifications that favor the sponsor's product (Safer, 2002). This author discusses the consequences of marketing influences on comparative psychopharmacology trials in terms of conflicts of interest, the integrity of the scientific literature, costs to consumers and their impact on physician practice.

A clear example of the interaction of the pharmaceutical industry and the search for effective treatments for psychiatric illnesses can be found in the lithium story. Lithium was found to be effective for cyclical mood disorders in the 1960s by several well-designed and controlled clinical trials in the USA and in Europe and Australia. Because it was an orphan drug (not patented and thus pharmaceutical firms could not profit from funding studies on its use), pharmaceutical houses were reluctant to fund and undertake a clinical trial of its use for manic-depressive illnesses. After several years of discourse, the study of lithium's efficacy and toxicity was undertaken by various psychopharmacologists associated with the Institutes of Health in Bethesda as well as by investigators in the Veterans Health Administration. Today, after numerous well-designed and well-controlled clinical trials, lithium stands firmly as an agent that is effective for bipolar disorders. Its various side effects, some of which can be severe, have been studied such that patients can now be treated and comfortably managed, getting maximal benefit with reasonable control of its side effects.

Research funded by pharmaceutical firms is fraught with complexities having to do with the confidential nature of the information gleaned by the industry. History has taught us that the less than scrupulous practice of terminating funding for a study that appears to be yielding negative results when positive results are being sought, will skew findings away from true negative outcomes toward possible false positive outcomes. This same issue obtains in the intensely competitive environment of academic research centers where promotions up the academic ladder often are dependent on positive findings. Oversight and supervision of the research that is conducted and the nature of the data generated can often be dependent on "investigator honor". Although there are checks and balances evident in all research environments, the nature of the rewards and of the setting will yield a higher percentage of false positive reports and minimize true negative results. As a result of these concerns, a group of journal editors has lobbied successfully to have a publicly accessible database of all clinical trials established. This group of editors has insisted that trials not put into this database prior to commencement of the study will ultimately not be accepted for publication in these specific journals. It is hoped this will restore confidence in the clinical trials approach by ensuring all data, both efficacy and safety, will be open to scrutiny. Most pharmaceutical companies have agreed that this is a worthwhile project and have indicated that they will comply.

A limited review of evidence for antidepressants in various clinical populations and presentations

We have done a limited review of several large database reports to glimpse at what these composite analyses can teach us about the pharmacological treatment of depression and depression that is seen in specific clinical settings such as in geriatric care, primary care, substance abuse and schizophrenia.

General comments on clinical trials to treat depressive illnesses

Depression in its various forms is among the top five illnesses worldwide accounting for disability, loss of function, and the cost associated with these factors (disability-adjusted life years), and at its present rate of increase, it is expected to be ranked second within 20 years. With the development of novel SSRIs over the past 20 years and with the increased currency of alternative medicine's herbal agents such as St. John's wort, the clinician and patient are faced with a dizzying array of choices, prices and often-conflicting claims as to short- and long-term efficacy and toxicity. A fundamental question that persists in searching for scientific evidence to support claims of the antidepressant efficacy of any intervention is the relative utility of (1) the well-designed and controlled single clinical trial versus (2) the meta-analyses of specialized study registries that compile data from many clinical trials. An oft-repeated story is that of John Cade, the Australian investigator, who, having concluded that lithium was responsible for a calming effect in a rodent model, tried lithium salts in 10 manic patients and concluded on the basis of this very limited trial, that this monovalent cation had anti-manic properties. It took more than 25 years and various very large-scale trials in America and Europe for lithium to finally be "confirmed" as a valid treatment for manic-depressive illness.

Various groups have analyzed large bodies of literature recently to better understand what evidence can be brought to bear on the pharmacotherapy of depression. Here we summarize the findings of several of these reports to illustrate the criteria used to validate a clinical research finding and to identify for the reader the conclusions that can legitimately be drawn when this literature is assessed.

In one report, pertinent literature from 1980 to January 1998 was reviewed from a specialized registry of controlled trials, meta-analyses and experts yielding 1277 records with a list of 32 specific antidepressants and herbal treatments. The following criteria were applied to these records:

(1) The trial was a minimum of 6 weeks in duration.
(2) The trial compared a 'newer' antidepressant with another antidepressant (newer or older), placebo or psychosocial intervention.
(3) Participants in the trials were diagnosed with depressive disorders.
(4) A specific metric was used to record clinical outcome.

Two or more independent reviewers identified 315 trials from the original group that met these criteria. Data were synthesized descriptively, with attention being paid to participant and diagnostic descriptors, intervention characteristics, study designs and clinical outcomes. Primary outcomes were response rate (50% or greater improvement rates), total discontinuation rates (dropouts) and discontinuation rates due to adverse events. The conclusions were that newer antidepressants were more effective than placebo in treating major depression and dysthymia in older adults and primary care patients with no significant differences in efficacy or overall discontinuation rates between newer and older agents. St. John's wort was more effective than placebo in treating mild to moderate depressive disorders (Mulrow et al., 1998).

Relative efficacy of older versus newer antidepressants

The question of the relative efficacy and toxicity of the older antidepressants, particularly the tricyclics, as compared with the newer SSRIs, is important when considering the economic burden of treatment for these often chronic and disabling diseases. Amitriptyline, introduced in the 1960s, has been considered a reference compound for the pharmacological treatment of depression until the arrival of the SSRIs with their claims of a more favourable tolerability/efficacy profile. The methods employed analyzed Cochrane Registers, key journals, conference and abstract searches as well as contact with pharmaceutical firms. The review indicated that amitriptyline was as efficacious as other tricyclics and more efficacious than the newer SSRI compounds. However, the burden of side effects was greater in the amitriptyline-treated patients. The authors concluded that although amitriptyline was less well tolerated than SSRIs, this was counterbalanced by a higher proportion of responders rendering the differences between the two classes of drugs overall as not being statistically significant (Guaiana et al., 2003).

Addressing the same question as to use of older antidepressants vs. the newer compounds, both English-language and non-English-language literature from 1980 to January 1998 was reviewed. The review identified 315 trials that used a randomized, placebo-controlled study design conducted among outpatients examining acute-phase treatment. Both newer and older antidepressants demonstrated similar profiles for efficacy and toxicity, and both classes of compounds should be considered when making treatment decisions for adult outpatient, depressed populations (Williams et al., 2000). Another publication by this same group in which the same criteria for selection of studies was applied to the registry reported that when data from 28 randomized controlled trials involving 5940 adult primary care patients with major depression were analyzed, the response rates were 63% for newer agents, 35% for placebo and 60% for tricyclic agents. Dropout rates as a result of adverse effects were 8% with newer agents and 13% with tricyclic agents ($P < 0.05$) (Mulrow et al., 2000).

Antidepressants for older primary care patients

Another study focused on the rates and predictors of lifetime and recent depression treatment in depressed older primary care patients. These authors reviewed cross-sectional data collected from 1999 to 2001 in 18 primary care clinics belonging to eight organizations in five states. Clinic users ($n = 1801$) aged 60 and older who met diagnostic criteria for major depression or dysthymia were identified. Lifetime depression treatment was defined as ever having received a prescription medication, counseling or psychotherapy for depression. Potentially effective recent depression treatment was defined as 2 or more months of antidepressant medications or four or more sessions of counseling or psychotherapy for depression in the past 3 months. Most study participants (83%) reported depressive symptoms for 2 or more years, and most (71%) reported two or more prior depressive episodes. About 65% reported any lifetime depression treatment, and 46% reported some depression treatment in the past 3 months, although only 29% reported potentially effective recent depression treatment. Most of the treatment provided consisted of antidepressant medications, with newer antidepressants such as SSRIs constituting the majority (78%) of antidepressants used. Most participants indicated a preference for counseling or psychotherapy over antidepressant medications, but only 8% had received such treatment in the past 3 months, and only 1% reported four or more sessions of counseling. Men, African Americans, Latinos, those without two or more prior episodes of depression, and those who preferred counseling to antidepressant medications, reported significantly lower rates of depression care (Unutzer et al., 2003).

Antidepressant use in the elderly

This group of investigators sought to determine whether antidepressant medications were effective compared with placebo in treating depression in older patients. It is known that depression sufficiently severe to warrant treatment is evident in approximately 10% of those over the age of 60. There are data to suggest that mortality among older, depressed people is higher than for comparable

non-depressed populations, and that depression in these more senior age groups differs regarding etiology, presentation, treatment and outcome. Performing a meta-analysis of the available literature to find randomized, placebo-controlled trials with antidepressants in patients described as elderly or geriatric, these investigators compiled data from electronic databases held by the Cochrane Collaboration Depression, Anxiety and Neurosis Review Group (CCDAN), reference lists of related reviews and references of located studies, as well as direct contact with authors working in the field. Seventeen trials contributed data to the analyses comparing the efficacy of antidepressant treatment and placebo including 245 patients treated with TCAs (223 with placebo), 365 patients treated with SSRIs (372 with placebo) and 58 patients treated with monoamine oxidase inhibitors (MAOIs) (63 with placebo). The authors concluded that TCAs, SSRIs and MAOIs are effective in the treatment of older community patients and inpatients when treated for at least 6 weeks with antidepressant compounds. There was little evidence that low dose TCA treatment was effective for depressive symptoms in this elderly population, and they recommended further trials to address this question (Wilson et al., 2001).

Another group studied the efficacy and toxicity of antidepressants in medically ill populations using two Cochrane Registers reporting on 18 studies with data on 838 patients with a range of physical diseases (cancer, diabetes, head injury, heart, HIV, lung, multiple sclerosis, renal, stroke and mixed). This group concluded that patients treated with antidepressants were significantly more likely to improve than those given placebo, and both tricyclics and SSRIs (15 trials) produced a small but significant increase in dropouts from study. Relative to placebo, antidepressants produced no change in cardiovascular function in heart disease, in respiratory function in lung disease, or in vital signs or laboratory tests in cancer with a trend toward tricyclics being more effective than SSRIs, but also more likely to produce dropouts. The authors noted in their discussion and conclusions that there is also a possibility of undetected negative trials which were not included in their database (Gill & Hatcher, 2000).

Depression in schizophrenic patients

The use of antidepressants in patients with schizophrenia is a critically important question because of the high rate of depression among patients diagnosed with schizophrenia. This group sought to determine the clinical effects of antidepressant medication for the treatment of depression in schizophrenic populations using various sources including the Cochrane Schizophrenia Group's Register (October

2000), ClinPsych (1988–2000), The Cochrane Library (Issue 3, 2000), EMBASE (1980–2000) and MEDLINE (1966–2000) supplemented by citation searches, contact with authors and pharmaceutical firms. Although 11 clinical trials that compared antidepressant medication with placebo for depressed schizophrenic or schizoaffective patients met inclusion criteria, all these reports had small numbers of subjects usually reporting depression following the acute psychotic phase using a wide range of antidepressants. For the outcome of "no important clinical response," antidepressants were significantly better than placebo, and there was no evidence that antidepressant treatment led to a deterioration of psychotic symptoms. The authors conclude rather grimly that "the literature was of poor quality, and only a small number of trials made useful contributions. Though our results provide some evidence to indicate that antidepressants may be beneficial for people with depression and schizophrenia, the results, at best, are likely to overestimate the treatment effect, and, at worst, could merely reflect selective reporting of statistically significant results and publication bias. At present, there is no convincing evidence to support or refute the use of antidepressants in treating depression in people with schizophrenia" (Whitehead et al., 2002, p. 10).

Depression and substance abuse disorders

This group of investigators conducted a systematic review and meta-analysis to assess the efficacy of antidepressant medications for the treatment of combined depression and substance use disorders using PubMed, MEDLINE and Cochrane database search (1970–2003). Among inclusion criteria used for study selection were prospective, parallel group, double-blind, controlled clinical trials with random assignment to an antidepressant medication or placebo. Trial patients met standard diagnostic criteria for current alcohol or other drug use and a current unipolar depressive disorder. Forty-four trials were placebo-controlled clinical trials, 14 of which were selected for this analysis and included 848 patients. The principal finding was that antidepressant medications exerted a modest beneficial effect for patients with combined depressive and substance-use disorders. But the use of antidepressants is not a stand-alone treatment, and concurrent therapy directly targeting the addiction is also indicated (Nunes & Levin, 2004).

Efficacy of treatments in psychiatry as compared with other illnesses

A common perception in the media and some branches of the medical profession is that the fact that there are no objective diagnostic tests for psychiatric disorders means that the evidence of treatment efficacy in these disorders is therefore less than in disorders with clearly known and identified etiologies such as cancer, tuberculosis or sickle cell anemia. Psychiatric diagnoses and treatments are hampered by the lack of ability to make a positive tissue diagnosis, as with cancer, or to have a definitive molecule to identify a disease, such as sickle cell anemia, or the ability to use Koch's Postulates to establish the cause of a disease, as with tuberculosis. This notwithstanding, for many psychiatric disorders the value of treatments in improving the disorder and improving quality of life can be very profound. We have already mentioned the Geddes et al. (2003) analysis of the efficacy of antidepressants to reduce relapse with a number needed to treat (NNT) of 3–4 in high-risk cases. Other examples of remarkable value can be given. For instance acamprosate in the treatment of alcohol dependence shows an NNT of around 10, which compares very favourably with figures in other branches of medicine. For instance, the statins, which are used to reduce myocardial infarction in people who have not had a prior infarction, has an NNT of about 30 (Soyka & Chick, 2003).

Another way of estimating the value of a treatment is in terms of quality of life years (QALYs). The cost of achieving a gain of one QALY can be used to compare the cost-efficacy of treatments and is one of the major factors that the UK-based National Institute of Clinical Excellence (NICE) uses to determine if a treatment should be recommended in the NHS. Recently (NICE, 2005) it reported that the use of cholinesterase inhibitors in dementia was not cost-effective and recommended their use not be sanctioned from the public purse. This decision was in part based on the estimate that the cost of gaining one QALY with these drugs was about £40 thousand per year which is a little more than their threshold of value which is thought to be about £35 thousand. In contrast, the NICE review of the use of the stimulant methylphenidate for attention-deficit hyperactivity disorder in children gave a QALY of about one-tenth of that which makes it a remarkably cost-effective treatment (NICE, 2006).

Conclusions

While enormous strides have been made in clinical psychopharmacologic research during the past 50 years, fundamental improvements in methodological and experimental designs are needed. The model used to test compounds for the treatment of psychiatric conditions essentially involves a comparison of the new agent with either an old agent known to be effective, or a placebo agent that is identical in all ways (size, shape, taste, frequency administered, etc.) except that it is an inert substance. This essential comparison of assumed dissimilar agents in people with the same condition, disorder or disease, is the fundamental model applied to determine efficacy. Stories and legends attesting to effective treatments and cures for the many diseases that afflict us, abound. Through the ages, the ability to treat and cure human suffering, especially behavioral, emotional or affective conditions, has been highly regarded and rewarded. Yet psychiatry continues to find it difficult to reproduce or to generalize many of its findings to other settings or other populations.

Unquestionably, the greatest weakness in psychiatric therapeutics and in our study of pharmacologic methods to treat these disease is our lack of an etiology for the diseases we treat, be it tissue, molecule, infectious agent or toxic substance. Allopathic medicine is based on identification of an etiology for a disease, understanding the pathophysiology, and subsequently developing treatments to control, reverse or eliminate the causative agent. Absent the definitive causative agent for the illnesses we treat, psychopharmacology has improved its ability to reliably identify behavioral, affective and cognitive syndromes that can be successfully treated by various compounds. That has led, in an iterative process, to improved nosology and to ever-more scientific, neurobiological hypotheses that help our understanding of the psychiatric illnesses we treat.

The most promising discipline to help us better understand the etiology of psychiatric diseases is likely to be genetics. Studying psychiatric illnesses such as bipolar disorder and unipolar depression, which are known to be highly heritable, using genetic strategies will most likely render sound biological hypotheses for the etiology of these illnesses. With this understanding in hand, we can then apply the classic principles of allopathic medicine to develop treatments and/or medicines to reduce, reverse or eliminate the pathophysiological causes of these crippling psychiatric illnesses.

REFERENCES

Bell, C. J., Hood, S. D. & Nutt, D. J. (2005). Acute tryptophan depletion part 2: Australia and New Zealand. *Journal of Psychiatry*, **39**, 565–74.

Feighner, J. P., Robins, E., Guze, S. B. *et al.* (1972). Diagnostic criteria for use in psychiatric research. *Archives of General Psychiatry*, **26**, 57–63.

Geddes, J., Carney, S., Davies, C. *et al.* (2003). Relapse prevention with antidepressant drug treatment in depressive disorders: a systematic review. *Lancet*, **361**, 653–61.

Gill, D. & Hatcher, S. (2000). Antidepressants for depression in medical illness. *Cochrane Database of Systematic Reviews*, **4**, CD001312. Oxford: Update Software Ltd.

Guaiana, G., Barbui, C. & Hotopf, M. (2003). Amitriptyline versus other types of pharmacotherapy for depression. *Cochrane Database of Systematic Reviews*, **2**, CD004186. Oxford: Update Software Ltd.

Guess, H., Kleinman, A., Kusek, J. & Engel, L. (2002). *The Science of Placebo: Towards an Interdisciplinary Research Agenda*. London: BMJ Books.

Hughes, J. R., Stead, L. F., Lancaster, T. Antidepressants for smoking cessation. *Cochrane Database of Systematic Reviews* 2004, Issue 4. Art. No.: CD000031. DOI: 10.1002/14651858.CD000031.pub2. Oxford: Update Software Ltd.

March, J., Kratochvil, C., Clarke, G. *et al.* (2004). AACAP 2002 research forum: placebo and alternatives to placebo in randomized controlled trials in pediatric psychopharmacology. *Journal of the American Academy of Child and Adolescent Psychiatry*, **43**, 1046–56.

Mulrow, C. D., Williams, J. W. Jr, Trivedi, M. *et al.* (1998). Treatment of depression – newer pharmacotherapies. *Psychopharmacology Bulletin*, **34**, 409–95.

Mulrow, C. D., Williams, J. W. Jr, Chiquette, E. *et al.* (2000). Efficacy of newer medications for treating depression in primary care patients. *American Journal of Medicine*, **108**, 54–64.

NICE (2005) http://www.nice.org.uk/page.aspx?o=appraisals. inprogress.dementianonalzheimer

NICE (2006) Methylphenidate, atomoxetine and dexamfetamine for attention deficit hyperactivity disorder in children and adolescents – guidance. www.nice.org.uk/uk

Nunes, E. V. & Levin, F. R. (2004). Treatment of depression in patients with alcohol or other drug dependence: a meta-analysis. *Journal of the American Medical Association*, **291**, 1887–96.

Nutt, D. J. (2003). Death and dependence: current controversies over the selective serotonin reuptake inhibitors. *Journal of Psychopharmacology*, **17**, 355–64.

Overall, J. E. & Rhoades, H. M. (1982). Refinement of phenomenological classification in clinical psychopharmacology research. *Psychopharmacology (Berlin)*, **77**, 24–30.

Safer, D. J. (2002). Design and reporting modifications in industry-sponsored comparative psychopharmacology trials. *Journal of Nervous and Mental Disease*, **190**, 583–92.

Soyka, M. & Chick, J. (2003). Use of acamprosate and opioid antagonists in the treatment of alcohol dependence: a European perspective. *American Journal of Addiction*, **12**, S69–80.

Unutzer, J., Katon, W., Callahan, C. M. *et al.* (2003). Depression treatment in a sample of 1,801 depressed older adults in primary care. *Journal of the American Geriatric Society*, **51**, 505–14.

Whitehead, C., Moss, S., Cardno, A. & Lewis, G. (2002). Antidepressants for people with both schizophrenia and depression. *Cochrane Database of Systematic Reviews*, **2**, CD002305. Oxford: Update Software Ltd.

Williams, J. W. Jr, Mulrow, C. D., Chiquette, E., Noel, P. H., Aguilar, C. & Cornell, J. (2000). A systematic review of newer pharmacotherapies for depression in adults: evidence report summary. *Annals of Internal Medicine*, **132**, 743–56.

Wilson, K., Mottram, P., Sivanranthan, A. & Nightingale, A. (2001). Antidepressant versus placebo for depressed elderly. *Cochrane Database of Systematic Reviews*, **2**, CD000561. Oxford: Update Software Ltd.

Section I – The efficacy and safety of electroconvulsive therapy

Daniel Maixner and Michael A. Taylor

Editor's note

Electroconvulsive therapy has the longest track record of a successful treatment in psychiatry and it would be unwise to cast it aside. Maixner and Taylor do the opposite. They are enthusiasts for the treatment and feel it is significantly underused. They give most attention to bilateral ECT and in terms of efficacy there is no doubt that this is more effective than unilateral treatment despite the advantages unilateral treatment has for likely cognitive disturbance. For more severe forms of depression bilateral ECT has definite advantages and it is in this group, both in general and old age psychiatry, that it is most widely recommended. Other disorders, apart from catatonia and neuroleptic malignant syndrome, have a much lower evidence base for treatment. Electroconvulsive treatment in the future is likely to come under threat from other newer physical treatments involving magnetic manipulations (see Chapter 4, Part II) and many more comparisons are needed between ECT and these new treatments to determine the therapeutic place of each. This chapter does not have a UK author; the differences between UK and Europe and the USA are not great, but a comparison can be made by reading.

Introduction

Electroconvulsive therapy (ECT) is the oldest continuous medical treatment for psychiatric disease. When introduced in 1938 it achieved remissions that were considered miraculous in patients who had been ill in mental hospitals for years (Endler, 1988). (Also see pp. 27–31.) As with all successful treatments it was eventually used beyond its understood indications. Until the mid-1950s it was administered without anesthesia, muscle relaxation, maintenance of 100% blood oxygen saturation and monitoring

of vital signs and electroencephalogram (EEG). These modifications were made to diminish patient discomfort and side effects. They were not introduced to enhance efficacy. Through the 1940s it was given to patients who also received multiple insulin comas and prefrontal lobotomies – two discarded procedures that adversely affect brain function, including memory. Public opinion lumped the three procedures, and concluded none was appropriate (Frankel, 1973). Electroconvulsive therapy's early overuse, side effects from unmodified and sometimes prolonged seizures, and association with substandard large state hospital systems where patients were often mistreated led to negative images of ECT that were intensified by films like *The Snake Pit*. The public perception of ECT has been further eroded by a few anti-ECT proselytizers (Breggin, 1991; Boodman, 1996), a vocal anti-psychiatry movement that ranges from opposition to all medical psychiatric treatments to the view that psychiatric illness is not disease but societal stigmatization (see www.cchr.com) and an entertainment industry that dramatizes ECT as a punitive attack on patients, as in the film *One Flew Over the Cuckoo's Nest*.

The public perception of ECT, however, differs substantially from professional opinion. Major psychiatric associations world-wide recognize the efficacy and safety of ECT (Freeman, 2000; APA, 2001; AETMIS, 2002). Indeed, since the 1980s, ECT usage has increased in response to the growing number of patients not adequately responding to antidepressant drugs. It is estimated that 100 000 patients in the USA and 20 000 in the UK receive ECT annually (Hermann *et al.*, 1995; Department of Health, 1999). Its usage in Europe varies widely across regions (Lauter & Sauer, 1987). Availability of ECT, however, remains below estimated need (Hermann *et al.*, 1995). Surveys also find that most patients that receive ECT in the USA meet practice guidelines for diagnosis and indications (Hermann *et al.*, 1998). Electroconvulsive therapy in the USA is not overused or misused. It is underused.

For a treatment that is almost 70 years old, the ECT literature, however, is relatively small. For example, the PubMed term "electroconvulsive therapy" yields fewer than 7000 citations, whereas the term "melancholia" generates over 43 000 references. In addition, the drug trial model of comparing active and placebo treatments has been long discarded in addressing ECT efficacy for ethical reasons because ECT is considered to have a powerful antidepressant effect while simulated-ECT has no benefit but its anesthesia risks remain. Thus, there are only a handful of controlled studies with randomized patient assignment and ECT versus placebo-ECT. However, these trials are supported by many clinical series and case reports (APA, 2001). Head-to-head studies comparing ECT with medication are also old, and mostly present small samples. However, ECT efficacy in these studies is consistently found to be superior for the treatment of depression and equivalent to drugs for acute mania, so that comparisons of acute treatment effects are no longer felt appropriate and the focus has shifted to continuation treatment (The UK ECT Review Group & Geddes, 2003).

Recent research has also stressed technical rather than clinical issues so that there are only a few assessments of present practice. These investigations indicate the response rates are less in community settings than in clinical trials conducted at university medical centers. Willingness to treat a greater diversity of patients and not fully employing optimal technical conditions account for much of the variance in practice (Prudic *et al.*, 2004). In addition, over the last 25 years the taxonomy of depression has changed so that "major depression," the most common diagnostic indication for ECT, has become an overly broad and heterogeneous classification category, making comparisons of studies from different eras more difficult (see Taylor & Fink, 2006). Nevertheless, despite the above literature limitations, the efficacy and safety findings for ECT are remarkably consistent.

In this chapter we review the evidence that supports the profession's recognition of the value of ECT. We discuss the efficacy of ECT for its main indications and in special patient populations. We review the safety of ECT and its acute and long-term effects on brain function. We also address technical issues that relate to efficacy and side effects, such as electrode placement, electrical wave form parameters, and clinical and EEG predictors of response. We review the procedures of ECT administration that appear to achieve the best therapeutic effect while maintaining safety. The efficacy and safety of proposed adjuncts and substitutes for ECT (vagal nerve and deep brain stimulation, transcranial magnetic and seizure stimulation) are not discussed here, except where a direct comparison to ECT is made (also see Chapter 4).

Efficacy in mood disorders

Major depression

Randomized controlled studies

Historically, real versus sham ECT studies demonstrate superiority for real ECT (Taylor, 1982). These studies vary in design, clinical outcome measures, and definition of depression making detailed interpretation difficult. Since the mid 1970s there have been only a few randomized studies with a placebo/sham arm in which participants are administered anesthesia without electrical stimulation.

Freeman *et al.* (1978) studied 40 patients who received either simulated ECT for their first two sessions followed by a continued course of bilateral ECT, or a full course of bilateral ECT. Patients receiving real ECT throughout their course demonstrated significantly lower scores on the Hamilton Rating Scale of Depression (HRS-D) after two sessions and ultimately had a lower number of treatments. Lambourn & Gill (1978) randomized 32 patients to receive either six real ECT or six sham sessions. Low dose right unilateral ECT was used in the active arm. The HRS-D ratings failed to show a significant difference between the two groups at the end of the six sessions. However, low-energy unilateral ECT is not considered effective for most patients (Sackeim *et al.*, 1987). The Northwick Park ECT trial (Johnstone *et al.*, 1980) studied 70 patients who received eight real or eight sham ECT sessions over 4 weeks; HRS-D ratings were used to assess outcome. At the end of 4 weeks, improvement was greater in the patients who received real ECT. In a smaller study, West (1981) randomized 22 patients to either six real or sham ECT over a 3-week period. After six sessions, patients were allowed to cross over to the alternate treatment if clinically indicated. Patients receiving real ECT showed significant improvement on three measures including physician, nursing and Beck Rating Scale scores and 10 of 11 of the sham ECT patients switched to real ECT while none of the patients receiving real ECT switched to the sham treatment.

The Leicestershire trial (Brandon *et al.*, 1984) is the largest of the randomized trials and included 95 subjects who received eight real or eight sham ECTs given twice weekly; HRS-D scores showed significantly greater improvement for the group receiving real ECT. The Nottingham ECT study (Gregory *et al.*, 1985) randomized 60 depressed patients to receive right unilateral, bilateral or sham ECT.

Both active treatment groups showed greater improvement as measured by depression rating scales than the group receiving sham ECT.

Although in these studies sample sizes were small, the sham groups experienced some improvement, study designs differed (varied number of ECT administered or cross-over strategies), and outcome measures varied, all but one study reports the superiority of real ECT over sham ECT. The study showing no significant difference in depression ratings between groups, Lambourn & Gill (1978), used low dose unilateral ECT and a short course of only six treatments. Both are factors that are known to adversely influence outcome.

Other recent studies

A three-site study examining relapse rates among ECT remitters who were given two different antidepressant regimens or placebo post ECT had 290 subjects complete an acute bilateral or right unilateral ECT course. Fifty-five percent of these subjects met the definition of remission with at least a 60% reduction in HRS-D scores and a total HRS-D of ≤ 10 (Sackeim et al., 2001). In another large multi-site trial designed to study maintenance medications versus maintenance ECT, the acute outcome data of 253 subjects were examined prior to randomization to maintenance treatments. Bitemporal electrode placement was used. Seventy-nine percent of patients obtained an improvement of sustained response defined as 50% reduction in HRS-D-24 item scores, and 75% of patients achieved remission defined as a HRS-D-24 item score of ≤ 10 (Husain et al., 2004).

Psychotic depression

Most patients with psychotic depression do not receive adequate pharmacotherapy (Mulsant et al., 1997), and those that do have a poor response to antipsychotic medications or antidepressants alone (Chan et al., 1987; Parker et al., 1992). Depression with delusions, however, predicts a good response to ECT (Hickie et al., 1996). In a review of a large 1964 study by DeCarolis, Avery & Lubrano (1979) identified 181 of 437 subjects as having psychotic depression. Only 40% responded to imipramine, while 83% (91/109) of the antidepressant non-responders were successfully treated with ECT. Buchan et al. (1992) combined data from the Northwick Park and Leicester controlled trials of ECT and reported significantly improved outcomes in HRS-D measures in those subjects with psychomotor retardation and delusions who received real ECT versus the sham ECT.

Recent studies also confirm the excellent response of psychotic depression to ECT. In a retrospective study of 55 depressed patients (26 delusional and 29 non-delusional) receiving right unilateral or bilateral ECT, Birkenhager et al. (2003) reported greater rates of response (50% reduction on HRS-D scores) and remission (score of < 7 on HRS-D ratings) for those with delusional depression. In the large prospective CORE (Consortium for Research in ECT) study of continuation ECT, Petrides et al. (2001) reported on the acute outcomes of psychotic depressed patients (n = 67) versus non-psychotic patients (n = 153). All subjects received bilateral ECT at 1.5 times seizure threshold. Remission was defined as a score of < 10 on the 24-item HRS-D. The entire sample had a remission rate of 87%, and the psychotic depressed patients had a remission rate of 96% (64/67), and with faster response.

Psychotic depression is a condition that is associated with a high risk of suicide. Loss of appetite coupled with severe weight loss or the development of catatonia can be life threatening. Electroconvulsive therapy has a profound and rapid effect for these patients and is a first-line treatment for these patients.

Effect on suicide risk

Suicide rates in patients with mood disorder are estimated at 4–20% and 50–70% of persons who kill themselves do so when depressed (Conwell et al., 2002; Bostwick & Pankratz, 2000). Antidepressant drugs have minimal or no acute effect on these rates, but may lower rates in the long term by reducing the frequency of recurrences (Khan et al., 2000; Baldessarini, 2001; Hall et al., 2003). Lithium, however, has a substantial and direct long-term effect on lowering rates whereas other mood stabilizers do not (Tondo et al., 1998; Baldessarini & Tondo, 2003). Although the literature is based primarily on case series, the effect of ECT on long-term rates is unclear, but likely minimal, whereas its effect in the short run (over the course of the episode and the next 6 months) is substantial. This effect is particularly striking as ECT patients are severely ill and often suicidal.

In a naturalistic study, Avery & Winokur (1978) examined the 6 months post-depression of 519 patients and found that 0.8% of ECT patients and 4–7% of patients treated with medication made a subsequent suicide attempt during this very high-risk period. Tsuang et al. (1979) reported a similar finding for patients identified as "schizoaffective." Tanney (1986) reviewed studies comparing ECT and tricyclic antidepressant drug use in different decades, and reported suicide frequency to be lower in the decades when ECT was the predominant treatment. A study of 1397 suicides in a 12-month period in Helsinki found that only two patients who had received ECT subsequently committed suicide, and in both cases the ECT was deemed inadequate and the suicides 3 months post last treatment (Isometsa *et al.*, 1996).

In contrast, in a naturalistic study, Roy & Draper (1995) could not find a difference in suicide rates between patients receiving or not receiving ECT. Sharma (1999) examined hospital records from 1969–1995 and identified 45 inpatients who had killed themselves. He compared them with a matched group of 45 inpatients who did not kill themselves, and reported no between-group difference in the use of ECT. The ECT, however, was not described, although electrode placement was variable and other parameters unknown. Recognizing these and other limitations of the study, Sharma (2001) reviewed the literature and reached the different conclusion that ECT has a short-term, but not a long-term, effect on reducing suicide rates in depressed patients. Bradvik & Berglund (2000) confirmed this conclusion in their study of the records of severely depressed patients, 89 of whom had killed themselves and 89 who had not. No between-group differences were found for acute treatment ECT use or antidepressant drug prescription. However, none of the patients who committed suicide during the 6 months post acute treatment had received any continuation treatment, and these outcomes suggested that suicide following relapse was likely. Prudic & Sackeim (1999) examined changes in suicidality as measured by the HRS-D in 148 patients who received ECT. Suicide and mortality rates were reduced. They also reviewed the literature and concluded that ECT has a substantial acute effect, particularly as patients that receive ECT are usually at the highest risk.

The most recent report comes from the CORE multicenter study of ECT. They report the effect of ECT in 131 patients who received ECT and had a pre-treatment HRS-D suicide score of 3 or the maximum score of 4. Scores decreased to zero after 1 week in 38.2% of patients, after 2 weeks (six ECT) in 61.1% of patients and in 80.9% at the end of the course of treatment. A total of 444 severely depressed patients were treated and of these two committed suicide after hospital discharge following their course of ECT and while waiting for assignment to continuation treatment (Kellner *et al.*, 2005).

The risk of suicide is high in patients with mood disorders. When that risk warrants hospitalization, medications have likely failed to elicit relief, and ECT becomes the treatment of choice as the only intervention that has demonstrated direct efficacy in reducing acute risk.

Acute mania

There are three prospective studies of ECT in the treatment of acute mania. None compare real ECT with sham ECT alone. Medications were used in comparison to ECT or in combination with real or sham ECT study arms. Despite the small sample sizes in the prospective studies, ECT was found to have significant benefit in treating patients in acute mania.

Small *et al.* (1988) studied 34 acutely manic patients who received either ECT or lithium treatment. Antipsychotic agents were used as needed in both groups. Electroconvulsive therapy patients received on average nine bilateral treatments. Raters unaware of the treatments received observed greater reductions in mania symptoms during the initial 8 weeks of monitoring for both treatment groups. At the end of the study period all of the 17 ECT patients were rated as in remission or only mildly ill.

Mukherjee *et al.* (1988, 1994) investigated whether left unilateral, right unilateral or bilateral ECT were superior to a combination of haloperidol and lithium in the treatment of acute mania. Twenty-two manic patients received ECT and 13 met stringent criteria for response and maintenance of remission 1 week after ECT treatments. None of the five who received pharmacotherapy alone were deemed responders. Sikdar (1994) randomized 30 manic patients to either eight ECT sessions or eight sham sessions. Both groups received 600 mg of chlorpromazine until the sixth session. The ECT-medication combination group responded significantly better than the medication only group. In a review of ECT in mania including prospective and retrospective studies from 1942 to 1994, Mukherjee *et al.* (1994) concluded that remission or marked clinical improvement was reported in 80% (470 of 589) of manic patients. Although large randomized trials are lacking, the ECT literature for mania consistently finds that ECT is effective in the treatment of acute mania. When the mania cannot be controlled by medication, or the risk of medication use is high, ECT is a reasoned treatment.

Catatonia/neuroleptic malignant syndrome (NMS)

Catatonia is a syndrome characterized by motor dysregulation that can result in prolonged posturing, stereotypy, mutism and other speech abnormalities, and stimulus bound motor responses (echolalia, echopraxia, Gegenhalten, automatic obedience). Stupor may be present. Catatonia is the clinical expression of many conditions, the most common being mood disorder (Fink & Taylor, 2003). The first patient in modern times to receive convulsive therapy was catatonic and he was successfully treated in 1934 with intramuscular camphor-in-oil (Fink, 1984). The first patient to receive ECT was a manic patient with catatonic features who was successfully treated in 1938 (Fink, 1979). Systematic assessments of acutely hospitalized adult psychiatric patients find 8–14% of samples exhibiting two or more catatonic features for 24 hours or longer (Fink & Taylor, 2003).

There are no double-blind, randomized controlled studies of ECT in the treatment of catatonia. Hawkins *et al.* (1995), however, reviewed the treatments for catatonia, commenting on 178 patients in 270 episodes. Benzodiazepines alone achieved a resolution in symptoms in 70% of patients. Lorazepam alone elicited a 76% remission rate in the dose ranges of 8–24 mg. Electroconvulsive therapy was used alone in 55 cases and 85% remitted. Of the 40 patients treated with an antipsychotic alone, 7.5% remitted. Case reports also describe ECT to be effective for catatonics not responding to benzodiazepines or sedatives (Petrides *et al.*, 2004). Suzuki *et al.* (2003) report nine catatonic patients age 45 or older who were intractable to medications but who then responded to ECT. Takaoka & Takata (2003) found ECT to be of benefit in their review of children and teens who were catatonic.

Malignant catatonia is a life-threatening condition characterized by severe catalepsy with rigidity, fever, autonomic instability and delirium. Creatinine phosphokinase levels can be markedly elevated while serum iron levels are commonly low. First described in the nineteenth century, 50–100% of patients died before the advent of modern life-supporting measures and ECT (Mann *et al.*, 1986, 1990). The similarity of malignant catatonia to neuroleptic malignant syndrome has led to a growing consensus that the two descriptors represent the same syndrome (Fink & Taylor, 2003; Mann *et al.*, 2004). For example, it is difficult to distinguish the two conditions on clinical features or laboratory tests. Both respond to benzodiazepines and to ECT. Neuroleptic malignant syndrome can be considered to be the drug-induced version of malignant catatonia, and there are other drugs that can induce it. Delirious mania and many oneroid states, which are dream-like and semistuporous, such as in Ganser's syndrome, are other forms of catatonia.

An early report claimed that bilateral ECT one to three times daily relieved malignant catatonia in 15 of 18 patients treated by day 3 of onset. Of 16 patients treated after day 5 of onset only one survived (Arnold & Stepan, 1952). Mann *et al.* (1986, 1990) identified 292 published cases of malignant catatonia/NMS with an overall mortality rate of 60%. Of 41 patients who received ECT 40 survived. Davis *et al.* (1991) reported 29 patients with NMS who received ECT. Three died. However, antipsychotic drugs were continued in these patients and ECT had been delayed. Philbrick & Rummans (1994) identified another 18 cases. Of the 13 who received ECT, 11 recovered and two died. Trollor & Sachdev (1999) examined 55 published cases identified as having NMS and who received ECT. Forty patients responded (73%), and of these 25 (63%) remitted and 11 (28%) had a partial recovery.

Continuation ECT in mood disorders

Electroconvulsive therapy is usually discontinued after successful treatment of the acute episode and maintenance pharmacotherapy prescribed. However, Sackeim *et al.* (2001) note that naturalistic studies indicate pharmacotherapy initiated after the acute (index) ECT course results in relapse rates of 50% or greater within 6–12 months. Patients who fail pharmacotherapy prior to beginning index ECT relapse more rapidly, despite medication treatment (Petrides *et al.*, 1994). Continuation (the next 6 months) or maintenance (after 6 months) ECT beyond the index episode is considered a means to maintain remission and prevent these high relapse rates (Monroe, 1991; Grunhaus *et al.* 1995). Continued ECT treatments are typically prescribed in a taper from weekly to monthly intervals over a few months to one year.

The use of continuation ECT has been described in the literature for over a half-century for various psychiatric conditions (Geoghegan & Stevenson, 1949; Bourne, 1954; Karliner & Wehrheim, 1965). For mood disorders, good outcomes are reported with continuation ECT (C-ECT). Clarke *et al.* (1989) in a naturalistic study design of 27 bipolar or unipolar depressed patients receiving monthly C-ECT reported that at 5 months those who continued treatment were at a significantly reduced risk of re-hospitalization. Vanelle *et al.* (1994) studied 22 patients with refractory mood disorders (unipolar and bipolar disorders) who received C-ECT for 18 months or longer. Before the C-ECT, these resistant patients spent 44% of the year in the hospital. During the C-ECT period, patients spent only 7% of the year in the hospital. Schwarz *et al.* (1995) compared a group of 21 C-ECT patients with similarly matched controls who were either treated with index ECT combined with maintenance pharmacotherapy, or treated with initial and maintenance pharmacotherapy alone. They noted that the C-ECT patients had more medication trials and hospitalizations and were more treatment resistant. Although the C-ECT patients did not differ significantly from the comparison group in rate of relapse, the rate of re-hospitalization was reduced by 67%. Petrides *et al.* (1994) studied retrospectively 21 patients who received an average of 33 treatments of C-ECT (approximately one treatment every 10 days for 10 weeks) and noted that 66% of patients did not require re-hospitalization during the one year post C-ECT. Gagne *et al.* (2000) conducted a retrospective chart review, identifying 29 depressed patients who responded to index

ECT and who received C-ECT, and they compared them with a matched group of 29 depressed patients who did not receive C-ECT. They found the probability of surviving without relapse or recurrence was 93% for the C-ECT patients and 52% for the medication-treated patients. Finally, numerous other smaller studies and case reports and series highlight that C-ECT can assist in providing sustained benefits in the treatment of manic or depressive symptoms (Decina *et al.*, 1987; Duncan *et al.*, 1990; Grunhaus *et al.*, 1990; Thienhaus *et al.*, 1990; Thornton *et al.*, 1990; Loo *et al.*, 1991; Husain *et al.*, 1993; Kramer, 1999; Fox, 2001; Kho, 2002; Vaidya *et al.*, 2003; Tsao *et al.*, 2004).

More systematic study of continuation ECT is needed, and data from the four-center Consortium for Research in ECT (CORE) are emerging. Patients who had successfully completed an index ECT course (n = 184) were assigned to continuation ECT (n = 89) or pharmacotherapy with nortriptyline and lithium (n = 95). Patients were followed for 6 months and relapse rates were tracked. Preliminary results suggest that patients who received continuation ECT sustained similar remission rates to those who received the maintenance medication combination of a tricyclic antidepressant and lithium. A significant limitation of this study includes a rigid continuation ECT taper over 6 months (Fink, personal communication) rather than the more flexible scheduling used in clinical practice.

Predictors of ECT response in mood disorders

Duration of illness and resistance to medication
A number of studies have shown that patients with longer durations of continuous depressive illness are less likely to respond to ECT (Kukopulos *et al.*, 1977; Dunn & Quinlan, 1978; Magni *et al.*, 1988). Black *et al.* (1989) studied 1087 unipolar depressed patients who were treated with ECT, medications, or treated with therapies other than ECT or medications. They found that ECT elicited significantly better recovery except when the depressive illness lasted > 2 years. In a smaller study, Kindler *et al.* (1991) reviewed the records of 52 patients receiving bilateral ECT. The non-responders had a longer duration of illness and greater severity of symptoms.

Another factor that may impact response to ECT is medication resistance. Prudic *et al.* (1990) studied 53 patients with depression receiving various ECT stimulation dosing strategies and electrode placements (bilateral and unilateral). Two clinicians then rated the adequacy of medication trials. Patients were placed in either adequate treatment group (n = 24) indicating resistance or inadequate treatment group (n = 29). Despite the various forms of ECT used, the total sample showed a response rate of 57% with a stringent remission definition of a HRS-D score of < 9. The adequately treated group (resistant) showed a 42% response rate versus a 69% response for the inadequate treatment group. In a larger multi-site trial, Prudic *et al.* (1996) evaluated medication resistance and ECT response in 100 subjects with unipolar, non-psychotic depression. The Antidepressant Treatment History Form (ATHF) was used to assess duration, dose, compliance and outcome of medications used during and prior to ECT. Patients who were rated as having at least one adequate medication trial were classified as resistant (n = 65). The other subjects were rated as having inadequate treatment trials (n = 35). Response was defined as 60% reduction in HRS-D scores and HRS-D maximum score of 10. The resistant depressed patients had a response rate of 63% compared with 91% of the inadequate medication treatment group. In a more recent study, Dombrovski *et al.* (2005) reviewed the predictors of non-remission (remission defined as HRS-D < 10) in 328 patients treated with ECT. Medication resistance and chronicity of depression again were associated with lower remission rates. Overall, these findings suggest that ECT can still provide significant benefit for patients who are resistant to medication, but the degree of response may be less than in depressed patients who are not considered to have such resistance.

Laboratory and ECT-related EEG parameters
Post-ictal suppression and ictal amplitude, two main features of EEG changes from ECT treatment, have been suggested as being associated with ECT efficacy. Post-ictal suppression refers to the acute fall in EEG amplitude immediately after the ECT-induced seizure terminates. Nobler *et al.* (1993) using a visual rating scale of EEGs first reported that low-dose right unilateral ECT was least likely to elicit EEG suppression compared with high-dose bilateral ECT. In their earlier studies, low-dose unilateral ECT was associated with poor antidepressant effects compared with bilateral ECT, offering the conclusion that EEG suppression may be a useful marker of treatment efficacy. Krystal *et al.* (1995) reported similar preliminary evidence of a relationship between post-ictal suppression and outcome in a study of low-dose unilateral versus moderately suprathreshold right unilateral ECT. Nobler *et al.* (2000) in a larger study of 62 patients, used quantitative EEG analysis of ECT-induced seizures and found a significant association between post-ictal suppression and outcome, although they comment that the effect was small. In another study using quantitative EEG assessments, Perera *et al.* (2004) report similar findings with post-ictal suppression being modestly associated with outcome. Finally,

Suppes et al. (1996) studied 33 patients receiving ECT in a university setting and manually rated post-ictal suppression. They found a significant association between degree of suppression and likelihood of clinical improvement.

Ictal EEG amplitude or power is measured as voltage and is felt to be related to seizure strength or intensity. In two separate studies, Folkerts (1996) and Hrdlicka et al. (1996) visually rated EEG manifestations of ECT-induced seizures and reported higher amplitude associated with greater improvement. Many studies previously cited for post-ictal suppression also highlight a correlation between clinical outcome and EEG intensity (Krystal et al., 1995; Nobler et al., 1993, 2000; Perera et al., 2004).

Some authors question the current utility of these findings in developing treatment algorithms based on EEG findings because of the reported modest effect size (Perera et al., 2004; Nobler et al., 2000). However, it is possible that these markers may have clinical importance, and visual observations of these parameters during ECT may provide early detection of responders, and suggest strategies of electrical dosing that maximize efficacy. Future study is needed of these and other EEG variables (e.g. inter-treatment slowing and interhemisphere seizure coherence).

Electrode placement
The sole reason for the development of alternatives to the bi-frontotemporal electrode placement (BL-ECT) was to reduce ECT-related cognitive changes while maintaining efficacy. Although there have been many recommendations, the right unilateral d'Elia temporal-vertex positioning (RUL-ECT) is the standard alternative to BL-ECT (d' Elia, 1970). A left frontal, right temporal electrode placement, or LART, is also in some use, but there are no systematic studies of it (Swartz, 1994). Direct comparison systematic studies repeatedly find that when controlling for current parameters, RUL-ECT is associated with somewhat less anterograde and clearly less retrograde amnesia than observed with BL-ECT. Subjective retrograde memory complaints are also less following RUL-ECT (Squire & Slater, 1983; Rosenberg & Pettinati, 1984; Sackeim et al., 1987, 2000; Sobin et al., 1995; Sackeim et al., Lisanby et al., 2000).

Sackeim et al.'s study (2000) brings this literature into focus. They examined the cognitive effects of brief-pulse, RUL-ECT at three dosage levels: 1.5, 2.5 and 6 times seizure threshold estimated by titration. A comparison group receiving high dose BL-ECT did worse on a retrograde verbal memory task than the lowest dose RUL-ECT, but about the same as patients receiving the other UL-ECT doses. There were no significant differences across groups on other cognitive tests. Relief of depression, however, was only equivalent when BL-ECT was compared with high-dose UL-ECT. Thus, the only cognitive advantage to UL-ECT was at a dose that was not as effective as BL-ECT.

In the modern era of ECT post 1980, researchers began to discern that all seizures are not created equal with respect to different electrode placements and outcome. Sackeim et al. (1987) in studying 52 patients discovered that an electrical stimulus dose at barely threshold levels for RUL-ECT could generate a 20–25 second seizure but with a poorer response rate versus BL-ECT. A follow-up study (Sackeim et al., 1993) randomized 96 patients with depression into four treatment arms: low-dose (RUL-ECT 1 × threshold or BL-ECT 1 × threshold) or high dose (RUL-ECT 2.5 × threshold or BL-ECT 2.5 × threshold). Response was defined as a 60% reduction in HRS-D scores. The response rates were 17% for low-dose RUL-ECT, 43% for high-dose RUL-ECT, 65% for low-dose BL-ECT and 63% for high-dose BL-ECT. Because the response of high-dose RUL-ECT lagged behind BL-ECT, a third study was designed with even an higher RUL-ECT dosing strategy included. Sackeim et al. (2000) randomized 80 patients with depression into four electrical stimulation dosings: 1.5 × threshold RUL-ECT, 2.5 × threshold RUL-ECT, 2.5 × threshold BL-ECT, or 6 × threshold RUL-ECT. Response rates were 65% for the BL-ECT and highest dose RUL-ECT while the lowest and moderate dosed RUL-ECT showed response rates of 35% and 30% respectively. In another study of high-dose RUL-ECT, McCall et al. (2000) randomized depressed patients to titrated moderate-dose (2.25 times threshold RUL-ECT) or fixed high-dose (70% of the maximum ECT device output). They reported a 67% response rate for fixed high-dose RUL-ECT versus 39% response rate for moderate-dose RUL-ECT (response defined as 60% reduction in the 21-item HRS-D). As a group, the low-dose RUL-ECT response rates are similar to placebo rates observed in clinical antidepressant drug trials (Taylor & Fink, 2006, Chapters 9 and 10).

Some experts feel that to conclude that RUL-ECT at very high suprathreshold dosages is equivalent to BL-ECT is erroneous because of the small sample sizes used in comparing the different modalities, and because the evidence for efficacy for RUL-ECT with other psychiatric disorders such as schizophrenia and mania is lacking. They also caution that in the USA the electrical output of ECT devices is limited by the FDA, precluding most patients from receiving the ultra high RUL-ECT doses that are now considered effective (Fink et al., 2001; Taylor, 2001).

Hypothalamic-pituitary axes functioning and the dexamethasone suppression test
Neuroendocrine function is perturbed in melancholia and psychotic depression, and these, and other severe depressions, reflect an abnormal stress-response state

(Sapolsky, 2000; Holsboer, 2001; Heim & Nemeroff, 2001). Some antidepressant medications and ECT resolve these abnormalities in the stress-response system (Lopez *et al.*, 1998; Serra *et al.*, 2002), and these abnormalities have been investigated as possible predictors of outcome for treatments of depression.

The dexamethasone suppression test (DST) is used to assess neuroendocrine function and has been applied to identify patients with endogenous depression or melancholia with 50–75% of patients being non-suppressors (Fink, 1986). The DST is reported to normalize over a course of ECT (Albala *et al.* 1981). Coryell (1982) studied 42 depressed patients who were grouped as either non-suppressors or normal suppressors to the DST. Patients with abnormal DSTs (non-suppression) showed better results on global ratings but did not differ in change on HRS-D ratings. Katona *et al.* (1987) attempted and failed to predict outcome with the DST in 26 depressed ECT patients, while others (Grunhaus *et al.*, 1987) studying 22 depressed patients with weekly DSTs and HRS-D assessments noted that most patients had a "normalization" of the DST, with moderately high correlations between DST and HRS-D assessments. Others have had less success in showing a positive correlation of DST findings and response to ECT (Coppen *et al.*, 1985; Lipman *et al.*, 1986; Devanand *et al.*, 1987). However, in a review of the literature of ECT and depression relapse, Bourgon & Kellner (2000) noted six of nine studies of the DST and one study of cortisol hypersecretion showing that post-ECT DST non-suppressors were at higher risk of relapse. Thus, although the response to the DST does not predict ECT response, abnormalities of the HPA axis after successful ECT may assist in prediction of relapse of the depression.

Direct comparisons with other treatments

ECT versus medication
Most studies comparing ECT with medication treatments for depression date from the early 1960s to the 1980s. During this period, 18 studies were reported (UK ECT Review Group & Geddes, 2003). They vary widely in design, subject inclusion criteria, ECT delivery and scheduling methods, and concomitant medication prescription and dosages. The comparisons include tricyclic antidepressants, monoamine oxidase inhibitors and tryptophan. The reports found ECT to be superior to all three agents in relieving depressive illness. The references for these trials can be found at http://image.thelancet.com/extras/02art8375webtable2.pdf.

Dinan & Barry (1989) randomized 30 medication-resistant patients with depressive illness to either six ECT treatments over 3 weeks or to lithium augmentation of a tricyclic antidepressant. Over the study period 21 of 30 patients significantly improved but no significant difference in response was noted between the ECT and the dual medication groups. Folkerts *et al.* (1997) randomized 39 participants resistant to two or more medication trials to either moderately suprathreshold (2.5 × ST) right unilateral ECT or a titration of paroxetine (dose range 20–50 mg). Response was defined as 50% reduction in HRS-D scores. In the ECT group, 71% (n = 21) met the response criteria while in the paroxetine group (n = 18) 28% responded. The authors concluded that ECT produced a greater and faster response compared with paroxetine in medication-resistant depressed patients. Evaluating the benefits of a rhythmic hyperventilation type of yoga for melancholic depression, Janakiramaiah *et al.* (2000) randomized 45 subjects to bilateral ECT, imipramine or yoga. Remission was defined as HRS-D score of 7 or less. Remission rates were 93% for ECT (n = 15), 73% for imipramine (n = 15) and 67% for yoga (n = 15). Further details from this study are not available. However, it is difficult to reconcile the substantial remission rates with all treatment modalities in the same depressed patient sample. There was no identified placebo group, but there is no other support for yoga in the treatment of severe depression making it likely that its use was equivalent to placebo. From that perspective, the diagnostic validity of the sample is questionable as most would then be considered placebo responders.

Despite earlier ECT versus medication trials having several methodologic limitations (Rifkin, 1988), recent meta-analyses evaluating the evidence for ECT in the treatment of depression conclude that ECT is more effective than medications. The UK ECT Review Group & Geddes (2003) report "treatment with ECT was significantly more effective than pharmacotherapy." Pagnin *et al.* (2004) also concluded that the randomized controlled trials revealed a significant superiority for ECT versus antidepressants.

Electroconvulsive therapy versus transcranial magnetic stimulation (also see Chapter 4)
Transcranial magnetic stimulation (TMS) was first introduced in 1985 as a non-invasive method of stimulating the brain (Barker *et al.*, 1985). It directs a magnetic field into the cortex inducing electrical activation of neurons. Since the mid 1990s many reports using TMS to stimulate the left prefrontal cortex have suggested antidepressant effects of TMS (Conca *et al.*, 1996; Pascual-Leone *et al.*, 1996; George *et al.*, 1997; Figiel *et al.* 1998). Researchers have considered TMS a potential non-convulsive option for the treatment of depression (George & Wasserman, 1994; Zyss *et al.*, 1997). Meta-analyses of this literature

mostly reach the conclusion that the antidepressant effects of TMS are marginal and no better than placebo for patients with severe depressive illness, and that larger better designed randomized trials are required (Burt *et al.*, 2002; Martin *et al.*, 2003; Couturier, 2005). Nevertheless, TMS has been compared to ECT.

Comparison studies between TMS and ECT mostly employ RUL-ECT at or modestly above seizure threshold which is a weak form of the treatment (Sackeim *et al.*, 2000). The proper comparison is with BL-ECT. Grunhaus *et al.* (2000) conducted an open trial with 40 depressed patients referred for ECT. Patients were randomized to either RUL-ECT twice weekly (with the potential to switch to BL-ECT if inadequately responding) or TMS treatments five times weekly for 4 weeks. Nineteen patients had psychotic depression. Using the HRS-D, Grunhaus reports that the non-psychotic depressed patients responded similarly to both treatment modalities, but for the psychotic depressed patients ECT provided response in all ten subjects versus only two of nine subjects in the TMS group. In a follow-up study, Grunhaus *et al.* (2003) randomized 40 patients with non-psychotic depression to either five times weekly TMS or twice weekly RUL-ECT. The overall response rate, defined as a 50% reduction in HRS-D and HRS-D < 10, was 58 % in both groups (12/20 ECT group and 11/20 TMS group). The authors concluded that ECT and TMS provide similar results in non-psychotic depression. In another study comparing ECT with TMS with unlimited number of treatment sessions, Pridmore *et al.* (2000) reported that the remission rates or HRS-D-17 item score of < 8 were the same for TMS and RUL-ECT. These studies, however, do not provide adequate comparisons.

Janicak *et al.* (2002) conducted a trial of 22 patients with depressive illness referred for ECT. Thirteen received TMS and nine received BL-ECT. Patients were treated from 2–4 weeks depending upon response, defined as a HRS-D improvement of 50% and final score < 8. The authors reported a response rate of 46% (6/13) for TMS and 56% (5/9) for the ECT group and concluded that TMS and ECT produced comparable therapeutic effects in severely depressed patients. In contrast, others (Kellner *et al.*, 2002) argue that the small sample size and unequal cohorts are inadequate to draw this conclusion.

The efficacy of ECT in psychotic disorders

Schizophrenia

Few controlled studies compare ECT to sham treatment in patients with schizophrenia. Methodological issues and diagnostic concerns are prominent in many of the older studies. The administration of ECT and the procedures to assess outcome varied during that era. The duration of psychotic illness was also not appreciated as a possible confound. Patients with mood disorder symptoms were not excluded and the classification of schizophrenia was not as specific as it is today. In the few well-designed sham, controlled trials conducted primarily in patients with chronic schizophrenia, ECT did not show significant benefit over sham treatment (Miller *et al.*, 1953; Brill *et al.*, 1959; Heath *et al.*, 1964).

The emergence of antipsychotic agents in the 1950s elicited comparisons of ECT alone to ECT in combination with medication treatment. Taylor & Fleminger (1980) studied 20 schizophrenic patients who failed a 2-week trial of an antipsychotic agent. Patients remained on medication and were randomized to a course of 8–12 ECT or sham sessions. Using the Comprehensive Psychiatric Rating Scale, patients receiving real ECT had lower rating scores acutely, but this result did not persist after one month from discontinuing treatments. As part of the Leicester ECT study, Brandon *et al.* (1985) studied 19 schizophrenic patients on stable medication dosages who received either 8 sham or 8 real ECT over 4 weeks. Using the Montgomery-Åsberg Schizophrenia Scale, raters unaware of the treatment received found significant improvement in scores for the patients receiving real ECT compared with the sham group. Bagadia *et al.* (1983) randomized 38 patients to receive six ECT treatments plus an oral placebo or six sham ECTs plus chlorpromazine. Brief Psychiatric Rating Scale (BPRS) scores did not significantly change in either group indicating that at least for a short course of ECT, medication and ECT results were similar.

Recent studies in ECT and schizophrenia

A number of recent prospective studies and small case series provide mixed results. Tang & Ungvari (2003) in an open prospective trial, treated 30 medication-resistant schizophrenic patients with a combination of antipsychotic medication and ECT or medication alone. The ECT/medication combination group (n = 15) received 8–20 ECT sessions. The authors reported ECT augmentation of medications was of marginal efficacy. In another small study of 20 schizophrenic patients, Ukpong *et al.* (2002) report that improvement with real ECT was not significantly different from sham ECT, although contrary to the clinical lore that 12 or more treatments are needed in these patients, only six ECT sessions were offered. In contrast, Chanpattana and colleagues (Chanpattana *et al.*, 1999; Chanpattana, 2000; Chanpattana & Chakrabhand, 2001; Chanpattana & Kramer, 2003) report that ECT in combination with medication provides improvement in psychopathology and quality of life acutely, and a sustained benefit for some who receive continuation ECT. Recent case literature also supports the finding that ECT combined with antipsychotic drugs (e.g. clozapine) provides acute benefit to medication-resistant schizophrenia patients (Cardwell & Nakai, 1995; Benatov et al., 1996; Bhatia et al., 1998; Kales et al., 1999; Kupchik et al., 2000).

Overall, the evidence to date suggests that ECT is not a first-line treatment for chronic schizophrenic patients who have substantial negative symptoms. For schizophrenic patients who have not responded to medications and who have a sparing of personality and some affective features, ECT offers some benefit.

ECT in special circumstances

Pregnancy

Pregnant women who suffer from psychiatric illness face difficult treatment choices. Prenatal exposure to psychotropic agents is associated with teratogenic complications, perinatal syndromes and neonatal toxicity, and postnatal behavioral problems (Altshuler et al., 1996). Exposure to benzodiazepines, phenothiazines, lithium and some anticonvulsants in the first trimester increases the risk for congenital abnormalities. Because of these dangers, ECT becomes a first-line treatment option, especially for pregnant women suffering from a severe episode of depression, mania or psychosis.

The case literature of over 300 pregnant women who received ECT supports the use of ECT as relatively safe and effective during pregnancy (Ferrill et al., 1992; Miller, 1994; Walker & Swartz, 1994). Ferrill et al. (1992) reviewed 69 cases between 1942 and 1991, detailing history and outcome information. Two (2.9%) fetal deaths and three (4.3%) birth defects occurred in these reports but the role of ECT in the complications was difficult to assess. Other more recent reports (Moreno et al., 1998; Bhatia et al., 1999) highlight the occurrence of a miscarriage in the first trimester in one patient and the development of uterine contractions requiring tocolytics in one of two patients in their third trimesters.

The risks to mother and fetus during ECT, however, must be weighed against the risks of a parapartum psychiatric illness episode as such episodes are associated with severe maternal malnutrition and aggression toward the newborn (Walker & Swartz, 1994). Prepartum depression is also a high stress response state and stress response hormones (e.g. glucocorticoids, vasopressin) cross the placenta (Glover et al., 1998). Children who are exposed as fetuses to this stress-related intrauterine environment exhibit neuromotor growth delays, neuroendocrine and neurotransmitter abnormalities, and disorganized sleep patterns that may permanently alter circadian rhythms (Field et al., 2002 O'Connor et al., 2002). Maternal blood flow to the fetus is also reduced in depressed women, leading to newborn low birth weight (Glover, 1999).

Newborns of women depressed during pregnancy have increased rates of premature birth and low birth weight (Copper et al., 1996; Hedegaard et al., 1996). They respond less to stimuli than comparison infants (as if they had higher thresholds), are hypoactive, and are less robust and sustained in their movements (Field, 1998). They cry excessively and appear inconsolable. The more severe the prepartum depression, the more likely the infant will express these behaviors, and the more severe they are likely to be (Zuckerman et al., 1990). Prepartum depression may also increase the risk for pre-eclampsia (Kurki et al., 2000). Rapid and effective antidepressant treatment is essential. The prolonged treatment trials seen in practice today are contraindicated.

Because of the potentially dire consequences of a lingering prepartum depression, and the relative safety and strong efficacy of ECT in depression, the APA Task Force on ECT (2001) recommended that ECT can be administered in all three trimesters. Evaluation by an obstetrician should be obtained. Modifications to the ECT procedure should be made to diminish aspiration risk and may include antacids or intubation. Non-invasive fetal heart monitoring before and after ECT is recommended after 14 weeks gestational age.

ECT in children and adolescents

The use of ECT in child and adolescent patients is uncommon and to some controversial. Many factors contribute to the reluctance to use ECT in this age group including public and media attitudes against ECT, and the lack of knowledge of psychiatric professionals in treating the young with ECT (Walter et al., 1999). Surveys find about 50% of mental health professionals feel they have limited knowledge of ECT in treatment for minors with psychiatric illness (Walter et al., 1997; Ghaziuddin et al., 2001).

Electroconvulsive therapy, however, has been used for over 60 years in the young, but no large systematic investigation has been done. Small retrospective studies were conducted in the 1990s. Schneekloth et al. (1993) treated 20 patients (10 male and 10 female) diagnosed as having schizophrenia, schizophreniform disorder, bipolar disorder (depressed or manic) or major depression. They reported that in 13 of 20 patients, target symptoms responded to ECT with preferential responses in the patients diagnosed with schizophreniform psychosis, depression without character pathology, mania and catatonia. Cohen *et al.* (1997) assessed 21 adolescents treated with ECT who were diagnosed with depressive, manic or catatonic symptoms. Sixteen patients were reported as improved. The subset of patients diagnosed as schizophrenic or schizoaffective fared less well, with only three of seven deemed responders. Kutcher & Robertson (1995) reported better outcomes for young bipolar patients receiving ECT than for those receiving only medications, with 50% of the ECT patients responding, many achieving remission. Ghaziuddin *et al.* (1996) studied 11 medication-resistant depressed adolescents who then received ECT. All 11 patients significantly improved on the Children Depression Rating Scale-Revised (CDRS-R) and 7 of 11 met CDRS-R criteria for remission. Safety findings included prolonged seizures (> 2.5 minutes) and one episode of a seizure post ECT treatment, suggesting that adolescents have a lower seizure threshold and should be monitored closely during a course of ECT. Moise & Petrides (1996) reviewed the treatment of 13 adolescents (age 16 to 18) from 1983 to 1993 in a university hospital setting. Diagnoses included depression, psychosis, catatonia and bipolar disorder. Response was defined as remission of target symptoms and sustained benefit one month following hospital discharge. Ten of 13 met their criteria for response. Strober *et al.* (1998) studied 10 adolescents receiving ECT for depression. Prospectively evaluating patients with the 17-item HRS-D, nine of ten patients met criteria for response (50% reduction on HRS-D) and six patients were in remission (HRS-D < 8) by the end of the study. Of the nine responders, six were still free of significant mood disorder at 1-year follow-up.

In a literature review of ECT use in young people, Rey & Walter (1997) assessed the quality and outcome of 396 patients. Thirty-nine percent (154) had sufficient information about diagnosis and outcome. The authors concluded that 53% showed marked improvement. Response rates were 63% for depression, 80% for mania, 42% for schizophrenia and 80% for catatonia. No fatalities directly related to ECT were found. Prolonged seizures were noted in 11 patients.

Thus, ECT in the young has been found to be similar in effectiveness and side effects to ECT in adults. More systematic study of ECT in this age group, however, is needed.

Geriatric patients

The elderly make up a large subset of patients treated with ECT. Thompson *et al.* (1994) found individuals 65 years of age and older receive ECT at a higher rate than other age groups. Some authors stressed that ECT in the elderly may be associated with greater memory side effects, cardiorespiratory problems and falls (Alexopoulos *et al.*, 1984; Burke *et al.*, 1987; Cattan *et al.*, 1990).

In the last decade, however, a number of studies have found ECT to be safe and effective in the elderly. Tomac *et al.* (1997) retrospectively studied 34 older adults over 85 and found ECT to be safe and effective with transient post-ECT confusion as the most common side effect. In a chart review, Gormley *et al.* (1998) evaluated the outcome of patients over 75 years of age during the period 1995–1997 treated at three psychiatric hospitals in Dublin and London. Sixty-seven older adult patients received a total of 93 courses of ECT. Ten patients had adverse effects with six experiencing confusion that cleared in 2 weeks after treatment ended. Four bipolar patients developed hypomania. (It should be noted that a switch rate of 5–6% is well within the switch rate for bipolar disorder when treated with antidepressants [Altshuler *et al.*, 1995], and since ECT is effective in both hypomania and mania, the treatment should be continued.) Eighty-five percent of patients were rated as having a marked or moderately good response. Manly *et al.* (2000) studied 39 patients treated with ECT matched with 39 medication-treated patients in a retrospective design. Medical co-morbidity was similar in both groups. The ECT patients had a 77% response rate of "Good," versus 33% in the medication group. The ECT group also had fewer total adverse events including falls, but ten ECT patients versus five medication patients had confusion.

Tew *et al.* (1999), in a large multi-site trial investigating ECT response and subsequent medication treatment and relapse, stratified 268 subjects into adult (59 and younger), young-old (60–74 years) and old-old (75 and older) who had received an index ECT course and follow-up. Response was defined as a HRS-D-24 score of < 10. Most patients received moderately supra-threshold RUL-ECT initially. Response rates were 54% for adults, 73% for the young-old and 67% for the old-old. The authors concluded that, despite a higher general medical illness burden and cognitive impairment, even the oldest patients with depression demonstrate similar or better rates of acute response to ECT.

A similar longitudinal multi-site study investigating continuation ECT versus medication maintenance and relapse initially began in 1997 (Consortium for Research in ECT – CORE). As part of this study O'Connor *et al.* (2001) stratified 253 patients with major depression acutely treated with BL-ECT. Analysis was done on 217 patients who were defined as completers (symptoms remitted or patients remained in the study through the required 10 ECT treatments without remission). Age groups were defined as < 45 years, 46–64 years and > 65 years old. Remission was defined as a 60% reduction on the HRS-D-24 item scale and < 10 on the HRS-D-24. Remission rates were 75% (< 45 years), 93% (46–64 years) and 90% (65 and older). Despite using two different types of ECT (right uni-lateral versus bilateral ECT), these two well-designed studies are impressive in their consistent results of showing strong effectiveness for ECT in elderly patients.

Persons with developmental disorders

In the past, mental retardation and mental illness have been regarded as mutually exclusive conditions (Addington et al., 1993). However, psychiatric disorders occur in 30–70% of patients with mental retardation (Roberts, 1986). Schizophrenia occurs at a rate of two to three times greater than the general population and mood disorders are also common (Bergman & Harris, 1998). Mentally retarded persons are also exposed to psychotropic agents such as antipsychotics for aggressive and destructive behaviors (Poindexter, 1989; Burd et al., 1991; Hancock et al., 1991), and these agents can lead to malignant catatonic states in these patients that require ECT for relief (Fink et al., 2006).

Because of the high occurrence of psychiatric disorders and exposure to medications capable of inducing malignant catatonia (i.e. the neuroleptic malignant syndrome), ECT is a treatment option for mentally retarded persons with ECT responsive conditions. Case report literature is the primary source of the ECT experience in such patients. Aziz et al. (2001) described one mentally retarded patient with bipolar disorder who developed malignant catatonia/neuroleptic malignant syndrome (NMS) after exposure to risperidone and haloperidol. He responded to six bilateral treatments. Aziz et al. (2000) also reported 11 bilateral ECT treatments used to counter psychosis and catatonia in a 39-year-old woman with mental retardation and schizoaffective dis-order. Thuppal & Fink (1999) reported five patients with various psychiatric illnesses all of whom responded to ECT and another three who were stabilized without relapse. Cutjar & Wilson (1999) described eight mentally retarded patients with major depression. Seven patients showed rapid response in mood symptoms with only one patient not responding after eight ECTs. Many other reports of ECT used to treat severe psychosis and depression highlight that ECT can be used safely and effectively in patients with mental retardation (Bates & Smeltzer, 1982; Guze et al., 1987; Kearns, 1987; Goldstein & Jensfold, 1989; Lazarus et al., 1990; Merrill, 1990; Karvounis et al., 1992; Puri et al., 1992; Bebchuck et al., 1996; Chanpattana, 1999).

Electroconvulsive therapy in the treatment of patients with neurological disorders

Epilepsy

Electroconvulsive therapy has long been known to have anticonvulsant properties and to raise seizure threshold (Sackeim et al., 1983; Sackeim, 1999), and the use of ECT as a successful treatment for epilepsy has been reported since the 1940s (Kalinowsky & Kennedy, 1943; Caplan, 1945, 1946). The ECT literature for status epilepticus or intractable seiz-ures, however, arises mainly from case reports (Schnur et al., 1989; Viparelli & Viparelli, 1992; Gonzales et al., 1997; Griesemer et al., 1997; Regenold et al., 1998; Lisanby et al., 2001). Intractable epilepsy and status epilepticus may be associated with incomplete seizures that are unable to elicit an effective anti-seizure brain response to terminate the seizures. In contrast, ECT-induced seizures are complete seizures assisting in raising the seizure threshold, and ECT has been recommended for inclusion in the treatment algor-ithm for status and intractable seizures before inducing barbiturate coma with its high mortality (Fink et al., 1999).

Parkinson's disease

Case literature dating back to 1959 describes the use of ECT in treating patients with Parkinson's disease. These reports mostly find ECT to be safe and effective. In a review of 25 studies, Kellner & Bernstein (1993) noted substantial improvement in movement symptoms with a response rate of 64% (61/95 patients). A few noteworthy studies from this period include Balldin et al. (1981), Andersen et al. (1987) and Douyon et al. (1989). In these larger case series a total of 27 patients with Parkinson's disease were treated with ECT. All but two patients had improved movement symptoms.

Since 1990, another 21 reports including over 100 patients receiving ECT for Parkinson's symptoms or mood symptoms are available in the literature (Kennedy et al., 2003). They provide considerable evidence that ECT improves motor symptoms of Parkinson's disease.

Most ECT clinicians treat patients with Parkinson's dis-ease for the co-morbid depression often associated with movement disorders. Nonetheless, ECT shows benefit for both mood and Parkinson's symptoms. A growing case literature suggests that some patients with Parkinson's disease benefit from continuation ECT (Aarsland et al., 1997; Wengel et al., 1998; Shulman, 2003).

Delirium

In the case literature, ECT also has been found to be safe and effective in treating some patients with delirium due to various etiologies including barbiturate overdose, delirium tremens, uremia, head injury, acute intermittent porphyria, Wilson's disease and pernicious anemia (Krystal & Coffey, 1997). The treatment of delirious states with ECT may be more common in Europe (Kramp & Bolwig, 1981).

Stroke

Depression occurs in 30–40% of patients within two years post-stroke (Robinson *et al.*, 1987). Murray *et al.* (1986) conducted a retrospective review of ECT patients at a university setting over a 12-year period. Fourteen of 193 patients received ECT specifically for depression post-stroke and 12/14 patients had marked improvement in mood symptoms. In another retrospective study, Currier *et al.* (1992) reviewed the outcome of 20 depressed patients post-stroke treated with ECT. They reported a 95% (19/20) response rate. Most recently, Weintraub & Lippmann (2000) described the successful treatment of depression in a post-stroke patient still in the acute phase of stroke recovery (7–14 days).

Dementia

Depression is identified in as many as 87% of patients with dementia (Fischer *et al.*, 1990). Often these depressions are severe and unresponsive to medications. The case literature contains many reports of successful ECT treatment of depression in patients with dementia (Frances *et al.*, 1989; Liang *et al.*, 1988; Benbow, 1988; Weintraub & Lippmann, 2001). Rasmussen *et al.* (2003) treated seven patients with suspected Lewy Body dementia and depression and reported substantial relief of depression with ECT. Mania in conjunction with dementia has also been successfully treated with ECT by McDonald & Thompson (2001) in a case series of three elderly patients. Behavioral symptoms related to dementia (e.g. pathologic screaming) and agitation, which at times may be life threatening, are also reported to respond to ECT (Carlyle *et al.*, 1991; Roccaforte *et al.*, 2000; Grant & Mohan, 2001).

Other neurological conditions

Psychiatric syndromes are present in many other neurological conditions. The case literature identifies numerous reports indicating that ECT is safe and effective for depressed patients also suffering from multiple sclerosis, brain tumors, subdural hematomas, intracranial arachnoid cyst, normal pressure hydrocephalus, cerebral aneurysm, cerebral palsy, traumatic brain injury, Huntington's chorea,

myasthenia gravis and CNS systemic lupus erythematosus (Krystal & Coffey, 1997).

ECT safety and side effects

Mortality

From a review of older studies, the mortality rate for patients receiving ECT was estimated to be four deaths per 100 000 treatments (Abrams, 1997). Kramer (1985) in a descriptive study of the use of ECT in California between 1977 and 1983 found a death rate of two deaths per 100 000 treatments. Since 1993, Texas law has required the reporting of deaths within 14 days of an ECT treatment. Shiwach *et al.* (2001) reviewed this database from 1993 to 1998. They also contacted the treatment sites to obtain more details about the death reports. Over the 5-year period, 8148 patients received 49 048 treatments. No deaths occurred during an ECT session. Thirty patients died within 14 days and seven died within 48 hours of a treatment. A review of the circumstances of the seven deaths proximal to the ECT (48 hours) found one death due to laryngospasm, one due to pneumonitis, two myocardial infarctions, two deaths from sepsis and one unknown death. The authors report a conservative death rate of 2–10 per 100 000 treatments because as many as 5–6 deaths were not related to anesthesia or ECT. This low mortality rate is similar to the mortality rate for those receiving general anesthesia alone which is in the range of 3.3–3.7 deaths per 100 000 inductions (Roy & Overdyk, 1997).

Common side effects and their tolerability

Electroconvulsive therapy is a procedure under general anesthesia and an intravenous line is required to deliver medications. These needed efforts elicit some discomfort. Outpatient ECT, primarily used during continuation treatment, carries the same requirements as minor day surgery. Electroconvulsive therapy may also be an expensive procedure. In our hospital, ECT is administered in a post-anesthesia recovery unit and can be billed at $1500–$2000 per treatment.

Common complaints after ECT treatments include headache, nausea and muscle aches. Patients almost never discontinue treatment because of these problems when properly managed. Post-ECT headaches occur in 40% of patients (Devanand *et al.*, 1995; Freeman & Kendell, 1980). The etiology of this headache is unknown, but Weiner *et al.* (1994) suggest it may be similar to a vascular headache, and in our clinical experience, it appears to be more frequent in people who experience migraines.

Electroconvulsive therapy may also induce headache by its direct stimulation of the temporalis muscle. Treatment is symptomatic, using non-steroidal anti-inflammatory agents (NSAIDS) or other standard analgesics (Leung *et al.*, 2004; Markowitz *et al.*, 2001; Fantz *et al.*, 1998; Oms *et al.*, 1998)

Nausea immediately following ECT is an uncommon side effect of anesthesia and is treated symptomatically. The use of dopamine blocking agents such as prochlorperazine or droperidol to treat post-ECT nausea is too risky because these agents can cause a prolonged QTc on ECG and acute extrapyramidal side effects. 5-HT3 antagonists such as ondansetron and dolasetron are preferred. Muscle pain following a treatment results from strong fasciculations during depolarizing muscle relaxation, from excessive muscle contractions during the seizure from under-dosing the muscle relaxant, or from manipulations of the neck and jaw to maintain an airway. Once observed, both concerns are readily managed, especially by premedicating with a low-dose non-polarizing curare-like muscle relaxant. Alternatively, optimizing the succinylcholine dose treats the excessive convulsive movements.

Cognition

A main concern with ECT is its short- and long-term effects on memory and other cognitive functions. Reaching a conclusion about such effects with present-day standard usage ECT, however, is complicated by the fact that studies span half a century, use different assessment instruments that measure different aspects of memory, and that early ECT practice used high-dose sine-wave machines. Today, ECT is mostly given through machines that deliver brief pulses of lower energy. Cognitive effects of ECT are also dependent on electrode placement and frequency of administration.

There is widespread agreement that brief-pulse, RUL-ECT rather than sine-wave or BL-ECT is associated with less cognitive problems (Abrams, 2002). The following discussion, however, is an overview of the likely cognitive effects of present day ECT. The specifics of electrode placement and waveform are discussed below.

Anterograde amnesia

Some transient disorientation and anterograde amnesia, i.e. the rapid forgetting of newly learned information, during the morning following a treatment is common (Sackeim *et al.*, 1986). Depending on patient variables (e.g. age, neurologic status before ECT) and treatment factors (e.g. electrode placement, stimulus parameters, numbers of stimulations and treatments, concurrent medications, anesthesia effects), some degree of anterograde amnesia may be experienced during the course of

treatment and for a variable period of time after the acute treatment course has ended (Calev *et al.*, 1989). Retrospective studies report rates from 4% to 58% (van der Wurff *et al.*, 2003). One study reports that patients with "high cognitive reserve," determined by more years of education and higher occupational attainment, while not differing in pre-ECT new verbal memory, forgot significantly less than a comparison group with "low" cognitive reserve (Legendre *et al.*, 2003). No study, however, has demonstrated anterograde amnesia to persist more than a few weeks after the course of ECT (APA, 2001). In contrast, many studies have shown cognitive performance to improve immediately after successful ECT (Sackeim *et al.*, 1992, 1993, 2000; Rossi *et al.*, 1990).

Retrograde amnesia

Following a course of ECT some patients experience retrograde amnesia. This amnesia is typically spotty and greater for public events than for personal information and experiences (Lisanby *et al.*, 2000). Patients with pre-existing neurologic disease or who are taking drugs with substantial anticholinergic properties are most likely to experience retrograde amnesia during a course of ECT (APA, 2001). However, the greater the cognitive impairment from depression before ECT, as measured by the MMSE, the greater the likelihood of *improved* cognition after successful ECT, although persistent spotty retrograde amnesia for personal memories is also more likely. However, MMSE scores are not strongly correlated with specific assessment of anterograde and retrograde amnesia (Sobin *et al.*, 1995). The emotional valence of autobiographical information (e.g. sad or happy event) does not relate to what is forgotten (McElhiney *et al.*, 1995).

Some retrograde amnesia persists for weeks after ECT. Permanent loss can also occur for some events that took place during the few months preceding treatment (McElhiney *et al.*, 1995; Sobin *et al.*, 1995; Lisanby *et al.*, 2000). The subjective reports of permanent substantial retrograde amnesia are anecdotal (APA, 2001; Reisner, 2003).

Two controlled trials have directly compared the acute memory effects of ECT and tricyclic antidepressant treatment. Both studies used ECT devices delivering a sinusoidal wave current that today is not optimal in its effect on cognition (APA, 2001). One study (McDonald *et al.*, 1966) found no significant difference between treatments and the other (Gangadhar *et al.*, 1982) found that more patients who received ECT complained of memory loss.

Other cognitive functions

The effect of ECT on other cognitive functions has also been examined. There is no evidence that ECT results in any lasting impairment in general intelligence, executive functions, abstract thinking, visual-spatial function, creativity, semantic memory, implicit memory or the learning of new skills (Frith *et al.*, 1983; Squire *et al.*, 1984; Taylor and Abrams, 1985; Jones *et al.*, 1988; Sackeim *et al.*, 1992).

Studies of maintenance ECT (M-ECT) are few, samples are small and findings are mixed. One study reports poorer new learning and "frontal function" in 11 recovered depressed patients receiving M-ECT compared with 11 who had not received ECT (Rami-Gonzales *et al.*, 2003). Another study reports no differences between 11 patients receiving M-ECT versus 13 receiving maintenance pharmacotherapy (Vothknecht *et al.*, 2003).

Long-term cognitive function

There are few studies of the long-term cognitive effects of ECT. Abrams and Taylor (1985) followed a small cohort of successfully treated ECT patients who had received either UL- or BL-sine wave ECT. Patients were assessed pre-ECT and immediately post-ECT, and again at 1, 6, 12 and 24 months post-treatment on an extensive neuropsychological test battery. Compared with normal controls, ECT patients had more global impairment regardless of electrode placement immediately post-ECT, but were no different in performance from controls at all follow-up assessments. The scores of ECT patients improved over the follow-up period, and by 12 and 24 months were substantially better than pre-ECT levels. More recently, Devanand *et al.* (1991) compared eight patients who had each received over 100 lifetime BL-ECT sine wave treatments with a matched control group. There were no significant between-group differences in objective or subjective memory testing.

Subjective experience for most patients is consistent with systematic memory assessment. Shortly after a course of ECT, following the resolution of any anterograde amnesia, most patients report improvement in cognitive functioning compared to pre-ECT levels (Coleman *et al.*, 1996). The best predictor of the self-rating of cognitive functioning is the degree of recovery from depression (Mattes *et al.*, 1990; Calev *et al.*, 1991a, 1991b; Coleman *et al.*, 1996).

However, there are a few case reports of patients who subjectively experience substantial cognitive decline that they attribute to ECT (Freeman & Kendell, 1980; Donahue, 2000). Much of this experience can be explained by continuing or recurrent psychiatric illness affecting cognition, older patients who received ECT during the early stages of a dementing process unrecognized at the time of treatment, and patients incorrectly attributing the normal cognitive changes of aging to ECT (Sackeim, 1992; Coleman *et al.*, 1996; Devanand *et al.*, 1996; Chen *et al.*, 1999).

Brain structural, metabolic and neurochemical effects

The public discourse concerning adverse effects of ECT on the brain is no longer based on science, and there is no evidence that properly administered ECT has adverse effects on the brain. Because present-day ECT administration maintains oxygenation and cardiovascular function while minimizing the motor convulsion, any adverse effect on the brain would occur by heat from the direct flow of electricity through the brain, the direct effects of the seizure, or from high blood or cerebral spinal fluid pressures damaging brain tissue. No data suggest any of these possibilities. At maximum output ECT machines deliver a current that might raise brain tissue temperature one tenth of a degree centigrade, eliminating the possibility of electrical damage (Swartz, 1989).

Direct damage to brain tissue from induced seizures (electroconvulsive stimulation or ECS) has been studied in laboratory animals. Damage results primarily from anoxia. For baboons to sustain hippocampal damage, the brain area most sensitive to anoxia, they must experience sustained generalized seizures lasting more than 90 minutes, more than 26 recurrent seizures in an 8-hour interval, or continuous limbic seizures lasting more than 3 hours. When seizures are modified, as is done during ECT, a continuous seizure needed to produce damage must be several hours longer (Meldrum, 1986). Seizures during ECT rarely last longer than a minute and are stopped after 2 minutes.

Studies using neurotoxic chemicals (O'Connell *et al.*, 1988) or electrical doses far beyond what are used in ECT to induce unmodified seizures in laboratory animals are not relevant models. Most of these studies were also done in the 1940s and 1950s and their tissue fixation methods, lack of controls and other factors have made their conclusions doubtful. Intracerebral petechial hemorrhages found in some studies of laboratory animals undergoing unmodified electrically induced seizures appear due to unrestrained head movement (Weiner, 1984; Abrams, 2002). Modern ECT eliminates this possibility.

Repeated subconvulsive electrical stimulation in laboratory animals can result in lowering the seizure threshold leading to spontaneous seizures even when the electrical stimulations have stopped (Post *et al.*, 1988). Electroconvulsive therapy does not induce this kindling process. In studies of kindled animals, the administration of an electroconvulsive stimulus (ECS) induced seizure before the animal is induced to seize by the kindled stimulus reduces the seizure response to the kindling stimulus (Babington & Wedeking, 1975; Handforth, 1982). Once-daily ECS protects against additional kindling for a week or more, and if administered before the kindling process is started, prevents its occurrence (Post *et al.*, 1984). Electroconvulsive therapy raises the seizure threshold and is anti-kindling. Dosing over the course of treatment often needs to be increased because of this seizure threshold increase (Abrams, 2002).

Both kindling and ECT, however, are associated with neurogenesis in the rat (Scott *et al.*, 2000; Vaidya *et al.*, 2000). Hippocampal neuronal loss occurs in kindling (Dalby *et al.*, 1996). Electroconvulsive stimulus is associated with mossy fiber sprouting but not cell loss (Vaidya *et al.*, 2000; Dalby *et al.*, 1996). New cell formation can occur with ECS (Scott *et al.*, 2000); ECS also increases the expression of brain-derived neurotrophic factor and its receptor, a process associated with neurogenesis and increased neural plasticity and resistance to neural stressors (Lindefors *et al.*, 1995; Nibuya *et al.*, 1995; Smith *et al.*, 1997).

Brain imaging studies of ECT patients are few but are consistent with ECS studies in laboratory animals. These studies demonstrate that the blood pressure and other transient cardiovascular changes seen during an ECT treatment session do not cause microvascular insult. Increased blood–brain barrier permeability following ECT returns to baseline within 24 hours (Mander *et al.*, 1987; Scott & Turnbull, 1990). In a prospective, blind MRI study of seven severely depressed patients receiving RUL-ECT, Pande *et al.* (1990) showed no differences from baseline one week post-ECT. Coffey *et al.* (1991) also showed that in 35 patients 6 months post-ECT any MRI changes from baseline were from other causes and not from ECT. Using MRI spectroscopy, Ende *et al.* (2000) showed that there were no changes consistent with hippocampal cell loss in 14 severely depressed patients who had received RUL-ECT. A number of individual case reports also fail to find brain-damaging effects from many ECT treatments (Abrams, 2002).

Neurochemical studies assessing brain factors associated with brain damage fail to find an association with ECT. Increased myelin basic protein immunoreactivity in serum associated with stroke and traumatic brain injury is not elevated in patients undergoing ECT (Hoyle *et al.*, 1984). Serum neuron-specific enolase, elevated after stroke, anoxia and epileptic seizures is also unchanged after ECT (Berrouschot *et al.*, 1997). Tau protein, neurofilament and S-100 beta protein, markers of neuronal and glial damage are also unchanged after ECT (Zachrisson *et al.*, 2000).

Conclusions and recommendations

ECT can be considered "neuroconversion." Like cardioconversion, electricity is used to temporarily stop the organ's rhythms permitting it to naturally "re-boot." In

Table 4.1. American Psychiatric Association ECT Taskforce practice guidelines

---

First-line usage
When speed of action is a major consideration
When a high probability of response is needed
When it is safer to use ECT than other treatments
When ECT is clearly the treatment of choice

Secondary usage
When side effects from other treatments are intolerable
When an ECT responsive condition has not responded to
    other treatments
When the patient's condition deteriorates
When suicidality emerges

---

cardioconversion 200–400 joules are delivered in a split second, sometimes several times. In ECT typically 40–50 joules are needed (maximum about 110), delivered over several seconds. About 6–15 administrations are needed over a 2–5 week period in the acute treatment of most patients.

Scientific evidence supports the use of ECT in many disorders and conditions including mood disorders, psychosis and catatonia. Psychiatric illness knows no age limit, and ECT is safe and effective in the young as well as the very old. When co-occurring general medical or neurologic conditions preclude pharmacotherapy or markedly increase the risks of further morbidity or mortality, ECT is a reasoned alternative treatment (Table 4.1). No antidepressant treatment offers faster full relief of depression. While first trials of SSRIs, lasting 12 weeks or more, yield remission rates in depressive illness of 30–40%, and first trials of TCAs with blood level monitoring yield remission rates of 60–70%, 6 to 12 bilateral ECT (2–4 weeks) can achieve remission in 80–95% of patients with depressive illness. No proposed novel treatment for depression offers the benefit of ECT.

Electroconvulsive therapy is often successfully used for patients who have not responded to pharmacotherapy, but many psychiatric conditions such as catatonia or severe depression are life threatening. For patients with severe depression associated with psychosis, stupor, catatonic features and high suicide risk, ECT is the treatment of choice. In these situations, ECT is not the "last choice" it is the first choice. The APA ECT practice guidelines are consistent with this conclusion, and define primary and secondary usage of ECT (see Table 4.1) (APA, 2001, pp. 5–6).

The relatively few well-controlled randomized studies of ECT reflect its success and the ethical consensus that the anesthesia risks with sham-ECT were unacceptable. The collective evidence of nearly 70 years of ECT use points to

Table 4.2. Indications for use of ECT in psychiatric disorder

Treatment	Form of treatment	Psychiatric disorder	Level of evidence for efficacy	Comments
Bilateral ECT	6–12 treatments	Depression	Ia	Undoubtedly effective as an antidepressant treatment
Bilateral ECT	6–12 treatments	Delusional and suicidal depression	Ia	Undoubtedly effective and may be of greater superiority to antidepressants in this group
Bilateral ECT	6–12 treatments (sometimes more than three times weekly)	Mania	IIIa	No randomized trials but consistent evidence of efficacy from cohort studies
Bilateral ECT	6–12 treatments	Catatonia (including malignant catatonia)	IV	May be life saving in neuroleptic malignant syndrome but low level of evidence
Bilateral ECT	6–18 treatments	Schizophrenia	IV	No substantial evidence of efficacy, particularlry for negative symptoms
Unilateral ECT	6–12 treatments	Depression	Ib	Controlled trials show treatment is less effective than bilateral ECT and cognitive gains not strong enough for unilateral preference
Bilateral ECT	10 weeks	Childhood depression	IV	Limited evidence of efficacy
Bilateral ECT	6–12 treatments	Depression in old age psychiatry	IIa IV	Consistent evidence of improvement from cohort studies (possibly more effective than in younger patients with depression)
Bilateral ECT	Up to 12 months given once per week/month	Maintenance treatment (mainly for depression)	IIb	Several good cohort studies

the fact that ECT is safe and highly effective for many conditions, most prominently mood disorders. However, more systematic study of laboratory and clinical predictors of outcome and techniques to optimize efficacy is needed. Studies of the mechanism of action of ECT might also lead to further understanding of the pathophysiology of mood disorders.

The level of evidence for each of the interventions discussed in this chapter is summarized in Table 4.2.

REFERENCES

Aarsland, D., Larsen, J. P., Waage, O. & Langeveld, J. H. (1997). Maintenance electroconvulsive therapy for Parkinson's disease. *Convulsive Therapy*, **13**, 274–7.

Abrams, R. (1997). The mortality rate with ECT. *Convulsive Therapy*, **13**, 125–7.

Abrams, R. (2002). *Electroconvulsive Therapy*, 4th edn. New York: Oxford University Press.

Abrams, R. & Taylor, M. A. (1985). A prospective follow-up study of cognitive functions after ECT. *Convulsive Therapy*, **1**, 4–9.

Addington, D., Addington, J. M. & Ens, I. (1993). Mentally retarded patients on general hospital psychiatric units. *Canadian Journal of Psychiatry*, **38**, 134–42.

AETMIS (2002). *The Use of Electroconvulsive Therapy in Quebec*. Montreal: AETMIS.

Albala, A. A., Greden, J. F., Tarika, J. & Carroll, B. J. (1981). Changes in serial dexamethasone suppression tests among unipolar depressive patients receiving electroconvulsive treatment. *Biological Psychiatry*, **16**, 551–60.

Alexopoulos, G. S., Shamoian, C. J., Lucas, J., Weiser, N. & Berger, H. (1984). Medical problems of geriatric psychiatric patients and younger controls during electroconvulsive therapy. *Journal of the American Geriatrics Society*, **32**, 651–4.

Altshuler, L. L., Post, R. M., Leverich, G. S., Mikalauskas, K., Rosoff, A. & Ackerman, L. (1995). Antidepressant-induced mania and cycle acceleration: a controversy revisited. *American Journal of Psychiatry*, **152**, 1130–8.

Altshuler, L. L., Cohen, L., Szuba, M. P., Burt, V. K., Gitlin, M. & Mintz, J. (1996). Pharmacologic management of psychiatric illness during pregnancy: dilemmas and guidelines. *American Journal of Psychiatry*, **153**, 592–606.

American Psychiatric Association Committee on Electroconvulsive Therapy (2001). *The Practice of Electroconvulsive Therapy: Recommendations for Treatment, Training, and Privileging*, 2nd edn. Washington, DC: American Psychiatric Association.

Andersen, K., Balldin, J., Gottfries, C. G. *et al.* (1987). A double-blind evaluation of electroconvulsive therapy in Parkinson's disease with "on-off" phenomena. *Acta Neurologica Scandinavica*, **76**, 191–9.

Arnold, O. H. & Stepan, H. (1952). Untersuchungen zur Frage der akuten todlichen, Katatonie. *Wiener Zeitschrift fur Nervenheilkunde und Deren Grenzgebiete*, **4**, 235–58.

Avery, D. & Lubrano, A. (1979). Depression treated with imipramine and ECT: the DeCarolis study reconsidered. *American Journal of Psychiatry*, **136**, 559–62.

Avery, D. & Winokur, G. (1978). Suicide, attempted suicide, and relapse rates in depression. *Archives of General Psychiatry*, **35**, 749–53.

Aziz, M., Maixner, D. F., DeQuardo, J., Aldridge, A. & Tandon, R. (2001). ECT and mental retardation: a review and case reports. *Journal of ECT*, **17**, 149–52.

Babington, R. G. & Wedeking, P. W. (1975). Blockade of tardive seizures in rats by electroconvulsive shock. *Brain Research*, **88**, 141–4.

Bagadia, V. N., Abhyankar, R. R., Doshi, J., Pradhan, P. V. & Shah, L. P. (1983). A double blind controlled study of ECT vs chlorpromazine in schizophrenia. *Journal of the Association of Physicians of India*, **31**, 637–40.

Baldessarini, R. J. (2001). Drugs and the treatment of psychiatric disorders: antidepressant and antianxiety agents. In *Goodman and Gilman's The Pharmacological Basis of Therapeutics, 10th edn*, ed. J. G. Hardman, L. E. Gilman & A. G. Gilman, pp. 447–83. New York: McGraw-Hill.

Baldessarini, R. J. & Tondo, L. (2003). Suicide risk and treatments for patients with bipolar disorder. *Journal of the American Medical Association*, **290**, 1517–19.

Balldin, J., Granerus, A. K., Lindstedt, G., Modigh, K. & Walinder, J. (1981). Predictors for improvement after electroconvulsive therapy in parkinsonian patients with on-off symptoms. *Journal of Neural Transmission*, **52**, 199–211.

Barker, A. T., Jalinous, R. & Freeston, I. L. (1985). Non-invasive magnetic stimulation of human motor cortex. *Lancet*, **1**, 1106–7.

Bates, W. J. & Smeltzer, D. J. (1982). Electroconvulsive treatment of psychotic self-injurious behavior in a patient with severe mental retardation. *American Journal of Psychiatry*, **139**, 1355–6.

Bebchuck, J. M., Barnhill, J. & Dawkins, K. (1996). ECT and mental retardation. *American Journal of Psychiatry*, **153**, 1231.

Benatov, R., Sirota, P. & Megged, S. (1996). Neuroleptic-resistant schizophrenia treated with clozapine and ECT. *Convulsive Therapy*, **12**, 117–21.

Benbow, S. M. (1988). ECT for depression in dementia. *British Journal of Psychiatry*, **152**, 859.

Bergman, J. D. & Harris, J. C. (1998). Mental retardation. In *Comprehensive Textbook of Psychiatry*, ed. S. Kaplan & B. Sadock, p. 2224. Baltimore, MD: Williams & Wilkins.

Berrouschot, J., Rolle, K., Kuhn, H. J. & Schneider, D. (1997). Serum neuron-specific enolase levels do not increase after electroconvulsive therapy. *Journal of Neurological Science*, **150**, 173–6.

Bhatia, S. C., Bhatia, S. K. & Gupta, S. (1998). Concurrent administration of clozapine and ECT: a successful therapeutic strategy for a patient with treatment-resistant schizophrenia. *Journal of ECT*, **14**, 280–3.

Bhatia, S. C., Baldwin, S. A. & Bhatia, S. K. (1999). Electroconvulsive therapy during the third trimester of pregnancy. *Journal of ECT*, **15**, 270–4.

Birkenhager, T. K., Pluijms, E. M. & Lucius, S. A. (2003). ECT response in delusional versus non-delusional depressed inpatients. *Journal of Affective Disorders*, **74**, 191–5.

Black, D. W., Winokur, G. & Nasrallah, A. (1989). Illness duration and acute response in major depression. *Convulsive Therapy*, **5**, 338–43.

Boodman, S. G. (1996). Shock therapy … it's back. *The Washington Post*, p. 24.

Bostwick, J. M. & Pankratz, V. S. (2000). Affective disorders and suicide risk: a reexamination. *American Journal of Psychiatry*, **157**, 1925–32.

Bourgon, L. N. & Kellner, C. H. (2000). Relapse of depression after ECT: a review. *Journal of ECT*, **16**, 19–31.

Bourne, H. (1954). Convulsion dependence. *Lancet*, **2**, 1193–6.

Bradvik, L. & Berglund, M. (2000). Treatment and suicide in severe depression: a case-control study of antidepressant therapy at last contact before suicide. *Journal of ECT*, **16**, 399–408.

Brandon, S. P., Cowley, C., McDonald, P., Neville, R., Palmer, R. & Wellstood-Eason, S. (1984). Electroconvulsive therapy: results in depressive illness from the Leicestershire trial. *British Medical Journal*, **288**, 22–5.

Brandon, S., Cowley, P., McDonald, C., Neville, P., Palmer, R. & Wellstood-Eason, S. (1985). Leicester ECT trial: Results in schizophrenia. *British Journal of Psychiatry*, **146**, 177–83.

Breggin, P. R. (1991). *Toxic Psychiatry: Why Therapy, Empathy, and Love Must Replace the Drugs, Electroshock, and Biochemical Theories of the "New Psychiatry"*. New York: St. Martin's Press.

Brill, N. O., Crumpton, E., Eiduson, S., Crayson, H. M., Hellman, L. I. & Richards, R. A. (1959). Relative effectiveness of various components of electroconvulsive therapy. *Archives of Neurology and Psychiatry*, **81**, 627–35.

Buchan, H., Johnstone, E., McPherson, K., Palmer, R. L., Crow, T. J. & Brandon, S. (1992). Who benefits from electroconvulsive therapy? Combined results of the Leicester and Northwick Park trials. *British Journal of Psychiatry*, **160**, 355–9.

Burd, L., Fisher, W., Vesely, B. N., Williams, M., Kerbeshian, J. & Leech, C. (1991). Prevalence of psychoactive drug use among North Dakota group home residents. *American Journal of Mental Retardation*, **96**, 119–26.

Burke, W. J., Rubin, E. H., Zorumski, C. F. & Wetzel, R. D. (1987). The safety of ECT in geriatric psychiatry. *Journal of the American Geriatrics Society*, **35**, 516–21.

Burt T., Lisanby, S. H. & Sackeim, H. (2002). Neuropsychiatric applications of transcranial magnetic stimulation: a meta-analysis. *International Journal of Neuropsychopharmacology*, **5**, 73–103.

Calev, A., Ben-Tzvi, E., Shapira, B., Drexler, H., Carasso, R. & Lerer, B. (1989). Distinct memory impairments following electroconvulsive therapy and imipramine. *Psychology Medicine*, **19**, 111–19.

Calev, A., Kochavlev, E., Tubi, N. *et al.* (1991a). Change in attitude toward electroconvulsive therapy: effects of treatment, time since treatment, and severity of depression. *Convulsive Therapy*, **7**, 184–9.

Calev, A., Nigal, D., Shapira, B. *et al.* (1991b). Early and long-term effects of electroconvulsive therapy and depression on memory and other cognitive functions. *Journal of Nervous and Mental Disorders*, **179**, 526–33.

Caplan, G. (1945). Treatment of epilepsy by electrically induced convulsions. A preliminary report. *British Medical Journal*, **1**, 511–12.

Caplan, G. (1946). Electrical convulsion therapy in treatment of epilepsy. *Journal of Mental Science*, 784–93.

Carlyle, W., Killick, L. & Ancill, R. (1991). ECT: an effective treatment in the screaming demented patient. *Journal of the American Geriatrics Society*, **39**, 637.

Cardwell, B. A. & Nakai, B. (1995). Seizure activity in combined clozapine and ECT: a retrospective view. *Convulsive Therapy*, **11**, 110–13.

Cattan, R. A., Barry, P. P., Mead, G., Reefe, W. E., Gay, A. & Silverman, M. (1990). Electroconvulsive therapy in octogenarians. *Journal of the American Geriatrics Society*, **38**, 753–8.

Chan, C. H., Janicak, P. G., Davis, J. M., Altman, E., Andriukaitis, S. & Hedeker, D. (1987). Response of psychotic and nonpsychotic depressed patients to tricyclic antidepressants. *Journal of Clinical Psychiatry*, **48**, 197–200.

Chanpattana, W., Chakrabhand, M. L., Sackeim, H. A. *et al.* (1999). Continuation ECT in treatment-resistant schizophrenia: a controlled study. *Journal of ECT*, **15**, 178–92.

Chanpattana, W. & Chakrabhand, M. L. (2001). Combined ECT and neuroleptic therapy in treatment-refractory schizophrenia: prediction of outcome. *Psychiatry Research*, **105**, 107–15.

Chanpattana, W. & Kramer, B. A. (2003). Acute and maintenance ECT with flupentixol in refractory schizophrenia: sustained improvements in psychopathology, quality of life, and social outcomes. *Schizophrenia Research*, **63**, 189–93.

Chanpattana, W. (1999). Maintenance ECT in mentally retarded, treatment-resistant schizophrenic patients. *Journal of ECT*, **5**, 150–3.

Chanpattana, W. (2000). Maintenance ECT in treatment-resistant schizophrenia. *Journal of the Medical Association of Thailand*, **83**, 657–62.

Chen, P., Ganguli, M., Mulsant, B. H. & DeKosky, S. T. (1999). The temporal relationship between depressive symptoms and dementia: a community-based prospective study. *Archives in General Psychiatry*, **56**, 261–6.

Clarke, T. B., Coffey, C. E., Hoffman, G. W. & Weiner, R. D. (1989). Continuation therapy for depression using outpatient electroconvulsive therapy. *Convulsive Therapy*, **5**, 330–7.

Coffey, C. E., Weiner, R. D., Djang, W. T. *et al.* (1991). Brain anatomic effects of ECT: a prospective magnetic resonance imaging study. *Archives in General Psychiatry*, **48**, 1013–21.

Cohen, D., Paillere-Martinot, M. L. & Basquin, M. (1997). Use of electroconvulsive therapy in adolescents. *Convulsive Therapy*, **13**, 25–31.

Coleman, E. A., Sackeim, H. A., Prudic, J., Devanand, D. P., McElhiney, M. C. & Moody, B. J. (1996). Subjective memory complaints before and after electroconvulsive therapy. *Biological Psychiatry*, **39**, 346–56.

Conca, A., Koppi, S., Konig, P., Swoboda, E. & Krecke, N. (1996). Transcranial magnetic stimulation: a novel antidepressive strategy? *Neuropsychobiology*, **34**, 204–7.

Conwell, Y., Duberstein, P. R. & Caine, E. D. (2002). Risk factors for suicide in later life. *Biological Psychiatry*, **52**, 193–204.

Copper, R. L., Goldenberg, R. L., Das, A. *et al.* (1996). The preterm prediction study: maternal stress is associated with spontaneous preterm birth at less than thirty-five weeks gestation. *American Journal of Obstetrics and Gynecology*, **175**, 1286–92.

Coppen, A., Milln, P., Harwood, J. & Wood, K. (1985). Does the dexamethasone suppression test predict antidepressant treatment success? *British Journal of Psychiatry*, **146**, 294–6.

Coryell, W. (1982). Hypothalamic-pituitary-adrenal axis abnormality and ECT response. *Psychiatry Research*, **6**, 283–91.

Couturier, J. L. (2005). Efficacy of rapid-rate repetitive transcranial magnetic stimulation in the treatment of depression: a systematic review and meta-analysis. *Journal of Psychiatry and Neuroscience*, **30**, 83–90.

Currier, M. B., Murray, G. B. & Welch, C. C. (1992). Electroconvulsive therapy for post-stroke depressed geriatric patients. *Journal of Neuropsychiatry and Clinical Neurosciences*, **4**, 140–4.

Cutjar, P. & Wilson, D. (1999). The use of ECT in intellectual disability. *Journal of Intellectual Disability Research*, **43**, 421–7.

Davis, J. M., Janicak, P. G., Sakkas, P., Gilmore, C. & Wang, Z. (1991). Electroconvulsive therapy in the treatment of the neuroleptic malignant syndrome. *Convulsive Therapy*, **7**, 111–20.

d'Elia, G. (1970). Unilateral electroconvulsive therapy. *Acta Psychiatrica Scandinavica*, **215** (Suppl.), 1–98.

Dalby, N. O., Tonder, N., Wolby, D. P., West, M., Finsen, B. & Bolwig, T. G. (1996). No loss of hippocampal hilar somatostatinergic neurons after repeated electroconvulsive shock: a combined stereological and in situ hybridization study. *British Journal of Psychiatry*, **169**, 68–74.

Decina, P., Guthrie, E. B., Sackeim, H. A., Kahn, D. & Malitz, S. (1987). Continuation ECT in the management of relapses of major affective episodes. *Acta Psychiatrica Scandinavica*, **75**, 559–62.

Devanand, D. P., Fitzsimons, L., Prudic, J. & Sackeim, H. A. (1995). Subjective side effects during electroconvulsive therapy. *Convulsive Therapy*, **11**, 232–40.

Devanand, D. P., Decina, P., Sackeim, H. A., Hopkins, N., Novacenko, H. & Malitz, S. (1987). Serial dexamethasone suppression tests in initial suppressors and non-suppressors treated with electroconvulsive therapy. *Biological Psychiatry*, **22**, 463–72.

Devanand, D. P., Sano, M., Tang, M. X. *et al.* (1996). Depressed mood and the incidence of Alzheimer's disease in the elderly living in the community. *Archives in General Psychiatry*, **53**, 175–82.

Devanand, D. P., Verma, A. K., Tirumalasetti, F. & Sackeim, H. A. (1991). Absence of cognitive impairment after more than 100 lifetime ECT treatments. *American Journal of Psychiatry*, **148**, 929–32.

Dinan, T. G. & Barry, S. (1989). A comparison of electroconvulsive therapy with a combined lithium and tricyclic combination among depressed tricyclic nonresponders. *Acta Psychiatrica Scandinavica*, **80**, 97–100.

Department of Health (1999). *Electroconvulsive Therapy: Survey Covering the Period from January 1999 to March 1999. England. Bulletin 1999/22*. London: Government Statistical Service.

Dombrovski, A. Y., Mulsant, B. H., Haskett, R. F., Prudic, J., Begley, A. E. & Sackeim, H. A. (2005). Predictors of remission after electroconvulsive therapy in unipolar depression. *Journal of Clinical Psychiatry*, **66**, 1043–9.

Donahue, J. C. (2000). Electroconvulsive therapy and memory loss: anatomy of a debate. *Journal of ECT*, **16**, 133–43.

Douyon, R., Serby, M., Klutchko, B. & Rotrosen, J. (1989). ECT and Parkinson's disease revisited: a "naturalistic" study. *American Journal of Psychiatry*, **146**, 1451–5.

Duncan, A. J., Ungvari, G. S., Russell, R. J. & Seifert, A. (1990). Maintenance ECT in very old age. *Annals of Clinical Psychiatry*, **2**, 139–44.

Dunn, C. G. & Quinlan, D. (1978). Indicators of ECT response and non-response in the treatment of depression. *Journal of Clinical Psychiatry*, **39**, 620–2.

Ende, G., Braus, D. F., Walter, S., Walter, S., Weber-Fahr, W. & Henn, F. A. (2000). The hippocampus in patients treated with electroconvulsive therapy: a proton magnetic resonance spectroscopic imaging study. *Archives in General Psychiatry*, **57**, 937–43.

Endler, N. S. (1988). The origins of electroconvulsive therapy (ECT). *Convulsive Therapy*, **4**, 5–23.

Ferrill, M. J., Kehoe, W. A. & Jacisin, J. J. (1992). ECT during pregnancy: physiologic and pharmacologic considerations. *Convulsive Therapy*, **8**, 186–200.

Field, T. M. (1998). *Depressed Mothers and their Newborns*. Paper presented at the 11th Biennial Conference on Infant Studies, Atlanta, GA.

Field, T., Diego, M., Hernandez-Reif, M., Schanberg, S. & Kuhn, C. (2002). Relative right versus left frontal EEG in neonates. *Developmental Psychobiology*, **41**, 147–55.

Figiel, G. S., Epstein, C., McDonald, W. M. *et al.* (1998). The use of rapid-rate transcranial magnetic stimulation (rTMS) in refractory depressed patients. *Journal of Neuropsychiatry and Clinical Neurosciences*, **10**, 20–25.

Fink, M. (1979). *Convulsive Therapy: Theory and Practice*. New York: Raven Press.

Fink, M. (1984). Meduna and the origins of convulsive therapy. *American Journal of Psychiatry*, **141**, 1034–41.

Fink, M. (1986). Neuroendocrine predictors of electroconvulsive therapy outcome. Dexamethasone suppression test and prolactin. *Annals of the New York Academy of Sciences*, **462**, 30–6.

Fink, M., Kellner, C. & Sackeim, H. A. (1999). Intractable seizures, status epilepticus, and ECT. *Journal of ECT*, **15**, 282–4.

Fink, M., Bailine, S. & Petrides, G. (2001). Electrode placement and electroconvulsive therapy: a search for the chimera. *Archives of General Psychiatry*, **58**, 607–9.

Fink, M. & Taylor, M. A. (2003). *Catatonia: A Clinician's Guide to Diagnosis and Treatment*. Cambridge: Cambridge University Press.

Fink, M., Taylor, M. A. & Ghaziuddin, N. (2006). Catatonia in autistic spectrum disorders: a medical treatment algorithm. In *Catatonia in Autism Spectrum Disorders*, ed. D. M. Dhossche, L. Wing, M. Ohta & K-J. Neumarker, pp. 233–44. Amsterdam: Elsevier/Academic Press.

Fischer, P., Simanyi, M. & Danielczyk, W. (1990). Depression in dementia of the Alzheimer type and in multi-infarct dementia. *American Journal of Psychiatry*, **147**, 1484–7.

Folkerts, H. (1996). The ictal electroencephalogram as a marker for the efficacy of electroconvulsive therapy. *European Archives of Psychiatry and Clinical Neuroscience*, **246**, 155–64.

Folkerts, H. W., Michael, N., Tolle, R., Schonauer, K., Mucke, S. & Schulze-Monking, H. (1997). Electroconvulsive therapy vs. paroxetine in treatment-resistant depression – a randomized study. *Acta Psychiatrica Scandinavica*, **96**, 334–42.

Fox, H. A. (2001). Extended continuation and maintenance ECT for long-lasting episodes of major depression. *Journal of ECT*, **17**, 60–4.

Frances, A., Weiner, R. D. & Coffey, C. E. (1989). ECT for an elderly man with psychotic depression and concurrent dementia. *Hospital and Community Psychiatry*, **40**, 237–38, 242.

Frankel, F. H. (1973). Electro-convulsive therapy in Massachusetts: a task force report. *Massachusetts Journal of Mental Health*, **3**, 3–29.

Fantz, R. M., Markowitz, J. S. & Kellner, C. H. (1998). Sumatriptan for post-ECT headache. *Journal of ECT*, **14**, 272–4.

Freeman, C. P. (2000). *The ECT Handbook*. London: Royal College of Psychiatrists.

Freeman, C. P. & Kendell, R. E. (1980). ECT: I. Patients' experiences and attitudes. *British Journal of Psychiatry*, **137**, 8–16.

Freeman, C. P. L., Basson, J. V. & Crichton, A. (1978). Double-blind controlled trial of electroconvulsive therapy (ECT) and simulated ECT in depressive illness. *Lancet*, **I**, 738–40.

Frith, C. D., Stevens, M., Johnstone, E. C., Deakin, J. F., Lawler, P. & Crow, T. J. (1983). Effects of ECT and depression on various aspects of memory. *British Journal of Psychiatry*, **142**, 610–17.

Gagne, G. G. Jr., Furman, M. J., Carpenter, L. L. & Price, L. H. (2000). Efficacy of continuation ECT and antidepressant drugs compared to long-term antidepressants alone in depressed patients. *American Journal of Psychiatry*, **157**, 1960–5.

Gangadhar, B. N., Kapur, R. L. & Kalyanasundarum, S. (1982). Comparison of electroconvulsive therapy with imipramine in endogenous depression: a double blind study. *British Journal of Psychiatry*, **141**, 367–71.

Geoghegan, J. J. & Stevenson, G. H. (1949). Prophylactic electroshock. *American Journal of Psychiatry*, **105**, 494–5.

George, M. S. & Wassermann, E. M. (1994). Rapid-rate transcranial magnetic stimulation and ECT. *Convulsive Therapy*, **10**, 251–4.

George, M. S., Wassermann, E. M., Kimbrell, T. A. et al. (1997). Mood improvement following daily left prefrontal repetitive transcranial magnetic stimulation in patients with depression: a placebo-controlled crossover trial. *American Journal of Psychiatry*, **154**, 1752–6.

Ghaziuddin, N., Kaza, M., Ghazi, N., King, C., Walter, G. & Rey, J. M. (2001). Electroconvulsive therapy for minors: experiences and attitudes of child psychiatrists and psychologists. *Journal of ECT*, **17**, 109–17.

Ghaziuddin, N., King, C. A., Naylor, M. W. et al. (1996). Electroconvulsive treatment in adolescents with pharmacotherapy-refractory depression. *Journal of Child and Adolescent Psychopharmacology*, **6**, 259–71.

Glover, V. (1999). Maternal stress or anxiety during pregnancy and the development of the baby. *Practising Midwife*, **2**, 20–2.

Glover, V., Teixeira, J., Gitau, R. & Fisk, N. (1998). *Links between Antenatal Maternal Anxiety and the Fetus*. Paper presented at the 11th Biennial Conference on Infant Studies, Atlanta, GA.

Goldstein, M. Z. & Jensfold, M. F. (1989). ECT treatment of an elderly mentally retarded man. *Psychosomatic*, **30**, 104–6.

Gonzales, M. D. C., Palomar, M. & Rovira, R. (1997). Electroconvulsive therapy for status epilepticus. *Annals of Internal Medicine*, **127**, 247–8.

Gormley, N., Cullen, C.. Walters, L., Philpot, M. & Lawlor, B. (1998). The safety and efficacy of electroconvulsive therapy in patients over age 75. *International Journal of Geriatric Psychiatry*, **13**, 871–4.

Grant, J. E. & Mohan, S. N. (2001). Treatment of agitation and aggression in four demented patients using ECT. *Journal of ECT*, **17**, 205–9.

Gregory, S., Shawcross, C. R. & Gill, D. (1985). The Nottingham ECT Study. A double-blind comparison of bilateral, unilateral and simulated ECT in depressive illness. *British Journal of Psychiatry*, **146**, 520–4.

Griesemer, D. A., Kellner, C. H., Beale, M. D. & Smith, G. M. (1997). Electroconvulsive therapy for treatment of intractable seizures. Initial findings in two children. *Neurology*, **49**, 1389–92.

Grunhaus, L., Zelnik, T., Albala, A. A. et al. (1987). Serial dexamethasone suppression tests in depressed patients treated only with electroconvulsive therapy. *Journal of Affective Disorders*, **13**, 233–40.

Grunhaus, L., Pande, A. C. & Haskett, R. F. (1990). Full and abbreviated courses of maintenance electroconvulsive therapy. *Convulsive Therapy*, **6**, 130–8.

Grunhaus, L., Dolberg, O. & Lustig, M. (1995). Relapse and recurrence following a course of ECT: reasons for concern and strategies for further investigation. *Journal of Psychiatric Research*, **29**, 165–72.

Grunhaus, L., Dannon, P. N., Schreiber, S. et al. (2000). Repetitive transcranial magnetic stimulation is as effective as electroconvulsive therapy in the treatment of non-delusional major depressive disorder: an open study. *Biological Psychiatry*, **47**, 314–24.

Grunhaus, L., Schreiber, S., Dolberg, O. T., Polak, D. & Dannon, P. N. (2003). A randomized controlled comparison of electroconvulsive therapy and repetitive transcranial magnetic stimulation in severe and resistant nonpsychotic major depression. *Biological Psychiatry*, **53**, 324–31.

Guze, B., Weinman, B. & Diamond, R. (1987). Use of ECT to treat bipolar depression in a mentally retarded with cerebral palsy. *Convulsive Therapy*, **3**, 60–4.

Hall, W. D., Mant, A., Mitchell, P. B., Rendle, V. A., Hickie, I. B. & McManus, P. (2003). 1991–2000. Association between antidepressant prescribing and suicide in Australia, trend analysis. *British Medical Journal*, **326**, 1008–11.

Hancock, R. D., Weber, S. L., Kaza, R. & Her, K. S. (1991). Changes in psychotropic drug use in long-term residents of an ICF/MR facility. *American Journal of Mental Retardation*, **96**, 137–41.

Handforth, A. (1982). Postseizure inhibition of kindled seizures by electroconvulsive shock. *Experimental Neurology*, **78**, 483–91.

Hawkins, J. M., Archer, K. J., Strakowski, S. M. & Keck, P. E. (1995). Somatic treatment of catatonia. *International Journal of Psychiatry in Medicine*, **25**, 345–69.

Heath, E. S., Adams, A. & Wakeling, P. L. G. (1964). Short courses of ECT and simulated ECT in chronic schizophrenia. *British Journal of Psychiatry*, **110**, 800–7.

Hedegaard, M., Henriksen, T. B., Secher, N. J., Hatch, M. C. & Sabroe, S. (1996). Do stressful life events affect duration of gestation and risk of preterm delivery? *Epidemiology*, **7**, 339–45.

Heim, C. & Nemeroff, C. B. (2001). The role of childhood trauma in the neurobiology of mood and anxiety disorders: preclinical and clinical studies. *Biological Psychiatry*, **49**, 1023–30.

Hermann, R. C., Ettner, S. L., Dorwart, R. A., Hoover, C. W. & Young, E. (1998). Characteristics of psychiatrists who perform ECT. *American Journal of Psychiatry*, **155**, 889–94.

Hermann, R. C., Dorwart, R. A., Hoover, C. W. & Brody, J. (1995). Variation in ECT use in the United States. *American Journal of Psychiatry*, **152**, 869–75.

Hickie, I., Mason, C., Parker, G. & Brodaty, H. (1996). Prediction of ECT response: validation of a refined sign-based (CORE) system for defining melancholia. *British Journal of Psychiatry*, **169**, 68–74.

Holsboer, F. (2001). Stress, hypercortisolism and corticosteroid receptors in depression: implications for therapy. *Journal of Affective Disorder*, **62**, 77–91.

Hoyle, N. R., Pratt, R. T. & Thomas, D. G. (1984). Effects of electroconvulsive therapy on serum myelin basic protein immunoreactivity. *British Medical Journal*, **288**, 1110–11.

Hrdlicka, M., Moran, M., Vachutka, J. et al. (1996). EEG correlates of therapeutic effects of electroconvulsive therapy. *Ceska a Slovenska Psychiatrie*, **92**, 32–40.

Husain, M. M., Meyer, D. E., Muttakin, M. H. & Weiner, M. (1993). Maintenance ECT for treatment of recurrent mania. *American Journal of Psychiatry*, **150**, 985.

Husain, M. M., Rush, A. J., Fink, M. et al. (2004). Speed of response and remission in major depressive disorder with acute electroconvulsive therapy (ECT): a Consortium for Research in ECT (CORE) report. *Journal of Clinical Psychiatry*, **65**, 485–91.

Isometsa, E. T., Henriksson, M. M., Heikkinen, M. E. & Lonnqvist, J. K. (1996). Completed suicide and recent electroconvulsive therapy in Finland. *Convulsive Therapy*, **12**, 152–5.

Janakiramaiah, N., Gangadhar, B. N., Naga, V. *et al.* (2000). Antidepressant efficacy of Sudarshan Kriya Yoga (SKY) in melancholia: a randomized comparison with electroconvulsive therapy (ECT) and imipramine. *Journal of Affective Disorders*, **57**, 255–9.

Janicak, P. G., Dowd, S. M., Martis, B. *et al.* (2002). Repetitive transcranial magnetic stimulation versus electroconvulsive therapy for major depression: preliminary results of a randomized trial. *Biological Psychiatry*, **51**, 659–67.

Johnstone, E. C., Deakin, J. F., Lawler, P. *et al.* (1980). The Northwick Park electroconvulsive therapy trial. *Lancet*, **2**, 1317–20.

Jones, B. P., Henderson, M. & Welch, C. A. (1988). Executive functions in unipolar depression before and after electroconvulsive therapy. *International Journal of Neuroscience*, **38**, 287–97.

Kales, H. C., Dequardo, J. R. & Tandon, R. (1999). Combined electroconvulsive therapy and clozapine in treatment-resistant schizophrenia. *Progress in Neuro-Psychopharmacology & Biological Psychiatry*, **23**, 547–56.

Kalinowsky, L. B. & Kennedy, F. (1943). Observations in electric shock therapy applied to problems of epilepsy. *Journal of Nervous Mental Disease*, **98**, 56–67.

Karliner, W. & Wehrheim, H. K. (1965). Maintenance convulsive treatments. *American Journal of Psychiatry*, **121**, 1113–15.

Karvounis, S., Holt, G. & Hodgkiss, A. (1992). Outpatient ECT for depression in a man with moderate learning disability. *British Journal of Psychiatry*, **161**, 426–7.

Katona, C. L., Aldridge, C. R., Roth, M. & Hyde, J. (1987). The dexamethasone suppression test and prediction of outcome in patients receiving ECT. *British Journal of Psychiatry*, **150**, 315–18.

Kearns, A. (1987). Cotard's syndrome in a mentally retarded man. *British Journal of Psychiatry*, **150**, 112–14.

Kellner, C. H. & Bernstein, H. J. (1993). ECT as a treatment for neurologic illness. In *Clinical Science of Electroconvulsive Therapy*, ed. C. E. Coffey, pp. 183–210. Washington, DC: American Psychiatric Press.

Kellner, C. H., Husain, M., Petrides, G., Fink, M. & Rummans, T. (2002). Comment on "Repetitive transcranial magnetic stimulation versus electroconvulsive therapy for major depression: preliminary results of a randomized trial". *Biological Psychiatry*, **52**, 1032–3.

Kellner, C. H., Fink, M., Knapp, R. *et al.* (2005). Relief of expressed suicidal intent by ECT: a consortium for research in ECT study. *American Journal of Psychiatry*, **162**, 977–82.

Kennedy, R., Mittal, D. & O'Jile, J. (2003). Electroconvulsive therapy in movement disorders: an update. *Journal of Neuropsychiatry and Clinical Neurosciences*, **15**, 407–21.

Khan, A., Warner, H. A. & Brown, W. A. (2000). Symptom reduction and suicide risk inpatients treated with placebo in antidepressant clinical trials: an analysis of the Food and Drug Administration database. *Archives in General Psychiatry*, **57**, 311–17.

Kho, K. H. (2002). Treatment of rapid cycling bipolar disorder in the acute and maintenance phase with ECT. *Journal of ECT*, **18**, 159–61.

Kindler, S., Shapira, B., Hadjez, J., Abramowitz, M., Brom, D. & Lerer, B. (1991). Factors influencing response to bilateral electroconvulsive therapy in major depression. *Convulsive Therapy*, **7**, 245–54.

Kramer, B. A. (1985). Use of ECT in California, 1977–1983. *American Journal of Psychiatry*, **142**, 1190–2.

Kramer, B. A. (1999). A naturalistic review of maintenance ECT at a university setting. *Journal of ECT*, **15**, 262–9.

Kramp, P. & Bolwig, T. G. (1981). Electroconvulsive therapy in acute delirious states. *Comprehensive Psychiatry*, **22**, 368–71.

Krystal, A. D. & Coffey, C. E. (1997). Neuropsychiatric considerations in the use of electroconvulsive therapy. *Journal of Neuropsychiatry and Clinical Neurosciences*, **9**, 283–92.

Krystal, A. D., Weiner, R. D. & Coffey, C. E. (1995). The ictal EEG as a marker of adequate stimulus intensity with unilateral ECT. *Journal of Neuropsychiatry and Clinical Neurosciences*, **7**, 295–303.

Kutcher, S. & Robertson, H. A. (1995). Electroconvulsive therapy in treatment resistant bipolar youth. *Journal of Child and Adolescent Psychopharmacology*, **5**, 167–75.

Kukopulos, A., Reginaldi, D., Tondo, L., Bernabei, A. & Caliari, B. (1977). Spontaneous length of depression and response to ECT. *Psychological Medicine*, **7**, 625–9.

Kupchik, M., Spivak, B., Mester, R. *et al.* (2000). Combined electroconvulsive-clozapine therapy. *Clinical Neuropharmacology*, **23**, 14–16.

Kurki, T., Hiilesmaa, V., Raitasalo, R., Mattila, H. & Ylikorkala, O. (2000). Depression and anxiety in early pregnancy and risk for preeclampsia. *Obstetric Gynecology*, **95**, 487–90.

Lambourn, J. & Gill, D. (1978). A controlled comparison of simulated and real ECT. *British Journal of Psychiatry*, **133**, 514–19.

Lauter, H. & Sauer, H. (1987). Electroconvulsive therapy: a German perspective. *Convulsive Therapy*, **3**, 204–9.

Lazarus, A., Jaffe, R. & Dubin, W. (1990). Electroconvulsive therapy and major depression in Down's syndrome. *Journal of Clinical Psychiatry*, **51**, 422–5.

Legendre, S. A., Stern, R. A., Solomon, D. A., Furman, M. J. & Smith, K. E. (2003). The influence of cognitive reserve on memory following electroconvulsive therapy. *Journal of Neuropsychiatry and Clinical Neurosciences*, **15**, 333–9.

Leung, M., Hollander, Y. & Brown, G. R. (2004). Pretreatment with ibuprofen to prevent electroconvulsive therapy-induced headache. *Journal of Clinical Psychiatry*, **64**, 551–3.

Liang, R. A., Lam, R. W. & Ancill, R. J. (1988). ECT in the treatment of mixed depression and dementia. *British Journal of Psychiatry*, **152**, 281–4.

Lindefors, N., Brodin, E. & Metsis, M. (1995). Spatiotemporal selective effects on brain-derived neurotrophic factor and trkB messenger RNa in rat hippocampus by electroconvulsive shock. *Neuroscience*, **65**, 661–70.

Lipman, R. S., Backup, C., Bobrin, Y. *et al.* (1986). Dexamethasone suppression test as a predictor of response to electroconvulsive therapy. I. Inpatient treatment. *Convulsive Therapy*, **2**, 151–60.

Lisanby, S. H., Bazil, C. E., Resor, S. R., Nobler, M. S., Finck, D. A. & Sackeim, H. A. (2001). ECT in the treatment of status epilepticus. *Journal of ECT*, **17**, 210–15.

Lisanby, S. H., Maddox, J. H., Prudic, J., Devanand, D. P. & Sackeim, H. A. (2000). The effects of electroconvulsive therapy on memory of autobiographical and public events. *Archives in General Psychiatry*, **57**, 581–90.

Loo, H., Galinowski, A., De Carvalho, W., Bourdel, M. C. & Poirier, M. F. (1991). Use of maintenance ECT for elderly depressed patients. *American Journal of Psychiatry*, **148**, 810.

Lopez, J. F., Chalmers, D. T., Little, K. Y., Watson, S. J. & Bennett, A. E. (1998). Regulation of serotonin1 A, glucocorticoid, and mineralocorticoid receptor in rat and human hippocampus: implications for the neurobiology of depression. *Biological Psychiatry*, **43**, 547–73.

Magni, G., Fisman, M. & Helmes, E. (1988). Clinical correlates of ECT-resistant depression in the elderly. *Journal of Clinical Psychiatry*, **49**, 405–7.

Mander, A. J., Whitfield, A., Kean, D., Smith, M. A., Douglas, R. H. & Kendell, R. E. (1987). Cerebral and brain stem changes after ECT revealed by nuclear magnetic resonance imaging. *British Journal of Psychiatry*, **151**, 69–71.

Manly, D. T., Oakley, S. P. Jr & Bloch, R. M. (2000). Electroconvulsive therapy in old-old patients. *American Journal of Geriatric Psychiatry*, **8**, 232–6.

Mann, S. C., Caroff, S. N., Bleier, H. R., Welz, W. K., Kling, M. A. & Hayashida, M. (1986). Lethal catatonia. *American Journal of Psychiatry*, **143**, 1374–81.

Mann, S. C., Caroff, S. N., Bleier, H. R., Antelo, R. E. & Un, H. (1990). Electroconvulsive therapy of the lethal catatonia syndrome. *Convulsive Therapy*, **6**, 239–47.

Mann, S. C., Caroff, S. N., Fricchione, G. L. & Greenstein, R. A. (2004). Malignant catatonia. In *Catatonia: from Psychopathology to Neurobiology*, ed. S. N. Caroff, S. C. Mann, A. Francais & G. L. Fricchione, pp. 105–19. Washington, DC: American Psychiatric Publishing, Inc.

Markowitz, J. S., Kellner, C. H., DeVane, C. L. *et al.* (2001). Intranasal sumatriptan in post-ECT headache: results of an open-label trial. *Journal of ECT*, **17**, 280–3.

Martin, J. L., Barbanoj, M. J., Schlaepfer, T. E. *et al.* (2003). Repetitive transcranial magnetic stimulation for the treatment of depression. Systematic review and meta-analysis. *British Journal of Psychiatry*, **182**, 480–91.

Mattes, J. A., Pettinati, H. M., Stephens, S., Robin, S. E. & Willis, K. W. (1990). A placebo-controlled evaluation of vasopressin for ECT-induced memory impairment. *Biological Psychiatry*, **27**, 289–303.

McCall, W. V., Reboussin, D. M., Weiner, R. D. & Sackeim, H. A. (2000). Titrated moderately suprathreshold vs fixed high-dose right unilateral electroconvulsive therapy: acute antidepressant and cognitive effects. *Archives of General Psychiatry*, **57**, 438–44.

McDonald, I. M., Perkins, G., Marjerrison, G. & Podilsky, M. (1966). A controlled comparison of amitriptyline and electroconvulsive therapy in the treatment of depression. *American Journal of Psychiatry*, **122**, 1427–31.

McDonald, W. M. & Thompson, T. R. (2001). Treatment of mania in dementia with electroconvulsive therapy. *Psychopharmacology Bulletin*, **35**, 72–82.

McElhiney, M. C., Moody, B. J., Steif, B. L., Prudic, J., Devanand, D. P. & Nobler, M. S. (1995). Autobiographical memory and mood effects of electroconvulsive therapy. *Neuropsychology*, **9**, 501–17.

Meldrum, B. S. (1986). Neuropathological consequences of chemically and electrically induced seizures. *Annals of the New York Academy of Sciences*, **462**, 186–93.

Merrill, R. D. (1990). ECT for a patient with profound mental retardation. *American Journal of Psychiatry*, **147**, 256–7.

Miller, D. H., Clancy, J. & Cummings, F. (1953). A comparison between unidirectional current nonconvulsive electrical stimulation, alternating current electroshock and pentothal in chronic schizophrenia. *American Journal of Psychiatry*, **109**, 617–20.

Miller, L. J. (1994). Use of electroconvulsive therapy during pregnancy. *Hospital and Community Psychiatry*, **45**, 444–50.

Moise, F. N. & Petrides, G. (1996). Case study: electroconvulsive therapy in adolescents.[see comment]. *Journal of the American Academy of Child and Adolescent Psychiatry*, **35**, 312–18.

Moreno, E. M., Martin, M. J., Sanchez, V. J. & Vazquez, G. T. (1998). Electroconvulsive therapy in the first trimester of pregnancy. *Journal of ECT*, **14**, 251–4.

Monroe, R. R., Jr (1991). Maintenance electroconvulsive therapy. *Psychiatric Clinics of North America*, **14**, 947–60.

Mukherjee, S., Sackeim, H. A. & Lee, C. (1988). Unilateral ECT in the treatment of manic episodes. *Convulsive Therapy*, **4**, 74–80.

Mukherjee, S., Sackeim, H. A. & Schnur, D. B. (1994). Electroconvulsive therapy of acute manic episodes: a review of 50 years' experience. *American Journal of Psychiatry*, **151**, 169–76.

Mulsant, B. H., Haskett, R. F., Prudic, J. *et al.* (1997). Low use of neuroleptic drugs in the treatment of psychotic major depression. *American Journal of Psychiatry*, **154**, 559–61.

Murray, G. B., Shea, V. & Conn, D. K. (1986). Electroconvulsive therapy for poststroke depression. *Journal of Clinical Psychiatry*, **47**, 258–60.

Nibuya, M., Morinobu, S. & Duman, R. S. (1995). Regulation of BDNF and trkB mRNS in rat brain by chronic electroconvulsive seizure and antidepressant drug treatments. *Journal of Neuroscience*, **15**, 7539–47.

Nobler, M. S., Sackeim, H. A., Solomou, M., Luber, B., Devanand, D. P. & Prudic, J. (1993). EEG manifestations during ECT: effects of electrode placement and stimulus intensity. *Biological Psychiatry*, **34**, 321–30.

Nobler, M. S., Luber, B., Moeller, J. R. *et al.* (2000). Quantitative EEG during seizures induced by electroconvulsive therapy: relations to treatment modality and clinical features. I. Global analyses. *Journal of ECT*, **16**, 211–28.

O'Connell, B. K., Towfighi, J., Kofke, W. A. & Hawkins, R. A. (1988). Neuronal loss in mercaptopropionic acid-induced status epilepticus. *Acta Neuropathologica*, **77**, 47–54.

O'Connor, M. K., Knapp, R., Husain, M. *et al.* (2001). The influence of age on the response of major depression to electroconvulsive therapy: a C.O.R.E. Report. *American Journal of Geriatric Psychiatry*, **9**, 382–90.

O'Connor, T. G., Heron, J., Golding, J., Beveridge, M. & Glover, V. (2002). Maternal antenatal anxiety and children's behavioural/

emotional problems at 4 years. Report from the Avon Longitudinal Study of Parents and children. *British Journal of Psychiatry*, **180**, 502–8.

Oms, A., Miro, E. & Rojo, J. E. (1998). Sumatriptan was effective in electroconvulsive therapy (ECT) headache. *Anesthesiology*, **89**, 1291–2.

Pagnin, D., de Queiroz, V., Pini, S. & Cassano, G. B. (2004). Efficacy of ECT in depression: a meta-analytic review. *Journal of ECT*, **20**, 13–20.

Pande, A. C., Grunhaus, L. J., Aisen, A. M. & Haskett, R. F. (1990). A preliminary magnetic resonance imaging study of ECT-treated depressed patients. *Biological Psychiatry*, **27**, 91–3.

Parker, G., Hadzi-Pavlovic, D., Brodaty, H., Boyce, P., Mitchell, P., Wilhelm, K. & Hickie, I. (1992). Predicting the course of melancholic and nonmelancholic depression. A naturalistic comparison study. *Journal of Nervous and Mental Disease*, **180**, 693–702.

Pascual-Leone, A., Rubio, B., Pallardo, F. & Catala, M. D. (1996). Rapid-rate transcranial magnetic stimulation of left dorsolateral prefrontal cortex in drug-resistant depression. *Lancet*, **348**, 233–7.

Perera, T. D., Luber, B., Nobler, M. S., Prudic, J., Anderson, C. & Sackeim, H. A. (2004). Seizure expression during electroconvulsive therapy: relationships with clinical outcome and cognitive side effects. *Neuropsychopharmacology*, **29**, 813–25.

Petrides, G., Dhossche, D., Fink, M. & Francis, A. (1994). Continuation ECT: relapse prevention in affective disorders. *Convulsive Therapy*, **10**, 189–94.

Petrides, G., Fink, M., Husain, M. M. *et al.* (2001). ECT remission rates in psychotic versus nonpsychotic depressed patients: a report from CORE. *Journal of ECT*, **17**, 244–53.

Petrides, G., Malur, C. & Fink, M. (2004). Convulsive therapy. In *Catatonia: from Psychopathology to Neurobiology*, ed. S. N. Caroff, S. C. Mann & G. L. Fricchione, pp. 151–60. Washington, DC: American Psychiatric Publishing, Inc.

Philbrick, K. L. & Rummans, T. A. (1994). Malignant catatonia. *Journal of Neuropsychiatry and Clinical Neurosciences*, **6**, 1–13.

Poindexter, A. R. (1989). Psychotropic drug patterns in a large ICF/MR facility: a ten-year experience. *American Journal of Mental Retardation*, **93**, 624–6.

Post, R. M., Weiss, S. R. B. & Pert, A. (1988). Cocaine-induced behavioral sensitizations and kindling: implications for emergence of psychopathology and seizures. *Annals of the New York Academy of Sciences*, **537**, 292–308.

Post, R. M., Putnam, F., Contel, N. R. & Goldman, B. (1984). Electroconvulsive seizures inhibit amygdala kindling: implications for mechanisms of action in affective illness. *Epilepsia*, **25**, 234–9.

Pridmore, S., Bruno, R., Turnier-Shea, Y., Red, P. & Rybak, M. (2000). Comparison of unlimited numbers of rapid transcranial magnetic stimulation (rTMS) and ECT treatment sessions in major depressive episode. *International Journal of Neuropharmacology*, **3**, 129–34.

Prudic, J. & Sackeim, H. A. (1999). Electroconvulsive therapy and suicide risk. *Journal of Clinical Psychiatry*, **60** (Suppl. 2), 104–10.

Prudic, J., Sackeim, H. A. & Devanand, D. P. (1990). Medication resistance and clinical response to electroconvulsive therapy. *Psychiatry Research*, **31**, 287–96.

Prudic, J., Haskett, R. F., Mulsant, B. *et al.* (1996). Resistance to antidepressant medications and short-term clinical response to ECT. *American Journal of Psychiatry*, **153**, 985–92.

Prudic, J., Olfson, M., Marcus, S. C., Fuller, R. B. & Sackeim, H. A. (2004). Effectiveness of electroconvulsive therapy in community settings. *Biological Psychiatry*, **55**, 301–12.

Puri, B. K., Langa, A., Coleman, R. M. & Singh, I. (1992). The clinical efficacy of maintenance electroconvulsive therapy in a patient with a mild mental handicap. *British Journal of Psychiatry*, **161**, 707–9.

Rami-Gonzales, L., Salamero, M., Boget, T., Catalan, R., Ferrer, J. & Bernardo (2003). Pattern of cognitive dysfunction in depressive patients during maintenance electroconvulsive therapy. *Psychiatry in Medicine*, **33**, 345–50.

Rasmussen, K. G. Jr, Russell, J. C., Kung, S., Rummans, T. A., Rae-Stuart, E. & O'Connor, M. K. (2003). Electroconvulsive therapy for patients with major depression and probable Lewy body dementia. *Journal of ECT*, **19**, 103–9.

Regenold, W. T., Weintraub, D. & Taller, A. (1998). Electroconvulsive therapy for epilepsy and major depression. *American Journal of Geriatric Psychiatry*, **6**, 180–3.

Reisner, A. D. (2003). The electroconvulsive therapy controversy: evidence and ethics. *Neuropsychological Review*, **13**, 199–219.

Rey, J. M. & Walter, G. (1997). Half a century of ECT use in young people. *American Journal of Psychiatry*, **154**, 595–602.

Rifkin, A. (1988). ECT versus tricyclic antidepressants in depression: a review of the evidence. *Journal of Clinical Psychiatry*, **49**, 3–7.

Roberts, J. K. A. (1986). Neuropsychiatric complications of mental retardation. *Psychiatric Clinics of North America*, **9**, 647–57.

Robinson, R. G., Bolduc, P. L. & Price, T. R. (1987). Two-year longitudinal study of poststroke mood disorders: diagnosis and outcome at one and two years. *Stroke*, **18**, 837–943.

Roccaforte, W. H., Wengel, S. P. & Burke, W. J. (2000). ECT for screaming in dementia. *American Journal of Geriatric Psychiatry*, **8**, 177.

Rosenberg, J. & Pettinati, H. M. (1984). Differential memory complaints after bilateral and unilateral ECT. *Amerian Journal of Psychiatry*, **141**, 1071–4.

Rossi, A., Stratta, P., Nistico, R., Sabatini, M. D., Di Michele, V. & Casacchia, M. (1990). Visuospatial impairment in depression: a controlled ECT study. *Acta Psychiatrica Scandinavica*, **81**, 245–9.

Roy, A. & Draper, R. (1995). Suicide among psychiatric hospital in-patients. *Psychological Medicine*, **25**, 199–202.

Roy, C. R. & Overdyk, F. J. (1997). The adult patient. In *Patient Safety in Anesthetic Practice*, ed. R. C. Morell & J. H. Eichorn. St. Louis, MI: Churchill Livingstone.

Sackeim, H. A. (1986). Acute cognitive side effects of ECT. *Psychopharmacological Bulletin*, **22**, 482–548.

Sackeim, H. A. (1992). The cognitive effects of electroconvulsive therapy. In *Cognitive Disorders: Pathophysiology and Treatment*, ed. W. H. Moos, E. R. Gamzu & L. J. Thal. New York: Marcel Dekker.

Sackeim, H. A. (1999). The anticonvulsant hypothesis of the mechanisms of action of ECT: current status. *Journal of ECT*, **15**, 5–26.

Sackeim, H. A., Decina, P., Prohovnik, I., Malitz, S. & Resor, S. R. (1983). Anticonvulsant and antidepressant properties of electroconvulsive therapy: a proposed mechanism of action. *Biological Psychiatry*, **18**, 1301–10.

Sackeim, H. A., Portnoy, S., Neeley, P., Steif, B. L., Decina, P. & Malitz, S. (1987). Cognitive consequences of low-dose electroconvulsive therapy. *Annals of the New York Academy of Sciences*, **462**, 326–40.

Sackeim, H. A., Decina, P., Kanzler, M., Kerr, B. & Malitz, S. (1987). Effects of electrode placement on the efficacy of titrated, low-dose ECT. *American Journal of Psychiatry*, **144**, 1449–55.

Sackeim, H. A., Freeman, J., McElhiney, M. C., Coleman, E., Prudic, J. & Devanand, D. P. (1992). Effects of major depression on estimates of intelligence. *Journal of Clinical and Experimental Neuropsychology*, **14**, 268–88.

Sackeim, H. A., Prudic, J., Devanand, D. P. et al. (1993). Effects of stimulus intensity and electrode placement on the efficacy and cognitive effects of electroconvulsive therapy. *New England Journal of Medicine*, **328**, 839–46.

Sackeim, H. A., Prudic, J., Devanand, D. P. (2000). A prospective, randomized, double-blind comparison of bilateral and right unilateral ECT at different stimulus intensities. *Archives of General Psychiatry*, **57**, 425–34.

Sackeim, H. A., Haskett, R. F., Mulsant, B. H. et al. (2001). Continuation pharmacotherapy in the prevention of relapse following electroconvulsive therapy: a randomized controlled trial. *Journal of the American Medical Association*, **285**, 1299–307.

Sapolsky, R. M. (2000). Glucocorticoids and hippocampal atrophy in neuropsychiatric disorders. *Archives of General Psychiatry*, **57**, 925–35.

Shiwach, R. S., Reid, W. H. & Carmody, T. J. (2001). An analysis of reported deaths following electroconvulsive therapy in Texas, 1993–1998. *Psychiatric Services*, **52**, 1095–7.

Schneekloth. T. D., Rummans, T. A. & Logan, K. M. (1993). Electroconvulsive therapy in adolescents. *Convulsive Therapy*, **9**, 158–66.

Schnur, D. B., Mukherjee, S., Silver, J., Degreef, G. & Lee, C. (1989). Electroconvulsive therapy in the treatment of episodic aggressive dyscontrol in psychotic patients. *Convulsive Therapy*, **5**, 353–61.

Schwarz, T., Loewenstein, J. & Isenberg, K. E. (1995). Maintenance ECT: indications and outcome. *Convulsive Therapy*, **11**, 14–23.

Scott, A. I. & Turnbull, L. W. (1990). Do repeated courses of ECT cause brain damage detectable by MRI? *American Journal of Psychiatry*, **147**, 371–2.

Scott, B. W., Wojtowicz, J. M. & Burnham, W. M. (2000). Neurogenesis in the dentate gyrus of the rat following electroconvulsive shock seizures. *Experimental Neurology*, **165**, 231–6.

Serra, M., Pisul, M. G., Dazzi, L., Purdy, R. H. & Biggio, G. (2002). Prevention of the stress-induced increase in the concentration of neuroactive steroids in rat brain by long-term administration of mirtazapine but not of fluoxetine. *Journal of Psychopharmacology*, **16**, 133–8.

Sharma, V. (1999). Retrospective controlled study of inpatient ECT; does it prevent suicide? *Journal of Affective Disorders*, **56**, 183–7.

Sharma, V. (2001). The effect of electroconvulsive therapy on suicide risk in patients with mood disorders. *Canadian Journal of Psychiatry*, **46**, 704–9.

Shulman, R. B. (2003). Maintenance ECT in the treatment of PD. Therapy improves psychotic symptoms, physical function. *Geriatrics*, **58**, 43–5.

Sikdar, S., Kulhara, P., Avasthi, A. & Singh, H. (1994). Combined chlorpromazine and electroconvulsive therapy in mania. *British Journal of Psychiatry*, **164**, 806–10.

Small, J. G., Klapper, M. H., Kellams, J. J. et al. (1988). Electroconvulsive treatment compared with lithium in the management of manic states. *Archives of General Psychiatry*, **45**, 727–32.

Smith, M. A., Zhang, L. X., Lyons, W. E. & Mamounas, L. A. (1997). Anterograde transport of endogenous brain-derived neurotrophic factor in hippocampal mossy fibers. *NeuroReport*, **8**, 1829–34.

Sobin, C., Sackeim, H. A., Prudic, J., Devanand, D. P., Moody, B. J. & McElhiney, M. C. (1995). Predictors of retrograde amnesia following ECT. *American Journal of Psychiatry*, **152**, 995–1001.

Squire, L. R., Cohen, N. & Zouzounis, J. (1984). Preserved amnesia and bilateral electroconvulsive therapy. Long-term follow-up. *Archives of General Psychiatry*, **38**, 89–95.

Squire, L. R. & Slater, P. C. (1983). Electroconvulsive therapy and complaints of memory dysfunction: a prospective three-year follow-up study. *British Journal of Psychiatry*, **142**, 1–8.

Strober, M., Rao, U., DeAntonio, M. et al. (1998). Effects of electroconvulsive therapy in adolescents with severe endogenous depression resistant to pharmacotherapy. *Biological Psychiatry*, **43**, 335–8.

Suppes, T., Webb, A., Carmody, T. et al. (1996). Is postictal electrical silence a predictor of response to electroconvulsive therapy? *Journal of Affective Disorders*, **41**, 55–8.

Suzuki, K., Awata, S. & Matsuoka, H. (2003). Short-term effect of ECT in middle-aged and elderly patients with intractable catatonic schizophrenia. *Journal of ECT*, **19**, 73–80.

Swartz, C. M. (1989). Safety and ECT stimulus electrodes: I. Heat liberation at the electrode skin interface. *Convulsive Therapy*, **5**, 171–5.

Swartz, C. M. (1994). Asymmetric bilateral right frontotemporal left frontal stimulus electrode placement for electroconvulsive therapy. *Neuropsychobiology*, **29**, 174–8.

Takaoka, K. & Takata, T. (2003). Catatonia in childhood and adolescence. *Psychiatry and Clinical Neuroscience*, **57**, 129–37.

Tang, W. K. & Ungvari, G. S. (2003). Efficacy of electroconvulsive therapy in treatment-resistant schizophrenia: a prospective open trial. *Progress in Neuro-Psychopharmacology and Biological Psychiatry*, **27**, 373–9.

Tanney, B. L. (1986). Electroconvulsive therapy and suicide. *Suicide and Life Threatening Behavior*, **16**, 116–40.

Taylor, M. A. (1982). Indications for electroconvulsive therapy. In *Electroconvulsive Therapy: Biological Foundations and Clinical Applications*, ed. R. Abrams & W. B. Essman, pp. 7–40. New York: Spectrum Publications.

Taylor, M. A. (2001). Use of suprathreshold electroconvulsive therapy. *Archives of General Psychiatry*, **58**, 607.

Taylor, M. A. & Abrams, R. (1985). Short-term cognitive effects of unilateral and bilateral ECT. *British Journal of Psychiatry*, **146**, 308–11.

Taylor, M. A. & Fink, M. (2006). *Melancholia: The Diagnosis, Pathophysiology, and Treatment of Depressive Illness.* Cambridge: Cambridge University Press.

Taylor, P. J. & Fleminger, J. J. (1980). ECT for schizophrenia. *Lancet*, **I**, 380–82.

Tew, J. D., Jr, Mulsant, B. H., Haskett, R. F. *et al.* (1999). Acute efficacy of ECT in the treatment of major depression in the old-old. *American Journal of Psychiatry*, **156**, 1865–70.

Thienhaus, O. J., Margletta, S. & Bennett, J. A. (1990). A study of the clinical efficacy of maintenance ECT. *Journal of Clinical Psychiatry*, **51**, 141–4.

Thompson, J. W., Weiner, R. D. & Myers, C. P. (1994). Use of ECT in the United States in 1975, 1980, and 1986. *American Journal of Psychiatry*, **151**, 1657–61.

Thornton, J. E., Mulsant, B. H., Dealy, R. & Reynolds, C. F. (1990). Retrospective study of maintenance electroconvulsive therapy in a university-based psychiatry practice. *Convulsive Therapy*, **6**, 121–9.

Thuppal, M. & Fink, M. (1999). Electroconvulsive therapy and mental retardation. *Journal of ECT*, **15**, 140–9.

Tomac, T. A., Rummans, T. A., Pileggi, T. S. & Li, H. (1997). Safety and efficacy of electroconvulsive therapy in patients over age 85. *American Journal of Geriatric Psychiatry*, **5**, 126–30.

Tondo, L., Baldessarini, R. J., Hennen, J., Floris, G., Silvetti, F. & Tohen, M. (1998). Lithium treatment and risk of suicidal behavior in bipolar disorder patients. *Journal of Clinical Psychiatry*, **59**, 405–14.

Trollor, J. N. & Sachdev, P. S. (1999). Electroconvulsive treatment of neuroleptic malignant syndrome: a review and report of cases. *Australia and New Zealand Journal of Psychiatry*, **33**, 650–9.

Tsao, C. I., Jain, S., Gibson, R. H., Guedet, P. J. & Lehrmann, J. A. (2004). Maintenance ECT for recurrent medication-refractory mania. *Journal of ECT*, **20**, 118–19.

Tsuang, M. T., Dempsey, G. M. & Fleming, J. A. (1979). Can ECT prevent premature death and suicide in 'schizoaffective' patients? *Journal of Affective Disorders*, **1**, 167–71.

UK ECT Review Group & Geddes, J. (2003). Efficacy and safety of electroconvulsive therapy in depressive disorders: a systematic review and meta-analysis. *Lancet*, **361**, 799–808.

Ukpong, D. I., Makanjuola, R. O. & Morakinyo, O. (2002). A controlled trial of modified electroconvulsive therapy in schizophrenia in a Nigerian teaching hospital. *West African Journal of Medicine*, **21**, 237–40.

Vaidya, N. A., Maableshwarkar, A. R. & Shahid, R. (2003). Continuation and maintenance ECT in treatment-resistant bipolar disorder. *Journal of ECT*, **19**, 10–16.

Vaidya, V. A., Terwilliger, R. Z. & Duman, R. S. (2000). Alterations in heavy and light neurofilament proteins in hippocampus following chronic ECS administration, *Synapse*, **35**, 137–43.

Van der Wurff, F. B., Stek, M. L., Hoogendijk, W. J. G. & Beekman, A. T. F. (2003). The efficacy and safety of ECT in depressed older adults, a literature review. *International Journal of Geriatric Psychiatry*, **18**, 894–904.

Vanelle, J. M., Loo, H., Galinowski, A. *et al.* (1994). Maintenance ECT in intractable manic-depressive disorders. *Convulsive Therapy*, **10**, 195–205.

Viparelli, U. & Viparelli, G. (1992). ECT and grand-mal epilepsy. *Convulsive Therapy*, **8**, 39–42.

Vothknecht, S., Kho, K. H., van Schaick, H. W., Zwinderman, A. H., Middelkoop, H. & Blansjaar, B. A. (2003). Effects of maintenance electroconvulsant therapy on cognitive functions. *Journal of ECT*, **19**, 151–7.

Walker, R. & Swartz, C. M. (1994). Electroconvulsive therapy during high-risk pregnancy. *General Hospital Psychiatry*, **16**, 348–53.

Walter, G., Rey, J. M. & Starling, J. (1997). Experience, knowledge and attitudes of child psychiatrists regarding electroconvulsive therapy in the young. *Australian and New Zealand Journal of Psychiatry*, **31**, 676–81.

Walter, G., Rey, J. M. & Mitchell, P. B. (1999). Practitioner review: electroconvulsive therapy in adolescents. *Journal of Child Psychology and Psychiatry and Allied Disciplines*, **40**, 325–34.

Weiner, R. D. (1984), Does electroconvulsive therapy cause brain damage? *Behavioral and Brain Sciences*, **7**, 1–53.

Weiner, S. J., Ward, T. N. & Ravaris, C. L. (1994). Headache and electroconvulsive therapy. *Headache*, **34**, 155–9.

Weintraub, D. & Lippmann, S. B. (2000). Electroconvulsive therapy in the acute poststroke period. *Journal of ECT*, **16**, 415–18.

Weintraub, D. & Lippmann, S. B. (2001). ECT for major depression and mania with advanced dementia. *Journal of ECT*, **17**, 65–7.

Wengel, S. P., Burke, W. J., Pfeiffer, R. F., Roccaforte, W. H. & Paige, S. R. (1998). Maintenance electroconvulsive therapy for intractable Parkinson's disease. *American Journal of Geriatric Psychiatry*, **6**, 263–9.

West, E. D. (1981). Electroconvulsive therapy in depression: a double blind controlled trial. *British Medical Journal*, **282**, 355–7.

Zachrisson, O. C., Balldin, J., Ekman, R. *et al.* (2000). No evident neuronal damage after electroconvulsive therapy. *Psychiatry Research*, **96**, 157–65.

Zuckerman, B., Bauchner, H., Parker, S. & Cabral, H. (1990). Maternal depressive symptoms during pregnancy, and newborn irritability. *Journal of Developmental and Behavioral Pediatrics*, **11**, 190–4.

Zyss, T., Gorka, Z., Kowalska, M. & Vetulani, J. (1997). Preliminary comparison of behavioral and biochemical effects of chronic transcranial magnetic stimulation and electroconvulsive shock in the rat. *Biological Psychiatry*, **42**, 920–4.

4

Section II – Focal brain stimulation approaches to psychiatric treatment: Transcranial magnetic stimulation (TMS), magnetic seizure therapy (MST), vagus nerve stimulation (VNS), deep brain stimulation (DBS) and transcranial direct current stimulation (tDCS)

Antonio Mantovani, Arielle D. Stanford, Peter Bulow and Sarah H. Lisanby

Editor's note

This chapter illustrates how fast-growing are effective treatments in psychiatry. Twenty years ago the contents of this chapter would hardly be understood by the average clinician; now each new treatment is hammering on the door of clinical practice demanding to be let in. The most researched treatment is transcranial magnetic stimulation (TMS); this has been shown clearly to have antidepressant efficacy and, although not as effective as ECT in severe depression, has fewer adverse effects. All the other treatments are really at the early stage of clinical experience and are not first-line treatments. Magnetic seizure therapy and vagus nerve stimulation may have a role in treatment-resistant depression and deep brain stimulation (DBS) is likely to replace the various forms of leucotomy still practiced in some parts of the world, mainly because DBS can be controlled and directed so much more specifically than the older treatments. Transcranial direct current stimulation (tDCS) may also have antidepressant effects but more studies are needed. We will all be hearing more about these new treatments which have the potential to replace ECT, leucotomy and related treatments entirely.

Introduction

Advances in the science and technology of neuromodulation over the past two decades have led to several interventions that have rekindled clinical and research interest in nonpharmacological somatic therapies.

Although electroconvulsive therapy (ECT) remains the only somatic treatment with widespread acceptance and application based upon 70 years of clinical use, transcranial magnetic stimulation (TMS), magnetic seizure therapy (MST), vagus nerve stimulation (VNS), deep brain stimulation (DBS) and transcranial direct current stimulation (tDCS), all offer novel means of potentially treating neuropsychiatric conditions and may provide a better understanding of the brain pathophysiology of these disorders. This chapter describes some of these newer somatic interventions now available and reviews the evidence of their effectiveness and future potential in psychiatric treatment (Table 4.II.1).

Lessons from ECT and the rationale for focal brain stimulation

Despite the excellent efficacy of ECT in severe major depression, its use is limited by its cognitive side effects that decrease its acceptance by patients and some clinicians (Lisanby *et al.*, 2000; Prudic *et al.*, 2000; American Psychiatric Association, 2001). The antidepressant properties of ECT and its effects on cognition are separable (Sackeim, 1992; Lerer *et al.*, 1995; McElhiney *et al.*, 1995; Lisanby *et al.*, 2000), and considerable progress has been made in altering the ECT technique to maintain efficacy while reducing cognitive side effects (Benbow, 2005). Nonetheless, the forms of ECT with the most well-established efficacy/side-effect profile reviewed elsewhere in this volume still result in a substantial side-effect burden (Sackeim *et al.*, 1993, 2000; Bailine *et al.*, 2000; Delva *et al.*,

2000; McCall *et al.*, 2000). This reality highlights the need to develop novel somatic approaches to psychiatric treatment.

The development of these novel somatic approaches has been guided to a large degree by the evidence provided by the ECT literature regarding the relations among site of stimulation, electrical dosage and clinical outcome. A growing body of evidence suggests that electrical dosage and the intracerebral pathway of the electrical current are critical for determining both efficacy and side effects (Sackeim *et al.*, 1986, 1993, 1996, 2000; Abrams *et al.*, 1991; Nobler *et al.*, 1994; McCall *et al.*, 2000). Depending on the combination of stimulus intensity and electrode position, antidepressant response rates with ECT vary from below 20% to 70% or higher (Sackeim *et al.*, 1993, 2000; McCall *et al.*, 2000). Right unilateral (RUL) ECT results in less intense and persistent adverse cognitive effects than bilateral (BL) ECT, but RUL ECT can either be highly ineffective or effective, depending upon the electrical dosage relative to the seizure threshold (Sackeim *et al.*, 1993, 2000; Ng *et al.*, 2000). Supporting these clinical findings, dissociable alterations in regional brain activity, as reflected in regional cerebral blood flow (rCBF) (Awata *et al.*, 2002; Nobler *et al.*, 1994), glucose cerebral metabolic rate (Henry *et al.*, 2001; Nobler *et al.*, 2001), and electroencephalographic (EEG) measures (Sackeim *et al.*, 1996, 2000), correlate with the efficacy and objective cognitive side effects of ECT. For example, antidepressant response has been linked to increased EEG power and decreased rCBF in prefrontal regions, while retrograde amnesia for autobiographical memories has been linked to increased left frontotemporal EEG τ power (Luber *et al.*, 2000; Sackeim *et al.*, 1996, 2000). These findings suggest that a technique that can target the induced current to regions implicated in antidepressant response, while sparing regions implicated in adverse cognitive effects, would maintain efficacy and have a superior side-effect profile. This advantage would be accentuated if such a focal brain stimulation technique also offered better control not only over intracerebral current pathways (i.e. spatial targeting of regions) but also over intracerebral current density (i.e. dosage).

The transcranial application of an electrical stimulus is a fundamental limitation in making brain stimulation more focal. The high impedance of the skull (Geddes & Baker, 1967; Rush & Driscoll, 1968; Driscoll, 1970) shunts 80–97% of the electrical stimulus away from the brain (Smitt & Wegener, 1944; Hayes, 1950; Law, 1993). There are various ways to avoid this problem by indirectly inducing electricity in the brain using magnetic fields (as in TMS and MST), electrically stimulating a cranial nerve that in turn changes brain function (VNS), implanting electrodes directly in the brain (DBS), and polarizing the brain with direct currents (transcranial direct current stimulation, tDCS). Each of these approaches is reviewed below.

Transcranial magnetic stimulation (TMS) and magnetic seizure therapy (MST)

Stimulating the brain with repetitive transcranial magnetic stimulation (rTMS) could obviate some of the limitations of electrical stimulation by inducing intra-cerebral current non-invasively using rapidly alternating magnetic fields (Barker *et al.*, 1985; Pascual-Leone *et al.*, 1993). The scalp and skull are transparent to magnetic fields and then a major source of individual differences in the intensity and spatial distribution of intra-cerebral current density is removed. In addition, depending principally on coil geometry, the magnetic field can be spatially targeted, and this offers further control over intra-cerebral current paths (Maccabee *et al.*, 1990, 1991; Brasil-Neto *et al.*, 1992; Mills *et al.*, 1992). However, the electrical field induced by rTMS is capable of neural depolarization only to about 2 cm below the scalp (i.e. grey–white matter junction), so direct effects are limited to the superficial cortex (Epstein, 1990). When rTMS is given at high dosages, it can induce seizures. This is termed magnetic seizure therapy (MST). Measurements in nonhuman primates with intracerebral multicontact electrodes support the hypothesis that rTMS-induced current and MST-induced seizures are more focal than those obtained with ECT (Lisanby *et al.*, 1998a, 1998b, 2003a; Lisanby & Sackeim, 2002). Thus, magnetic stimulation holds the promise of more precise control over current pathways and current density in neural tissue.

A growing number of studies have examined the effects of subconvulsive levels of rTMS in depression, mania, schizophrenia, obsessive-compulsive disorder, post-traumatic stress disorder and panic disorder (for reviews, see George *et al.*, 1999; Lisanby & Sackeim, 2000; Wassermann & Lisanby, 2001; Burt *et al.*, 2002). While prior work had shown that subconvulsive levels of ECT are not effective for depression (Gottesfeld *et al.*, 1944; Hargrove *et al.*, 1953; Ulett *et al.*, 1956), it was not known whether the same would be true for rTMS, particularly since a single electrical train was applied for subconvulsive ECT while repeated trains were given with subconvulsive rTMS. Indeed, work with subconvulsive rTMS challenges the view that a seizure is necessary for brain stimulation techniques to exert antidepressant effects (George & Wassermann, 1994).

Evidence for the effectiveness of rTMS in psychiatry

Major depression

Major depression has been the focus of the bulk of the clinical trials with rTMS to date. Initial work used nonfocal coils positioned over the vertex and found some suggestions of clinical benefit. Based on evidence for prefrontal abnormalities in depression, it was thought that rTMS over prefrontal cortex could produce a more profound antidepressant effect than over other cortical areas. To test this hypothesis, using a within-subject crossover design, Pascual-Leone et al. (1996) reported that high frequency left dorsolateral prefrontal cortex (DLPFC) rTMS for 5 days had marked antidepressant effects even in psychotic depression while stimulation at other sites (right DLPFC, vertex) and sham had no effect. Other studies that followed could not replicate the same magnitude or speed of response using similar parameters and length of stimulation, but extending the treatment to 10 days and increasing the number of pulses per day, a 50% response rate was reported in medication-resistant unipolar depressed patients in an open trial (Triggs et al., 1999). A double-blind, sham-controlled, single-crossover study of fast left DLPFC rTMS in medication-resistant outpatients found improvements with 10 days of active rTMS but the degree of improvement was modest (George et al., 1997). Herwig et al. (2003) reported similar findings with a 30% response rate to real rTMS, and no response with sham.

There are suggestions that longer duration of treatment may result in more significant improvement. Pridmore et al. (1999) was the first to extend the period of treatment to 3 or 4 weeks. Patients with melancholic depression referred for ECT treated with rTMS to the left DLPFC resulted in remission in 88% of cases in an open study. More recently patients with medication-resistant depression were randomized to receive 15 sessions of active or sham rTMS delivered to the left DLPFC (Avery et al., 2006). The response rate for the TMS group was 30.6%, significantly greater than the 6.1% rate in the sham group. The remission rate for the TMS group was 20%, significantly greater than the 3% rate in the sham group. The authors concluded that although all the patients in this study had medication resistance and over half the sample met DSM–IV criteria for chronic depression, rTMS can still produce clinically significant antidepressant effects. An ongoing double-blind sham-controlled multicenter study on the efficacy of rTMS applied to the left DLPFC for 6 weeks will test whether longer periods of stimulation are more effective in a controlled setting, according to data regarding the application of rTMS to treat major depression that a longer period of stimulation could be required to evoke a clinical response (Gershon et al., 2003).

It is still an open question as to whether the antidepressant effects of rTMS are region or frequency-dependent. Klein et al. (1999) randomized depressed outpatients to 2 weeks of active or sham slow (1 Hz) rTMS over right prefrontal cortex using a round, nonfocal coil. In the active group 41% of patients responded compared with 17% with sham. This study suggested that right-sided stimulation might be effective. A much smaller double-blind study replicated these results with the active group showing a better clinical response compared with the sham (Kauffmann et al., 2004).

If lower frequencies are indeed as effective as higher frequencies, this would have significant safety implications, as lower frequencies carry a lower risk of seizure. When low and high frequency have been compared in the same study, there are suggestions that individuals treated with lower frequencies may actually fare better. Kimbrell et al. (1999) found a trend toward better improvement following 2 weeks of 1 Hz rTMS compared with 20 Hz to the left DLPFC in a cross-over design. There were suggestions that baseline metabolic activity in the DLPFC correlated with response. Similarly, Padberg (1999) tested nonpsychotic depressed patients with sham treatment, slow rTMS, or fast rTMS, over the left prefrontal cortex. After 5 days, 83% in the slow group and 50% in the fast group improved, with no change in the sham group. A parallel-design, blinded study from George et al. (2000) suggests that slower (5 Hz) left prefrontal TMS may be as effective as faster (20 Hz) stimulation. Despite these percentages, statistically the results show a trend but do not reach significance, and perhaps different measures of improvement or outcome may improve the significance of the differences. Fitzgerald et al. (2003) demonstrated that both high-frequency left-rTMS and low-frequency right-rTMS have benefits in patients with medication-resistant major depression. They concluded that treatment for at least 4 weeks is necessary for clinically meaningful benefits to be achieved. A four-center NIMH sponsored trial is currently underway which will examine the utility of 1 Hz rTMS to the right prefrontal cortex in patients who fail to respond to high frequency to the left DLPFC. Further, over what period of time rTMS ought to be applied remains a matter of some discussion.

There has been great interest in determining whether rTMS could offer an alternative to ECT for severe or treatment-resistant depression, particularly since the adverse effect profile of rTMS is relatively benign. Using a parallel-group, non-blinded design, Grunhaus et al. (2000) randomly assigned inpatients to treatment with fast left DLPFC rTMS or ECT. Among nonpsychotic patients, up to 4 weeks of daily rTMS was not different in efficacy to ECT, but ECT was superior among psychotically depressed patients. Dannon *et al.* (2002) demonstrated that patients treated with rTMS or ECT showed the same percentage of clinical stabilization at 3 and 6 months of follow-up. Janicak *et al.* (2002) randomized severely depressed patients to be treated with rTMS or ECT. No significant difference in efficacy was found between the two treatments (rTMS, 55%; ECT, 64%). All of these studies have the unavoidable limitation that the patients were not blinded to the form of treatment, and some have questioned whether the ECT comparison group represented optimal ECT practice. Nevertheless, this magnitude of clinical response in ECT referrals is impressive, but we need to look more closely at the type of ECT (uni- versus bilateral), threshold of ECT, and possible effect size before we assume no difference between the two treatments. But it is promising that there is some effort, even early on with this treatment, for head-to-head, so to speak, comparisons, a type of methodology often missing in psychopharmacologic trials.

Several meta-analyses have examined the antidepressant efficacy of rTMS (Holtzheimer *et al.*, 2001; Martin *et al.*, 2002, 2003), and concluded that there is definite evidence for benefit of rTMS; nevertheless, the effect size could only be described as moderate and so of limited clinical significance. For example, Burt *et al.* (2002) found the average percent improvement with active TMS was 28.94% (SD = 23.19) and with sham was 6.63% (SD = 25.56). Relatively few patients met standard criteria for response or remission. It is also true, however, that the meta-analyses are heavily weighted towards the earlier studies that used what may now be considered inadequate dosage and duration of rTMS, in terms of number of pulses per day and number of days of treatment.

Further work using controlled designs is needed to determine whether the antidepressant effects of rTMS are region, frequency, or intensity dependent, and to test the efficacy of more robust parameters in a sample large enough to provide adequate statistical power. Such work is presently under way, with multicenter trials sponsored both by industry and by the NIMH. In particular, an industry-sponsored double-blind sham-controlled multicenter study carried out in 20 centers on the efficacy of high-frequency rTMS applied to the left DLPFC for 6 weeks has tested in 301 patients that more pulses per day (3000 pulses/day) and longer periods of stimulation are effective to evoke a clinical response (results are unpublished at this time).

Mania

Belmaker & Grisaru (1999) tested the hypothesis that the laterality of mania may be opposite to that of depression by randomly assigning manic patients to fast rTMS to the left or right DLPFC as an add-on to standard pharmacological care. After 2 weeks, the group treated on the right DLPFC did better, but they could not replicate the anti-manic effect in a subsequent follow-up study of right active rTMS versus right sham rTMS. It is possible that the previous results were due to an effect of left rTMS to worsen mania, as an antidepressant would. Alternatively, it is noted that the patient group had much more psychosis than the previous study of rTMS in mania, and depression studies have reported that psychosis is a poor prognostic indicator of rTMS response (Kaptsan *et al.*, 2003). A more recent study found 4 weeks of rTMS produced a sustained reduction of manic symptoms in all patients (Michael & Erfurth, 2004). Due to the open and add-on design of the study, a clear causal relationship between rTMS treatment and reduction of manic symptoms cannot be established.

Schizophrenia

As in the case of the early studies in depression, the first rTMS studies in schizophrenia patients employed rTMS administered with a large round coil to the vertex, thereby stimulating broad regions of bilateral prefrontal and parietal cortices. In 1997, Geller *et al.* reported that 60% of medicated chronic schizophrenia patients showed some transient improvement following a single session of rTMS in an open study. Using 2 weeks of 1 Hz rTMS with a smaller round coil positioned on the right prefrontal cortex, Feinsod *et al.* (1998) reported that 70% of treated schizophrenia patients were moderately or markedly improved as evidenced by significant reductions in anxiety and restlessness, but not core schizophrenia symptoms (e.g. psychosis). When the same group followed up their findings with a sham-controlled trial, rTMS did not differ from sham on measures of psychosis (Klein *et al.*, 1999).

Hoffman *et al.* (1999) had more success with 1 Hz rTMS when the coil was positioned over the left temporal-parietal cortex, a region that has shown selective activation during auditory hallucinations (Silbersweig *et al.*, 1995). This trial was based upon the hypothesis that low frequency rTMS may dampen excitability in the region implicated in this specific symptom (Chen *et al.*, 1997). In an initial cross-over study, significant reductions in hallucinations were noted with 4 days of active rTMS compared with sham (Hoffman *et al.*, 1999). Two of three patients experienced a near total cessation of hallucinations for at least 2 weeks. Significant reductions in auditory hallucinations were replicated in larger open (d'Alfonso *et al.*, 2002) and randomized cross-over and parallel designed trials (Hoffman *et al.*, 2000, 2003, 2005). Poulet *et al.* (2005) found that responders maintained improvement for at least 2 months of follow-up. Not all studies have replicated these findings (McIntosh *et al.*, 2004; Schonfeldt-Lecuona *et al.*, 2004; Fitzgerald *et al.*, 2005), although treatment duration was reduced (McIntosh *et al.*, 2004; Schonfeldt-Lecuona *et al.*, 2004) in two of these studies.

Other groups have examined the effects of high frequency rTMS applied to the prefrontal cortex as fronto-temporal loops have been implicated in the pathophysiology of positive symptoms. Early case reports demonstrated improvement in catatonia with high frequency rTMS (Grisaru *et al.*, 1998; Saba *et al.*, 2002). In a 2-week cross-over randomized controlled study high frequency active rTMS significantly decreased psychotic symptoms as well (Rollnik *et al.*, 2000).

Since decreased activity in this region has also been associated with negative symptoms, it was hypothesized that the activating effects of high frequency rTMS might reverse this hypofrontality. Cohen *et al.* (1999) completed an open study of patients who received 20 Hz rTMS to midline prefrontal cortex for at least 2 weeks. They observed a significant reduction in negative symptoms, but tests of frontal cognitive function were essentially unchanged. Other open studies have since replicated this finding (Jandl *et al.*, 2004; Sachdev *et al.*, 2005). In 1999, Nahas administered a single session of 20 Hz rTMS to the left DLPFC in the first sham-controlled cross-over trial. Improvement in negative symptoms was noted the day following treatment. In a longer study, Hajak *et al.* (2004) also found beneficial effects of high-frequency rTMS on negative as well as depressive symptoms, together with a trend for worsening positive symptoms. Interestingly, the improvement in depressive symptoms did not account for the improvement of negative symptoms. Negative results with a randomized trial design have also been reported (Holi *et al.*, 2004). More studies need to be done to determine whether high frequency rTMS will be helpful for negative symptoms.

Panic disorder

Limited studies, mostly case series, have been conducted on the therapeutic applications of rTMS in anxiety disorders. The majority of neuroimaging studies have shown elevated right-sided activity in the frontal and hippocampal-parahippocampal regions in fear paradigms and in anxiety disorders. This has led to the hypothesis that low frequency rTMS may be helpful in dampening the lateralized hyperexcitability, similar to the rationale behind using 1 Hz rTMS for the positive symptoms of schizophrenia.

Zwanzger *et al.* (2002) demonstrated a reduction in panic symptoms with a marked improvement of anxiety in an open case study of a patient treated for two weeks with slow rTMS to the right DLPFC. Anxiety symptoms decreased 78%, and panic/agoraphobia symptoms decreased 59%. Improvements lasted at 1 month follow up. Interestingly, there was a reduction in CCK-4 induced panic attacks, associated with blunting of the CCK-4 induced elevation of ACTH and cortisol usually found with panic attacks. These data demonstrate the downstream biological effects of rTMS. In another open case series, three patients with treatment-resistant panic disorder showed modest improvement with ten rTMS sessions (1 Hz, 110% motor threshold, 30 trains, 60 second duration) to the right DLPFC (Garcia-Toro *et al.*, 2002). Alternating low frequency rTMS to the right DLPFC with 20 Hz rTMS to the left DLPFC failed to produce further benefits.

We recently reported a case series of six patients with panic disorder and comorbid depression showing improvements in both panic and depression and decreases in motor cortex excitability following 2 weeks of 1 Hz rTMS to the right DLPFC (Mantovani *et al.*, 2007). There has yet to be a properly controlled trial of rTMS in the treatment of panic.

Post-traumatic stress disorder

McCann *et al.* (1998) treated two patients with treatment-resistant post-traumatic stress disorder (PTSD), both of whom showed elevated baseline cerebral metabolism on PET. Slow rTMS to the right DLPFC reduced post-traumatic symptoms and reversed the cerebral hyper-metabolism, most markedly in the right prefrontal cortex.

In line with symptom provocation studies that have demonstrated significantly greater activity in patients with PTSD in brain regions associated with motor preparedness in response to threat, Grisaru *et al.* (1998) applied 0.3 Hz rTMS bilaterally to motor cortex of PTSD patients. Although PTSD scores improved transiently, this finding may underestimate the value of such an approach since the stimulation parameters were highly conservative (only 60 pulses per day). Rosenberg *et al.* (2002) hypothesized that left frontal rTMS (either 1 or 5 Hz, 90% of motor threshold, total 6000 stimuli) could mimic the beneficial effect of antidepressant medications in patients with combat PTSD and comorbid major depression. They found that 75% of patients had at least a 50% decrease in depression, but just a minimal improvement in PTSD symptomatology. At the 2-month follow-up, the antidepressant effects were maintained in half the patients. Finally, Cohen *et al.* (2004) found beneficial effects of 10 Hz, but not 1 Hz or sham rTMS, to the right DLPFC in PTSD patients PTSD core symptoms (re-experiencing, avoidance) and other anxiety symptoms in a double-blind sham controlled trial. The frequency specificity of these effects, demonstrated in the context of a well-controlled study, support further exploration of the use of rTMS in this disorder.

Obsessive-compulsive disorder

Neurophysiological data suggest that obsessive-compulsive disorder (OCD) may be associated with reduced cortico-cortical inhibition and a higher than normal level of cortical excitability (Rossi *et al.*, 2005). Using paired-pulse TMS, Greenberg *et al.* (1998, 2000) found that OCD patients, like those with Tourette's syndrome (TS), had markedly decreased intracortical inhibition. Patients with "tic-related" OCD showed the most profound deficit in intracortical inhibition. Additionally, the OCD patients had lower resting and active motor thresholds than healthy volunteers.

Imaging studies of OCD also implicate hyperactivity in a circuit involving orbitofrontal cortex and basal ganglia. To test whether modulating activity in this network could influence OCD symptoms, Greenberg *et al.* (1997) administered rTMS to the right lateral prefrontal, left lateral prefrontal, and a midoccipital (control) site on separate days in a blinded trial. Compulsive urges decreased significantly for 8 hours after right lateral prefrontal rTMS. A short-lasting, modest, and nonsignificant reduction in compulsive urges occurred after left lateral prefrontal rTMS. A recent open study in a group of OCD patients refractory to standard treatments who were randomly assigned to right or left prefrontal fast rTMS found that clinically significant and sustained improvement was observed in one third of patients (Sachdev *et al.*, 2001). Not all studies have produced positive results. A double-blind study using right prefrontal 1 Hz rTMS and a less focal coil failed to find significant effects greater than sham (Alonso *et al.*, 2001).

More work will be needed to clarify whether rTMS will be helpful in OCD, but the availability of a defined neural circuitry should guide the design of such trials. For example, we recently reported improvements in OCD symptoms and normalization of motor cortex excitability following 1 Hz to the supplementary motor area, a selection based upon motor-limbic loops implicated in OCD (Mantovani *et al.*, 2006).

Evidence for the effectiveness of MST in major depression

Magnatic stimulation therapy refers to the use of rTMS to induce a seizure under anesthesia for therapeutic purposes (Sackeim, 1994; Lisanby *et al.*, 2001a; Lisanby, 2004). The goal of MST is to couple the superior spatial precision of magnetic fields with the unparalleled antidepressant action of seizures to create a more tolerable form of convulsive therapy. Forty patients have received MST worldwide since the first patient was treated in 2000 (Lisanby *et al.*, 2001b; Lisanby *et al.*, 2003b). In general, MST has been well-tolerated with no significant adverse events or unanticipated side effects.

In the context of a proof of concept case study, the first depressed patient to receive MST had a 50% drop in Hamilton Depression Ratings Scale (HRSD$_{24}$) scores following four MST sessions; MST was well tolerated with no significant side effects (Lisanby *et al.*, 2001b). A second patient with medication-resistant depression received 12 MST sessions and experienced remission with an 82% drop in HRSD$_{24}$ and final HRSD$_{24} = 6$ (Kosel *et al.*, 2003). Clinical testing with MST in the USA commenced first with a study contrasting MST and ECT in their acute cognitive side effects (Lisanby *et al.*, 2003a) followed by a two-center trial of the antidepressant efficacy of MST (Lisanby *et al.*, 2003b).

Our double-masked, randomized, within-subject trial contrasting the acute cognitive side effects of MST with ultrabrief pulse RUL ECT (selected for its exceptionally low cognitive side-effect burden), found MST was well tolerated with fewer side effects than unilateral ECT and faster recovery of orientation, a measure that predicts the magnitude of long-term retrograde amnesia (Lisanby *et al.*, 2003a; Sobin *et al.*, 1995). Masked neuropsychological assessments revealed advantages of MST relative to ECT. Consistent with the differential impact of MST and ECT on seizure expression and hippocampal effects, the cognitive domains where ECT showed greater impairment than MST were those implicating temporal lobe structures (i.e. memory for recent events, new list learning, category fluency). In contrast, MST and ECT did not differ on tasks more heavily dependent on prefrontal lobe function (i.e. memory for temporal order, verbal fluency).

Marked differences in the nature of the seizures induced by MST and ECT were seen, although both ECT and MST seizures were generalized and resulted in motor convulsion. Compared with ECT, MST seizures had shorter duration, lower ictal EEG amplitude, and less postictal suppression. Subsequent work will need to determine whether these differences have clinical significance. Of note, lower ictal EEG amplitude and less postictal suppression are also seen with ultrabrief pulse RUL ECT, treatment that has strong antidepressant action. Differences were also seen between MST and ECT in their effects on deeper brain structures, as indexed by the seizure-induced surge in serum prolactin and vagally mediated post-stimulation bradycardia (Morales *et al.*, 2003). Less intense ictal expression also has the benefit of requiring lower doses of succinylcholine to protect the body from the motor convulsion.

To examine the antidepressant efficacy of MST, we recently completed a randomized, double-masked, two-center (New York State Psychiatric Institute and University of Texas Southwestern Medical Center) study comparing two forms of MST in their antidepressant properties and side effects (Lisanby *et al.*, 2003b). This work established the feasibility and tolerability of MST in clinical settings, and provided the first controlled data on the antidepressant efficacy of MST. More work needs to be done to characterize the long-term side-effect profile and antidepressant efficacy of MST relative to ECT, but these early studies are promising and are being followed up with another multicenter trial.

Vagus nerve stimulation

Based on a large body of literature demonstrating that stimulation of the vagus nerve and its sensory afferent connections through the nucleus tractus solitarius (NTS) could produce slowing of the EEG (Bailey & Bremer, 1938; Dell & Olson, 1951), Zabara (1985) demonstrated an anticonvulsant action of VNS on experimental seizures in dogs. Zabara hypothesized that vagus nerve stimulation (VNS) could prevent or control the motor and autonomic components of epilepsy. Since the mid-1990s, VNS has been used in the treatment of resistant partial-onset seizures (Penry & Dean, 1990; Uthman *et al.*, 1993).

The vagus nerve is composed mostly of sensory afferents carrying information to the brain from the thorax, abdomen, head and neck. The vagal sensory afferent cell bodies are located in the nodose ganglion and convey information to the NTS, which sends projections along three pathways: an autonomic feedback loop, direct projections to the medullary reticular formation and ascending projections to the forebrain. The latter travels via the parabrachial nucleus (PBN) and locus coeruleus (LC), which have direct connections with the forebrain, thalamus, hypothalamus, amygdala and stria terminalis, regions important in the modulation of mood (George *et al.*, 1997; Van Bockstaele *et al.*, 1999).

The electrical pulse generator is implanted in the left chest wall and delivers electrical signals via a bipolar lead to an electrode that is wrapped around the left vagus nerve in the neck (Amar *et al.*, 1998). The pulse generator is programmed telemetrically. The adverse effects of VNS are those associated with the surgical implantation and those that are related to the stimulation, including pain, coughing, vocal cord paralysis, hoarseness, nausea and very occasionally infection. The majority of these are transient and are described by most patients as moderate (Schachter & Saper, 1998).

Initial reports of mood changes in patients receiving VNS for the treatment of epilepsy prompted speculation that VNS may have antidepressant activity (Harden *et al.*, 1999; Elger *et al.*, 2000). In support of this hypothesis there are reports that VNS increases central noradrenergic, serotonergic, and dopaminergic neurotransmission (Krahl *et al.*, 1998; Jobe *et al.*, 1999; Carpenter *et al.*, 2004), and that like other effective antidepressant therapies, it alters frontal, limbic (particularly the cingulate) and thalamic blood flow (Henry *et al.*, 1999; Devous, 2001; Conway *et al.*, 2002). Depending upon the frequency of stimulation, Lomarev *et al.* (2002) found that VNS increased BOLD-fMRI response in the orbitofrontal cortex, frontal pole, hypothalamus, left pallidum, and less significantly, the thalamus, confirming the previous study by Bohning *et al.* (2001).

Evidence for the effectiveness of VNS in psychiatry

Major depression

In a multicenter study open-label trial, 30 depressed patients underwent 10 weeks of VNS, and 40% of patients reported a significant reduction in mood, and several aspects of neuropsychological function improved (Sackeim *et al.*, 2001a). Adding 30 patients to the original open-label cohort, it was reported that VNS was ineffective in patients who had not satisfactorily responded to seven or more adequate antidepressant trials during the current major depressive episode (Sackeim *et al.*, 2001b). Longer-term follow-up studies suggest that improvements are largely sustained over time. Responders at 3 months (acute study exit) largely remained responders at 12 months (91%). More recently a 10-week, acute, randomized, controlled, masked trial compared adjunctive VNS with sham treatment in 235 outpatients with nonpsychotic major depressive disorder or nonpsychotic, depressed phase, bipolar disorder (Rush *et al.*, 2005a). There was no difference between active and sham VNS at 10 weeks (response rates were 15.2% for the active and 10.0% for the sham group). A naturalistic follow-up study revealed a response rate of 27.2%, with a remission rate of 15.8% following 1 year of open-label VNS (Rush *et al.*, 2005b). When VNS outcomes were compared with those from treatment as usual (TAU) in a separately recruited group of medication-resistant depressed patients, the response rates at

12 months were 27% for VNS + TAU and 13% for TAU (George *et al.*, 2005). At 2-years follow-up of the initial open-label trial, response rates were 42% and remission rates were 22%. At 2 years, 81% of the study participants were still receiving VNS. Benefits seen at 1 year were largely sustained for the group at 2 years (Nahas *et al.*, 2005). These studies are necessarily confounded by the lack of blinding, but based upon these results, the US Food and Drugs Administration (FDA) approved VNS for the adjunctive long-term treatment of chronic or recurrent depression in patients 18 years or older who are experiencing a major depressive episode and have not had an adequate response to four or more adequate antidepressant treatments.

Deep brain stimulation

The observation that chronic high-frequency electrical stimulation of the brain could result in clinical benefits similar to those achieved by surgical lesioning (Benabid *et al.*, 1987, 1991) transformed the use of functional neurosurgery for the treatment of movement disorders and opened the door for the potential uses of deep brain stimulation (DBS) in psychiatric disorders as well (Gross & Lozano, 2000). Thalamic DBS for intractable tremor has virtually replaced ablative lesions (Benabid *et al.*, 1996), and DBS of the subthalamic nucleus (STN) or globus pallidus internus has largely replaced pallidotomy for Parkinson's disease (Obeso *et al.*, 2001). Studies have begun to examine the utility of DBS for dystonia (Coubes *et al.*, 2000; Yianni *et al.*, 2003), epilepsy (Hodaie *et al.*, 2002), obsessive-compulsive disorder (Gabriels *et al.*, 2003) and depression (Aouizerate *et al.*, 2004).

Deep brain stimulation involves delivering a current using implanted quadripolar electrodes connected to a battery-powered pulse-generating device. Stimulation can be adjusted by varying electrode selection and polarity and by altering frequency, amplitude and pulse width. Serious adverse effects of the surgical procedure include intracerebral haemorrhage (< 2% of cases), which can result in a range of deficits and even death. Confusion is a more common perioperative adverse effect. The stimulation itself can result in speech disturbances, paraesthesias, eye movement difficulties and motor contractions. The mechanism of action is unknown, but may be related to direct disruption of neuronal activity, increased GABA-mediated inhibitory neurotransmission, or stimulation-induced modulation of pathological network activity (McIntyre *et al.*, 2004).

Evidence for the effectiveness of DBS in psychiatry

Obsessive-compulsive disorder and major depression

Work to date with DBS in psychiatry has been limited but encouraging. Stereotactic lesioning has been of some benefit in severe intractable OCD cases (Schmidek & Sweet 1995; Greenberg *et al.*, 2003), suggesting that DBS of these surgical targets may have a clinical role as an alternative to lesioning (Devinsky *et al.*, 1995; Zald & Kim, 1996). Gabriels *et al.* (2003) prospectively investigated the impact of DBS in the anterior limbs of the internal capsules on psychopathology and neuropsychological functioning in three patients with chronic, severe, treatment-resistant OCD and found improvement in two cases. In another study, Aouizerate *et al.* (2004) examined the utility of DBS of the ventral caudate nucleus in a patient with intractable severe OCD and concomitant major depression. Depression and anxiety improved 6 months after the start of stimulation and remission of OCD was observed after 1 year, with a progressive increase in the level of functioning. No neuropsychological deterioration was observed.

Recently, based on a preliminary observation that the subgenual cingulate region (Brodmann area, BA 25) is metabolically overactive in treatment-resistant depression, Mayberg *et al.* (2005) studied whether DBS of BA25 could reduce this elevated activity and produce clinical benefit in six patients with severe medication-resistant depression. Chronic stimulation of white matter tracts adjacent to the subgenual cingulate gyrus produced a striking and sustained remission of depression in four of six patients. Antidepressant effects were associated with a marked reduction in local cerebral blood flow as well as changes in downstream limbic and cortical sites as measured with positron emission tomography (PET). While this work may be confounded by a placebo effect, the association of clinical benefit with metabolic changes in the stimulated circuitry is suggestive with respect to attribution. More controlled trials in larger samples will be needed to test the utility of this approach which carries the strength of being able to focally target and chronically stimulate the implicated circuitry.

Transcranial direct current stimulation

Transcranial direct current stimulation (tDCS) is a non-invasive means of electrically polarizing neurons in the human cerebral cortex. Also called direct current polarization, tDCS administers 1–3 mA of direct current through scalp electrodes. It has been shown to exert a polarity-dependent effect on cortical neurons locally and downstream of stimulation sites, with anodal stimulation facilitating cortical function and cathodal stimulation inhibiting it. Transcranial direct current stimulation is thought to affect brain function via a non-synaptic mechanism involving NMDA and other receptors to modulate resting membrane potentials (Liebetanz *et al.*, 2002). Lasting polarity-dependent changes in cortical excitability persist after the current is turned off, with duration of after-effects dependent on length of stimulation (lasting for more than an hour if current is given for 10 or more minutes; Lang *et al.*, 2005). Safety studies have shown no deleterious side effects within established limits of current strength and electrode placement and subjects are unaware of current flowing except for a slight tingling beneath the electrodes for the first few minutes that current is turned on (Iyer *et al.*, 2005).

Early, uncontrolled studies in Britain in the 1960s on subjects with a variety of psychiatric diagnoses claimed lasting relief from symptoms that ranged from depressed mood to mutism, excited and catatonic states (Redfearn *et al.*, 1964). These results have never been adequately replicated, though work with tDCS in the last 20 years has yielded data suggesting that tDCS may be able to enhance verbal fluency, improve word recall, and facilitate recovery from hand paresis in stroke patients (Hummel *et al.*, 2005). A recent double-blind, randomized, sham-controlled trial of the efficacy of tDCS in treating depression reported significant antidepressant effect after anodal stimulation over the dorsolateral prefrontal cortex was given 20 minutes a day for 5 alternated days (Fregni *et al.*, 2006). Its low cost and good safety profile may make it an attractive modality relative to other more invasive and costly procedures (Nitsche, 2002), but further clinical trials of longer duration involving more subjects will be required to determine if tDCS can live up to its promise.

Conclusions

We will soon know whether routine clinical use of rTMS in psychiatric disorders will become a reality as the results of large well-controlled trials become available within the next few years. Depression is the condition with the most consistent evidence, but encouraging work is also emerging in schizophrenia and anxiety disorders. Though subject to the usual concerns about sample comparability and the reliability of assessment, the early results with rTMS raise the possibility that focal modulation of cortical excitability can have therapeutic properties in psychiatric

disorders and that rTMS may prove informative about the anatomy and physiology of the neural systems involved in achieving therapeutic effects.

While this work with rTMS is encouraging, there may remain a role for convulsive therapy for more resistant cases. The enhanced control over both dosage and focality of stimulation, which may be achieved with MST, offers the capacity to restrict seizure induction to specific cortical areas, such as prefrontal cortex regions, and perhaps improve the efficacy and/or reduce the adverse effects of traditional convulsive treatment. Studies to date support the feasibility and safety of MST. More work will be needed to define its optimal dosing paradigms and determine its efficacy. Work with focal seizure induction treatments such as MST will also help to further define the mechanisms of action of convulsive treatments.

Vagus nerve stimulation is now FDA approved for the long-term adjunctive management of treatment-resistant severe depression. The establishment of predictive factors for treatment response to VNS is particularly important since VNS involves a surgical implant and the onset of action appears slow and to build over time. Relatively little is known about the relationships among stimulation parameters and outcome, and this makes dose finding and mechanistic studies important to guide the ultimate clinical usage of VNS for depression.

Deep brain stimulation has revolutionized the practice of neurosurgery, particularly in the realm of movement disorders. It is not surprising that DBS is now being studied in the treatment of treatment-resistant psychiatric disorders. Deep brain stimulation has inherent advantages over previous lesioning procedures. It is reversible, and stimulation can be adjusted according to a patient's changing symptoms and disease progression. Unlike TMS, DBS can reach deep brain structures, and stimulation is provided on a long-term basis. The few published studies on DBS for OCD and major depression are encouraging and warrant further controlled work to define its safety and efficacy.

Transcranial direct current stimulation is the least invasive of the procedures discussed here, and work with tDCS in psychiatry is in its infancy. More work is required to elucidate its unique mechanisms of action and shed light on its potential role in psychiatry.

This is a time of renewed interest in the entire area of device-based approaches to neuropsychiatric disorders. From well-established ECT to TMS, MST, VNS, DBS, and tDCS, these modalities greatly differ in their degree of invasiveness and their method of influencing brain function. They share in common the use of electrical stimulation of neurons, either directly or indirectly, as a

Table 4.II.1. Focal brain stimulation: treatments and their efficacy

Treatment	Form of treatment	Psychiatric disorder	Level of evidence for efficacy	Comments
Repetitive transcranial magnetic stimulation (rTMS)	10 days 15 days 28 days	Depression	Ia	Clinically effective but no advance on ECT in terms of efficacy; uncertainty about value of increased length of treatment
rTMS	Variable	Mania	IV	Experimental stage only
rTMS	Variable	Schizophrenia	IIb	Inconsistent results indicate no clear recommendation over efficacy
rTMS	Variable	Obsessive-compulsive disorder (OCD), Tourette's syndrome, PTSD and panic disorder	IV	Some encouraging findings but no controlled studies
Magnetic seizure therapy (MST)	12 sessions	Depression	IIIb	Controlled trials not yet compared with sham treatments
Vagus nerve stimulation (VNS)	10 weeks	Resistant depression	IIb	Limited evidence of efficacy but some encouraging findings
Deep brain stimulation (DBS)	Stereotactic lesioning	Resistant depression OCD	IV	More work needed but evidence difficult to accumulate as numbers so low
Transcranial direct current stimulation (tDCS)	20 minutes daily for 5 (alternate) days	Depression	IIb	One trial only; more needed

route to therapeutic change and to better understand the pathophysiology of psychiatric disorders. With this proliferation of tools, our understanding of the brain basis of psychiatric disorders can only increase.

The level of evidence for each of the interventions discussed in this chapter is summarized in Table 4.II.1.

REFERENCES

Abrams, R., Swartz, C. M. & Vedak, C. (1991). Antidepressant effects of high-dose right unilateral electroconvulsive therapy. *Archives of General Psychiatry*, **48**, 746–8.

Alonso, P., Pujol, J., Cardoner, N. *et al.* (2001). Right prefrontal repetitive transcranial magnetic stimulation in obsessive-compulsive disorder: a double-blind, placebo-controlled study. *American Journal of Psychiatry*, **158**, 1143–5.

Amar, A. P., Heck, C. N., Levy, M. L. *et al.* (1998). An institutional experience with cervical vagus nerve trunk stimulation for medically refractory epilepsy: rationale, technique, and outcome. *Neurosurgery*, **43**, 1265–80.

American Psychiatric Association (2001). *The Practice of ECT: Recommendations for Treatment, Training and Privileging*, 2nd edn. Washington, DC: American Psychiatric Press.

Aouizerate, B., Cuny, E., Martin-Guehl, C. *et al.* (2004). Deep brain stimulation of the ventral caudate nucleus in the treatment of obsessive-compulsive disorder and major depression. Case report. *Journal of Neurosurgery*, **101**, 682–6.

Avery, D. H., Holtzheimer, P. E., Fawaz, W. (2006). A controlled study of repetitive transcranial magnetic stimulation in medication-resistant major depression. *Biological Psychiatry*, **59**, 187–94.

Awata, S., Konno, M., Kawashima, R. *et al.* (2002). Changes in regional cerebral blood flow abnormalities in late-life depression following response to electroconvulsive therapy. *Psychiatry and Clinical Neuroscience*, **56**, 31–40.

Bailey, P. & Bremer, F. (1938). A sensory cortical representation of the vagus nerve. *Journal of Neurophysiology*, 405–12.

Bailine, S. H., Rifkin, A., Kayne, E. *et al.* (2000). Comparison of bifrontal and bitemporal ECT for major depression. *American Journal of Psychiatry*, **157**, 121–3.

Barker, A. T., Jalinous, R. & Freeston, I. L. (1985). Non-invasive magnetic stimulation of human motor cortex. *Lancet*, **1**, 1106–7.

Belmaker, R. H. & Grisaru, N. (1999). Antibipolar potential for transcranial magnetic stimulation. *Bipolar Disorder*, **1**, 71–2.

Benabid, A. L., Pollak, P., Gao, D. *et al.* (1996). Chronic electrical stimulation of the ventralis intermedius nucleus of the thalamus as a treatment of movement disorders. *Journal of Neurosurgery*, **84**, 203–14.

Benabid, A. L., Pollak, P., Gervason, C. *et al.* (1991). Long-term suppression of tremor by chronic stimulation of the ventral intermediate thalamic nucleus. *Lancet*, **337**, 403–6.

Benabid, A. L., Pollak, P., Louveau, A., Henry, S. & de Rougemont, J. (1987). Combined (thalamotomy and stimulation) stereotactic surgery of the VIM thalamic nucleus for bilateral Parkinson disease. *Applied Neurophysiology*, **50**, 344–6.

Benbow, S. M. (2005). Adverse effects of ECT. In *The ECT Handbook*, 2nd edn, ed. A. Scott. London: Royal College of Psychiatrists.

Bohning, D. E., Lomarev, M. P., Denslow, S., Nahas, Z., Shastri, A. & George, M. S. (2001). Feasibility of vagus nerve stimulation-synchronized blood oxygenation level-dependent functional MRI. *Investigative Radiology*, **36**, 470–9.

Brasil-Neto, J. P., Cohen, L. G., Panizza, M., Nilsson, J., Roth, B. J. & Hallett, M. (1992). Optimal focal transcranial magnetic activation of the human motor cortex: effects of coil orientation, shape of the induced current pulse, and stimulus intensity. *Journal of Clinical Neurophysiology*, **9**, 132–6.

Burt, T., Lisanby, S. H. & Sackeim, H. A. (2002). Neuropsychiatric applications of transcranial magnetic stimulation: a meta analysis. *International Journal of Neuropsychopharmacology*, **5**, 73–103.

Carpenter, L. L., Moreno, F. A., Kling, M. A. *et al.* (2004). Effect of vagus nerve stimulation on cerebrospinal fluid monoamine metabolites, norepinephrine, and gamma-aminobutyric acid concentrations in depressed patients. *Biological Psychiatry*, **56**, 418–26.

Chen, R., Classen, J., Gerloff, C. *et al.* (1997). Depression of motor cortex excitability by low-frequency transcranial magnetic stimulation. *Neurology*, **48**, 1398–403.

Cohen, E., Bernardo, M., Masana, J. *et al.* (1999). Repetitive transcranial magnetic stimulation in the treatment of chronic negative schizophrenia: a pilot study. *Journal of Neurology, Neurosurgery and Psychiatry*, **67**, 129–30.

Cohen, H., Kaplan, Z., Kotler, M., Kouperman, I., Moisa, R. & Grisaru, N. (2004). Repetitive transcranial magnetic stimulation of the right dorsolateral prefrontal cortex in posttraumatic stress disorder: a double-blind, placebo-controlled study. *American Journal of Psychiatry*, **161**, 515–24.

Conway, C. R., Chibnall, J. T., Li, X. & George, M. S. (2002). Changes in brain metabolism in response to chronic vagus nerve stimulation in depression. *Biological Psychiatry*, **51**, 8S–544.

Coubes, P., Roubertie, A., Vayssiere, N., Hemm, S. & Echenne, B. (2000). Treatment of DYT1-generalised dystonia by stimulation of the internal globus pallidus. *Lancet*, **355**, 2220–1.

d'Alfonso, A. A., Aleman, A., Kessels, R. P. *et al.* (2002). Transcranial magnetic stimulation of left auditory cortex in patients with schizophrenia: effects on hallucinations and neurocognition. *Journal of Neuropsychiatry and Clinical Neuroscience*, **14**, 77–9.

Dannon, P. N., Dolberg, O. T., Schreiber, S. & Grunhaus, L. (2002). Three and six-month outcome following courses of either ECT or rTMS in a population of severely depressed individuals – preliminary report. *Biological Psychiatry*, **51**, 687–90.

Dell, P. & Olson, R. (1951). Projections secondaires mesencéphaliques, diencéphaliques et amygdaliennes des afférents viscérales vagales. *Comptes Rendus de Société de Biologie*, **145**, 1088–91.

Delva, N. J., Brunet, D., Hawken, E. R., Kesteven, R. M., Lawson, J. S. & Waldron, J. J. (2000). Electrical dose and seizure threshold: relations to clinical outcome and cognitive effects in bifrontal, bitemporal, and right unilateral ECT. *Journal of ECT*, **16**, 361–9.

Devinsky, O., Morrell, M. J. & Vogt, B. A. (1995). Contributions of anterior cingulated cortex to behaviour. *Brain*, **11**, 8279–306.

Devous, M. D. (2001). Effects of VNS on regional cerebral blood flow in depressed subjects. Vagus Nerve Stimulation (VNS) for Treatment-Resistant Depression. Satellite Symposium in conjunction with the 7th World Congress of Biological Psychiatry. Berlin, Germany.

Driscoll, D. A. (1970). An investigation of a theoretical model of the human head with application to current flow calculations and EEG interpretation. Ph.D. Thesis, University of Vermont.

Elger, G., Hoppe, C., Falkai, P., Rush, A. J. & Elger, C. E. (2000). Vagus nerve stimulation is associated with mood improvements in epilepsy patients. *Epilepsy Research*, **42**, 203–10.

Epstein, C. M. (1990). Localizing the site of magnetic brain stimulation in humans. *Neurology*, **40**, 666–70.

Feinsod, M., Kreinin, B., Chistyakov, A. & Klein, E. (1998). Preliminary evidence for a beneficial effect of low-frequency, repetitive transcranial magnetic stimulation in patients with major depression and schizophrenia. *Depression and Anxiety*, **7**, 65–8.

Fitzgerald, P. B., Brown, T. L., Marston, N. A., Daskalakis, Z. J., De Castella, A. & Kulkarni, J. (2003). Transcranial magnetic stimulation in the treatment of depression: a double-blind, placebo-controlled trial. *Archives of General Psychiatry*, **60**, 1002–8.

Fitzgerald, P. B., Benitez, J., Daskalakis, J. Z. *et al.* (2005). A double-blind sham-controlled trial of repetitive transcranial magnetic stimulation in the treatment of refractory auditory hallucinations. *Journal of Clinical Psychopharmacology*, **25**, 358–62.

Fregni, F., Boggio, P. S., Nitsche, M., Marcolin, M. A., Rigonatti, S. P. & Pascual-Leone, A. (2006). Treatment of major depression with transcranial direct current stimulation. *Bipolar Disorders*, **8**, 203–4.

Gabriels, L., Cosyns, P., Nuttin, B., Demeulemeester, H. & Gybels, J. (2003). Deep brain stimulation for treatment-refractory obsessive-compulsive disorder: psychopathological and neuropsychological outcome in three cases. *Acta Psychiatrica Scandinavica*, **107**, 275–82.

Garcia-Toro, M., Salva Coll, J., Crespi Font, M. *et al.* (2002). Panic disorder and transcranial magnetic stimulation. *Actas Espagnola de Psiquiatria*, **30**, 221–4.

Geddes, L. A. & Baker, L. E. (1967). The specific resistance of biological material – a compendium of data for the biomedical engineer and physiologist. *Medical and Biological Engineering*, **5**, 271–93.

Geller, V., Grisaru, N., Abarbanel, J. M., Lemberg, T. & Belmaker, R. H. (1997). Slow magnetic stimulation of prefrontal cortex in depression and schizophrenia. *Progress in Neuropsychopharmacology and Biological Psychiatry*, **21**, 105–10.

George, M. S. & Wassermann, E. M. (1994). Rapid-rate transcranial magnetic stimulation and ECT. *Convulsive Therapy*, **10**, 251–4.

George, M. S., Post, R. M., Ketter, T. A., Kimbrell, T. A. & Speer, A. M. (1997). Neural mechanisms of mood disorders. *Current Review of Mood and Anxiety Disorders*, **1**, 71–83.

George, M. S., Lisanby, S. H. & Sackeim, H. A. (1999). Transcranial magnetic stimulation: applications in neuropsychiatry. *Archives of General Psychiatry*, **56**, 300–11.

George, M. S., Nahas, Z., Molloy, M. *et al.* (2000). A controlled trial of daily left prefrontal cortex TMS for treating depression. *Biological Psychiatry*, **48**, 962–70.

George, M. S., Rush, A. J., Marangell, L. B. *et al.* (2005). One-year comparison of vagus nerve stimulation with treatment as usual for treatment-resistant depression. *Biological Psychiatry*, **58**, 364–73.

Gershon, A. A., Dannon, P. N. & Grunhaus, L. (2003). Transcranial magnetic stimulation in the treatment of depression. *American Journal of Psychiatry*, **160**, 835–45.

Grisaru, N., Chudakov, B., Yaroslavsky, Y. & Belmaker, R. H. (1998). Catatonia treated with transcranial magnetic stimulation. *American Journal of Psychiatry*, **155**, 1630.

Gottesfeld, B. H., Lesse, S. M. & Herskovitz, H. (1944). Studies in subconvulsive electric shock therapy effect of varied electrode applications. *Journal of Nervous and Mental Disorders*, **99**, 56–64.

Greenberg, B. D., George, M. S., Martin, J. D. *et al.* (1997). Effects of prefrontal repetitive transcranial magnetic stimulation (rTMS) in obsessive-compulsive disorder: a preliminary study. *American Journal of Psychiatry*, **154**, 867–9.

Greenberg, B. D., Ziemann, U., Harmon, A., Murphy, D. L. & Wassermann, E. M. (1998). Decreased neuronal inhibition in cerebral cortex in obsessive-compulsive disorder on transcranial magnetic stimulation. *Lancet*, **352**, 881–2.

Greenberg, B. D., Ziemann, U., Cora-Locatelli, G. *et al.* (2000). Altered cortical excitability in obsessive-compulsive disorder. *Neurology*, **54**, 142–7.

Greenberg, B. D., Price, L. H., Rauch, S. L. (2003). Neurosurgery for intractable obsessive-compulsive disorder and depression: critical issues. *Neurosurgery Clinics of North America*, **14**, 199–212.

Gross, R. E. & Lozano, A. M. (2000). Advances in neurostimulation for movement disorders. *Neurology Research*, **22**, 247–58.

Grunhaus, L., Dannon, P. N., Schreiber, S. *et al.* (2000). Repetitive transcranial magnetic stimulation is as effective as electroconvulsive therapy in the treatment of nondelusional major depressive disorder: an open study. *Biological Psychiatry*, **47**, 314–24.

Hajak, G., Marienhagen, J., Langguth, B., Werner, S., Binder, H. & Eichhammer, P. (2004). High-frequency repetitive transcranial magnetic stimulation in schizophrenia: a combined treatment and neuroimaging study. *Psychological Medicine*, **34**, 1157–63.

Harden, C. L., Pulver, M. C., Nikolov, B., Halper, J. P. & Labar, D. R. (1999). Effect of vagus nerve stimulation on mood in adult epilepsy patients. *Neurology*, **52** (Suppl. 2), A238-P03122.

Hargrove, E. A., Bennett, A. E. & Ford, F. R. (1953). The value of subconvulsive electrostimulation in the treatment of some emotional disorders. *American Journal of Psychiatry*, **109**, 612–16.

Hayes, K. J. (1950). The current path in ECS. *Archives of Neurology and Psychiatry*, **63**, 102–9.

Henry, M. E., Schmidt, M. E., Matochik, J. A., Stoddard, E. P. & Potter, W. Z. (2001). The effects of ECT on brain glucose: a pilot FDG PET study. *Journal of ECT*, **17**, 33–40.

Henry, T. R., Votaw, J. R., Pennell, P. B. *et al.* (1999). Acute blood flow changes and efficacy of vagus nerve stimulation in partial epilepsy. *Neurology*, **52**, 1166–73.

Herwig, U., Lampe, Y., Juengling, F. D. *et al.* (2003). Add-on rTMS for treatment of depression: a pilot study using stereotaxic coil-navigation according to PET data. *Journal of Psychiatric Research*, **37**, 267–75.

Hodaie, M., Wennberg, R. A., Dostrovsky, J. O. & Lozano, A. M. (2002). Chronic anterior thalamus stimulation for intractable epilepsy. *Epilepsia*, **43**, 603–8.

Hoffman, R. E., Boutros, N. N., Berman, R. M. *et al.* (1999). Transcranial magnetic stimulation of left temporoparietal cortex in three patients reporting hallucinated "voices". *Biological Psychiatry*, **46**, 130–2.

Hoffman, R. E., Boutros, N. N., Hu, S., Berman, R. M., Krystal, J. H. & Charney, D. S. (2000). Transcranial magnetic stimulation and auditory hallucinations in schizophrenia. *Lancet*, **355**, 1073–5.

Hoffman, R. E., Hawkins, K. A., Gueorguieva, R. *et al.* (2003). Transcranial magnetic stimulation of left temporoparietal cortex and medication-resistant auditory hallucinations. *Archives of General Psychiatry*, **60**, 49–56.

Hoffman, R. E., Gueorguieva, R., Hawkins, K. A. *et al.* (2005). Temporoparietal transcranial magnetic stimulation for auditory hallucinations: safety, efficacy and moderators in a fifty patient sample. *Biological Psychiatry*, **58**, 97–104.

Holi, M. M., Eronen, M., Toivonen, K., Toivonen, P., Marttunen, M. & Naukkarinen, H. (2004). Left prefrontal repetitive transcranial magnetic stimulation in schizophrenia. *Schizophrenia Bulletin*, **30**, 429–34.

Holtzheimer, P. E. 3rd, Russo, J. & Avery, D. H. (2001). A meta-analysis of repetitive transcranial magnetic stimulation in the treatment of depression. *Psychopharmacological Bulletin*, **35**, 149–69.

Hummel, F., Celnik, P., Giraux, P. *et al.* (2005). Effects of non-invasive cortical stimulation on skilled motor function in chronic stroke. *Brain*, **128**, 490–9.

Iyer, M. B., Mattu, M. A., Grafman, J., Lomarev, M., Sato, M. & Wassermann, E. (2005). Safety and cognitive effects of frontal DC brain polarization in healthy individuals. *Neurology*, **64**, 872–5.

Jandl, M., Bittner, R., Sack, A. *et al.* (2004). Changes in negative symptoms and EEG in schizophrenic patients after repetitive transcranial magnetic stimulation (rTMS): an open-label pilot study. *Journal of Neural Transmission*, **112**, 955–67.

Janicak, P. G., Dowd, S. M., Martis, B. *et al.* (2002). Repetitive transcranial magnetic stimulation versus electroconvulsive therapy for major depression: preliminary results of a randomised trial. *Biological Psychiatry*, **51**, 659–67.

Jobe, P. C., Dailey, J. W. & Wernicke, J. F. (1999). A noradrenergic and serotonergic hypothesis of the linkage between epilepsy and affective disorders. *Critical Reviews in Neurobiology*, **13**, 317–56.

Kaptsan, A., Yaroslavsky, Y., Applebaum, J., Belmaker, R. H. & Grisaru, N. (2003). Right prefrontal TMS versus sham treatment of mania: a controlled study. *Bipolar Disorder*, **5**, 36–9.

Kauffmann, C. D., Cheema, M. A. & Miller, B. E. (2004). Slow right prefrontal transcranial magnetic stimulation as a treatment for medication-resistant depression: a double-blind, placebo-controlled study. *Depression and Anxiety*, **19**, 59–62.

Kimbrell, T. A., Little, J. T., Dunn, R. T. *et al.* (1999). Frequency dependence of antidepressant response to left prefrontal repetitive transcranial magnetic stimulation (rTMS) as a function of baseline cerebral glucose metabolism. *Biological Psychiatry*, **46**, 1603–13.

Klein, E., Kolsky, Y., Puyerovsky, M., Koren, D., Chistyakov, A. & Feinsod, M. (1999). Right prefrontal slow repetitive transcranial magnetic stimulation in schizophrenia: a double-blind sham-controlled pilot study. *Biological Psychiatry*, **46**, 1451–4.

Klein, E., Kreinin, I., Chistyakov, A. *et al.* (1999). Therapeutic efficacy of right prefrontal slow repetitive transcranial magnetic stimulation in major depression: a double-blind controlled study. *Archives of General Psychiatry*, **56**, 315–20.

Kosel, M., Frick, C., Lisanby, S. H., Fisch, H. U. & Schlaepfer, T. E. (2003). Magnetic seizure therapy improves mood in refractory major depression. *Neuropsychopharmacology*, **28**, 2045–8.

Krahl, S. E., Clark, K. B., Smith, D. C. & Browning, R. A. (1998). Locus coeruleus lesions suppress the seizure-attenuating effects of vagus nerve stimulation. *Epilepsia*, **39**, 709–14.

Lang, N., Siebner, H. R., Ward, N. S. *et al.* (2005). How does transcranial DC stimulation of the primary motor cortex alter regional neuronal activity in the human brain? *European Journal of Neuroscience*, **22**, 495–504.

Law, S. K. (1993). Thickness and resistivity variations over the upper surface of the human skull. *Brain Topography*, **6**, 99–109.

Lerer, B., Shapira, B., Calev, A. *et al.* (1995). Antidepressant and cognitive effects of twice- versus three-times-weekly ECT. *American Journal of Psychiatry*, **152**, 564–70.

Liebetanz, D., Nitsche, M., Tergau, F. & Paulus, W. (2002). Pharmacological approach to the mechanisms of transcranial DC-stimulation-induced after-effects of human motor cortex excitability. *Brain*, **125**, 2238–47.

Lisanby, S. H., Luber, B. L., Schroeder, C. *et al.* (1998a). rTMS in primates: intracerebral measurement of rTMS and ECS induced voltage *in vivo*. *Electroencephalography and Clinical Neurophysiology*, **107**, 79P.

Lisanby, S. H., Luber, B., Schroeder, C. *et al.* (1998b). Intracerebral measurement of rTMS and ECS induced voltage *in vivo*. *Biological Psychiatry*, **43**, 100S.

Lisanby, S. H., Maddox, J. H., Prudic, J., Devanand, D. P. & Sackeim, H. A. (2000). The effects of electroconvulsive therapy on memory of autobiographical and public events. *Archives of General Psychiatry*, **57**, 581–90.

Lisanby, S. H. & Sackeim, H. A. (2000). TMS in major depression. In *Transcranial Magnetic Stimulation (TMS): Applications in Neuropsychiatry*, ed. M. S. George & R. H. Belmaker, pp. 185–200. Washington, DC: American Psychiatric Press.

Lisanby, S. H., Luber, B., Fincle, A. D., Schroeder, C. & Sackeim, H. A. (2001a). Deliberate seizure induction with repetitive transcranial magnetic stimulation in nonhuman primates. [Erratum appears in *Archives of General Psychiatry*, (2001) **58**(5), 515]. *Archives of General Psychiatry*, **58**, 199–200.

Lisanby, S. H., Schlaepfer, T. E., Fisch, H. U. & Sackeim, H. A. (2001b). Magnetic seizure therapy of major depression. *Archives of General Psychiatry*, **58**, 303–5.

Lisanby, S. H. & Sackeim, H. A. (2002). Transcranial magnetic stimulation and electroconvulsive therapy: similarities and differences. In *Handbook of Transcranial Magnetic Stimulation*, ed. A. Pascual-Leone, N. Davey, J. Rothwell, E. Wassermann & B. K. Puri, pp. 376–95. London: Arnold Publishers.

Lisanby, S. H., Luber, B., Schlaepfer, T. E. & Sackeim, H. A. (2003a). Safety and feasibility of magnetic seizure therapy (MST) in major depression: randomized within-subject comparison with electroconvulsive therapy. *Neuropsychopharmacology*, **28**, 1852–65.

Lisanby, S., Husain, M., Morales, O. G. *et al.* (2003b). Controlled clinical trial of the antidepressant efficacy of magnetic seizure therapy in the treatment of major depression. *ACNP Annual Meeting Abstracts*, 166.

Lisanby, S. H. (2004). Magnetic seizure therapy: development of a novel convulsive technique. In *Brain Stimulation in Psychiatric Treatment*, ed. S. H. Lisanby, pp. 77–116. Arlington, VA: American Psychiatric Publishing.

Lomarev, M., Denslow, S., Nahas, Z., Chae, J. H., George, M. S. & Bohning, D. E. (2002). Vagus nerve stimulation (VNS) synchronized BOLD fMRI suggests that VNS in depressed adults has frequency/dose dependent effects. *Journal of Psychiatric Research*, **36**, 219–27.

Luber, B., Nobler, M. S., Moeller, J. R. *et al.* (2000). Quantitative EEG during seizures induced by electroconvulsive therapy: relations to treatment modality and clinical features. II. Topographic analyses. *Journal of ECT*, **16**, 229–43.

Maccabee, P. J., Amassian, V. E., Eberle, L. P. *et al.* (1991). Measurement of the electric field induced in inhomogeneous volume conductors by magnetic coils: application to human spinal neurogeometry. *Electroencephalography and Clinical Neurophysiology*, **81**, 224–37.

Maccabee, P. J., Eberle, L., Amassian, V. E., Cracco, R. Q., Rudell, A. & Jayachandra, M. (1990). Spatial distribution of the electric field induced in volume by round and figure '8' magnetic coils: relevance to activation of sensory nerve fibers. *Electroencephalography and Clinical Neurophysiology*, **76**, 131–41.

Mantovani, A., Lisanby, S. H., Pieraccini, F., Ulivelli, M., Castrogiovanni, P. & Rossi, S. (2006). Repetitive transcranial magnetic stimulation (rTMS) in the treatment of obsessive-compulsive disorder (OCD) and Tourette's syndrome (TS). *International Journal of Neuropsychopharmacology*, **9**, 95–100.

Mantovani, A., Lisanby, S. H., Pieraccini, F., Ulivelli, M., Castrogiovanni, P. & Rossi, S. (2007). Repetitive transcranial magnetic stimulation (rTMS) in the treatment of panic disorder (PD) with comorbid major depression. *Journal of Affective Disorders*, in Press.

Martin, J. L., Barbanoj, M. J., Schlaepfer, T. E. *et al.* (2002). Transcranial magnetic stimulation for treating depression. *Cochrane Database System Review*, **2**, CD003493.

Martin, J. L., Barbanoj, M. J., Schlaepfer, T. E., Thompson, E., Perez, V. & Kulisevsky, J. (2003). Repetitive transcranial magnetic stimulation for the treatment of depression. Systematic review and meta-analysis. *British Journal of Psychiatry*, **182**, 480–91.

Mayberg, H.S., Lozano, A.M., Voon, V. *et al.* (2005). Deep brain stimulation for treatment-resistant depression. *Neuron*, **45**, 651–60.

McCall, W.V., Reboussin, D.M., Weiner, R.D. & Sackeim, H.A. (2000). Titrated moderately suprathreshold vs fixed high-dose right unilateral electroconvulsive therapy: acute antidepressant and cognitive effects. *Archives of General Psychiatry*, **57**, 438–44.

McCann, U.D., Kimbrell, T.A., Morgan, C.M. *et al.* (1998). Repetitive transcranial magnetic stimulation for post-traumatic stress disorder. *Archives of General Psychiatry*, **55**, 276–9.

McElhiney, M.C., Moody, B.J., Steif, B.L. *et al.* (1995). Autobiographical memory and mood: effects of electroconvulsive therapy. *Neuropsychology*, **9**, 501–17.

McIntosh, A.M., Semple, D., Tasker, K. *et al.* (2004). Transcranial magnetic stimulation for auditory hallucinations in schizophrenia. *Psychiatry Research*, **127**, 9–17.

McIntyre, C.C., Savasta, M., Kerkerian-Le Goff, L. & Vitek, J.L. (2004). Uncovering the mechanism(s) of action of deep brain stimulation: activation, inhibition, or both. *Clinical Neurophysiology*, **115**, 1239–48.

Michael, N. & Erfurth, A. (2004). Treatment of bipolar mania with right prefrontal rapid transcranial magnetic stimulation. *Journal of Affective Disorder*, **78**, 253–7.

Mills, K.R., Boniface, S.J. & Schubert, M. (1992). Magnetic brain stimulation with a double coil: the importance of coil orientation. *Electroencephalography and Clinical Neurophysiology*, **85**, 17–21.

Morales, O., Luber, B., Kwan, E., Ellsasser, R., Sackeim, H.A. & Lisanby, S.H. (2003). Prolactin response to convulsive therapy: Magnetic seizure therapy (MST) versus electroconvulsive shock (ECS) in nonhuman primates. *Journal of ECT*, **19**, 58A.

Nahas, Z., Marangell, L.B., Husain, M.M. *et al.* (2005). Two-year outcome of vagus nerve stimulation (VNS) for treatment of major depressive episodes. *Journal of Clinical Psychiatry*, **66**, 1097–104.

Ng, C., Schweitzer, I., Alexopoulos, P. *et al.* (2000). Efficacy and cognitive effects of right unilateral electroconvulsive therapy. *Journal of ECT*, **16**, 370–9.

Nitsche, M.A. (2002). Transcranial direct current stimulation: a new treatment for depression? *Bipolar Disorders*, **4**, 98–9.

Nobler, M.S., Oquendo, M.A., Kegeles, L.S., Campbell, C., Sackeim, H.A. & Mann, J.J. (2001). Decreased regional brain metabolism after ECT. *American Journal of Psychiatry*, **158**, 305–8.

Nobler, M.S., Sackeim, H.A., Prohovnik, I. *et al.* (1994). Regional cerebral blood flow in mood disorders, III. Treatment and clinical response. *Archives of General Psychiatry*, **51**, 884–97.

Obeso, J.A., Olanow, C.W., Rodriguez-Oroz, M.C., Krack, P., Kumar, R. & Lang, A.E. (2001). Deep-brain stimulation of the subthalamic nucleus or the pars interna of the globus pallidus in Parkinson's disease. *New England Journal of Medicine*, **345**, 956–63.

Padberg, F., Zwanzger, P., Thoma, H. *et al.* (1999). Repetitive transcranial magnetic stimulation (rTMS) in pharmacotherapy-refractory major depression: comparative study of fast, slow and sham rTMS. *Psychiatry Research*, **88**, 163–71.

Pascual-Leone, A., Houser, C.M., Reese, K. *et al.* (1993). Safety of rapid-rate transcranial magnetic stimulation in normal volunteers. *Electroencephalography and Clinical Neurophysiology*, **89**, 120–30.

Pascual-Leone, A., Rubio, B., Pallardo, F. & Catala, M.D. (1996). Beneficial effects of rapid-rate transcranial magnetic stimulation of the left dorsolateral prefrontal cortex in drug resistant depression. *Lancet*, **248**, 233–7.

Penry, J.K. & Dean, J.C. (1990). Prevention of intractable partial seizures by intermittent vagal nerve stimulation in humans: preliminary results. *Epilepsy*, **31**, S40–S43.

Poulet, E., Brunelin, J., Bediou, B. *et al.* (2005). Slow transcranial magnetic stimulation can rapidly reduce resistant auditory hallucinations in schizophrenia. *Biological Psychiatry*, **57**, 188–91.

Pridmore, S., Rybak, M., Turnier-Shea, P., Reid, P., Bruno, R. & Couper, D. (1999). A naturalistic study of response in melancholia to transcranial magnetic stimulation (TMS). *German Journal of Psychiatry*, **2**, 13–21.

Prudic, J., Peyser, S. & Sackeim, H.A. (2000). Subjective memory complaints: a review of patient self-assessment of memory after electroconvulsive therapy. *Journal of ECT*, **16**, 121–32.

Redfearn, J.W., Lippold, O.C. & Costain, R. (1964). A preliminary account of the clinical effects of polarizing the brain in certain psychiatric disorders. *British Journal of Psychiatry*, **110**, 773–85.

Rollnik, J.D., Huber, T.J., Mogk, H. *et al.* (2000). High frequency repetitive transcranial magnetic stimulation (rTMS) of the dorsolateral prefrontal cortex in schizophrenic patients. *Neuroreport*, **11**, 4013–15.

Rosenberg, P.B., Mehndiratta, R.B., Mehndiratta, Y.P., Wamer, A., Rosse, R.B. & Balish, M. (2002). Repetitive transcranial magnetic stimulation treatment of comorbid posttraumatic stress disorder and major depression. *Journal of Neuropsychiatry and Clinical Neurosciences*, **14**, 270–6.

Rossi, S., Bartalini, S., Ulivelli, M. *et al.* (2005). Hypofunctioning of sensory gating mechanisms in patients with obsessive-compulsive disorder. *Biological Psychiatry*, **57**, 16–20.

Rush, A.J., Marangell, L.B., Sackeim, H.A. *et al.* (2005a). Vagus nerve stimulation for treatment-resistant depression: a randomized, controlled acute phase trial. *Biological Psychiatry*, **58**, 347–54.

Rush, A.J., Sackeim, H.A., Marangell, L.B. *et al.* (2005b). Effects of 12 months of vagus nerve stimulation in treatment-resistant depression: a naturalistic study. *Biological Psychiatry*, **58**, 355–63.

Rush, S. & Driscoll, D. (1968). Current distribution in the brain from surface electrodes. *Anesthesie et analgesie*, **47**, 717–23.

Saba, G., Rocamora, J.F., Kalalou, K. *et al.* (2002). Catatonia and transcranial magnetic stimulation. *American Journal of Psychiatry*, **159**, 1794.

Sachdev, P.S., McBride, R., Loo, C.K., Mitchell, P.B., Malhi, G.S. & Croker, V.M. (2001). Right versus left prefrontal transcranial magnetic stimulation for obsessive-compulsive disorder: a preliminary investigation. *Journal of Clinical Psychiatry*, **62**, 981–4.

Sachdev, P., Loo, C., Mitchell, P. & Malhi, G. (2005). Transcranial magnetic stimulation for the deficit syndrome of schizophrenia: a pilot investigation. *Psychiatry and Clinical Neuroscience*, **59**, 354–7.

Sackeim, H. A. (1992). The cognitive effects of electroconvulsive therapy. In *Cognitive Disorders: Pathophysiology and Treatment*, ed. W. H. Moos, E. R. Gamzu & L. J. Thal, pp. 183–228. New York: Marcel Dekker.

Sackeim, H. (1994). Magnetic stimulation therapy and ECT. *Convulsive Therapy*, **10**, 255–8.

Sackeim, H. A., Portnoy, S., Neeley, P., Steif, B. L., Decina, P. & Malitz, S. (1986). Cognitive consequences of low-dosage electroconvulsive therapy. *Annals of the New York Academy of Sciences*, **462**, 326–40.

Sackeim, H. A., Prudic, J., Devanand, D. P. *et al.* (1993). Effects of stimulus intensity and electrode placement on the efficacy and cognitive effects of electroconvulsive therapy. *New England Journal of Medicine*, **328**, 839–46.

Sackeim, H. A., Luber, B., Katzman, G. P. *et al.* (1996). The effects of electroconvulsive therapy on quantitative electroencephalograms. Relationship to clinical outcome. *Archives of General Psychiatry*, **53**, 814–24.

Sackeim, H. A., Prudic, J., Devanand, D. P. *et al.* (2000). A prospective, randomized, double-blind comparison of bilateral and right unilateral electroconvulsive therapy at different stimulus intensities. *Archives of General Psychiatry*, **57**, 425–34.

Sackeim, H. A., Keilp, J. G., Rush, A. J. *et al.* (2001b). The effects of vagus nerve stimulation on cognitive performance in patients with treatment-resistant depression. *Neuropsychiatry, Neuropsychology, and Behavioral Neurology*, **14**, 53–62.

Sackeim, H. A., Rush, A. J., George, M. S. *et al.* (2001a). Vagus nerve stimulation (VNS) for treatment-resistant depression: efficacy, side effects, and predictors of outcome. *Neuropsychopharmacology*, **25**, 713–28.

Schachter, S. C. & Saper, C. B. (1998). Vagus nerve stimulation. *Epilepsia*, **39**, 677–86.

Schmidek, H. H. & Sweet, W. H., ed. (1995). *Operative Neurosurgical Techniques*, 4th edn. Philadelphia, PA: WB Saunders Co.

Schonfeldt-Lecuona, C., Gron, G., Walter, H. *et al.* (2004). Stereotaxic rTMS for the treatment of auditory hallucinations in schizophrenia. *Neuroreport*, **15**, 1669–73.

Silbersweig, D. A., Stern, E., Frith, C. *et al.* (1995). A functional neuroanatomy of hallucinations in schizophrenia. *Nature*, **378**, 176–9.

Smitt, J. W. & Wegener, C. F. (1944). On electric convulsive therapy with particular regard to a parietal application of electrodes, controlled by intracerebral voltage measurements. *Acta Psychiatrica Neurologica*, **19**, 529–49.

Sobin, C., Sackeim, H. A., Prudic, J., Devanand, D. P., Moody, B. J. & McEthiney, M. C. (1995). Predictors of retrograde amnesia following ECT. *American Journal of Psychiatry*, **152**, 995–1001.

Triggs, W. J., McCoy, K. J., Greer, R. *et al.* (1999). Effects of left frontal transcranial magnetic stimulation on depressed mood, cognition, and corticomotor threshold. *Biological Psychiatry*, **45**, 1440–6.

Ulett, G., Smith, K. & Gleser, G. (1956). Evaluation of convulsive and subconvulsive shock therapies utilizing a control group. *American Journal of Psychiatry*, **112**, 795–802.

Uthman, B. M., Wilder, B. J., Penry, J. K. *et al.* (1993). Treatment of epilepsy by stimulation of vagus nerve. *Neurology*, **43**, 1338–45.

Van Bockstaele, E. J., Peoples, J. & Valentino, R. J. (1999). Anatomic basis for differential regulation of the rostrolateral peri-locus coeruleus region by limbic afferents. *Biological Psychiatry*, **46**, 1352–63.

Wassermann, E. M. & Lisanby, S. H. (2001). Therapeutic application of repetitive transcranial magnetic stimulation: a review. *Clinical Neurophysiology*, **112**, 1367–77.

Yianni, J., Bain, P., Giladi, N. *et al.* (2003). Globus pallidus internus deep brain stimulation for dystonic conditions: a prospective audit. *Movement Disorders*, **18**, 436–42.

Zabara, J. (1985). Time course of seizure control to brief, repetitive stimuli. *Epilepsia*, **26**, 518.

Zald, D. H. & Kim, S. W. (1996). Anatomy and function of the orbital frontal cortex: II. Function and relevance to obsessive–compulsive disorder. *Journal of Neuropsychiatry and Clinical Neuroscience*, **82**, 49–61.

Zwanzger, P., Minov, C., Ella, R. *et al.* (2002). Transcranial magnetic stimulation for panic. *American Journal of Psychiatry*, **159**, 315–16.

5

The effectiveness of psychological treatments in psychiatry

Peter Fonagy and Joel Paris

Editor's note

Psychotherapy appears to be effective when compared to naturalistic outcome. While the benefits of psychotherapy may differ across different disorders and different types of psychotherapy may be more effective for certain disorders and less effective for other disorders, repeatedly psychotherapy has shown itself to be more effective than naturalistic outcome. While there are many different types of psychotherapy, they essentially fall into two large classes, the psychodynamic therapies, which includes interpersonal psychotherapy, and the behavioral and cognitive-behavioral therapies. There are also a number of other therapies classified as supportive therapy and experiential therapy. Group and systems, including family, therapy can be subsumed under the above groupings. Currently, there is great attention being paid to both the behavioral (including cognitive-behavioral) and the interpersonal psychotherapies because these seem amenable to study via randomized control methodology. These therapies are also time-limited which facilitates their empirical study because there is a specified time limit or time point at which outcome can be measured. What the essential ingredients are that contribute to a successful therapy remain speculative, but client factors, therapist factors, and the maintenance of a healthy and positive alliance between client and therapist appear to be major influences. Others factors include a well-defined contract, encouraging openness in the patient, and maintaining a focus on current life problems and relationships. There is little evidence to support long-term open-ended therapy no matter what the approach. Most therapists in practice probably use an eclectic mix of different therapies or therapeutic styles rather than strictly adhering to one psychotherapeutic approach.

Introduction

Psychological treatments, usually termed *psychotherapies*, involve the management of emotional or behavioral symptoms through psychological means. These therapies are designed to modify beliefs, emotional states, or interpersonal conflicts related to mental disorders. Psychological treatment, when conducted on a one-on-one basis between therapist and patient, is usually referred to as individual psychotherapy (Table 5.1). While there is also an extensive literature on group and family psychotherapies, the largest amount of research and practice has focused on individual therapy, which will be the focus of this chapter.

There are many methods of conducting psychotherapy. They are sometimes estimated to be in the hundreds. But this profusion of techniques is actually an artefact. It results from the tendency of writers about psychotherapy to give their own approach a "brand name". Moreover, one can exclude from discussion therapies that have never been studied empirically. Thus, in practice, individual psychotherapies can be divided into two broad categories, the psychodynamic-related psychotherapies and the cognitive-behavior-related psychotherapies.

Psychodynamic therapies

The psychodynamic approach derives from the work of Freud and his followers. While modern psychoanalysis has departed significantly from the models developed a hundred years ago, all these therapies share certain characteristics (Westen, 1998).

First, psychodynamic therapy is concerned with exploring the unconscious mind. Free association and dream analysis are assumed to provide a window into the unconscious. At the same time, therapists examine defense

Cambridge Textbook of Effective Treatments in Psychiatry, ed. Peter Tyrer and Kenneth R. Silk. Published by Cambridge University Press.
© Cambridge University Press, 2008.

mechanisms, which are believed to guard against the direct expression of unconscious wishes (Vaillant, 1977). Second the psychodynamic approach is characterized by an interest in childhood experience. Psychoanalytic theory is based on the concept that early experiences shape adult behavior, and therapy aims to examine these relationships as a way of changing maladaptive patterns. Third, psychodynamic therapists are interested in interpreting links between past, present, and transference (Malan, 1979). Particular to the psychoanalytic approach is the concept that the analysis of childhood experience, as well as of problems in the therapist–patient relationship, sheds light on unconscious conflicts, which are believed to be a crucial element in effective therapy.

Psychodynamic therapy has classically been open-ended and long-term. But today it is rare for patients to be seen several times a week in formal psychoanalysis (Gabbard *et al.*, 2002). Instead, therapy is most often provided once or twice a week for periods of months to years. The psychodynamic approach has also been adapted for use as a short-term or time-limited method (Malan, 1979). More pertinent to providing managed care services are the focal therapies (see Alexander & French, 1946; Sifneos, 1972; Mann, 1973; Malan, 1976; Davanloo, 1978; Luborsky, 1984; Strupp & Binder, 1984). Focal approaches no longer aim at pervasive transformations of the personality, but assume that cognitive understanding of personal problems may initiate symptomatic change, which continues after termination of the formal treatment. Long-term exploratory psychodynamic psychotherapy may span 1 year or more. Its focal implementation is more likely to compromise 4 to 6 months of once- or twice-weekly sessions. Whereas long-term exploratory therapy aims to consider a wide variety of transference distortions, focal therapy tends to be aimed at circumscribed character change. Both exploratory and focused treatment have the resolution of unconscious conflict as their goal. Unlike cognitive and behavioral psychotherapies, these are not primarily or only concerned with achieving symptomatic change.

Interpersonal therapy (IPT; Klerman & Weissman, 1993) is an empirically validated adaptation of time-limited dynamic therapy. But IPT avoids exploration of childhood and transference and focuses instead on current problems in intimate relationships. Interpersonal psychotherapy is based on the ideas of the interpersonal school (Sullivan, 1953), and was initially formulated as a time-limited weekly therapy for depressed patients. It makes no assumptions about etiology but uses the connection between the onset of depressive symptoms and current interpersonal problems as a focus for treatment. It therefore focuses on current relationships rather than enduring aspects of the personality, and therapists take an active and supportive stance.

Interpersonal therapy is normally a brief treatment, usually administered in the acute phase of depression. Therapy starts with a diagnostic phase, where the patient's disorder is identified and explained. The therapist highlights the ways in which the patient's current functioning, social relationships, and expectations within these relationships may have been causal in the depression. In the second phase of treatment, the therapist pursues strategies specific to one of these problem areas. For example, the therapist may facilitate mourning and help the patient to find new relationships and activities to compensate for the loss. Role disputes may be tackled by helping the patient explore problem relationships and consider options available to resolve them. In the final phase of the treatment, the patient is helped to focus on therapeutic gains and to develop ways of identifying and countering depressive symptoms, should they arise in the future. Though originally intended for application only to depression, IPT has more recently been adapted for use with a wider range of populations (e.g. Weissman & Markowitz, 1994; Agras *et al.*, 2000).

Behavioral and cognitive-behavioral therapies

These approaches use methods designed to modify dysfunctional behaviors, cognitions, and emotions. The original concept of behavior therapy (BT) (Eysenck, 1969) involved the application of classical and operant conditioning methods to modify behavioral patterns. Wolpe's systematic desensitization method was probably the first rigorous attempt to adapt Pavlovian conditioning to a clinical situation. At the same time, Skinner and colleagues used operant conditioning techniques to modify the behavior of psychotic inpatients.

Largely for epistemological reasons, behavioral approaches ignore the importance of cognitive processes. Under the influence of Bandura, Ellis, Meichenbaum, and Beck, the balance has been redressed, and cognitions (both conscious and unconscious) have come to occupy an increasingly prominent role in models of psychopathology (as indeed is the case in the academic discipline of psychology as a whole). Today, this approach has been largely replaced by cognitive-behavioral therapy (Beck, 1986), which focuses on the modification of abnormal thoughts and emotional responses. Emotion-focused therapy (Greenberg, 2002) is a related method designed to target emotional dysregulation.

Although BT might seem to have little in common with psychoanalytic therapy, it actually shares several elements. Both approaches apply methods of re-education related to pathological patterns of behavior (Wachtel, 1977). Cognitive-behavioral therapy has even more commonality with psychodynamic therapy, in its concept of schema thought patterns that emerge early in life and drive pathology (Young *et al.*, 2003). However, the techniques used in BT and CBT are very different. Instead of simply listening and talking to the client, therapists intervene, and the model tends to resemble education. Within cognitive therapy, cognitions are seen as having been learned and to be maintained through reinforcement. Challenges to these assumptions may therefore be made directly rather than via unconscious determinants as implied by dynamic theory. In addition, the proposed links between symptomatology and specific cognitions are somewhat less complex in cognitive than in dynamic approaches. The goals of intervention tend to be clear, and the patient's motivation is strongly reinforced by suggestion and support from the therapist.

Other approaches

While psychodynamic and cognitive therapies have dominated the theoretical, clinical, and empirical literature, in practice, most psychotherapists seem to make use of multiple methods in an eclectic mix (Lambert, 2004). Moreover, many patients, particularly those who suffer from chronic symptoms, require maintenance or supportive therapy (Rockland, 1992), which makes use of techniques derived from both methods. Supportive therapists reject intellectual solutions and suggest interventions which reinforce and validate spontaneous and immediate experience. Supportive approaches, whilst encouraging self-awareness, are phenomenological, focusing on enhanced awareness of experience. The therapist achieves his or her aim of enhancing the integrity of the self and undoing inhibition of a self-actualizing tendency by remaining a facilitating observer, offering support to clients in their natural striving towards self-determination, personal meaning and self-awareness.

While the intellectual roots of supportive and experiential therapies are in the humanistic, existential and phenomenological ideas proposed by Nietzsche, Sartre, and Husserl, another alternative to behavioral-psychodynamic hegemony was the systemic orientation with its roots in anthropology and cybernetics (Bateson, Haley, and Erickson). The basic assumption of the systemic orientation is that problem behaviors are best addressed in the context of the system which generated them. The family system is the prototypical example but other human systems such as schools can also produce behavioral

problems that are best addressed by correcting their malfunction. The therapist's role is to identify the way in which the processes that generate a problem may be corrected by identifying and modifying dysfunctional aspects of the system. Systemic therapists use a range of interventions including psycho-education, suggestion, marking of boundaries, the prescribing of symptoms as ways of bringing about change to the family system.

Some approaches aim deliberately to integrate orientations. Within a clinical setting, the approach taken by a clinician is likely to depend on the characteristics of the client rather than on the therapist's own training and orientation. Mostly the two will interact, with specific behaviors of particular patients eliciting specific reactions from a particular therapist based on his or her prior training and experience. There have been attempts at systematizing these largely arbitrary processes by integrative psychotherapies. In the UK, cognitive analytic therapy (CAT) has gained increasing acceptance (Ryle, 1990, 1995). This integrates psychodynamic therapy with a more structured approach reflecting personal construct therapy and CBT. In the USA, cognitive therapists working with individuals with personality disorders are in the process of expanding cognitive therapy using schema theory. A particularly significant contribution has been made with borderline patients by Young & Lindemann (1992), whose approach extends the traditional cognitive framework in terms of both theory and technique. There is considerable cross-fertilization between treatment approaches in terms of both theory and technique. Ultimately, theoretical orientations will have to be integrated, since they are all approximate models of the same phenomenon: the human mind in distress. For the moment, however, integration may well be counterproductive as theoretical coherence is the primary criterion for distinguishing false and true assertions in many psychotherapeutic domains. To the extent that it removes the applicability of this criterion, integration would create confusion rather than clarify controversies. This objection does not apply to the desirability of integration at the level of technique. In everyday clinical practice there is much that is "borrowed" from different orientations by all practitioners. From the point of view of evaluation, what remains crucial is that all such borrowed techniques should make sense in the context of the theory into which they are borrowed.

Historical overview

At one time, the public image of psychiatrists was tied to their expertise in psychotherapy. This perception reflected an era in North American society in which psychiatry was dominated by psychoanalysis (Shorter, 1998). In this context, psychological treatments were more of an art than a science. Since the time of Freud, therapists have been publishing clinical papers and books describing their methods without subjecting them to formal clinical trials. This tradition of case study continues even today. Some therapists are more interested in convincing narrative than in quantitative data. Yet the outcome of psychotherapy is an empirical issue, no less so than the effectiveness of psychopharmacology. Research has demonstrated that psychological treatments are powerful tools that are consistently effective in a wide variety of clinical problems (Lambert, 2004). But many of the findings of psychotherapy research have contradicted beliefs commonly held by clinicians.

Three phases can be identified in the emergence of psychological therapy research. The first phase covers 35 years from about the midpoint of the last century. Over 50 years ago, Eysenck (1952), a German-born British clinical psychologist, challenged psychiatrists and psychotherapists to prove that their treatments were actually effective. Reviewing the scant literature at the time on therapy outcome, Eysenck concluded that people recover naturalistically from symptoms at the same rate as patients undergoing psychological treatment. During this time the psychology profession stood alone in decrying non-evidence-based treatments and in promoting empirically based psychological interventions.

Eysenck got the ball rolling by demanding the application of tightly controlled experimental designs to evaluate the usefulness of specific psychological treatments for particular conditions (Eysenck, 1952). Behind this initiative was the promotion of the recently introduced behavioral therapies, though it should be noted that this approach was backed by data which, by current standards, would hardly be considered compelling. Eysenck (1969) later claimed that behavior therapy was the only approach that could demonstrate consistent results. Whilst behavioral therapies such as systematic desensitization and token economies claimed experimental support, these were predominantly to be found in small sample or even single case studies. These initiatives were handicapped by several factors. First was the simplistic (even naïve) application of experimental/laboratory concepts and findings to clinical problems. A good example is provided by a particularly inappropriate study applying operant conditioning principles to auditory hallucinations in schizophrenia (Fonagy & Slade, 1982). These workers were happy to accept the diminished reporting of voices by people with schizophrenia following an aversive stimulus as evidence for an actual decrease in auditory hallucinations, rather than a reluctance to indicate to the experimenter when they heard the voice in order to avoid the aversive stimulus. Second was the trenchantly anti-medical ideology of early clinical psychology that in many instances led to a partial isolation of the profession and to limited access to research resources, which to a significant measure remained under medical control. Thus early studies of the effectiveness of psychological therapies administered by psychologists often suffered from being under-powered and flawed in terms of flaunting diagnostic considerations (Chambless & Ollendick, 2001).

But Eysenck's challenge echoed across the Atlantic. It had a positive effect on North American psychiatry and clinical psychology and stimulated a large body of research. A number of periodicals (e.g., *The Journal of Consulting and Clinical Psychology*) published empirical studies of psychotherapy. Eventually, there were enough data to fill a rather large volume, the *Handbook of Psychotherapy and Behavior Change*. Bergin and Garfield's text has remained the standard book on the subject in North America and a fifth edition has appeared (Lambert, 2004). Unfortunately, this large volume of psychotherapy research has not had a great effect on practice. Surveys repeatedly demonstrate that clinicians are often ill informed about, and have limited interest in, findings from psychotherapy research (Cohen *et al.*, 1986; Morrow-Bradley & Elliott, 1986).

The limited impact of research on services is perhaps understandable. Clinicians are experts in their field, but there is a tendency for them to limit their interest to the studies which apply directly to their current practice and to selectively disregard findings that would require of them substantial modification of their mode of work. This appears to be as true of CBT therapists as of psychodynamic clinicians (Raw, 1993; Suinn, 1993). On this basis it is clear that evidence cannot be expected to "speak for itself" (Chilvers *et al.*, 2002; Higgitt & Fonagy, 2002). This is as much the failing of researchers as of clinicians.

Associated with an unrealistic insistence on experimental rigor, a gulf quickly opened between university-based researchers and teachers and practitioners. The gap, while considerably reduced, remains to the present day. A partially successful attempt was made to bridge this gap in clinical psychology by the so-called Boulder model in training clinical psychologists that identified clinician psychologists as "scientist practitioners" and prescribed a systematic method of practice couched in the cannons of contemporary science. Nevertheless, many practitioners in the field remained skeptical about the relevance of research findings in everyday work and were disinclined to apply procedures recommended by their university-based colleagues even when these appeared to be superior to methods in general use (Davison, 1998). One reason is that clinicians who apply psychological treatments tend to rely more on their clinical acumen than on hard data. (To be fair, this can be as true of psychiatrists who prescribe psychopharmacology.) In addition, while research shows that psychotherapy works, it does not tell the practitioner how to conduct treatment.

Nonetheless, important changes have taken place in how psychological treatments are prescribed. The second phase of the development of the practice of effective psychological therapy is marked by a far better integration of psychotherapy practitioners with their academic colleagues. In part, this is undoubtedly attributable to the latter embracing aspects of the value system (developed initially in clinical psychology) to govern general health care practice. The last 15 years have seen a powerful increase in concern with the evidence base of all medical procedures including mental health interventions such as psychological therapies (Sackett et al., 1996).

In an increasing number of areas of medicine throughout the late 1980s and early 90s, the desirability of replacing clinical opinion with reliable, empirically sound observation ideally based in randomized controlled trials (RCTs) took hold. A hierarchy of evidence has been developed (Sheldon et al., 1993) which usefully distinguishes studies according to their susceptibility to bias. It is beyond our scope to consider the longstanding controversy concerning the balance between internal and external validity in RCTs. There can be no doubt that by imposing methodological rigor to attain high levels of internal validity trials can lose generalizability, because of biased samples and a highly coherent and controlled treatment protocol. Yet, RCTs of psychological therapies suddenly became the essential basis for the viability of widely offered procedures and indeed entire professions. Largely due to their greater suitability for RCT methodology as well as economic factors, briefer treatments have become standard, with longer-term therapies being offered less often (Lambert, 2004; Lambert, et al., 2004). In response to this demand, reviews of "the evidence base" have almost become a cottage industry, whether or not the authors of such reviews fully understand the limitations of the research on which their reviews are based (Roth & Parry, 1997). Psychoanalysis and psychoanalytically oriented psychotherapies are no longer dominant, and have often been replaced, both in practice and in the mind of the public, by other methods, most particularly cognitive-behavioral therapy.

The development of evidence-based psychological treatments owes a debt to Aaron Beck, the founder of CBT. Beck (1986) developed a method of psychotherapy that included built-in evaluations. Studies of treatment efficacy were conducted from the very beginning, and its methods have been consistently refined using empirical data. Cognitive-behavioral therapy, with its emphasis on cognitive change with practical methods for rapid symptom resolution, has a comprehensive theoretical basis allowing it to fill a niche formerly occupied by BT. Moreover, while CBT was originally developed for the treatment of depression and anxiety disorders, its range of application has become wider. Some therapists (e.g. Linehan, 1993) have applied its methods to personality disorders, and others have developed techniques for the management of psychotic patients (Kingdon et al., 1994; Rector & Beck, 2001).

The other method of therapy that has gained a strong evidence base is IPT (Klerman & Weissman, 1993), a technique that has been shown to be effective in treating depression and dysthymia when compared with CBT (Elkin, 1994) or medication (Kupfer et al., 1992; Schulberg et al., 1996; Frank et al., 2000). It is offered to couples (Baucom et al., 1998; Beach et al., 1998), groups (Wilfley et al., 2002), or individuals, in both therapeutic or prophylactic form (Frank et al., 1990) and in cultural settings as diverse as that of Uganda (Bolton et al., 2003; Bass et al., 2000). The method offers a brief and practical approach to common symptoms other than depression such as bulimia (Agras et al., 2000).

In other psychodynamic therapies, research has focused on short-term approaches, which have also been shown to be effective for many common psychological symptoms (Crits-Christoph & Siqueland, 1996; Westen & Morrison, 2001; Leichsenring et al., 2004). There is still a lack of evidence from controlled clinical trials that long-term open-ended therapy can accomplish more than briefer interventions (Nathan & Gorman, 2002). However, this conclusion must be tempered by a serious lack of empirical data addressing this question (Cummings & Cicchetti, 1990; Westen et al., 2004).

As the psychological therapies delivered by clinical psychologists were frequently the only methods of intervention subjected to research trials, trainers and practitioners of evidence-based psychological therapies were in line to experience a significant boom. Sadly, at the same time (and particularly in the USA), there was a growing awareness that mental health services consumed a substantial proportion of third party payments for health care, and the amount of reimbursement available for psychological therapies decreased dramatically. Managed care has attempted to change clinician behavior through the greater use of clinical protocols for reimbursement decisions (Cummings, 1991). Concurrent reimbursement reviews caused clinicians deep concern about their ability to provide optimal treatment (Gabbard *et al.*, 1991), and psychological therapy practices were felt to be particularly vulnerable (Cummings, 1987), although in practice this era has also brought significant new roles for some practitioners (Sanchez & Turner, 2003). Imaginative readings of the evidence base enabled a number of healthcare systems to shorten the period of fully reimbursed psychological interventions.

There is an irony and a paradox in the conjunction of scientific and finance-driven governance of service provision in psychological therapy. In most cases the evidence points to clear dose-effect relationships for psychological therapies (Howard *et al.*, 1986; Barkham *et al.*, 1996), and the fully reimbursed treatment duration falls below the clinically effective dose. Sadly, all too often reviews of the evidence base were applied naïvely and in the service of cutting relatively expensive treatments in favor of apparently cheaper therapies.

All this of course begs the question of the nature of the evidence. Contrary to the declared aims of evidence-based medicine, in reality the limitations of the experimental evidence, particularly in terms of generalizability, disempowered rather than empowered the practicing clinician, (Sackett *et al.*, 1996). For example, as it is known that the percentage of people excluded before randomization correlates strongly with effect size (Westen & Morrison, 2001), it is clear that claims made on the basis of the most dramatically successful studies are also most likely to be suspect in terms of their generalizability. Roth & Parry (1997) cautioned us that clinicians may be alienated from the evidence-based practice endeavor if they see it as a justification for favoring cheap, short-term interventions (where the research is easier to conduct) over longer-term therapies. In the USA, where these controversies are far more dramatically played out than in the UK, there has been a major move away from so-called efficacy studies to studies in psychological therapy which, at least in principle, are more generalizable because they provide a better analogue to everyday practice. It is not evident that the simple expedient of removing rigorous procedural complaints will itself generate data with clearer implications. In our view, considerable further intellectual work remains to be done before treatment choice in psychological therapy will truly be made on the basis of empirical data alone.

Closing the gap between practice and evidence brings us to the third phase in the development of clinical psychology. This phase is arguably just beginning and entails another quantum leap in the sophistication with which evidence for psychotherapeutic clinical psychological services is considered. It is increasingly recognized that evidence does not speak for itself, and to be usefully applied, evidence needs to be reviewed and integrated by a group of unbiased experts, including individuals whose expertise is as users and carers. Pressures to examine value for money and cost-effectiveness led to the debate that took place in the USA in the early 1980s being recapitulated in Britain in the 1990s. Concerns about efficacy and cost-effectiveness of psychotherapy and counseling led to some UK health authorities examining more closely the types and lengths of psychological treatments they purchase. A National Institute for Health and Clinical Excellence (NICE) was established to produce nationally authoritative guidance to the NHS, with systematic and formal processes for health technology assessments, cost-effectiveness review and guideline commissioning. There is a growing number of NICE mental health guidelines on depression, schizophrenia, anxiety disorders, and others, each incorporating recommendations on psychological therapies (www.nice.org. uk). "Clinical guidelines" that integrate evidence and front-line experience drawn up by multidisciplinary panels, which as a collection of individuals have full awareness of the limitations of everyday clinical practice, is a key step that has all too often been omitted in the past when the sole experience applied to the interpretation of evidence was one of management. A good example of the replacement of competition between mental health professionals by a collaboration, charged with the responsibility of developing evidence-based guidelines for a range of common psychological disorders, is the Mental Health National Collaborating Centre set up by the National Institute for Clinical Excellence.

Research, with its focus on selected patient populations, cannot, of course, tell clinicians what to do with specific individuals. Clinicians have to ask the research database specific questions with an individual patient in mind. How to pose this massive accumulation of data such questions and, even more difficult, how to obtain meaningful answers remains a challenge. These are far more complex skills than that of generating a systematic review. Many hope that clinical guidelines can and will perform the role of translation of research into practice increasingly well. The controversy that surrounds this issue is beyond the scope of this chapter. It is perhaps sufficient for us to say that we cannot see guidelines, however sophisticated, ever substituting for clinical skill and experience any more than the Highway Code can substitute for skilled driving. Future research needs look also at the skill with which clinicians implement particular treatments and the relationship of that to patient outcome (see below).

Overall efficacy of treatment

The doubts expressed by Eysenck (1952) about the overall efficacy of psychotherapy have now been thoroughly addressed. In an influential and widely quoted meta-analysis of the psychotherapy research literature, Smith *et al.* (1980) examined 475 studies measuring the outcome of many forms of therapy. They found a considerable effect size (.85) between treatment and no treatment. This may be something of an overestimate, and when Shadish *et al.* (1997) re-examined the same data, weighting the analysis to take sample size into account, the average effect size was reduced to .60. Lipsey & Wilson (1993) conducted a separate meta-analysis of 303 studies, yielding an overall effect size of .47. But as Lambert (2004) has pointed out, effect sizes tend to be higher in the diagnostic groups for which psychotherapy is most effective, i.e. depression and anxiety. In summary, there is broad agreement that psychotherapy is more effective for most patients than naturalistic recovery. As Smith *et al.* (1980) put it, "Psychotherapy benefits people of all ages as reliably as school educates them, medicine cures them, or business turns a profit" (p. 183). And as most of us are born dualists at heart and believe in psychological changes only when these are demonstrated at the level of the brain (Bloom, 2004), it is reassuring for us to know that effective psychotherapy has been shown to produce measurable changes in brain blood flow (Martin *et al.*, 2001).

The major meta-analyses of therapy outcome have been drawn from well-controlled studies. However, psychotherapy researchers recognize a difference between efficacy studies, using controlled trials, and effectiveness studies, where data are drawn from naturalistic designs (Lambert, 2004; Lambert *et al.*, 2004). While randomized controlled trials are the gold standard in evidence-based medicine, they are not always fully generalizable to practice. The main reason for this is that subjects who enter clinical trials do not always resemble the patients clinicians normally see (Westen & Morrison, 2001). Effectiveness studies use larger and more representative samples. One widely discussed report (Seligman, 1995) examined data obtained from thousands of readers of the magazine *Consumers Report*.

The tension between naturalistic assessment of outcome and experimental measures of efficacy is a real one, and it should be recognized that the bridge between research trials and routine treatment is difficult to span. It is reasonably clear that in general "research therapy" appears more effective than everyday clinical practice (Weisz *et al.*, 1995; Shadish *et al.*, 1997). There are many reasons why this could be. Some of the more obvious

relate to methodological issues such as the use of focused and structured treatments, regular access to supervision, participants recruited by advertisement rather than through clinical services, and greater exclusion rates. However, the vicissitudes of biology and individual psychological differences in treatment response may also be relevant. Psychotherapy is a highly complex interchange in which a large number of factors, any one of which could significantly influence outcome, interact. Patients differ along many dimensions, including their socioeconomic circumstances, the stage of their disorder at the time of presentation, and in their premorbid psychological functioning. Similarly, therapists vary in their personality, their skills, their motivation, their ability to comprehend their patients' problems, and their adherence to treatment modalities. Service provision also varies in important ways, including the length of treatment offered, the quality of liaison with other services, the support and supervision offered to practitioners, and the physical resources available.

Another difficulty is that the outcome of psychological treatments can be assessed in more than one way. Each way has its own advantages and disadvantages (Lambert, 2004). If the goal of therapy is symptomatic relief, patient self-reports are the simplest measure. However, many forms of psychotherapy aim to modify interpersonal behaviors, in which case patients are not always the best judge of meaningful change. Meta-analyses have demonstrated that evaluation of treatments solely in terms of their impact on core symptoms leads to a potentially misleading overestimation of the effect of the treatment, at least in terms of effect size (Weisz *et al.*, 1995). By and large, the kind of clinical ratings used in psychopharmacological studies are less useful for psychotherapy outcome, since they are likely to reflect observer bias. In some cases, observations from significant others in the patient's life may provide a more balanced picture although such individuals are also likely to have their vested interests in specific outcomes, for example, depending on their involvement in the client's treatment.

Common factors in psychotherapy

Psychological treatments work, but by what mechanism? Does it make a difference which method (or which theory) is the basis for treatment? This issue can only be addressed by conducting comparative trials in which different forms of treatment are studied "head to head".

A number of such studies, comparing a wide range of therapies, including psychodynamic, behavioral, cognitive, interpersonal, and client-centered methods, have been published. The results are surprisingly consistent: with notable exceptions, research has failed to show that any one method is more potent than any other. Almost 70 years ago, Rosenzweig (1936) wittily quoted Lewis Carroll to conclude that these comparisons elicit a "Dodo bird verdict" ("all have won and all shall have prizes"). Reviewing formal research literature 40 years later Luborsky et al. (1975) came to precisely the same conclusion. More recently, Wampold et al. (1997) examined a much larger number of studies and formal meta-analyses and concluded that the data still support a dodo bird verdict. Some reviews have claimed that effect sizes associated with CBT for depression were greater than alternative psychological treatments (e.g. Gloaguen et al., 1998). However, closer scrutiny of this kind of finding reveals that large effect sizes for psychological therapies tend to be associated with comparisons when the control or comparison therapy is not a bona fide treatment with a sound theoretical rationale, e.g. relaxation therapy (Wampold et al., 2002). Differences tend to be on "fringes", around issues of practicability. For example, group therapy for depression is only slightly less effective than individual therapy, but dropouts tend to be more common (McDermut et al., 2001). There are relatively fewer trials of psychodynamic (psychoanalytically orientated) therapies but at least one review of studies comparing cognitive-behavior therapy with short-term psychodynamic therapy suggests that their effectiveness is comparable (Leichsenring, 2001).

To summarize, psychotherapy research over the past decades has demonstrated repeatedly that a substantial proportion of the variability in therapeutic outcomes is not explained by differences between formally defined therapeutic procedures, differences between client groups, or (though less well examined) the interaction between these two factors (Garfield, 1994; Beutler et al., 1994; Beutler et al., 2004; Clarkin & Levy, 2004b). The absence of differences between procedures based on entirely different theories provides an important clue as to what are the most effective ingredients in psychological treatments. If success depends on factors common to all methods, therapy must work in part due to "non-specific" or "common" factors. (These factors are only called "non-specific" because we do not yet know how to specify them.)

Frank & Frank (1991) proposed an influential explanation of how common factors in therapy actually work. Patients come in to therapy hopeless and demoralized; treatment helps them to re-mobilize their inner resources. Thus, therapists' theories are less important than their capacity to make patients feel hopeful. This concept is in accordance with data showing that a good relationship

with a therapist is a crucial factor in the outcome of treatment (Lambert, 2004; Luborsky et al., 1988).

Short-term therapy may depend more strongly on non-specific factors while specific technical interventions could be more important in longer treatments. However, we do not know if this is the case. Strupp et al. (1969) conducted an interesting study of open-ended treatment, in which researchers asked therapists and patients what had been most helpful. While therapists stressed accurate technical interventions, patients talked mainly about the relationship to the therapist. Similar findings were obtained in a study of how psychotherapists themselves view their own therapy experiences (Buckley et al., 1981). Thus, it remains possible that long-term therapy is, as suggested long ago by Alexander & French (1946), a "corrective emotional experience".

Patient/client factors in therapy outcome
Some patients seem to do better in therapy than others. To make rational decisions about prescribing treatment, it would be useful to establish prognosis at the very beginning. Yet diagnosis is not generally of great help in predicting therapy outcome. Instead, the most consistent findings are that severity of symptoms, as well as functional levels in work and relationships, are correlated with the outcome of psychotherapy (Clarkin & Levy, 2004a). Patients with higher functioning are more involved in psychotherapy and form a stronger therapeutic alliance. This relationship has sometimes been described as "the rich get richer and the poor get poorer" (Horwitz, 1974).

On the other hand, the correlations between functional levels and outcome, while statistically significant, are not high (usually less than .30). Other factors intrinsic to the client predict psychotherapy outcome. Low socioeconomic and educational levels are associated with higher drop-outs and poorer results (Clarkin & Levy, 2004a). The presence of any personality disorder, in addition to other symptoms, has often been shown to predict a negative outcome (Shea et al., 1990).

Yet no single patient variable is a strong predictor of outcome. This is why the effects of psychotherapy, good or bad, can sometimes be surprising. However, attempts to identify a demographic or characteristic that enables prospective assignment may be unproductive. As Garfield (1994) suggested some years ago, even if we can predict about two-thirds of the variance in therapy outcomes by applying formal measures, that is not much better than most of us could do without such measures, simply by applying clinical intuition. The most interesting studies in this area tend to describe the impact of a process rather than a category. For example, variations in quality of object relations seems a more powerful predictor of treatment response than qualities, such as gender, class, ethnicity, etc. This observation also applies to issues such as the therapist's or patient's contribution to outcome, where it seems less likely that the characteristics of each party will emerge as obvious determinants of outcome than the way these factors operate in therapy.

Therapist factors in therapy outcome

Studies have shown that although some therapists appeared to achieve consistently better outcomes, even those who performed poorly overall had some patients with good outcomes (Luborsky *et al.*, 1986). More detailed examination suggested that individual therapists achieved better effects in some domains than others. For example, some therapists achieved better impacts on target symptoms, whereas others were more successful at increasing levels of interpersonal functioning. A further study (Luborsky *et al.*, 1997) examined outcomes from 22 therapists working across seven samples of substance-abusing and depressed patients and found that there were differences in rates of improvement across therapists, and that these differences did not appear to relate to patient severity or to patient attributes. Further, three therapists took part in more than one study, showing similar levels of efficacy with different patient samples and as they applied different manualized techniques. Wampold (2001) points out that the importance of common factors clearly points to the importance of therapist skill. Some therapists are more naturally talented than others, but what contributes to that talent? Beutler *et al.* (1994, 2004) carefully reviewed studies of the impact of therapist characteristics on outcome. There appears to be little overall impact of therapist's age, gender or ethnicity, or differences in outcome when therapist and client are matched on these variables. Assessment of the impacts of therapist personality variables is limited, with some studies attempting post hoc atheoretical analysis, and others a more theory-driven approach, with no consistent or robust findings. There are indications that therapists with better levels of adjustment have better outcomes, though there is some inconsistency across studies.

One might expect that therapist experience would predict outcome. However, the empirical findings on this relationship have been equivocal. The best-known test was the Vanderbilt study (Strupp & Hadley, 1979). When patients were assigned either to experienced therapists or to college professors chosen for relationship skills, both groups did equally well. The generalizability of that study was limited by the patient population, a well-defined but not very disturbed group of university students. Smith &

Glass's (1977) large-scale meta-analysis yielded a correlation of zero between experience and outcome, though since most therapists were rather inexperienced, few contrasts were available for analysis. All the same, other attempts to show the effects of experience have yielded only weak or unreplicated positive findings (Propst *et al.*, 1994; Beutler *et al.*, 2004). Wierzbicki & Pekarik's (1993) meta-analysis of 125 studies found no correlation between dropout and either the number of years of therapist experience or the professional degree gained by the therapist. A meta-analysis by Stein & Lambert (1995) reached the most definitive conclusions so far. These authors note that the codings of experience used by most studies make it difficult to distinguish between experience and training. For example, researchers frequently classify experience using global criteria, such as the type of degree held by a therapist. However, this may be misleading, since categorizing in this way will treat as homogeneous both newly qualified therapists and those who have been practicing for many years. These classificatory problems are likely to reduce the variance attributable to experience. Nonetheless, on the basis of 36 studies, moderate effect sizes were found for the relationship between experience and outcome, as measured both by pre-post measures of symptoms (0.3) and by clients (0.27). Given the problems of coding 'experience', it is surprising that studies should attribute any variance to therapist experience. It may also be the case that experience is less relevant than expertise, and a number of studies have linked this variable to outcomes. There is some evidence that experience becomes a more important predictor of outcome with patients who are more disturbed. The tendency for more experienced therapists both to have less dropout and to retain more difficult patients in therapy may lead them to show apparently poorer average outcomes relative to inexperienced therapists. Experience may therefore be important in dealing with cases where the patient's attitude is predominantly negative to the therapy.

The possession of a professional qualification is (at best) only weakly associated with better outcomes, a conclusion which, if robust, would have obvious and profound implications for training and accreditation of psychological therapists. However, this is a difficult area to survey, since different levels of professional qualification are often conflated with level of experience. Further (and as noted by Atkins & Christensen, 2001) the criteria used to distinguish between professionals and paraprofessionals varies across studies and reviews, and classification as a paraprofessional often indicates the absence of a formal qualification rather than a lack of experience, training or skillfulness. These findings do not prove that technique makes no difference. In fact the literature clearly indicates that training and supervision appear to be helpful for the effectiveness of both CBT and dynamic therapies.

Howard (1999) contrasted 20 specialists and 27 non-specialists treating 86 patients with anxiety disorders using CBT. A "specialist" was defined as an individual who not only have training in CBT, but also in the specific application of CBT to anxiety disorders (on which basis the term non-specialists may be misleading, since it does not imply that these therapists are untrained). Results were clear. Patients seen by the specialist group were seen for a shorter period of time, had better post-therapy outcomes and lower relapse rates over 2 years, and fewer sought additional treatment after therapy had ended.

Hilsenroth et al. (2002) randomized 68 patients to receive short-term psychodynamic therapy either from a trainee receiving highly structured supervision or from a trainee receiving "supervision-as-usual". Though alliance levels were high in both groups, there was significant additional benefit to structured training in relation to the alliance. A potential confound is that while only one supervisor therapist offered the structured supervision, "supervision-as-usual" was offered by 14 supervisors. Findings from Henry et al. (1993), suggest that generalization beyond the impacts of particular supervisors carries some risk. These results however do not negate the potential importance of non-specific technical factors in explaining between therapist differences in outcome. Therapists who are empathic and good at promoting a strong therapeutic alliance probably get better results (Beutler et al., 2004). But these findings may depend on the therapist's ability to elicit non-specific factors.

The foregoing suggests that manuals of psychotherapy may have much to contribute to the training of psychotherapists, and that models of good training practice would include formally assessing their capacity to adhere to these. However, it also suggests that while good knowledge of the key components of a technique is an important foundation for effective practice, expert practitioners may be those who are able to use technical recommendations flexibly and deviate and go beyond them at times when the clinical situation seems to require this. Since there are indications that the level and type of skills defining competence vary across therapies, it is difficult to know if studies which consider the impact of skillfulness in delivering different therapies are commensurate. The more demanding the therapy, the more critical issues of competence are likely to be. As an example, it seems unlikely that performing exposure therapy for a specific phobia requires the same skill level as delivering complex CBT to individuals with multiple disabilities (for example,

implementing schema-focused work, or CBT focused on the modification of delusional beliefs). It is at least an interesting possibility that studies which find an apparent lack of difference between simpler and more elaborate therapies may be detecting the wider variation in competence associated with the latter. That is an issue which is rarely specifically examined.

The role of the therapeutic alliance

Client and therapist factors intersect in the concept of a therapeutic alliance. This term describes the collaborative relationship between patient and therapist. One of the most consistent findings in the research literature is that the quality of the alliance is one of the better predictors of outcome (Luborsky & Crits-Christoph, 1990; Orlinksy et al., 2004). Whether therapy will ultimately succeed is often apparent in the first few sessions, depending on the extent to which patients feel understood, and by the extent to which patients feel they are working (Horvath & Simmonds, 1991) well with their therapists. When therapy starts well, it is likely to continue well.

While a number of measures have been used to assess the quality of the alliance, the California Scale (CALPAS; Gaston, 1991) is the most widely used. Interestingly, while the CALPAS has both patient and therapist versions, it is the patient version that predicts the results of therapy. The patient's subjective experience appears to be a better guide than that of the therapist (Horvath & Simmonds, 1991). After all, it is the consumer who needs to feel better, not the service provider. However, Martin et al.'s (2000) more substantive review did not support these observations because no further variance was accounted for by type of rater (patient, therapist, or observer), time or type of alliance rating (early, middle, late, or averaged across sessions), type of therapy, or methodological quality. However, there were some indications that patient-rated alliance is stable over sessions, whereas therapist- or observer-rated alliance is more variable.

Ackerman and Hilsenroth (2001, 2003) identify a number of therapist characteristics associated with the development of the alliance, noting that these are consistent across therapeutic orientations. Positive alliances tend to be fostered by therapist empathy, warmth and understanding, perceived trustworthiness, experience and confidence and perceived investment in the treatment relationship. Perhaps unsurprisingly, therapists perceived to be rigid, uncertain, critical and uninvolved are more likely to have negative alliances. Client factors contributing to the alliance include their motivation, their psychological status and quality of object relations, the quality of their social and family relations, and indices of stressful life events. Both intrapersonal and interpersonal factors appear to play a part. At the intrapersonal level, lack of hope, poor intrapsychic representations of others, and lack of psychological mindedness are often associated with poor outcome in terms of treatment alliance and therapeutic efficacy (Ryan, 1985; Piper *et al.*, 1991). Individuals rated as securely attached had higher scores on the goal subscale of the Working Alliance Inventory (Satterfield & Lyddon, 1998). While anxiety about intimacy may impede the development of the alliance, the impact of specific attachment patterns on the alliance is probably complex (Mallinckrodt *et al.*, 1995; Eames & Roth, 2000), and may be partly dependent on the interaction between therapist and patient attachment styles (Dozier *et al.*, 1994; Tyrell *et al.*, 1999; Rubino *et al.*, 2000).

While this account might suggest some stability in alliance level once it has developed, in reality variations from session to session are likely and common. For some researchers these variations in alliance level are in themselves important, since the process of "repairing" significant challenge to, and deterioration in, the alliance (denoted as alliance rupture) could be seen as therapeutic in its own right (e.g. Safran *et al.*, 1990; Safran & Muran, 2000). Though this notion is interesting and potentially important, rather few studies have directly examined this possibility (e.g. Bennett *et al.*, 1998; Safran & Muran, 1996).

The studies of how alliance evolves are somewhat inconsistent in their findings. Some studies suggest that alliance is the consequence of change in the client associated with the start of therapy (DeRubeis & Feeley, 1990; Gaston *et al.*, 1991; Barber *et al.*, 1999; Feeley *et al.*, 1999), while others controlling for this possibility continue to demonstrate that good alliance predicts outcome irrespective of initial symptom change (Barber *et al.*, 2000; Klein *et al.*, 2003). While it would be misleading to reduce the alliance to a proxy for improvement, the notion of the alliance as a common relationship factor, exerting impact independent of therapeutic progress, may equally be an over-simplification. At the very least it seems appropriate to question the assumption that the alliance represents a homogenous variable. It might be more useful to think of it as a complex set of processes which vary across stages of therapy, especially because the limited available literature on temporal relationship suggest that at different points in the therapy it acts in different ways. Perhaps a failing with these studies is that their definition of stages of therapy relates to time rather than therapeutic context. By way of illustration, the procedures used to engage a client in the initial stages of therapy are very different from those deployed in the management of alliance ruptures, and these shifts in focus and process are difficult for statistical techniques to capture and to account for.

Process research

Process research examines whether specific interventions lead to progress. In an extensive review, Orlinksy *et al.* (2004) examined research on over 50 different variables describing the process of psychotherapy in relation to its outcome. Their conclusions support the primacy of the "non-specific" factors in treatment. The factors that helped most in all forms of psychotherapy were: (1) a well-defined contract; (2) creating a strong alliance; (3) encouraging openness in the patient; (4) maintaining a focus on current life problems and relationships. Notably, this list does not include many technical interventions. Orlinksy *et al.* (2004) have proposed a "generic model" of psychotherapy describing the common factors in all methods, from psychoanalysis to behavior therapy.

One way to examine the role of specific interventions is to carry out a "dismantling" strategy, i.e. to take an effective treatment and remove its elements one by one to determine if it remains effective (Miranda & Borkovec, 1999). Given the time and expense of this method, this approach has not often been used. Thus, we do not know whether methods that therapists believe to be most effective have specific effects. Is the modification of false beliefs and schemata, considered to be crucial in CBT, actually its most effective element? Is the exploration of links between past, present, and transference, considered to be crucial in psychodynamic therapy, actually the most important aspect of that treatment?

This question can also be addressed by examining the impact of specific interventions. A large literature on this subject has been developed for various techniques associated with CBT (Beck, 1986). Not all of these support the expectations of the originators about what may be the effective component of their intervention. For example, in a study of CBT, the extent of focus on "parental issues" turned out to be positively associated with outcome (Hayes *et al.*, 1996). A major embarrassment to CBT is the rapid nature of change that tends to take place in this type of therapy. The change may be evident after a few sessions, at least in some patients (Tang & DeRubeis, 1999; Tang *et al.*, 2002; Stiles *et al.*, 2003). This occurs before most of the so-called effective components of the treatment, such as cognitive restructuring, have been introduced. In another study of CBT and dynamic therapy, the differences between the success of either intervention appeared to be correlated with the use of interventions prototypically considered "pychoanalytic" (Ablon & Jones, 1998). However, similar evidence can be readily mustered to support CBT.

Using the same instrument (Enrico Jones' Psychotherapy Q-sort) on tapes of the NIMH treatment of depression trial, Ablon and Jones demonstrated the superiority of therapies where process codings of both IPT or CBT more closely resembled the CBT prototype (Ablon & Jones, 1999, 2002).

In psychodynamic therapy research, researchers have attempted to examine the value of interpretation and of focusing on transference. Studies of psychodynamic psychotherapy process and outcome have not thus far demonstrated powerful associations between change and putative mechanism of action. For example, Piper et al. (1991) found that in sicker patients in whom the alliance is shaky, the use of transference interpretations to deal with problems between therapist and patient made outcome worse, not better. In another study, a negative association has been reported between the number of transference interpretations and therapy outcome, indicating that the overuse of this technique, frequently regarded by clinicians as essential to therapeutic success, may even have iatrogenic results (Connolly et al., 1999).

Luborsky (Luborsky et al., 1975; Luborsky & Crits-Christoph, 1990) developed a method of scoring for psychodynamic issues using the Core Conflict Relationship Theme Method (CCRT). This research showed that therapy had a better outcome if the therapist consistently follows the CCRT. However, these findings might also be interpreted as showing that patients are more likely to improve when therapists listen accurately to the themes the patients present and when therapists are consistent in following their own rules. Thus, what looks like a specific effect may only be another reflection of a strong alliance.

The length of therapy

One of the great debates in psychotherapy research has concerned the length of treatment. Almost all research in the literature has been conducted on therapy lasting for months rather than years. While brief courses of therapy are most common in practice, many psychotherapists continue to prescribe open-ended treatment. A formal psychoanalysis can last, on average, 7 years (Doidge et al., 2002).

Longer courses of therapy have become less common in recent years. There is less demand for open-ended therapy as potential patients seek out briefer therapies and/or psychopharmacological interventions (Shorter, 1998). Moreover, in the last few decades, psychiatrists in the USA have had to adjust their practice to the demands and the scrutiny of third party payers. Insurers tend to be skeptical about extended periods of therapy. This has led some Health Maintenance Organizations to go overboard in the other direction (Lambert, 2004; Lambert et al.,

2004). Current policies, in which only a handful of sessions are paid for, are not based on existing evidence.

Several naturalistic studies have examined length of therapy in relation to outcome. Some (Bovasso et al., 1999; Luborsky et al., 1997) have found relationships between a greater number of sessions and recovery. The only study to measure a precise dose–response relationship was conducted at Northwestern University where a sample of 2400 patients was followed over time (Howard et al., 1986). On average, 50% of patients show clinical improvement by 8 sessions, and 75% by 26 sessions. These findings support the usefulness of briefer forms of therapy in clinical settings as the default condition. However, they also suggest that 6 months (not 6 weeks) of therapy should be the standard for insurance companies. A limitation of this study was that it relied on pre- and post-data to estimate the likely "shape" of change across sessions rather than examining session-by-session change directly. Recent reports have employed survival analysis to derive a more direct estimate of the number of sessions required to achieve clinically significant change. Anderson & Lambert (2001) tracked outcomes for 75 clients, estimating the number of sessions required for 50% of clients to achieve clinically significant change. For their sample, a median of 11 sessions was required. The combination of this with a sample of 47 patients from Kadera et al. (1996) indicated that while less distressed individuals required a median of 12 sessions, more distressed patients required 20. A larger trial by Hansen & Lambert (2003) examined outcomes for 4761 patients seen in standard treatment settings (including HMOs, employee assistance programs and community mental health centers). These individuals required a median of between 15 and 19 sessions, depending on the setting, to achieve this level of change.

Yet every therapist knows that patients often do not respond in a few months. What are the characteristics of this treatment-resistant group? In a second study by the Northwestern group (Kopta et al., 1994), the dose-effect relationship was broken down according to the nature of presenting symptoms. A multi-site study of 854 patients in which patients were seen weekly in open-ended therapy showed that the number of sessions needed depended on whether patients presented acute distress, chronic distress, or characterological problems. Acute distress, such as acute anxiety or depression, improved rapidly, usually within a few months, although complete recovery could take up to a year. Chronic distress, such as chronic anxiety or depression, or interpersonal sensitivity and loneliness, improved more slowly, requiring a year to obtain significant clinical improvement in 75% of the cases. In another study of outpatients with personality disorders (Hoglend, 1993), similar findings were obtained in that patients with personality pathology only improved when treatments lasted for 50 sessions.

Thus, "characterological" symptoms, such as hostility, paranoid ideas, or chronic sleep disturbances, tend to require longer therapy. In the Kopta *et al.* (1994) study, the symptoms for which over 2 years of therapy were needed to achieve improvement included unusual levels of irritability and an inability to get close to other people. The problem was that only about 50% of these cases actually showed improvement, even after a year. This raises questions about the cost-effectiveness of routinely continuing therapy in patients who do not show an initial response.

We have almost no data concerning the value of open-ended psychological treatments. The few reports that have been published have been naturalistic and uncontrolled. One of the most famous studies was carried out at the Menninger Clinic in the 1950s (Wallerstein, 1990). The Menninger Study had serious limitations: it examined only 42 subjects, had no control group, failed to make precise diagnoses, and used measures that were out of date by the time the data analyses were conducted. Its most consistent finding was that patients with higher initial levels of functioning had the best outcome (Kernberg *et al.*, 1972). But there was great variability in outcome in relation to functional levels. Higher functioning patients did poorly if they failed to form a strong alliance, whereas lower functioning patients did better than expected when they had a good therapeutic alliance (Horwitz, 1974). Again, these results tend to support the importance of non-specific factors in therapy.

Long-term psychotherapy is often prescribed for patients with personality disorders. A few naturalistic studies have evaluated the efficacy of this approach in that population. Both Stevenson & Meares (1992) studying a cohort with borderline personality, and Monsen *et al.* (1995) studying a cohort with several categories of personality disorder, found that most patients achieved clinical improvement after 2 years of therapy. However, these cohorts lacked a control group for comparison. But a study by Winston *et al.* (1994) that did use a control group reported that, after 40 sessions of therapy, patients with anxious cluster disorders or histrionic personality disorder showed significantly greater improvement than those left untreated on a waiting list.

An extensive and influential study of the psychotherapy of patients with borderline personality disorder was conducted over a 1-year period by Linehan (1993). Linehan's "dialectical behavior therapy" was found to be superior to "treatment as usual" in reducing parasuicidal behaviors, findings that have since been confirmed in other cohorts (Koerner & Linehan, 2000) and in a replication study with

some methodological refinements that has been recently published (Linehan *et al.*, 2006). While improvement was only partial (most patients continued to suffer from affective dysregulation), achieving lasting results required a full year of treatment. In another controlled trial of treatment for patients with borderline personality, Bateman & Fonagy (1999) found that psychodynamically oriented day treatment, lasting 18 months, was effective against the core symptoms of the disorder. However, it was not clear whether these results derived from the structure of a day hospital or from specific components of treatment. It was notable that many of the achievements in this study were attained after the completion of the formal day-hospital treatment (Bateman & Fonagy, 2001). It is not unusual that psychodynamic treatment should be associated with so called 'sleeper effects' when the impact of the treatment does not fully emerge until it is over (Kolvin *et al.*, 1988).

Conclusions

One can draw several conclusions from the psychotherapy research literature:

(1) There is overwhelming evidence for the efficacy and effectiveness of psychotherapy in a wide variety of clinical conditions, with results often equal to those for pharmacological agents.
(2) The therapeutic alliance (i.e., the quality of the relationship between therapist and patient) is a key factor in effective therapy.
(3) Therapist skill is important in establishing this relationship, but skill has not consistently been shown to depend on experience.
(4) Factors within the patient predict therapy outcome; not so much diagnosis, but level of functioning and ability to form an alliance.
(5) Common factors are crucial in therapy, while there is little evidence that specific interventions are as important.
(6) Most patients benefit from psychotherapy within 6 months; there is little evidence that long-term therapy can accomplish what short-term cannot.

Yet in spite of the success in psychotherapy research over the last half century, this complex subject requires much more investigation. The overwhelming evidence for common factors suggests that research needs to focus less on technique, and more on how alliances are built in therapy. On the other hand, evidence may be gathered in the future supporting the use of more focused and more precise techniques, expanding the range of applications for psychotherapy. Finally, research is needed to

Table 5.1. Effectiveness of psychotherapy

Treatment	Form of treatment	Psychiatric disorder/target audience	Level of evidence for efficacy	Comments
Psychotherapeutic	All types of psychotherapy	Multiple psychiatric disorders	Ia	Effect sizes range from 0.45–0.85

determine whether long-term open-ended psychotherapy is consistently effective for the populations for which it is currently prescribed.

The level of evidence for the interventions discussed in this chapter is summarized in Table 5.1.

REFERENCES

Ablon, J. S. & Jones, E. E. (1998). How expert clinicians' prototypes of an ideal treatment correlate with outcome in psychodynamic and cognitive-behavior therapy. *Psychotherapy Research*, **8**, 71–83.

Ablon, J. S. & Jones, E. E. (1999). Psychotherapy process in the National Institute of Mental Health Treatment of Depression Collaborative Research Program. *Journal of Consulting and Clinical Psychology*, **67**, 64–75.

Ablon, J. S. & Jones, E. E. (2002). Validity of controlled cinical trials of psychotherapy: findings from the NIMH Treatment of Depression Collaborative Research Program. *American Journal of Psychiatry*, **159**, 775–83.

Ackerman, S. J. & Hilsenroth, M. J. (2001). A review of therapist characteristics and techniques negatively impacting the therapeutic alliance. *Psychotherapy: Theory, Research, Practice, Training*, **38**, 171–85.

Ackerman, S. J. & Hilsenroth, M. J. (2003). A review of therapist characteristics and techniques positively impacting the therapeutic alliance. *Clinical Psychology Review*, **23**, 1–33.

Agras, W. S., Walsh, T., Fairburn, C. G., Wilson, G. T. & Kraemer, H. C. (2000). A multicenter comparison of cognitive-behavioral therapy and interpersonal psychotherapy for bulimia nervosa. *Archives of General Psychiatry*, **57**, 459–66.

Alexander, F. & French, T. (1946). *Psychoanalytic Therapy*. New York: Ronald.

Anderson, E. M. & Lambert, M. J. (2001). A survival analysis of clinically significant change in outpatient psychotherapy. *Journal of Clinical Psychology*, **57**, 875–88.

Atkins, D. C. & Christensen, A. (2001). Is professional training worth the bother? A review of the impact of psychotherapy training on client outcome. *Australian Psychologist*, **36**, 122–30.

Barber, J. P., Connolly, M. B., Crits-Christoph, P., Gladis, L. & Siqueland, L. (2000). Alliance predicts patients' outcome beyond in-treatment change in symptoms. *Journal of Consulting and Clinical Psychology*, **68**, 1027–32.

Barber, J. P., Luborsky, L., Crits-Christoph, P. *et al.* (1999). Therapeutic alliance as a predictor of outcome in treatment of cocaine dependence. *Psychotherapy Research*, **9**, 54–73.

Barkham, M., Rees, A., Shapiro, D. A. *et al.* (1996). Outcomes of time-limited psychotherapy in applied settings: replicating the Second Sheffield Psychotherapy Project. *Journal of Consulting and Clinical Psychology*, **64**, 1079–85.

Bateman, A. W. & Fonagy, P. (1999). The effectiveness of partial hospitalization in the treatment of borderline personality disorder – a randomised controlled trial. *American Journal of Psychiatry*, **156**, 1563–9.

Bateman, A. W. & Fonagy, P. (2001). Treatment of borderline personality disorder with psychoanalytically oriented partial hospitalization: an 18-month follow-up. *American Journal of Psychiatry*, **158**, 36–42.

Baucom, D. H., Shoham, V., Mueser, K. T., Daiuto, A. D. & Stickle, T. R. (1998). Empirically supported couple and family interventions for marital distress and adult mental health problems. *Journal of Consulting and Clinical Psychology*, **66**, 53–88.

Bass, J., Neugebauer, R., Clougherty, K. F. *et al.* (2006). Group interpersonal psychotherapy for depression in rural Uganda: 6-month outcomes: randomised controlled trial. *British Journal of Psychiatry*, **188**, 567–73.

Beach, S. R., Fincham, F. D. & Katz, J. (1998). Marital therapy in the treatment of depression: toward a third generation of therapy and research. *Clinical Psychology Review*, **18**, 635–61.

Beck, T. (1986). *Cognitive Therapy and the Emotional Disorders*. New York: Basic Books.

Bennett, K. J., Lipman, E. L., Racine, Y. & Offord, D. R. (1998). Annotation: Do measures of externalising behaviour in normal populations predict later outcome? Implications for targeted interventions to prevent conduct disorder. *Journal of Child Psychology and Psychiatry*, **39**, 1059–70.

Beutler, L., Malik, M., Alimohamed, S. *et al.* (2004). Therapist variables. In *Bergin and Garfield's Handbook of Psychotherapy and Behavior Change*, ed. M. Lambert, pp. 227–306. New York: Wiley.

Beutler, L. E., Machado, P. P. P. & Neufeldt, S. A. (1994). Therapist variables. In *Handbook of Psychotherapy and Behavior Change*, 4th edn, ed. A. E. Bergin & S. L. Garfield. New York: Wiley.

Bloom, P. (2004). *Descartes' Baby*. New York: Basic Books.

Bolton, P., Bass, J., Neugebauer, R. *et al.* (2003). Group interpersonal psychotherapy for depression in rural Uganda: a randomized controlled trial. *Journal of the American Medical Association*, **289**, 3117–124.

Bovasso, G. B., Eaton, W. W. & Armenian, H. K. (1999). The long-term outcomes of mental health treatment in a population-based study. *Journal of Consulting and Clinical Psychology*, **67**, 529–38.

Buckley, P., Karasu, T. B. & Charles, E. (1981). Psychotherapists view their personal therapy. *Psychotherapy*, **18**, 299–305.

Chambless, D. L. & Ollendick, T. H. (2001). Empirically supported psychological interventions: controversies and evidence. *Annual Review of Psychology*, **52**, 685–713.

Chilvers, R., Harrison, G., Sipos, A. & Barley, M. (2002). Evidence into practice: application of psychological models of change in evidence-based implementation. *British Journal of Psychiatry*, **181**, 99–101.

Clarkin, J. & Levy, K. L. (2004a). The influence of client variables on psychotherapy. In *Bergin and Garfield's Handbook of Psychotherapy and Behavior Change*, 5h edn, ed. M. Lambert, pp. 227–308. New York: Wiley.

Clarkin, J. F. & Levy, K. N. (2004b). The influence of client variables on psychotherapy. In *Bergin & Garfield's Handbook of Psychotherapy and Behavior Change*, 5th edn, ed. M. Lambert, pp. 194–226. New York: Wiley.

Cohen, L. H., Sargent, M. M. & Sechrest, L. B. (1986). Use of psychotherapy research by professional psychologists. *American Psychologist*, **41**, 198–206.

Connolly, M. B., Crits-Christoph, P., Shappell, S., Barber, J. P., Luborsky, L. & Shaffer, C. (1999). Relation of transference interpretations to outcome in the early sessions of brief supportive-expressive psychotherapy. *Psychotherapy Research*, **9**, 485–95.

Crits-Christoph, P. & Siqueland, L. (1996). Psychosocial treatment for drug abuse: selected review and recommendations for national health care. *Archives of General Psychiatry*, **53**, 749–56.

Cummings, E. M. & Cicchetti, D. (1990). Towards a transactional model of relations between attachment and depression. In *Attachment in the Preschool Years: Theory, Research, and Intervention*, ed. D. Cicchetti, M. T. Greenberg & E. M. Cummings, pp. 339–72. Chicago, IL: University of Chicago Press.

Cummings, N. A. (1987). The future of psychotherapy: one psychologist's perspective. *American Journal of Psychotherapy*, **61**, 349–60.

Cummings, N. A. (1991). Brief intermittent therapy throughout the life cycle. In *Psychotherapy in Managed Health Care: The Optimal Use of Time and Resources*, ed. C. S. Austad & W. H. Berman, pp. 35–45. Washington, DC: American Psychological Association.

Davanloo, H. (Ed.). (1978). *Basic Principles and Techniques in Short-Term Dynamic Psychotherapy*. New York: Spectrum Publications.

Davison, C. G. (1998). Being bolder with the boulder model: the challenge of education and training in empirically supported treatments. *Journal of Consulting and Clinical Psychology*, **66**, 163–7.

DeRubeis, R. J. & Feeley, M. (1990). Determinants of change in cognitive therapy for depression. *Cognitive Therapy and Research*, **14**, 469–82.

Doidge, N., Simon, B., Brauer, L. *et al.* (2002). Psychoanalytic patients in the U.S., Canada, and Australia: I. DSM-III-R disorders, indications, previous treatment, medications, and length of treatment. *Journal of the American Psychoanalytic Association*, **50**, 575–614.

Dozier, M., Cue, K. & Barnett, L. (1994). Clinicians as caregivers: role of attachment organization in treatment. *Journal of Consulting and Clinical Psychology*, **62**, 793–800.

Eames, V. & Roth, A. D. (2000). Patient attachment orientation and the early working alliance – a study of patient and therapist reports of alliance quality and ruptures. *Psychotherapy Research*, **10**, 421–34.

Elkin, I. (1994). The NIMH treatment of depression collaborative research program: where we began and where we are. In *Handbook of Psychotherapy and Behaviour Change*, ed. A. E. Bergin & S. L. Garfield, pp. 114–39. New York: Wiley.

Eysenck, H. (1952). The effects of psychotherapy: an evaluation. *Journal of Consulting Psychology*, **16**,319–24.

Eysenck, H. (1969). *The Effects of Psychotherapy*. New York: Science House.

Feeley, M., DeRubeis, R. J. & Gelfand, L. A. (1999). The temporal relation of adherence and alliance to symptom change in cognitive therapy for depression. *Journal of Consulting and Clinical Psychology*, **67**, 578–82.

Fonagy, P. & Slade, P. (1982). Punishment vs negative reinforcement in the aversive conditioning of auditory hallucinations. *Behaviour Research and Therapy*, **20**, 483–92.

Frank, E., Grochocinski, V. J., Spanier, C. A. *et al.* (2000). Interpersonal psychotherapy and antidepressant medication: evaluation of a sequential treatment strategy in women with recurrent major depression. *Journal of Clinical Psychiatry*, **61**, 51–7.

Frank, E., Kupfer, D. J., Perel, J. M. *et al.* (1990). Three year outcomes for maintenance therapies in recurrent depression. *Archives of General Psychiatry*, **47**, 1093–9.

Frank, J. D. & Frank, J. B. (1991). *Persuasion and Healing*. Baltimore, MD: Johns Hopkins University Press.

Gabbard, G. O., Takahashi, T., Davidson, J., Bauman-Bork, M. & Ensroth, K. (1991). A psychodynamic perspective on the clinical impact of insurance review. *American Journal of Psychiatry*, **148**, 318–23.

Gabbard, G. O., Gunderson, J. G. & Fonagy, P. (2002). The place of psychoanalytic treatments within psychiatry. *Archives of General Psychiatry*, **59**, 505–10.

Garfield, S. L. (1994). Research on client variables in psychotherapy. In *Handbook of Psychotherapy and Behavior Change*, ed. S. L. Garfield & A. E. Bergin, pp. 190–228. New York: Wiley.

Gaston, L. (1991). Reliability and criterion-related validity of the California Psychotherapy Alliance Scales-Patient Version. *Psychological Assessment*, **3**, 68–74.

Gaston, L., Marmar, C. R., Gallagher, D. & Thomson, L. W. (1991). Alliance prediction of outcome beyond in-treatment symptomatic change as psychotherapy progresses. *Psychotherapy Research*, **1**, 104–12.

Gloaguen, V., Cottraux, J., Cucherat, M. & Blackburn, I. (1998). A meta-analysis of the effects of cognitive therapy in depressed patients. *Journal of Affective Disorders*, **49**, 59–72.

Greenberg, L. S. (Ed.). (2002). *Emotion-focused Therapy: Coaching Clients to Work through their Feelings*. Washington, DC: American Psychological Association.

Hansen, N. B. & Lambert, M. J. (2003). An evaluation of the dose-response relationship in naturalistic treatment settings using survival analysis. *Mental Health Services Research*, **5**, 1–12.

Hayes, A. M., Castonguay, L. G. & Goldfried, M. R. (1996). Effectiveness of targeting the vulnerability factors of depression in cognitive therapy. *Journal of Consulting and Clinical Psychology*, **64**, 623–7.

Henry, R. W., Schacht, T. E., Strupp, H. H. *et al.* (1993). Effects of training in time-limited psychotherapy: mediators of therapists responses to training. *Journal of Consulting and Clinical Psychology*, **61**, 441–7.

Higgitt, A. & Fonagy, P. (2002). Clinical effectiveness. *British Journal of Psychiatry*, **181**, 170–4.

Hilsenroth, M. J., Ackerman, S. J., Clemence, A. J., Strassle, C. G. & Handler, L. (2002). Effects of structured clinician training on patient and therapist perspectives of alliance early in psychotherapy. *Psychotherapy: Theory, Research, Practice, Training*, **39**, 309–23.

Hoglend, P. (1993). Personality disorders and long-term outcome after brief dynamic psychotherapy. *Journal of Personality Disorders*, **7**, 168–81.

Horvath, A. O. & Simmonds, B. D. (1991). Relation between working alliance and outcome in psychotherapy: a meta-analysis. *Journal of Consulting and Clinical Psychology*, **38**, 139–49.

Horwitz, L. (1974). *Clinical Prediction in Psychotherapy*. New York: Aronson.

Howard, K. I., Kopta, S. M., Krause, M. S. & Orlinsky, D. E. (1986). The dose-effect relationship in psychotherapy. Special Issue: Psychotherapy research. *American Psychologist*, **41**, 159–64.

Howard, R. C. (1999). Treatment of anxiety disorders: Does specialty training help? *Professional Psychology: Research and Practice*, **30**, 470–3.

Kadera, S. W., Lambert, M. J. & Andrews, A. A. (1996). How much therapy is really enough? A session-by-session analysis of the psychotherapy dose-effect relationship. *Journal of Psychotherapy: Practice and Research*, **5**, 1–20.

Kernberg, O. F., Coyne, L., Appelbaum, A., Horwitz, L. & Voth, H. (1972). Final report of the Menninger Psychotherapy Research Project. *Bulletin of the Menninger Clinic*, **36**, 1–275.

Kingdon, D., Turkington, D. & John, C. (1994). Cognitive behaviour therapy of schizophrenia. *British Journal of Psychiatry*, **164**, 581–7.

Klein, D. N., Schwartz, J. E., Santiago, N. J. *et al.* (2003). Therapeutic alliance in depression treatment: controlling for prior change and patient characteristics. *Journal of Consulting and Clinical Psychology*, **71**, 997–1006.

Klerman, G. L. & Weissman, M. M. (Eds) (1993). *New Applications of the Interpersonal Therapy of Depression*. Washington, DC: American Psychiatric Press.

Koerner, K. & Linehan, M. M. (2000). Research on dialectical behavior therapy for patients with borderline personality disorder. *Psychiatric Clinics of North America*, **23**, 151–67.

Kolvin, I., MacMillan, A. & Wrate, R. M. (1988). Psychotherapy is effective. *Journal of the Royal Society of Medicine*, **81**, 261–6.

Kopta, S. M., Howard, K. I., Lowry, J. L. & Beutler, L. E. (1994). Patterns of symptomatic recovery in psychotherapy. *Journal of Consulting and Clinical Psychology*, **62**, 1009–16.

Kupfer, D. J., Frank, E., Perel, J. M. *et al.* (1992). Five year outcome for maintenance therapies in recurrent depression. *Archives of General Psychiatry*, **49**, 769–73.

Lambert, M. (ed.) (2004). *Bergin and Garfield's Handbook of Psychotherapy and Behavior Change*. New York: Wiley.

Lambert, M. J., Bergin, A. E. & Garfield, S. L. (2004). Introduction and historical overview. In *Bergin and Garfield's Handbook of Psychotherapy and Behavior Change*, ed. M. Lambert, pp. 3–15. New York: Wiley.

Leichsenring, F. (2001). Comparative effects of short-term psychodynamic psychotherapy and cognitive-behavioral therapy in depression: a meta-analytic approach. *Clinical Psychology Review*, **21**, 401–19.

Leichsenring, F., Rabung, S. & Leibing, E. (2004). The efficacy of short-term psychodynamic psychotherapy in specific psychiatric disorders: a meta-analysis. *Archives of General Psychiatry*, **61**, 1208–16.

Linehan, M. M. (1993). *Dialectical Behavioral Therapy of Borderline Personality Disorder*. New York: Guilford Press.

Linehan, M. M., Comtois, K. A., Murray, A. M. *et al.* (2006). Two-year randomized controlled trial and follow-up of dialectical behavior therapy vs therapy by experts for suicidal behaviors and borderline personality disorder. *Archives of General Psychiatry*, **63**, 757–66.

Lipsey, M. W. & Wilson, D. B. (1993). The effficacy of psychological, educational, and behavioral treatment; confirmation from metaanalysis. *American Psychologist*, **48**, 1181–209.

Luborsky, L. (1984). *Principles of Psychoanalytic Psychotherapy: A Manual for Supportive-Expressive (SE) Treatment*. New York: Basic Books.

Luborsky, L. & Crits-Christoph, P. (1990). *Understanding Transference: the Core Conflict Relationship Theme Method*. New York: Basic Books.

Luborsky, L., Crits-Christoph, P., McLellan, T. *et al.* (1986). Do therapists vary much in their success? Findings from four outcome studies. *American Journal of Orthopsychiatry*, **51**, 501–12.

Luborsky, L., Crits-Christoph, P., Mintz, J. & Auerbach, A. (1988). *Who will Benefit from Psychotherapy? Predicting Therapeutic Outcomes*. New York: Basic Books.

Luborsky, L., McLellan, A. T., Diguer, L., Woody, G. & Seligman, D. (1997). The psychotherapist matters: comparison of outcome across twenty-two therapists and seven patient samples. *Clinical Psychology: Science and Practice*, **4**, 53–65.

Luborsky, L. Singer, B. & Luborsky, L. (1975). Comparative studies of psychotherapy: is is true that "everyone has won and all shall have prizes"? *Archives of Genernal Psychiatry*, **41**, 165–80.

Malan, D. H. (1976). *Toward the Validation of Dynamic Psychotherapy: A Replication*. New York: Plenum Press.

Malan, D. H. (1979). *Individual Psychotherapy and the Science of Psychodynamics*. Boston: Butterworth.

Mallinckrodt, B., Gantt, D. & Coble, H. (1995). Attachment patterns in the psychotherapy relationship: development of a client attachment to the therapist scale. *Journal of Counselling Psychology*, **42**, 307–17.

Mann, J. (1973). *Time-limited Psychotherapy*. Cambridge, MA: Harvard University Press.

Martin, D. J., Garske, J. P. & Davis, M. K. (2000). Relation of the therapeutic alliance with outcome and other variables: a meta-analytic review. *Journal of Consulting Clinical Psychology*, **68**, 438–50.

Martin, S. D., Martin, E., Rai, S. S., Richardson, M. A. & Royall, R. (2001). Brain blood flow changes in depressed patients treated with interpersonal psychotherapy or venlafaxine hydrochloride: preliminary findings. *Archives of General Psychiatry*, **58**, 641–8.

McDermut, W., Miller, I. W. & Brown, R. A. (2001). The efficacy of group psychotherapy for depression: a meta-analysis and review of the empirical research. *Clinical Psychology: Science and Practice*, **8**, 98–116.

Miranda, J. & Borkovec, T. D. (1999). Reaffirming science in psychotherapy research. *Journal of Clinical Psychology*, **55**, 191–200.

Monsen, J. T., Odland, T., Faugli, A., Daee, E. & Eilertsen, D. E. (1995). Personality disorders: changes and stability after intensive psychotherapy focusing on affect consciousness. *Psychotherapy Research*, **5**, 33–48.

Morrow-Bradley, C. & Elliott, R. (1986). Utilization of psychotherapy research by practicing psychotherapists. *American Psychologist*, **41**, 188–97.

Nathan, P. E. & Gorman, J. M. (2002). *A Guide to Treatments that Work*. New York: Oxford University Press.

Orlinksy, D. E., Ronnestad, M. H. & Willutski, U. (2004). Fifty years of psychotherapy process-outcome research: continuity and change. In *Bergin and Garfield's Handbook of Psychotherapy and Behavior Change*, ed. M. Lambert, pp. 307–90. New York: Wiley.

Piper, W. E., Azim, H. A., Joyce, A. S. & McCallum, M. (1991). Transference interpretations, therapeutic alliance, and outcome in short-term individual psychotherapy. *Archives of General Psychiatry*, **48**, 946–53.

Propst, A., Paris, J. & Rosberger, Z. (1994). Do therapist experience, diagnosis and functional level predict outcome in short-term psychotherapy? *Canadian Journal of Psychiatry*, **39**, 178–83.

Raw, S. D. (1993). Does psychotherapy research teach us anything about psychotherapy? *Behavior Therapist*, March, 75–6.

Rector, N. A. & Beck, A. T. (2001). Cognitive behavioral therapy for schizophrenia: an empirical review. *Journal of Nervous and Mental Disease*, **189**, 278–87.

Rockland, L. H. (1992). *Supportive Therapy for Borderline Patients: A Dynamic Approach*. New York: Guilford Press.

Rosenzweig, S. (1936). Some implicit common factors in diverse methods of psychotherapy. *American Journal of Orthopsychiatry*, **6**, 412–15.

Roth, A. & Parry, G. (1997). The implications of psychotherapy research for clinical practice and service development: lessons and limitations. *Journal of Mental Health*, **6**, 367–80.

Rubino, G., Barker, C., Roth, A. D. & Fearon, P. (2000). Therapist empathy and depth of interpretation in response to potential alliance ruptures: the role of therapist and patient attachment styles. *Psychotherapy Research*, **10**, 408–20.

Ryan, E. R. (1985). Predicting the quality of alliance in the initial psychotherapy interview. *Journal of Nervous and Mental Disease*, **12**, 717–25.

Ryle, A. (1990). *Cognitive Analytic Therapy: Active Participation in Change*. Chichester: Wiley.

Ryle, A. (1995). Research relating to CAT. In *Cognitive Analytic Therapy: Developments in theory and practice*, ed. A. Ryle, pp. 175–89. Chichester: Wiley.

Sackett, D. L., Rosenberg, W. M., Gray, J. A. M., Haynes, R. B. & Richardson, W. S. (1996). Evidence based medicine: what it is and what it isn't. *British Medical Journal*, **312**, 71–2.

Safran, J. D. & Muran, J. C. (1996). The resolution of ruptures in the therapeutic alliance. *Journal of Consulting and Clinical Psychology*, **55**, 379–84.

Safran, J. D. & Muran, J. C. (2000). *Negotiating the Therapeutic Alliance*. New York: Guilford Press.

Safran, J. D., Crocker, P., McMain, S. & Murray, P. (1990). The therapeutic alliance rupture as a therapy event for empirical investigation. *Psychotherapy*, **27**, 154–65.

Sanchez, L. M. & Turner, S. M. (2003). Practising psychology in the era of managed care. Implications for practice and training. *American Psychologist*, **58**, 116–29.

Satterfield, W. A. & Lyddon, W. J. (1998). Client attachment and the working alliance. *Counselling Psychology Quarterly*, **11**, 407–15.

Schulberg, H. C., Block, M. R., Madonia, M. J. *et al.* (1996). Treating major depression in primary care practice. Eight-month clinical outcomes. *Archives of General Psychiatry*, **53**, 913–19.

Seligman, M. E. P. (1995). The effectiveness of psychotherapy: the Consumer Report study. *American Psychologist*, **50**, 965–74.

Shadish, W. R., Matt, G. E., Navarro, A. M. *et al.* (1997). Evidence that therapy works in clinically representative conditions. *Journal of Consulting and Clinical Psychology*, **65**, 355–65.

Shea, M. T., Pilkonis, P. A., Beckham, E. *et al.* (1990). Personality disorders and treatment outcome in the NIMH Treatment of Depression Collaborative Research Program. *American Journal of Psychiatry*, **147**, 711–18.

Sheldon, T. A., Song, F. & Davey-Smith, G. (1993). Critical appraisal of the medical literature: how to assess whether health care interventions do more good than harm. In *Purchasing and Providing Cost Effective Health Care*, ed. M. F. Drummond & A. Maynard, pp. 31–48. London: Churchill Livingstone.

Shorter, E. (1998). *A History of Psychiatry*. New York: Wiley.

Sifneos, P. E. (1972). *Short-Term Psychotherapy and Emotional Crisis*. Cambridge, MA: Harvard University Press.

Smith, M. L. & Glass, G. V. (1977). Meta-analysis of psychotherapy outcome studies. *American Psychologist*, **32**, 752–60.

Smith, M. L., Glass, G. V. & Miller, T. I. (1980). *The Benefits of Psychotherapy*. Baltimore, MD: Johns Hopkins University Press.

Stein, D. M. & Lambert, M. J. (1995). Graduate training in psychotherapy: are therapy outcomes enhanced? *Journal of Consulting and Clinical Psychology*, **63**, 182–96.

Stevenson, J. & Meares, R. (1992). An outcome study of psychotherapy for patients with borderline personality disorder. *American Journal of Psychiatry*, **149**, 358–62.

Stiles, W. B., Leach, C., Barkham, M. *et al.* (2003). Early sudden gains in psychotherapy under routine clinic conditions: practice-based evidence. *Journal of Consulting and Clinical Psychology*, **71**, 14–21.

Strupp, H. & Hadley, S. (1979). Specific vs. non-specific factors in psychotherapy. *Archives of General Psychiatry*, **36**, 1125–36.

Strupp, H. H. & Binder, J. L. (1984). *Psychotherapy in a New Key: A Guide to Time-limited Dynamic Psychotherapy*. New York: Basic Books.

Strupp, H. H., Fox, R. E. & Lesser, K. (1969). *Patients View Their Psychotherapy*. Baltimore, MD: Johns Hopkins University Press.

Suinn, R. M. (1993). Psychotherapy: can the practitioner learn from the researcher? *Behavior Therapist*, February, 47–9.

Sullivan, H. S. (1953). *The Interpersonal Theory of Psychiatry*. New York: Norton.

Tang, T. Z. & DeRubeis, R. J. (1999). Sudden gains and critical sessions in cognitive-behavioral therapy for depression. *Journal of Consulting and Clinical Psychology*, **67**, 894–904.

Tang, T. Z., Luborsky, L. & Andrusyna, T. (2002). Sudden gains in recovering from depression: are they also found in psychotherapies other than cognitive-behavioral therapy? *Journal of Consulting and Clinical Psychology*, **70**, 444–7.

Tyrell, C. L., Dozier, M., Teague, G. B. & Fallott, R. B. (1999). Effective treatment relationships for persons with severe psychiatric disorders: the importance of attachment states of mind. *Journal of Consulting and Clinical Psychology*, **67**, 725–33.

Vaillant, G. E. (1977). *Adaptation to Life*. Cambridge, MA: Little Brown.

Wachtel, P. L. (1977). *Psychoanalysis and Behavior Therapy*. New York: Basic Books.

Wallerstein, R. S. (1990). Psychoanalysis: the common ground [see comments]. *International Journal of Psychoanalysis*, **71**, 3–20.

Wampold, B., Minami, T., Baskin, T. & Callen-Tierney, S. (2002). A meta-(re)analysis of the effects of cognitive therapy versus 'other therapies' for depression. *Journal of Affective Disorders*, **68**, 159–65.

Wampold, B. E. (2001). *The Great Psychotherapy Debate: Models, Methods, and Findings*. Mahwah, NJ: Laurence Erlbaum.

Wampold, B. E., Mondin, G. W., Moody, M., Stich, F., Benson, K. & Ahn, H. (1997). A meta-analysis of outcome studies comparing bona fide psychotherapies: empiricially, "all must have prizes". *Psychological Bulletin*, **122**, 203–15.

Weissman, M. M. & Markowitz, J. (1994). Interpersonal psychotherapy – current status. *Archives of General Psychiatry*, **51**, 599–606.

Weisz, J. R., Donenberg, G. R., Han, S. S. & Kauneckis, D. (1995). Child and adolescent psychotherapy outcomes in experiments versus clinics: why the disparity? *Journal of Abnormal Child Psychology*, **23**, 83–106.

Weisz, J. R., Weiss, B., Han, S. S., Granger, D. A. & Morton, T. (1995). Effects of psychotherapy with children and adolescents revisited: a meta-analysis of treatment outcome studies. *Psychological Bulletin*, **117**, 450–68.

Westen, D. (1998). The scientific legacy of Sigmund Freud: towards a psychodynamically informed psychological science. *Psychological Bulletin*, **124**, 360–70.

Westen, D. & Morrison, K. (2001). A multidimensional meta-analysis of treatments for depression, panic, and generalized anxiety disorder: an empirical examination of the status of empirically supported therapies. *Journal of Consulting and Clinical Psychology*, **69**, 875–99.

Westen, D., Novotny, C. M. & Thompson-Brenner, H. (2004). The empirical status of empirically supported psychotherapies: assumptions, findings, and reporting in controlled clinical trials. *Psychology Bulletin*, **130**, 631–63.

Wierzbicki, M. & Pekarik, G. (1993). A meta-analysis of psychotherapy dropout. *Professional Psychology: Research and Practice*, **24**, 190–5.

Wilfley, D. E., Welch, R. R., Stein, R. I. *et al.* (2002). A randomized comparison of group cognitive-behavioral therapy and group interpersonal psychotherapy for the treatment of overweight individuals with binge-eating disorder. *Archives of General Psychiatry*, **59**, 713–21.

Winston, A., Laikin, M., Pollack, J., Samstag, L. W., McCullough, L. & Muran, J. C. (1994). Short-term dynamic psychotherapy of personality disorders. *American Journal of Psychiatry*, **15**, 190–4.

Young, J. E., Klosko, J. S. & Weishaar, M. E. (2003). *Schema Therapy: A Practitioner's Guide*. New York: Guilford Press.

Young, J. E. & Lindemann, M. D. (1992). An integrative schema-focused model for personality disorders. *Journal of Cognitive Psychotherapy*, **6**, 11–23.

6

Educational interventions

Christopher Dowrick, Nancee Blum and Bruce Pfohl

Editor's note

The place for psycho-education in the treatment of psychiatric disorders appears to be growing. While lip service has often been paid to educational interventions for psychiatric patients, it is really only in the last decade that evidence has been systematically gathered as to its role(s) and effectiveness. Overall educational interventions appear to improve primary care medical workers' (general practitioners, nurse practitioners and the like) detection of, as well as attitudes towards, mental illness, though there is little evidence, with respect especially to 'milder' mood disorders, that these interventions change the ultimate outcome of the disorder. Further, they do not, at this time, appear to impact patients' and their families' dislike of pharmacological treatment. Educational interventions in severe and persistent mental illness, especially if patients themselves are involved in the education either as teachers or participants, will reduce stigma towards the illness, but again the reduction in stigma does not translate into better or improved health outcomes. But in severe mental illness, psycho-education, particularly involving problem-solving and motivational interviewing, delivered to patients, other care workers and families appears to reduce rates of relapse and readmission to hospital.

With regard to common affective disorders:

- There is evidence of effectiveness, particularly in reducing symptoms and severity of depression, for psycho-education delivered to patients through a variety of means.
- Public education can change some attitudes towards the illness itself though antipathy to drug treatment appears difficult to alter.
- Extensive educational interventions for health professionals can alter professional attitudes and behaviours, but to date they have demonstrated little specific impact on health outcomes.

With regard to severe and enduring mental illness:

- Psycho-educational approaches for patients and carers can reduce rates of relapse and readmission to hospital, particularly if the approaches include problem-solving techniques and motivational interviewing.
- Public education can reduce stigma, particularly if people with severe mental illness are directly involved in delivering the education.
- Education for health professionals may improve early detection rates but in itself has a limited impact on case management in primary care.

Educational interventions will only be effective if they are closely allied to the delivery of other effective treatments. The role of patients as educators is of potential importance for the future.

Summary

Educational interventions for mental illness may be provided for patients and carers, the general public or health professionals. They may seek to affect knowledge, skills or attitudes.

Introduction

Educational interventions for mental illnesses may be concerned with acquiring knowledge, developing skills or changing attitudes. They are commonly aimed at patients,

Cambridge Textbook of Effective Treatments in Psychiatry, ed. Peter Tyrer and Kenneth R. Silk. Published by Cambridge University Press.
© Cambridge University Press, 2008.

their families and informal care providers. They may also be offered to healthcare professionals and the general public. They are distinguished from other forms of psychiatric intervention in that they do not focus on the unique problems of the individual.

Much of the literature in this field is concerned with psycho-education, which may be defined as the education of a person with psychiatric disorder in subject areas that serve the goals of treatment and rehabilitation. The terms 'patient education', 'patient teaching', and 'patient instruction' have also been used for this process. All imply that there is a focus on knowledge, although learning involves much more than this. Learning involves cognitive, affective and psychomotor processes (Rankin & Stallings, 1996). Patient education can take a variety of forms depending upon the abilities and interest of the patient and family. For example, the education may take place in small groups or on a one-to-one basis, it may involve the use of videotapes or pamphlets or a combination of these.

The goal of patient education may be economic, to try to prevent hospitalisation, or personal, to manage the illness or condition in such a way that patients may attain their maximum degree of health. Many patients feel stigmatised by their illness and may deny its existence. The extent to which people with serious or persistent mental illness comply with prescribed treatment regimes is of great concern to health professionals and is often a focus of patient education (Falvo, 1994).

It may be useful to bear in mind the semantic distinction between education and instruction, although both will be considered in this chapter. Education contains elements of 'leading forth' of the culture, drawing out or development of the powers and capacities inherent in all those involved in the process while paying attention to the position and perspectives of the participants. In contrast instruction is concerned with the imparting of knowledge or skill; it is more likely to be didactic, derived from prior principles or evidence, designed to inform its recipients of answers and attitudes which are presumed to be correct.

This chapter is constructed as follows: educational interventions concerning affective disorders, severe and enduring mental illness and other psychiatric problems will be considered in three discrete sections; within each of these sections, interventions will be categorized into three groups, depending on whether they are concerned with patients and informal carers, the general public, or health professionals. The principles involved in each type of intervention will be described, followed by an assessment of their efficacy and (where available) their cost effectiveness. In the final section of the chapter, we consider the potential role of patients as educators.

Educational interventions for affective disorders

Interventions for patients and carers

Psycho-education

Psycho-education is derived from a model which views affective disorders, mainly depression and anxiety, as a product of multiple risk factors acting together to transform the emotions, actions and thought processes of individuals facing adverse conditions (Lewinsohn *et al.*, 1985). It incorporates techniques drawn from cognitive-behavioural therapy and strategies found to be effective in the treatment of depression, and it offers these elements in a structured group format. The aim is to treat the disorder through encouragement of relaxation, positive thinking, pleasant activities and improvement in social skills. There is a clear emphasis on instruction rather than therapy, with the participants being described as teachers and pupils rather than therapists and clients or patients. The intention is to reach people who otherwise may not seek formal healthcare treatment.

The most common format for psycho-education is the coping with depression course which involves twelve 2-hour sessions over 8 weeks, with class reunions 1 and 6 months later (Lewinsohn, 1989). Modified versions include the eight session depression prevention course that is intended for people who are at high risk of developing depression (Muñoz & Ying, 1993).

Psycho-educational approaches have been used in both healthcare and community settings with the aim of prevention as well as treatment. Two large-scale studies provide evidence for the benefits of such approaches. In the USA, Wells and colleagues effectively employed a modified version of the coping with depression course in a primary care trial of quality improvement programmes for depression (Wells *et al.*, 2000). The ODIN study also tested the depression prevention course in urban and rural community settings in three European countries. Although participants were less likely to take up the offer of this intervention than they were to accept the offer of individual problem-solving treatment, the study demonstrated that the depression prevention course was effective over a 6-month period in reducing the number of cases of depression, and in improving participants' subjective function (Dowrick *et al.*, 2000).

Self-help materials

Self-help materials may be presented in the form of written materials, such as booklets or leaflets, audiocassettes or – increasingly – as computer-aided packages delivered either directly or via the internet. These materials commonly contain information about anxiety and depression, offer advice on techniques for self-monitoring including diaries, instructions in managing worrying thoughts, lifestyle changes, coping strategies, and provide accessible diagrams and self-test quizzes. Self-help materials may be offered as stand-alone materials or provided in conjunction with limited access to a health professional, usually a nurse, either by telephone or through brief face-to-face meetings.

A systematic review of trials of self-help interventions for patients with anxiety and depression in primary care identified eight studies examining written interventions based mostly on behavioural principles. Although the majority of trials reported some significant advantages in outcome associated with self-help treatments, the number of included studies was limited and important methodological limitations were identified. There were no data concerning long-term clinical benefits or cost-effectiveness. The authors of the review concluded that self-help treatments may have the potential to improve the overall cost-effectiveness of mental health service provision. However, they considered that the available evidence is limited in quantity and quality and more rigorous trials are required to provide more reliable estimates of the clinical and cost-effectiveness of these treatments (Bower et al., 2001).

Computer-aided self-help for people with anxiety and depression shows promise. In one study a clinic that gave immediate computer-aided cognitive behavioural therapy self-help plus brief advice from a therapist achieved significant and clinically meaningful improvements among their patients, while substantially reducing per-patient therapist time (Marks et al., 2003). In Australia, a randomized controlled trial evaluated the efficacy for community-dwelling individuals with symptoms of depression of two internet interventions offered to the general public. One was a psycho-education website offering information about depression (BluePages); the other was an interactive website offering cognitive-behaviour therapy (MoodGYM). Over 500 people were interested enough in using these services to take part in the trial. Both cognitive-behaviour therapy and psycho-education delivered via the internet were found to be effective in reducing symptoms of depression when compared with a credible community control group. MoodGYM reduced dysfunctional thinking and increased knowledge of cognitive-behaviour therapy. BluePages significantly improved participants' understanding of effective evidence-based treatments for depression (Christensen et al., 2004).

It is also important to remember that many people with symptoms of psychological distress do not seek professional help at all. A postal survey in New South Wales assessed actions taken to cope with depression at different levels of psychological distress in a community sample. Actions taken to cope with depression could be classified as intensification of everyday strategies, initiation of new self-help (including complementary therapies, non-prescription medication and dietary changes) and seeking professional help. Use of everyday strategies peaked with mild psychological distress, new self-help showed a peak in moderate distress, while professional help-seeking peaked in severe distress. The authors concluded that these 'genuine' self-help strategies are very commonly used, particularly in mild-moderate psychological distress. More evidence is needed to evaluate their effectiveness so that optimal self-help can be encouraged (Jorm et al., 2004).

Interventions for the general public

Public awareness campaigns, focused mainly on depression, have been a common feature of governmental health policy in many western countries during the past decade. These include 'Keep your Chin Up' in Finland, and the 'Beyond Blue' in Australia.

In the UK, the aims of the Defeat Depression Campaign (1992–1996) included the reduction of stigma associated with depression, education of the public about the disorder and its treatment, and encouragement of earlier treatment-seeking. Newspaper and magazine articles, radio and television programmes and other media activities were employed. Surveys of public attitudes were conducted by a national polling organisation before, during and after the campaign. Each survey covered about 2000 subjects who were sampled to be representative of the population of the UK.

These surveys found that attitudes to depression and to treatment by counselling were very favourable, whereas antidepressants were regarded by the majority of respondents as addictive and less effective. They also found significant positive changes regarding public attitudes to depression and reported experience of it, and a shift of attitudes in favour of antidepressant medication, all in the order of 5–10% (Paykel et al., 1998). A similar set of surveys in Nuremburg, Germany noted a shift in public attitudes towards a favourable view of depression following a public information campaign, but no change in attitudes towards pharmacotherapy (Hegerl et al., 2003).

Interventions for health professionals

Finding effective educational strategies to increase the knowledge and skills of doctors and other health professionals in relation to affective disorders has been a major concern for health policy makers during the past two decades.

Box 6.1 The range of professional educational interventions intended to improve the quality of care for depression

Distribution of educational material: published or printed recommendations for clinical care including clinical practice guidelines, provided personally or through mass mailings.

Educational meetings: healthcare practitioners who have participated in conferences, lectures, workshops or traineeships.

Local consensus processes: inclusion of participating practitioners in discussion to ensure that they agreed the chosen clinical problem was important and the approach to managing the problem was appropriate.

Educational outreach visits and academic detailing: use of a trained person who met with practitioners in their practice settings to give information with the intent of changing the practitioners' practice; the information given may have included feedback on the performance of practitioners.

Local opinion leaders: use of practitioners nominated by their colleagues as educationally influential; the investigators must have explicitly stated that their colleagues identified the opinion leaders.

Patient-mediated interventions: new clinical information collected directly from patients and given to the practitioners, e.g. depression scores from an instrument.

Audit and feedback: any summary of clinical performance of healthcare during a specified period; the summary must have included recommendations for clinical action; the information may have been obtained from medical records, computerized databases or observations from patients.

Reminders: patient- or encounter-specific information, provided verbally, on paper or on computer screens, which is designed or intended to prompt a health professional to recall information, including computer-aided decision support and drug dosages.

Marketing: a survey of targeted practitioners to identify barriers to change and subsequent design of an intervention that addresses identified barriers.

A wide variety of educational interventions for health professionals have been employed, and these are summarized in Box 6.1. In this section we will describe in some detail two main types of intervention, direct education and construction of complex care pathways and then summarize the evidence for effectiveness in this field.

Direct educational intervention

The archetypal educational intervention was the one conducted in the 1980s on the Swedish island of Gotland, with a population of some 60 000. A series of seminars on diagnosing and managing depression was provided for the island's 18 primary care physicians. This was followed by a decrease in suicide rates, sickness absence and hospital referrals for depression, and an increase in the rate of antidepressant prescribing (Rutz *et al.*, 1989).

Following the Gotland study there has been considerable interest in the potential utility of providing training programmes for general practitioners (GPs) in the assessment and management of depression. This study was not a controlled trial, and it is unclear what proportion of the changes reported reflected a real reduction in psychiatric morbidity, rather than simply an alteration in the doctor's management behaviours.

It has been difficult to replicate these findings in relation to the management of depression. Several well-conducted randomized controlled trials testing the effects of training family doctors, nurses and other primary healthcare professionals on outcomes for depressed patients have subsequently been published. None has been able to replicate the positive findings from Gotland. By way of examples I will describe three of these studies undertaken in England.

The Hampshire Depression Project assessed the effectiveness of an educational programme based on a depression clinical practice guideline, using a randomized controlled trial in a sample of 60 primary care practices. Education was delivered to all members of the primary healthcare teams in the intervention group. The main outcomes were recognition of depression by doctors, and clinical improvement as measured by the hospital anxiety and depression scale.

The education was well received by the participants, 80% of whom thought it would change their management of patients with depression. Over 20 000 patients were subsequently screened, of whom 4192 were classified as depressed on the basis of scores on the hospital anxiety and depression scale. This practice programme was designed to convey the current consensus on best practice for the care of depression, and was well received by the health professionals who took part. However it did not deliver improvements in recognition of or recovery from depression. The educational programme did not increase the sensitivity of the doctors to depressive symptoms. Nor did the outcome of depressed patients as a whole improve significantly, either at 6 weeks or 6 months after the assessment (Thompson *et al.*, 2000). In part this was due to patients' concerns about the addictive potential of antidepressants, which led many of them to discontinue treatment within a few weeks (Kendrick *et al.*, 2001).

Eighty-four GPs from London took part in a randomized controlled trial involving a training package of four half days on brief cognitive-behaviour therapy. Half of the doctors received the training at the beginning of the study, and the other half received it at the end. The researchers then examined two outcomes: whether the training had any effect on doctors' attitudes towards depression; and whether this in turn affected the depressive symptoms of 272 patients attending these doctors, as measured by their scores on the Beck Depression Inventory. They found that the training had no significant effect on doctors' knowledge of depression or attitudes towards its treatment. Nor did it have any discernable impact on patient outcomes (King *et al.*, 2002).

A study in the north-west of England set out to measure the health gain from providing GPs with additional skills in the assessment and management of depression (Gask *et al.*, 2004). Thirty-eight doctors took part. First, they were assessed for their ability to recognize psychological disorders, their attitudes to depression, prescribing patterns and their experience of psychiatry and communication skills training. Then they were randomly allocated to receive 10 hours of training either at the start or at the end of the study, using a training programme which has been thoroughly tested and demonstrated to have a positive effect on doctors' knowledge and skills (see Box 6.2).

All the doctors in this study went on to identify patients whom they considered to be depressed. They identified 318 people, of whom 189 agreed to take part in the study. These patients were assessed for depressive diagnoses and symptoms, quality of life, satisfaction with consultations, and their health service use and costs. After 3 months there were no significant differences in the depression status or quality of life scores between patients who were treated by doctors who had received the training programme and those treated by untrained doctors. After a year there was some evidence of a beneficial effect of training on patients' quality of life, but none on depression status or on health-care costs. There were no significant differences in patients' levels of satisfaction with their medical care, although patients reported that the doctors who had received the training were better at listening and understanding.

Training programmes such as these can improve the skills of doctors and other primary care health professionals in assessing and managing depression. However, increasing these skills does not appear to translate into improved health for depressed patients. Nor does it lead to more effective use of health services.

Box 6.2 The assessment and management of depression in primary care a 10-hour course for general practitioners (Gask *et al.*, 1998)

Aims: to improve the assessment and management of depression in general practice by effective use of pharmacological, physical and social interventions that are realistic within the confines of the consultation.
Training methods: The key focus of the course is on the acquisition of appropriate clinical skills. Each of the five 2-hour sessions includes:

- A brief presentation/lecture on each topic, viewing specially developed videotapes.
- The opportunity for each GP to role-play consultations as both GP and patient.
- Discussion of the videotaped role-plays in small feedback groups.
- Written materials to support each session.

Course timetable
Week 1: assessing depression.
Week 2: negotiating the treatment contract and drug treatment of depression.
Week 3: problem solving therapy and social interventions.
Week 4: the question of suicide.
Week 5: cognitive and behavioural skills.

There may be more success with educational programmes concentrating on the identification and management of patients at risk of suicide. In England such a programme was organized for all frontline staff in primary care, accident and emergency units and community mental health teams in one health district. There was a 14% drop in suicide in the following year in this health district, compared with an increase of about 4% in the suicide rate for the UK as a whole (Appleby *et al.*, 2000).

Educational interventions as part of organized care pathways
There is an emphasis on considering how best to restructure the ways in which healthcare services are delivered and to create organized care pathways for depression. In the USA there is an increasing tendency to promote depression as a chronic illness, like asthma, diabetes and hypertension, which would benefit from a multifactorial approach to management (Wagner *et al.*, 1996; Katon *et al.*, 2001). The essential components of successful care pathways are seen as having information systems

adequate to support organized care, restructuring practice to provide adequate follow-up, creating appropriate access to evidence-based expert systems whether electronic or human, and developing strong support for patient self-management.

Several studies have been undertaken in the USA to determine the efficacy and cost-effectiveness of formal, systematic approaches to the management of depression in primary care. Wells and colleagues put together a complex package of care aimed at quality improvement, and evaluated it in a randomized controlled trial. The package of care involved patient screening, clinician education, specific reminders for patients, case management undertaken by trained nurses, and enhanced integration between primary and specialist care (Wells *et al.*, 2000). Quality improvement was targeted at either increasing concordance between doctor and patient with regard to antidepressant medication, or else at increasing uptake of cognitive-behavioural therapy. The interventions were effective in improving concordance and depression outcomes over 12 months, although this effect had disappeared by 2 years. The incremental cost of providing these interventions for each patient was calculated at $419 for the drug arm and $485 for the therapy arm of the trial (Schoenbaum *et al.*, 2001).

In Washington state, Wayne Katon and colleagues set up a multifaceted organized treatment programme for depression in primary care clinics. They provided depressed patients with booklets and videotapes, involved GPs in training sessions and case conferences, and introduced a structured series of extended visits with family doctors and psychiatrists. This programme was effective in treating cases of major depression, though it did not appear to affect the outcome of mild and moderate depression. It involved extra treatment costs of between $260 and $540 per patient, which raised resource concerns within the US insurance-based healthcare system (Katon *et al.*, 1995).

Greg Simon and colleagues reported significant benefits at lower cost from a telephone care management system. Patients starting antidepressant treatment were randomized in a trial to receive either GP usual care, treatment feedback to GPs or feedback to GPs plus care management. The latter was delivered by a care manager with no specific training in antidepressant drug treatment. It included two 10–15 minute telephone assessments of each patient, 8 and 16 weeks after the initial prescription, followed by sophisticated treatment recommendations for the GP and support for the doctors in implementing these recommendations. At an incremental cost of $80 per patient, those patients in the 'feedback plus care management' arm of the trial had a higher probability of receiving at least a moderate dose of antidepressants. They also had a 50% improvement in depression checklist scores, and a lower probability of a diagnosis of major depression at follow up (Simon *et al.*, 2000).

This group has extended its activities by introducing IMPACT, a collaborative care management programme for late-life depression. This intervention involves a depression care manager, supervised by a psychiatrist and a primary care expert, who offered education, care management and support for either antidepressant medication or problem-solving treatment. In a randomized controlled trial involving 18 primary care clinics from five different states, they found that IMPACT produced substantial benefits in terms of reduction in depressive symptoms and functional impairment, and improvements in access to treatment, satisfaction with depression care and greater quality of life (Unutzer *et al.*, 2002).

Care management by nurses has also been positively evaluated as an intervention to improve treatment of depression in primary care. In 12 primary care practices across the USA, Rost and colleagues enrolled 211 adults who were beginning a new treatment episode for major depression in a trial designed to encourage them to engage in active treatment. They employed practice nurses to provide care management over 2 years. They found that ongoing intervention significantly improved both symptoms and functioning after 2 years: rates of remission increased by a third, emotional functioning improved by a quarter and physical functioning improved by almost a fifth. By 2 years 74% of patients in the enhanced care group reported remission, with emotional functioning exceeding 9% of population norms and physical functioning approaching 75% of population norms (Rost *et al.*, 2002).

Hunkeler and colleagues compared usual care with tele-healthcare provided by nurses, and tele-healthcare plus peer support from other patients who had recovered from depression, in the treatment of 302 people starting antidepressant drug therapy. Tele-healthcare took the form of emotional support and focused behavioural interventions, provided in 10 brief phone calls over 4 months. Although they found no evidence that peer support made any difference, the tele-healthcare intervention was associated with improved clinical outcomes and greater patient satisfaction (Hunkeler *et al.*, 2000).

Conclusions

A number of professional education strategies to improve the management of affective disorders have been proposed. Simple guideline implementation and educational strategies appear to be generally ineffective. Strategies more likely to prove effective in improving patient outcome are complex organizational interventions that incorporate combinations of clinician education, an enhanced role of the nurse, a greater degree of integration between primary and secondary care, and monitoring of medication adherence (Gilbody *et al.*, 2003).

The active ingredients of these complex packages are by definition difficult to establish. Nurse case management, effective integration between primary and secondary care and telephone medication counselling appear to be of importance. However, it is not clear how important the direct educational components may be.

What they all have in common is a commitment to regular routine management of patients with diagnosed depression, in contrast to the irregular and often haphazard approaches taken by family doctors. Doctors tend to rely on patients' own initiative in remembering to come back when they need a renewal of their prescription for antidepressant medication. The ability to establish a clear organizational framework within which doctors and patients can operate is likely to bring with it a sense of security and purpose, often conspicuously lacking in patients who feel low in mood, hopeless and without motivation, and whose poor self-esteem may lead them to worry about bothering the doctor with their trivial concerns (Gask *et al.*, 2003). Providing this sense of security and purpose may be intrinsically therapeutic. This, rather than any specific educational intervention, could be the key to the relative success of these programmes.

Educational interventions for severe and enduring mental illness

Interventions for patients and carers

Schizophrenia and bipolar disorders can be severe and chronic illnesses, often characterized by lack of insight and poor compliance with treatment. Psycho-educational approaches have been developed to increase patients' and their families' knowledge of, and insight into, their illness and its treatment. Interventions common to family psycho-education include empathic engagement, education with ongoing support, clinical resources during periods of crisis, social network enhancement, and problem solving and communication skills (McFarlane *et al.*, 2003). It is assumed that such educational approaches will enable people with severe and enduring mental illness to cope in a more effective way with their condition, thereby improving prognosis.

Bipolar disorders

For patients with bipolar disorders, reviews of the available literature indicate evidence of the effectiveness of psycho-educational approaches, particularly those which provide training in the identification of early manic symptoms in combination with pharmacological treatment (Perry *et al.*, 1999; Gonzalez-Pinto *et al.*, 2004).

Colom and colleagues conducted randomized controlled trial of group psycho-education involving 120 patients with bipolar disorders in Barcelona, Spain. The programme, aimed at improving four main issues, illness awareness, treatment compliance, early detection of prodromal symptoms and recurrences, and lifestyle regularity, was composed of 21 sessions of 90 minutes each (see Box 6.3). It was conducted by two experienced psychologists and provided to groups of 8–12 patients (Colom *et al.*, 2003).

This trial demonstrated that group psycho-education significantly reduced the number of patients who relapsed and the number of recurrences per patient. For example, 60% of control subjects fulfilled criteria for recurrence, compared with only 38% in the psycho-education group. It also increased the time to depressive, manic, hypomanic and mixed recurrences over 2 years of follow-up. The

---

Box 6.3 Content of the Barcelona Bipolar Disorders Programme (Colom *et al.*, 2003)

1. Introduction.
2. What is bipolar illness?
3. Causal and triggering factors.
4. Symptoms (1): mania and hypomania.
5. Symptoms (2): depression and mixed episodes.
6. Course and outcome.
7. Treatment (1): mood stabilizers.
8. Treatment (2): antimanic agents.
9. Treatment (3): antidepressants.
10. Serum levels: lithium, carbamazepine and valproate.
11. Pregnancy and genetic counselling.
12. Psychopharmacology vs alternative therapies.
13. Risks associated with treatment withdrawal.
14. Alcohol and street drugs: risks in bipolar illness.
15. Early detection of manic and hypomanic episodes.
16. Early detection of depressive and mixed episodes.
17. What to do when a new phase is detected?
18. Regularity.
19. Stress management techniques.
20. Problem-solving techniques.
21. Final session.

number and length of hospitalizations per patient was also lower in patients who received psycho-education. Psycho-education patients had 0.30 admissions per person over 2 years, significantly fewer than the 0.78 admissions per person in the control group.

As with affective disorders such as depression, it is not yet clear what the active ingredients are in psycho-education for bipolar disorders. It may be reasonable to hypothesize that teaching lifestyle regularity and the early detection of prodromal symptoms are important, particularly with regard to mania. Enhancement of cognitive function may also be protective (Martinez-Aran *et al.*, 2004), and involvement in an education programme over a substantial period of time may in itself promote treatment adherence. Further studies are needed to determine the specific content of these programmes that elicit more favourable responses.

Schizophrenia

Pekkala and Merinder have undertaken a systematic review of the effects of psycho-educational interventions in schizophrenia compared with standard levels of knowledge provision (Pekkala & Merinder, 2004). They included 10 studies of group or individual programmes. These programmes address the illness from a multidimensional viewpoint, including familial, social, biological and pharmacological perspectives. All studies of group education included family members. They provided patients and family members with support, information and management strategies.

An example of a brief psycho-education intervention for schizophrenia is that offered by Macpherson and colleagues, who gave patients a single individualized educational session following manual guidelines based on the psycho-education literature and principles of general health education (Macpherson *et al.*, 1996). An example of a longer intervention is the programme for relapse prevention tested by Herz and colleagues. This provided education for patients and family members about the process of relapse in schizophrenia and how to recognize prodromal symptoms and behaviours. It included active monitoring for prodromal symptoms and clinical intervention within 48 hours when prodromal episodes were detected. Participants were offered 1-hour weekly supportive group or individual therapy emphasizing improving coping skills and 90-minute multi-family psycho-education groups. These were held twice a week for 6 months and monthly thereafter (Herz *et al.*, 2000).

The main conclusion from this systematic review was that psycho-educational interventions for schizophrenia were associated with a small but significantly decreased risk of relapse and readmission rates at 9–18 months follow-up when compared with standard care. The relative risk of relapse was 0.8, with a 95% confidence interval of 0.7 to 0.9, compared with standard care. In a 'number needed to treat' analysis, nine patients needed to be offered psycho-education in order to prevent one relapse.

Compliance with medication was significantly improved in a single study using brief group intervention, but other studies produced equivocal or skewed data. Several secondary outcomes were measured, and these included knowledge gain, mental state, global level of functioning and expressed emotion in family members. Pekkala and Merinder's general conclusions were that research to date is consistent with the possibility that psycho-education has a positive effect on a person's well-being. However, they consider that there are very few adequate studies in this field, and that there is as yet insufficient evidence to support the contention that psycho-education has a significant impact on insight, medication, related attitudes or on overall satisfaction with services of patients or relatives. Health economic outcome was only measured in the Herz study, which found no significant difference in combined costs of hospital and ambulatory services between intervention and control groups.

This systematic review excluded interventions which had elements of behavioural training, such as social skills or life skills training, or education performed by patient peers. These factors may go some way to explaining the relatively limited success of interventions which concentrate primarily on instruction. Zygmunt and colleagues consider that effective psycho-educational interventions must include both behavioural components and supportive services. They see particular promise for interventions which include problem-solving techniques, principles of motivational interviewing, and models of care such as assertive community treatment (Zygmunt *et al.*, 2002).

Family education

While most studies on family psycho-education have focused primarily on its role in improving patient outcomes, family education programmes have also been developed not only to help empower family members but also to reduce the burden of caregiving when a family member has a severe mental disorder. These latter programmes may differ in that they are more likely to be led by trained volunteers rather than professionals. The setting is also more likely to be community-based rather than in a hospital or clinic. These programmes are often more accessible to family members because there is generally no or minimal cost (Solomon, 1996).

The Family-to-Family Education programme (FFEP) is a free 12-week programme (2–3 hours per week) developed by the National Alliance for the Mentally Ill (NAMI). It provides psycho-education taught by trained family members of those with a serious and persistent mental illness (Burland, 1998). The programme uses a structured, scripted manual to present information about several mental disorders and their treatments (e.g. schizophrenia, major depression, bipolar disorder, obsessive-compulsive disorder, borderline personality disorder and addictive disorders). There is an emphasis on teaching family members self-care, communication skills and problem-solving. Advocacy strategies are also included.

A non-randomized efficacy study of 37 family members who participated in the programme found respondents significantly more empowered in their community, their family, and in interactions with the service system than at baseline. The participating family members also experienced less displeasure and worry about their ill family member. These outcomes remained stable at 6-month follow-up (Dixon et al., 2001). A second study with 95 participants utilized a waiting list as a control group and again found that Family-to-Family participants felt a greater sense of empowerment in coping both with the mental health system and their ill family member. These gains were maintained at 6-month follow-up. Those on the waiting list did not improve, suggesting that the FFEP programme was responsible for the improvement (Dixon et al., 2004).

Psycho-educational approaches to severe and enduring mental illness need to be culturally sensitive. In rural China, for example, family interventions may be more effective if they focus primarily on relatives' recognition of illness and have a strong social skills component (Ran et al., 2003; Chien et al., 2006). Amongst members of the Latino community with schizophrenia in California, an intensive culturally relevant emphasis on training in social skills showed beneficial results in terms both of personal functioning and rates of rehospitalization (Kopelowicz et al., 2003).

There is also early evidence of benefit from an approach which focuses on the promotion of self-determination in young adults with schizophrenia, through the development of a therapeutic alliance with experienced community mental health nurses (McCann & Clark, 2004).

Interventions for the general public

In 1996 the World Psychiatric Association launched 'Open the Doors', an international programme to fight stigma and discrimination because of schizophrenia. The programme is designed to increase the awareness and knowledge of the nature of schizophrenia and treatment options, improve public attitudes about those who have or have had schizophrenia and their families, and generate action to eliminate discrimination and prejudice. The programme has developed a variety of materials to improve public information, facilitate community involvement, enhance knowledge of healthcare professionals, educate and support family and friends, and change legislation to ensure equitable healthcare coverage. It is not yet clear what impact this programme will have at a community level (see www.openthedoors.com for reports of initiatives at the national level).

Researchers in Canada evaluated a media intervention designed to improve one newspaper's portrayal of schizophrenia. The intervention attempted to influence news content by providing reporters with more accurate background information and helping them develop more positive story lines. The evaluation compared story content and length over a 24-month period: 8 months prior to the anti-stigma intervention and 16 months afterwards. Positive stories were more common than negative stories in both periods. Stories about schizophrenia increased by a third after the intervention, but their word count declined by 10%. However, there was also an increase in negative news about schizophrenia: stigmatizing stories about schizophrenia increased by 46%, and their length increased from 300 to 1000 words per story per month (Stuart, 2003).

Corrigan and colleagues have evaluated the effects of three strategies for changing stigmatizing attitudes: education, which replaces myths about mental illness with accurate conceptions; contact, which challenges public attitudes about mental illness through direct interactions with persons who have these disorders; and protest, which seeks to suppress stigmatizing attitudes about mental illness. One hundred and fifty-two students at a community college were randomly assigned to one of these three strategies or a control condition. They found that education led to improved attributions with regard to people with psychotic disorders. Contact produced the most positive changes, and exceeded education effects in attributions about depression and psychosis. However, protest yielded no significant changes in attributions (Corrigan et al., 2001).

Simple public education may also be effective. Giving information on the association between violent behaviour and schizophrenia can reduce impressions of the dangerousness of this condition. People who report previous contact with individuals with a mental illness rate individuals with mental illness as less dangerous than those without previous contact. People who receive information summarizing the prevalence rates of violent behaviour among individuals with schizophrenia rate them as less dangerous than those who do not receive this information (Penn *et al.*, 1999). Secondary school students who meet a young person with schizophrenia show a marked reduction in negative stereotypes and a positive trend regarding social distance (Schulze *et al.*, 2003).

Interventions for health professionals

Early detection

Timing of treatment may be important in that some studies of first-episode schizophrenia correlate shorter duration of untreated psychosis with better prognosis (Falloon *et al.*, 1998).

A three-site prospective clinical trial in Scandinavia has investigated the effect of the timing of treatment in first-episode psychosis. The major independent intervention variable is a comprehensive education and detection system to change the duration of untreated first-onset psychosis. It includes targeted information towards the general public, schools and health professionals, and early detection teams to recruit appropriate patients into treatment as soon as possible.

Specific information was imparted to primary healthcare workers and specialized psychiatric healthcare networks on how to recognize the early signs of psychosis and access early help for developing psychosis. Educational programmes tailored for GPs, psychiatric nurses and other professionals working within the general health system and psychiatry were introduced. This included checklists and a rating manual for prodromal symptoms to be used with a video demonstrating a patient experiencing psychiatric symptoms. All this, including clinical case discussions, was delivered within a 3–4 hour training seminar. The GPs also received a letter twice each year updating the results of the study with an appeal to refer patients as soon as possible when they suspected a possible serious psychiatric disorder.

These measures, in combination with easy access to psychiatric services, systematically changed referral patterns of first-episode schizophrenia. The mean duration of untreated psychosis was significantly reduced from 114 weeks to 26 weeks. The yearly costs associated with the educational initiatives was in the region of $200 000. The researchers concluded that educational and clinical interventions must be closely linked. Educational efforts to raise consciousness about psychosis will survive only so long as identified clients receive what that education says is necessary (Johannessen *et al.*, 2001).

Case management

During the past two decades there has been considerable interest in educational interventions for health professionals in primary care settings, with the aim of enabling them to take a more active and effective role in the case management of patients with severe and enduring mental illness. This interest has arisen as a result of the major shift in emphasis from hospital-based to community-based care for this vulnerable group of patients combined with an awareness that primary care teams have often lacked the skills (and sometimes the motivation) to provide effective care management. However, the evidence to date regarding the efficacy of such educational interventions is inconsistent.

Nazareth and colleagues evaluated the feasibility, acceptability and effectiveness of training GPs and practice nurses to undertake a structured approach to the management of schizophrenia. They recruited all patients with non-affective psychoses in four inner-city practices. In two of these practices doctors and nurses are trained in the use of a checklist and a set of outcome measures to apply when reviewing these patients. In these intervention practices there was a significant increase in consultation rates, significant improvements in global clinical assessments, and improvements in the behaviour, speech and 'other syndromes' subscales of the Present State Examination (Nazareth *et al.*, 1996).

Kendrick and colleagues tested the effectiveness of teaching GPs how to undertake structured assessments of their long-term mentally ill patients. They found that changes in treatment with neuroleptic drugs and referrals to community psychiatric nurses were significantly more frequent in the intervention group, but few patients received the assessments after the first 6 months. They concluded that teaching GPs about these problems can increase their involvement in psychiatric care, but regular structured assessments were not feasible in routine medical examination appointments (Kendrick *et al.*, 1995).

The impact of a similar structured assessment, this time delivered by practice nurses after a one-day training course, was also evaluated. The result demonstrated a high rate of consultation as well as uncovering a clinical need in this patient group. The practice nurses were more diligent than general practitioners in carrying out assessment, but there was no impact on treatment patterns or clinical outcome (Burns *et al.*, 1998).

The implications of these research studies appear to be that structured assessments by GPs and nurses with this patient group may well be feasible and may identify a previously unidentified group of patients in need, but further training is needed if this intervention is to be translated into health gain and improved outcome.

Educational interventions for other psychiatric problems

Borderline personality disorder

Interventions for patients and carers

A treatment programme for borderline personality disorder (BPD) called Systems Training for Emotional Predictability and Problem Solving (STEPPS™) was developed by Blum and colleagues at the University of Iowa. The 20-week group treatment programme combines a psycho-education component designated as *Awareness of Illness* with cognitive-behavioural therapy and skills training. Pilot data (non-RCT) suggest that patients experience improvement in BPD and mood-related symptoms. A survey of patients and therapists suggested moderate to high levels of satisfaction for the treatment. Early results from a randomized controlled trial are also encouraging (Blum *et al.*, 2002; Black *et al.*, 2004). An important part of the STEPPS program includes psycho-education sessions for family members, significant others, healthcare professionals and others who regularly interact with the patient to improve their self-efficacy and effectiveness in responding consistently to the individual with borderline personality disorder in ways that reinforce the STEPPS materials (Black *et al.*, 2004).

The National Education Alliance for Borderline Personality Disorder has a free 12-week programme called Family CONNECTIONS for people with a family member who has been diagnosed with BPD. The course is based on theories and skills from dialectical behaviour therapy, offers current information about the disorder and teaches new skills. The skills training component was added in response to an earlier study which showed that simply increasing family members' knowledge of BPD without teaching skills was associated with greater levels of perceived burden, distress and depression (Hoffman *et al.*, 2003a). Trained family members follow a structured, tested curriculum. Initial results reported significantly lowered levels of depression, grief and perceived burden of care after participating in the programme (Hoffman *et al.*, 2003b). A recent review has also supported these findings with other personality disorders (Hubard *et al.*, 2007).

Substance abuse

Interventions for patients

Kaminer and colleagues report on a randomized comparison of cognitive behavioral therapy vs. psycho-educational therapy for a consecutive series of 88 adolescents with substance abuse. Most patients had a dual diagnosis. Both subgroups received 8 weeks of the specified therapy with follow-up at 3 and 9 months using both urine drug screens and a substance use rating scale. Similar reductions in substance use were found in both subgroups (Kaminer *et al.*, 2002). However, the lack of an untreated control group limits any conclusions about effectiveness.

Bibliotherapy – the production of written self-help materials – may also be helpful with this group of patients. A controlled study found this approach decreased harmful drinking in individuals seeking help for alcohol abuse (Apodaca & Miller, 2003).

Interventions for the public

Psycho-educational programmes have been designed to prevent or stop substance abuse in children and adolescents. Some programmes are designed for a specific grade level, some for an entire school population, and some target high-risk students. Many of those studies compare outcome for a large sample of students by matching or randomizing schools that receive the intervention with those that do not. Use of substances at intake and follow-up is usually measured by anonymous self-report questionnaires.

For example, Eisen and colleagues studied the results of an intensive psycho-educational programme called 'Skills for Adolescence' in a sample of 6239 seventh grade students one year after the intervention. The programme consisted of forty 35-minute sessions focusing on building self-confidence, peer relationships, refusal skills and healthy, drug-free living. At 2-years follow-up, after controlling for baseline substance abuse scores and other variables, students from schools where the programme was given had a lower history of marijuana abuse. There was no significant treatment effect for alcohol use and other substances (Eisen *et al.*, 2003).

Obsessive-compulsive disorder

Although behaviour therapy utilizing exposure and ritual prevention for obsessive-compulsive disorder (OCD) has been shown repeatedly to be very effective, it is not widely available and is usually quite costly in those places that offer it. BT STEPS uses a treatment manual and interactive voice response telephone calls to carry out OCD self-assessment and then to assist patients in designing and implementing self-help behaviour therapy. This method was studied in 65 patients in two trials. Both trials reported substantial reduction in severity of OCD symptoms as measured by the Yale-Brown Obsessive Compulsive Scale. Patients assessed the programme positively and 71% considered their lives improved as a result of the programme. BT STEPS offers the potential to make OCD behaviour therapy available to anyone with a touch-tone telephone. The programme is intended for use in conjunction with a clinician (Baer & Griest, 1997).

An 8-site randomized controlled trial with nearly 200 patients compared BT STEPS, clinician-administered behaviour therapy, and systematic relaxation in a 12-week study. BT STEPS and clinician-administered behaviour therapy were significantly more helpful than relaxation (Greist *et al.*, 1998).

Final thought: patients as educators

It would be unwise to assume that education is all one way, from professionals and specialists to patients and generalists. Patients themselves can make excellent teachers.

In the context of undergraduate medical education, patients offer unique qualities that can improve the acquisition of examination and communication skills and instil confidence and reduce anxiety among students. Patients with mental health problems have successfully become involved with undergraduate medical education (Coodin & Chisholm, 2001), and with continuing professional development for primary care professionals, with specific roles in enabling health professionals to define effectiveness and to consider how they can best care for and treat patients (Fisher & Gilbert, 2001).

For example, the National Alliance for the Mentally Ill (NAMI) Provider Education Program is currently being taught in 13 of the United States. The 10-week course is led by a team that includes two patients who are knowledgeable about their mental illness, two family members who have been trained as teachers in the NAMI Family-to-Family Education Program, and a mental health professional who is either a family member of someone with a mental illness or someone who has a mental illness him/herself. The team works with staff at public agencies who serve people with severe and persistent mental disorders to increase provider awareness of the emotional and day-to-day practical consequences of these disorders. In written evaluations and focus-group surveys, providers report the experience as very helpful and leading to changes in how they view families and patients (see http://www.nami.org/).

In general, patient educators engender more positive attitudes in doctors, encouraging them to see patients as experts in their own conditions who should be actively involved in their own treatment and care (Wykurz & Kelly, 2002).

The level of evidence for each of the interventions discussed in this chapter is summarized in Table 6.1.

Table 6.1. Effectiveness of educational interventions

Treatment	Form of treatment	Psychiatric disorder/target audience	Level of evidence for efficacy	Comments
Psycho-education: Quality Improvement (QI) education	Designed course	Depression/care givers	Ia	Educational QI programmes increased compliance and functioning. Significant level of evidence from randomized controlled studies but overall impact on depression is probably less than what is hoped for.
Psycho-education: depression prevention and problem solving	Designed course	depression/patients	IIa	Problem solving more acceptable than depression prevention with better functioning with either intervention. Consistent level of evidence.
Self-help materials	NA	Anxiety, depression/patients	IIIa	Existing studies are few with methodological limitations but trend towards being cost-effective.
Computer-aided self-help	NA	Depression/patients	IIa	There is evidence for cognitive-behavioural therapy training to be helpful in decreasing dysfunctional thinking and knowledge of CBT, but more studies of computer-aided psycho-education are clearly needed.
Public awareness campaigns	NA	Depression/general public	IV	Survey methodology primarily here. There is evidence that public awareness campaigns can increase public awareness about depression itself but does not change peoples' negative impressions of antidepressant medications.
Direct educational intervention for health professionals	NA	Depression/professional care-givers	IIc	There is inconsistent evidence here that educational interventions may make physicians more aware of depression but they do not improve outcome or drastically change utilization of resources.

Table 6.1. (cont.)

Treatment	Form of treatment	Psychiatric disorder/target audience	Level of evidence for efficacy	Comments
Educational intervention utilizing organized care pathways combined with clinician education and co-operation among caregivers	NA	Depression/professional care-givers	IIc	The results are inconsistent here. There is some evidence pointing towards better outcomes and better adherence to medications though not necessarily greater patient satisfaction with treatment. The key factor appears to be an organizing process in the routine management of depression. Clinical care pathways alone do not have much impact.
Patient psycho-education to recognized early signs of mania	10–21 sessions	Bipolar disorder/patients and family members	IIa	There are still few studies here, but they uniformly reveal a significant decrease in the number of subsequent manic episodes and decreased number and frequency of hospitalisations.
Psycho-education	NA	Schizophrenia/patients	IIa	Systematic review suggests that psycho-education when family members are included has a beneficial effect but does not impact insight, satisfaction with services, or attitudes towards medications.
Family education	NA	Schizophrenia/family members	IIIa	Few well-controlled studies and outcome measures are not consistent. Overall family members feel more empowered and less anxious in managing and dealing with the ill relative.
Public campaigns	NA	Schizophrenia/general public	IIIa	Only one controlled trial that suggested that direct contact with people who have mental illness can improve attributions made about the illness. Other non-controlled studies support a similar positive effect of real-life contact with patients as a way to reduce stigma.
Direct educational intervention for health professionals	3–4 hours training session	Schizophrenia/healthcare professionals	IIIa	One ongoing controlled study to try to have healthcare professionals identify and refer first-break psychosis at the earliest possible time. Early results are somewhat encouraging.
Educational intervention utilizing organized care pathways combined with clinician education and cooperation among caregivers	NA	Schizophrenia/healthcare professionals	IIb	Several good cohort studies suggest that nurses and non-physicians are better at following a structured intervention, but that it is difficult for general practitioners to follow or fit in the structured assessment into the way that patients are currently scheduled.
Psycho-education for patients and families regarding borderline personality disorder	10–21 sessions	Borderline personality disorder/patients and caregivers	IIIb	Controlled trials have yet to be done but early results suggest that there is less caregiver burden and less depression in caregivers.
Psycho-education for patients and families regarding substance abuse	NA	Decrease use of alcohol	IV	There are no good controlled studies. Studies look at outcome but in no systematic way. Results are not consistent as to whether there is a measurable decrease in substance use after psycho-education compared with 'treatment as usual'.
Self-help for patients with Obsessive-compulsive disorder (OCD) using a manual and a telephone	NA	Obsessive-compulsive disorder/patients	IIIa	No good controlled studies, but case studies reveal that this intervention may be useful in reducing OCD symptoms and helping with relaxation.

REFERENCES

Apodaca, T. & Miller, W. (2003). A meta-analysis of the effectiveness of bibliotherapy for alcohol problems. *Journal of Clinical Psychology*, **59**, 289–304.

Appleby, L., Morriss, R., Gask, L. *et al.* (2000). An educational intervention for front-line health professionals in the assessment and management of suicidal patients (the STORM Project). *Psychological Medicine*, **30**, 805–12.

Baer, L. & Greist, J. H. (1997). An interactive computer-administered self-assessment and self-help program for behavior therapy. *Journal of Clinical Psychiatry*, **58** Suppl. 12, 23–8.

Black, D. W., Blum, N., Pfohl, B. & St. John, D. (2004). The STEPPS group treatment program for outpatients with borderline personality disorder. *Journal of Contemporary Psychotherapy*, **34**, 193–210.

Blum, N., Pfohl, B., St. John, D., Monahan, P. & Black, D. W. (2002). STEPPS: a cognitive-behavioral systems-based group treatment for outpatients with borderline personality disorder – a preliminary report. *Comprehensive Psychiatry*, **43**, 301–10.

Bower, P., Richards, D. & Lovell, K. (2001). The clinical and cost-effectiveness of self-help treatments for anxiety and depressive disorders in primary care: a systematic review. *British Journal of General Practice*, **51**, 838–45.

Burland, J. (1998). Family-to-family: a trauma and recovery model of family education. *New Directions for Mental Health Services*, **77**, 33–44.

Burns, T., Millar, E., Garland, C., Kendrick, T., Chisolm, B. & Ross, F. (1998). Randomized controlled trial of teaching practice nurses to carry out structured assessments of patients receiving depot antipsychotic medication. *British Journal of General Practice*, **48**, 1845–8.

Chien, W-T., Chan, S. W. C. & Thompson, D. R. (2006). Effects of a mutual support group for families of Chinese people with schizophrenia: 18-month follow-up. *British Journal of Psychiatry*, **189**, 41–9.

Christensen, H., Griffiths, K. M. & Jorm, A. F. (2004). Delivering interventions for depression by using the internet: randomised controlled trial. *British Medical Journal*, **328**, 265–8.

Colom, F., Vieta, E., Martinez-Aran, A. *et al.* (2003). A randomized trial on the efficacy of group psychoeducation in the prophylaxis of recurrences in bipolar patients whose disease is in remission. *Archives of General Psychiatry*, **60**, 402–7.

Coodin, S. & Chisholm, F. (2001). Teaching in a new key: effects of a co-taught seminar on medical students' attitudes towards schizophrenia. *Psychiatric Rehabilitation Journal*, **24**, 299–302.

Corrigan, P. W., River, L. P., Lundin, R. K. *et al.* (2001). Three strategies for changing attributions about severe mental illness. *Schizophrenia Bulletin*, **27**, 187–95.

Dixon, L., Lucksted, A., Stewart, B. *et al.* (2004). Outcomes of the peer-taught 12-week family-to-family education program for severe mental illness. *Acta Psychiatrica Scandinavica*, **109**, 207–15.

Dixon, L., Stewart, B., Burland, J., Delahanty, J., Lucksted, A. & Hoffman, M. (2001). Pilot study of the effectiveness of the family-to-family education program. *Psychiatric Services*, **52**, 965–7.

Dowrick, C., Dunn, G., Ayuso-Mateos, J. *et al.* (2000). Problem solving treatment and group psychoeducation for depression: multicentre randomised controlled trial. *British Medical Journal*, **321**, 1450–4.

Eisen, M., Zellman, G. L. & Murray, D. M. (2003). Evaluating the Lions-Quest "Skills for Adolescence" drug education program. Second-year behavior outcomes. *Addictive Behaviors*, **28**, 883–97.

Falloon, J. R., Coverdale, J. H., Laidlaw, T. M., Merry, S., Kidd, R. R. & Morosini, P. (1998). Early intervention for schizophrenic disorders: implementing optimal strategies in routine clinical services. *British Journal of Psychiatry*, **172** Suppl. 33, 33–8.

Falvo, D. R. (1994). *Effective Patient Education. A Guide to Increased Compliance*. Gaithersburg, MD: Aspen Publication Inc.

Fisher, B. & Gilbert, D. (2001). Patient involvement and clinical effectiveness. In *New Beginnings: Towards Patient and Public Involvement in Primary Health Care*, ed. S. Gillam & F. Brooks, pp. 119–31. London: King's Fund.

Gask, L., Usherwood, T., Thompson, H. & Williams, B. (1998). Evaluation of a training package in the assessment and management of depression in primary care. *Medical Education*, **32**, 190–8.

Gask, L., Rogers, A., Oliver, D., May, C. & Roland, M. (2003). Qualitative study of patients' perceptions of the quality of care in general practice. *British Journal of General Practice*, **53**, 278–83.

Gask, L., Dowrick, C., Dixon, C. *et al.* (2004). A pragmatic cluster randomised controlled trial of an educational intervention for general practitioners in the assessment and management of depression. *Psychological Medicine*, **34**, 63–72.

Gilbody, S., Whitty, P., Grimshaw, J. & Thomas, R. (2003). Educational and organizational interventions to improve the management of depression in primary care: a systematic review. *Journal of the American Medical Association*, **289**, 3145–51.

Gonzalez-Pinto, A., Gonzalez, C., Enjuto, S. *et al.* (2004). Psychoeducation and cognitive-behavioral therapy in bipolar disorder: an update. *Acta Psychiatrica Scandinavica*, **109**, 83–90.

Greist, J. H., Marks, I. M., Baer, L. *et al.* (1998). Self-treatment for obsessive-compulsive disorder using a manual and a computerized telephone interview: A US-UK study. *MD Computing*, **15**, 149–57.

Hegerl, U., Althaus, D. & Stefanek J. (2003). Public attitudes towards treatment of depression: effects of an information campaign. *Pharmacopsychiatry*, **36**, 288–91.

Herz, M. I., Lamberti, J. S., Minz, J. *et al.* (2000). A program for relapse prevention in schizophrenia: a controlled study. *Archives of General Psychiatry*, **57**, 277–83.

Hoffman, P., Buteau, E., Hooley, J. M., Fruzzetti, A. E. & Bruce M. L. (2003a). Family members' knowledge about borderline personality disorder: correspondence with their levels of depression, burden, distress, and expressed emotion. *Family Process*, **42**, 469–78.

Hoffman, P. D., Fruzzetti, A. E., Buteau, E. *et al.* (2003b). Family connections: a dialectical support and educational approach for families of persons with borderline personality disorder. Paper presented at the meeting of the International Society for the Investigation and Teaching of Dialectical Behavior Therapy, Boston, MA, November 2003.

Huband, N., Duggan, C., Evans, C. et al. (2007). Social problem-solving plus psychoeducation for adults with personality disorder. Pragmatic randomised controlled trial. *British Journal of Psychiatry*, **190**, 307–13.

Hunkeler, E. M., Meresman, J. F., Hargreaves, W. A. et al. (2000). Efficacy of nurse telehealth care and peer support in augmenting treatment of depression in primary care. *Archives of Family Medicine*, **9**, 700–8.

Johannessen, J. O., McGlashan, T. H., Larsen, T. K. et al. (2001). Early detection strategies for untreated first-episode psychosis. *Schizophrenia Research*, **51**, 39–46.

Jorm, A. F., Griffiths, K. M., Christensen, H., Parslow, R. A. & Rogers, B. (2004). Actions taken to cope with depression at different levels of severity: a community survey. *Psychological Medicine*, **34**, 293–9.

Kaminer, Y., Burleson, J. A. & Goldberger, R. (2002). Cognitive-behavioral coping skills and psychoeducation therapies for adolescent substance abuse. *Journal of Nervous and Mental Disease*, **190**, 737–45.

King, M., Davidson, O., Taylor, F., Haines, A., Sharp, D. & Turner, R. (2002). Effectiveness of teaching general practitioners skills in brief cognitive behaviour therapy to treat patients with depression: randomised controlled trial. *British Medical Journal*, **324**, 947–50.

Lewinsohn, P. (1989). The Coping with Depression Course: review and future directions. *Canadian Journal of Behavioural Science*, **21**, 470–93.

Lewinsohn, P., Hoberman, H., Teri, L. & Hautzinger, M. (1985). An integrative theory of depression. In *Theoretical Issues in Behaviour Therapy*, ed. S. Reiss & R. Bootzin, pp. 331–59. New York: Academic Press.

Katon, W., von Korff, M., Lin, E. et al. (1995) Collaborative management to achieve treatment guidelines. Impact on depression in primary care. *Journal of the American Medical Association*, **273**, 1026–31.

Katon, W., Von Korff, M., Lin, E. & Simon G. (2001). Rethinking practitioner roles in chronic illness: the specialist, primary care physician and the practice nurse. *General Hospital Psychiatry*, **23**, 138–44.

Kendrick, T., Burns, T. & Freeling, P. (1995). Randomised controlled trial of teaching general practitioners to carry our structured assessments of their long term mentally ill patients. *British Medical Journal*, **311**, 93–8.

Kendrick, T., Stevens, L., Bryant, A. et al. (2001). Hampshire Depression Project: changes in the process of care and cost consequences. *British Journal of General Practice*, **51**, 911–13.

Kopelowicz, A., Zarate, R., Gonzalez Smith, V., Mintz, J. & Liberman, R. P. (2003). Disease management in Latinos with schizophrenia: a family assisted, skills training approach. *Schizophrenia Bulletin*, **29**, 211–27.

Marks, I. M., Mataix-Cols, D., Kenwright, M., Cameron, R., Hirsch, S. & Geda, L. (2003). Pragmatic evaluation of computer aided self-help for anxiety and depression. *British Journal of Psychiatry*, **183**, 57–65.

Martinez-Aran, A., Vieta, E., Reinares, M. (2004). Cognitive function across manic or hypomanic, depressed, and euthymic states in bipolar disorder. *American Journal of Psychiatry*, **161**, 262–70.

McCann, T. V. & Clark, E. (2004). Advancing self-determination with young adults who have schizophrenia. *Journal of Psychiatric and Mental Health Nursing*, **11**, 12–20.

McFarlane, W. R., Dixon, L., Lukens, E. & Lucksted, A. (2003). Family psychoeducation and schizophrenia: a review of the literature. *Journal of Marital and Family Therapy*, **29**, 223–45.

Macpherson, R., Jerrom, B. & Hughes, A. (1996). A controlled study of education about drug treatment in schizophrenia. *British Journal of Psychiatry*, **168**, 709–17.

Muñoz, R. & Ying, Y. (1993). *The Prevention of Depression: Research and Practice* Baltimore, MD: Johns Hopkins University Press.

Nazareth, I., King, M. & Tai, S. S. (1996). Monitoring psychosis in general practice: a controlled trial. *British Medical Journal*, **169**, 475–82.

Paykel, E. S., Hart, D. & Priest, R. G. (1998). Changes in public attitudes to depression during the Defeat Depression Campaign. *British Journal of Psychiatry*, **173**, 519–22.

Pekkala, E. & Merinder, L. (2004). Psychoeducation for schizophrenia (Cochrane Review). In *The Cochrane Library*, **1** Chichester, UK: John Wiley & Sons, Ltd.

Penn, D. L., Kommana, S., Mansfield, M. & Link, B. G. (1999). Dispelling the stigma of schizophrenia: II. The impact of information on dangerousness. *Schizophrenia Bulletin*, **25**, 437–46.

Perry, A., Tarrier, N., Morris, R., McCarthy, E. & Limb, K. (1999). Randomised controlled trial of the efficacy of teaching patients with bipolar disorder to identify early symptoms of relapse and obtain treatment. *British Medical Journal*, **318**, 149–53.

Ran, M. S., Xiang, M. Z., Chan, C. L. et al. (2003). Effectiveness of psychoeducational intervention for rural Chinese families experiencing schizophrenia – a randomised controlled trial. *Social Psychiatry and Psychiatric Epidemiology*, **38**, 69–75.

Rankin, S. H. & Stallings, K. D. (1996). *Patient Education: Issues, Principles, Practices*. Philadelphia, PA: Lippincott-Raven.

Rost, K., Nutting, P., Smith, J., Elliott, C. & Dickinson, M. (2002). Managing depression as a chronic disease: a randomised trial of ongoing treatment in primary care. *British Medical Journal*, **325**, 934–7.

Rutz, W., Walinder, J., Eberhard, G. et al. (1989). An education programme for depressive disorders on Gotland: background and evaluation. *Acta Psychiatrica Scandinavica*, **79**, 19–26.

Schoenbaum, M., Unutzer, J., Sherbourne, C. et al. (2001). Cost-effectiveness of practice-initiated quality improvements for depression: results of a randomized controlled trial. *Journal of the American Medical Association*, **286**, 1325–30.

Schulze, B., Richter-Werling, M., Matschinger, H. & Angermeyer, M. C. (2003). Crazy? So what! Effects of a school project on students' attitudes towards people with schizophrenia. *Acta Psychiatrica Scandinavica*, **107**, 142–50.

Simon, C. E., Von Korff, M., Rutter, C. & Wagner, M. (2000). Randomised trial on monitoring, feedback, and management of care by telephone to improve treatment of depression in primary care. *British Medical Journal*, **320**, 550–4.

Solomon, P. (1996). Moving from psychoeducation to family education for families of adults with serious mental illness. *Psychiatric Services*, **47**, 1364–70.

Stuart, H. (2003). Stigma and the daily news: evaluation of a newspaper intervention. *Canadian Journal of Psychiatry*, **48**, 651–6.

Thompson, C., Kinmonth, A. L., Stevens, L. (2000). Effects of a clinical-practice guideline and practice-based education on detection and outcome of depression in primary care: Hampshire Depression Project randomised controlled trial. *Lancet*, **355**, 185–91.

Unutzer, J., Katon, W., Callahan, C. *et al.* (2002). Collaborative care management of late-life depression in the primary care setting: a randomized controlled trial. *Journal of the American Medical Association*, **288**, 2836–45.

Wagner, E. T., Austin, B. T. & Von Korff, M. (1996). Organizing care for patients with chronic illness. *Milbank Quarterly*, **74**, 511–44.

Wells, K., Sherbourne, C., Schoenbaum, M. *et al.* (2000). Impact of disseminating quality improvement programs for depression in managed primary care: a randomized controlled trial. *Journal of the American Medical Association*, **283**, 212–20.

Wykurz, G. & Kelly, D. (2002). Developing the role of patients as teachers: literature review. *British Medical Journal*, **325**, 818–23.

Zygmunt, A., Olfson, M., Boyer, C. A. & Mechanic, D. (2002). Interventions to improve medication adherence in schizophrenia. *American Journal of Psychiatry*, **159**, 1653–64.

7

Complementary and alternative medicine

Sally Guthrie and George Lewith

Editor's note

While many claims are made for the effectiveness of treatment with herbs, minerals, homeopathy and acupuncture, the data that support their effectiveness are sparse. Regulations that govern these compounds and these treatments are much more lax than those laws and regulations governing other forms of treatment, and it is this lack of regulations that often can lead to claims that are not at all substantiated. The careful review presented here suggests that perhaps St John's wort has effectiveness in mild depression and kava in anxiety, though there is always the risk of liver damage. S-adenosyl-l-methionine (SAMe) is probably not effective. Valerian may, over a long period of time, provide some effectiveness for insomnia, and omega-3 fatty acids do appear effective in depression. Homeopathy has absolutely no data to support any effectiveness other than perhaps the relationship of the homeopath to the patient. Acupuncture may be helpful in nicotine dependence and alcohol withdrawal, but again the role of the relationship between the acupuncturist and the patient may be the key ingredient for any claims made to the effectiveness of this treatment.

Introduction

Complementary and alternative medicine (CAM) encompasses a wide array of methods for treating illness and maintaining health. Perhaps the only thing consistent amongst these approaches is their lack of absolute acceptability as conventional medicine. Complementary medicine refers to practices or types of medicine used in combination with conventional medicine. An example of a complementary therapy is using massage therapy or acupuncture in addition to conventional medicine to treat back pain. Alternative medicine is used in place of conventional medicine. An example of an alternative therapy is using homeopathy or a special diet to treat depression instead of taking prescription antidepressants or undergoing ECT that might be recommended by a psychiatrist practising conventional medicine. What is considered CAM has to always be considered relative to the local cultural context. For instance, while Traditional Chinese Medicine or Ayurveda are considered as 'alternative' medical practices in Western countries they could be considered conventional medical practice in China and India, respectively.

Since it is estimated that approximately 25–50% of people in industrialized countries use forms of CAM (Schaffer et al., 2003; Dello Buono et al., 2001; MacLennan et al., 1996) it is a rather gross form of denial to ignore them completely. It is unfortunate that in many instances such therapies have not been subjected to rigorous scientific study, and it is in fact very difficult to apply the standard scientific study design to some of these therapies.

In this chapter we have attempted to address some of the CAM therapies that have been used to treat various psychiatric disorders. We will discuss herbal (St John's wort, kava, valerian) and nonherbal (SAMe, omega-3 fatty acids) dietary supplements, as well as acupuncture and homeopathy.

Legislation regarding herbal and nonherbal dietary supplements

Dietary supplements, especially herbals, have been used for millennia. Unfortunately this generally has not translated into a sizeable body of scientific knowledge regarding the efficacy, adverse effects, or the likelihood and incidence of food or drug interactions. A large portion of the public uses herbal and nonherbal dietary supplements

Cambridge Textbook of Effective Treatments in Psychiatry, ed. Peter Tyrer and Kenneth R. Silk. Published by Cambridge University Press.
© Cambridge University Press, 2008.

and may or may not elect to tell their physicians about their use of these agents. A recent population-based telephone survey conducted in 1998–1999 in the USA found that 14% of the 2590 persons interviewed had taken a herbal supplement within a week of the interview (Kaufman *et al.*, 2002). Additionally, 16% of those taking prescription drugs had also taken one or more herbal supplements within a week of the interview.

In the USA the Dietary Supplement Health and Education Act (DSHEA) was enacted in 1994. This law restricted the FDA regulation of dietary supplements. The act allows the availability of dietary supplements, including herbals and nonherbals, without the constraints placed on prescription drugs such as proof of efficacy for a specific disease state. Because these supplements are often not patentable, there has been little incentive for the pharmaceutical industry to conduct extensive efficacy trials. Most of these products have not been extensively evaluated and some have only anecdotal or traditional reports to substantiate their usefulness. This DSHEA allows the consumer the freedom to choose amongst a wide variety of available supplements, but the regulation of these products is largely in the hands of those who manufacture them. Although manufacturers have established guidelines, no governmental body has been established to oversee compliance with these guidelines.

In the European Union (EU) there is no legal category like the US Dietary Supplement classification between a food or a medicine. The main EU medicines law (Directive 2001/83/EC) has a wide definition of a medicine based on its function (i.e. it is perceived to have a medicinal function) and/or its presentation (i.e. it is marketed as having medicinal properties or packaged to look like a medicine). Previously herbal medicines had difficulty in satisfying stringent and expensive EU licensing requirements and so in 2004, in order to provide a legislative home for herbal medicines, the EU passed a new Directive on Traditional Herbal Medicinal Products (DTHMP). Herbal products registered under the DTHMP must demonstrate 30 years' safe use, at least 15 years of which, controversially, must be within the EU, and are required to carry indications (restricted to simple self-limiting conditions) and contraindications. They must also meet simple standards of good manufacturing practice (GMP). In the UK, herbal medicines prepared on an individual basis by herbal practitioners on their own premises are exempt from EU licensing and are regulated by Section 12.1 of the 1968 Medicines Act. In 2002, a separate Food Supplements Directive (FSD) was enacted within the EU. Although the timetable on its implementation allows a degree of negotiation on detail, the FSD is contentious since only a limited range of nutrient forms are allowed on a 'positive list' of food supplements and there are time and financial implications in providing dossiers to support products included on such a list. In addition, it is likely that high dose vitamin and mineral formulations may not be acceptable for registration under the FSD. Within the EU there is therefore some confusion and continuing negotiation in relation to future legislation for herbals and nutritional supplements.

The rather confusing laws regulating herbals have resulted in difficulties in enforcement. For example, the DSHEA indicates that dietary supplement products may include 'structure or function' statements relating to the promotion of general well-being, but any claims of efficacy for a specific disease state would move the product from the supplement category to the drug category. In this case, the supplement manufacturer would be required to meet the same stringent requirements necessary for producing and marketing of prescription drugs. However, a recent evaluation of internet marketing of dietary supplements in the USA found that of 338 websites devoted to selling herbal products, 81% made one or more health claims in their marketing (Morris & Avorn, 2003). This indicates that many internet retailers may not be complying with the DSHEA requirements.

While this is a bothersome finding, it merely reflects the ethical standards of a portion of the distributors of these products and serves to confuse the issue by further polarizing consumers and healthcare providers into those who 'believe' supplements are effective and helpful and those who do not. However, this does not address the questions of efficacy and safety that consumers and healthcare practitioners have concerning these products. Many of these supplements may be effective treatments for particular ailments. After all, digoxin, psyllium seed, and acetylsalicylic acid have all been derived from plant products, but until more well-designed studies are funded and completed, we simply cannot know whether these supplements might be effective.

In the following section we have attempted to summarize the available information regarding several herbal and nonherbal dietary supplements that are commonly used for psychiatric indications.

Herbal supplements

St. John's wort

Background

St. John's wort (*Hypericum perforatum*) is a perennial plant, native to Europe, but now found widely in Canada and the USA, especially in the western USA where it has been viewed as an annoying invasive species. It is a member of the family *Clusiaceae* (or *Hypericaceae*), genus *Hypericum*, which contains approximately 370 species (Natural Medicine Comprehensive Database; Review of Natural Products eFacts St. John's wort). The plant is called St. John's wort because it generally blooms around June 24th, the date traditionally celebrated as the birth date of John the Baptist. The plant is harvested during flowering. Approximately the upper third of the above-ground part of the plant is harvested and most of the active components of the plant probably reside in the flowers and buds (Chavez & Chavez, 1997).

Medicinal use of St. John's wort dates back to the time of Hippocrates, when it was recommended for its wound-healing and diuretic properties. Although used extensively through the Middle Ages, it fell out of use in the late nineteenth century. Recently it has been rediscovered and administered orally as a 'nerve tonic' for the treatment of anxiety, depression or insomnia (Review of Natural Products, eFacts, 2000). Also, it is still used externally as an aid to wound healing and for relief of inflammation.

Uses

Most recently, St. John's wort has become quite popular as a treatment for depression, especially in Germany. Sales of St. John's wort increased markedly in the USA and the UK following the publication of a meta-analysis of studies of St. John's wort for the treatment of depression by Linde *et al.* (1996) in the *British Medical Journal*. Inclusion criteria for this meta-analysis included: randomization or quasi-randomization of subjects, a diagnosis of a depressive disorder, the use of placebo or other antidepressant comparators, and the presence of outcome measures such as depression scales. Twenty-three trials met their criteria (15 with placebo comparator, 8 with an antidepressant comparator) and were included. The authors concluded that St. John's wort was more effective than placebo in the treatment of depression but the evidence was insufficient to conclude if St. John's wort was as effective as other standard antidepressants. From these trials they also concluded that it appeared to cause fewer short-term side effects than other antidepressants. Most comparator antidepressants were tricyclic antidepressants and none were serotonin specific reuptake inhibitors (SSRIs).

Three subsequent meta-analyses of St. John's wort trials were published, one by an American group (Gaster & Holroyd, 2000), the second by a group from the UK (Whiskey *et al.*, 2001), and the third an update of the earlier (1996) study by Linde *et al.* (2005). The results were inconsistent. Both the Gaster and the Whiskey review concluded that St. John's wort appeared to be more effective than placebo. However, the American group concluded that tricyclic antidepressants were more effective than St. John's wort, whereas the group from the UK concluded that St. John's wort displayed effectiveness similar to standard antidepressants. Both called for additional large-scale studies to evaluate the efficacy of St. John's wort compared with newer antidepressants such as the SSRIs. Linde *et al.* (2005) conducted a systematic review and meta-analysis of 37 double-blind randomized controlled trials that compare clinical effects of *Hypericum* monopreparation with either placebo or a standard antidepressant in adults with depressive disorders, including six trials of St. John's wort with SSRIs. Taking these latter trials alone, there was no difference in response rate; the rate ratio (ratio of St. John's wort responders to SSRI responders) was 0.98 (95% CI 0.85–1.12).

Recently, the results of two multicentre studies and one study with dual study sites, conducted in the USA were published. The first (Shelton *et al.*, 2001) compared 900 mg/day St John's wort (LI-160 brand) to placebo for an 8-week trial in 11 different centres. In this study response was defined a priori as > 50% reduction in HRS-D, a HRS-D score 12 or less, and Clinical Global Impression Improvement Scale (CGI-I) of 1 or 2, while remission was defined as HRS-D score of 7 or less, and CGI-I of 1 or 2. The intention-to-treat sample did not yield a significant difference in response between the group receiving St. Johns' wort (n = 98) and the placebo group (n = 102). However, a significantly greater percentage of the St. John's wort group achieved remission (14.3% St. John's wort vs 4.9% placebo). The authors concluded that there 'currently is no credible evidence to support the efficacy of St. John's wort for people with depression'. The second study (*Hypericum* Depression Trial Study Group, 2002) compared three treatment arms over an 8-week study period: 900–1500 mg/day of St. John's wort (LI-160), 50–100 mg/day of sertraline, and placebo. The primary outcome measures were a change in HRS-D from baseline and the rate of full response, defined as a CGI of 1 or 2 and a HRS-D score of less than eight. Surprisingly, with regard to change in HRS-D over time or rate of full response, neither the St. John's wort nor sertraline groups performed better than placebo. The only statistically significant difference was in a secondary outcome variable, CGI-I, which was significant in favour of sertraline in comparison to both placebo (*P* = 0.02) and St. John's wort (*P* = 0.01). In spite of the lack of response noted with the standard antidepressant in this study, the authors concluded that the weight of available data indicates that St. John's wort should not be substituted for other antidepressants in persons with moderate depression. The third study (Fava *et al.*, 2005) was conducted at two study sites. A total of 135 depressed individuals were randomized to receive St. John's wort (900 mg/day), fluoxetine (20 mg/day), or placebo for 12 weeks. The group receiving St. John's wort displayed a significantly lower HRS-D-17 score at 12 weeks in comparison to the group receiving fluoxetine, although results were not significantly better than placebo. Unfortunately, the study sponsor withdrew support for this study prior to the recruitment of the proposed study population of 180 patients and, as a result, the study population was probably too small to conclude that St. John's wort is the superior treatment, since it did not separate from placebo.

Unfortunately these two studies did not provide a definitive answer to the question of whether St. John's wort is effective for the treatment of depression. Although many of the earlier studies of St. John's wort reported positive findings, their methodologies were often flawed. Often the duration of treatment was short (4–6 weeks), the investigators usually failed to specify prior drug therapy for depression or other current drugs taken by the subjects, and patients were generally not well characterized with regard to diagnosis and duration of illness. Additionally, it is possible that the study personnel were, in some cases, not well trained. However, the two larger American studies (Shelton *et al.*, 2001; *Hypericum* Depression Trial Study Group, 2002) included patients that were chronically ill and some were suffering from severe depression, which is not considered an indication for the use of St. John's wort in Germany (where it is most widely used). The most recent conclusions of Linde & Mulrow (2004) (a review that will continue to be updated as it is a Cochrane review) summarize the aura of uncertainty over what was regarded initially as an excellent example of a complementary medicine proving its efficacy. 'Current evidence regarding *Hypericum* extracts is inconsistent and confusing. In patients who meet criteria for major depression, several recent placebo-controlled trials suggest that *Hypericum* has minimal beneficial effects while other trials suggest that *Hypericum* and standard antidepressants have similar beneficial effects' (Linde *et al.*, 2005).

Active components

St. John's wort contains a variety of pharmacologically active components including phenylpropanes, flavonol derivatives, biflavones, proanthrocyanidines, xanthones, phloroglucinols, naphthodianthrones, and essential oil constituents (Bombardelli & Morazzoni 1995). It was initially assumed that hypericin was probably the active antidepressant component and most products were standardized to contain a specific amount of this ingredient.

However, subsequent studies attributed the antidepressant activity not only to the naphthodianthrones (hypericin and pseudohypericin), but also to the phloroglucinols (hyperforin and adhyperforin), as well as to various other flavinoids (Chatterjee *et al.*, 1998; Jensen *et al.*, 2001). Most recently, animal models have revealed that a combination of active components may confer an additive antidepressant effect (Butterweck *et al.*, 2003). Regardless of the active component, or components, the proportion of different ingredients is likely to vary considerably between different lots of St. John's wort due to differences in growing conditions such as climate, light, fertilizer, soil, etc. An analysis of wild populations of *Hypericum perforatum* in the northwestern USA found that the hypericin content varied from 0.0003–0.1250% and pseudohypericin from 0.0019–0.8458%, and that the ratio of hypericin to pseudohypericin varied considerably from site to site (Sirvent *et al.*, 2002).

The antidepressant mechanism of action for St. John's wort is not known. Initially it was thought to inhibit monoamine oxidase, but this is not likely (Bladt & Wagner, 1994; Thiede & Walper, 1994). A variety of in vitro studies have documented that whole St. John's wort extracts, as well as specific components, may inhibit vesicular uptake of monoamines, or bind to different neurotransmitter receptor subtypes. However, most of these actions require relatively high concentrations of St. John's wort or its components (Cott, 1997; Singer *et al.*, 1999). While a limited number of studies on pharmacokinetics and bioavailability have been conducted with hypericin/pseudohypericin and hyperforin/adhyperforin, the pharmacokinetic parameters of many of the components of the hypericum extract have not been determined (Staffeldt *et al.*, 1994; Brockmöller *et al.*, 1997; Biber *et al.*, 1998; Jacobson *et al.*, 2001). Additionally, it is unclear what fraction of any of the components of St. Johns' wort is able to cross into the brain. Following an extensive evaluation of the interactions of pure constituents of St. John's wort with gene-protein-coupled receptors (including serotonin, dopamine, opioid, norepinephrine, oxytocin, vasopressin, NMDA and benzodiazepine), one group of investigators found that the affinity for most components was very weak; they concluded that rather than a single component, the additive or synergistic effects of multiple components of St. John's wort may contribute to the antidepressant effect (Butterweck *et al.*, 2002).

Despite the lack of certainty about the specific active component (or components), most preparations are standardized to either hypericin or hyperforin. However, when preparations available in the USA have been assayed the actual amount of the standardized compound has varied widely from that stated on the label. In one study only two of eight products were within 10% of the amount of hypericin stated on the label (De Los Reyes & Koda, 2002). It is possible that either manufacturing or storage may result in significant degradation of hypericin and hyperforin (Bilia *et al.*, 2001).

Adverse effects

St. John's wort causes few adverse effects. The adverse effects reported in clinical trials include insomnia, restlessness, anxiety, agitation, irritability, gastrointestinal upset, anorgasmia, fatigue, dry mouth, dizziness and headache. In general, the incidence of side effects is similar to that produced by placebo. In the multicentre comparison with placebo and sertraline, only anorgasmia, frequent urination, and swelling occurred more often with St. John's wort than placebo (*Hypericum* Depression Trial Study Group, 2002). Case reports have also indicated allergic skin rash and neuropathy are possible rare adverse effects (Woelk *et al.*, 1994; Bove, 1998; Ernst & White, 1998). Photosensitivity was initially reported in livestock that had grazed on St. John's wort. The adverse effect is dose-related and may also occur in humans (Brockmöller *et al.*, 1997). Fair-skinned individuals should be cautioned to use sunscreen or wear protective clothing when they are likely to encounter intense sunlight. As with most other antidepressants, St. John's wort has also been associated with the induction of manic episodes in bipolar patients (Moses & Mallinger, 2000).

Herb–drug interactions

St. John's wort interacts with a considerable number of commonly used drugs. It induces the expression of both CYP450 3A4 and the ATP-dependent transport protein, p-glycoprotein (Durr *et al.*, 2000). CYP3A4 is responsible for oxidative metabolism of greater than 50% of all drugs. While some CYP3A4 drugs are also transported by p-glycoprotein, other drugs such as digoxin are transported by p-glycoprotein but not metabolized by CYP3A4. Table 7.1 lists reported drug interactions. Since St. John's wort may have serotonergic effects, it may interact with other drugs with serotonergic effects to cause the 'serotonin syndrome'. Other commonly used serotonergic compounds include SSRIs, nefazodone, venlafaxine, duloxetine, merperidine (pethidine) and dextromethorphan. There have been case reports of a hypertensive reaction or a 'serotonin syndrome' when such agents have been combined with St. John's wort. Although these reports commonly note hypertension, nausea, dizziness, vomiting, headache, anxiety and restlessness, none have reported hyperthermia and none have resulted in a fatality

(Dannawi, 2002; Patel *et al.*, 2002; Zullino & Borgeat, 2003). It is difficult to know if this represents an actual serotonin syndrome because the serotonergic activities of St. John's wort are actually quite weak. However, caution would dictate close monitoring of patients who opt to take both serotonergic compounds and St. John's wort.

Kava

Background

Kava (*Piper methysticum*) is a perennial shrub, growing between 150–300 cm tall, that is native to the South Pacific, possibly originating in Vanuatu. It belongs to the family Piperaceae, and its name means 'intoxicating pepper'. It produces glossy green heart-shaped leaves that are up to 28 cm long (Review of Natural Products eFacts, 2003). The roots and rhizomes of the plant were collected, crushed and mixed with coconut juice or water by indigenous peoples in the South Pacific islands. The kava drinking ceremony varied from island to island, but most of the traditional religious or ceremonial events were restricted to the men and sometimes to royalty and priests. Although Captain James Cook wrote about kava use during his travels in the late 1700s, it had been introduced into Europe at least 150 years earlier by Dutch explorers (Cawte, 1985; Norton & Ruze, 1994). In spite of its early introduction to Europe, large-scale use in Europe and the USA is a recent phenomenon. It requires a warm and moist climate for growth and it would not thrive in most of Europe. In the late 1990s kava was associated with several cases of fulminant hepatic failure and its sale has been restricted in Switzerland, Germany, Canada, Australia and France. In the USA the FDA has advised consumers and healthcare providers of the risk of liver injury (Blumenthal, 2002).

Uses

Kava is most commonly used as an anxiolytic. Although it has been used as an antidepressant, there are no studies evaluating the use of kava as an antidepressant. A meta-analysis of studies utilizing kava for the treatment of anxiety has recently been published (Pittler & Ernst, 2003). While 21 studies were identified, only 11 met inclusion criteria which included randomization of patients; a placebo-control, double-blind design; the study preparation contained kava as the single ingredient (all used the same preparation, WS1490); and the study participants were suffering from anxiety. Of the 11 identified studies, six used a common outcome measure, the Hamilton Rating Scale-Anxiety (HRSA). The results from the 345 patients in these six studies were included in the meta-analysis. Four

Table 7.1. St. John's wort – drug interactions

Drug	Interaction	Clinical significance
Digoxin	Decreased absorption	Reduction of AUC by 18% (?)
Alprazolam	Increased clearance	Increases clearance by 100%, shortens half-life from 12.4 to 6 hours, might see decreased effect
Amitriptyline	Increased clearance	Serum concentrations of amitriptyline decreased by 22%, nortriptyline by 42%
Selective serotonin reuptake inhibitors	Serotonin syndrome	This been reported with paroxetine and sertraline, but has not been associated with fatalities in these cases. Many patients probably combine St. John's wort with their antidepressants
Cyclosporine	Decrease absoption and increase clearance	Decreases of plasma cyclosporine levels by 30–70%. Transplant rejections have occurred due to this interaction
Irinotecan	Increased clearance	Decrease parent drug levels by 50%, decrease active metabolite AUC by 42%
Nefazodone	Serotonin syndrome	A case report, associated with nausea, vomiting and restlessness, but not fatal
Nervirapine	Increased clearance	Increased oral clearance by 35%, could be very significant, associated with treatment failure, development of resistance to drug/class. Only reported with nevirapine but might also happen with delavirdine and efavirenz
Oral contraceptives	Increased clearance	Increases clearance of oestrogen, unwanted pregnancies have been reported due to this interaction
Phenprocoumon	Increased clearance	Decreases anticoagulant effect, monitor INR
Indinavir	Increased clearance	Decreases indinavir AUC by 57%. Likely to also decrease AUC of amrenavir, nelfinavir, ritonavir and saquinavir. May result in therapeutic failure
Simvastatin	Increased clearance	Reduces plasma concentrations of active metabolite (simvastatin hydroxy acid) by 28%. Could also reduce concentrations of atorvastatin and lovastatin. Monitor cholesterol levels
Tacrolimus	Increased clearance	Dose increases of 60% have been necessary to maintain therapeutic tacrolimus levels in patients taking St. John's wort
Theophylline	Increased clearance	Use of St. John's wort might decrease serum theophylline levels resulting in a necessary dose increase. Monitor theophylline levels
Warfarin	Increased clearance and possible decreased absorption	Use of St. John's wort has caused a significant drop in INR. Monitor INR.

AUC, area under plasma concentration versus time curve; INR, International Normalized Ratio.

of the six studies required that patients score > 19 on the HRSA at baseline. Most patients (72%) met DSM–III–R criteria for anxiety but the type of anxiety varied and patients with agoraphobia, specific phobia, social phobia, generalized anxiety disorder or adjustment disorder with anxiety were included in studies. The resulting pooled data indicated a significant reduction of HRSA score in the patients receiving kava in comparison to placebo

$(P = 0.002)$. Although they acknowledged that the effect was not robust, the authors concluded that kava extract seemed to be more effective than placebo in the treatment of symptomatic anxiety.

Most of the studies of kava for the treatment of anxiety possess significant shortcomings. Often diverse patient populations are included, making it difficult to determine which group might benefit most from kava. The duration of treatment in most of these studies is quite short. Prior medications used by the patients, or even current medications, are usually not specified. The data, to date, support the conclusion that kava has anxiolytic effects in comparison to placebo. To establish kava as a first-line anxiolytic, additional comparison studies with standard anxiolytics, as well as dose-ranging studies, should be conducted. Due to the controversy regarding the connection between kava and hepatotoxicity these studies may never be conducted.

Active components

The activity of kava is thought to be due to several arylethylene pyrones that bear a structural resemblance to myristicin (found in nutmeg). A group of substituted dihydropyrones that possess central nervous system activity has been described. These are also known as kava lactones. Usually kava lactones comprise at least 3.5% of the dried root and 14 kava lactones have been identified in the urine of those who have taken kava orally (Duffield et al., 1989; Natural Medicines Comprehensive Database, 2004). One of the most popular products used in Europe (Laitan® WS; WS1490) is a concentrated root extract that may contain up to 70% kava lactones (Blumenthal, 2002).

Kava causes muscle relaxation, that is dissimilar to that caused by curare, and it possesses a local anaesthetic effect. Strychnine-induced convulsions may be antagonized by some kava lactones (Review of Natural Products, eFacts, 2003). Although it may possess analgesic effects, these are not reversed by naloxone, indicating that it does not induce analgesia via actions at mu opiate receptors. Kava can cause sedation, but the mechanism is not established at this time. Studies evaluating kava binding to gamma-aminobutyric acid (GABA) or benzodiazepine receptors are conflicting (Pepping, 1999a).

Adverse effects

In general, kava causes few adverse effects. At lower doses, mild gastrointestinal effects are possible and at higher doses sedation, fatigue, hangover effects, ataxia and papillary dilation may occur.

A well-known adverse effect associated with chronic kava use is a dose- and time-related dermopathy, characterized as an acquired reversible ichthyosis. Skin changes are described as generalized, shiny, fine polygonal scaly eruptions involving the neck, torso, arms, legs and dorsum of the hands, possibly accompanied by reddened eyes. The cause of the dermopathy is unknown (Ruze, 1990; Norton & Ruze, 1994).

Even though traditional use of kava dates back many years it has only recently been associated with any significant toxicity. In 1998 case reports of hepatic toxicity began to appear in the European literature (Strahl et al., 1998; Stevinson et al., 2002). The reports described elevations of liver enzymes, cholestatic hepatitis, liver necrosis and irreversible liver failure. Several cases have required liver transplant (Center for Disease Control, 2002). The basis of the hepatotoxicity is unknown at this time but it is often associated with an eosinophilia, suggesting the possibility that it is an idiosyncratic hypersensitivity reaction. Although it was initially hypothesized that hepatotoxic reactions occur only in those with a deficiency of CYP2D6, it appears that kava-induced hepatotoxicity is not limited to that subgroup (Russman et al., 2001; Blumenthal, 2002; Stevinson et al., 2002). Regardless of the aetiology, it would be reasonable to monitor liver enzymes in all patients taking kava.

Valerian

Background

Valerian (Valeriana officinalis) is a tall (30–150 cm) herbaceous perennial that has been used for thousands of years for digestive problems, flatulence and urinary tract disorders. Use of valerian as a sleep aid dates to about the sixteenth century (Plushner, 2000). It is native to Europe and Asia and naturalized to the USA and Great Britain. Valerian produces clusters of white or pink flowers. There are over 200 valeriana species and many have pharmacologically active components, but the roots and rhizomes of Valeriana officinalis are most commonly used for medicinal purposes. The roots and rhizomes are harvested in the autumn when the plant is 2 years old (Foster & Tyler, 1999).

Uses

A review of the randomized clinical trials conducted using valerian for insomnia was published in 2000 (Stevinson & Ernst, 2000). At the time of evaluation the authors were able to find 19 clinical trials. Of these, four used combination valerian products, three did not include randomization procedures and an additional three did not measure sleep parameters. Of the nine remaining studies, two found no significant differences from placebo in any sleep parameters measured. Conversely, one found an improvement in slow wave sleep, while another found a decrease in stage 4 sleep. Of the remaining five studies, four found improvements in sleep latency, and one found improvements in all sleep parameters measured. The authors concluded that the trials were contradictory. They also concluded that additional rigorous, well-designed trials were needed to determine if valerian was effective for the treatment of insomnia.

Unfortunately, the studies published following this review have done little to resolve the controversy. Part of the difficulty may lie in the fact that many of the studies used combination products. Additionally, it is possible that valerian does not exhibit acute effects on sleep. In studies that have used chronic dosing of valerian it has been noted that the sleep-enhancing effects of valerian may require a period of time (from 4 days to several weeks) to manifest. In the doses normally administered, valerian does not appear to induce acute hypnotic effects in humans. A recent comparison of single doses of diphenhydramine (50 and 75 mg), temazepam (15 and 30 mg), valerian (400 and 800 mg) and placebo found that valerian caused no significant difference in psychomotor effects or subjective sedation in comparison with either diphenhydramine or placebo (Glass *et al.*, 2003). Although a lack of acute sedative effect has been noted in this and other studies, subjects often report improved quality of sleep in placebo-controlled studies with valerian, even in the absence of convincing effects on polysomnography.

Active components

Traditionally, valerian was ingested in the form of a tea. Currently, probably due to its somewhat unpleasant penetrating odour, it is usually taken in tablet form. Components of valerian that may confer sedative properties include mono- and sesquiterpenes (valerenic acid and congeners), iridoid esters (valepotriates) and pyridine alkaloids. While considerable research has been devoted to the valepotriates, they are rather unstable and mostly destroyed in the preparation process, such that dosage forms composed of crude extract contain very few valepotriates (Natural Medicines Comprehensive Database, valerian, 2004). Marketed valerian root products are generally standardized to the content of valerenic and acetoxyvalerenic acids (0.08 to 0.3%) (Bisset & Wichtl, 1994). Because most of the valepotriates are probably destroyed during the manufacturing process, it has been hypothesized that the sedative properties of valerian root may be partially due to the breakdown products of valepotriates, termed baldrinals. Another component of valerian, valerenic acid, has shown activity as a muscle relaxant and antispasmodic. Valerenic acid also inhibits GABA-transaminase, in animal studies (Houghton, 1999). This should increase the availability of GABA by blocking its catabolism. However, because pharmacokinetic studies of valerenic acid have not been conducted in humans, it is unknown if enough valerenic acid is present following oral administration to cause clinically significant inhibition of GABA-transaminase in humans.

Side effects

Few side effects have been associated with valerian. Gastric discomfort, dry mouth, and vivid dreams have been reported (Plushner, 2000; Wheatley, 2001). Several cases of hepatotoxicity have been reported but it is difficult to ascribe these to valerian because in most cases combination products were taken and the content of valerian in the product taken was not determined in any of the cases. If the reported hepatotoxicity is due to valerian it is likely an idiosyncratic effect because it is very rarely reported in relation to the amount of valerian that is sold. Additionally, the fact that overdoses involving up to 20 times the recommended dose have not been associated with any elevations of the liver enzymes indicates that if this effect occurs it is most likely idiosyncratic (Chan, 1998). A single case report hypothesized that valerian may be associated with a withdrawal syndrome but the case was complicated by the variety of other medications being taken by the patient (Garges *et al.*, 1998).

Herb–drug interactions

There are no data in humans evaluating the effect of valerian on drug metabolism. There are some in vitro data suggesting that valerian may moderately inhibit CYP3A4 (Budzinski *et al.*, 2000).

Omega-3 fatty acids

Background

Fatty acids are classified into three main groups: saturated, monounsaturated and polyunsaturated (PUFAs). The PUFAs are further divided into three series (the oleic acid or $C18:2\omega9$, the linoleic or $C18:2\omega6$, and the α-linolenic or $C18:3\omega3$ series). In humans, oleic acid is considered nonessential but both linoleic and α-linolenic acids are 'essential' fatty acids that have to be ingested in the diet because they cannot be synthesized. Linoleic and α-linolenic acids are precursors to a variety of ω-6 and ω-3 fatty acids. The primary $\omega3$ derived fatty acids are eicosapentanoic acid (EPA) and docosahexanoic acid (DHA), and the primary $\omega6$ derived fatty acid is arachidonic acid (AA). It is necessary to maintain a balanced intake of linoleic and α-linoleic acids because they both compete for the same desaturase and elongase enzymes and an overabundance of one will lead to a relative deficiency of the derived fatty acids from the competing series. Forty-five per cent of synaptic membrane is composed of essential fatty acids and DHA is an especially important component. Biomembranes are very selective and efficient in their incorporation of DHA and it is critical for maintenance of normal neural functions (Horrocks & Yeo, 1999; Pepping, 1999b; Bruinsma & Taren, 2000).

The ratio of ω-6 to ω-3 fatty acids in the US diet today is estimated at 10:1. This leads to an overabundance of ω-6 derived fatty acids (principally AA) at the expense of ω-3 derived fatty acids (EPA and DHA). The World Health Organization now recommends a ratio of ω-6 to ω-3 fatty acids ranging from 3:1 to 4:1 (Horrocks & Yeo, 1999). Linoleic acid is found in a wide variety of foods, such as lean meats, margarine, and eggs. Most vegetable oils (safflower, soy bean, corn) contain predominantly linoleic acid. The precursor to ω-3 fatty acids, α-linolenic acid, predominates in fish oil (especially oily fish such as mackerel or salmon), wild game, canola oil, flaxseed oil and walnuts. However, humans have a limited capacity for conversion of α-linolenic acid to EPA, and subsequently to DHA. Fish oil is a particularly good source of ω-3 fatty acids because it contains a high content of both EPA and DHA.

In 1998, Hibbeln published a letter in the *Lancet* showing a significant association between fish consumption and depression; societies with a high consumption of fish appear to have a lower prevalence of depression (Hibbeln, 1998). Other studies have supported a relationship between an imbalance of ω-3 and ω-6 fatty acids and depression. Depressed patients have exhibited an increased ratio of AA to EPA in serum phospholipids and cholesteryl esters, and the total fraction of ω-3 fatty acids in serum cholesteryl esters is decreased (Maes *et al.*, 1996, 1999). Also, the ratio of AA to EPA in serum phospholipids and red blood cells is correlated with the severity of depression and a significant decrease in the overall sum of ω-3 fatty acids (especially DHA) in red blood cell membranes has been found in depression (Adams *et al.*, 1996).

Proposed mechanism of action

Alteration of the biomembrane phospholipids composition, especially DHA (since so much of the membrane is composed of DHA), will alter the stabilization and viscosity of the membrane. Docosahexanoic acid also appears to play an important role in the functioning of neurotransmitters, including serotonin. Rats with low brain concentrations of DHA exhibited a 44% increase in serotonin-2A receptors in the frontal cortex (Delion *et al.*, 1994). This upregulation of serotonin-2A receptors may reflect decreased serotonin function, and is hypothesized to have a role in the pathophysiology of depression (Maes & Meltzer, 1995).

Also, depression appears to be associated with an activation of the inflammatory response system, in part mediated by AA, which is a precursor to prostaglandins

and related eicosanoids through the cyclooxygenase and lipooxygenase pathways (Babcock *et al.*, 2000). Conversely, when human diets are supplemented with DHA and EPA, the monocyte production of IL-1, IL-2, IL-6 and TNF-α is suppressed (Meydani *et al.*, 1991; Meydani *et al.*, 1993; Calder, 1997; Kelley *et al.*, 1999). An increase in the ratio of ω-6 to ω-3 fatty acids in biomembranes may lead to an overabundance of mediators of inflammation.

Uses

Few rigorous studies of ω-3 fatty acids in mood disorders have been conducted, but the studies that have been conducted have been largely positive. Stoll *et al.* (1999) randomized 30 bipolar-I or -II patients to treatment with either 10 g of fish oil per day or placebo. The fish oil was a partially purified combination of ω-3 fatty acid esters; ethyl-eicosapentanoate and ethyl docosahexanoate. Treatment was initially designed to continue for 9 months or relapse, which was defined as the occurrence of either a manic or depressive episode. The study was concluded early because (1) the supplier for their fish oil formulation discontinued production, and (2) an interim analysis conducted when 30 patients had either failed treatment or completed 4 months of treatment indicated that the group receiving fish oil was significantly more likely to remain free of mood symptoms. Interestingly, the only patients relapsing in the fish oil group suffered from manic, hypomanic or mixed states.

In a subsequent study 70 depressed patients received 500 mg capsules of pure EPA ethyl-ester for 12 weeks (Peet & Horrobin, 2002). Three different doses of EPA ethyl-ester (1 g/day, 2 g/day or 3 g/day) and placebo were compared. At baseline all patients were also taking standard antidepressants but remained depressed with a HRSD-17 rating of at least 15. A better outcome on all depression scales was achieved in the group receiving 1 g/day EPA ethyl-ester in comparison with placebo. Interestingly the other two doses were not associated with a significant effect in comparison with placebo. In another study (Marangell *et al.*, 2003), 36 depressed patients were randomly assigned to receive either placebo or DHA (2 g/day) for 6 weeks. The group receiving DHA did no better than the group receiving placebo. However, these patients were not receiving concomitant standard antidepressants. Finally, in a study conducted by Su *et al.* (2003), 28 depressed patients were randomized to receive either omega-3 fatty acids (n = 14) or placebo (n = 14) for 8 weeks. The fish oil capsules contained both EPA acid (440 mg) and DHA acid (220 mg) and the dose was five capsules twice daily. Based on decrease in the 28-item HRS-D scale, those receiving omega-3 fatty acids responded significantly better

($P < 0.001$) than those receiving placebo. Only one patient in each group was not receiving concomitant standard antidepressants during the study, but the results were not affected by either the dose or duration of antidepressant medication.

Based on the studies presented above it appears that EPA may be more effective than DHA for the treatment of depression. This is somewhat unexpected since, based on the role of DHA in neurotransmitter functioning, one would predict that it might be the key compound, rather than EPA. It is also possible that EPA acts as an augmenting agent in the presence of standard antidepressants, rather than being effective on its own, since in most of the positive studies, patients were also taking other standard antidepressants. Few studies have been conducted and all of these studies contained relatively small populations. However, a recent well-controlled trial was conducted by Frangon et al. (2006).

Side effects and formulations

Fish oil capsules contain a combination of EPA and DHA. The amount and ratio of these ω-3 fatty acids probably vary considerably depending on the manufacturer and lot. Studies of ω-3 fatty acids for the treatment of depression have all used specific amounts of EPA, DHA or a combination of both. It is unknown if the dose of these components is crucial for ensuring a therapeutic effect. The single study that used different dose ranges found that a low dose of EPA (1 g/day) was more effective than higher doses (2 g/day or 4 g/day) (Peet & Horrobin, 2002).

Fish oil capsules (as well as the EPA and/or DHA capsules) have been well tolerated in general. The most common complaint has been diarrhoea, followed by gastric distress. Another common complaint is a faint 'fishy' aftertaste or belching (Pepping, 1999b; Marangell et al., 2003).

S-adenosyl-methionine (SAMe)

Background

Unlike most alternative/complementary treatments, S-adenosyl-methionine (SAMe) does not have a history dating to antiquity; it was first described in 1953 (Cantoni, 1953). S-adenosyl-l-methionine is endogenously synthesized by the body when methionine is converted to cysteine, taurine, glutathione and various other polyamine compounds. Both adenosine triphosphate and the enzyme methionine-adenosyl-transferase are necessary for the synthesis of SAMe. In its role as the main methyl donor within the body, SAMe is instrumental in the synthesis of many different compounds including catecholamines

and other neurotransmitters, proteins, membrane phospholipids, fatty acids, nucleic acids, porphyrins, choline, carnitine and creatinine. Following donation of its methyl group, SAMe is converted to S-adenosyl-homocysteine, which acts as a competitive inhibitor of further SAMe methyl donation reactions. S-adenosyl-methionine probably crosses the blood–brain barrier. Following intravenous or oral administration of SAMe, the cerebral spinal fluid (CSF) concentrations of the serotonin metabolite, 5-HIAA, and the dopamine metabolite, HVA, increase. Also SAMe concentrations measured in the CSF increase. It has been hypothesized that SAMe's therapeutic effect in depression may arise from its ability to concomitantly blunt the effects of norepinephrine while increasing the concentrations of serotonin and dopamine (Fetrow & Avila, 2001). Interestingly there is some documentation of low SAMe levels in the CSF of depressed persons (Bottiglieri & Hyland, 1994). Also, a correlation between increases in SAMe in plasma and improvement of depressed symptoms has been noted by some (Bell et al., 1994).

Use

Reports of clinical efficacy of SAMe in depression date back as far as the early 1970s. Approximately 40 clinical trials have evaluated SAMe use for the treatment of depression. A meta-analysis published in 1994 (Bressa, 1994) concluded that SAMe is more effective than placebo. It produced an effect size from 17% to 38%. They also concluded that it was equivalent to standard tricyclic antidepressants (doses ranging between 75 and 250 mg/day). Many of these studies used very small populations and diagnostic criteria are often inconsistent from one study to the next. Some of these studies used an intravenous formulation of SAMe (not available in the USA), while others used oral preparations. Most studies were conducted for 4 weeks or less (the longest are for 6 weeks), and long-term data with regard to relapse prevention are not available. Comparisons were generally to low-dose tricyclic antidepressants or placebo.

Side effects, formulations and pharmacokinetics

S-adenosyl-methionine has relatively poor bioavailability, possibly related to a significant first-pass effect (Stramentinoli et al., 1979). Oral doses range from 400 to 1600 mg/day (most commonly 1600 mg/day) in comparison with the typical IV/IM doses of 200 to 400 mg/day. Following IV administration, the drug's half-life is 80 minutes (Stramentinoli, 1987). It is generally well tolerated although gastrointestinal distress, including nausea, vomiting, diarrhoea and dizziness are reported. Also, insomnia, lack of appetite, constipation, sweating and nervousness have been reported. A switch from depression to mania has also been reported (Friedel *et al.*, 1989).

For oral administration, three salt forms are available, the sulphate, sulphate-p-toluenesulphonate (also called tosylate) and butanedisulphonate. The bioavailability of the butanedisulphonate is larger (5%) than that of the tosylate (1%). Additionally, the tosylate may not be as stable as the butanedisulphonate, which is stable for 2 years at room temperature (Natural Medicines Comprehensive Database, SAMe, 2004).

Homeopathy: what is it and can it be used effectively in psychiatric illness?

Introduction

The word homeopathy is derived from two Greek words: 'homoios', meaning similar, and 'pathos', meaning suffering. The combination of these two words defines the practice of homeopathy. The main governing principle of this form of medicine is summed up by the Latin phrase 'simila, similibus curentur' – like cures like.

This approach contrasts with the principles of conventional medicine, which are allopathic – the Greek word *allos* meaning different. An appropriate remedy produces symptoms different (or opposite) from those of the disease – for instance, the suppression of a fever by aspirin.

'Like cures like' means, simply, that a homeopathic substance producing certain symptoms in a healthy person will treat similar symptoms in an ill person. For example, the medicine *Belladonna*, derived from deadly nightshade and containing atropine, causes mania and confusion, a flushed red face, dilated pupils, a high fever and a dry mouth. If a person had similar symptoms, for instance as a result of an upper respiratory tract infection, a homeopath would assume that an infinitesimal dose of *Belladonna* might relieve the complaint. In other words, a homeopathic remedy can use the toxic effects produced by a herbal remedy as a "symptom picture", to select the appropriate homeopathic medication.

Principles of homeopathy

The basic principles of homeopathy were first defined by the German physician, Dr Samuel Hahnemann (1755–1843). He seems to have based many of his original thoughts on Hippocratic principles that suggested symptoms were an expression of nature's healing powers. A German physician, George Stahl, also stumbled across and used homeopathic principles about a century before Hahnemann's birth.

Hahnemann developed homeopathy by carefully observing in detail the effects of specific medicines, both in healthy people and in ill people. The first clearly defined by him was that of Peruvian cinchona bark (quinine). During the eighteenth century this remedy was commonly used to treat many infections, including malaria and intermittent fever. On dosing himself with cinchona bark, Hahnemann found that he was able to mimic many of the symptoms of malaria. It occurred to him that the bark reduced this febrile (fever-producing) disease by producing its own self-limiting fever. Similarly, mercury was used as a treatment for syphilis, and Hahnemann noted that mercurial fever was in many ways similar to the symptoms with which syphilis presented. He began to test other substances. He either took them in tiny doses himself or one of his friends or students took them. He made detailed records (drug pictures) of the mental and physical symptoms that occurred over the following week or two. Homeopathic prescribing, from its initial inception, was based on the whole picture the drug created with all the individuals' 'systems' so it is as much based on mental symptoms as it is on physical complaints.

Hahnemann slowly began to build a detailed 'library' of drug pictures which was subsequently recorded in the various homeopathic *materia medicas*. Each drug was associated with a long list of symptoms in many different systems or locations. If a patient required any homeopathic treatment, then a detailed history was (and still is) taken, so that the symptoms can be fitted into the most appropriate drug picture, and then the required remedy prescribed. An initial homeopathic consultation for a chronic complaint will often take an hour or possibly longer and will involve a history that encompasses every physical bodily system as well as a detailed understanding of the patient's mental state. A homeopath is required to listen to the patient at some length and explore their constitution in great detail and many homeopaths have observed that this in itself may be very therapeutic for a whole range of minor psychiatric and psychological complaints.

The prescription of homeopathic medication has tended to be divided into two main approaches: the constitutional and the symptomatic. Constitutional remedies are designed to rebalance the whole – body, mind and emotions. For instance, if an individual is suffering from recurrent attacks of indigestion, they may be given a remedy based on their general manner and personality, with the idea of controlling both symptoms in the short term and cause in the long term. Symptomatic prescribing is based on the immediate presenting symptoms and designed to control acute and minor illnesses such as viral infections. Constitutional and symptomatic remedies are sometimes given together in order to obtain the 'best' therapeutic results, according to classical Hahnemannian homeopathy.

Homeopathic preparations

Homeopathic medicines are largely made from naturally occurring substances and are so dilute that they frequently contain none of the original substance. The term ultra-molecular is used to describe these infinitesimal dilutions that are below the Avogadro number. The manufacture of homeopathic medicines involves two techniques: dilution and succussion. Homeopathic pharmacies dilute the medicines in two main ways – decimal or D (in ratios of 1:10 – one drop of tincture in 10 drops of water) and centesimal or C (in ratios of 1:100 – one drop of tincture in 100 drops of water). For example, 30 C is the original mother tincture diluted one in a hundred, 30 times; none of the original substance remains in the homeopathic medicine once the dilution exceeds 12 C. Between each dilution it is necessary actively to shake the medication for a period of at least 10 seconds. This agitation, or succussion, appears to be an essential part of what makes homeopathic medicines effective. Usually only a small drop of medicine is taken once or twice a day, the exact dose dependent on the dilution being used. In general terms homeopaths consider the more dilute the medicine, the more 'potent' it is and that stronger (in homeopathic terms, more dilute medicines) should be given to the patients less frequently.

Homeopaths also talk about therapeutic aggravations, as do most complementary therapists. These imply that if a complementary medicine is going to be effective, there will often be a worsening of the initial presenting symptoms prior to the effect becoming apparent. Many complementary therapists therefore seek symptomatic deterioration as an important precursor to improvement rather than thinking of it as an unwanted adverse reaction, as one might in conventional medicine.

Does homeopathy work?

Linde & Jonas (1998) have published the most recent and comprehensive systematic review of randomized controlled trials within homeopathy. While they have unequivocally demonstrated, through their meta-analysis, that homeopathic medicines do not seem to be placebos, they are unable to demonstrate that homeopathy is specifically efficacious for any particular condition. The combined odds ratio of the 89 studies reviewed was 2.45 with 95% confidence intervals of 2.05–2.93 in favour of homeopathy. Studies with better internal validity, and therefore better scientific quality, showed an odds ratio of 1.66 with 95% confidence intervals of 1.33–2.08. These outcomes appear to provide a solid argument for homeopathy's value, but unfortunately there is not a single study in this meta-analysis which has assessed the use of homeopathy in the treatment of anxiety, depression or indeed any other psychiatric illness. The fact of the matter is, however, that homeopaths treat many individuals with a whole range of largely minor psychiatric complaints with remedies that would appear to be, in a general pragmatic sense, effective. However, objectively, the use of homeopathy for psychiatric illness is best described as an 'evidence-free zone' that is common for many CAM interventions.

On a philosophical level, the absence of such studies does not necessarily mean that one should not use this approach, providing of course that the patient is managed in a safe and responsible clinical environment. For instance, mild anxiety may be very likely to respond to the whole process of homeopathy that involves a combination of the consultation and subsequent prescription associated with repeated visits. This may in many ways be similar to the process of psychotherapy, indeed the broad nature and principles of the homeopathic consultation have frequently been compared with a variety of psychotherapeutic techniques. While it is essential to create an evidence base for all treatments, it is not practical to do so, immediately, and for everything. It is also vital not to confuse the issue of 'a lack or absence of evidence' with the implication that the treatment is ineffective.

How does homeopathy work?

If homeopathic remedies appear to be more effective than placebo, but at the same time contain no molecules of the original substance, how might they work? Hahnemann's initial explanation centred around the concept of vitalism, a sort of ill-defined energetic concept. Somehow, in illness, the flow of vital energy through the body was abnormal, and homeopathic medicines were thought, in some ill-defined manner, to normalize this as part of their healing mechanism. More recently mechanistic research has concentrated on the manner in which water may transmit information. There have been a number of suggestions implying that the hydrogen bonding in water may be modified by the process of dilution and succussion, or potentisation, as the homeopaths describe it. Recently, work by Roy et al. (2005) suggests that homeopathic medicines have particular and distinct thermoluminescence properties which implies that theories around 'the memory of water' may have some substance. Somehow information may be stored and transmitted through mechanisms that have previously evaded conventional pharmacological investigation, but how this might be effective in the treatment of illness within biological systems is entirely unclear.

How do we evaluate the effects of homeopathy?

The situation pertaining to the use of homeopathy in minor psychiatric illness is similar to that which faces many of the CAM therapies. Homeopathy is practiced by a number of registered physicians, both in the UK and the USA. While there may possibly be a mechanism of action that underpins homeopathy, and while it may possibly prove to be effective in some conditions, in the context of psychiatric illness there is very little evidence. A patient presenting with mild depression or mild free-floating anxiety, may require any one of 50 or 60 remedies. The whole process of therapeutic contact and consultation that leads to the prescription of an individualized remedy may in itself provide an important therapeutic intervention without the need for any homeopathic medication. Therefore, conducting randomized clinical trials within this context is complex.

If one randomized patients, post-consultation, to receive either verum or placebo, then it could be argued that the whole homeopathic process may be altered by the doubt in both the homeopath's and patient's mind as to whether the patient had received a verum remedy with respect to their subsequent therapeutic response. Consequently, there is an argument for pragmatic comparative studies within homeopathy, with clear health economic and quality-of-life endpoints, perhaps with associated qualitative studies. This process may be entirely scientifically sustainable when considering the complexities of the homeopathic interaction, however, it will not provide answers as to the specific efficacy of an individualized homeopathic prescription. These issues are illustrative of the whole field of CAM research. We have long-established therapeutic interventions within both conventional and complementary medicine which are 'believed' by patients and therapists alike. This can create entrenched positions and all the problems that brings in the context of an evaluative culture.

Should the use of homeopathy be recommended in psychiatric illness?

It is probably sensible to accept a combination of pragmatism and professionalism in regard to this particular issue. Provided the patient is managed by a competent practitioner and is aware of the dangers and issues inherent within the individual's psychiatric diagnosis, then homeopathy may provide an effective complement or even a safe alternative to conventional psychiatry. If an individual wishes to choose a homeopathic approach, then this whole process may empower and enable them within the context of their own self-management. The difficulties inherent in CAM research and the lack of evidence within this area should be looked upon as a challenge. The development of a CAM research agenda may help us understand how we may differentiate between the therapeutic relationship and a specific intervention within complementary medicine, and indeed may provide insight into similar conundrums within the conventional field. On balance, and providing the patient is managed responsibly, it would seem sensible to encourage patients to be managed homeopathically should they be interested in pursuing this option. It would not, however, be ethical to recommend any treatment as the intervention of choice without appropriate evidence to sustain that opinion.

Acupuncture, its history and philosophy

Introduction

Acupuncture has probably been practiced in China for around 3500 years, but the exact date of its origin is difficult to determine. The first medical textbook on acupuncture was called the Nei Ching Su Wen; this literally means the 'Yellow Emperor's Classical of Internal Medicine' and it dates from about 400 BC. Acupuncture has been known to Western doctors since the Jesuits first went to China in the seventeenth century, and it was used extensively by physicians in this country in the early part of the nineteenth century. The first edition of the *Lancet* in 1823 carried a detailed report of the use of acupuncture in timpani (ear infections and/or deafness) and rheumatism, praising the virtues of this technique. The author, John Elliotson, was a consultant physician at St Thomas's Hospital in central London.

Traditional Chinese medicine

The first recorded therapeutic success with acupuncture occurred in the 'historical records' of some 2000 years ago. Pein Chueh, a physician, used acupuncture to revive a dying patient already in a coma. The practice of acupuncture was progressively developed and refined throughout Chinese history until the Ching dynasty (1644–1911 AD). During this period, acupuncture fell into disrepute and was discouraged in favour of Western medicine. However, since the Communist revolution of 1948 acupuncture has been revitalized and is now widely used in China.

Acupuncture is one of the therapeutic techniques used in traditional Chinese medicine (TCM), which has its own complete system of anatomy, physiology and diagnosis: the main concepts are described in detail in the Nei Ching Su Wen. The traditional Chinese viewed the human body as a balance between two opposing forces, yin and yang: yin represents placidity or water, while yang represents activity or fire. If yin or yang are deficient or in gross excess, the balance between them is distorted and disease results. The Chinese concept of health can best be defined as a normal fluctuating balance between yin and yang. Their system of diagnosis and therapy is designed to determine the imbalance of yin and yang and to correct it, therefore restoring the person's health. To produce this change, the Chinese insert needles into acupuncture points. Most of the important acupuncture points are on 14 channels running over the body, each representing an internal organ. Qi, or vital energy, is said to flow through these channels. In disease the flow of qi is altered and the insertion of an acupuncture needle into an appropriate point is said to correct the flow of vital energy, thereby restoring the body to good health.

The Chinese also developed a sophisticated idea of physiology and specific functions were defined for each of the 12 main organs. The Nei Ching Su Wen states that: 'the heart fills the pulse with blood …. And the force of the pulse flows into the arteries, and the force of the arteries ascends into the lungs'. This describes the double circulation of blood some 2000 years before William Harvey demonstrated the function of the heart and the circulation of blood in the seventeenth century. The anatomy (acupuncture points and channels) and physiology of TCM, along with a detailed examination of the pulse and tongue, provides the basis for a TCM diagnosis. A practitioner then follows a set of empirical rules to select the appropriate acupuncture points to treat the disease and correct the imbalances dispersing any pathogens.

Not all acupuncturists use a traditional Chinese approach. Some just treat the tender points that arise in various musculoskeletal diseases, such as arthritis. A number of clinical trials have shown that acupuncture in tender trigger points, which are also frequently acupuncture points, is both effective and efficacious in painful musculoskeletal conditions. In the treatment of pain, it is not yet clear which approach is the best – the traditional Chinese diagnosis or simply treating tender trigger points. However, in non-painful diseases, such as asthma or irritable bowel syndrome (IBS), trigger points do not usually occur, so to perform effective acupuncture, a traditional diagnosis must be made and the points selected within the context of TCM.

Traditional Chinese medicine and emotional well-being
As with many traditional Chinese systems, TCM can be described as a 'whole system'. This in effect means the combination of acupuncture, herbal medicine and dietary intervention is a complete system of diagnosis and therapy, bringing with it many strengths and limitations as well as a clearly different perspective to that employed by conventional medicine. Within TCM the emotions are attributable to the function of various organs and there is no Cartesian division between the mind and body. The organs within TCM are equivalent and overlap our conventional physiological and diagnostic paradigms, but also sustain a uniquely TCM view of physiology with each organ having an 'energetic component' and an attributable emotion. For instance, anxiety is often attributed to an imbalance in the paired lung and large intestine meridians, worry and over-thinking to an imbalance of the spleen and paired stomach meridian and anger to an imbalance in the liver and paired gall bladder meridian (Lewith & Lewith, 1980). While this at first may seem bizarre to the conventional physician, the implications of this unique diagnostic process have a substantial impact on the manner in which psychiatric disease is managed. Those practicing TCM do not see mental illness as separate from physical disease. This not only permeates some aspects of medical practice in China, but it also has cultural implications. If anxiety and depression can be managed, after an appropriate diagnosis, through the needling of acupuncture points on the liver, spleen or heart meridian, then this in itself suggests that the mind and body are part of a whole that interact and can respond to physical intervention. The neurophysiology of acupuncture (vide infra) suggests that the mechanism for this may be mediated through sustained changes in neurotransmission that may be produced by the act of acupuncture. The specificity of particular acupuncture points remains in doubt, but overall the effects of acupuncture appear to support the TCM model. If emotional problems can be diagnosed and treated, and at least in part effectively managed, within a system that relates them to bodily dysfunction, then this represents a different cultural and historical perspective when compared with our understanding and treatment of mental illness in the West.

The neurophysiological mechanisms of acupuncture
While TCM practitioners can explain how and why acupuncture works, as well as the underlying principles behind the selection of specific acupuncture points, TCM is not firmly grounded in modern conventional science. There is, nevertheless, considerable evidence to suggest

that acupuncture does have important and well-investigated underlying physiological mechanisms.

Acupuncture is used in the West primarily for painful conditions; therefore most research into its mechanism has been directed at the treatment and management of pain. Melzack and Wall's gate control theory was the first coherent theory of pain that proposed a sophisticated balance between pain excitation and inhibition (Melzack & Wall, 1965). They suggested that the input of pain via small diameter demyelinated nerve fibres can be inhibited, within the spinal cord, by the peripheral stimulation of large myelinated fibres. This appeared to 'close the gate to pain' and early work by Melzack and others in the 1970s suggested that acupuncture may be providing pain relief through this mechanism (Lewith & Kenyon, 1984). Furthermore, Melzack was able to show, again in the 1970s, that over 70% of local trigger points were in fact acupuncture points (Fox & Melzack, 1976). Travell & Rinzler (1946) had already established that the injection of local trigger points could be used to relieve both musculoskeletal and cardiac pain and the observation this might effectively be a therapy based on the stimulation of acupuncture points suggests that acupuncture may have been 'rediscovered' in a Western context.

The connection between acupuncture and endorphins was initially noted by Wen, a Chinese neurosurgeon, in 1973. He observed that opium addicts being treated with electroacupuncture for post-surgical analgesia reported substantial relief from withdrawal symptoms (Wen & Cheung, 1973). Subsequent research involved combining naloxone with electroacupuncture (EA) and yielded a 51% drug-free rate among heroin and opium addicts at one year post-surgical follow-up. Wen's research then stimulated colleagues in London, who were just beginning to assay endorphins and enkephalins in the CSF and serum, to evaluate whether acupuncture could affect these substances. Clement-Jones's seminal work in this area has demonstrated clearly that CSF endorphin levels rose substantially in heroin addicts and that this rise facilitated a substantial amelioration of withdrawal symptoms (Clement Jones et al., 1979). In the 1970s various studies by both Han and Pomeranz demonstrated that in both human and animal models, acupuncture could promote the release of endorphins and enkephalins (Pomeranz & Chin, 1976; Han & Terenius, 1982; Han, 1986). Blockade of the analgesic effect by opiate antagonists, such as naloxone, further supported the connection between acupuncture and the body's natural opiate system (Kosten et al., 1986). Steiner then went on to report that acupuncture has been shown to alter the levels of various other central neurotransmitters, including serotonin and norepinephrine, and also to affect the regulation of other hormones, such as prolactin, oxytocin, corticosteroids and insulin (Steiner et al., 1982). There is now a substantial body of evidence to demonstrate that acupuncture may have a wide range of effects, both on the neurotransmitters directly and on various hormone-releasing factors acting on the pituitary (Lewith & Kenyon, 1984). While there is no coherent theory as to how acupuncture may be acting in the treatment of mood disorder and depression, there is substantial evidence to demonstrate that it may be affecting many of the central pathways that we think are involved in these conditions. Current theory suggests that exogenous opiates bind at endogenous endorphin sites and downregulate the production and action of natural endorphins (Berg et al., 1991). It appears that acupuncture may enhance the production of endogenous endorphins which then compete for the receptor sites from which they have been displaced. This may be the mechanism through which acupuncture may have an effect in aiding drug withdrawal. In alcohol addiction, endogenous opiate receptor sites can be occupied by alcohol metabolites which may promote the addictive potential of acupuncture. Enhancing the production of endogenous opiates may therefore allow competition for these binding sites and can potentially help not only with substance abuse but alcohol withdrawal as well. While this provides an acceptable but by no means conclusive theoretical foundation for the widespread use of acupuncture in many conditions, its clinical value must depend on the outcome of appropriate and rigorous clinical trials.

Acupuncture and its clinical applications

In the West acupuncture has mainly been used for the treatment of pain. Systematic reviews suggest that it is almost certainly effective in the treatment of back pain; a recent meta-analysis indicated an odds ratio of 2.3 in favour of acupuncture with 95% confidence intervals of 1.28–4.13 (Ernst & White, 1998; Van Tulder et al., 1999). There is also increasingly positive evidence to sustain the clinical use of acupuncture in other areas, but in common with many CAM therapies, the evaluation of acupuncture has been bedeviled by inadequate research funding and poor quality clinical trials. However, there is a clear suggestion that acupuncture may be effective for neck pain (White et al., 2002) and in osteoarthritis (Ernst, 1997); although in both these conditions more research is mandatory.

While acupuncture has at least had some investigative rigour applied to its use in pain and arthritis, there have been very few clinical trials that have evaluated its use in non-painful conditions such as irritable bowel and asthma, with the exceptions being nausea and headache/ migraine. The seminal systematic review by Vickers (1996) clearly demonstrated that acupuncture could have an effect in nausea produced by a whole range of different stimuli from early morning sickness to chemotherapy. The situation in relation to migraine is less clear with somewhat inconclusive reviews and conflicting positive and negative studies. Acupuncture therefore represents a CAM therapy in which there is much interest, a plausible physiological mechanism and some evidence of specific clinical efficacy.

Acupuncture for anxiety, depression and insomnia

There is no doubt that acupuncture is widely and pragmatically used in the treatment of these conditions. Both patients and practitioners perceive it to be an effective treatment and indeed the underlying neurophysiological mechanisms would suggest that it might be (vide supra). However, there is clearly inadequate clinical evidence to sustain the use of acupuncture in these three conditions. While it is certainly valuable to look at the effects of acupuncture versus a placebo control, in any given condition, it may be equally valuable to compare acupuncture with appropriate standard conventional treatments in order to evaluate whether these interventions are equally effective and to compare the adverse reaction profiles of both conventional medicine and acupuncture in mood disorder. Cost effectiveness must also be an issue, particularly as acupuncture is a very labour intensive intervention. Finally, there is now little doubt that acupuncture is a safe treatment when carried out by appropriately regulated professionals (MacPherson et al., 2001).

Depression

There have been at least six clinical trials of acupuncture in depression. Three of them are Chinese in origin and are randomized controlled trials which have compared electroacupuncture with tricyclic antidepressants (Luo et al., 1985; Luo et al., 1990; Yang, 1994). Usually, acupuncture for depression would be carried out using careful point selection in accordance with TCM guidelines and manual, not electrical, stimulation of the acupuncture needles. In these three studies, although the points were selected on the basis of a TCM diagnosis, the use of electroacupuncture makes generalizable conclusions difficult. Electroacupuncture may well serve to enhance endorphin release and thus provide a 'non-point specific effect'. Nevertheless, these three studies do indicate that acupuncture is probably as effective as tricyclic

antidepressants and certainly appears to have far fewer side effects. There are three further studies involving 164 patients which look at manual acupuncture compared with sham acupuncture (Allen et al., 1998; Eich et al., 2000; Roschke et al., 2000). It has been suggested previously (Lewith & Vincent, 1995) that acupuncture, particularly electroacupuncture, at almost any body site including non-acupuncture points, may elicit endorphin release and thus in theory may help to modify the process of both depression and anxiety. In one study (Allen et al., 1998), specific TCM-based acupuncture was compared with waiting list control and sham acupuncture in 38 patients. Using standard outcome measures, it was very clear that patients benefited from the process of specific acupuncture. A further German study involving 56 patients who received 10 manual acupuncture sessions over 2 weeks also reported similar outcomes (Eich et al., 2000). When manual acupuncture was used as an adjunct to treatment with conventional antidepressants (in this case, mianserin), the group who received specific traditional Chinese acupuncture were again reported to have better depression outcomes than with conventional medicine (Roschke et al., 2000). The conclusions that one can draw from these studies are tentative as they involve small numbers and some major design faults. However, the sum of the evidence is certainly positive overall.

Anxiety

While there is no doubt that all acupuncture practitioners will report that acupuncture appears to relieve anxiety, there are unfortunately no clinical trials in this area. The neurophysiological mechanisms that appear to underpin acupuncture provide a sound basis for suggesting that acupuncture may be effective. Furthermore, the whole process of acupuncture may in itself be anxiolytic as patients need to come for a consultation which is often caring and frequently quite prolonged (MacPherson et al., 2001).

Insomnia

There is limited evidence for the use of acupuncture in insomnia which includes four studies. One study involved 40 patients and compared traditional Chinese acupuncture with sham acupuncture and found, using a variety of outcomes, that patients' sleep improved significantly more with real acupuncture than with sham treatment (Montakab, 1999). In a further study which involved patients choosing their treatment, sleep improved with both needle and laser acupuncture, but unfortunately there was no difference between those receiving acupuncture and those on the waiting list control (Becker-Carus *et al.*, 1985). The largest study involved 84 patients and looked at the use of acupressure versus sham acupressure in elderly insomniacs (Chen *et al.*, 1999). Acupressure produced significantly better results than sham treatment, and the authors suggested that this might provide a safe and side effect free option for those who would be best advised to take as few medications as possible. A final very small study involving six patients receiving acupressure versus sham acupressure in a crossover model noted positive effects (Buguet *et al.*, 1995). Overall, it seems that acupuncture techniques may have some effect in insomnia, but further work is undoubtedly required in this area.

Use of acupuncture in the treatment of substance abuse, alcoholism and smoking

The evidence for the use of acupuncture in these areas is particularly confused. Acupuncture as a treatment for all forms of addiction is a relatively recent phenomenon, having first been observed by Wen in the mid 70s (Wen & Cheung, 1973; Wen & Teo, 1975). This was a serendipitous observation and is not firmly grounded in clinical practice in the same way as much of TCM. Consequently there is almost no clinical literature that helps us define either the ideal acupuncture points to use in these situations or the ideal dose and type of acupuncture (manual stimulation or electro acupuncture). Therefore, to begin by assuming that these chance observations and the subsequent empirical treatment packages have somehow been defined rigorously would be quite incorrect. There may therefore be a substantial misunderstanding of the whole process of acupuncture and its evaluation within the area of addiction as the effects of acupuncture in these conditions may be entirely non-specific (Lewith & Vincent, 1995).

It may matter very little where the acupuncture needle is placed as long as acupuncture is given, possibly ideally with some electro-stimulation. Studies that evaluate the use of acupuncture versus a sham acupuncture treatment fail to recognize these important assumptions that are inherently espoused by acupuncture enthusiasts, so many studies have been based on very poor scientific foundations and have used approaches that would be entirely unacceptable in the context of the development of a new medication. To our knowledge, no phase I or II studies have ever been conducted on the use of acupuncture in the treatment of addictions. To add to this, many of the studies have been under-powered and poorly designed with inadequate follow-up. Overall, therefore, the conclusions that we can draw are limited, however acupuncture and smoking withdrawal offers an interesting case study.

Acupuncture and smoking withdrawal

It is probably fair to say that no addiction can be adequately treated by any single therapeutic approach, so advocating the treatment of smoking withdrawal solely with acupuncture is a priori a poor idea. If acupuncture has a place in the treatment of this condition, it is likely that it would be as part of a whole treatment programme. Nevertheless, White *et al.* (2002) published a systematic review of acupuncture for smoking cessation and were able to identify 22 randomized controlled trials. These studies compared acupuncture or an acupuncture-based technique, such as acupressure, laser acupuncture or electro-stimulation, with either sham treatment, another intervention or no intervention for smoking cessation. Unfortunately the majority of the studies had poor long-term follow-up so the systematic review did not enable a clear medium- or long-term conclusion (at 6 or 12 months). The odds ratio for the early outcome (immediately after treatment) was 1.22 in favour of acupuncture with 95% confidence intervals of 0.99–1.94. At 6 months an odds ratio of 1.5 with confidence intervals of 0.99–2.27 was obtained and similar results were obtained at 12 months. Clearly these failed to detect any specific effect from acupuncture over and above other control interventions. Consequently we must conclude that acupuncture techniques did not demonstrate superiority to any of the control or comparative interventions. Interestingly, only one of the studies involved no intervention when in fact a waiting list control was used. All the other control or comparative interventions involved either sham acupuncture, comparison with nicotine gum or 'group therapy'. Overall, the cessation rates, irrelevant of treatment, appeared to be roughly equivalent to that which one would expect from conventional and appropriately licensed interventions, such as the use of nicotine gum. It is clear that within the context and question posed by this Cochrane systematic review, that the so-called 'correct acupuncture points' offer no definite benefit over treatment with either 'incorrect acupuncture points' or appropriately delivered control/comparative treatments. Possibly the correct conclusion to be drawn from this review is that acupuncture does not have a point-specific effect but that its non-specific effect may be equivalent to all other single interventions used to aid smoking cessation. As such, it may be worthy of further consideration and possible inclusion in a comprehensive anti-smoking programme. Certainly, within the UK, acupuncture is still being used to aid smoking withdrawal in the NHS, in spite of this apparent lack of evidence. While one would not wish to argue with the conclusion of White *et al.*'s review, it is vital to place it in context. The only conclusion that one can draw from these data is that more pragmatic studies are required with appropriate health economic and abstinence outcomes. In particular these studies should focus not on the specific efficacy of acupuncture but its pragmatic and overall effectiveness in comparison with other widely available treatments that claim and are indeed limited as aids to smoking cessation.

Alcohol withdrawal

Another interesting case in point is the use of acupuncture among alcoholics. One particular study by Bullock *et al.* (1989) used a traditional Chinese medical approach to diagnosis and treatment of alcoholics among a group of recidivist homeless alcoholics in Minnesota. This group was compared with an equivalent group of patients who were equally recidivist and were given sham acupuncture (i.e. inappropriate acupuncture points were used). The treatment was intensive and the patients received 10 treatments over 2 weeks in the first phase of the study, then treatments 3 times a week for a further 4 weeks and finally treatments twice a week for 2 weeks. There was a very significant total abstinence effect at 6 months when comparing the patients receiving real acupuncture with sham. This study illustrates that acupuncture was not simply given with the intent of enhancing endorphin release and minimizing addiction, but rather in an attempt to balance the patient's individualized energetic dysfunction according to TCM principles. The therapeutic investment was intensive, but these individuals were severely disabled by their addiction. The process proved to be effective but represents only one relatively small study. A non-systematic review presented by Ernst (2001) suggests that Bullock *et al.*'s initial reports may have been ill founded. However, the study models involved in the majority of the other trials reviewed by Ernst were different, and a number of them did not use a traditional Chinese approach. This makes it difficult to systematize the data and draw generalizable conclusions. Furthermore, treatment in some of the studies was far less intense than that reported by Bullock *et al.* (1989). In some studies the groups were not entirely comparable; in one instance the patients had already been withdrawn from alcohol prior to treatment while the other three studies quoted by Ernst (2001) involved patients who were still clearly dependent.

Substance abuse

The use of acupuncture in the treatment of heroin addiction must remain at the centre of the discovery of the endorphin/enkephalin hypothesis as it applies to the use of acupuncture in pain (Wen & Cheung, 1973). While there is every

reason to suppose that, in theory, acupuncture may help drug withdrawal, the clinical trial results are varied. This may be because acupuncture could have been used, inappropriately, as a sole therapy. It may also relate to the search for efficacy rather than overall effectiveness and the difficulty of defining 'best practice' in this context as far as acupuncture treatment is concerned. What is clear is that acupuncture is widely available, and indeed widely used, as part of cocaine and opiate withdrawal treatment programmes in both the USA and the UK (Culliton *et al.*, 1997). Schwartz *et al.* (1999) suggest that acupuncture is a valuable adjunct in these treatment programmes but rigorous randomized controlled trials of real versus sham acupuncture do not consistently support this assertion. In one study involving 60 subjects entering a methadone maintenance programme, cravings were greater in the group that had real acupuncture when compared with those given 'placebo acupuncture' with all the potential confounding that placebo acupuncture may involve (Wells *et al.*, 1995). Drop-out rates in these very dependent and difficult patients are a real cause for concern; Washburn *et al.* (1993) were able to demonstrate that the addition of acupuncture to 100 subjects with heroin dependence increased the rate in which these patients remained in the treatment programme, the problem was that only six subjects completed the 21-day study. Bullock *et al.* (1999) were not able to demonstrate that acupuncture was efficacious as compared with placebo, in drug withdrawal in 236 cocaine addicts and this negative finding was reduplicated by Richard *et al.* in a larger study involving 277 cocaine-dependent individuals when acupuncture was compared with cognitive-behavioural therapy (Richard *et al.*, 1995). However, Avants *et al.* (2000) report that acupuncture was more effective than sham needling and relaxation in 82 cocaine addicts when measuring as their primary outcome urinary drug concentrations.

Conclusion

The place of acupuncture in the treatment of addictions must therefore be open to some doubt. There is an underlying suggestion that in all these situations acupuncture may be providing non-specific and beneficial effects and indeed this would be consistent with the underlying neurophysiological mechanisms that may be triggered by acupuncture. However, the point-specific assumptions that are made by acupuncturists in the context of their training and treatment provision must be in doubt when the evidence is examined carefully.

Table 7.2. Licensing and training of major complementary and alternative medicine therapies in the USA

Therapy	Licensure as of 2000	Appropriate training	Professional organizations
Acupuncture	All states except Alabama, Delaware, Kansas, Kentucky, Michigan, Mississippi, Nevada, Oklahoma, South Dakota and Wyoming	Minimum 3-year master's or doctorate degree, variable postgraduate training for medical providers Board exams	American Association of Oriental Medicine American Academy of Medical Acupuncture National Acupuncture Foundation Accreditation Commission for Acupuncture and Oriental Medicine National Certification Commission for Acupuncture and Oriental Medicine
Chiropractic	50 states	3–4-year doctorate program at an accredited university Board exams	American Chiropractic Organization Foundation for Chiropractic Education and Research
Massage therapy	Alabama, Arkansas, Connecticut, Delaware, District of Columbia, Florida, Hawaii, Iowa, Louisiana, Maine, Maryland, Mississippi, Missouri, Nebraska, Nevada, New Hampshire, New Jersey, New Mexico, New York, North Carolina, Ohio, Oregon, Rhode Island, South Carolina, Tennessee, Texas, Utah, Virginia, Washington, West Virginia and Wisconsin	Minimum of 500 hours, usually from an accredited program Board exams	American Massage Therapy Association Commission on Massage Training Accreditation National Certification Board for Therapeutic Massage and Bodywork
Herbalism	None; often practiced under another health-care license	Apprenticeship program or 3-year degree	American Herbalist's Guild American Botanical Council Herb Research Foundation
Naturopathy	Arkansas, Arizona, Connecticut, Hawaii, Maine, Montana, New Hampshire, Oregon, Utah, Vermont and Washington	4-year accredited doctorate programme Board exams	American Association of Naturopathic Physicians North American Board of Naturopathic Examiners
Homeopathy	Arizona, Connecticut and Nevada, often practiced under another healthcare license	Naturopathic program, postgraduate training for medical providers, homeopathic universities abroad	National Center for Homeopathy American Board of Homeotherapeutics Homeopathic Academy of Naturopathic Physicians Council for Homeopathic Certification

Licensing laws vary widely from state to state in terms of eligibility, examination, scope of practice and autonomy; moreover, many states have introduced statutes that have yet to take effect. Training is highly variables; the minimum training required for professional competency is listed here. Contact the appropriate professional organization for information on qualified practitioners in your area. *Source: Rheumatology*, 3rd edn. (2003). Ed. M. C. Hochberg *et al.*, p. 513. Mosby.

Addendum: referral to a CAM practitioner

Above all, physicians need to initiate an open dialogue with their patients about CAM therapies, particularly as more than 70% of patients who use CAM do not inform their physician (Eisenberg *et al.*, 1998). In the context of psychiatric illness, some patients may present with inappropriate expectations and frankly delusional requests and these need to be managed appropriately. In general terms CAM approaches can be supportive in severe and potentially suicidal depression, severe anxiety and various psychoses, but they should not be used as the primary treatment options. Probably the single most important issue is that the CAM therapist(s) and those providing conventional care should be working as a team with the patient's interest at heart. From here patients and physicians can make responsible decisions about treatment options and monitor progress together with the CAM provider. Table 7.2 provides information about the licensing and professional training of CAM practitioners in the USA. The situation in the UK is much less definite than the USA. Medical homeopaths are usually members or fellows of the Faculty of Homeopathy in the UK and simultaneously medically registered and indemnified. Osteopaths, chiropractors and herbalists all have 3–5 years university-based training courses in order for them to first register and then practice in their chosen profession. Osteopaths and chiropractors are currently statutorily registered in the UK and herbalists and acupuncturists (who also have a 3 year training course) are in the process of becoming nationally registered with Department of Health co-operation. The qualification and registration for many other CAM therapists, such as non-medically qualified homeopaths, is very variable. Issues of public safety, regulation and indemnity are important for the CAM professions to resolve in order that they may progress within the UK medical environment and these are very clearly articulated in a House of Lords Select Committee Report published in 2000 (House of Lords Select Committee Report, 2000).

General considerations

It is impossible to provide specific guidelines for the training and practice of CAM on a worldwide basis. As a consequence, we have provided some general questions that should be asked by physicians thinking of referring patients to CAM or patients thinking of seeking CAM treatment.

How do I know the therapist is competent?

- Do you think that the practitioner is technically competent? This usually means, are they a member of an appropriate organization and have they adequate training in the field in which they practice?
- Might they advise the patient to change their conventional medical treatment without seeking the advice of their doctor?
- Can the proposed treatment be provided safely? If you are discussing referral to an herbalist, are you sure they are aware of the potential cross-reactions between herbal medicine and your conventional medications?
- Will the complementary practitioner set guidelines at the first appointment for how they think the treatment should progress? Should the patient expect a response to treatment after three or four acupuncture sessions or would it be more reasonable to assess the treatment after eight or ten sessions?

Is the therapist a professional?

- Is the environment in which treatment is provided safe and appropriate?
- Does the therapist have professional indemnity?
- Does the therapist have a code of ethics and are the data they hold legally protected and will they treat the information given to them in a confidential manner?
- Do the therapists have an organization which employs a process of self-regulation and will remove members from their lists if they are not behaving ethically?
- Are the therapists aware of, and do they have a process of reporting, adverse reactions to the treatments they provide?

Is CAM treatment appropriate?

- Has a clear diagnosis of the problem been made? If such a diagnosis cannot be made, have other common problems been excluded? Is the patient missing out on an appropriate conventional medical treatment?
- If the patient has a chronic condition which is relatively stable, then it may be reasonable to try a CAM approach, either to help symptoms or minimize the use of potentially damaging long-term conventional medications.
- You may know a competent complementary therapist to whom you regularly refer, are you sure that they are a safe, professional and competent person?
- You may wish to refer a patient to another doctor practising some form of CAM; this kind of referral should be treated in exactly the same manner as referral to any other properly medically qualified specialist.

In general, we have so little information about whether complementary medicine works it is usually impossible to make an evidence-based decision. In our view, it is reasonable to embark on CAM treatment as long as it is safe and provided in the context of proper professional practice associated with clear clinical guidelines.

ACKNOWLEDGMENTS

We would like to thank Michael McIntyre, President of the European Herbal Practitioners Association for his contributions to the text. We would also like to acknowledge Jackie Burnham for providing secretarial skills. Dr Lewith's post is funded by a grant from the Rufford Maurice Lange Foundation.

The level of evidence for each of the interventions discussed in this chapter is summarized in Table 7.3.

Table 7.3. Effectiveness of complementary and alternative medicines

Treatment	Form of treatment	Psychiatric disorder	Level of evidence for efficacy	Comments
Herbal	St. John's wort	Depression	Ia–Ib	Conflicting evidence. Some studies show no difference from placebo; others show no difference from 'standard' antidepressants, but overall its effectiveness has not been proved. If effective, probably would be in mild depression
Herbal	St. John's wort	Anxiety	IIa	One meta-analysis found it better than placebo. Hepatic failure is a caution
Herbal	Valerian	Insomnia	IIa or IIb	Contradictory. Different studies suggest improvement in different stages of sleep. May need to be taken over several days to weeks to begin to work.
Herbal	Omega-3 fatty acids	Depression	Ia	Data are not conclusive but appear to support use in depression, especially as an adjunct to regular pharmacologic treatment
Herbal	S-adenosyl-l-methionine (SAMe)	Depression	IIb	A meta-analysis concluded that it is more effective than placebo though most studies had significant methodological flaws
Homeopathy	Homeopathy	Various psychiatric illnesses	IV	No evidence for effectiveness. Whatever benefit that is attributed to the treatment may lie in the relationship of the homeopath to the patient
Acupuncture	Acupuncture	Depression	Ia	Evidence that it is more effective than placebo and equal to antidepressants though studies have methodological flaws
Acupuncture	Acupuncture	Anxiety	IV	While there is strong belief it is effective, there is no evidence and whatever effectiveness there is may be in the relationship of the acupuncturist to the patient
Acupuncture	Acupuncture	Insomnia	III	Some evidence but weak
Acupuncture	Acupuncture	Addiction	IV	No real evidence
Acupuncture	Acupuncture	Nicotine dependence	IIa	May be equivalent to other single interventions
Acupuncture	Acupuncture	Alcohol use disorders	III	Because of the nature of acupuncture, difficult to do placebo-controlled trials. Evidence is contradictory and plagued by methodological issues

REFERENCES

Adams, P. B., Lawson, S., Sanigorski, A. & Sinclair, A. J. (1996). Arachidonic to eicosapentaenoic acid ratio in blood correlates positively with clinical symptoms of depression. *Lipids*, **31** (suppl.), 157–61.

Allen, J. J. B., Schnyer, R. N. & Hitt, S. K. (1998). The efficacy of acupuncture in the treatment of major depression in women. *Psychological Science*, **9**, 397–401.

Astin, J. A. Why patients use alternative medicine. *Journal of the American Medical Association*, **279**, 1548–53.

Avants, S. K., Margolin, A., Holford, T. R. & Kosten, T. R. (2000). A randomized controlled trial of auricular acupuncture for cocaine dependence. *Archives of Internal Medicine*, **160**, 2305–12.

Babcock, T., Helton, W. S. & Espat, N. J. (2000). Eicosapentaenoic acid (EPA): an anti-inflammatory – 3 fat with potential clinical applications. *Nutrition*, **16**, 1116–18.

Becker-Carus, C., Heyden, T. & Kelle, A. (1985). Die Wirksamkeit von Akupunktur und Einstellungs-Entspannungstraining zur Behandlung primarer Schlafstorungen. *Zeitschrift für Klinische Psychologie und Psychopathologie*, **33**, 161–72.

Bell, K. M., Potkin, S. G., Carreon, D. & Plon, L. (1994). S-adenosylmethionine blood levels in major depression: changes with drug treatment. *Acta Neurologica Scandinavica*, **Suppl. 154**, 15–18.

Berg, B. J., Volpicelli, J. R., Alterman, A. I. & O'Brien, C. P. (1991). The relationship between endogenous opioids and alcohol drinking: the opioid compensation hypothesis. In *Novel Pharmacological Interventions for Alcoholism*, ed. C. A. Naranjo & E. M. Sellars. New York: Springer-Verlag.

Biber, A., Fischer, H., Romer, A. & Chatterjee, C. C. (1998). Oral bioavailability of hyperforin from hypericum extracts in rats and human volunteers. *Pharmacopsychiatry*, **31** (Suppl.), 36–43.

Bilia, A. R., Bergonzi, M. C., Morgenni, F., Mazzi, G. & Vincieri, F. F. (2001). Evaluation of chemical stability of St. John's wort commercial extract and some preparations. *International Journal of Pharmaceuticals*, **213**, 199–208.

Bisset, N. G. & Wichtl, M. (ed.) (1994). Valerianae radix. In *Herbal Drugs and Phytopharmaceuticals*, pp. 513–16. Stuttgart: Medpharm GmbH Scientific Publishers.

Bladt, S. & Wagner, H. (1994). Inhibition of MAO by fractions and constituents of hypericum extract. *Journal of Geriatric Psychiatry and Neurology*, 7(Suppl. 1), S57–9.

Blumenthal, M. (2002). Kava safety questioned due to case reports of liver toxicity. *HerbalGram*, **55**, 26–32.

Bombardelli, E. & Morazzoni, P. (1995). *Hypericum perforatum*. *Fitoterapia*, **66**, 43–68.

Bottiglieri, T. & Hyland, K. (1994). S-adenosylmethionine levels in psychiatric and neurological disorders: a review. *Acta Neurologica Scandinavica*, **Suppl. 154**, 19–26.

Bove, G. M. (1998). Acute neuropathy after exposure to sun in a patient treated with St. John's wort. *Lancet*, **352**, 1121–2 (Letter).

Bressa, G. M. (1994). S-adenosyl-l-methionine (SAMe) as antidepressant: meta-analysis of clinical studies. *Acta Neurologica Scandinavica*, **Suppl. 154**, 7–14.

Brockmöller, J., Reum, T., Bauer, S., Kerb, R., Hübner, W.-D. & Roots, I. (1997). Hypericin and pseudohypericin: pharmacokinetics and effects on photosensitivity in humans. *Pharmacopsychiatry*, **30** (Suppl.), 94–101.

Bruinsma, K. A. & Taren, D. L. (2000). Dieting, essential fatty acid intake, and depression. *Nutrition Review*, **58**, 98–108.

Budzinski, J. W., Foster, B. C., Vandenhoek, S. & Arnason, J. T. (2000). An in vitro evaluation of human cytochrome P450 3A4 inhibition by selected commercial herbal extracts and tinctures. *Phytomedicine*, **7**, 273–82.

Buguet, A., Sartre, M. & LeKerneau, J. (1995). Continuous nocturnal automassage of an acupuncture point modifies sleep in healthy subjects. *Neurophysiologie Clinique*, **25**, 78–83.

Bullock, M. L., Culliton, P. D. & Olander, R. T. (1989). Controlled trial of acupuncture for severe recidivist alcoholism. *Lancet*, **8652**, 1435–9.

Bullock, M. L., Kiresuk, T. J., Pheley, A. M. et al. (1999). Auricular acupuncture in the treatment of cocaine abuse. *Journal of Substance Abuse and Treatment*, **16**, 31–8.

Butterweck, V., Nahrstedt, A., Evans, J. (2002). In vitro receptor screening of pure constituents of St. John's wort reveals novel interactions with a number of GPCRs. *Psychopharmacology*, **162**, 193–202.

Butterweck, V., Christoffel, V., Nahrstedt, A., Petereit, F., Spengler, B. & Winterhoff, H. (2003). Step by step removal of hyperforin and hypericin: activity profile of different *Hypericum* preparations in behavioral models. *Life Science*, **73**, 627–39.

Calder, P. C. (1997). n-3 polyunsaturated fatty acids and cytokine production in health and disease. *Annals of Nutrition and Metabolism*, **41**, 203–34.

Cantoni, G. L. (1953). S-Adenosylmethionine: a new intermediate formed enzymatically from L-methionine and adenosinetriphosphate. *Journal of Biological Chemistry*, **204**, 403–16.

Cawte, J. (1985).Psychoactive substances of the south seas: betel, kava and pituri. *Australia and New Zealand Journal of Psychiatry*, **19**, 83–7.

Chatterjee, S. S., Nsldner, M., Koch, E. & Erdelmeier, C. (1998). Antidepressant activity of *Hypericum perforatum* and hyperforin: the neglected possibility. *Pharmacopsychiatry*, **31** (Suppl.), 7–15.

Chavez, M. L. & Chavez, P. I. (1997). Saint John's wort. *Hospital Pharmacy*, **32**, 1621–32.

Chen, M. L., Lin, L. C., Wu, S. C. & Lin, J. G. (1999). Effectiveness of acupressure in improving the quality of sleep of institutionalised residents. *Journals of Gerontology. Series A, Biological Sciences and Medical Sciences*, **54A**, M389–94.

Chan, T. Y. K. (1998). An assessment of the delayed effects associated with valerian overdose. *International Journal of Clinical Pharmacology and Therapy*, **36**, 569 (letter).

Clement-Jones, V., McLoughlin, L., Lowry, P. J., Besser, G. M., Rees, L. H. & Wen, H. L. (1979). Acupuncture in heroin addicts; changes in Met-enkephalin and beta-endorphin in blood and cerebrospinal fluid. *Lancet*, **2** (8139), 380–3.

Cott, J. M. (1997). In vitro receptor binding and enzyme inhibition by *Hypericum perforatum* extract. *Pharmacopsychiatry*, **30** (Suppl.), 108–12.

Culliton, P. D., Boucher, T. A. & Carlson, G. A. (1997). Substance misuse. In *Mind-Body Medicine. A Clinicians's Guide to Psychoneuroimmunology*, ed. A. Watkins, pp. 221–50. Churchill Livingstone, Edinburgh.

Dannawi, M. (2002). Possible serotonin syndrome after combination of buspirone and St. John's wort. *Journal of Psychopharmacology*, **16**, 401 (Letter).

De Los Reyes, G. C. & Koda, R. T. (2002). Determining hyperforin and hypericin content in eight brands of St. John's wort. *American Journal of Health Systems and Pharmacy*, **59**, 545–7.

Delion, S., Chalon, S., Herault, J., Fuilloteau, D., Besnard, J. C. & Durand, G. (1994). Chronic dietary alpha-linolenic acid deficiency alters dopaminergic and serotonergic neurotransmission in rats. *Journal of Nutrition*, **124**, 2466–75.

Dello Buono, M., Urciuoli, O., Marietta, P., Padoani, W. & De Leo, D. (2001). Alternative medicine in a sample of 655 community-dwelling elderly. *Journal of Psychosomatic Research*, **50**, 147–54.

Duffield, A. M., Jamieson, D. D., Lidgard, R. O., Duffield, P. H. & Bourne, D. J. (1989). Identification of some human urinary metabolites of the intoxicating beverage kava. *Journal of Chromatography*, **475**, 273–81.

Durr, D., Stieger, B., Kullak-Ublick, G. A. et al. (2000). St. John's wort induces intestinal p-glycoprotein/MDR1 and intestinal and hepatic CYP3A4. *Clinical Pharmacology and Therapeutics*, **68**, 598–604.

Eich, H., Agelink, M. W., Lehmann, E., Lemmer, W. & Klieser, E. (2000). Acupuncture in patients with minor depressive episodes and generalized anxiety. Results of an experimental study. *Fortschritte des Neurologie-Psychiatrie*, **68**, 137–44.

Eisenberg, D. M., Davis, R. B. & Ettner, S. L. (1998). Trends in alternative medicine use in the United States. *Journal of the American Medical Association*, **280**, 246–52.

Ernst, E. (2001). *The Desktop Guide to Complementary and Alternative Medicine*. Edinburgh: Mosby.

Ernst, E. (1997). Acupuncture as a symptomatic treatment of osteoarthritis. A systematic review. *Scandinavian Journal of Rheumatology*, **26**, 444–7.

Ernst, E. & White, A. R. (1998). Acupuncture for back pain. A meta-analysis of randomized controlled trials. *Archives of Internal Medicine*, **158**, 2235–41.

Fava, M., Alpert, J., Nierenberg, A. A. *et al.* (2005). A double-blind, randomized trial of St. John's wort, fluoxetine, and placebo in major depressive disorder. *Journal of Clinical Psychopharmacology*, **25**, 441–7.

Fetrow, C. W. & Avila, J. R. (2001). Efficacy of the dietary supplement S-adenosyl-L-methionine. *Annals of Pharmacotherapy*, **35**, 1414–25.

Foster, S. & Tyler, V. E. (1999). *Tyler's Honest Herbal. A Sensible Guide to the Use of Herbs and Related Remedies*, 4th edn. New York: Hayworth Herbal Press.

Fox, E. J. & Melzack, R. (1976). Transcutaneous electrical stimulation of acupuncture; comparison of treatment for low back pain. *Pain*, **2**, 141–8.

Frangou, S., Lewis, M. & McCrone, P. (2006). Efficacy of ethyl-eicosapentaenoic acid in bipolar depression: randomised double-blind placebo-controlled study. *British Journal of Psychiatry*, **188**, 46–50.

Friedel, H. A., Goa, Kl. & Benfield, P. (1989). S-adenosyl-L-methionine. A review of its pharmacological properties and therapeutic potential in liver dysfunction and affective disorders in relation to its physiological role in cell metabolism. *Drugs*, **38**, 389–416.

Garges, H. P., Varia, I. & Doraiswamy, P. M. (1998). Cardiac complications and delirium associated with valerian root withdrawal. *Journal of the American Medical Association*, **280**, 1566–7 (letter).

Gaster, B. & Holroyd, J. (2000). St. John's wort for depression. *Archives of Internal Medicine*, **160**, 152–6.

Glass, J. R., Sproule, B. A., Herrmann, N., Streiner, D. & Busto, U. E. (2003). Acute pharmacological effects of temazepam, diphenhydramine, and valerian in healthy elderly subjects. *Journal of Clinical Psychopharmacology*, **23**, 260–8.

Han, J. S. & Terenius, L. (1982). Neurochemical basis of acupuncture analgesia. *Annual Review of Pharmacology and Toxicology*, **22**, 193–220.

Han, J. S. (1986). Electroacupuncture: an alternative to antidepressants for treating affective diseases? *International Journal of Neuroscience*, **29**, 79–92.

Center for Disease Control (2002). Hepatic toxicity possibly associated with kava-containing products–United States, Germany, and Switzerland, 1999–2002. *Morbidity and Mortality Weekly Report*, **51**, 1065–7.

Hibbeln, J. R. (1998). Fish consumption and major depression. *Lancet*, **351**, 1213 (letter).

Horrocks, L. A. & Yeo, Y. K. (1999). Health benefits of docosahexanoic acid (DHA). *Pharmacological Research*, **40**, 211–25.

Houghton, P. J. (1999). The scientific basis for the reputed activity of valerian. *Journal of Pharmaceutical Pharmacology*, **51**, 505–12.

House of Lords Select Committee on Science and Technology (2000). 6th Report, Session 1999–2000. *Complementary and Alternative Medicine*. London: House of Lords.

Hypericum Depression Trial Study Group (2002). Effect of *Hypericum perforatum* (St. John's wort) in major depressive disorder. A randomized controlled trial. *Journal of the American Medical Association*, **287**, 1807–14.

Jacobson, J. M., Feinman, L., Liebes, L. *et al.* (2001). Pharmacokinetics, safety, and antiviral effects of hypericin, a derivative of St. John's wort plant, in patients with chronic hepatitis C virus infection. *Antimicrobial Agents and Chemotherapy*, **45**, 517–24.

Jensen, A. G., Hansen, S. H. & Nielsen, E. (2001). Adhyperforin as a contributor to the effect of *Hypericum performaturm* L. in biochemical models of antidepressant activity. *Life Science*, **68**, 1593–605.

Kaufman, D. W., Kelly, J. P., Rosenberg, L., Anderson, T. E. & Mitchell, A. A. (2002). Recent patterns of medication use in the ambulatory adult population of the United States. *Journal of the American Medical Association*, **287**, 337–44.

Kelley, D. S., Taylor, P. C., Nelson, G. J. *et al.* (1999). Docosahexaenoic acid ingestion inhibits natural killer cell activity and production of inflammatory mediators in young healthy men. *Lipids*, **34**, 317–24.

Kosten, T. R., Kreck, M. J., Ragunath, J. & Kleber, H. B. (1986). A preliminary study of beta-endorphin during chronic naltrexon maintenance treatment in ex-opiate addicts. *Life Science*, **31**, 55–9.

Lewith, G. T. & Lewith, N. R. (1980). *Modern Chinese Acupuncture*. Wellingborough, UK: Thorsons Publishers.

Lewith, G. T. & Kenyon, J. N. (1984). Physiological and psychological explanations for the mechanism of acupuncture as a treatment for chronic pain. *Social Science and Medicine*, **19**, 1367–78.

Lewith, G. T. & Vincent, C. (1995). The evaluation of the clinical effects of acupuncture. A problem reassessed and a framework for future research. *Pain Forum*, **4**, 29–39.

Linde, K. & Jonas, W. B. (1998). Meta-analysis of homoeopathy trials. *Lancet*, **351**, 367–8.

Linde, K. & Mulrow, C. D. (2004). St. John's wort for depression. *Cochrane Systematic Database of Reviews*, **3**. Oxford: Update Software Ltd.

Linde, K., Ramirez, G., Mulrow, C. D., Pauls, A., Weidenhammer, W. & Melchart, D. (1996). St. John's wort for depression – an overview and meta-analysis of randomized clinical trials. *British Medical Journal*, **313**, 253–8.

Linde, K., Berner, M., Egger, M. & Mulrow, C. (2005). St. John's wort for depression. Meta-analysis of randomised controlled trials. *British Journal of Psychiatry*, **186**, 11–17.

Luo, H., Jia, Y., Wu, X. & Dai, W. (1990). Electro-acupuncture in the treatment of depressive psychosis. *International Journal of Clinical Acupuncture*, **1**, 7–13.

Luo, H., Jia, Y. & Zhan, L. (1985). Electro-acupuncture vs amitriptyline in the treatment of depressive states. *Journal of Traditional Chinese Medicine*, **5**, 3–8.

MacLennan, A. H., Wilson, D. H. & Taylor, A. W. (1996). Prevalence and cost of alternative medicine in Australia. *Lancet*, **347**, 569–73.

MacPherson, H., Thomas, K., Walters, S. & Fitter, M. (2001). The York acupuncture safety study: prospective survey of 34000 treatments by traditional acupuncturists. *British Medical Journal*, **323**, 486–7.

Maes, M. & Meltzer, H. Y. M. (1995). The serotonin hypothesis of major depression. In *Psychopharmacology, The Fourth Generation of Progress*, ed. F. E. Bloom & D. J. Kupfer, pp. 933–41. New York: Raven Press.

Maes, M., Christophe, A., Delanghe, J., Altamura, C., Neels, H. & Meltzer, H. Y. (1999). Lowered 3 polyunsaturated fatty acids in serum phospholipids and cholesteryl esters of depressed patients. *Psychiatry Research*, **85**, 275–91.

Maes, M., Smith, R., Christophe, A., Cosyns, P., Desnyder, R. & Meltzer, H. Y. (1996). Fatty acid composition in major depression: decreased 3 fractions in cholesteryl esters and increased C20:46/C20:53 ratio in cholesteryl esters and phospholipids. *Journal of Affective Disease*, **38**, 35–46.

Marangell, L. B., Martinez, J. M., Zboyan, H. A., Kertz, B., Kim, H. F. S. & Puryear, L. J. (2003). A double-blind, placebo-controlled study of the omega-3 fatty acid docosahexaenoic acid in the treatment of major depression. *Archives of General Psychiatry*, **160**, 996–8.

Melzack, R. & Wall, P. D. (1965). Pain mechanisms, a new theory. *Science*, **150**, 971–9.

Meydani, S. N., Endres, S., Woods, M. M. *et al.* (1991). Oral (n-3) fatty acid supplementation suppresses cytokine production and lymphocyte proliferation; comparison between young and older women. *Journal of Nutrition*, **121**, 547–55.

Meydani, S. N., Lichtenstein, A. H., Cornwall, S. *et al.* (1993). Immunologic effects of national cholesterol education panel step-2 diets with and without fish-derived N-3 fatty acid enrichment. *Journal of Clinical Investigation*, **92**, 105–13.

Montakab, H. (1999). Acupuncture and insomnia. *Forsch Komplementarmed*, **1** (Suppl.), 29–31.

Morris, C. A. & Avorn, J. (2003). Internet marketing of herbal products. *Journal of the American Medical Association*, **290**, 1505–9.

Moses, E. L. & Mallinger, A. G. (2000). St. John's wort: three cases of possible mania induction. *Journal of Clinical Psychopharmacology*, **20**, 115–17 (Letter).

Natural Medicines Comprehensive Database. Kava (2004). http://www.naturaldatabase.com/monograph.

Natural Medicines Comprehensive Database. SAMe (2004). http://www.naturaldatabase.com/monograph.

Natural Medicines Comprehensive Database. St. John's wort (2004). http://www.naturaldatabase.com/monograph.

Natural Medicines Comprehensive Database. Valerian (2004). http://www.naturaldatabase.com/monograph.

Norton, S. A. & Ruze, P. (1994). Kava dermopathy. *Journal of the American Academy of Dermatology*, **31**, 89–97.

O'Breasail, A. M. & Argouarch, S. (1998). Hypomania and St. John's wort. *Canadian Journal of Psychiatry*, **43**, 746–7 (Letter).

Patel, S., Robinson, R. & Burk, M. (2002). Hypertensive crisis associated with St. John's wort. *American Journal of Medicine*, **112**, 507–8 (Letter).

Peet, M. & Horrobin, D. F. (2002). A dose-ranging study of the effects of ethyl-eicosapentanoate in patients with ongoing depression despite apparently adequate treatment with standard drugs. *Archives of General Psychiatry*, **59**, 913–19.

Pepping, J. (1999a). Kava: *Piper methysticum. American Journal of Health-System Pharmacy*, **56**, 957–60.

Pepping, J. (1999b). Omega-3 essential fatty acids. *American Journal of Health-System Pharmacy*, **56**, 719–24.

Pittler, M. H. & Ernst, E. (2003). Kava extract for treating anxiety (Cochrane Review). In *The Cochrane Library*, Issue 4. Chichester: John Wiley & Sons.

Plushner, S. L. (2000). Valerian: *Valeriana officinalis. American Journal of Health-System Pharmacy*, **57**, 328–35.

Pomeranz, B. & Chiu, D. (1976). Naloxone blocks acupuncture analgesia and causes hyperalgesia: endorphin is implicated. *Life Science*, **19**, 1757–62.

Review of Natural Products, efacts. Kava, 2003. http://efactsweb.com.

Review of Natural Products, efacts. St. John's wort, 2000. http://efactsweb.com.

Richard, A. J., Montoya, I. D., Nelson, R. & Spencer, R. T. (1995). Effectiveness of adjunct therapies in crack cocaine treatment. *Journal of Substance Abuse Treatment*, **12**, 401–13.

Roschke, J., Wolf, C., Muller, M. J. *et al.* (2000). The benefit from whole body acupuncture in major depression. *Journal of Affective Disorders*, **57**, 73–81.

Roy, R., Tiller, W. A., Bell, I. & Hoover, M. R. (2005). The structure of liquid water; novel insights from materials research; potential relevance to homeopathy. *Materials Research and Innovations*, **9**, 93–124.

Russman, S., Lauterburg, B. H. & Helbling, A. (2001). Kava hepatotoxicity. *Annals of Internal Medicine*, **135**, 68–9 (letter).

Ruze, P. (1990). Kava-induced dermopathy: a niacin deficiency? *Lancet*, **335**, 1442–5.

Schwartz, M., Saitz, R., Mulvey, K. *et al.* (1999). The value of acupuncture detoxification programs in a substance abuse treatment system. *Journal of Substance Abuse Treatment*, **17**, 305–12.

Schaffer, D. M., Gordon, N. P., Jensen, C. D. & Avins, A. L. (2003). Nonvitamin, nonmineral supplement use over a 12-month period by adult members of a large health maintenance organization. *Journal of the American Dietetic Association*, **103**, 1500–5.

Shelton, R. C., Keller, M. B., Gelenberg, A. *et al.* (2001). Effectiveness of St. John's wort in major depression, a randomized controlled trial. *Journal of the American Medical Association*, **285**, 1978–86.

Singer, A., Wonnemann, M. & Müller, W. E. (1999). Hyperforin, a major antidepressant constituent of St. John's wort, inhibits serotonin uptake by elevating free intracellular Na^+. *Journal of Pharmacology and Experimental and Therapeutics*, **290**, 1363–8.

Sirvent, T. M., Walker, L., Vance, N. & Gibson, D. M. (2002). Variation in hypericins from wild populations of *Hypericum perforatum* L. in the Pacific northwest of the U.S.A. *Economic Botany*, **56**, 41–8.

Staffeldt, B., Kerb, R., Brockmüller, J., Ploch, M. & Roots, I. (1994). Pharmacokinetics of hypericin and pseudohypericin after oral intake of the *Hypericum perforatum* extract LI 160 in healthy volunteers. *Journal of Geriatric Psychiatry and Neurology*, **7** (Suppl. 1), S47–53.

Steiner, R. P., May, D. L. & Davis, A. W. (1982). Acupuncture therapy for the treatment of tobacco smoking addiction. *American Journal of Chinese Medicine*, **10**, 107–21.

Stevinson, C. & Ernst, E. (2000). Valerian for insomnia: a systematic review of randomized clinical trials. *Sleep Medicine*, **1**, 91–9.

Stevinson, C., Huntley, A. & Ernst, E. (2002). A systematic review of the safety of kava extract in the treatment of anxiety. *Drug Safety*, **25**, 251–61.

Stoll, A. L., Severus, W. E., Freeman, M. P. *et al.* (1999). Omega 3 fatty acids in bipolar disorder. A preliminary double-blind, placebo-controlled trial. *Archives of General Psychiatry*, **56**, 407–12.

Strahl, S., Ehret, V., Dahm, H. H. & Maier, K. P. (1998). Necrotizing hepatitis after taking herbal remedies (in Dutch). *Deutsche Medizinische Wochenschrift*, **123**, 1410–14.

Stramentinoli, G., Gualano, M. & Galli-Kienle, M. (1979). Intestinal absorption of S-adenosyl-L-methionine. *Journal of Pharmacology Experimental Therapeutics*, **209**, 323–6.

Stramentinoli, G. (1987). Pharmacologic aspects of S-adenosyl-methionine. Pharmacokinetics and pharmacodynamics. *American Journal of Medicine*, **83**, 35–42.

Su, K.-P., Huang, S.-Y., Chiu, C.-C. & Shen, W. W. (2003). Omega-3 fatty acids in major depressive disorder. A preliminary double-blind, placebo-controlled trial. *European Journal of Neuropsychopharmacology*, **13**, 267–71.

Thiede, H. M. & Walper, A. (1994). Inhibition of MAO and COMT by hypericum extracts and hypericin. *Journal of Geriatric Psychiatry and Neurology*, **7** (Suppl. 1), S54–6.

Travell, J. & Rinzler, S. H. (1946). Relief of cardiac pain by local block of somatic trigger areas. *Proceedings of the Society of Experimental and Biological Medicine*, **63**, 480–2.

Van Tulder, M. W., Cherkin, D. C., Berman, B., Lao, L. & Koes, B. V. (1999). Acupuncture for low back pain. *Cochrane Database of Systematic Reviews*. Oxford: Update Software Ltd.

Vickers, A. J. (1996). Can acupuncture have specific effects on health? A systematic review of acupuncture antiemesis trials. *Journal of the Royal Society of Medicine*, **89**, 303–11.

Washburn, A. M., Fullilove, R. E., Fullilove, M. T. *et al.* (1993). Acupuncture heroin detoxification: a single-blind clinical trial. *Journal of Substance Abuse Treatment*, **10**, 345–51.

Wells, E. A., Jackson, R., Dias, O. R. *et al.* (1995). Acupuncture as an adjunct to methadone treatment services. *American Journal of Addiction*, **4**, 169–214.

Wen, H. & Cheung, S. (1973). Treatment of drug addiction by acupuncture and electrical stimulation. *Asian Journal of Medicine*, **9**, 138–41.

Wen, H. & Teo, S. (1975). Experience in the treatment of drug addiction by electro-acupuncture. *Modern Medicine in Asia*, **11**, 23–4.

Wheatley, D. (2001). Kava and valerian in the treatment of stress-induced insomnia. *Phytotherapy Research*, **15**, 549–51.

Whiskey, E., Werneke, U. & Taylor, D. (2001). A systematic review and meta-analysis of *Hypericum perforatum* in depression: a comprehensive clinical review. *International Journal of Clinical Psychopharmacology*, **16**, 239–52.

White, A. R., Rampes, H. & Ernst, E. (2002). Acupuncture for smoking cessation. *Cochrane Database of Systematic Reviews*, **4**. Chichester: John Wiley & Sons Ltd.

White, P., Lewith, G. T., Berman, B. & Birch, S. (2002). Reviews of acupuncture for chronic neck pain: pitfalls in conducting systematic reviews. *Rheumatology*, **41**, 1224–31.

Woelk, H., Burkard, G. & Grunwald, J. (1994). Benefits and risks of the hypericum extract LI 160: drug monitoring study with 3250 patients. *Journal of Geriatric Psychiatry and Neurology*, **7** (Suppl. 1), S34–8.

Yang, X. (1994). Clinical observation on needling extra channel points in treatment of mental depression. *Journal of Traditional Chinese Medicine*, **14**, 14–18.

Zullino, D. & Borgeat, F. (2003). Hypertension induced by St. John's wort. *Pharmacopsychiatry*, **36**, 32 (Letter).

8

Complex interventions

Peter Tyrer and Karen Milner

Editor's note

We have included a chapter on complex interventions in this section because we feel it is necessary to introduce the subject before the fuller accounts in Part III of this book. Evidence is often difficult to obtain in psychiatry, not just because the collection of data involves harder work than in many other subjects but also because so many of our interventions are complex ones, and the interpretation of data from them so much more difficult than those of simple interventions. We hope it helps making interpretations here a little more cautious. There is also an important element of effectiveness included in this chapter; the evaluation of different types of service delivery in psychiatry, and these too usually represent very complex interventions.

Introduction

A complex intervention is easily understood at one level. According to Samuel Johnson, the originator of the first Dictionary of English, a complex intervention is 'an agency between antecedents and consecutives including many particulars', and this is as good a definition as any. In the evaluation of treatment, complex interventions are the most difficult one has to undertake. Let me give one example to make it clear that we are not exaggerating. We do not yet have good evidence of the effectiveness of a treatment that has been with us for over 60 years, collectively called 'therapeutic communities'. This contains at least five possible active elements, at least for the original residential form of the treatment; (a) the internal motivation to take part in a group intervention with people you do not know in a strange place, (b) the general milieu of the environment, (c) the ability of the therapeutic groups to work together effectively, (d) the quality of external supervision

and support, and (e) the extent to which fidelity of the treatment programme follows the principles of attachment (sense of belonging), containment (safety), communication (openness), involvement (participation) and agency (empowerment) (Haigh, 1999). There are also different types of therapeutic community and so the complexity of evaluation becomes even greater (see also Chapter 26). If we had a control group in such an evaluation how would we begin to decide which of the elements was essential and specific to the therapeutic community? Which of the five principles are absolutely essential and which can be discarded? Are there important positive interactions between any aspects of therapeutic community treatment that are not present with them separately? Do people need a full course of treatment and do they do worse if they leave the programme prematurely? Is the treatment only suitable for those with a certain diagnosis or can it be more general? If we assume there are around 10 elements that could all be evaluated separately as well as together in any combination there are 3 628 800 possible interactions that in theory could be evaluated separately. So although a randomized trial of the essential elements of the therapeutic community is feasible (Rutter & Tyrer, 2003), it has to ask the right question(s) to be of value (see Chapters 16 and 28 for further discussion on this form of treatment).

This is where a system for evaluating complex interventions becomes necessary. The term was rarely used until a few years ago, but the Medical Research Council in the UK promoted its development and it is now generally accepted to have five separate elements. However, the study of complex interventions in mental health is still at a very early stage. The blueprint adopted by the Medical Research Council for the study of complex interventions (Campbell et al., 2000) is already out of date as the notion of a carefully sequenced series of stages in the

Cambridge Textbook of Effective Treatments in Psychiatry, ed. Peter Tyrer and Kenneth R. Silk. Published by Cambridge University Press.

investigation of an intervention is very rarely possible with most mental health issues, principally because the precise research question for so many interventions is either very elusive or not possible to identify with proper precision.

Range of complex interventions

Non-medical intervention in poor countries

The exigencies of life in very poor countries, where less than 1% of the Gross National Product is spent on health, makes it impossible to provide adequate primary care for mental health problems. In many countries native healers have taken the part of conventional medically qualified doctors but are now joining forces with them. These include phytotherapies in France, acupuncturists in China, the native healers of Tanzania (Ngoma *et al.*, 2003) and a variety of native witch doctors ranging from the Maori healers of New Zealand to the njanga of Central Africa (of which one author (PT) is an honorary member but has taken no examinations) (Nzimakwe, 1996).

In almost all these interventions there is frequently a standardized form of the treatment linked to a great deal of ritual, and particularly when this involves members of the family or sometimes a whole village, this can have a powerful therapeutic effect. This can of course be regarded as a placebo effect but we do not have sufficient knowledge of its persistence to decide whether this is the right way of describing it. However, it is unlikely to be entirely without efficacy and this type of intervention remains a common pathway of care even when conventional treatment becomes the norm in ordinary practice.

What is of particular interest is that Western forms of treatment can often be accommodated within this general structure to produce extra benefit. This has been shown particularly in a randomized trial of group cognitive inter-personal psychotherapy in Uganda, in which powerful and persistent therapeutic effects in the treatment of depression were reported (Bolton *et al.*, 2003; Bass *et al.*, 2006). This was a classical example of a complex intervention. In this cluster randomized clinical trial 30 villages in rural Uganda were randomly assigned for studying men and 15 for women. In each village, those adult men or women believed by themselves and others to have depressive illness were interviewed and randomized to interpersonal psychotherapy (16 group sessions) or control treatment. The results showed a staggering improvement of 17.5 depression points for the intervention groups and only 3.6 points for the controls ($P < 0.001$), and after 6 months

these differences were almost exactly maintained (14 points intervention, 5 points control) (Bass *et al.*, 2006).

This study could be the first to meld together traditional and modern healing methods in a positive way and in this study it is hard to avoid the speculative conclusion that the intervention between the treatment and the other people in each village interacted in a positive way to maximize improvement.

Secondary care

Hospital and community services

It is hard to believe now that in the 1940s and 1950s almost all secondary care for mental illness took place in isolated mental hospitals where for many years their doctors were called 'alienists' to emphasize their detachment from the rest of medicine. Then, for no apparent reason, between 1954 and 1960 the demand for beds stopped growing in all Western countries and then, dramatically, started to lessen. There are arguments about why this took place – the introduction of antipsychotic drugs, the exposure of the perils of institutionalism (Barton, 1959; Goffman, 1961), a more enlightened view of mental illness – but, whatever the reason, it was almost universal. This was highlighted in the UK by Tooth & Brooke (1961) who first showed that the rate of decline was so great that the future of the asylums could not be sustained.

The change was postulated as an epic struggle by Enoch Powell, the Birmingham born and educated classical scholar who became Minister of Health and whose speeches were beautifully presented, even if they were somewhat marred by the background whine of the characteristic accent of the city, so that even a call to arms sounded like a complaint about an error in a bank statement. His famous 'water towers' speech adumbrated the battle ahead.

I have intimated to the hospital authorities who will be producing the constituent elements of the national hospital plan that in 15 years' time there may well be needed not more than half as many places in hospitals for mental illness as there are today. Expressed in numerical terms, this would represent a redundancy of no fewer than 75 000 hospital beds. Even so, I would say that if we err, we would rather err on the side of underestimating the provision which ought to be required in hospitals 15 years from now. This 50 per cent reduction itself is only a statistical projection by the General Register Office of the fall in demand based upon present trends. Yet there is not a person present whose ambition is not to speed up those present trends. So if we are to have the courage of our ambitions, we ought to pitch the estimate lower still, as low as we dare, perhaps lower. But that 50 per cent or less of present places in hospitals for the mentally sick – what will they look like and where will they be? We know already what ought to be the answer to that question: they ought for the most part to be in wards and wings of general hospitals. Few ought to be in great isolated institutions or clumps of institutions, though I neither forget nor underestimate the continuing requirements of security for a small minority of patients.

They imply nothing less than the elimination of by far the greater part of this country's mental hospitals as they exist today. This is a colossal undertaking, not so much in the new physical provision which it involves, as in the sheer inertia of mind and matter which it requires to be overcome. There they stand, isolated, majestic, imperious, brooded over by the gigantic water-tower and chimney combined, rising unmistakable and daunting out of the countryside – the asylums which our forefathers built with such immense solidity to express the notions of their day. Do not for a moment underestimate their powers of resistance to our assault. (The full speech can be read at http://www.mdx.ac.uk/www/study/xpowell).

Isn't that stirring? In fact, Enoch Powell, and most others who predicted long battles, got it wrong, and it was only in Italy, where the famous Law 180 was passed in 1978, abolishing mental hospitals at a stroke, that the change was a revolutionary one. Most people working in traditional mental hospitals were quite happy for their premises to be taken away, usually swallowed up by grateful general hospitals with a need to expand, but where he was right is in predicting a revolution in care, and unbeknown at that time, the growth of complex interventions.

Unfortunately, the growth of community care was not accompanied by the large-scale randomized controlled trial that the well-known epidemiologist, Sir Richard Doll, wanted to carry out, in which he hoped to randomize a significant proportion of all inpatients to continued hospital or community care (Cook, 2004), so we cannot really say that community care has a good evidence base. However, we have some indications from later trials.

The outpatient department, originally alongside the mental hospital, or more commonly, in more appropriate facilities in towns or other centres, has now become an accepted form of treatment in most parts of the world. In the USA what is commonly called 'office psychiatry' is basically the outpatient consultation and this could be in private or public facilities. This is an acceptable and appropriate setting for most treatments to be carried out in psychiatry for common illnesses, mainly those in which the sufferer recognizes the presence of unpleasant symptoms or behaviour and wants to have them treated.

However, in most Western countries, psychiatric services have increasingly become focused on severe mental illness, a term that is rarely defined but should be. It is now often interpreted as 'most psychotic disorders, any non-

organic psychosis; a duration of treatment of 2 years or more; and persistent dysfunction' (Schinnar et al., 1990; Ruggeri et al., 2000). The problem with so many of these patients, particularly the ones with psychotic disorders, is that insight is limited and treatment seeking is unpredictable. More simply, many of the patients being seen will do anything possible to avoid having contact with the psychiatric services.

This phenomenon has been tackled in different ways in different countries and it is unfortunate that, because of this, direct comparisons of the different models have not usually been made.

Assertive community treatment

Assertive community treatment (ACT) and two very similar overlapping interventions, intensive case management and assertive outreach, are becoming increasingly popular ways of delivering treatment to those with severe mental illness in many Western countries. Although there have been several other similar models for providing such care in the last 25 years the assertive community treatment model has been the most durable. It began in the early 1970s in Dane County in Wisconsin, USA. It is worth reminding ourselves that at this time community psychiatry in the USA was in a bad way. The Community Mental Health Center Movement that had been promoted heavily by President J. F. Kennedy in the early 1960s, was running into serious trouble. Most of the centres that had been set up with the intention of helping the more severely ill ended up by providing psychological treatment for what became known as the 'worried well' (Goldman et al., 1980). At the same time funding for state hospitals was being reduced because of the expansion of these new community centres. The main consequence of this is that community care for the severely mentally ill became almost non-existent. It was in this climate of a desert of resources that Len Stein and Mary Test in Dane County decided on the bold step of providing almost total care in the community for those who had serious mental illness, mainly schizophrenia and related psychoses. After considerable resistance at first, outlined well by Stein & Santos (1998) in a recent book, the benefits of this approach, originally called PACT (Programme for Assertive Community Treatment) and concentrating on improving activities of daily living, became clear. Instead of languishing in a state mental hospital with limited rehabilitative resources the patients were seen by enthusiastic committed therapists working for a range of disciplines, in their home environment and with a clear understanding of their important needs. A randomized controlled trial published in 1980 (Stein & Test, 1980; Weisbrod *et al.*, 1980) confirmed the effectiveness of this approach, but the design used was really more appropriate for a crisis intervention service than an assertive community one. Patients considered appropriate to be admitted to hospital were randomized at this point to the ACT approach or to standard hospital treatment. Not surprisingly in retrospect but strikingly for the time, the patients in the ACT treatment arm improved to a somewhat greater extent but not dramatically so in terms of symptoms, but more significantly, spent much less time in hospital over the subsequent period and as a consequence consumed much fewer resources. This attracted the attention of service planners and before long assertive community teams were being developed in all parts of the USA. However, it is worth noting that very few states have a comprehensive network of assertive community teams, with Texas only having one team and with only Michigan getting close to state-wide cover with a total of 86 such teams (Stein & Santos, 1998).

It is helpful to get the US system of mental health care into context when comparing assertive community treatment across countries in those with severe mental illness. Public mental health care for these individuals in the USA has been described in terms of a cyclical pattern of institutional reforms. Each reform has been characterized by a new environmental approach to treatment and an innovative type of facility or locus of care. The first cycle was based on 'moral treatment' and the development of the asylum in the early nineteenth century. The second cycle was associated with the mental hygiene movement and based in the psychopathic hospital (early twentieth century); the third the community mental health movement and the community mental health centre (mid-twentieth century). As described by Morrisey & Goldman (1984), each reform began with the promise that treatment in the new locus of care would 'prevent the personal and societal problems associated with severe and persisting mental illness'. Although successful at addressing the needs of those with acute or milder forms of mental illness, each cycle failed when it was unable to address the needs of individuals at the severe end of the spectrum.

What was different about the fourth cycle of reform, the community support programme, is that it recognized and targeted the needs of individuals with severe mental illness, thus breaking the cycle of innovation and failure. The community support programme proposed a network or system of care that included crisis care services (i.e. public and private hospitals, day programmes, crisis residential facilities, mobile crisis teams), psychosocial rehabilitation services, supportive living and working arrangements,

medical and mental health care, and case management for individuals with severe, persistent mental illness (SPMI). It drew on existing community agencies and programmes rather than the construction of a new institution or facility.

In this model, individuals with SPMI are provided with the clinical services that they require to live successfully in the community. Stein & Diamond (1985) suggest that seven characteristics determine what kind of programming is best suited to the needs of individual consumers: willingness to come in for services, medication compliance, need for structured daily activities, ability to self-monitor, frequency of crises, need for professional psychological support, and degree of case management services required. A majority of consumers function adequately in the community with individual case management and medication monitoring. Additional programming may include time-limited crisis intervention; coping skills, co-occurring, and/or psychoeducation groups, and supported employment.

Patients who only satisfy some of these requirements are ideally placed to benefit from assertive community treatment, with its five key components:

(1) low caseload (staff/consumer ratio of 1/10 as opposed to 1/30 or more in traditional case management),
(2) provision of services in the consumers' environment,
(3) direct provision of services,
(4) 24-hour coverage, and
(5) team case management (caseload is shared across team members as opposed to case managers each having his/her own caseload).

The desired outcomes include reduced hospitalization, increased community tenure, meaningful reintegration into the community, and progress toward recovery or self-determination. Administrative cost-effectiveness is derived from the reduction in hospital stays as well as the enhanced consumer satisfaction and quality of life.

Shortly after the publication of Stein and Test's seminal trial, John Hoult and colleagues in New South Wales, Australia, carried out a similar study. There was a great saving on hospital care as a consequence of the new approach, but this study approached crisis intervention even more closely than the original Stein and Test study. Patients were seen at the point of admission to hospital and, if allocated to the active treatment arm, could also be admitted to boarding houses staffed by members of the team rather than going into a psychiatric hospital as well as having a 24-hour crisis team available. During the 12 months of the study period, 96% of controls were admitted, 51% more than once. In the active treatment arm 60% were not admitted at all and only 8% were admitted more than once, with the control group spending 53.5 days in psychiatric hospitals compared with the active group who spent an average of 8.4 days. This study also attracted considerable world attention although it was difficult to summarize this treatment as typical ACT (Hoult, 1986).

The summary of the US and rest of world studies and those confined to the UK can be split into two halves. The first half, mainly of studies carried out between 1980 and 1992 in the USA, show large differences in favour of ACT. For example, a systematic review in 1997 found 14 randomized controlled trials involving 2647 people aged 18–65 (Marshall *et al.*, 1997). This review found that patients receiving ACT were less likely to be admitted to hospital that those receiving standard care (RR 0.75, 95% CI 0.64–0.87, NNT – one admission saved per 10 patients treated) and spent less time in hospital (weighted average from eight trials showed a 42% reduction). They were also more likely to remain in contact with the psychiatric services (RR 0.61, 95% CI 0.50–0.73, NNT 8.9).

The second half is dominated by trials in the UK and Australia between 1998 and 2006. In all five of these (Holloway & Carson, 1998; Burns *et al.*, 1999; Issakidis *et al.*, 1999; Harrison-Read *et al.*, 2002; Killaspy *et al.*, 2006), there was no difference in number or duration of admissions, or in rates of loss of contact with psychiatric services, although in one study loss of contact with the case manager was greater in the intensive treatment group (Burns *et al.*, 1999). This has led to a change in attitudes towards ACT so that even in countries such as Australia, which has been one of the most vocal in support of this intervention a recent review has concluded that 'both clinical and cost effectiveness of ICM may be weakening' (King, 2006). It is also worthwhile mentioning that, although bed usage is not reduced in the recently reported studies, engagement with services and satisfaction with care is greater with the assertive approach than in standard teams. This should not be forgotten when considering the future role of such teams (Tyrer, 2007). The collective findings have led to a reaction from what is often called the recovery movement. The recovery movement in mental health has been defined as the belief that all individuals, even those with severe mental illness, can develop hope for the future, participate in meaningful activities, exercise self-determination, and live in a society without stigma and discrimination (Resnick *et al.*, 2005). The recovery movement's focus on subjective experience has been seen as conflicting with the emphasis on the empirical evidence that forms the basis of evidence-based practice. Resnick argues that better evidence-based practice may help to identify interventions that support the recovery movement and its propagation.

Taken together, these three movements in the USA provide a snapshot of the American perspective on complex interventions for individuals with severe mental illness. The community support movement creates a system of care fashioned from community providers to address the needs of individuals with severe mental health problems; evidence-based practices provide the technology (i.e. expertise and tools) to ensure the success of the community support movement (Dixon & Goldman, 2004), and the recovery movement, informed by evidence-based practice, ensures that consumer self-determination and recovery are the focus of care. Unfortunately, there is one other variable, cost, that is not taken into account here, and it is likely that interventions will oscillate considerably as evidence of similar outcomes at lower cost become available.

The main difference between the USA and the UK, and to a great extent in New Zealand also, is that, ever since 1948, there has been a socialized health service (the National Health Service) in all parts of the UK in which every individual receives treatment free at the point of need (although this is beginning to change with dental and other services that are not considered to be concerned with life-threatening illness). This means that there is an automatic safety net for all who fall through conventional service provision and all political parties in the UK are committed to its future (Tempest, 2006).

When the differences between the outcomes of UK and USA studies became known there was a great debate over two possible hypotheses:
(1) the assertive treatment has not been given correctly in the UK so does not satisfy the fidelity characteristics of the model,
(2) the comparison service in the UK is the community mental health team, and this has already been shown to be an effective form of intervention for those with severe mental illness in the community.

Although there are supporters in favour of the first explanation (Marshall & Creed, 2000), there are probably stronger arguments in favour of the alternative one (Burns *et al.*, 2001; Fiander *et al.*, 2003), as a systematic review of community mental health teams shows that they confer the same advantages over hospital-orientated care, with fewer deaths, less drop out from care and somewhat lower bed occupancy (Simmonds *et al.*, 2001).

The results can be interpreted as ACT conferring no advantage in well-developed psychiatric services. This can be compared to the phenomenon of plant succession in botany, whereby the highly specialized plant (synonymous with ACT) is very successful in colonizing new territory which has no other competitors, but when the soil conditions become more favourable as a consequence of the pioneer plants thriving, other plants become established and gradually squeeze out the pioneers (Tyrer, 1999). However, there is clear evidence that some groups do particularly well with assertive community treatment even in a well-developed service. Those with personality disorders and severe mental illness and those with learning disability (Hassiotis *et al.*, 2001) occupy fewer hospital beds after treatment with ACT than with standard care. This is not just a question of those with more complex needs doing well; these do not fare very differently from those with ordinary needs (Metcalfe *et al.*, 2005). What it suggests is that the assertive approach, with its frequent contacts with the patient in the community, may have particular advantages only in certain special groups, *which may vary from country to country* (my italics), but for others community mental health teams can serve those with severe mental illness equally well.

The future of assertive treatment is far from certain. It seems to be highly appropriate for new services that have not really yet developed the full range of community treatment but its place in well-developed services is much less certain. What is clear is that attitudes about the nature of assertive treatment differ depending on experience of local conditions, with the original ACT approach being more suited to new community services and a softer, more sensitive approach with a less macho attitude to assertiveness in the more established ones (Tyrer *et al.*, 2007). There certainly does not appear to be any major advantage in terms of use of hospital beds (and this is often the main aim of planners when they introduce new services) but the general finding that greater satisfaction and better engagement occurs with assertive treatment is a positive advantage as there is increasing evidence that such indices are proxy measures of quality of care (Shipley *et al.*, 2000). What also needs to be reviewed is the requirements for the assertive approach. These were developed in the 1970s and they are hardly appropriate for the twenty-first century, yet they seem to have been followed with slavish enthusiasm by many people without questioning whether they are all still necessary.

Liaison psychiatry in primary care

The notion of providing specialized psychiatric care in primary care services has been an aspect of service delivery in the UK for many years, with one in five psychiatrists in England in the early 1980s spending at least some time in primary care services (Strathdee & Williams, 1984), and later an actual majority (56%) of those in Scotland doing

the same (Pullen & Yellowlees, 1988). This type of service has spread to Canada (Farrar *et al.*, 2001) and Australia (Carr *et al.*, 1997). Although it seems to be popular among the practitioners who are involved in these initiatives (which by and large have come about without any external pressure), the level of evaluation has been low and it has also been noted that a proportion of primary care physicians avoid all involvement with such community initiatives (Puri *et al.*, 1996). Case-control and matched population comparisons showed some slight superiority with regard to satisfaction and hospital admission (Tyrer *et al.*, 1990; Carr *et al.*, 1997), but these were accompanied by greater numbers of referrals and it could be argued that such a service was not cost-effective. This was confirmed in a controlled study (not a randomized controlled trial) of a psychiatric team being placed in a primary care setting, when there was significant benefit in symptom improvement compared with a control practice (Jackson *et al.*, 1993) but at much greater cost as so many more patients were being treated (Goldberg *et al.*, 1996). The only truly randomized trial of a liaison psychiatric service provided by link workers (not psychiatrists) showed some slight superiority for the liaison service with regard to social functioning (Emmanuel *et al.*, 2002), but no other clear differences.

In many countries that have opted for community care for severe mental illness there has been a shift in emphasis in services towards severe mental illness. Liaison psychiatry, which is most popular with primary care physicians for non-psychotic illness, has therefore been squeezed out and tensions have developed in services (Gask *et al.*, 1997). The best model of providing good liaison to general practice that is cost-effective and which can work in tandem with community mental health teams, remains currently out of our grasp.

Day hospitals

The notion of day hospitals is relatively new in the history of psychiatry. The first one was opened in Russia in 1933, the first in North America in 1946 (in Montreal) (Cameron, 1947) and in 1948 in the UK by Joshua Bierer, whom incidentally was the first person to coin the term 'social psychiatry'. Initially their main purpose was to provide comprehensive treatment rather like a therapeutic community (Bierer, 1959) and also to treat refractory disorders. The evidence for their effectiveness for this purpose compared with outpatient care for acute, long-term refractory disorders, or as an option for early discharge from hospital, is very slim. A systematic review of all randomized studies in 2001 found only one trial showing benefit of day hospital care in improving psychiatric symptoms and similar outcomes for all other variables, and there was some evidence that day hospital care was more expensive (Marshall *et al.*, 2001a).

Subsequently in many Western countries devoted to the reduction of hospital beds, day hospitals were used as supplementary to inpatient admission. The largest systematic review carried out in 2001 identified nine randomized controlled trials of acute day hospital treatment including 2268 patients; but such was the bewildering array of trial designs, admission criteria, follow up methods, and outcomes that it was necessary to collect and reanalyse data from individual patients. The review found that treatment in day hospitals was feasible for at least 23%, and at most 38%, of patients currently admitted to hospital and led to cost reductions ranging from 20.9% to 36.9% over inpatient care. Unexpectedly, patients at day hospitals showed a more rapid improvement in mental state than patients randomized to inpatient care, a finding not shown for any other alternative to admission. There was also evidence of increased satisfaction of patients and no evidence of an increased burden on carers. Two randomized trials suggested that this was effective in reducing bed usage with no loss of therapeutic benefit, and as day hospitals were cheaper than inpatient care, they should be preferred.

Since this review there has been a more recent randomized trial in which day hospital care was provided exclusively as an alternative to inpatient care. A total of 206 voluntarily admitted patients were allocated to either day hospital or inpatient treatment. Day hospital patients showed significantly more favourable changes in psychopathology and greater satisfaction with treatment at discharge but not at follow-up after a year. Mean costs were higher for those treated at the day hospital (Priebe *et al.*, 2006).

These data in combination do not make an especially strong case for day hospitals as alternatives to hospital admission, and the data show that even in the most favourable settings less than 2 out of every 5 patients presenting for admission can be treated as day patients. Success also depends on a reasonable degree of co-operation with the patients attending regularly. For those with the most severe forms of illness this degree of adherence to treatment is difficult to achieve and some day hospitals provide outreach services to bring patients in for treatment if they do not come in on their own. The principles of assertive outreach may be useful in this exercise.

In recent years, new personality disorder services have developed (see Chapter 43) which may be particularly useful for basing at a day hospital. Providing care for those with borderline personality disorder depends on a coherent plan of management in which all those involved work closely together. Placing such teams in the setting of a day hospital may be the preferred way of ensuring coherence and consistency and at least one important randomized study has shown the benefits of this (Bateman & Fonagy, 2001). However, at present this treatment appears to be best suited for those with borderline personality disorder, who unlike many others with personality disorder, are treatment seeking (Type S) (Tyrer *et al.*, 2003) and who therefore are more reliable in attending the day hospital setting. What is important is for the day hospital setting to be flexible to the needs of those attending and to cater for relatively homogeneous groups in a systematic fashion (Rosie *et al.*, 1995). The relative neglect of the day hospital in the USA (not in Canada, which has always embraced them enthusiastically) is largely due to the funding arrangements for care, in which day hospital attendance comes out badly in comparison with inpatient care.

Rehabilitation and employment

One of the aims of the old mental hospital movement was to return every patient to some form of useful work activity, and this was one of the main aims of the mental hygiene movement of the early twentieth century. Indeed, those hospitals that were considered to be advanced and progressive were the ones that devoted so much energy to improving work opportunities (Kidd, 1965) and, even today, several still exist and have proud defenders (Wells, 2006). However, the work in these ITUs (Industrial Therapy Units) was often at a low level of skill and seldom developed into purposive paid employment and so the ITUs were replaced in many areas by sheltered workshops away from the hospital, and it was quickly recognized that once people developed to the point at which they could work in open employment their self-esteem and competence improved greatly (Early, 1975).

However, in the early days of rehabilitation progress was made by far-sighted charismatic individuals and did not depend on evidence from controlled studies. The notion of employment also fell somewhat into abeyance and even today less than 20% of those with severe mental illness are gainfully employed (Marwaha & Johnson, 2004). Studies have subsequently been carried out and a recent systematic review of 18 randomized controlled trials showed that a period of sheltered employment (pre-vocational training) is not necessary for most people and immediate supported open employment leads to a better outcome (defined by the number of people in paid competitive employment at various time points) with no advantages for pre-vocational training for any secondary measure (Marshall *et al.*, 2001b). Since this time there have been several more studies of the individual placement and support (IPS) model of supported employment in the USA and a recent randomized controlled trial in Canada showed that after 12 months 47% of clients in the supported employment group obtained at least some competitive work compared with 18% in those receiving standard vocational services. The overall message is clear. If a patient is capable of working they should go for employment in the open market.

Home treatment

Home treatment is not usually regarded as a specific service in its own right because it is part of the philosophy of assertive community teams and many community mental health ones.

However, in recent years special home treatment services have been set up in some countries and for these every intervention is in the home environment. However, one systematic review (Catty *et al.*, 2002) demonstrated no added benefit of home treatment beyond those achieved by good outpatient or team monitoring in other settings, and so this form of management cannot be considered to have a good evidence base. However, home treatment also may often be essential for those with severe learning disability or dementia, and when patients are unable to leave their houses for any reason then home treatment is clearly the only option if hospital management is to be avoided.

Crisis resolution teams

Crisis resolution has been part of psychiatric services for over 50 years but only recently has been formulated into general service strategies. It was first introduced by Gerald Caplan (1951) in child psychiatric services in Israel. Caplan noted that problems presenting acutely (i.e. crises) were often best dealt with by intensive input in the setting in which they occurred rather than taking the traditional form of management which was to remove the individual concerned from the setting and place them somewhere else, often in hospital, where resolution of the problem took a great deal longer. The original principles of crisis resolution are encapsulated in five service principles:
(1) identifying the risk factors for mental disorder,
(2) linking the mental disorder to those risks,
(3) identifying the stresses that have provoked the crisis,

(4) assessment of the level of competence of coping with these stresses,
(5) identifying relevant social supports (Caplan, 1980).

In the last 20 years the principles of crisis resolution have been employed aggressively in adult psychiatry in the treatment of the severely mentally ill and in the early days of assertive community treatment there was a great deal of overlap between the two approaches. The evidence for the effectiveness of crisis resolution teams is limited and only one randomized controlled trial has been carried out (Johnson *et al.*, 2005), although the earlier studies by Stein & Test (1980) and Hoult *et al.* (1983) were also controlled. The recent trial showed that a crisis resolution team significantly reduced admissions compared with a control group both in the short (8 weeks) and medium term (6 months) with more than twice the admissions and bed days in the control group (Johnson *et al.*, 2005). Client satisfaction was also just significantly improved but compulsory admissions were no different between the groups.

In a recent national survey in the UK areas with established crisis (and home treatment) teams were shown to have a 10% reduction in admissions compared with areas without these teams, although the duration of bed usage was only reduced by 5% (Glover *et al.*, 2006). These changes were most marked in women aged between 35 and 64.

It is difficult to know how to interpret these preliminary results. Patients in general prefer to be seen at home rather than in hospital and this is an important consideration. The suggestion that the risks of continuing to see people in a crisis at home might be too great for this to be maintained have not generally been realized. However, there may be an increased burden on carers and this needs closer evaluation.

In summary it is not surprising that crisis resolution teams prevent admission in the first instance as this is their *raison d'être*. However, the important issue is what happens in the longer term, and, as yet, data are not available. However, because of the benefit with regard to admissions, even in well-developed services it is likely that these will come to replace the assertive community teams at least until more data are available.

Feedback of outcomes of care

A complex intervention not dealt with elsewhere in this book is the impact of giving information about outcomes of progress to patients during the course of treatment. Outcomes in mental health are much less defined than in other medical disciplines, but increasingly general measures such as the CORE-OM, and needs assessments such as the Camberwell Assessment of Need (CAN) (Phelan *et al.*, 1995) are being recorded in routine practice and are regarded as reasonably robust. Feedback of this information has been tested in a randomized controlled trial in which the active treatment arm were given feedback and those in the control group were not. The results showed that giving feedback had no impact on the primary outcomes of patient-rated unmet need and of quality of life but that, rather surprisingly, inpatient stay was reduced (Slade *et al.*, 2006) and so the intervention was cost-effective.

Problems of interpretation

Complex interventions are likely to become much more sophisticated, larger and more frequent in the coming years, but the interpretation of their results is much more difficult than for simple interventions. Because the effect of a complex intervention may be a consequence of a combination of treatments, neither of which is effective alone, and conversely, a single intervention that is effective may be counteracted by the negative effect of a second, one can never be sure what is the mechanism behind positive or negative results. Nevertheless it is important to carry out studies, preferably with large numbers, because at present service policy is governed almost entirely by non-evidence; this is a combination of the effects of product champions, cost pressures, fashion and expediency. There are seldom opportunities to test out whether national policy decisions are appropriate in randomized controlled studies because, once a policy has been implemented nationally, there is no adequate control group to compare it with. When the opportunity does become available the results are often of considerable interest. For example, the introduction of the Care Programme Approach in the UK in 1990 was a little-heralded initiative that was only adopted piecemeal at first. It introduced a modified form of case management, the policy of maintaining contact with patients over a specified period and providing care 'packages' that could also be monitored closely. The expectation was that this programme would ensure the patients did not 'fall through the net' of continuing care, and because relapses could be detected at an earlier stage, that admission to hospital would be reduced. A randomized trial of nearly 400 patients in which this new approach was compared with existing care showed that it was highly effective in stopping people from dropping out of care but increased the duration of admission by a mean of 68% (Tyrer *et al.*, 1995).

The likely explanation for this was that the Care Programme Approach was not implemented on a team basis but nominated individual practitioners, often of a junior level, to carry out the monitoring. It is therefore not surprising that when there was evidence of a deterioration of symptoms the option of admission to hospital was considered more readily even when the collective decision could be shared. However, it is also possible that patients were indeed admitted appropriately and that in the standard approach their needs were missed and neglected. Whatever the explanation, the unintended impact of introducing the Care Programme Approach was an increase in admissions leading to tremendous pressures on beds, particularly in London (Lamont *et al.*, 2000) and fragmentation of care when patients could not be admitted to beds in their place of residence (Bindman *et al.*, 1999).

This example also illustrates a common consequence of the evaluation of complex interventions; although the primary outcome may be in the direction desired the secondary outcomes may often be not. Everyone supports the notion of continuity of care and reducing drop-out. However, if this is accompanied by an increase in resources used the results are much less palatable. In interpreting studies of this nature it is often valuable to incorporate a qualitative component to the study to be carried out at the same time as the randomized trial. Although this is somewhat at variance of the advice given above it is worth emphasizing that the process of evaluating a complex intervention is rarely a smooth graded one. Initial studies are seldom replicated exactly, and then other studies carried out to decide on the validity of important differences. By combining qualitative and quantitative studies additional information can often be obtained that is extremely valuable in interpretation (Weaver *et al.*, 1996) and, in effect, flesh is put on the randomized controlled trial skeleton.

For many complex interventions the cluster randomized controlled trial is often appropriate. With cluster randomized trials the unit of randomization is not the patient but a setting such as a general practice or hospital. This is particularly appropriate when the individuals in the cluster unit (e.g. a support home) have close contact with each other and it is difficult to provide a 'pure' intervention to a single patient because it has an impact on others. Although cluster randomized trials are becoming increasingly popular their analysis is different from those of ordinary randomized trials and a large number of patients is required to show significant differences compared with the equivalent simple randomized trial. The details of the methodology of cluster randomized trials can be found elsewhere (Ukoumunne *et al.*, 1999).

Summary

Although the evidence from tightly controlled, well-regulated randomized trials of interventions constitute the main evidence base in this book, the interactions between even the simplest of interventions such as drug treatments with treatment setting, type of staff, frequency of monitoring and other influences (see Chapter 49), result in complex interventions in ordinary psychiatric practice. This is at the heart of the distinction between explanatory (highly controlled) and pragmatic (treatment in practice) clinical trials (Schwarz & Lellouch, 1967) and makes a case for very large studies being carried out in conditions of ordinary practice (Geddes & Goodwin, 2001). These are the ones that provide the best evidence on the ground and may often yield results that are very different from those of small explanatory trials. For example, the recently published CATIE and CutLass studies into the treatment of schizophrenia with atypical and typical antipsychotic drugs (described more fully in Chapter 48) illustrate this. These large studies cater for the impact of complex interventions, and if they demonstrate robust differences, these are ones that can be taken as the best available evidence for clinicians on the ground.

The level of evidence for each of the interventions discussed in this chapter is summarized in Table 8.1.

Table 8.1. Effectiveness of complex interventions in mental health

Treatment	Form of treatment	Psychiatric disorder	Level of evidence for efficacy	Comments
Community mental health teams	Multi-disciplinary personnel	Severe mental illness	Ia	Better than hospital-oriented care for mortality, loss to care and satisfaction
Assertive community treatment (intensive case management)	Autonomous multi-disciplinary teams	Severe mental illness	Ia (Ib for learning disability)	Certainly effective against standard hospital treatment but only superior to community mental health teams in satisfaction and engagement (except in learning disability)
Liaison psychiatry in general practice	Linked workers or team attached to primary care	All mental illness but mainly non-psychotic patients	Ib	Some evidence of symptom and functioning benefit but team attachment is not cost-effective
Home treatment	Dedicated teams	Severe mental illness	III	Not addressed specifically in randomized trials but no evidence that they are essential
Day hospitals	Separate centres but no inpatient care	Neurotic and related non-psychotic disorders	Ia	No evidence that day hospital is superior to other forms of care
Day hospitals	As above	Severe mental illness	Ia	Reduction of inpatient usage, greater satisfaction with care, possible improvement in psychopathology
Day hospital	As above	Borderline personality disorder	Ib	See Chapter 28 for full details
Vocational employment	Specific training for work	Severe mental illness	Ia	Unequivocal gains for policies aimed at getting those with severe mental illness into work
Crisis resolution	Specific multi-disciplinary teams	Severe mental illness or any condition thought to require hospital admission	I(b)	Evidence of bed reduction and greater satisfaction but data still limited
Complex interpersonal psychotherapy	Large group format	Depression	Ib	One very good study with follow-up
Outcome feedback	Multi-disciplinary teams	Mental illness in secondary care	Ib	No clear value but admissions may be reduced
Case management (care management)	Multi-discliplinary teams or external commissioner of services	Mental illness in secondary care	Ia	Convincing evidence that drop-out from care is reduced but inpatient care is increased
Native witch doctor	Variable depending on culture but usually with much ritual	Various psychiatric illnesses	III	Results not clear but certainly a very powerful non-specific effect that may not be entirely a placebo one

ACKNOWLEDGEMENT

I should like to thank Karen Milner for valuable material used in the preparation of this chapter.

REFERENCES

Barton, R. (1959). *Institutional Neurosis*. Bristol: John Wright.

Bass, J., Neugebauer, R., Clougherty, K. F. *et al.* (2006). Group interpersonal psychotherapy for depression in rural Uganda: 6-month outcomes: randomised controlled trial. *British Journal of Psychiatry*, **188**, 567–73.

Bierer, J. (1959). Theory and practice of psychiatric day hospitals. *Lancet*, **2**, 901–2.

Bindman, J., Beck, A., Glover, G. *et al.* (1999). Evaluating mental health policy in England – Care Programme Approach and supervision registers. *British Journal of Psychiatry*, **175**, 327–30.

Bolton, P., Bass, J., Neugebauer, R. *et al.* (2003). Group interpersonal psychotherapy for depression in rural Uganda: a randomized controlled trial. *Journal of the American Medical Association*, **289**, 3117–24.

Burns, T., Creed, F., Fahy, T., Thompson, S., Tyrer, P. & White, I. (1999). Intensive versus standard case management for severe psychotic illness: a randomised trial. *Lancet*, **353**, 2185–9.

Burns, T., Fioritti, A., Holloway, F., Malm, U. & Rössler, W. (2001). Case management and assertive community treatment in Europe. *Psychiatric Services*, **52**, 631–6.

Campbell, M., Fitzpatrick, R., Haines, A., Sandercock, P., Spiegelhalter, D. & Tyrer, P. (2000). A framework for the design and evaluation of complex interventions to improve health. *British Medical Journal*, **321**, 694–6.

Cameron, D. E. (1947). The day hospital. *Modern Hospital*, **69**, 60–2.

Caplan, G. (1951). A public-health approach to child psychiatry: an introductory account of an experiment. *Mental Hygiene*, **35**, 235–49.

Caplan, G. (1980). An approach to preventive intervention in child psychiatry. *Canadian Journal of Psychiatry*, **25**, 671–82.

Carr, V. J., Lewin, T. J., Reid, A. L. A., Walton, J. M. & Faehrmann, C. (1997). An evaluation of the effectiveness of a consultation-liaison psychiatry service in general practice. *Australian and New Zealand Journal of Psychiatry*, **31**, 714–25.

Cook, C. (2004). Oral history: Sir Richard Doll. *Journal of Public Health*, **26**, 327–36.

Dixon, L. & Goldman, H. (2004). Forty years of progress in community mental health: the role of evidence-based practices. *Administration and Policy in Mental Health*, **31**, 381–92.

Early, D. F. (1975). Sheltered groups in open industry. A new approach to training and to employment. *Lancet*, **i**, 1370–3.

Emmanuel, J. S., McGee, A., Ukoumunne, O. C. & Tyrer, P. (2002). A randomised controlled trial of enhanced key-worker liaison psychiatry in general practice. *Social Psychiatry and Psychiatric Epidemiology*, **37**, 261–6.

Farrar, S., Kates, N., Crustolo, A. M. & Nikolaou, L. (2001). Integrated model for mental health care – are health care providers satisfied with it? *Canadian Family Physician*, **47**, 2483–8.

Fiander, M., Burns, T., McHugo, G. J. & Drake, R. E. (2003). Assertive community treatment across the Atlantic: comparison of model fidelity in the UK and USA. *British Journal of Psychiatry*, **182**, 248–54.

Gask, L., Sibbald, B. & Creed, F. (1997). Evaluating models of working at the interface between mental health services and primary care. *British Journal of Psychiatry*, **170**, 6–11.

Geddes, J. & Goodwin, G. (2001). Bipolar disorder: clinical uncertainty, evidence-based medicine and large-scale randomised trials. *British Journal of Psychiatry*, **178**, 191–4.

Glover, G., Arts, G. & Suresh Babu, K. (2006). Crisis resolution/home treatment teams and psychiatric admission rates in England. *British Journal of Psychiatry*, **189**, 441–5.

Goffman, E. (1961) *Asylums*. New York: Doubleday.

Goldberg, D., Jackson, G., Gater, R., Campbell, M. & Jennett, N. (1996). The treatment of common mental disorders by a community team based in primary care: a cost effectiveness study. *Psychological Medicine*, **26**, 487–92.

Goldman, H. H., Regier, D. A., Taube, C. A., Redick, R. W. & Bass, R. D. (1980). Community mental health centers and the treatment of severe mental disorder. *American Journal of Psychiatry*, **137**, 83–6.

Haigh, R. (1999). The quintessence of a therapeutic environment: five universal qualities. In *Therapeutic Communities: Past, Present and future*, ed. P. Campbell & R. Haigh, pp. 246–57. London: Jessica Kingsley.

Harrison-Read, P., Lucas, B., Tyrer, P. (2002). Heavy users of acute psychiatric beds: randomised controlled trial of enhanced community management in an outer London borough. *Psychological Medicine*, **32**, 413–26.

Hassiotis, A., Ukoumunne, O. C., Byford, S. *et al.* (2001). Intellectual functioning and outcome of patients with severe psychotic illness randomised to intensive case management: report from the UK700 case management trial. *British Journal of Psychiatry*, **178**, 166–71.

Holloway, F. & Carson, J. (1998). Intensive case management for the severely mentally ill: controlled trial. *British Journal of Psychiatry*, **172**, 19–22.

Hoult, J. (1986) Community care of the acutely mentally ill. *British Journal of Psychiatry*, **149**, 137–44.

Hoult, J., Reynolds, I., Charbonneau-Powis, M., Weekes, P. & Briggs, J. (1983). Psychiatric hospital versus community treatment: the results of a randomised trial. *Australian and New Zealand Journal of Psychiatry*, **17**, 160–7.

Issakidis, C., Sanderson, K., Teesson, M., Johnston, S. & Buhrich, N. (1999). Intensive case management in Australia: a randomized controlled trial. *Acta Psychiatrica Scandinavica*, **99**, 360–7.

Jackson, G., Gater, R., Goldberg, D., Tantam, D., Loftus, L. & Taylor, H. (1993). A new community mental health team based in primary care: a description of the service and the effect on service use in the first year. *British Journal of Psychiatry*, **162**, 375–84.

Johnson, S., Nolan, F., Pilling, S. (2005). Randomised controlled trial of acute mental health care by a specialist crisis team: the north Islington crisis study. *British Medical Journal*, **331**, 599–602.

Kidd, H. B. (1965). Industrial units in psychiatric hospitals. *British Journal of Psychiatry*, **111**, 1205–9.

Killaspy, H., Bebbington, P., Blizard, R. *et al.* (2006). The REACT study: randomised evaluation of assertive community treatment in north London. *British Medical Journal*, **332**, 815–20.

King, R. (2006). Intensive case management: a critical re-appraisal of the scientific evidence for effectiveness. *Administration and Policy in Mental Health*, **33**, 529–35.

Lamont, A., Ukoumunne, O., Tyrer, P. *et al.* (2000). The geographic mobility of severely mentally ill residents in London. *Social Psychiatry and Psychiatric Epidemiology*, **35**, 164–9.

Marshall, M., Lockwood, A., Gray, A. & Green, R. (1997). Assertive community treatment. *Schizophrenia Module of the Cochrane Database of Systematic Reviews*. Oxford: Update Software Ltd.

Marshall, M. & Creed, F. (2000). Assertive community treatment – is it the future of community care in the UK? *International Review of Psychiatry*, **12**, 191–6.

Marshall, M., Crowther, R., Almaraz-Serrano, A. M. & Tyrer, P. (2001a). Day hospital versus out-patient care for psychiatric disorders. *Cochrane Database of Systematic Reviews*, **3**, CD003240. Oxford: Update Software Ltd.

Marshall, M., Crowther, R., Almaraz Serrano, A. *et al.* (2001b). Systematic reviews of the effectiveness of day care for people with severe mental disorders: (1) acute day hospital versus admission; (2) vocational rehabilitation; (3) day hospital versus outpatient care. *Health Technology Assessment*, **5**, 1–75.

Marwaha, S. & Johnson, S. (2004). Schizophrenia and employment: a review. *Social Psychiatry and Psychiatric Epidemiology*, **39**, 337–49.

Metcalfe, C., White, I. R., Weaver, T. *et al.* (2005). Intensive case management for severe psychotic illness: is there a general benefit for patients with complex needs? A secondary analysis of the UK700 trial data. *Social Psychiatry and Psychiatric Epidemiology*, **40**, 718–24.

Morrisey, J. P. & Goldman, H. H. (1984). Cycles of reform in the care of the chronically mentally ill. *Hospital and Community Psychiatry*, **35**, 785–93.

Ngoma, M. C., Prince, M. & Mann, A. (2003). Common mental disorders among those attending primary health clinics and traditional healers in urban Tanzania. *British Journal of Psychiatry*, **183**, 349–55.

Nzimakwe, D. (1996). Primary health care in South Africa: private practice nurse practitioners and traditional healers form partnerships. *Journal of Academic Nursing Practice*, **8**, 311–16.

Phelan, M., Slade, M., Thornicroft, G. *et al.* (1995). The Camberwell Assessment of Need: the validity and reliability of an instrument to assess the needs of people with severe mental illness. *British Journal of Psychiatry*, **167**, 589–95.

Priebe, S., Jones, G., McCabe, R. *et al.* (2006) Effectiveness and costs of acute day hospital treatment compared with conventional in-patient care: randomised controlled trial. *British Journal of Psychiatry*, **188**, 243–9.

Pullen, I. M. & Yellowlees, A. J. (1988). Scottish psychiatrists in primary health-care settings. a silent majority. *British Journal of Psychiatry*, **153**, 663–6.

Puri, B. K., Hall, A. D., Reefat, R., Mayer, R. & Tyrer, P. (1996). General practitoners' views of an open referral system to a community mental health service. *Acta Psychiatrica Scandinavica*, **94**, 133–6.

Resnick, S. G., Fontana, A., Lehman, A. F. & Rosenheck, R. A. (2005). An empirical conceptualization of the recovery orientation. *Schizophrenia Research*, **75**, 119–28.

Rosie, J. S., Azim, H. F., Piper, W. E. & Joyce, A. S. (1995). Effective psychiatric day treatment: historical lessons. *Psychiatric Services*, **46**, 1019–26.

Ruggeri, M., Leese, M., Thornicroft, G., Bisoffi, G. & Tansella, M. (2000). Definition and prevalence of severe and persistent mental illness. *British Journal of Psychiatry*, **177**, 149–55.

Rutter, D. & Tyrer, P. (2003). The value of therapeutic communities in the treatment of personality disorder: a suitable place for treatment? *Journal of Psychiatric Practice*, **9**, 291–302.

Schinnar, A. P., Rothbard, A. B., Kanter, R. & Jung, Y. S. (1990). An empirical literature review of definitions of severe and persistent mental illness. *American Journal of Psychiatry*, **147**, 1602–8.

Schwarz, D. & Lellouch, J. (1967). Explanatory and pragmatic attitudes in therapeutic trials. *Journal of Chronic Diseases*, **20**, 637–48.

Shipley, K., Hilborn, B., Hansell, A., Tyrer, J. & Tyrer, P. (2000). Patient satisfaction: a valid measure of quality of care in a psychiatric service. *Acta Psychiatrica Scandinavica*, **101**, 330–3.

Simmonds, S., Coid, J., Joseph, P., Marriott, S. & Tyrer, P. (2001). Community mental health team management in severe mental illness: a systematic review. *British Journal of Psychiatry*, **178**, 497–502.

Slade, M., McCrone, P., Kuipers, E., Leese, M., Cahill, S. & Parabiaghi, A. (2006). Use of standardised outcome measures in adult mental health services: randomised controlled trial. *British Journal of Psychiatry*, **189**, 330–6.

Stein, L. I. & Diamond, R. J. (1985). A program for difficult-to-treat patients. In *New Directions for Mental Health Services*, **26**, ed. L. I. Stein & M. A. Test. San Francisco, CA: Jossey-Bass.

Stein, L. I. & Test, M. A. (1980). Alternative to mental hospital treatment. I. Conceptual model, treatment program, and clinical evaluation. *Archives of General Psychiatry*, **37**, 392–7.

Stein, L. I. & Santos, A. B. (1998). *Assertive Community Treatment of Persons with Severe Mental Illness*. London: WW Norton.

Stein, L. I. & Santos, A. B. (1998). *Assertive Community Treatment of Persons with Severe Mental Illness*. New York: Norton.

Strathdee, G. & Williams, P. (1984). A survey of psychiatrists in primary care: the silent growth of a new service. *Journal of the Royal College of General Practitioners*, **34**, 615–18.

Tempest, M. (2006). *The Future of the NHS*. London: XPL Publishing.

Tooth, G. C. & Brooke, E. M. (1961). Trends in the mental hospital population and their effect on future planning. *Lancet*, **i**, 710–13.

Tyrer, P. (1999). What is the future of assertive community treatment? *Epidemiologia e Psichiatrica Sociale*, **8**, 16–18.

Tyrer, P. (2007). The future of specialist community teams in the care of those with severe mental illness. *Epidemiologia e Psichiatria Sociale*, **16**, 225–30.

Tyrer, P., Ferguson, B. & Wadsworth, J. (1990). Liaison psychiatry in general practice: the comprehensive collaborative model. *Acta Psychiatrica Scandinavica*, **81**, 359–63.

Tyrer, P., Morgan, J., Van Horn, E. *et al.* (1995). A randomised controlled study of close monitoring of vulnerable psychiatric patients. *Lancet*, **345**, 756–9.

Tyrer, P., Balod, A., Germanavicius, A., McDonald, A., Varadan, M. & Thomas, J. (2007). Perceptions of assertive community treatment in the UK and Lithuania. *International Journal of Social Psychiatry* (in press).

Ukoumunne, O.C., Gulliford, M.C., Chinn, S., Sterne, J.A.C., Burney, P.G.J. & Donner, A. (1999). Methods in health service research. Evaluation of health interventions at area and organisation level. *British Medical Journal*, **319**, 376–9.

Weaver, T., Renton, A., Tyrer, P. & Ritchie, J. (1996). Combining qualitative data with randomised controlled trials is often useful. *British Medical Journal*, **313**, 629.

Weisbrod, B.A., Test, M.A. & Stein, L.I. (1980). Alternatives to mental hospital treatment: II. Economic benefit-cost analysis. *Archives of General Psychiatry*, **37**, 400–5.

Wells, J.S. (2006). Hospital-based industrial therapy units and the people who work within them – an Irish case analysis using a soft-systems approach. *Journal of Psychiatric Mental Health Nursing*, **13**, 139–47.

Specific treatments

Organic disorders

Section editors

James Warner and Robert van Reekum

9

Delirium

Laura Gage and David K. Conn

Editor's note

Delirium is one of the forgotten areas of therapeutics. It is observed frequently, often misinterpreted and misunderstood, but often mercifully disappears just as uncertainty about what to do gets stronger. This probably explains the relative paucity of evidence available about preferred treatments; delirium is a prelude to focused intervention rather than a clarion call for action. This chapter nonetheless indicates the beginnings of an evidence base for intervention that is of definite value.

Introduction

Delirium is associated with increased rates of mortality and medical complications, prolonged hospitalization, as well as cognitive and functional impairment. Symptoms of delirium can also cause significant distress and discomfort to both patients and their families. Unfortunately, delirium is commonly underdiagnosed by physicians. Recognition and appropriate treatment of delirium is essential to minimize associated morbidity.

The treatment of delirium is to tackle the underlying cause. Identifying underlying aetiologies and their correction should always be foremost in the clinician's mind. The common causes include infection, drug intoxication, renal or hepatic insufficiency, vascular disease affecting the brain, and electrolyte disturbance, and the prevalence of the condition varies from 10% in young hospitalized medical patients to 80% in those who are terminally ill (Brown & Boyle, 2002).

Delirium may cause agitation or psychotic symptoms, which puts patients or others at risk, affects their treatment, or may cause significant distress. In addition to environmental interventions, pharmacological treatment may be necessary to control these symptoms.

Antipsychotics have been the mainstay of treatment for agitation and psychotic symptoms in delirium. The use of various other medications have also been reported in the literature, although not as widely as antipsychotic treatment. An exception to this is the treatment of alcohol or sedative-hypnotic withdrawal delirium for which benzodiazepines are the treatment of choice (APA, 1999).

Some authors have suggested that antipsychotics should be used not only for behavioural management, but that they may be disease-specific treatments for delirium that should be implemented even in the absence of agitation or psychosis (Hales & Yudofsky, 2003). There is some theoretical support that medications such as antipsychotics may treat an underlying common final neural pathway of delirium itself, such as elevated dopamine (Trzepacz, 2000). Some authors suggest therefore that the hypoactive subtype of delirium, which is characterized by psychomotor retardation, inattention and decreased mobility, should be treated, not for behavioural control but to treat the delirium itself. It has been suggested that the hypoactive subtype may be the most important to treat given their poor prognosis (Platt et al., 1994). Unfortunately, there are no controlled clinical trials to support this theory and the available guidelines do not specifically address this issue.

Studies of physician prescription patterns show that haloperidol is the most common medication used to treat delirium, as it is used in approximately two-thirds of cases (Olofsson et al., 1996; Someya et al., 2001; Carnes et al., 2003). The next most commonly used agents are the benzodiazepines either as monotherapy or in combination with haloperidol. According to one study, only 43% of respondents to a mail survey selected treatments that would correspond to 'best practice' in accordance with the American Psychiatric Association Practice Guidelines for the treatment of delirium (Carnes et al., 2003).

Cambridge Textbook of Effective Treatments in Psychiatry, ed. Peter Tyrer and Kenneth R. Silk. Published by Cambridge University Press.
© Cambridge University Press, 2008.

Although there is extensive clinical experience in the use of antipsychotics in the treatment of delirium, there remains a paucity of controlled trials. The best evidence available in the literature on the pharmacological treatment of delirium will be critically reviewed and current practice guidelines will be outlined. Evidence supporting non-pharmacological interventions will also be reviewed.

Pharmacological interventions

Typical antipsychotics

There has been only one randomized controlled trial comparing typical antipsychotics in delirium. Breitbart *et al.* (1996) investigated the effectiveness of chlorpromazine, haloperidol and lorazepam in hospitalized AIDS patients. These patients all met DSM–III–R criteria for delirium and scored 13 or greater on the Delirium Rating Scale (DRS). A total of 244 non-delirious patients were initially enrolled in the trial and were then followed prospectively for the onset of delirium. The 30 patients who subsequently developed delirium were then randomized and treated in a double-blind fashion with one of the three study medications. All delirious patients were included in the study, apparently irrespective of subtype (i.e. hyperactive, hypoactive or mixed), as the inclusion criteria was the overall DRS score, not specifically hyperactive symptoms.

The lorazepam arm of this study had to be stopped prematurely due to adverse effects. All six patients developed treatment-limiting side effects at a mean daily maintenance dose of 4.6 mg (a higher than usual dosage of this drug). Patients receiving lorazepam also showed an increase in cognitive impairment. Efficacy, as measured by the DRS, was equivalent for both haloperidol and chlorpromazine. In both cases, improvement was noted in the first 24 hours, usually before the initiation of interventions directed at the underlying medical etiologies of the delirium. Relatively low dosages of antipsychotics were required (e.g. average daily maintenance drug doses: haloperidol 1.4 mg, chlorpromazine 36 mg). Cognitive function in the chlorpromazine group decreased slightly from day two to the end of treatment, which may be related to its anticholinergic properties. The implications from this study are that haloperidol was equivalent to chlorpromazine in treating delirium, although chlorpromazine was associated with a slight decline in MMSE score. Lorazepam worsened cognition, did not improve other delirium symptoms and had significant side effects. The efficacy of the antipsychotics relative to placebo is not known, as there was no placebo control arm. The study infers their efficacy based on the rapid improvement in

delirium symptoms which usually occurred before the initiation of interventions directed at the medical etiologies of the delirium. The limitations of this study include its small sample size, particularly in the lorazepam arm which included only six patients, the limitation to AIDS patients, and the lack of placebo control.

The other studies investigating haloperidol in the treatment of delirium are methodologically weak. A prospective study by Moulaert (1989) followed six post-operative delirious patients who were treated with intravenous haloperidol without a control group. There was no standardized definition of delirium and the study did not use a validated delirium rating scale. An initial dose of 5 mg intravenous (IV) haloperidol was given and the dose was doubled every 30 minutes until the patient was calm. An average dose of 38 mg was used and no side effects were reported. Relatively lower haloperidol dosages were efficacious in a prospective study by Akechi *et al.* (1996). Ten cancer patients with delirium (as defined by DSM–III–R) were followed using the DRS and treated with either IV or oral (PO) haloperidol depending on the clinical situation. This was titrated according to a treatment protocol. They found that relatively low dosages of haloperidol were required to control patient target symptoms (e.g. agitation, disruptive behaviour) with 60% of the patients receiving less than 5 mg haloperidol/day. The dosage required during the first day of treatment was significantly related to the eventual maintenance dosage. There were no serious adverse effects reported.

The use of intravenous versus oral haloperidol was evaluated by Menza *et al.* (1987) in a prospective, naturalistic study where the raters were blinded to the route of administration. This was a mixed population with the majority of those receiving intravenous haloperidol (n = 4) having delirium and those receiving oral haloperidol (n = 6) suffering from a range of psychiatric disorders. The patients receiving IV haloperidol experienced fewer extrapyramidal symptoms compared with the patients receiving oral haloperidol. There was no difference in the rates of akathesia, which was present in half of the patients.

The combination of benzodiazepines and haloperidol in delirious patients was investigated in a prospective, naturalistic study with blinded raters by Menza *et al.* (1988). Although the patients receiving the IV haloperidol plus benzodiazepines (n = 14) had significantly higher dosages of haloperidol, they had fewer extrapyramidal symptoms (EPS) then those receiving IV haloperidol alone (n = 4). A retrospective case series by Adams *et al.* (1986) reviewed critically ill cancer patients with delirium who were treated with an extremely high-dosage combination of IV haloperidol (100–480 mg/24 hours) and lorazepam

(36–480 mg/24 hours). There was only one reported case of acute dystonia and no other reported extrapyramidal side effects. A contrasting study of intravenous haloperidol plus lorazepam showed much higher rates of EPS (Fernandez & Levy, 1989). This prospective study (without a comparison group) in terminally ill, delirious AIDS patients (n = 38) showed that half of the patients treated with a combination of IV haloperidol and lorazepam developed EPS. However, it is suggested that AIDS patients may be particularly sensitive to side effects from antipsychotics, including EPS. Several case reports have described the development of EPS (Blitzstein & Brandt, 1997), akathesia (Seneff & Mathews, 1995) and withdrawal dyskinesias (Riker et al., 1997) associated with the use of IV haloperidol specifically in delirium.

There have been two randomized, double-blind controlled trials comparing haloperidol to droperidol (Resnick & Burton, 1984; Thomas et al., 1992). These studies were not specific to delirium as they evaluated a mixed population. Both studies suggested that intramuscular droperidol may have a faster onset of action then intramuscular haloperidol in controlling agitation, but it is no longer available in the UK due to withdrawal for reasons of cardiotoxicity.

A retrospective chart review examined the use of haloperidol versus narcotics in delirium (Sanders et al., 1992). Of the 198 patient charts reviewed, 67 patients were identified retrospectively as having delirium following intra-aortic balloon pump therapy. Fifteen of those patients who were treated with haloperidol were compared with ten patients who were treated with narcotics. Patients treated with narcotics had a higher mortality rate (50% vs. 40%), higher rates of 'residual organic brain syndrome' (undefined in the article) (40% vs. 11%) and higher rates of complications. The APA guidelines do suggest opioids when pain is an aggravating factor in the delirium; however they caution that they can exacerbate delirium, particularly through their anticholinergic metabolites (American Psychiatric Association, 1999).

Few studies have investigated the role of antipsychotics specifically in the treatment of hypoactive delirium. A prospective, open trial which lacked a placebo-control group compared patients with hyperactive delirium (n = 9) to patients with hypoactive delirium (n = 11) who were treated with haloperidol or chlorpromazine (Platt et al., 1994). Patients were identified using the DSM–III–R criteria for delirium and followed using the DRS by non-blinded raters. Both groups had equivalent and significant improvement in DRS scores on the first day of treatment. The authors note that the improvement became evident within hours, well before medical interventions were initiated and suggest that this preliminary evidence supports a possible role for antipsychotics in the management of hypoactive delirium. The study also suggests that chlorpromazine is equivalent in efficacy to haloperidol. However, the use of chlorpromazine is discouraged by the American College of Critical Care Medicine Guidelines due to its strong anticholinergic, sedative and α-adrenergic antagonist effects.

In summary, there is only one randomized controlled trial (RCT) supporting the use of typical antipsychotics in the treatment of delirium, which has several limitations. Haloperidol is more effective than lorazepam monotherapy, which may worsen cognition. Chlorpromazine was found to be as effective as haloperidol but may cause a slight decline in cognition due to anticholinergic effects. The remainder of the evidence is very limited due to poor methodological design. There is some limited evidence to suggest lower rates of EPS with the use of IV haloperidol instead of oral, as well as lower rates of EPS with the addition of lorazepam to IV haloperidol. Further information regarding treatment strategies is reviewed in the guideline section of this chapter.

Atypical antipsychotics

Olanzapine

Olanzapine was compared with haloperidol in a randomized controlled trial in which only the evaluators were blinded to treatment group (Skrobik et al., 2004). All patients admitted to an intensive care unit (ICU), the majority post-operative patients, were screened periodically for delirium. Patients who scored ≥ 4 on the ICU Delirium Screening Checklist were then assessed for delirium using DSM–IV criteria. Seventy-three patients were enrolled and the groups were found to be similar at baseline, although the unconcealed allocation (patients were randomized on an even/odd day basis) resulted in uneven groups (haloperidol n = 45, olanzapine n = 28) and may have led to bias within the study. Patients were followed using the Delirium Index (DI). The mean dosage of haloperidol was 6.5 mg (range 1–28 mg) and olanzapine 4.54 mg (range 2.5–13.5 mg). Mild EPS developed in six of the patients receiving haloperidol, and in none of the olanzapine patients. There was no difference between the groups in the reduction of the DI over time. However, 'rescue' intravenous haloperidol was used in 10/28 (36%) of the olanzapine patients on the first day and in 5/28 (18%) of patients on the second, which likely contaminated the early DI evaluation between the groups. The need for the addition of haloperidol to the olanzapine group early in the study significantly affects the interpretation of the results, particularly since improvement in the first 24 hours after the addition of an antipsychotic is felt to be most supportive of efficacy in delirium.

There has been one other comparative trial investigating olanzapine and haloperidol for delirium (Sipahimalani & Masand, 1998). In a non-blinded, naturalistic study 22 delirious patients were assigned to haloperidol or olanzapine based on the treating clinician's preference. They were evaluated according to the DRS; however this was retrospectively assigned based on a chart review. In the olanzapine group 3/11 were on standing doses of other antipsychotics for psychotic illnesses, which could contaminate the results. The mean improvement in DRS was a reduction of 7.6 for the olanzapine group and 10 for the haloperidol group, but the statistical significance of this was not reported in the paper. Peak response time was similar in both groups and 45% of the olanzapine group and 54% of the haloperidol group showed significant improvement (> 50% score reduction). Of the haloperidol patients, 45% developed sedation or extrapyramidal symptoms and none of the patients on olanzapine had side effects.

In addition, there have been two open prospective trials with no control groups of olanzapine in the treatment of delirium (Kim *et al.*, 2001; Breitbart *et al.*, 2002). In the study by Kwang-Soo, 20 patients with delirium (as per DSM–IV criteria) were treated with olanzapine (8.8 mg $+/-$ 2.2 mg/day). The evaluator was blinded and patients were followed with the DRS. Seventy per cent of the patients had a 50% improvement in the DRS score. Side effects due to olanzapine, including dry mouth and sedation, were found in 10% of patients. Breitbart *et al.* (2002) prospectively followed 79 delirious hospitalized cancer patients treated with olanzapine (mean dose at end of study 6.3 mg, range 2.5–20 mg). Standardized measures were used for diagnosis and course of illness. Seventy-six per cent of patients scored ≤ 10 on the Memorial Delirium Assessment Scale (MDAS) after 4–7 days. Delirium of mild severity and hyperactive subtype had better response rates. Of note, 30% of patients developed sedation and two patients worsened after treatment with olanzapine.

In summary, there has been one RCT with methodological limitations and several open trials supporting the use of olanzapine in delirium. These preliminary trials suggest that olanzapine has similar efficacy to haloperidol and lower rates of extrapyramidal symptoms in the treatment of delirium.

Risperidone

There has been one randomized, double-blind controlled trial of risperidone compared with haloperidol in the treatment of delirium (Han & Kim, 2004). These were 24 patients with mixed medical aetiologies referred to consultation psychiatry and diagnosed with delirium based on the Structured Clinical Interview for DSM–III–R. The mean dose of haloperidol was 1.71 mg (range 1.0–3.0 mg) and the mean dosage of risperidone was 1.02 mg (range 0.5–2.0 mg). The Confusion Assessment Method (CAM), the DRS and the MDAS scales were used to follow the patients. There was no statistically significant difference in the frequency of response to the drugs between the two groups (haloperidol group response: 75%; risperidone group response: 42%). One patient in the initial haloperidol group dropped out of the study due to severe sedation and one developed mild akathisia. No patients in the risperidone group had significant side effects. No standardized scales were used to rate side effects of the medications. A significant limitation of this study is its small sample size and the possibility of type II error.

Three prospective, open studies with no control group have found similar response rates for risperidone in delirium. One study which was significantly limited by a small sample size ($n = 11$) and a lack of structured diagnostic interviews or rating scales, found a 72% response rate to risperidone with a maximum response seen at $5.1 +/- 4.3$ days, with one patient (9%) developing EPS (Sipahimalani *et al.*, 1997). A study of similar size ($n = 10$) found an efficacy rate of 80%, with the time to maximum effect averaging 7.1 days. Sedation occurred in 30% of patients and mild EPS in 10% (Horikawa *et al.*, 2003). A larger, multi-centre study ($n = 64$) with standardized diagnostic criteria and rating scales found a 90.6% response to treatment of patients with delirium with risperidone (defined as a DRS < 13 within 72 hours) (Parellada *et al.*, 2004). Improvement in DRS score was seen in the first 24–48 hours after administration of risperidone, before the underlying cause of the delirium symptomatology was treated. Sedation was reported in 3.1% of patients and there was no reported EPS.

A systematic retrospective chart review of all patients diagnosed with delirium (based on DSM–IV) during a discrete period revealed 41 patients who received treatment with risperidone and 36 who received haloperidol treatment (Liu *et al.*, 2004). The psychiatrists who retrospectively rated the severity and response rates to the medications were not blinded to the medication group and did not use standardized scales. The haloperidol group had more severe delirium symptoms at baseline, therefore a direct comparison between the groups could not be made. Subgroup comparisons of patients of similar severity showed similar efficacy between risperidone (mean daily doses of 1.91 mg) and haloperidol (mean daily dose of 2.84 mg). Anticholinergic adjunctive treatment was administered to 70% of the haloperidol group versus 7% of the risperidone group.

There has been one case report of delirium caused by risperidone (Tavcar) and three other case reports where risperidone may have contributed to delirium (Ravona-Springer *et al.*, 1998). There has also been one case report of torsades de pointes caused by risperidone in a delirious patient (Tei *et al.*, 2004).

In summary there has been one RCT which is limited by its small sample size and several open studies of risperidone in delirium. These preliminary studies suggest that risperidone has similar response rates to haloperidol and has lower rates of EPS.

Quetiapine

The study of quetiapine in delirium has been limited to two prospective, open studies without control arms (Kim *et al.*, 2003; Sasaki *et al.*, 2003) and a retrospective chart review (Schwartz & Masand, 2000). Kim *et al.* (2003) found in 12 patients the mean duration for stabilization was 5.91 days on a mean dose of 93.75 mg/day. No patients developed EPS, although sedation occurred in 16%. Sasaki *et al.* (2003) found that all of 12 patients treated with quetiapine (mean dose 44.9 mg/day) achieved response (DRS < 13) within several days (4.6 ± 3.5 days). There were no adverse effects reported.

The systematic retrospective chart review (Schwartz & Masand, 2000) identified all patients with delirium who had been treated with quetiapine (mean dose 211.4 mg/day) during a discrete period of time (n = 11). They were compared with a randomly selected, historical control group of delirious patients treated with haloperidol (mean dose 3.4 mg/day). The DRS scores were gathered directly from the charts and if no score was available, the chart was reviewed by an independent psychiatrist to assign a score retrospectively. Ten of 11 patients in both groups had > 50% improvement in DRS scores and there was no difference in onset of symptom resolution and duration of treatment. Two haloperidol-treated patients developed EPS leading to discontinuation of the drug and two quetiapine-treated patients developed sedation (leading to discontinuation of the drug in one patient).

To summarize, the very limited data available suggest that quetiapine may have similar efficacy to haloperidol, with sedation the most common side effect and fewer extrapyramidal side effects.

Ziprasidone

There are no published studies on the use of ziprasidone in delirium. A case report (Leso & Schwartz, 2002) showed improvement in delirium in a 34-year-old male; however the treatment had to be discontinued due to an 8.4% increase in the QTc interval as well as unstable levels of potassium and magnesium. Another case reported the successful use of intravenous ziprasidone for delirium refractory to haloperidol and benzodiazepine treatment (Young & Lujan, 2004).

Remoxipride

Remoxipride is an atypical antipsychotic drug with selective antagonism of dopamine D_2 receptors. One retrospective chart review of elderly patients with behavioural disturbances included 75 patients with delirium, 70 of whom had concurrent dementia (93%) (Robertson *et al.*, 1996). A 'good effect' from remoxipride, which was not clearly defined, was reported in 75% of the patients.

Benzodiazepines

As reviewed earlier, several studies have suggested the addition of benzodiazepines to intravenous haloperidol may lower the risk of extrapyramidal symptoms (Menza *et al.*, 1988; Adams *et al.*, 1986). The one randomized controlled trial of benzodiazepine monotherapy compared with antipsychotics (Breitbart *et al.*, 1996), already described, resulted in all benzodiazepine-treated patients developing treatment-limiting side effects and a worsening in cognitive impairment. A retrospective chart review of 39 delirious patients with advanced cancer found that 26% of the patients required sedation to control symptoms of delirium which were refractory to treatment with haloperidol and in 9/10 of these patients this was induced with a continuous infusion of midazolam (Stiefel *et al.*, 1992).

The American Psychiatric Association Guidelines do not recommend benzodiazepine monotherapy for delirium, other than for alcohol or sedative withdrawal (American Psychiatric Association, 1999). It is noted that the combination of benzodiazepines and antipsychotics may decrease medication side effects and potentially increase effectiveness in special populations and that open studies suggest that the combination of haloperidol plus lorazepam may be more efficacious, with a shorter duration of the delirium and fewer EPS than haloperidol. They suggest that when benzodiazepines are used, short-acting medications with no active metabolites (e.g. lorazepam) should be chosen and that the dose be titrated carefully as benzodiazepines may exacerbate delirium. The American College of Critical Care Medicine Guidelines comments that delirious patients may become more confused when treated with sedatives, which could cause a paradoxical increase in agitation.

In summary, the evidence shows no support for the use of benzodiazepine monotherapy in delirium (except in alcohol or sedative withdrawal delirium) and weak evidence that the addition of lorazepam to intravenous haloperidol may result in lower rates of EPS.

Cholinesterase inhibitors

The use of cholinesterase inhibitors in delirium is supported only by case reports, including the successful use of donepezil in post-operative delirium (Wengel et al., 1999) and delirium in dementia (Wengel et al., 1998). Improvement was noted in a case of rivastigmine in lithium toxicity delirium (Fischer, 2001) and in three elderly patients with prolonged delirium (Kalisvaart et al., 2004). In contrast, one case report described a delirium which appeared to be caused by the cholinesterase inhibitor tacrine (Trzepacz et al., 1996). There have been no reported cases of any other cholinesterase inhibitors causing delirium.

Mianserin

Mianserin is a tetracyclic compound which increases the duration of deep slow wave sleep and decreases the length of rapid eye movement periods in humans (Dugovic & Adrien, 1991). Its pharmacological profile shows potent antagonism of presynaptic α_2 receptors and post-synaptic 5-HT$_2$ receptors and weak antagonism of D$_2$ receptors (Coppen et al., 1976; Marshall, 1983; Pinder, 1983), as well as H$_1$ blocking action (Uchiyama et al., 1996). It is often used in Japan, where haloperidol is not covered by health insurance, to treat delirium, with one user survey indicating it was used in 14% of delirium cases (Someya et al., 2001).

One randomized, non-blinded trial compared mianserin (10–60 mg/day) to haloperidol (2–6 mg/day) in 40 patients with delirium as diagnosed by DSM–IV (Nakamura et al., 1997a). There was no difference in the improvement between the groups with 69.4% of the mianserin group responding (DRS improved by 50%) compared with 70.6% of the haloperidol group. Oversedation occurred in two mianserin patients and there were no adverse effects in the haloperidol group. In a prospective, open trial without a control group 49/62 (79%) of mianserin-treated patients were responders (improvement on > 4 items on DRS and aggravation of < 2) (Uchiyama et al., 1996). Patients whose symptoms worsened at night had a particularly good response. Hypoactive deliriums were included and they had the lowest response rate. Cognition only modestly improved relative to other symptom domains, which suggest that mianserin may not have

a direct therapeutic effect on cognitive improvement and may explain the drug's lesser effectiveness on hypoactive delirium. Excess sedation occurred in 6.5% of patients. Finally, an open trial of mianserin suppositories for delirious patients unable to take oral medications showed improvement in all 16 cases (Nakamura et al., 1997b).

In summary, there are no randomized, double-blind trials assessing the efficacy of mianserin. There is some weak evidence that mianserin improves delirious symptoms, although it may have limited effect at improving cognition and may cause excess sedation.

Electroconvulsive therapy

Electroconvulsive therapy (ECT) has not been shown to be an effective treatment for general cases of delirium and can itself carry a risk of exacerbating cognitive impairment. Case reports support the use of ECT as a treatment for particular cases of delirium due to specific aetiologies. In a review of case reports of ECT in neuroleptic malignant syndrome (NMS), delirium symptoms improved in 24 out of 29 patients (Davis et al., 1991) and in another review, 26 out of 31 of the patients improved (Scheftner & Shulman, 1992). It is difficult to draw conclusions from these studies, as published cases are likely biased towards those with positive outcomes.

Electroconvulsive therapy has also been suggested in the treatment of delirium tremens. A retrospective chart review found that 10 patients receiving ECT with conventional treatment had a shorter duration of delirium symptoms than 10 patients receiving conventional treatment alone (Dudley & Williams, 1972).

The American Psychiatric Association Practice Guidelines for the Treatment of Patients with Delirium counsels that ECT should be considered only very rarely for patients with delirium due to specific aetiologies such as neuroleptic malignant syndrome and should not be considered initially as a substitute for more conservative and conventional treatments.

Other medications

The use of methylphenidate in hypoactive delirium was examined in a prospective trial with no control group in 14 patients with advanced cancer (Gagnon et al., 2005). The patients were included in the study if the delirium persisted beyond one week in spite of aggressive efforts to reverse correctable causes. The median pretreatment MMSE score of 21 improved to a median score of 27 one hour following the first dose of methylphenidate. Patients improved in cognition and psychomotor activities upon reaching a stable dose of methylphenidate. Most patients were treated with a dose of 20–30 mg per day; the maximum effective daily dose was 50 mg. Higher doses were not associated with further improvement but, instead, with increased side effects. In addition to this positive study, there have been two case reports of the successful use of methylphenidate in the treatment of hypoactive delirium (Morita *et al.*, 2000; Meyers & Van Ojen, 2004).

A randomized prospective non-blinded study investigated a combination of pethidine (an opioid analgesic), diazepam and flunitrazepam as compared to those given treatment-as-usual in the *prevention* of post-operative delirium in the elderly following gastrointestinal surgery (Aizawa *et al.*, 2002). Although there was a treatment-as-usual control group, they did not receive placebo. The subsequent development of delirium was 7/20 (35%) in the control group compared with 5% in the treatment group. Morning lethargy was observed in 40% of the treatment group. Although these authors suggested the efficacy of benzodiazepines and opioids in the prevention of delirium, these agents are not generally recommended due to lack of further evidence and as they may exacerbate delirium symptoms (Jacobi *et al.*, 2002). There have also been two case reports of the use of melatonin (Hanania & Kitain, 2002) and a case series of seven patients treated with trazodone in delirium (Okamoto *et al.*, 1999).

Ondansetron is a $5-HT_3$ receptor antagonist which was studied in 35 post-cardiotomy delirious patients (Bayindir *et al.*, 2000). The serotonin system has been implicated in acute delirium (Van der Mast & Fekkes, 2000) and is affected by cardiopulmonary bypass (Bayindir *et al.*, 2000). Therefore, it was hypothesized that an agent, which was a serotonin receptor antagonist could ameliorate delirium. Bayindir *et al.* (2000) administered a single dose of ondansetron intravenously without patients being aware of the treatment. The patients were evaluated using a 'mental status scoring scale' which the study team had developed and were re-evaluated ten minutes following treatment. Eighty per cent of the patients dropped to a score of zero ('normal') in 10 minutes. The study was obviously limited with a lack of placebo group, lack of blinding, the lack of a standardized assessment scale and the extremely brief follow-up period of 10 minutes.

Guidelines

The American Psychiatric Association Practice Guidelines for the Treatment of Patients with Delirium

The American Psychiatric Association Practice Guidelines for the Treatment of Patients with Delirium (American Psychiatric Association, 1999) supports the use of antipsychotics as the pharmacologic treatment of choice in delirium. Haloperidol is identified as most frequently used due to the different available routes of administration, lack of anticholinergic side effects, few active metabolites and the low likelihood of causing sedation and hypotension. Because antipsychotic medications have occasionally been found to lengthen the QT_c interval, possibly leading to torsades de pointes, a baseline ECG is suggested, as well as the monitoring of serum levels of magnesium and potassium in critically ill patients. The guidelines acknowledge the lack of data in guiding dosing strategies and suggest initiating haloperidol at 1–2 mg every 2–4 hours as needed (0.25–0.50 mg every 4 hours as needed in the elderly). For patients that require higher dosages, intravenous (IV) infusions are suggested, for example, haloperidol bolus 10 mg IV followed by continuous intravenous infusion of 5–10 mg/hour. This dosing strategy has been criticized for being based on only one case series and for recommending overly high dosages (Tauscher *et al.*, 2000). Droperidol may be considered when a more rapid onset of action is required. The atypical antipsychotics are mentioned as being used by some physicians, but as having no controlled evidence supporting their use.

These guidelines counsel the avoidance of benzodiazepines as monotherapy, with the exception of delirium due to withdrawal from alcohol or sedative-hypnotics or delirium caused by seizures. The combination of benzodiazepines with an antipsychotic is proposed for patients who can only tolerate lower dosages of antipsychotic medications or who have prominent anxiety or agitation. For initiating combined therapy, lorazepam 0.5–1.0 mg IV is suggested as an addition to haloperidol 3.0 mg IV.

Cholinergic medications are mentioned in the guidelines primarily for use in reversing anticholinergic delirium with physostigmine. The use of cholinesterase inhibitors is not specifically endorsed due to lack of data. The guidelines state that ECT has not been shown to be an effective treatment for general cases of delirium and proposes that it should be considered only rarely for patients with delirium due to specific causes such as neuroleptic malignant syndrome and should not be considered initially as a substitute for more conservative measures.

The American College of Critical Care Medicine Clinical Practice Guidelines for the Sustained Use of Sedatives and Analgesics in the Critically Ill Adult

Haloperidol is recommended as the preferred agent of choice in the treatment of delirium in critically ill patients.

Physicians are cautioned to monitor patients for electrocardiogram changes when receiving haloperidol. A dosing strategy of intravenous haloperidol is outlined: an initial dose of 2 mg, followed by repeated doses (double the previous dose) every 15–20 minutes while agitation persists. It is cautioned that the optimal dose and regimen of haloperidol have not been defined. This dosing strategy was later criticized as being excessive, likely leading to an excess of 60% D_2 receptor blockade (Skrobik, 2002). The authors of these guidelines have clarified that they advocate the use of the least amount of haloperidol that achieves the desired outcomes (Jacobi et al., 2002).

The guidelines advise against the use of chlorpromazine due to its strong anticholinergic, sedative and α-adrenergic antagonist effects. Droperidol is also discouraged due to its association with frightening dreams, vasodilation effects, anti-adrenergic effects and because it has been less studied than haloperidol in the ICU population. Sedatives are not suggested as they may lead to further cognitive impairment and can cause a paradoxical increase in agitation.

Non-pharmacological interventions

Non-pharmacological approaches and supportive care are widely recommended for the management of patients with delirium. Although many of these interventions make common sense, the evidence that they reduce symptoms is limited. Many of these interventions aim at providing a consistent environment with an optimal level of stimulation. Attempts are made to provide orienting cues for the patient to encourage social interaction, to limit the number of staff involved in the care of the patient, to ensure adequate sleep, to remove unnecessary and excessive stimuli, to alternate periods of rest and activity, to communicate clearly and simply so that information is easily understandable (Foreman et al., 1999). Supportive care also includes adequate oral intake, safe mobility, psychosocial support and the prevention of falls, aspiration and cubitus ulcers (Cole, 2004).

Budd & Brown (1974) carried out a randomized study of 31 patients following open-heart surgery in an intensive care unit. They utilized a specific reorientation procedure, which focused on time, place, person and physical status. This was administered post-operatively by intensive care unit nurses. Patients who received the reorientation procedure subsequently demonstrated a significantly lower instance of total symptoms of delirium, had significantly fewer post-operative complications and were discharged from the hospital an average of 4 days earlier compared to control group patients. Williams et al. (1985) carried out a study of elderly patients with hip fractures. Interpersonal and environmental nursing interventions were carried out with 57 patients on orthopaedic units in three hospitals. They were compared with a non-intervention group of 170 patients. The incidence of delirium was lower in the intervention group throughout the 5 post-operative days, but this was most pronounced during the first 3 days. The study involved an intervention phase and a non-intervention phase. Importantly, project funds enabled modest supplementation of staffing when a study patient was on the unit. For part of the study a clinical specialist in psychiatric nursing was involved. Interventions that were carried out most consistently were: orientation; keeping patients informed about and giving rationale for treatments and procedures; and, correcting sensory deficits. Chatham (1978) studied the effect of family involvement in patients with 'post-cardiotomy psychosis'. Family members were instructed to use eye contact, frequent touch and verbal orientation to time, person and place. Twenty patients were randomized into intervention and control groups. Patients receiving the intervention were significantly more oriented to time, person and place, were more appropriate and less confused, had fewer delusions and had longer periods of sleep as compared with subjects in the control group. The author noted that for too long family members had been shut out of the ICU. She encouraged healthcare professionals to treat the patient and family as a functional entity.

Numerous studies have attempted to improve outcomes through systematic detection and treatment of delirium. The interventions generally evaluate the effectiveness of early detection, treatment of possible causal factors and special nursing interventions. Milisen et al. (2001) studied a nurse-led interdisciplinary intervention programme for delirium in elderly hip fracture patients. The intervention consisted of education of nursing staff, systematic cognitive screening, consultative services by a delirium resource nurse, a geriatric nurse specialist or a psychogeriatrician and the use of a scheduled pain protocol. Although there was no significant effect on the incidence of delirium, the duration of delirium was significantly shorter and the severity of delirium was reduced in the intervention cohort. A trend toward decreased length of stay post-operatively was noted for the delirious patients in the intervention cohort. Cole et al. (1994) carried out a randomized controlled trial to assess a systematic intervention in cases of delirium in elderly inpatients. The intervention consisted of consultation by a geriatric internist or psychiatrist and follow-up by a liaison nurse. The intervention appeared to result in a small improvement in cognition and functioning, but there were no significant differences between the groups in length of hospital stay, discharge settings or mortality rate. A similar study with more subjects by Cole *et al.* (2002) found no significant benefits. In a non-randomized trial of 214 elderly orthopaedic patients, who received careful monitoring and intervention post-operatively, there was a large decrease in the incidence of severe confusion and a decreased length of stay (Gustafson *et al.*, 1991). A review by Cole (2004) concluded that systematic interventions appear to be somewhat more effective with older surgical patients as compared with patients on medical units. He suggests that the larger effect among surgical patients may have been related to more specific putative causes (e.g. post-operative hypoxia) and as a result, more readily treatable conditions.

It is important also to recognize that delirium can be an extremely distressing condition for both patients and their caregivers. Breitbart *et al.* (2002) conducted a systematic examination of the experience of delirium in a sample of 154 hospitalized patients with cancer. Of the 154 patients assessed, 101 had complete resolution of their delirium and were administered the Delirium Experience Questionnaire (DEQ), which is a valid measure that assesses delirium recall and distress related to an episode of delirium. Spouse/caregivers and primary nurses were also administered the DEQ to assess distress related to caring for a delirious patient. Of the 101 patients, 53.5% recalled their delirium experience. Mean delirium distress levels (on a 0–4 numerical rating score of the DEQ) were 3.2 for patients who recalled delirium, 3.75 for spouses/caregivers and 3.09 for nurses. The most significant predictor of patient distress was the presence of delusions (OR = 7.9). Patients with hypoactive delirium were just as distressed as patients with hyperactive delirium. This paper highlighted the importance of prompt recognition and treatment of delirium, but also the need for psychosocial support for patients during and after their episode of delirium.

A recent Cochrane Review of multidisciplinary team interventions for delirium in patients with chronic cognitive impairment concluded that although nine controlled trials were identified for possible inclusion in the review, only one met the inclusion criteria. They were unable to analyse the data from that study and concluded that delirium is currently managed empirically and that there was no evidence in the literature to support changes to current practice (Britton & Russell, 2004).

Guidelines

The American Psychiatric Association published guidelines for the management of delirium in 1999. It concluded that while there are no large rigorous randomized controlled trials, environmental interventions are widely endorsed because of clinical experience and the lack of adverse effects. It also noted that although the value of environmental interventions is widely recognized, they remain substantially under utilized (American Psychiatric Association, 1999; Meagher *et al.*, 1996). The potential sensory deprivation in hospital intensive care units is highlighted as well as its apparent contribution to disorganized sleep/wake cycles, which in turn can aggravate fatigue and confusion. It is also noted that the ICU can be a very noisy environment and that patients with delirium may become over-stimulated by too much noise. Under-stimulation can also be a problem and the guidelines emphasize the importance of providing an optimal level of modest stimulation. The need to correct underlying sensory impairment including visual and auditory impairment is also emphasized. The guidelines emphasize the need for staff to provide emotional support with the goal of reducing anxiety and fear. It is suggested that all individuals who come in contact with the patient should provide reorientation, which entails reminding the patient in an unpressured manner of where he or she is, the date and time and what is happening to him or her. The patient should be told that the symptoms are temporary and reversible and do not reflect a persistent psychiatric disorder. The guidelines note that at that time there were no large clinical trials examining the efficacy of cognitive and emotional support in delirium. However, as with environmental interventions, increased use of these currently under-utilized supportive measures has been encouraged on the basis of clinical experience, common sense and the lack of adverse effects. The need for support and education for the family is also highlighted. Educating the patient's friends and family about delirium is extremely helpful since they may have the same worries as the patient and become frightened and demoralized, instead of being hopeful and encouraging. It is also suggested that it may be useful to recommend that family and friends spend time in the patient's room and bring familiar objects from home to help orient the patient and help him or her feel secure.

The level of evidence for each of the interventions discussed in this chapter is summarized in Table 9.1.

Table 9.1. Evidence base for interventions in delirium

Treatment	Form of treatment	Psychiatric disorder	Level of evidence for efficacy	Comments
Typical antipsychotic drugs	Haloperidol in low dosage, either in tablet or IV form	Delirium of all types, including hypoactive delirium	Ib	Effective but adverse effects may preclude use
	Chlorpromazine		IIb	
Atypical vs typical antipsychotic drugs	Olanzapine and haloperidol	Post-operative delirium	Ib	Better results, at least initially, with haloperidol
Atypical antipsychotic drugs	Olanzapine	Delirium of all types	III	Claimed equivalent efficacy to haloperidol with fewer unwanted effects but data unsound to conclude efficacy
Atypical antipsychotic drugs	Riperidone vs haloperidol	Delirium	Ib	Risperidone better but in spite of small numbers suggested repeat study not carried out yet
	Quetiapine	Delirium (general)	III	No adequate studies
	Remoxipride	Delirium with dementia	III	Alleged benefit with inadequate support
Benzodiazepines	Lorazepam	Delirium of all types	Ib	Of limited efficacy, tends to impair cognition
Combined typical antipsychotic drugs and benzodiazepines	Haloperidol and lorazepam	Delirium	III	Slight evidence of similar efficacy to typical antipsychotic drugs at a lower dose and fewer extrapyramidal symptoms. This is a preferred pharmacological combination
Combined benzodiazepines and opioids	Diazepam and flunitrazepam, pethidine	Prevention of post-operative delirium	IIb	Results suggest benefit from combination but are at some variance from other data
5-HT$_3$ receptor antagonist	Odansetron	Post-operative delirium	III	Before–after study only with short time period
Cholinesterase inhibitors	Donepezil, Rivastigmine	Mixed causes of delirium	III	Case report success only
Tetracyclic antidepressants	Mianserin	Delirium of all types	IIa	Equivalent efficacy to haloperidol
Psychostimulants	Methylphenidate	Hypoactive delirium in terminal illness	III	Before–after study only
Electroconvulsive therapy	Bilateral (most cases)	Delirium tremens in particular	III	Weak evidence from case reports
Optimal environment manipulation in those at risk	Specific interventions by staff and creation of homely normalizing environments	Delirium of all types	Ib	One randomized trial supportive of intervention

REFERENCES

Adams, F., Fernandez, F. & Andersson, B. (1986). Emergency pharmacotherapy of delirium in the critically ill cancer patient. *Psychosomatics*, **27** (Suppl. 1), 33–7.

Aizawa, K., Kanai, T., Saikawa, Y. *et al.* (2002). A novel approach to the prevention of post-operative delirium in the elderly after gastrointestinal surgery. *Surgery Today*, **32**, 310–14.

Akechi, T., Uchitomi, Y., Okamura, H. *et al.* (1996). Usage of haloperidol for delirium in cancer patients. *Support Care Cancer*, **4**, 390–2.

American Psychiatric Association (1999). Practice guideline for the treatment of patients with delirium. *American Journal of Psychiatry*, **156** (May suppl.), 1–20.

Bayindir, O., Akpinar, B., Can, E. *et al.* (2000). The use of 5-HT$_3$ receptor antagonist ondansetron for the treatment of post-cardiotomy delirium. *Journal of Cardiothoracic and Vascular Anesthesia*, **14**, 288–92.

Blitzstein, S. M. & Brandt, G. T. (1997). Extrapyramidal symptoms from intravenous haloperidol in the treatment of delirium. *American Journal of Psychiatry*, **154**, 1474–5.

Breitbart, W., Marotta, R., Platt, M. *et al.* (1996). A double-blind trial of haloperidol, chlorpromazine and lorazepam in the treatment of delirium in hospitalized AIDS patients. *American Journal of Psychiatry*, **153**, 231–7.

Breitbart, W., Tremblay, A. & Gibson, C. (2002). An open trial of olanzapine for the treatment of delirium in hospitalized cancer patients. *Psychosomatics*, **43**, 175–82.

Britton, A. & Russell, R. (2004). Multidisciplinary team interventions for delirium in patients with chronic cognitive impairment. *Cochrane Database of Systematic Reviews*, **2**, CD000395.

Brown, T. M. & Boyle, M. F. (2002). Delirium. *British Medical Journal*, **325**, 644–7.

Budd, S. & Brown, W. (1974). Effect of a reorientation technique on postcardiotomy delirium. *Nursing Research*, **23**, 341–8.

Carnes, M., Howell, T., Rosenberg, M. *et al.* (2003). Physicians vary in approaches to the clinical management of delirium. *Journal of the American Geriatrics Society*, **51**, 234–9.

Chatham, M. A. (1978). The effect of family involvement on patients' manifestations of postcardiotomy psychosis. *Heart & Lung*, **7**, 995–9.

Cole, M. G. (2004). Delirium in elderly patients. *American Journal of Geriatric Psychiatry*, **12**, 7–21.

Cole, M. G., Primeau, F. J., Bailey, R. F. *et al.* (1994). Systematic intervention for elderly inpatients with delirium: a randomized trial. *Canadian Medical Association Journal*, **151**, 965–70.

Cole, M. G., McCusker, J., Bellavance, F. *et al.* (2002). Systematic detection and multidisciplinary care of delirium in older medical inpatients: a randomized trail. *Canadian Medical Association Journal*, **167**, 753–9.

Coppen, A., Gupta, R., Montgomery, S. *et al.* (1976). Mianserin hydrochloride: a novel antidepressant. *British Journal of Psychiatry*, **129**, 342–5.

Davis, J. M., Janicak, P. G., Sakkas, P. *et al.* (1991). Electroconvulsive therapy in the treatment of the neuroleptic malignant syndrome. *Convulsive Therapy*, **7**, 111–20.

Dudley, W. H. & Williams, J. G. (1972). Electroconvulsive therapy in delirium tremens. *Comprehensive Psychiatry*, **13**, 357–60.

Dugovic, C. & Adrien, J. (1991). 5-HT receptors involved in sleep regulation. In *Biological Psychiatry*, Vol. 2, ed. G. K. Racagni, N. Brunllo & T. Fukuda, pp. 710–12. Amsterdam: Elsevier.

Fernandez, F. & Levy, J. K. (1989). Management of delirium in terminally ill AIDS patients. *International Journal of Psychiatry in Medicine*, **19**, 165–72.

Fischer, P. (2001). Successful treatment of nonanticholinergic delirium with a cholinesterase inhibitor. *Journal of Clinical Psychopharmacology*, **21**, 118.

Foreman, M. D., Mion, L. C., Tryostad, L. *et al.* (1999). Standard of practice protocol: acute confusion/delirium. *Geriatric Nursing*, **20**, 147–52.

Gagnon, B., Low, G., Schreier, G. *et al.* (2005). Methylphenidate hydrochloride improves cognitive function in patients with advanced cancer and hypoactive delirium: a prospective clinical study. *Journal of Psychiatry and Neuroscience*, **30**, 100–7.

Gustafson, Y., Brannstrom, B., Berggren, D. *et al.* (1991). A geriatric-anesthesiologic program to reduce acute confusional states in elderly patients treated for femoral neck fractures. *Journal of the American Geriatrics Society*, **39**, 655–62.

Hales, R. E. & Yudofsky, S. C., ed. (2003). *Textbook of Clinical Psychiatry*. American Psychiatric Publishing Inc.

Han, C. & Kim, Y. (2004). A double-blind trial of risperidone and haloperidol for the treatment of delirium. *Psychosomatics*, **45**, 297–301.

Hanania, M. & Kitain, E. (2002). Melatonin for treatment and prevention of post-operative delirium. *Anesthesia and Analgesia*, **94**, 338–9.

Horikawa, N., Yamazaki, T., Miyamoto, K. *et al.* (2003). Treatment for delirium with risperidone: results of a prospective open trial with 10 patients. *General Hospital Psychiatry*, **25**, 289–92.

Jacobi, J., Fraser, G. L., Coursin, D. B. *et al.* (2002). Clinical practice guidelines for the sustained use of sedatives and analgesics in the critically ill adult. *Critical Care Medicine*, **30**, 119–41.

Kalisvaart, C. J., Boelaarts, L., DeJonghe, J. F. *et al.* (2004). Successful treatment of three elderly patients suffering from prolonged delirium using the cholinesterase inhibitor rivastigmine. *Nederlands Tijdschrift voor Geneeskunde*, **148**, 1501–4 (in Dutch).

Kim, K. Y., Bader, G. M., Kotlyar, V. *et al.* (2003). Treatment of delirium in older adults with quetiapine. *Journal of Geriatric Psychiatry and Neurology*, **16**, 29–31.

Kim, K., Pae, C., Chae, J. *et al.* (2001). An open pilot trial of olanzapine for delirium in the Korean population. *Psychiatry and Clinical Neurosciences*, **55**, 515–19.

Leso, L. & Schwartz, T. L. (2002). Ziprasidone treatment of delirium. *Psychosomatics*, **43**, 61–2.

Liu, C., Juang, Y., Liang, H. *et al.* (2004). Efficacy of risperidone in treating the hyperactive symptoms of delirium. *International Clinical Psychopharmacology*, **19**, 165–8.

Marshall, R. J. (1983). The pharmacology of mianserin – an update. *British Journal of Clinical Pharmacology*, **15**, 263S–8S.

Meagher, D. J., O'Hanlon, D., O'Mahoney, E. & Casey, P. R. (1996). The use of environmental strategies and psychotropic medication in the management of delirium. *British Journal of Psychiatry*, **168**, 512–15.

Menza, M. A., Murray, G. B., Holmes, V. F. *et al.* (1987). Decreased extrapyramidal symptoms with intravenous haloperidol. *Journal of Clinical Psychiatry*, **48**, 278–80.

Menza, M. A., Murray, G. B., Holmes, V. F. *et al.* (1988). Controlled study of extrapyramidal reactions in the management of delirious, medically ill patients: intravenous haloperidol versus intravenous haloperidol plus benzodiazepines. *Heart and Lung*, **17**, 238–41.

Meyers, B. J. & Van Ojen, R. L. (2004). The treatment with methylphenidate of demoralisation, apathy and hypoactive delirium in patients with somatic illness. *Nederlands Tijdschrift voor Geneeskunde*, **148**, 1738–41 (in Dutch).

Milisen, K., Foreman, M. D., Abraham, I. L. *et al.* (2001). A nurse-led interdisciplinary intervention program for delirium in elderly hip-fracture patients. *Journal of the American Geriatrics Society*, **49**, 523–32.

Morita, T. Otani, H., Tsunoda, J. *et al.* (2000). Successful palliation of hypoactive delirium due to multi-organ failure by oral methylphenidate. *Support Care Cancer*, **8**, 134–7.

Moulaert, P. (1989). Treatment of nonspecific delirium with IV haloperidol in surgical intensive care patients. *Acta Anaesthesiologica Belgica*, **40**, 183–6.

Nakamura, J., Uchimura, N. & Yamada, S. (1997a). Does plasma free-3-methoxy-4-hydroxyphenyl (ethylene) glycol increase in the delirious state? A comparison of the effects of mianserin and haloperidol on delirium. *International Clinical Psychopharmacology*, **12**, 147–52.

Nakamura, J., Uchimura, N., Yamada, S. *et al.* (1997b). Mianserin suppositories in the treatment of post-operative delirium. *Human Psychopharmacology*, **12**, 595–9.

Okamoto, Y., Matsuoka, Y., Sasaki, T. *et al.* (1999). Trazodone in the treatment of delirium. *Journal of Clinical Psycho-pharmacology*, **19**, 280–2.

Olofsson, S. M., Weitzner, M. A., Valentine, A. D. *et al.* (1996). A retrospective study of the psychiatric management and outcome of delirium in the cancer patient. *Support Care Cancer*, **4**, 351–7.

Parellada, E., Baeza, I., de Pablo, J. *et al.* (2004). Risperidone in the treatment of patients with delirium. *Journal of Clinical Psychiatry*, **65**, 348–53.

Pinder, R. M. (1983). Antidepressants and α-adrenoreceptors. In *Clinical Pharmacology in Psychiatry: Bridging the Experimental–Therapeutic Gap*, ed. L. Gram, pp. 268–87. London: Macmillan.

Platt, M. M., Breitbart, W., Smith, M. *et al.* (1994). Efficacy of neuroleptics for hypoactive delirium. *Journal of Neuropsychiatry*, **6**, 66–7.

Ravona-Springer, R., Ramit, M. D., Ornah, T. *et al.* (1998). Delirium in elderly patients treated with risperidone: a report of three cases. *Journal of Clinical Psychopharmacology*, **18**, 171–2.

Resnick, M. & Burton, B. T. (1984). Droperidol vs. haloperidol in the initial management of acutely agitated patients. *Journal of Clinical Psychiatry*, **45**, 298–9.

Riker, R. R., Fraser, G. L., Gilles, L. *et al.* (1997). Movement disorders associated with withdrawal from high-dose intravenous haloperidol therapy in delirious ICU patients. *Chest*, **111**, 1778–81.

Robertson, B., Karlsson, I., Eriksson, L. *et al.* (1996). An atypical neuroleptic drug in the treatment of behavioural disturbances and psychotic symptoms in elderly people. *Dementia*, **7**, 142–6.

Sanders, K. M., Stern, T. A., O'Gara, P. T. *et al.* (1992). Delirium during intra-aortic balloon pump therapy. *Psychosomatics*, **33**, 35–44.

Sasaki, Y., Matsuyama, T., Inoue, S. *et al.* (2003). A prospective, open-label, flexible-dose study of quetiapine in the treatment of delirium. *Journal of Clinical Psychiatry*, **64**, 1316–21.

Scheftner, W. A. & Shulman, R. B. (1992). Treatment choice in neuroleptic malignant syndrome. *Convulsive Therapy*, **8**, 267–79.

Schwartz, T. L. & Masand, P. S. (2000). Treatment of delirium with quetiapine. *Primary Care Companion Journal of Clinical Psychiatry*, **2**, 10–12.

Seneff, M. G. & Mathews, R. A. (1995). Use of haloperidol infusions to control delirium in critically ill adults. *Annals of Pharmacotherapy*, **29**, 690–3.

Sipahimalani, A., Sime, R. M. & Masand, P. S. (1997). Treatment of delirium with risperidone. *International Journal of Geriatric Psychopharmacology*, **1**, 24–6.

Sipahimalani, A. & Masand, P. S. (1998). Olanzapine in the treatment of delirium. *Psychosomatics*, **39**, 422–30.

Skrobik, Y. (2002). Haloperidol should be used sparingly. *Critical Care Medicine*, **30**, 2613–14.

Skrobik, Y. K., Bergeron, N., Dumont, M. *et al.* (2004). Olanzapine vs haloperidol: treating delirium in a critical care setting. *Intensive Care Medicine*, **30**, 444–9.

Someya, T., Endo, Hara, T. *et al.* (2001). A survey on the drug therapy for delirium. *Psychiatry and Clinical Neurosciences*, **55**, 397–401.

Stiefel, F., Fainsinger, R. & Bruera, E. (1992). Acute confusional states in patients with advanced cancer. *Journal of Pain and Symptom Management*, **7**, 94–8.

Tauscher, J., Tauscher-Wisniewski, D. & Kasper, S. (2000). Treatment of patients with delirium. *American Journal of Psychiatry*, **157**, 1711.

Tei, Y., Morita, T., Inoue, S. *et al.* (2004). Torsades de pointes caused by a small dose of risperidone in a terminally ill cancer patient. *Psychosomatics*, **45**, 450–1.

Thomas, H., Schwartz, E. & Petrilli, R. (1992). Droperidol versus haloperidol for chemical restraint of agitated and combative patients. *Annals of Emergency Medicine*, **21**, 407–13.

Trzepacz, P. T., Ho, V. & Mallavarapu, H. (1996). Cholinergic delirium and neurotoxicity associated with tacrine for Alzheimer's dementia. *Psychosomatics*, **37**, 299–301.

Trzepacz, P. T. (2000). Is there a final common neural pathway in delirium? Focus on acetylcholine and dopamine. *Seminars in Clinical Neuropsychiatry*, **5**, 132–48.

Uchiyama, M., Tanaka, K., Isse, K. *et al.* (1996). Efficacy of mianserin on symptoms of delirium in the aged: an open trial study. *Progress in Neuro-Psychopharmacology & Biological Psychiatry*, **20**, 651–6.

Van der Mast, R. C. & Fekkes, D. (2000). Serotonin and amino acids: partners in delirium pathophysiology. *Seminars in Clinical Neuropsychiatry*, **5**, 125–31.

Wengel, S. P., Roccaforte, W. H. & Burke, W. J. (1998). Donepezil improves symptoms of delirium in dementia: implications for future research. *Journal of Geriatric Psychiatry and Neurology*, **11**, 159–61.

Wengel, S. P., Burke, W. J. & Roccaforte, W. H. (1999). Donepezil for post-operative delirium associated with Alzheimer's disease. *Journal of the American Geriatric Society*, **47**, 379–80.

Williams, M. A., Campbell, E. B., Raynor, W. J. *et al.* (1985). Reducing acute confusional states in elderly patients with hip fractures. *Research in Nursing and Health*, **8**, 329–37.

Young, C. C. & Lujan, E. (2004). Intravenous ziprasidone for treatment of delirium in the intensive care unit. *Anesthesiology*, **101**, 794–5.

10

Management of behavioural and psychological symptoms of dementia and acquired brain injury

Joel Sadavoy, Krista L. Lanctôt and Shoumitro Deb

Editor's note

The practical management of the behavioural symptoms of dementia is one of the most pressing subjects in psychiatry. It is this, more than any other form of treatment, that decides whether a sufferer from dementia stays at home, in supported accommodation, or in hospital. It is therefore a very important subject, and this chapter illustrates what tends to happen when many hard-working and well-meaning clinicians decide, more or less independently, to investigate the value of different treatments. We get a large number of rating scales for assessment that overlap considerably, many published studies and many controlled trials that are difficult to combine in meta-analyses. As a consequence we derive a relatively poor evidence base, particularly in acquired brain injury, that makes it very difficult for the practitioner to choose how to proceed. But we must not be too unfair. The diagnostic system has not helped clinicians in the management of these symptoms and the notion of BPSD (Behavioural and Psychological Symptoms of Dementia) is a relatively recent one. It appears to be a good foundation on which to build.

Introduction

Non-cognitive symptoms of dementia have been labelled in different ways depending on the focus of the observation: agitation (Cohen-Mansfield et al., 1989), behavioural disturbance (Baumgarten et al., 1990), and dysfunctional behaviour (Malloy et al., 1991), to name a few. A common and more comprehensive terminology was proposed in 1998 by the International Psychogeriatric Association, based on a series of consensus meetings, this being Behavioural and Psychological Symptoms of Dementia

or BPSD (Finkel et al., 1996; International Psychogeriatric Association, 1998, 2002). This term encompasses the array of behaviour and psychological disturbances that may emerge in the course of dementia. It is not a diagnostic term per se but is a useful short hand. Like BPSD, the term agitation has utility both theoretically and empirically. It has been defined by Cohen-Mansfield & Billig (1986) as inappropriate verbal, vocal or motor activity that is not judged by an outside observer to result directly from the needs or confusion of the agitated individual.

Behavioural disturbances associated with dementia are very common and at some points in the disease process close to universal; BPSD may emerge at any time in the course of dementia, with rates of emergence of symptoms ranging from 26–93% of patients (Zimmer et al., 1984; Cohen-Mansfield et al., 1989; Devanand et al., 1997; Lyketsos et al., 2000; Brodaty et al., 2001). In US nursing homes the prevalence of behavioural problems ranges between 53% and 83% (Zimmer et al., 1984; Swearer et al., 1988). Nagaratnam et al. (1998) studying 90 dementia patients in the community, found that 59% had aggression, 27% wandering and 22% had delusions. These symptoms led many to be institutionalized because of the degree of caregiver stress induced by these behaviours.

Rubin et al. (1988) described seven types of behaviour causing problems, namely memory disturbance, physical violence, hitting, incontinence, catastrophic reactions, suspiciousness and accusatory behaviour. Cohen-Mansfield et al. (1989, 1992) have summarized the clinical profile of the agitated patient in three categories: the aggressive resident – demented, married, male with poor interpersonal interactions, a history of aggressive behaviour prior to entry into the nursing home, and likely to fall; the verbally agitated resident – a non-demented or early dementia female, sicker than other nursing home residents (i.e. more medical diagnoses, more pain, greater

Cambridge Textbook of Effective Treatments in Psychiatry, ed. Peter Tyrer and Kenneth R. Silk. Published by Cambridge University Press.
© Cambridge University Press, 2008.

vision loss), depressed affect, negative interpersonal experiences and likely to fall; the *physically non-aggressive resident* – demented, relatively younger, has lived in the nursing home for a shorter period, healthier than the average resident, a history of more stress earlier in life, often described as being agitated prior to nursing home entry and tends to fall. The highest levels of physically non-aggressive behaviours are manifested by residents who have severe cognitive impairment yet retain some ability to perform activities of daily living (ADL). The majority of agitated behaviour is associated with comorbid states of psychosis and depression (Brodaty *et al.*, 2001).

Since the mid 1980s many rating scales have been developed to measure this important set of phenomena of dementia including Behavioural and Emotional Activities Manifested in Dementia (BEAM-D) (Sinha D *et al.*, 1992), Behavioural Pathology in Alzheimer's Disease Rating Scale (BEHAVE-AD) (Reisberg *et al.*, 1996), Brief Agitation Rating Scale (BARS) (Finkel *et al.*, 1993), Caretaker Obstreperous Behaviour Rating Scale (COBRA) (Drachman *et al.*, 1992), CERAD Behaviour Rating Scale for Dementia (Tariot *et al.*, 1996), Cohen-Mansfield Agitation Inventory (CMAI) (Cohen-Mansfield *et al.*, 1989), Dementia Behaviour Disturbance Scale (DBD) (Baumgarten *et al.*, 1990), Dysfunctional Behaviour Rating Instrument (DBR) (Malloy *et al.*, 1991), Global Assessment of Psychiatric Symptoms (GAPS) (Raskin *et al.*, 1988), Irritability/Apathy Scale (Burns *et al.*, 1990), Manchester and Oxford Universities Scale for the Psychopathological Assessment of Dementia (MOUSEPAD) (Allen *et al.*, 1996), Neurobehavioural Rating Scale (Levin *et al.*, 1987), Neuropsychiatric Inventory (NPI) (Cummings *et al.*, 1994), Pittsburgh Agitation Scale (Rosen *et al.*, 1994), and Revised Memory and behaviour Problems Checklist (Teri *et al.*, 1992). Use of the Minimum Data Set (MDS) is a systematic approach to recording behaviour in nursing home residents in the USA. It is commonly employed to assess behaviour problems and appears to have good interrater reliability coefficients and concurrent validity correlations (Snowden *et al.*, 2003).

While many scales have been developed to measure BPSD, relatively few controlled clinical trials of interventions have followed, this is surprising considering the clinical importance of these disturbances. What has emerged is that management of behavioural disturbances associated with dementia is complex and requires a full array of interventions including pharmacological and non-pharmacological approaches. This perspective is evident in the American Psychiatric Association Practice Guidelines for the treatment of patients with Alzheimer's disease and other dementias of late life (1997). The integrated approach they describe follows from the fact that the various presentations of BPSD are often of unknown or highly complex origin. For example, risk factors for harm due to self-neglect in cognitively impaired seniors who live alone include perception of fewer social resources, poorer performance on Mini-Mental State Examination (MMSE), presence of chronic obstructive pulmonary disease (COPD) and cerebrovascular disorders (Tierney *et al.*, 2004).

Pharmacotherapy in management of behaviour and psychological symptoms of dementia

Given the high prevalence and recognized impact of BPSD on both the patients and their caregivers, various drug treatments have been evaluated for efficacy and safety in treating these symptoms. There are five main therapeutic classes of medications that have varying degrees of evidence supporting their use in the treatment of BPSD: antipsychotics, cholinesterase inhibitors, antidepressants, benzodiazepines and mood stabilizers (Sink *et al.*, 2005). There are also additional pharmacotherapies ('other') with limited evidence that will be reviewed. The emphasis for this review will be on randomized controlled trials (RCTs) and meta-analyses. Safety issues of particular concern will also be highlighted.

Antipsychotics

Antipsychotics are the most frequently used medications for the control of moderate to severe BPSD (Grohmann *et al.*, 2004). Both conventional and atypical antipsychotics have been studied for BPSD in RCTs. Published guidelines (Herrmann, 2001; Howard *et al.*, 2001; International Psychogeriatric Association, 2002; Lawlor, 2004) list atypical or high potency conventional antipsychotics as a first-line treatment for BPSD. Treatment-responsive symptoms include psychotic symptoms (delusions and hallucinations), hostility, aggression, motor agitation and sleep-wake cycle disturbances (Rabinowitz *et al.*, 2004). Diagnostic criteria for psychosis in Alzheimer's disease have now been published (Jeste & Finkel, 2000).

In total, 17 RCTs involving about 500 patients on conventional antipsychotics and 235 controls have been published evaluating conventional antipsychotics (Lanctot *et al.*, 1998; De Deyn *et al.*, 1999). Meta-analysis of the randomized controlled trials have found that while antipsychotics have a response rate of about 64%, their therapeutic effect (drug placebo difference) is only 18–26% (Schneider *et al.*, 1990; Lanctôt *et al.*, 1998). Conventional antipsychotics have small but significant efficacy over placebo for treatment of BPSD, and the efficacy rate is equivalent to the side-effect rate (Schneider *et al.*, 1990; Lanctôt *et al.*, 1998). High potency antipsychotics such as haloperidol (0.5–2 mg/day) are currently recommended for BPSD.

There are also seven RCTs (1500 patients atypical, 560 placebo) that have been published utilizing the atypical antipsychotics risperidone (0.5 to 2 mg/day) (DeDeyn *et al.*, 1999; Katz *et al.*, 1999; Chan *et al.*, 2001; Brodaty *et al.*, 2003), olanzapine (5–10 mg/day) (Street *et al.*, 2000, 2001; De Deyn *et al.*, 2004) and quetiapine (25–150 mg/day) (Ballard *et al.*, 2005) in Alzheimer's disease and related dementias. Anxiety may respond also (Mintzer *et al.*, 2001). Together over 2000 patients have been studied in the RCTs of atypical antipsychotics. Overall, these RCTs confirm the efficacy of atypical antipsychotics for BPSD. Although efficacy may be similar, olanzapine is more anticholinergic than risperidone (Mulsant *et al.*, 2004) or quetiapine. In the two trials comparing risperidone to the conventional antipsychotic haloperidol (De Deyn *et al.*, 1999; Chan *et al.*, 2001), efficacy was similar. Olanzapine has also been shown to have efficacy for BPSD in dementia with Lewy bodies in one subanalysis (Cummings *et al.*, 2002), and the use of quetiapine supported in a case series (Takahashi *et al.*, 2003). With atypical antipsychotics in Lewy Body dementia (DLB), there has been no significant exacerbation of parkinsonian symptoms (Cummings *et al.*, 2002; Takahashi *et al.*, 2003).

Of concern, the RCTs of risperidone, olanzapine and quetiapine in elderly dementia patients suggested an approximate doubling of the risk of cerebrovascular adverse events compared with placebo (Wooltorton, 2002, 2004; Herrmann *et al.*, 2004b; De Deyn *et al.*, 2005). Subsequent warnings by drug regulatory authorities based on 17 published and unpublished studies have noted an increased risk of mortality with olanzapine, aripiprazole, risperidone and quetiapine compared with placebo (4.5% vs 2.6%) in those being treated for BPSD. The 1.6–1.7 times increase in mortality risk appeared to be related mainly to cardiovascular (e.g. heart failure, sudden death) or infectious (e.g. pneumonia) causes. While the role that vascular risk factors have played in this increase (Herrmann *et al.*, 2004b) is unclear, it is now suggested that care be taken in patients with vascular risk factors. Vascular dementia may account for 15–20% of all dementia cases (Nyenhuis & Gorelick, 1998) and Alzheimer's disease is commonly mixed with vascular dementia. Despite the fact that the recent evidence has concentrated on atypical antipsychotics, a large retrospective community-based database study found no difference between risk of stroke with atypical antipsychotics versus conventional typical ones (Herrmann *et al.*, 2004b). High potency conventional antipsychotics such as haloperidol are also associated with extrapyramidal symptoms (Lawlor, 2004), and are

contraindicated in Lewy Body dementia, and in general, their poor adverse-effect profile should make prescribers cautious in this population.

In summary, both atypical and conventional antipsychotics have demonstrated efficacy in BPSD. The decision to use these agents must be weighed against the possibility of extrapyramidal side effects, cerebrovascular adverse events and increased mortality.

Antidepressants

Antidepressants used in the treatment of BPSD include SSRIs (Cutler *et al.*, 1985; Dehlin *et al.*, 1985; Nyth & Gottfries, 1990; Olafsson *et al.*, 1992; Burke *et al.*, 1994; Auchus & Bissey-Black, 1997; Taragano *et al.*, 1997; Katona *et al.*, 1998; Lanctôt *et al.*, 2002; Pollock *et al.*, 2002), trazodone (Lawlor *et al.*, 1994; Sultzer *et al.*, 1997) and buspirone (Cantillon *et al.*, 1996; Lawlor *et al.*, 1994). The SSRIs studied in RCTs include fluoxetine (Auchus & Bissey-Black, 1997; Taragano *et al.*, 1997), paroxetine (Katona *et al.*, 1998), fluvoxamine (Olafsson *et al.*, 1992), sertraline (Finkel *et al.*, 2004; Lanctôt *et al.*, 2002; Lyketsos *et al.*, 2000, 2003) and citalopram (Nyth & Gottfries, 1990; Pollock *et al.*, 2002). Of these, citalopram shows the greatest efficacy in randomized controlled trials (Nyth & Gottfries, 1990; Pollock *et al.*, 2002). Pollock *et al.* (2005) showed that citalopram had efficacy similar to that of perphenazine. Besides depressive symptoms (Burke *et al.*, 1997; Taragano *et al.*, 1997; Katona *et al.*, 1998; Lyketsos *et al.*, 2000, 2003), agitation, irritability and aberrant motor behaviour may respond to SSRIs in non-depressed patients (Lanctot *et al.*, 2002; Pollock *et al.*, 2002). Additionally, sertraline was shown to have some efficacy over placebo in those stabilized on donepezil for the treatment of BPSD (Finkel *et al.*, 2004). The two trials with trazodone (Sultzer *et al.*, 1997) showed that repetitive behaviours, verbal aggression and oppositional behaviours were drug responsive (Lawlor *et al.*, 1994; Sultzer *et al.*, 1997). Additionally, trazodone can be used when sedation is required, although it is also associated with orthostatic hypotension. Buspirone has limited efficacy in BPSD. Venlafaxine (Oslin *et al.*, 2003) and mirtazapine (Schatzberg *et al.*, 2002) have been shown to be efficacious and safe for depression in the frail elderly (Rabheru, 2004), but there are no RCTs specifically for BPSD. The use of SSRIs has been associated with syndrome of inappropriate antidiuretic hormone secretion (SIADH) in the elderly (Jackson *et al.*, 1995). Tricyclic antidepressants have also been used for depression in dementia (Petracca *et al.*, 1996; Reifler *et al.*, 1989; Taragano *et al.*, 1997), but even the secondary amines (nortriptyline and desipramine) should be used with caution due to postural hypotension, anticholinergic effects and intracardiac conduction defects. Overall, there is strong support for treating depression in dementia with SSRIs, and so it is important to identify this disorder. In general, venlafaxine and mirtazapine are safe in the elderly, and there is some evidence supporting the use of citalopram specifically for BPSD, but more independent studies are needed.

Cognitive enhancers

The efficacy of the cholinesterase inhibitors in treating BPSD is supported by many open-label studies, but a limited number of RCTs. In other words, it is weak. One meta-analysis assessing efficacy of cholinesterase inhibitors in mild to moderate AD patients used six RCTs and found a small but statistically significant (95% CI, 0.87–2.57) improvement in total Neuropsychiatric Inventory (NPI) scores compared with placebo (Trinh et al., 2003). One factor undermining the results of that meta-analysis was the inclusion of metrifonate (not approved) (Herrmann & Knopman, 2004). Individually, the efficacy of donepezil (Feldman et al., 2001; Holmes et al., 2004), galantamine (Tariot et al., 2000) and rivastigmine (Rosler et al., 1998) are supported by RCTs, but inconsistently, with some negative trials (Rockwood et al., 2001; Tariot et al., 2001a). Similarly, meta-analyses support the efficacy of galantamine (Loy & Schneider, 2004) and donepezil (Birks & Harvey, 2003), although the results are not significant across all time points studied. While the majority of RCTs are in those with mild BPSD and mild to moderate AD, there is some evidence in those with moderate to severe AD (Feldman et al., 2001) and marked BPSD (Holmes et al., 2004). Patients with Alzheimer's disease who exhibit pretreatment delusions, agitation, depression, anxiety, apathy, disinhibition and irritability are more likely to improve with cholinesterase inhibitors, particularly if they have the symptoms of anxiety, delusions, depression and irritability (Mega et al., 1999).

Cholinesterase inhibitors have also been shown to have efficacy for BPSD with Lewy Body dementia (McKeith et al., 2000), with better response in those with delusions, hallucinations, apathy and anxiety. As well, BPSD may respond to cholinesterase inhibitor treatment in patients with vascular dementia or AD mixed with vascular dementia (Erkinjuntti et al., 2002; Erkinjuntti et al., 2004).

With memantine (20 mg/day), two RCTs totalling 650 patients showed a significant efficacy for BPSD in those with moderate to severe Alzheimer's disease (Reisberg et al., 2003; Tariot et al., 2004). One of these (Tariot et al., 2004) was in patients already stabilized on donepezil. In addition, a published meta-analysis confirmed the efficacy

of memantine for BPSD in Alzheimer's disease (Areosa et al., 2005) and vascular dementia (Areosa et al., 2005).

Anticonvulsants

The anticonvulsants carbamazepine (Tariot et al., 1994, 1998; Olin et al., 2001), valproate (Porsteinsson et al., 2001; Tariot et al., 2001b; Sival et al., 2002) and gabapentin (Moretti et al., 2003) have been studied for their efficacy in treating BPSD. For carbamazepine (100–300 mg daily) there have been three placebo controlled trials (Tariot et al., 1994, 1998; Olin et al., 2001) and a confirmatory washout (Tariot et al., 1999) supporting efficacy for BPSD over 6–12 weeks. Drug-responsive symptoms were agitation and aggression. Thus, placebo-controlled trials of carbamazepine support its efficacy in the treatment of aggression and agitation in dementia. The three RCTs for divalproex sodium (sodium valproate) (375–1375 mg daily) showed that agitation and aggression were drug-responsive symptoms, albeit in a limited number of patients (Porsteinsson et al., 2001; Tariot et al., 2001b; Sival et al., 2002). Unfortunately, at the dosages needed to achieve therapeutic effect, tolerability appears to be a concern. A recent meta-analysis concluded that low dose sodium valproate is ineffective in treating agitation among demented patients, and that high dose divalproex sodium is associated with an unacceptable rate of adverse effects (Lonergan et al., 2004). Thrombocytopaenia is now being recognized as a relatively frequent side effect of valproate treatment in the elderly, necessitating careful monitoring (Trannel et al., 2001; So & Wong, 2002). Current evidence does not support the use of this agent (Lonergan et al., 2004). For gabapentin, there are no randomized placebo-controlled trials as yet. The single open-label trial of gabapentin to date (Moretti et al., 2003) suggested that agitation, anxiety, aggressiveness and sleep disturbances were treatment responsive, and, while no serious adverse events were reported, sedation was noted to be a problem.

Benzodiazepines

The benzodiazepine class of drugs has been used for many years to reduce anxiety and promote sleep in the population with dementia. Benzodiazepines studied in RCTs to date include alprazolam (Ancill et al., 1991; Christensen & Benfield, 1998), diazepam (Covington, 1975; Stotsky, 1984), lorazepam (Sunderland et al., 1989; Ancill et al., 1991; Meehan et al., 2002) and oxazepam (Beber, 1965; Chesrow et al., 1965; Sanders, 1965; Coccaro et al., 1990; Herz et al., 1992). Drug-responsive symptoms include anxiety, tension, irritability and insomnia. For zolpidem, a non-benzodiazepine hypnotic, there have been case reports suggesting efficacy in BPSD (Jackson *et al.*, 1996; Shelton & Hocking, 1997) including one RCT for insomnia and night-time behaviours (Shaw *et al.*, 1992), but no RCTs specifically for BPSD. For acute control of BPSD, intramuscular lorazepam has shown efficacy (Meehan *et al.*, 2002). In comparative studies, benzodiazepines with different kinetics had similar efficacy (Ancill *et al.*, 1991) and efficacy of benzodiazepines was slightly less than (Covington, 1975; Stotsky, 1984; Herz *et al.*, 1992) or similar to (Coccaro *et al.*, 1990; Christensen & Benfield, 1998) that of conventional antipsychotics. Unfortunately, these agents may produce tolerance after long-term use as well as other side effects such as sedation, dizziness and ataxia. In summary, from the evidence to date, benzodiazepines can be useful in managing BPSD. The primary concern with these agents is the potential for adverse events, which may be augmented in an elderly population. Despite the frequent use of these medications (Grohmann *et al.*, 2004), benzodiazepine use is generally discouraged for BPSD and the decision to use them instead of other agents should be based as much on the balance of adverse effects as likely efficacy.

Beta-blockers

As mentioned previously, two very small controlled studies in brain injury patients originally suggested that β-blockers such as propranolol (Greendyke *et al.*, 1986) and pindolol (Greendyke & Kanter, 1986) may be effective for the treatment of behavioural disturbances such as aggression and agitation, with pindolol being better tolerated (Greendyke & Kanter, 1986). Subsequently, an RCT in patients with dementia found that aggression, agitation and anxiety were drug-responsive symptoms (Peskind *et al.*, 2005) to propranolol (mean dose 106 ± 38 mg/day). An RCT by Herrmann *et al.* (2004a) found that aggression was responsive to pindolol (up to 20 mg b.i.d.) in elderly institutionalized patients with dementia. Both RCTs in BPSD found limited efficacy and frequent contraindications to the use of β-blockers (Herrmann *et al.*, 2004a; Peskind *et al.*, 2005).

Other medications

Placebo-controlled RCTs in men with dementia by Kyomen *et al.* (1999) suggested that oestrogens can reduce aggressive behaviour. In uncontrolled trials, medroxyprogesterone (Cooper, 1987) and cyproterone (Nadal & Allgulander, 1993; Haussermann *et al.*, 2003) have also been reported to be effective in a small number of patients with dementia and sexually inappropriate

behaviours. Further trials are needed to confirm the efficacy of hormonal treatments in BPSD (Flynn, 1999).

In a single uncontrolled trial, Galynker *et al.* (1997) used methylphenidate in AD and vascular dementia patients. Individual cross-over, double-blinded, randomized ('N of 1') trials with methylphenidate (5 mg b.i.d.) (Jansen *et al.*, 2001) have also suggested efficacy in a very small number of patients with mixed diagnoses including dementia. While BPSD such as apathy appear to be drug-responsive, many more studies are needed to confirm the efficacy of methylphenidate in apathy associated with dementia.

Conclusions

From this review, it is clear that large randomized, placebo-controlled trials support the efficacy of atypical antipsychotics, conventional antipsychotics and cholinesterase inhibitors for BPSD. Furthermore, randomized controlled trials suggest that depressive symptoms should be treated with appropriate antidepressants in those with dementia. With the exception of treating depressive symptoms and possibly psychotic symptoms associated with dementia, there are no approved pharmacotherapies for the treatment of BPSD. When medications are warranted due to psychotic symptoms, agitation or aggressive behaviours that are moderate or severe, atypical antipsychotics should be considered in those who have not responded to cholinesterase inhibitors. While atypical antipsychotics have been associated with cerebrovascular adverse events, high potency conventional antipsychotics are associated with extrapyramidal symptoms and orthostatic hypotension. Benzodiazepines, while not recommended for long-term use, are effective for anxiety, tension, irritability and insomnia, but they contribute to risk of falls. Beta-blockers and mood stabilizers have some efficacy, but also have considerable safety issues and would be second line. Other medications such as oestrogen and methylphenidate may have efficacy in selected patients, or selected behavioural symptoms such as sexual inappropriateness and apathy.

Non-pharmacological management of non-cognitive symptoms of dementia

This section will address interventions for behavioural disturbances and non-cognitive symptoms associated with dementia and acquired brain injury. Depression and psychosis is addressed in Chapter 12 and will not be further discussed.

Medications are important for management of some BPSD, but many symptoms fail to respond well (Sadavoy,

2004). Behavioural symptoms unlikely to respond to medication and requiring greater emphasis on non-pharmacological interventions include: wandering, pacing and exit seeking, screaming and inappropriate verbalizing, resistance to toileting, inappropriate voiding or spitting, hoarding, withdrawal (to be distinguished from apathy which may be methylphenidate responsive) and some sexual behaviours (although SSRIs or oestrogen may be useful for some forms of disinhibition and aggressive sexuality). Behaviours more likely to be responsive to drugs include some Axis I disorders co-existing with dementia (such as mood disorders), sleep cycle disturbances, hostility and assaultiveness, hyperexcitability, hallucinations and delusions.

Over-reliance on pharmacological management of agitation and BPSD is not only likely to be of limited assistance, but its failure may lead to use of inappropriate management methods such as restraints. Restraint is known to carry risks – strangulation leading to death, bed sores and abrasions of the skin, and physiological and psychological consequences of prolonged immobilization (Evans & Strumpf, 1989). Kirkevold & Engedal (2004) interviewed 1362 carers of residents of nursing homes and 564 in special dementia care units in Norway about use of restraints. Reasons for their use included protection of patients or others and carrying out necessary care, but the key reason for use of force or pressure in medical treatment was patient non-compliance with staff-initiated procedures. Documentation of reasons and process were often not clear, and decisions to use restraints were made by the nurse in charge in most instances. Hence knowledge of appropriate non-pharmacological approaches to non-compliant, difficult to manage patients with dementia is essential, since lack of knowledge easily may lead to inappropriate and even dangerous interventions. This is especially true for front-line staff in chronic care institutions and those who care for demented individuals at home.

Research on non-pharmacologic management has most commonly focused on agitation (without specifying which form). Often medication management has continued while the non-pharmacological intervention is being tested, making effectiveness of the latter interventions even more difficult to interpret (Snowden *et al.*, 2003). Additionally, research has generally been targeted to modifying behaviours. This is problematic in that some behaviours may be more purposeful and communicative of interpersonal connection, distress or need, rather than just the result of neurological failure and cognitive impairments. If this is true then pure behavioural modification needs to be tempered and combined with attempts to understand the potential meaning of some forms of behaviour. For example, apparently aimless wandering may indicate boredom, attempts to get away from a stressful or abusive situation or a search for something familiar and comforting (Carlson *et al.*, 1995). In addressing agitation and other forms of BPSD, one may ask for whom the behaviour is disturbing, the patient or the caregiving environment.

Dementia and impaired psychological well-being

Emotional and psychological responses to dementia are varied and dependent on many possible factors such as premorbid personality (which can affect adaptive capacities), personality change (derived from dementing processes, notably fronto-temporal dementias), issues of abandonment associated with relocation in long-term care facilities, and both capacity for, and reaction to, insight into failing capacities.

From a psychodynamic perspective, all behaviour emerges as an expression of inner conflict, anxiety, experience of loss of others or the self and so on, and this concept has been applied to dementia and BPSD on occasion (Sadavoy, 1991; Jones, 1995). Theoretically the individual with a less maturely developed personality structure will have less effective defences with which to deal with the experience of the erosion of the self as the dementing disease progresses. This may cause some individuals to express their anxiety with increased levels of clinging, wandering attempts to find someone to connect to, demandingness, outcries for help, rage at being abandoned, panic at loss of self-sufficiency and so on. While the evidence-based literature is sparse on individual psychotherapeutic approaches to patients with dementia, data suggests it is needed because much of the therapeutic work with dementing elders in the community is some form of individual psychotherapy (Mosher-Ashley & Witkowski, 1999).

Premorbid personality may relate to the degree of expression of BPSD. Beck *et al.* (1983) theorized that certain personality traits, specifically highly sociotropic individuals, derive their sense of worth and efficacy from meaningful contacts with others, presenting with anxious behaviour when such contact is unavailable. Overly autonomous individuals need mastery and control. When the opportunity for personal achievement is denied by the environment, these individuals may develop behaviour of avoidance and hostility. Hilton & Moniz-Cook (2004) applied this theory to 63 demented patients evaluating them with the Sociotropy Autonomy Scale (SAS). They found that high scores on autonomy and sociotropy (>90) correlated with mood and behaviour difficulties in this sample. They concluded that aspects of personality (i.e. temperament) remain stable in dementia and that an instrument like the SAS can identify older people with dementia who are vulnerable to mood and behaviour problems. They hypothesized that emotion-based traits such as sociotropy and autonomy (similar to agreeableness and hostility) that seem to remain stable in dementia do so because they have a subcortical rather than cortical locus, thereby being spared from the dementia-related personality changes associated with characteristics that rely on cognitive function (Solms & Turnbull, 2002; Siegler *et al.*, 1994).

If these formulations and explanations for some of the expressions of BPSD are correct then they provide a model to caregivers and clinicians to understand the origin of symptoms at a deeper level and perhaps offer a basis for intervention strategies. Certainly, this perspective demands of the clinician and caregiver the need to understand the inner world of the individual patient in order to make sense of the apparently random BPSD expressions. Jones (1995) has proposed elements of interpersonal psychotherapy with demented elders based on a Sullivanian theoretical perspective: tailor interventions to the overall level of the patient's dementia and recognize that the level of impairment may fluctuate from one time to the next; address loss and mourning; deal with catastrophic reactions as the direct result of anxiety; begin the therapeutic relationship as early in the disease as possible to permit an effective therapeutic alliance to develop when the patient still has such a capacity and continue into the later stages of the impairment; attend to the therapist's emotional reactions such as anxiety or depression in dealing with a declining patient and recognize explicitly the frustrations and lack of traditional rewards in working with this type of condition; tailor technique to the level of dementia – confrontation and interpretation become increasingly less relevant as the dementia progresses.

Unfortunately, while psychodynamic and psychotherapeutic perspectives are intuitively attractive, they have been explored only in clinical case descriptions, not controlled research designs (Sadavoy & Robinson, 1989; Jones, 1995; Cohen, 1988; Hausman, 1991; Miller, 1989). However, some data have emerged from studies on the relationship of symptoms to defined personality types. For example, BPSD have been linked to specific personality features: higher premorbid neuroticism linked with increased depression and dysphoria, severity of anxiety and troublesome behaviour (Chaterjee *et al.*, 1992); lower premorbid extraversion and frustration tolerance linked with increased depression (Strauss *et al.*, 1997). Low *et al.* (2002) found higher neuroticism predicted delusions, higher agreeableness predicted hallucinations, aggressiveness, affective disturbance and overall behavioural disturbance; and higher openness predicted affective disorder. Not all studies have shown a relationship between premorbid personality traits and BPSD (Brandt *et al.*, 1998). Aitken *et al.* (1999) examined the prevalence and nature of personality changes in 60 subjects (mean age 79.8 years) with dementia of the Alzheimer type (DAT) and 39 subjects (mean age 80.2 years) with multi-infarct dementia, as well as the relationship of personality changes to other features of the dementia syndrome. Results indicated that personality characteristics were related to the patient's age and sex, duration of illness, degree of cognitive impairment, the presence of a grasp reflex, and extrapyramidal signs. Personality change was found to be almost universal and negative in nature and was particularly associated with severity of cognitive impairment, longer duration of illness, and neurological signs. These findings emphasize the biological basis of personality changes in dementia.

Early symptoms of dementia that are most notable to many caregivers are changes in personality-based behaviours rather than decline in cognitive symptoms. In a study of why families sought memory clinic referral, while cognitive symptoms were prominent reasons (Streams *et al.*, 2003), almost half the caregivers reported non-cognitive symptoms or a combination of cognitive and non-cognitive symptoms as the trigger for seeking diagnostic referral to memory clinics. Of these almost 40% specified at least one personality or behavioural change as the trigger – most common were depressive symptoms, violence and attitude problems, lack of initiative, paranoia and delusions, and decreased cleanliness.

Reminiscence therapy

Personality change is most likely a function of brain change, but some features of emotional response are probably associated with awareness of change in the self and anxiety associated with insight into loss of capacity to deal with the challenges of day-to-day life. To address the interplay between dementia, emotional expression and changes in self-perception, interventions for the emotional and psychological aspects of dementia have included an array of psychosocial techniques (Woods, 1996). Prominent among these are the reminiscence therapies. Comprehensive reviews of the effectiveness of reminiscence therapies in affecting behavioural disturbances of dementia have found that no firm conclusions can yet be drawn from the data (Pusey, 2000; Spector *et al.*, 2003) although recent clinical case study methods suggest emotional benefits for caregivers and patients, but not specific improvement in behavioural disturbances (Haight *et al.*, 2003). There was a trend in Spector *et al.*'s review of the effectiveness of reminiscence in modifying behavioural disturbances, in favour of improved behaviour but not cognition. In a carefully constructed study that took into account weaknesses in prior studies, Lai *et al.* (2004), using a single-blind parallel group randomized controlled trial method (n = 101), investigated the effectiveness of specific reminiscence therapy (defined life story approach) in promoting sustained social well-being in patients with dementia in a nursing home. The outcome was largely negative, but the study did improve some elements of well-being and social engagement so it remains premature to completely abandon this form of intervention at this time. A key question, as is true for all forms of psychotherapy, is which patient is most suited to a given intervention and who is most likely to respond. This question remains unanswered by data at this time.

Reminiscence group therapy, while often used, has not produced encouraging results. However, it is a mainstay of psychotherapeutic interventions despite the lack of positive effectiveness data. Techniques include structured and unstructured encouragement to retrieve past memories using aids such as pictures, with the theoretically based hope that such intervention will help the dementing patient utilize more intact past memories rather than less reliable recent memory. Rehearsing past memories strengthens them and thereby enhances sense of self and perhaps self-esteem. Some positive outcome trends have been found in cognitive performance but not depression or behavioural scores (Goldwasser *et al.*, 1987). Spector *et al.* (1999), in their review of the literature on reminiscence therapy, found only two randomized controlled studies and only one that met criteria for analysis (Baines *et al.*, 1987). Spector *et al.* (1999) concluded that there is insufficient evidence for the effectiveness of formal reminiscence therapy techniques for patients with dementia. In this therapy as in other psychotherapeutic interventions the point is emphasized by some, that subjects included in studies may need to be carefully chosen and intervention individualized, for example controlling for cognitive abilities in order to improve effectiveness (Goldwasser *et al.*, 1987; Ashton, 1993).

Group therapies

Group psychotherapy is perhaps the most common psychotherapeutic intervention used for people with dementia (Cheston, 1998). Key elements of group therapy that are theoretically important for effectiveness include learning new coping strategies and the therapeutic effect of group cohesion, generation of hope, enhancement of self-esteem and so on.

Scott & Clare (2003) reviewed the evidence for group therapy in cognitively impaired patients, beginning with

the perspective that cognitive limitations may reduce the impact of the putative influence of specific group-psychotherapeutic effects. The review focused particularly on reality orientation, validation and reminiscence therapies. Reality orientation (RO) may be implemented in a variety of ways including 24-hour orientation cuing (such as visible calendars, clocks and message boards plus staff reinforcement) or classroom interventions conducted in group formats. Orientation interventions, especially classroom models, incorporate other modalities inherent in the orientation process such as reminiscence and cognitive stimulation so outcomes are difficult to attribute to reality orientation per se (Bird, 2000). Hence studies of reality orientation are methodologically imprecise. Holden & Woods' (1995) review of 21 studies of reality orientation confirmed the wide variation in techniques studied and treatment and control conditions. Overall the review by Scott & Clare (2003) indicates that there may be modest improvement in behaviour, social interaction and functioning, although improvements appear to be largely transient, with the exception of some patients who may retain their improvement as long as the intervention is continued (Brook *et al.*, 1975; Hanley *et al.*, 1981; Baines *et al.*, 1987; Gerber *et al.*, 1991; Woods, 1996). The latter result was found by Reeve & Ivison (1985), using classroom reality orientation in a placebo-controlled outcome study. While methodological problems are evident (small sample size and concurrent environmental and interpersonal interventions) the classroom intervention over a period of one month did seem effective in inducing improved cognition and behaviour. Scott & Clare (2003) conclude that, overall, the results of the reality orientation data are encouraging although highly variable. A recent trial of 156 patients (Onder *et al.*, 2005) showed that reality orientation provided by caregivers, combined with donepezil, was more effective that donezepil alone in improving cognitive function. The reality orientation/donezepil group showed a slight improvement in MMSE scores (mean change + 0.2, s.e. = 0.4) compared with a decline in the control group (mean change −1.1) by the end of treatment after 25 weeks. There was no evidence that this improvement was lost or sustained after the end of treatment.

Validation therapy

Validation therapy derives from a similar perspective to that articulated by Moniz-Cook *et al.* (2003), in that it addresses the need for individual enhancement of personal identity. According to De Klerk-Rubin (1995), the goal of validation therapies is 'to stimulate energy and interaction both verbally and non-verbally, and increase each group member's sense of identity by calling up social roles from the past'. Validation groups include reminiscence, active support from therapists, and activities such as discussion and singing (Morton & Bleathman, 1991). Outcome studies are often poorly controlled so confident conclusions cannot be drawn although some studies are encouraging. One problem in interpretation lies in selection of subjects. Since this is an active intervention requiring patient participation not all patients are appropriate candidates.

Bright light therapy

Kim et al.'s (2003) review of 14 papers on the use of bright light for management of sleep and behavioural disturbance in dementia concluded that the utility of bright light therapy in these domains of dementia remains inconclusive. For example, in a small study (n = 15) Lyketsos et al. (1999) found that bright light therapy improved sleep in agitated elders with dementia but had no effect on behavioural disturbances. However, the debate will continue as marginal effects of different forms and doses of bright light are demonstrated on aspects of the sleep cycle, if not behaviour (Fetveit et al., 2003; Gasio et al., 2003). Ancoli-Israel et al. (2003) evaluated the effect of bright light therapy on agitated behaviour in 92 patients randomly assigned to morning bright light, morning dim red light, or evening bright light. Morning bright light delayed the acrophase of the agitation rhythm by over 1.5 hours. It was also associated with improved caregivers' ratings but had little effect on observational ratings of agitation. The authors suggest that severe AD may benefit less from bright light because of more degeneration of the suprachiasmatic nucleus and that milder forms of dementia may show more benefit. These results contrasted somewhat with an earlier study by the same group that suggested that bright light reduced agitation in demented nursing home residents (Lovell et al., 1995).

Pet therapy

Pet therapy has been used to enhance the experience of elders in long-term care institutions. But caring for pets may be problematic or impossible in a facility so Libin & Cohen Mansfield (2004) experimented with using a plush toy robotic cat and compared its effect with a live cat. There was no significant difference, widening the scope for creative non-pharmacological interventions and perhaps strengthening the theoretical position that dementia-related agitation, in part, is a communication reflecting needs for comfort and contact.

Symptom-specific approaches to general behaviour disturbances (BPSD)

Combined/non-specific approaches to treatment

Kruglov (2003) studied matched control and test groups (n = 95 in each group) to determine the effects of a non-specific array of supportive interventions for mildly disturbed behaviours associated with vascular dementia. In addition to psychotherapy and rehabilitation interventions the subjects were all treated with so-called 'vasoactive' medications (cinnarzine or vinpocetine) or a 'neurometabolical' agent ('pyracetam') or a combination (instenon). Multiple regression analysis showed that outcome was related to age, degree of premorbid, emotional stability, history of unfavourable exogenous factors such as head injury, and duration of dementia symptoms. The test group showed reduced intensity of cognitive-behavioural and psychological disturbance, suggesting that supportive interventions as a group may be useful for the broad array of BPSD. These include insight approaches, family therapy, activity and relaxation interventions, recreation, physical therapy and memory training exercises. However, the results also suggested that the medication was a factor in reducing the level of disturbance as measured by the Sandoz Clinical Assessment Geriatric Scale. This study is difficult to interpret with confidence as the groups are not adequately controlled for pharmacological interventions, supportive interventions and end points are not defined, and the measures employed questionable. Hence, as is true in many outcome trials of treatment intervention, the relationship between types of intervention and specific changes remain hard to confirm.

Laundreville et al. (1998) reviewed experimentally designed interventions for non-physical, non-aggressive behaviour such as wandering, self-injurious behaviour (scratching, bumping into objects, eating foreign objects), repetitive dawdling, stereotyped behaviours, inappropriate sexuality (genital exposure, public masturbation), inappropriate toileting and intrusive wandering. They concluded that effective interventions included:
- staff training plus token economy or stimulation programmes (such as activities) for self-injurious behaviours (Mishara & Kastenbaum, 1973);
- social and other reinforcers for returning dawdlers (Cuvo, 1976);
- training wandering residents to recognize hazardous areas by visual cues (such as two-dimensional horizontal grid patterns marked in front of exit doors or a large 'stop' sign posted at key points such as other patients'

rooms) and 'Do not Enter' signed areas (Hussian, 1982, 1988; Hussian & Brown, 1987);

• linking behaviour to a learned visual stimulus (such as a large orange disc) that signalled acceptable versus unacceptable actions and locations (e.g. masturbation) (Bird *et al.*, 1995).

With the exception of Mishara & Kastenbaum (1973) ($n = 135$), these were all small studies with numbers ranging from one to eight subjects. Hence the validity and certainly the generalizability are not strong. However, taken together they indicate that active interventions that involve environmental changes, coupled with expert, antecedent, staff-training interventions can ameliorate some difficult and possibly self-injurious behaviours even in patients with some degree of learning impairment secondary to dementia. They also support an active, creative interventive approach rather than a passive and nihilistic attitude. Some of these interventions demonstrated continued improvement for some time after the formal study ended. However, follow-up was generally short so the longer-term utility of interventions and necessary next levels of intervention are not addressed. De Young *et al.* (2002) described an array of interventions on a 32-bed behavioural management unit. In an uncontrolled study they found that verbal distraction time-outs, activity diversion, managing the environment and getting to know the patient well reduced the frequency of seven behaviours over 6 months. Clare *et al.* (2003) reviewed the effectiveness of cognitive rehabilitation and cognitive training for early-stage Alzheimer's disease and vascular dementia and found little effect of benefit.

Wandering poses significant challenges to clinical staff in nursing homes. Architectural approaches such as mazes, outdoor safe courtyards, endless corridor loops, alarms, locked doors and elevator key pad combinations are common methods of dealing with this issue. Lai & Arthur (2003) in a comprehensive review found that no specific interventions were demonstrably effective including enhancing the environment (Cohen-Mansfield & Werner, 1998b). Holmberg (1997) described a walking programme for demented nursing home residents to address the problem of wandering. The walkers' group was established as an ongoing programme in a 473-bed geriatric facility in western New York State. Criteria for participation in the walker's group included: (1) disruptive wandering behaviour; (2) dementia; (3) no history of unprovoked physical aggressiveness; (4) ability to respond to direction; and (5) ability to walk independently. The findings from this exploratory study suggest that taking a selected group of residents with a history of disruptive wandering behaviours off the unit for a walk had a positive effect on the

unit milieu. The author concluded that the finding of 30% fewer aggressive incidents during the 24-hour periods after these walking sessions suggests that this type of activity may reduce aggressive behaviours of elderly, institutionalized persons with dementia. However, the methodological limitations of the study (uncontrolled, non-randomized) restrict the generalizability of the findings. Other studies of activity programmes have been less positive (Zisselman *et al.*, 1996; Robichaud *et al.*, 1994).

Proctor *et al.* (1999) studied the effectiveness of a geriatric outreach team on inducing improvement in agitated residents of 12 randomly assigned nursing homes (six to active intervention and six to control conditions with a total of 120 subjects recruited). The active intervention consisted of staff training and of psychosocial management of residents' behavioural problems such as screaming, frequent and unnecessary toilet requests, aggressive behaviour, refusal to eat and low self-motivation. Seven 1-hour seminars were given by members of the outreach team based on skill-building topics selected by staff such as management of dementia, aggression or screaming. An experienced psychiatric nurse then visited each home every week to help workers in developing care-planning skills utilizing a 'goal planning' strategy which aimed to train staff in formulation of detailed and specific care plans based on each patient's strengths and needs as determined through careful observation and assessment. Outcomes were determined using an array of validated measures. The main findings were that residents were responsive to the intervention used by staff to achieve their goal plans. Depression scores and cognitive impairment measures both showed improvement but behavioural measures did not improve. Over 6 months, staff could be trained to develop skills in assessment and care planning, to implement the programme in everyday care, and to assess the efficacy of the programme. On the one hand the results are encouraging but with specific regard to non-pharmacological intervention for behavioural disturbance the results are in keeping with other similar studies in failing to demonstrate effectiveness.

Berger *et al.* (2004), in a 2-year controlled design study ($n = 18$ patient-carer dyads), evaluated a combination of weekly 1-hour, caregiver support group and memory training/music therapy in dementia patients on BPSD and caregiver burden. They found no significant differences between the intervention and control groups at any of the time periods measured. However, the authors caution that the usual care given to controls may have had enough impact that it reduced the significance of the treatment condition.

Other interventions have been systematically evaluated with subjects acting as their own controls. For example, the use of a glider swing improved emotional pleasure and relaxation in 34 residents. There was some decline in other behavioural disturbances during the period of swinging but these changes were all short-lived and did not persist past the time of active swinging.

Overall, the empirical data for the effectiveness of various interventions on BPSD is not strongly supportive of efficacy, with some exceptions. This leaves clinicians with the dilemma of needing to intervene but having no clearly effective method to do so and here the evidence base is clearly defective. While the statistical significance of interventions is not strong, impressions from many studies persist that individual patients many benefit even though the group effect did not emerge. Hence, clinicians continue to have to rely on individual clinical judgement tailored to each case when deciding on a therapeutic intervention.

Disruptive vocalizations
Persistent loud vocalizing can be very distressing to everyone in a long-term care environment and be very hard to modify. Vocalization or noise-making has received less attention than general agitation and studies do not often distinguish disruptive vocalizations (DV) from other forms of agitation. In the hospital setting the incidence ranges from 11–44% (Rosin, 1977; Gryle et al., 1986) and 25% in nursing homes (Cohen-Mansfield et al., 1990). Cohen Mansfield & Werner (1997) identified three main groups of verbal behaviours: (1) verbal behaviours associated with specific requests or needs, including behaviours associated with the performance of ADLs (such as chatting); or behaviours associated with pain, the need to be fed or put in bed (such as loud talk); (2) verbal behaviours not associated with specific requests but with general, undefined needs, including calling for attention or hallucinations (such as mumbling and disruptive talk); (3) verbal behaviours associated with self-stimulation, such as loud singing.

Verbal behaviours in general, but those associated with specific requests or needs in particular, were related to the cognitive functioning of the participants. As the cognitive abilities of the elderly residents deteriorated, their verbally disruptive behaviour became less verbal and seemed less related to specific needs or purposes. Non-verbal vocalizations included groaning, howling and sighing and do not relate to the factors associated with verbal vocalizations where meaning of some sort can be ascribed to the sounds. A recent study strongly supports the association between DV and depression, suggesting that interventions in some patients may be more effective if they include assessment for depression and address that issue concurrently (Dwyer & Byrne, 2000).

A number of interventions have been tried, some addressing the theoretical concept that these behaviours are the result of inadequate stimulation of the demented person (Allen-Burge et al., 1999). Interventions include differential reinforcement of other behaviour (Spayd & Smyer, 1988), reinforcement coupled with planned ignoring (Brink, 1980; Carstensen & Fremouw, 1981) or reinforcement coupled with redirection (Whelihan, 1978), as well as group interventions, and memory prompting using individualized written cues (Bourgeois et al., 1997). Results have been encouraging in some studies but no one method dominates. The importance of individualizing interventions is supported by earlier findings of Cohen-Mansfield et al. (1989) who reported that patterns of agitated behaviours tend to be specific to each resident studied.

Burgio and colleagues provided a variety of auditory and tactile stimuli to nursing home residents who displayed a clinically significant level of DV (Burgio et al., 1994). Auditory stimulation consisted of music or amplification of ambient sounds in the nursing home. Tactile stimulation consisted of providing some residents with a stuffed animal while others received a vibrating stuffed animal intended to increase the intensity of tactile stimulation. At the group level of analysis, none of these interventions were reliably associated with a decrease in DV; however, intrasubject analyses did show responders to each of the interventions. Other positive studies of music therapy of various types, usually with small numbers and uncontrolled, have shown some improvement in agitated behaviours (Ragneskog et al., 2001, Suzuki et al., 2004). Massage demonstrated significant reduction in noisiness using a combination of interventions including contingent reinforcement rewarding quiet behaviour, music, conversation, touch or visual aids.

Nagaratnam et al. (2003) studied noise-making behaviour in association with other behavioural and psychiatric manifestations, and dementia-related domains of cognitive impairment, severity of dementia, language dysfunction and overall disability. They also tried to correlate anatomic findings from neuroimaging with hypothesized brain mechanisms in order to formulate a neural substrate for noise-making. This was a retrospective small (n = 12) design. They categorized noise making into (i) persistent screaming, (ii) perseverative vocalization, (iii) continuous chattering, muttering, singing or humming and (iv) swearing, grunting and bizarre noise-making. They could not localize the behaviour to any anatomical brain lesion pattern although orbitofrontal pathways may be implicated including subcortical pathways in the right thalamus and caudate.

Controlled group intervention studies for 'difficult resident behaviour' have shown varied results (Proctor et al.,

1999; Ballard *et al.*, 2002) with the studies of Rovner *et al.* (1996) and Opie *et al.* (2002) among the small minority showing positive results. Moniz-Cook *et al.* (2003) suggests that this may be 'because these group-based interventions, which have become the hallmark for randomized controlled trials, may not be adequate to address the difficult behaviour'. They tried to remedy this methodological problem by using an individualized, multi-faceted intervention, incorporating theory derived from the concept that emotional and interpersonal needs (rather than or in addition to impact of the organic brain changes) are the drivers that produce difficult behaviours, as well as taking into account neuropsychological function. They selected five 'most difficult to manage' nursing home residents and analysed their emotional needs based on history and presumed effect of personality and other factors. Interventions were tailored to each profile. Reassurance, reinforcement of psychological needs and personal presence and interaction of staff are examples of tailored interventions with different cases in this small, elegant study. The results were positive in all five difficult cases.

Aggression

Physical and verbal aggression are among the most common BPSD (Hope *et al.*, 1999). There is considerable overlap between this problem in learning disability where the presentation is very similar (see Chapter 44). Some have found that it is most prevalent among patients with 'organic brain syndromes' (Wystanski, 2000), and there is conflicting data on whether aggression is associated with increased severity of dementia (Swearer *et al.*, 1988; Cohen Mansfield & Werner 1998a). Aggression is probably the principal management problem in nursing homes and is a predictor of admission (Cohen Mansfield, 1986; Aronson *et al.*, 1993; Gibbons *et al.*, 1997). Keene *et al.* (1999) found that verbal aggression was the most common and long-lasting form of aggression among 99 community-dwelling elders with dementia. Once aggressive resistance and physical aggression emerged it persisted until death. Intimate care was the most important factor in precipitating aggression. And physical aggression was more prevalent in those with more severe dementia. Psychosocial factors appear to trigger aggression as does emotional turmoil (Craig, 1982; Colenda & Hamer, 1991; Krakowsi & Czobor, 1997), suggesting possible intervention strategies.

Laundreville *et al.* (1998) reviewed six studies of interventions for physically aggressive behaviours in long-term care institutions. (Rosberger & MacLean, 1983; Vaccaro, 1988a, 1988b, 1990; Bourgeois & Vezina, 1998). Four of these studies had only one participant and two were small group interventions with six subjects each. Recognizing the very

limited generalizability of these studies, taken together, one may tentatively conclude that differential reinforcement of other behaviour (DRO) together with time-outs may be effective. These interventions aim to moderate aggressive behaviour by modifying its consequences.

Gormley *et al.* (2001) in a randomized, controlled trial evaluated behavioural management of aggression in dementia versus a control condition. The behavioural condition (n = 34) included training caregivers to view behavioural disturbance in the context of memory-impairing disease, and identifying factors that precipitate and maintain these problems. Four sessions were offered to caregivers over 8 weeks focusing on education and training in behavioural intervention that included avoiding precipitating factors, using appropriate communication techniques, acceptance of false statements made by patients and use of distraction. The control group (n = 28) had four sessions focused on advice and discussion of a variety of caregiving issues. The main outcome measure was the RAGE (Patel & Hope, 1992) as well as the BEHAVE-AD (Reisberg *et al.*, 1996). There was no significant difference between the aggression and behavioural scores in the behavioural and control groups although after statistical adjustment there was a trend toward effectiveness in the behavioural intervention group. Overall, in this group, behavioural training alone had little impact on aggressive behaviour or on carer burden. This result is counter-intuitive in some respects but is supported by other similarly negative outcomes on improving behaviour from staff-training interventions (Matthews *et al.*, 1996; Burgener *et al.*, 1998; McCallion *et al.*, 1999; Proctor *et al.*, 1999; Beck *et al.*, 2002) although a few positive results have also been reported for agitation and aggression (Hagen & Sayers, 1995; Haupt *et al.*, 2000).

Caregiver perceptions and behaviour may impair their ability to interact positively with demented aggressive elders thereby contributing to increased aggressive behaviour (Graneheim *et al.*, 2001). Skovdahl *et al.* (2004), in a qualitative observational study, concluded that caregivers who entered a 'negative spiral' were focused on accomplishing a task (in this case completing a shower) rather than on helping the individual with the task i.e. a person-centred approach, which seemed to avoid the negative spiral (Skovdahl *et al.*, 2003a, 2003b). Hagen & Sayers (1995) found that three half-hour educational sessions for all staff involved with residents of a nursing home reduced incidents of resident aggression. This finding is not strongly supported by other studies of effectiveness of staff education alone on altering patient behaviour.

Wystanski (2000) studied 29 patients in a psychogeriatric ward, dividing the group by diagnosis into organic vs non-organic diagnoses. Psychosocial events (e.g. admission to or discharge from the unit or transfers) and all medication changes were systematically recorded for each patient over 94 days (n = 612 organic and 784 non-organic). Assaultive behaviour occurred in 83% of organic patients compared with 29% of non-organic. Organic patients were also more likely to display aggressive behaviour in the absence of modifying events. A higher proportion of non-organic patients ceased aggressive behaviour in the absence of modifying factors. In general major psychosocial stimulation was ameliorating rather than aggravating. The data suggest that it is the course of underlying pathology that most influences emergence of aggressive behaviours rather than external factors.

Bathing, presumably because of the sometimes forced intimacy of the procedure, is associated with agitation and aggression. Sloane *et al.* (2004), in a randomized, controlled trial, evaluated effectiveness of two non-pharmacological interventions in reducing agitation, aggression and discomfort in nursing home residents with dementia in 15 different skilled nursing home facilities (n = 73 residents and 39 nursing assistants). Method included videotaped interactions, and standardized rating using the Care Recipient Behaviour Assessment, and Discomfort Scale for Dementia of the Alzheimer type. The two active interventions were person-centred bathing (i.e. focused on resident comfort and preferences, viewing behavioural disturbances as expressions of unmet need, use of communication techniques, problem-solving approaches and environmental modification as needed), and towel bath (i.e. an in-bed bath cleansing the resident with gentle massage) conducted by staff trained in the techniques. All measures of agitation and aggression declined in the intervention groups compared with the controls (53% in the person-centered shower group and 60% in the towel bath group). Whall *et al.* (1997) reduced agitation and aggression during bathing using nature sounds, bright pictures, trained staff and snacks during the procedure. Reducing the amount of forced interaction with staff may also reduce aggression (Negley & Manley, 1990).

Complementary therapies have been applied to dementia, with common techniques including hand and body massage (Snyder *et al.*, 1995; Smallwood *et al.*, 2001), music and aroma therapy. Sound and music intervention includes nature sounds (Burgio, 1996), audiotapes of family members (Woods & Ashley, 1995; Camberg *et al.*, 1999), preferred music (Tabloski *et al.*, 1995; Ragneskog *et al.*, 1996; Devereaux, 1997; Thomas *et al.*, 1997; Clark *et al.*, 1998; Remington, 1999; Gerdner, 2000), classical music (Denny, 1997). Reported results are generally positive while the music is playing but effects do not last beyond the period of immediate stimulation. Thorgrimsen *et al.* (2003) systematically reviewed the evidence in support of aromatherapy which has been employed for disturbed behaviour, sleep and to stimulate motivation. They found only two randomized controlled trials but the data could not be used for analysis. One study permitted reanalysis of the data which suggested that there may be benefits but more large-scale randomized controlled trials are needed before conclusions can be drawn. An uncontrolled, small (n = 7) study of audio presence nursing intervention (using the recorded voice of family) led to reduced agitation in some residents but unchanged or worsened behaviours in a minority of others, making clear conclusions impossible to draw (Miller *et al.*, 2001).

Clark *et al.* (1988) used a different strategy employing 'preferred music' during bathing episodes. In a controlled, small (18 severely demented subjects aged 55–95) cross-over design, patients were randomly assigned to either a control (no music) condition or an experimental condition in which recorded selections of preferred music were played via audiotape recorder during the bathing episode. After 2 weeks conditions were reversed. A total of 20 observations were recorded for each individual. Results of 20 observations per patient showed that the music condition significantly decreased aggressive behaviours with observed improvement in general co-operation and affect. Thomas *et al.* (1997) also found reduction in physical aggression using selected music based on patients preferences as reported by family members.

Feeding and hydration issues

Malnutrition is a common issue in dementia and is aggravated by lack of staff education, inadequate staffing, disregard for personal and culturally determined preferences, lack of assessment of comorbid health problems, intake of food and fluids, and dysphagia and oral hygiene (Amella, 2004). Studies by Kayser-Jones in this area led to changes in the regulation regarding staffing in nursing homes for assisting in feeding residents. While feeding is important, the way in which it is done is also important to enhance the social interaction and sense of nurturing that can also be part of eating.

Sleep and sundowning

Montgomery & Dennis (2004) conducted a systematic review of randomized controlled trials of three non-pharmacological interventions for sleep disturbance in non-demented elders: cognitive-behavioural therapy (CBT), bright light and physical exercise. Primary outcome measures were sleep quality, duration and efficiency. Cognitive-behavioural therapy (sleep hygiene, stimulus control, muscle relaxation therapy, sleep restriction therapy and cognitive therapy) produced a 'mild' positive effect on sleep maintenance. No conclusions on the effectiveness of bright light and exercise could be drawn from the very limited data. Sundowning is a diurnal agitation that emerges in demented individuals late in the day or early evening. Bright light therapy administered either in the morning or evening has had variable effect in reducing agitation associated with sundowning with some positive outcomes, but clinical utility and demonstrated effectiveness remain limited (Satlin *et al.*, 1992; Lovell *et al.*, 1995; Colenda *et al.*, 1997; Graf *et al.*, 2001).

Guidelines and recommendations

Behavioural approaches to BPSD and agitation were reviewed by Kazdin (1989) and described as sharing some common characteristics. These included operationalizing clinical problems on the basis of overt behavioural manifestations, using interventions that are directive, active and emphasize learning experience to alter behaviour, measuring treatment impact empirically, and implementing interventions in the patient's living environment utilizing the skills of carers to carry out the plan.

The consensus statement on improving quality of mental health care in US nursing homes (American Geriatrics Society and American Association for Geriatric Psychiatry, 2003) note that effective management requires adequate staffing levels, reimbursement of professional staff for delivering appropriate care and institutional commitment to this care at all levels. They further stated that management of behavioural symptoms requires comprehensive assessment including physical assessment (for pain, infections, dehydration, fecal impaction and injury), sensory deficits, drug effects, psychosis, depression and other psychiatric conditions associated with dementia, delirium, sleep disorders, other neurological conditions, substance misuse, withdrawal and environmental factors. The statement detailed the importance of staff education in observing for behavioural changes, interdisciplinary approaches, and family involvement as well as the need for referral for specialized mental health assessment if symptoms fail to respond to non-pharmacological intervention within 30 days or if behaviour is likely to be harmful to the patient or others. Treatment recommendations were based on a detailed and comprehensive review of the literature (Snowdon *et al.*, 2003). Non-pharmacological interventions were supported by various levels of evidence (I = randomized controlled study(s) and or meta-analyses, II = observational studies with control groups, III = expert opinion, case series/reports, or historical controls, IV = opinions of panel members without supporting

evidence). These recommendations included: observing new-onset non-dangerous behavioural changes and initially delaying specific intervention until the situation is clarified (III); using individualized interventions (IV); initial use of non-pharmacological intervention as long as there is no immediate danger to the patient and in the absence of psychosis (IV); employing the following array of non-pharmacological interventions – sensory therapy (II±), activities therapy (I±), modified activities of daily living routines based on patient need (I−), environmental modifications (II), behavioural theory treatments (II−), and social contact intervention (IV); interventions should be monitored at appropriate intervals (IV) using a validated scale (II), quantitative count of agitated behaviours (III) and global clinical impression of a trained staff (III).

Pharmacotherapy in the management of behaviour disorders in patients with acquired brain injury

This section presents a systematic review of the research published in English language on the effectiveness of drugs for the treatment of neurobehavioural disorders in patients with acquired brain injury. The evidence is primarily based on case studies rather than randomized controlled trials. There is no strong evidence either way to suggest that drugs are effective or ineffective in the treatment of behaviour disorders in patients with acquired brain injury. However, there is weak evidence, primarily based on case studies, that psychostimulants are effective in the treatment of apathy, inattention and slowness; anticonvulsants and antidepressants (particularly SSRIs) in the treatment of agitation and aggression, particularly in the context of an affective disorder; and possibly a specific neuroleptic methotrimeprazine in the treatment of agitation in the post-acute stage of acquired brain injury (ABI). Some drugs that are effective in some patients have been shown to be ineffective in others. Some drugs, particularly lithium and dopaminergic drugs can cause adverse effects and deterioration in some patients.

Introduction

After traumatic or acquired brain injury many patients develop neurobehavioural symptoms. Deb and colleagues (1999a) found the presence of neurobehavioural symptoms among 61.6% of 196 adults discharged from hospitals who were followed up 1-year post brain injury. About 40% had three or more symptoms; 30.5% showed impatience, 35.3% irritability, 28% mood swings, 18% slowness in thinking,

31.6% sleep problems, 24.8% socialization problems, 33.8% fatigue, 15% lack of initiative, 31.7% poor memory, 22% difficulty in planning, 3% socially disinhibited behaviour, 19.4% depressed mood and 15% verbal outbursts. Pre-morbid factors such as lower social class and lower educational achievement, brain-injury related factors such as a low Glasgow Coma Scale score (Jennett & Bond, 1975), and outcome related factors such as the presence of a disability according to the Edinburgh Rehabilitation Status Schedule (Affleck *et al.*, 1988) and psychiatric caseness according to the Clinical Interview Schedule – Revised (Lewis *et al.*, 1992) significantly influenced the rate and the pattern of behavioural symptoms. The pattern of behavioural symptoms varied between age groups and according to the severity of the brain injury. However, the causal relationship between traumatic brain injury and these neurobehavioural symptoms remains unclear.

Both pharmacological and non-pharmacological interventions have been used for the management of neurobehavioural symptoms, particularly agitation and aggression that occur after acquired brain injury.

We have excluded papers that used non-psychotropic drugs at the very acute stage of brain injury treatment. Apart from two studies on donepezil, we have not included studies on the use of other cognitive-enhancing agents (e.g. rivastigmine, CDP choline (citicoline) etc.) in this review. In the following section we present data under different drug group headings.

Lithium

There are no randomized controlled trials but six published case studies of use of lithium primarily for the treatment of agitation and aggression (Hale & Donaldson, 1982; Schiff *et al.*, 1982; Haas & Cope, 1985, Parmalee & O'Shanick, 1988; Glenn *et al.*, 1989; Bellus *et al.*, 1996) in patients with ABI. These case series included between one to eight cases ranging from mild to severe ABI. The time of treatment post-injury ranged from 6 weeks to up to 17 years. Patients with behaviours such as poor impulse control, mood change, decreased self-care, suicidal behaviour and behavioural dyscontrol were also included. Patients were followed up for periods varying from a few days to up to a few months. Most patients were treated with other drugs at the time of introduction of lithium. The daily dose of lithium varied from 600 mg to 1200 mg with a serum level of 0.44 to 1.4 ml/l. The overall finding from these six case studies is mixed, showing improvement in behaviour in some but deterioration in other cases.

At present there is no conclusive evidence to support lithium's effectiveness (but the information elsewhere in this book gives some support to its anti-aggressive action, for example, Chapter 44). It is, however, important to recognize that bipolar affective disorder may manifest as neurobehavioural symptoms in some patients with ABI. As lithium could be an effective prophylactic treatment for bipolar affective disorder, it could indirectly improve agitation and other behavioural problems in those ABI patients who have bipolar disorder. The adverse effect of lithium should be borne in mind and appropriate investigations should be carried out at regular intervals for those who are treated with lithium.

Antipsychotics

We found only four studies (Stanislav, 1997; Stanislav & Childs, 2000; Michals *et al.*, 1993; Maryniak *et al.*, 2001) on the use of antipsychotics. Stanislav's (1997) study included three patients treated with thioridazine 100 mg per day and haloperidol 20 mg per day. It is worth mentioning that thioridazine is no longer in regular use in the UK. Stanislav & Childs (2000) retrospectively examined case notes of 27 patients. The type of brain injury was not specified. It was not stated whether the patients were on other drugs at the time of initiation of antipsychotics. Authors compared the effect of intramuscular (IM) droperidol with IM lorazepam and IM haloperidol. The study showed that single doses of droperidol controlled agitation more often than single doses of comparative agents and caused less post-episode sedation. Droperidol is now withdrawn from the UK market. Michals *et al.* (1993) reported a case series of seven patients who were treated with clozapine with a mean dose of 500 mg per day with a range between 300–750 mg per day. Clozapine showed major adverse effects including seizures in two patients. Maryniak *et al.* (2001) reported a retrospective chart review of 56 patients discharged from an ABI unit. Most of these patients who were treated with methotrimeprazine 2–50 mg (average dose 25–50 mg) up to four times a day showed improvement in agitation but two patients developed significant adverse effects.

Antipsychotics are perhaps the most commonly used drugs for the control of aggression and agitation in ABI patients, yet there is a dearth of published literature on the use of antipsychotics in ABI patients. Therefore, at present, there is no convincing evidence to support the effectiveness of antipsychotics in the management of behaviour disorders in ABI patients. There is only one retrospective case series without a control group that lends weak support for the use of a specific antipsychotic drug, methotrimeprazine (this drug is not routinely used in the UK) in the treatment of agitation within the first few months of ABI. The sedating effects of some antipsychotics may further jeopardize the prospect of rehabilitation of ABI patients. Antipsychotics, however, do not always work by sedating patients. There is evidence that clozapine reduces aggression in psychotic patients without causing sedation.

Antidepressants

Eleven studies (Wroblewski *et al.*, 1990; Allman, 1992; Rowland *et al.*, 1992; Ranen *et al.*, 1996; Reinhard *et al.*, 1996; Muller *et al.*, 1999; Newburn *et al.*, 1999; Slaughter *et al.*, 1999; Fann *et al.*, 2000; Meythaler *et al.*, 2001) on the use of antidepressants for the management of neurobehavioural symptoms among ABI patients have been published. Of these, one is an RCT involving 11 patients, one is a non-randomized, single blind study of 15 patients, one is a non-blind open trial of 13 patients, one is a non-blind prospective trial of 26 patients, one is a retrospective review of 68 patients, one is a case series of 26 patients, one is a case report of one patient, two are case reports involving two patients each, one is a case report involving three patients, and one is a case report involving six patients. The first three studies used sertraline at a dose between 25–200 mg per day. The first study included patients with agitation, the second with major depression but the third study included patients with aggression and irritability. The first RCT involving a small cohort did not show any significant improvement in agitation and orientation in the group that was treated with sertraline. The third study showed significant reduction in irritability and aggressive outbursts but no significant change in depressive symptoms, whereas in the second study 87% had a decreased score on the Hamilton Rating Scale for Depression (Hamilton, 1960). The fourth study also included major depressive disorder, in which a high proportion responded. The fifth study, which was retrospective in nature and included a reasonable number of patients, only looked at the seizure potential of different antidepressants. The rest of the studies included either patients who had episodes of involuntary crying or exuberant and uncontrollable laughter. Other problem behaviours mentioned in the case reports included aggression associated with Huntington's disease, hypo-arousal, poor initiation, muteness and Kluver–Bucy syndrome. Most of these smaller case studies showed improvement in the target behaviour.

A proportion of studies in this section included a reasonable number of patients who were treated with the new generation antidepressants such as the SSRIs. Apart from one small-scale RCT that showed no improvement in agitation, alertness and arousal in the post-acute phase of traumatic brain injury, most studies have shown improvement in the target behaviour. However, the target behaviour that improved in most cases following the antidepressant treatment was affective in nature. This is not surprising considering the fact that antidepressants are primarily indicated for the treatment of depression. However, there is also some evidence to suggest that in certain cases antidepressants could be useful in the management of agitation and aggression. It is possible that depression and other affective disorders that are not uncommon following traumatic brain injury (Deb *et al.*, 1999b) may indirectly cause agitation and aggression. Therefore, by treating the underlying affective disorder, antidepressants may show an improvement in aggression and other neurobehavioural symptoms in these patients. It is worth noting that in clinical practice it is not always easy to differentiate between 'abulic' ('apathy') and 'depressive' symptoms among ABI patients.

Antidepressants, particularly the SSRIs, are used increasingly in the management of anxiety disorders (Den Boer *et al.*, 2000). It is possible that in certain ABI patients the manifestation of neurobehavioural symptoms is caused by an underlying anxiety disorder. Therefore, the improvement in aggression observed in ABI patients from the use of antidepressants may be due to the improvement in the underlying anxiety symptoms.

Psychostimulants

Eight studies (Evans *et al.*, 1987; Gualtieri & Evans, 1988; Wroblewski *et al.*, 1992; Mooney & Haas, 1993; Speech *et al.*, 1993; Hornstein *et al.*, 1995; Plenger *et al.*, 1996; Whyte *et al.*, 1997) are included in this section. Five studies used an RCT design that included 12, 38, 23, 19 and 15 patients. One study was a retrospective study of 30 patients, one was a case note review of 27 patients (who received dextro-amphetamine at 5–30 mg per day dose) and one was a single case report. Most studies used methylphenidate on average 0.3 mg/kg twice daily to 30 mg per day dose.

Target behaviours often included impaired vigilance and attention, impaired initiation and difficulty in concentrating. Some studies used anger and temper outbursts as primary target behaviours. When psychostimulants were compared with the control groups, some studies showed improvement, particularly in global mental functioning but others failed to do so. One study showed methylphenidate to be more effective than placebo in controlling anger. Some of these patients were treated with other drugs such as carbamazepine, clonazepam, desipramine, amitriptyline, baclofen, buspirone, sodium valproate, amantadine, dantrolene and carbi-L-dopa prior to the initiation of psychostimulants.

Because of these few controlled trials with small cohorts, the evidence for the effectiveness of psychostimulants in improving target behaviours in ABI patients is, at best, equivocal, and at worst, absent. These drugs seem to be particularly effective in treating symptoms such as slowness of behaviour, and lack of initiative and attention. There is also some evidence to suggest that these drugs might also be useful in the treatment of anger outbursts. The use of psychostimulants has to be monitored very closely because of the potential adverse events associated with their use. In the UK, psychostimulant drugs have only been licensed for the treatment of Attention Deficit Hyperactivity Disorder (ADHD) in children (www.nice.org.uk). Some patients following ABI may develop symptoms similar to that of the ADHD. It is also possible that some children and young adults with ADHD are prone to sustain ABI. However, their diagnosis may remain undetected in adult life and it is quite possible from extrapolating from a meta-analysis of similar studies in adult ADHD (Kessler et al., 2007) that psychostimulants may indirectly improve neurobehavioural symptoms by treating the underlying ADHD in these ABI patients.

Anticonvulsants

Thirteen studies (Pope et al., 1988; Stewart & Hemsath, 1988; Geracioti, 1994; Smith et al., 1994; Horne & Lindley, 1995; Chatham Showalter, 1996; Wroblewski et al., 1997; Azouvi et al., 1999; Chatham Showalter & Kimmel, 2000; Chatham Showalter & Netsky Kimmel, 2000; Dikmen et al., 2000; Perino et al., 2001; Kim & Humaran, 2002) are included in this section. Dikmen et al. (2000) is an RCT of prophylaxis with phenytoin versus sodium valproate among 279 patients, which did not show any significant adverse or beneficial neuropsychological effects of sodium valproate over phenytoin. Smith et al. (1994) is an RCT that used placebo to replace either phenytoin or carbamazepine in order to assess the effect of withdrawal of these two drugs. Perino et al. (2001), which is an open-label prospective study of combination treatment with citalopram and carbamazepine on 20 patients with traumatic brain injury, showed improvement in most target behaviours. Chatham Showalter & Kimmel (2000) retrospectively reviewed charts on 29 patients in the acute stage and Kim & Humaran (2002) included 11 patients with a remote history of ABI who were treated with divalproex sodium. The rest of the studies are case series including between 1 and 13 patients. In most studies agitation and aggression were the primary target behaviours for intervention, but two studies reported specifically the treatment effect on bipolar affective disorders. The majority of cases showed improvement in affective symptoms as well as anger and agitation. One study included 13 patients treated with lamotrigine on an average daily dose of 250 mg with a range of 150–400 mg per day and the rest of the studies used sodium valproate, divalproex sodium or carbamazepine. The dose of sodium valproate ranged between 750–2250 mg per day and that of carbamazepine between 200 mg and 900 mg per day.

There is, therefore, anecdotal evidence based on case reports that anticonvulsant/mood stabilizer drugs such as carbamazepine, sodium valproate, divalproex sodium and lamotrigine can reduce aggressive behaviour and agitation as well as treat affective disorder in ABI patients. As these drugs act as mood stabilizers, it is possible that their effect on aggression and agitation is mediated via an indirect effect on the patient's mood.

Buspirone

There are four case reports (Gualtieri, 1991a, 1991b; Ratey et al., 1992; Stanislav et al., 1994) of buspirone, a non-benzodiazepine anti-anxiety drug (see also Chapter 31), in the treatment of agitation and violent behaviour in ABI patients that included between 2–14 patients. The dosage ranged from 10–60 mg per day. The findings were mixed in that in some studies there was improvement in some patients but in one study there was no response to buspirone among seven patients with severe ABI, but 4 out of 7 mild ABI patients responded. When buspirone was first introduced into the market, it became quite popular because unlike benzodiazepine it does not cause tolerance, alcohol intolerance or withdrawal symptoms. However, lately its popularity has fallen because of its slow onset of action and low potency. It is possible that in some ABI patients the agitation is caused by an underlying anxiety, which may respond to buspirone or other anti-anxiety drugs.

Dopaminergic drugs

There are two (Schneider et al., 1999; Meythaler et al., 2002) prospective randomized double-blind, placebo-controlled, cross-over trial including 10 and 35 patients respectively, and three single case reports (Kraus & Maki, 1996; Karli et al., 1998; Zafonte et al., 1998) on the use of dopaminergic drugs in patients with traumatic brain injury. In the first RCT, involving only 10 patients, there was a general improvement in patients' cognition and behavioural function over time in both groups but no difference was observed between amantadine and placebo. The second RCT, involving 35 patients, showed a consistent trend toward a more rapid functional improvement among patients treated with amantadine than the placebo. The case reports have shown improvement in general condition including symptoms of frontal lobe dysfunction. However, one study reported deterioration in a patient who developed adverse effects like impulsivity, dysarthria and ataxia. Most studies are on amantadine, the dose of which ranged between 150 mg and 500 mg daily. In one single case study bromocriptine at 5 mg twice daily dose was added to amantadine.

There is currently equivocal evidence about the value of psychostimulants in ABI patients. Despite some weak anecdotal evidence that in certain cases these drugs may lead to general improvement in patients, the effect of dopaminergic drugs on aggression in ABI patients is far from clear. These drugs have potential significant adverse effects and therefore have to be monitored very closely and the dosage rationalized regularly. Also it is not known what possible adverse effects may be caused by the withdrawal of dopaminergic drugs.

Beta-blockers

Five studies (Greendyke *et al.*, 1984; Mattes, 1985; Greendyke *et al.*, 1986; Greendyke & Kanter, 1986; Brooke *et al.*, 1992) are reviewed under this section, of which three are RCTs that involved 4, 5 and 21 patients. In Brooke *et al.* (1992), a maximum daily dose of 420 mg propranolol produced significantly less intense but a similar frequency of episodes of agitation in the treatment group when compared with the placebo group. The rest of the studies in this section are single case reports. Drugs used were propranolol between 420–520 mg per day dose, pindolol up to 60 mg per day dose, and metoprolol 200 mg daily dose. In all cases there was significant improvement in temper outbursts and violent behaviour. It seems that there is very weak evidence based on a small number of very small-scale RCTs of beta-blockers' effectiveness in the reduction of violent behaviour and temper outbursts in ABI patients. However, often the dose of beta-blocker used is high, which makes patients vulnerable to adverse effects, and in these doses they act centrally and not by beta-blockade. In addition, the long-term effects of beta-blockers and particularly the effect of its withdrawal on ABI patients are not known.

Hormonal treatment

There are only three case reports (Arnold, 1993; Emroy *et al.*, 1995; Britton, 1998) including one to eight male patients on hormonal treatment of neurobehavioural symptoms of ABI patients. Medroxy-progesterone acetate at 300 mg weekly IM dose and oestrogen 1.25 mg per day dose have been used primarily to control sexually inappropriate social behaviour and aggression. At present there is no convincing evidence that hormonal therapy may be effective in the treatment of behavioural problem in patients with ABI. However, in a sub-group of patients where behaviour problems are particularly associated with sexual disinhibition, certain hormonal therapy may result in improvement.

Other medication

Medication such as vasopressin nasal spray (Eames & Liwood, 1999), donepezil 5 mg daily (Taverni *et al.*, 1997; Masanic *et al.*, 2001), and naltrexone 100 mg daily (Calvanio *et al.*, 2000) have been shown to improve cognitive and memory deficits in patients with ABI in case series involving one to 26 patients. None of these studies are controlled, and therefore it is difficult to comment on the effectiveness of these drugs. Donepezil is indicated in the treatment of early stage of Alzheimer's disease. Naltrexone has been tried in the treatment of self-injurious behaviour in patients with intellectual disability and lately in the treatment of alcohol dependence.

Conclusion

From the current review it is clear that there is no convincing evidence that any of the drugs described above is effective in the treatment of neurobehavioural problems in patients with ABI. However, as we have mentioned elsewhere in this book, absence of evidence is not evidence of absence. All we can say is that there is not enough evidence at present to either support or refute the use of drugs in clinical practice for the treatment of behavioural problems among patients with ABI.

The problem with the current evidence is that it overwhelmingly consists of case reports and there are very few data from properly controlled studies. The handful of studies that used control groups have included small numbers of patients, therefore giving very poor statistical power to these studies. Case reports can be misleading because, by and large, the positive findings rather than the negative ones are published in the literature. It is interesting to see that in many of these case reports patients have been treated with several other drugs before they have shown improvement on a particular drug. For example, some patients failed to respond to neuroleptics, anticonvulsant drugs and benzodiazepines before they responded to lithium. Similarly, there were examples of failure of response to tricyclics, benzodiazepine and anticonvulsants before patients improved on neuroleptics. It is therefore possible that there are subgroups of patients who tend to respond to certain drugs but not to others. There was also evidence of deterioration and adverse effects from the use of lithium (particularly when combined with carbamazepine) and dopaminergic drugs.

It appears that on the basis of mostly anecdotal evidence that a judicial use of pharmacotherapy could be justified in certain patients with ABI. Considering that most of the drugs reviewed in this chapter have potential severe adverse effects, their prescription will have to be very closely monitored. It is also important to keep in mind that pharmacological intervention alone will not solve the problem in most cases. A multidisciplinary approach to assessment and treatment is vital. Non-pharmacological interventions to treat behavioural problems such as aggression and agitation, which have been discussed in this chapter, should also be considered along with pharmacological treatment. The ultimate aim should not be to just control the target behaviour but to improve the quality of life of the patients and their carers.

Table 10.1. Evidence base for treatment of behavioural and related symptoms in conjunction with dementia and acquired brain injury

Treatment	Form of treatment	Psychiatric disorder	Level of evidence	Comments
Typical antipsychotic drugs (e.g. haloperidol)	Oral or intramuscular	BPSD	Ia	Large studies showing relative but small superiority over placebo (around 20%) but compromised by extrapyramidal and other adverse effects at higher doses (which are often necessary to show efficacy)
Atypical antipsychotic drugs (e.g. risperidone)	Oral	BSPD	Ia	Generally similar in efficacy to typical antipsychotic drugs with fewer extrapyramidal effects but some evidence of an increase in cerebrovascular complications with twice the mortality rate of placebo
Selective serotonin reuptake inhibitors (SSRIs)(e.g. citalopram)	Oral	BPSD	Ia	Reasonable level of evidence of equivalent efficacy to antipsychotic drugs with citalopram showing strongest evidence, which appears to be largely independent of depressive symptoms
Tricyclic antidepressants (amitriptyline)	Oral	BPSD	IIa	Less evidence than for SSRIs and concern over cardiotoxicity and other adverse effects
Trazodone	Oral	BPSD	Ib	Some evidence of efficacy for aggressive and challenging behaviour
Buspirone	Oral	BPSD	III	Limited evidence of relatively little value
Venlafaxine	Oral	BPSD	III	Open studies but no controlled ones suggesting some value
Mirtazapine	Oral	BPSD	III	Open studies but no controlled ones suggesting some value
Cholinesterase inhibitors (e.g. rivastigmine)	Oral	BPSD in Alzheimer's disease and Lewy body dementia	Ia	General evidence of efficacy at all stages of dementia, with possibly less evidence in severely advance cases
Anticonvulsants (e.g. carbamazepine)	Oral	BPSD	Ib	Carmazepine shows best evidence for efficacy, with no adequate evidence for gabapentin and weak support for sodium valproate offset by risk of thrombocytopaenia
Benzodiazepines (e.g. diazepam)	Oral or intramuscular injection	BPSD	Ia	Generally similar, or slightly inferior, in efficacy to antipsychotic drugs with sedating adverse effects
Beta-blocking drugs (e.g. propranolol)	Oral	BPSD	Ib	Some improvement in aggression but only with large doses
Oestrogens	Oral	BPSD	Ib	Some evidence of efficacy from controlled trials
Psychostimulants (e.g. methylphenidate)	Oral	BPSD	IIb	Some limited evidence from small studies
Individual psychotherapy	Individual	BPSD	IV	Strong belief of efficacy in some quarters but no real evidence
Reminiscence therapy	Individual or group	BPSD	Ib	One randomized trial showed very slight evidence of efficacy
Group therapy (including reality orientation)	Group	BPSD	Ib	Some evidence from controlled trials of effectiveness but doubts about sustainability
Validation therapy	Group	BPSD	III	No controlled studies but often highly supported by therapists
Light therapy	Individual	BPSD	IIb	Small controlled studies only with uncertain methodology
Walking therapy	Group	BPSD	IIb	May be of value but studies limited
Lithium salts	Oral	Traumatic brain injury	Ib	Of some value but effect size not clear

REFERENCES

Affleck, J. W., Aitken, R. C. B., Hunter, J. A. A. *et al.* (1988). Rehabilitation status: a measure of medicosocial dysfunction. *Lancet*, **I**, 230–3.

Aitken, L., Simpson, S. & Burns, A. (1999). Personality change in dementia. *International Psychogeriatrics*, **11**, 263–71.

Allen-Burge, R., Stevens, A. & Burgio, L. (1999). Effective behavioural interventions for decreasing dementia-related challenging behaviour in nursing homes. *International Journal of Geriatric Psychiatry*, **14**, 213–28.

Allen, N. H., Gordon, S., Hope, T. & Burns, A. (1996). Manchester and Oxford Universities Scale for the Psychopathological Assessment of Dementia (MOUSEPAD). *British Journal of Psychiatry*, **169**, 293–307.

Allman, P. (1992). Drug treatment of emotionalism following brain damage (letter). *Journal of the Royal Society of Medicine*, **85**, 423–4.

Amella, E. (2004). Feeding and hydration issues for older adults with dementia. *Nursing Clinics of North America*, **39**, 607–23.

American Geriatrics Society and American Association for Geriatric Psychiatry (2003). Consensus statement on improving the quality of mental health care in US nursing homes: management of depression and behavioural symptoms associated with dementia. *Journal of the American Geriatric Society*, **51**, 1287–98.

American Psychiatric Association (1997). Practice Guidelines for the treatment of patients with Alzheimer's disease and other dementias of late life. *American Journal of Psychiatry*, **154**, (suppl).

Ancill, R. J., Carlyle, W. W., Liang, R. A. & Holliday, S. G. (1991). Agitation in the demented elderly: a role for benzodiazepines? *International Clinical Psychopharmacology*, **6**, 141–6.

Ancoli-Israel, S., Martin, J. L., Gehrman, P. *et al.* (2003). Effect of light on agitation in institutionalized patients with severe Alzheimer disease. *American Journal of Geriatric Psychiatry*, **11**, 194–203.

Areosa, S. A., Sherriff, F. & McShane, R. (2005). Memantine for dementia. *Cochrane Database of Systematic Reviews*, CD003154. Oxford: Update Software Ltd.

Arnold, S. E. (1993). Estrogen for refractory aggression after traumatic brain injury. *American Journal of Psychiatry*, **150**, 1564–5.

Aronson, M. K., Post, D. C. & Guastadisegni, P. (1993). Dementia, agitation, and care in the nursing home. *Journal of the American Geriatric Society*, **41**, 507–12.

Ashton, D. (1993). Therapeutic work of reminiscence with the elderly. *British Journal of Nursing*, **2**, 894–8.

Auchus, A. & Bissey-Black, C. (1997). Pilot study of haloperidol, fluoxetine, and placebo for agitation in Alzheimer's disease. *Journal of Neuropsychiatry and Clinical Neurosciences*, **9**, 591–3.

Azouvi, P., Jokic, C., Attal, N. *et al.* (1999). Carbamazepine in agitation and aggressive behaviour following severe closed-head injury: results of an open trial. *Brain Injury*, **13**, 797–804.

Baines, S., Saxby, P. & Ehlert, K. (1987). Reality orientation and reminiscence therapy: a controlled cross-over study of elderly confused people. *British Journal of Psychiatry*, **151**, 222–31.

Ballard, C., Margallo-Lana, M., Juszczak, E. *et al.* (2005). Quetiapine and rivastigmine and cognitive decline in Alzheimer's disease: randomised double blind placebo controlled trial. *British Medical Journal*, **330**, 874.

Ballard, C., Powell, I., James, I. *et al.* (2002). Can psychiatric liaison reduce neuroleptic use and reduce health service utilization for dementia patients residing in care facilities. *International Journal of Geriatric Psychiatry*, **17**, 140–5.

Baumgarten, M., Backer, P. & Gauthier, S. (1990). Validity and reliability of the Dementia Behaviour Disturbance Scale. *Journal of the American Geriatric Society*, **38**, 221–6.

Beber, C. R. (1965). Management of behaviour in the institutionalized aged. *Diseases of the Nervous System*, **26**, 591–5.

Beck, C., Vogelpohl, T., Rasin, J. *et al.* (2002). Effects of behavioural interventions on disruptive behaviour and affect in demented nursing home residents. *Nursing Research*, **51**, 219–28.

Beck, A. T., Epstein, N., Harrision, R. P. & Emery, G. (1983). *Development of the Sociotropy-Autonomy Scale: A Measure of Personality Factors in Psychopathology*. Philadelphia: Center For Cognitive Therapy, University of Pennsylvania.

Behavioural and endocrinological evaluation of music therapy for elderly patients with dementia Nursing and Health Sciences (2004), **6**, 11–18.

Bellus, S. B., Stewart, D., Vergo, J. G. *et al.* (1996). The use of lithium in the treatment of aggressive behaviours with two brain-injured individuals in a state psychiatric hospital. *Brain Injury*, **10**, 849–60.

Berger, G. L., Bernhardt, T., Schramm, U. *et al.* (2004). No effects of a combination of caregivers support group and memory training/music therapy in dementia patients from a memory clinic population. *International Journal of Geriatric Psychiatry*, **19**, 223–31.

Bird, M., Alexopoulos, P. & Adamowicz, J. (1995). Success and failure in five case studies: use of cued recall to ameliorate behaviour problems in senile dementia. *International Journal of Geriatric Psychiatry*, **20**, 305–31.

Bird, M. J. (2000). Psychosocial rehabilitation for problems arising from cognitive deficits in dementia. In *Cognitive Rehabilitation in Old Age*, ed. R. D. Hill, L. Blackman & A. S. Neely, pp. 843–5. Oxford: Oxford University Press.

Birks, J. S. & Harvey, R. (2003). Donepezil for dementia due to Alzheimer's disease. *Cochrane Database of Systematic Reviews*, CD001190. Oxford: Update Software Ltd.

Bourgeois, S. & Vezina, J. (1998). L'extinction des comportements agressifs d'une personne agee souffrant de demence [Extinction for reducing aggressive behaviours in an older adult with dementia]. *Revue Francophone de Clinique Comportementale et Cognitive*, **2**, 1–5.

Bourgeois, M. S., Burgio, L. D., Schulz, R., Beach, S. & Palmer, B. (1997). Modifying repetitive verbalizations of community-dwelling patients with AD. *Gerontologist*, **37**, 30–9.

Brandt, J., Campodonico, J., Rich, J. *et al.* (1998). Adjustment to residential placement in Alzheimer's disease patients: does premorbid personality matter? *International Journal of Geriatric Psychiatry*, **13**, 509–15.

Brink, C. (1980). Urinary continence/incontinence: Assessing the problem. *Geriatric Nursing*, **1**, 241–5.

Britton, K. R. (1998). Medroxyprogesterone in the treatment of aggressive hypersexual behaviour in traumatic brain injury. *Brain Injury*, **12**, 703–7.

Brodaty, H., Draper, B., Saab, D. *et al.* (2001). Psychosis, depression and behavioural disturbances in Sydney nursing home residents: prevalence and predictors. *International Journal of Geriatric Psychiatry*, **16**, 504–12.

Brodaty, H., Ames, D., Snowdon, J. *et al.* (2003). A randomized placebo-controlled trial of risperidone for the treatment of aggression, agitation, and psychosis of dementia. *Journal of Clinical Psychiatry*, **64**, 134–43.

Brook, P., Degun, G. & Mather, M. (1975). Reality orientation, a therapy for psychogeriatric patients: a controlled study. *British Journal of Psychiatry*, **127**, 42–5.

Brooke, M. M., Patterson, D. R., Questad, K. A. *et al.* (1992). The treatment of agitation during initial hospitalization after traumatic brain injury. *Archives of Physical Medical Rehabilitation*, **73**, 917–21.

Burgener, S., Bakas, T., Murray, C., Dunahee, J. & Tossey, S. (1998). Effective caregiving approaches for patients with Alzheimer's disease. *Geriatric Nursing*, **19**, 121–6.

Burgio, L. (1996). Interventions for the behavioural complications of Alzheimer's disease: behavioural approaches. *International Journal of Psychogeriatrics*, **8** (Suppl. 1), 45–52.

Burgio, L. D., Scilley, K., Hardin, J. M. *et al.* (1994). Studying disruptive vocalization and contextual factors in the nursing home using computer-assisted real-time observation. *Journal of Gerontology*, **49**, P230–9.

Burke, W. J., Dewan, V., Wengel, S. P., Roccaforte, W. H., Nadolny, G. C. & Folks, D. G. (1997). The use of selective serotonin reuptake inhibitors for depression and psychosis complicating dementia. *International Journal of Geriatric Psychiatry*, **12**, 519–25.

Burke, W. J., Folks, D. G., Roccaforte, W. H. & Wengel, S. P. (1994). Serotonin reuptake inhibitors for the treatment of coexisting depression and psychosis in dementia of the Alzheimer type. *American Journal of Geriatric Psychiatry*, **2**, 352–4.

Burns, A., Folstein, S., Brandt, J. & Folstein, M. (1990). Clinical assessment of irritability, aggression, and apathy in Huntington and Alzheimer disease. *Journal of Nervous and Mental Disease*, **178**, 20–6.

Calvanio, R., Burke, D. T., Hyun Jung Kim *et al.* (2000). Naltrexone: effects on motor function, speech, and activities of daily living in a patient with traumatic brain injury. *Brain Injury*, **14**, 933–42.

Camberg, L., Woods, P., Ooi, W. L. *et al.* (1999). Evaluation of simulated presence: a personalized approach to enhance well-being in persons with Alzheimer's disease. *Journal of the American Geriatric Society*, **47**, 446–52.

Cantillon, M., Brunswick, R., Molina, D. & Bahro, M. (1996). Buspirone vs. haloperidol. A double-blind trial for agitation in a nursing home population with Alzheimer's disease. *American Journal of Geriatric Psychiatry*, **4**, 263–7.

Carlson, D., Fleming, K., Smith, G. & Evans, J. (1995). Management of dementia-related behavioural disturbances: a nonpharmacologic approach. *Mayo Clinic Proceedings*, **70**, 1108–15.

Carstensen, L. L. & Fremouw, W. J. (1981). The demonstration of a behavioural intervention for late life paranoia. *Gerontologist*, **21**, 329–33.

Chan, W. C., Lam, L. C., Choy, C. N., Leung, V. P., Li, S. W. & Chiu, H. F. (2001). A double-blind randomised comparison of risperidone and haloperidol in the treatment of behavioural and psychological symptoms in Chinese dementia patients. *International Journal of Geriatric Psychiatry*, **16**, 1156–62.

Chaterjee, A., Strauss, M., Smyth, K. & Whitehouse, P. (1992). Personality changes in Alzheimer's disease. *Archives of Neurology*, **49**, 486–91.

Chatham Showalter, P. E. & Kimmel, D. N. (2000). Agitated symptom response to divalproax following acute brain injury. *Journal of Neuropsychiatry and Clinical Neurosciences*, **12**, 395–7.

Chatham Showalter, P. E. (1996). Carbamazepine for combativeness in acute traumatic brain injury. *Journal of Neuropsychiatry and Clinical Neurosciences*, **8**, 96–9.

Chatham Showalter, P. E. & Netsky Kimmel, D. (2000). Stimulating consciousness and cognition following severe brain injury: a new potential clinical use for lamotrigine. *Brain Injury*, **14**, 997–1001.

Chesrow, E., Kaplitz, S., Veltra, H. & Breme, J. (1965). Blind study of oxazepam in the management of geriatric patients with behavioural problems. *Clinical Medicine*, **71**, 1001–5.

Cheston, R. (1998). Psychotherapy and dementia: a review of the literature. *British Journal of Medical Psychology*, **71**, 211–31.

Christensen, D. B. & Benfield, W. R. (1998). Alprazolam as an alternative to low-dose haloperidol in older, cognitively impaired nursing facility patients. *Journal of the American Geriatric Society*, **46**, 620–5.

Clare, L., Woods, R. T., Moniz Cook, E. D., Orrell, M. & Spector, A. (2003). Cognitive rehabilitation and cognitive training for early-stage Alzheimer's disease and vascular dementia. *Cochrane Database of Systematic Reviews*, CD003260. Oxford: Update Software Ltd.

Clark, M. E., Lipe, A. W. & Bilbrey, M. (1998). Use of music to decrease aggressive behaviours in people with dementia. *Journal of Gerontology Nursing*, **24**, 10–17.

Coccaro, E. F., Kramer, E., Zemishlany, Z. *et al.* (1990). Pharmacologic treatment of noncognitive behavioural disturbances in elderly demented patients. *American Journal of Psychiatry*, **147**, 1640–5.

Cohen, G. D. (1988). One psychiatrist's view. In *Treatment for the AlzheimerPatient: The Long Haul*, ed. L. Jarvik & C. Winograd, pp. 96–104. New York: Springer.

Cohen-Mansfield, J. (1986). Agitated behaviours in the elderly: II. Preliminary results in the cognitively deteriorated. *Journal of the American Geriatric Society*, **34**, 722–7.

Cohen-Mansfield, J. & Billig, N. (1986). Agitated behaviours in the elderly: 1. A conceptual review. *Journal of the American Geriatric Society*, **34**, 711–21.

Cohen-Mansfield, J. & Werner, P. (1997). Typology of disruptive vocalizations in older persons suffering from dementia. *International Journal of Geriatric Psychiatry*, **12**, 1079–91.

Cohen-Mansfield, J., Werner, P. (1998a). Longitudinal changes in behavioural problems in old age: A study in an adult day care population. *Journal of Gerontology, Biological Sciences, Medical Sciences*, **53**, M65–71.

Cohen-Mansfield, J. & Werner, P. (1998b). The effects of an enhanced environment on nursing home residents who pace. *The Gerontologist*, **38**, 199–208.

Cohen-Mansfield, J., Marx, M. & Rosenthal, A. (1989). A description of agitation in the nursing home. *Journal of Gerontology*, **44**, M77–84.

Cohen-Mansfield, J., Werner, P. & Marx M. S. (1990). Screaming in nursing home residents. *Journal of the American Geriatric Society*, **38**, 785–92.

Cohen-Mansfield, J., Man, M. & Werner, P. (1992). Agitation in Elderly Persons: An Integrative Report of Findings in a Nursing Home. *International Psychogeriatrics*, **4** (Suppl.), 221–40.

Colenda, C., Cohen, W., McCall, W. & Rosenquist, P. (1997). Phototherapy for patients with Alzheimer's disease with disturbed sleep patterns: results of a community-based pilot study. *Alzheimer Disease and Associated Disorders*, **11**, 175–8.

Colenda, C. C. & Hamer, R. M. (1991). Antecedents and interventions for aggressive behaviour of patients at a geropsychiatric state hospital. *Hospital and Community Psychiatry*, **42**, 287–92.

Cooper, A. J. (1987). Medroxyprogesterone acetate (MPA) treatment of sexual acting out in men suffering from dementia. *Journal of the Clinical Psychiatry*, **48**, 368–70.

Covington, J. S. (1975). Alleviating agitation, apprehension, and related symptoms in geriatric patients: a double-blind comparison of a phenothiazine and a benzodiazepine. *South Medical Journal*, **68**, 719–24.

Craig, T. J. (1982). An epidemiologic study of problems associated with violence among psychiatric inpatients. *American Journal of Psychiatry*, **139**, 1262–6.

Cummings, J. L., Street, J., Masterman, D. & Clark, W. S. (2002). Efficacy of olanzapine in the treatment of psychosis in dementia with lewy bodies. *Dementia and Geriatric Cognitive Disorders*, **13**, 67–73.

Cummings, J. L., Mega, M., Gray, K., Rosenberg-Thompson, S., Carusi, D. A. & Gornbein, J. (1994). The Neuropsychiatric Inventory: comprehensive assessment of psychopathology in dementia. *Neurology*, **44**, 2308–14.

Cutler, N. R., Haxby, J., Kay, A. D. *et al.* (1985). Evaluation of zimeldine in Alzheimer's disease: cognitive and biochemical measures. *Archives of Neurology*, **42**, 744–8.

Cuvo, A. J. (1976). Decreasing repetitive behaviour in an institutionalized mentally retarded resident. *Mental Retardation*, **24**, 22–5.

De Deyn, P. P., Carrasco, M. M., Deberdt, W. *et al.* (2004). Olanzapine versus placebo in the treatment of psychosis with or without associated behavioural disturbances in patients with Alzheimer's disease. *International Journal of Geriatric Psychiatry*, **19**, 115–26.

De Deyn, P. P., Katz, I. R., Brodaty, H., Lyons, B., Greenspan, A. & Burns, A. (2005). Management of agitation, aggression, and psychosis associated with dementia: a pooled analysis including three randomized, placebo-controlled double-blind trials in nursing home residents treated with risperidone. *Clinical Neurology and Neurosurgery*, **107**, 497–508.

De Deyn, P. P., Rabheru, K., Rasmussen, A. *et al.* (1999). A randomized trial of risperidone, placebo, and haloperidol for behavioural symptoms of dementia. *Neurology*, **53**, 946–55.

De Klerk-Rubin, V. (1995). A safe and friendly place to share feelings. *Journal of Dementia Care*, May/June, 22–24.

De Young, S., Just, G. & Harrison, R. (2002). Decreasing aggressive, agitated or disruptive behaviour: participation in a behaviour management unit. *Journal of Gerontology Nursing*, **28**, 22–31.

Deb, S., Lyons I. & Koutzoukis, C. (1999a). Neurobehavioural symptoms one year after a head injury. *British Journal of Psychiatry*, **174**, 360–5.

Deb, S., Lyons, I., Koutzoukis, C., Ali, I. & Mccarthy, G. (1999b). Rate of psychiatric illness one year after traumatic brain injury. *American Journal of Psychiatry*, **156**, 374–8.

Dehlin, O., Hedenrud, B., Jansson, P. & Nörgård, J. (1985). A double-blind comparison of alaproclate and placebo in the treatment of patients with senile dementia. *Acta Psychiatrica Scandinavica*, **71**, 190–6.

Den Boer, J. A., Bosker, F. J. & Slaap, B. R. (2000). Serotonergic drugs in the treatment of depressive and anxiety disorders. *Human Psychopharmacology*, **15**, 315–36.

Denny, A. (1997). Quiet music: an intervention for mealtime agitation? *Journal of Gerontology Nursing*, **52A**, M369–77.

Devanand, D., Jacobs, D., Tang, M. *et al.* (1997). The course of psychopathologic features in mild to moderate Alzheimer's disease. *Archives of General Psychiatry*, **54**, 257–63.

Devereaux, M. (1997). The effects of individualized music on cognitively impaired nursing home residents exhibiting agitation Unpublished master's thesis. College of St. Catherine St. Paul MN.

Dikmen, S. S., Machamer, M. A., Winn, H. R. *et al.* (2000). Neuropsychological effects of valproate in traumatic brain injury: a randomised trial. *Neurology*, **54**, 895–902.

Drachman, D. A., Swearer, J. M., O'Donnell, B. F., Mitchell, A. L. & Maloon, A. (1992). The Caretaker Obstreperous-Behavior Rating Assessment (COBRA) Scale. *Journal of the American Geriatrics Society*, **40**, 463–70.

Dwyer, M. & Byrne, G. (2000). Disruptive vocalization and depression in older nursing home residents. *International Psychogeriatrics*, **12**, 463–77.

Eames, P. & Liwood, R. (1999). Lysine vasopressin in post-traumatic memory disorders: an uncontrolled pilot study. *Brain Injury*, **13**, 255–60.

Emroy, L. E., Cole, C. M. & Meyer, W. J. (1995). Use of depo-provera to control sexual aggression in persons with traumatic brain injury. *Journal of Head Trauma Rehabilitation*, **10**, 47–58.

Erkinjuntti, T., Kurz, A., Gauthier, S., Bullock, R., Lilienfeld, S. & Damaraju, C. V. (2002). Efficacy of galantamine in probable vascular dementia and Alzheimer's disease combined with cerebrovascular disease: a randomised trial. *Lancet*, **359**, 1283–90.

Erkinjuntti, T., Roman, G. & Gauthier, S. (2004). Treatment of vascular dementia – evidence from clinical trials with cholinesterase inhibitors. *Journal of Neurological Science*, **226**, 63–6.

Evans, L. & Strumpf, N. (1989). Tying down the elderly: a review of the literature on physical restraint. *Journal of the American Geriatrics Society*, **37**, 65–79.

Evans, R. W., Gualtieri, C. T. & Patterson, D. (1987). Treatment of chronic closed head injury with psychostimulant drugs: a controlled case study and an appropriate evaluation procedure. *Journal of Nervous and Mental Disorders*, **175**, 106–10.

Fann, J. R., Uomoto, J. M. & Katon, W. J. (2000). Sertraline in the treatment of major depression following mild traumatic brain injury. *Journal of Neuropsychiatry and Clinical Neurosciences*, **12**, 226–32.

Feldman, H., Gauthier, S., Hecker, J., Vellas, B., Subbiah, P. & Whalen, E. (2001). A 24-week, randomized, double-blind study of donepezil in moderate to severe Alzheimer's disease. *Neurology*, **57**, 613–20.

Fetveit, A., Skjerve, A. & Bjorvatn, B. (2003). Bright light treatment improves sleep in institutionalized elderly – an open trial. *International Journal of Geriatric Psychiatry*, **18**, 520–6.

Finkel, S. I., Lyons, J. S. & Anderson, R. L. (1993). A brief agitation rating scale (BARS) for nursing home elderly. *Journal of the American Geriatrics Society*, **41**, 50–2.

Finkel, S., Costa e Silva, J., Cohen, G. *et al.* (1996). Behavioural and psychological signs and symptoms of dementia: a consensus statement on current knowledge and implications for research and treatment. *International Psychogeriatrics*, **8** (Suppl. 3), 497–500.

Finkel, S. I., Mintzer, J. E., Dysken, M., Krishnan, K. R., Burt, T. & McRae, T. (2004). A randomized, placebo-controlled study of the efficacy and safety of sertraline in the treatment of the behavioural manifestations of Alzheimer's disease in outpatients treated with donepezil. *International Journal of Geriatric Psychiatry*, **19**, 9–18.

Flynn, B. L. (1999). Pharmacologic management of Alzheimer disease, Part I: hormonal and emerging investigational drug therapies. *Annals of Pharmacotherapy*, **33**, 178–87.

Galynker, I., Ieronimo, C., Miner, C., Rosenblum, J., Vilkas, N. & Rosenthal, R. (1997). Methylphenidate treatment of negative symptoms in patients with dementia. *Journal of Neuropsychiatry and Clinical Neurosciences*, **9**, 231–9.

Gasio, P., Krauchi, K., Cajochen, C. *et al.* (2003). Dawn–dusk simulation light therapy of disturbed circadian rest–activity cycles in demented elderly. *Experimental Gerontology*, **38**, 207–16.

Geracioti, T. D. (1994). Valproic acid treatment of episodic explosiveness related to brain injury. *Journal of Clinical Psychiatry*, **55**, 416–17.

Gerber, G. J., Prince, P. N., Snider, H. G., Atchison, K., Dubios, L. & Kilgour, J. A. (1991). Group activity and cognitive improvement among patients with Alzheimer's disease. *Hospital and Community Psychiatry*, **42**, 843–5.

Gibbons, P., Gannon, M. & Wrigley, M. (1997). A study of aggression among referrals to a community-based psychiatry of old age service. *International Journal of Geriatric Psychiatry*, **12**, 384–8.

Glenn, M. B., Wroblewski, B., Parziale, J. *et al.* (1989). Lithium carbonate for aggressive behaviour or affective instability in ten brain-injured patients. *American Journal of Physical Medical Rehabilitation*, **68**, 221–6.

Goldwasser, N., Auerbach, S. M. & Harkins, S. W. (1987). Cognitive, affective and behavioural effects of reminiscence group therapy on demented elderly. *International Journal of Aging and Human Development*, **25**, 209–22.

Gormley, N., Lyons, D. & Howard, R. (2001). Behavioural management of aggression in dementia: a randomized controlled trial. *Age and Aging*, **30**, 141–5.

Graf, A., Wallner, C. & Schunnert, V. (2001). The effects of light therapy on mini-mental state examination scores in demented patients. *Biological Psychiatry*, **50**, 725–7.

Graneheim, U. H., Norberg, A. & Jansson, L. (2001). Interaction relating to privacy, identity, autonomy and security. An observational study focusing on a woman with dementia and "behavioural disturbances", and her care providers. *Journal of Advanced Nursing*, **36**, 256–65.

Greendyke, R. M. & Kanter, D. R. (1986). Therapeutic effects of pindolol on behavioural disturbances associated with organic brain disease: a double-blind study. *Journal of Clinical Psychiatry*, **47**, 423–6.

Greendyke, R. M., Kanter, D. R., Schuster, D. B. *et al.* (1986). Propranolol treatment of assaultative patients with organic brain disease. A double-blind crossover, placebo-controlled study. *Journal of Nervous and Mental Disorders*, **174**, 290–4.

Greendyke, R. M., Schuster, D. B. & Woonton, J. A. (1984). Propranolol in the treatment of assaultative patients with organic brain disease. *Journal of Clinical Psychopharmacology*, **4**, 282–5.

Grohmann, R., Engel, R. R., Geissler, K. H. & Ruther, E. (2004). Psychotropic drug use in psychiatric inpatients: recent trends and changes over time-data from the AMSP study. *Pharmacopsychiatry*, **37** (Suppl. 1), S27–38.

Gryle, D., Friedman, R., Tal, D. & Frendman, M. (1986). The noisy patient. Prevalence, assessment and management. *Abstracts of Clinical and Investigative Medicine*, **9**, 75.

Gualtieri, C. T. (1991a). Buspirone for the behaviour problems of patients with organic brain disorder. (letter) *Journal of Clinical Psychopharmacology*, **11**, 280–1.

Gualtieri, C. T. (1991b). Buspirone: neuropsychiatric effects. *Journal of Head Trauma Rehabilitation*, **6**, 90–2.

Gualtieri, C. T. & Evans, R. W. (1988). Stimulant treatment for the neurobehavioural sequelae of traumatic brain injury. *Brain Injury*, **2**, 273–90.

Haas, J. P. & Cope, D. V. (1985). Neuropharmacologic management of behavioural sequelae in head injury: a case report. *Archives of Physical Medical Rehabilitation*, **66**, 472–4.

Hagen, B. & Sayers, D. (1995). When caring leaves bruises: the effects of staff education on resident aggression. *Journal of Gerontology Nursing*, **21**, 7–16.

Haight, B., Bachman, D., Hendrix, S., Wagner, M., Meeks, A. & Johnson, J. (2003). Life review: treating the dyadic family unit with dementia. *Clinical Psychology and Psychotherapy*, **10**, 165–74.

Hale, M. S. & Donaldson, J. (1982). Lithium carbonate in the treatment of organic brain syndrome. *Journal of Nervous and Mental Disorders*, **170**, 362–5.

Hamilton, M. (1960). A rating scale for depression. *Journal of Neurology, Neurosurgery, and Psychiatry*, **23**, 56–62.

Hanley, I. G., McGuire, R. J. & Boyd, W. D. (1981). Reality orientation and dementia: a controlled trial of two approaches. *British Journal of Psychiatry*, **138**, 10–14.

Haupt, M., Karger, A. & Janner, M. (2000). Improvement of agitation and anxiety in demented patients after psychoeducative group intervention with their caregivers. *International Journal of Geriatric Psychiatry*, **15**, 1125–9.

Hausman, C. P. (1991). Dynamic psychotherapy with elderly demented patients. In *Caregiving in Dementia*, ed. G. Jones & B. Miesen. Amsterdam: Routledge.

Haussermann, P., Goecker, D., Beier, K. & Schroeder, S. (2003). Low-dose cyproterone acetate treatment of sexual acting out in men with dementia. *International Psychogeriatrics*, **15**, 181–6.

Herrmann, N. (2001). Recommendations for the management of behavioural and psychological symptoms of dementia. *Canadian Journal of Neurological Science*, **28** (Suppl. 1), S96–107.

Herrmann, N. & Knopman, D. (2004). Donepezil therapy for neuropsychiatric symptoms in AD: methods make the message. *Neurology*, **63**, 200–1.

Herrmann, N., Lanctot, K. L., Eryavec, G. & Khan, L. R. (2004a). Noradrenergic activity is associated with response to pindolol in aggressive Alzheimer's disease patients. *Journal of Psychopharmacology*, **18**, 215–20.

Herrmann, N., Mamdani, M. & Lanctôt, K. L. (2004b). Atypical antipsychotics and risk of cerebrovascular accidents. *American Journal of Psychiatry*, **161**, 1113–15.

Herz, L. R., Volicer, L., Ross, V. & Rheaume, Y. (1992). A single-case-study method for treating resistiveness in patients with Alzheimer's disease. *Hospital Community Psychiatry*, **43**, 720–4.

Hilton, C. & Moniz-Cook, E. (2004). Examining the personality dimensions of sociotropy and autonomy in older people with dementia: their relevance to person centered care. *Behavioural and Cognitive Psychotherapy*, **32**, 457–65.

Holden, U. P. & Woods, R. T. (1995). *Positive Approaches to Dementia Care*, 3rd edn. Edinburgh: Churchill Livingstone.

Holmberg, S. (1997). Evaluation of a clinical intervention for wanderers on a geriatric nursing unit. *Archives of Psychiatric Nursing*, **11**, 21–8.

Holmes, C., Wilkinson, D., Dean, C. *et al.* (2004). The efficacy of donepezil in the treatment of neuropsychiatric symptoms in Alzheimer disease. *Neurology*, **63**, 214–19.

Hope, T., Keene, J., Fairburn, C. *et al.* (1999). Natural history of behavioural changes and psychiatric symptoms in Alzheimer's disease. *British Journal of Psychiatry*, **174**, 39–44.

Horne, M. & Lindley, S. E. (1995). Divalproex sodium in the treatment of aggressive behaviour and dysphoria in patients with organic brain syndromes (letter). *Journal of Clinical Psychiatry*, **56**, 430–1.

Hornstein, A., Lennihan, L., Seliger, G. *et al.* (1995). Amphetamine in recovery from brain injury. *Brain Injury*, **10**, 145–8.

Howard, R., Ballard, C., O'Brien, J. & Burns, A. (2001). Guidelines for the management of agitation in dementia. *International Journal of Geriatric Psychiatry*, **16**, 714–17.

Hussian, R. A. (1982). Stimulus control in the modification of problematic behaviour in elderly institutionalized patients. *International Journal of Behavioural Geriatrics*, **2**, 33–46.

Hussian, R. A. (1988). Modification of behaviours in dementia via stimulus manipulation. *Clinical Gerontologist*, **8**, 37–43.

Hussian, R. A. & Brown, D. C. (1987). Use of two-dimensional grid patterns to limit hazardous ambulation in demented patients. *Journal of Gerontology*, **42**, 558–60.

International Psychogeriatric Association (2002). *Behavioural and Psychological Symptoms of Dementia* (pp. 1–20). www.ipa-online.org/ipaonlinev3/ipaprograms/bpsdarchives/bpsdrev/6BPSDfinal.pdf: International Psychogeriatric Association.

International Psychogeriatric Association (1998). *Behavioural and Psychological Symptoms of Dementia*. Chicago: International Psychogeriatric Association.

Jackson, C. W., Pitner, J. K. & Mintzer, J. E. (1996). Zolpidem for the treatment of agitation in elderly demented patients. *Journal of Clinical Psychiatry*, **57**, 372–3.

Jackson, C., Carson, W., Markowitz, J. & Mintzer, J. (1995). SIADH associated with fluoxetine and sertraline therapy. *American Journal of Psychiatry*, **152**, 809–10.

Jansen, I. H., Olde Rikkert, M. G., Hulsbos, H. A. & Hoefnagels, W. H. (2001). Toward individualized evidence-based medicine: five "N of 1" trials of methylphenidate in geriatric patients. *Journal of the American Geriatric Society*, **49**, 474–6.

Jennett, B. & Bond, M. (1975). Assessment of outcome after severe brain injury: a practical scale. *Lancet*, **I**, 480–5.

Jeste, D. V. & Finkel, S. I. (2000). Psychosis of Alzheimer's disease and related dementias. Diagnostic criteria for a distinct syndrome. *American Journal of Geriatric Psychiatry*, **8**, 29–34.

Jones, S. (1995). An interpersonal approach to psychotherapy with older persons with dementia. *Professional Psychology Research and Practice*, **26**, 602–7.

Karli, D. C., Burke, D. T., Hyun Jung Kim *et al.* (1998). Effects of dopaminergic combination therapy for frontal lobe dysfunction in traumatic brain injury rehabilitation. *Brain Injury*, **13**, 63–8.

Katona, C., Hunter, B. & Bray, J. (1998). A double-blind comparison of the efficacy and safety of paroxetine and imipramine in the treatment of depression with dementia. *International Journal of Geriatic Psychiatry*, **13**, 100–8.

Katz, I. R., Jeste, D. V., Mintzer, J. E., Clyde, C., Napolitano, J. & Brecher, M. (1999). Comparison of risperidone and placebo for psychosis and behavioural disturbances associated with dementia: a randomized, double-blind trial. Risperidone Study Group. *Journal of Clinical Psychiatry*, **60**, 107–15.

Kayser-Jones, J. (1997). Inadequate staffing at mealtime. Implications for nursing and health policy. *Journal of Gerontology Nursing*, **23**, 14–21.

Kayser-Jones, J. & Pengilly, K. (1999). Dysphagia among nursing home residents. *Geriatric Nursing*, **20**, 77–82.

Kayser-Jones, J., Schell, E. S., Porter, C. *et al.* (1998). A prospective study of the use of liquid oral dietary supplements in nursing homes. *Journal of the American Geriatric Society*, **46**, 1378–86.

Kayser-Jones, J., Schell, E. S., Porter, C., Barbaccia, J. C. & Shaw, H. (1999). Factors contributing to dehydration in nursing homes:

inadequate staffing and lack of professional supervision. *Journal of the American Geriatrics Society*, **47**, 1187–94.

Kazdin, A. (1989). *Behavioural Modification in Applied Settings*, 4th edition. Pacific Grove, CA: Brooks/Cole.

Keene, J., Hope, T., Fairburn, C. G., Jacoby, R., Gedling, K. & Ware, C. (1999). Natural history of aggressive behaviour in dementia. *International Journal of Geriatric Psychiatry*, **14**, 541–8.

Kessler, R. C. *et al.* (2007), Meta-analysis of effects of methylphenidate in adult attention deficit hyperactivity disorder (ADHD).

Kim, S., Song, H. & Yoo, S. (2003). The effect of bright light on sleep and behaviour in dementia: An Analytic Review. *Geriatric Nursing*, **24**, 239–43.

Kim, E. & Humaran, T. J. (2002). Divalproax in the management of neuropsychiatric complications of remote acquired brain injury. *Journal of Neuropsychiatry and Clinical Neurosciences*, **14**, 202–5.

Kirkevold, O. & Engedal, K. (2004). A study into the use of restraint in nursing homes in Norway. *British Journal of Nursing*, **13**, 902–5.

Krakowski, M. & Czobor, P. (1997). Violence in psychiatric patients. *Comprehensive Psychiatry*, **38**, 230–6.

Kraus, M. F. & Maki, P. (1996). The combined use of amantadine and l-dopa/carbidopa in the treatment of chronic brain injury. *Brain Injury*, **11**, 455–60.

Kruglov, L. (2003). The early stage of vascular dementia: significance of a complete therapeutic program. *International Journal of Geriatric Psychiatry*, **18**, 402–6.

Kyomen, H. H., Satlin, A., Hennen, J. & Wei, J. Y. (1999). Estrogen therapy and aggressive behaviour in elderly patients with moderate-to-severe dementia: results from a short-term, randomized, double-blind trial. *American Journal of Geriatric Psychiatry*, **7**, 339–48.

Lai, C., Chi, I. & Kayser-Jones, J. (2004). A randomized controlled trial of a specific reminiscence approach to promote the well-being of nursing home residents with dementia. *International Psychogeriatrics*, **16**, 33–49.

Lai, C. K. Y. & Arthur, D. G. (2003). Wandering behaviour in people with dementia. *Journal of Advanced Nursing*, **44**, 173–82.

Lanctôt, K. L., Best, T. S., Mittmann, N. *et al.* (1998). Efficacy and safety of neuroleptics in behavioural disorders associated with dementia. *Journal of Clinical Psychiatry*, **59**, 550–61; quiz 562–3.

Lanctôt, K. L., Herrmann, N., van Reekum, R., Eryavec, G. & Naranjo, C. A. (2002). Gender, aggression and serotonergic function are associated with response to sertraline for behavioural disturbances in Alzheimer's disease. *International Journal of Geriatric Psychiatry*, **17**, 531–41.

Laundreville, P., Bordes, M., Dicaire, L. & Verrault, R. (1998). Behavioural approaches for reducing agitation in residents of long-term-care facilities: critical review and suggestions for future research. *International Psychogeriatrics*, **10**, 397–419.

Lawlor, B. A. (2004). Behavioural and psychological symptoms in dementia: the role of atypical antipsychotics. *Journal of Clinical Psychiatry*, **65** (Suppl. 11), 5–10.

Lawlor, B. A., Radcliffe, J., Molchan, S. E., Martinez, R. A., Hill, J. L. & Sunderland, T. (1994). A pilot placebo-controlled study of

trazodone and buspirone in Alzheimer's disease. *International Journal of Geriatric Psychiatry*, **9**, 55–9.

Lewis, G., Pelosi A. J., Araya, R. C. *et al.* (1992). Measuring psychiatric disorder in the community: a standardized assessment for use by lay interviewers. *Psychological Medicine*, **22**, 465–86.

Levin, H. S., High, W. M., Goethe, K. E. *et al.* (1987). The neurobehavioural rating scale: assessment of the behavioural sequelae of head injury by the clinician. *Journal of Neurology, Neurosurgery and Psychiatry*, **50**, 183–93.

Libin, A. & Cohen-Mansfield, J. (2004). Therapeutic robocat for nursing home residents with dementia: preliminary inquiry. *American Journal of Alzheimer's Disease and Dementia*, **19**, 111–16.

Lonergan, E. T., Cameron, M. & Luxenberg, J. (2004). Valproic acid for agitation in dementia. *Cochrane Database of Systematic Reviews*, CD003945. Oxford: Update Software Ltd.

Lovell, B., Ancoli-Israel, S. & Gervirtz, R. (1995). Effect of bright light treatment on agitated behaviour in institutionalized elderly subjects. *Psychiatry Research*, **57**, 7–12.

Low, L., Brodaty, H. & Draper, B. A. (2002). Study of premorbid personality and behavioural and psychological symptoms of dementia in nursing home residents. *International Journal of Geriatric Psychiatry*, **17**, 779–83.

Loy, C. & Schneider, L. (2004). Galantamine for Alzheimer's disease. *Cochrane Database of Systematic Reviews*, CD001747. Oxford: Update Software Ltd.

Lyketsos, C., Veiel, L., Baker, A. & Steele, C. (1999). A randomized, controlled trial of bright light therapy for agitated behaviours in dementia patients residing in long-term care. *International Journal of Geriatric Psychiatry*, **14**, 520–5.

Lyketsos, C. G., Sheppard, J. M., Steele, C. D. *et al.* (2000). Randomized, placebo-controlled, double-blind clinical trial of sertraline in the treatment of depression complicating Alzheimer's disease: initial results from depression in Alzheimer's Disease study. *American Journal of Psychiatry*, **157**, 1686–9.

Lyketsos, C. G., DelCampo, L., Steinberg, M. *et al.* (2003). Treating depression in Alzheimer disease: efficacy and safety of sertraline therapy, and the benefits of depression reduction: the DIADS. *Archives of General Psychiatry*, **60**, 737–46.

Malloy, D., McIlroy, W., Guyatt, G. & Lever, J. (1991). Validity and reliability of the Dysfunctional Behaviour Rating Instrument. *Acta Psychiatrica Scandinavica*, **84**, 103–6.

Maryniak, O., Manchanda, R. & Velani, A. (2001). Methotrimeprazine in the treatment of agitation in acquired brain injury patients. *Brain Injury*, **15**, 167–74.

Masanic, C., Bayley, M. T., van Reekum, R. & Simard, M. (2001). Open-label study of donepezil in traumatic brain injury. *Archives of Physical Medicine and Rehabilitation*, **82**, 896–901.

Mathews, E., Farrell, G. & Blackmore, A. (1996). Effects of an environmental manipulation emphasizing client-centered care on agitation and sleep in dementia sufferers in a nursing home. *Journal of Advanced Nursing*, **24**, 439–47.

Mattes, J. A. (1985). Metoprolol for intermittent explosive disorder. *American Journal of Psychiatry*, **142**, 1108–9.

McCallion, P., Toseland, R., Lacey, D. et al. (1999). Educating nursing assistants to communicate more effectively with nursing home residents with dementia. Gerontologist, 39, 546–58.

McKeith, I., Del Ser, T., Spano, P. et al. (2000). Efficacy of rivastigmine in dementia with Lewy bodies: a randomised, double-blind, placebo-controlled international study. Lancet, 356, 2031–6.

Meehan, K. M., Wang, H., David, S. R. et al. (2002). Comparison of rapidly acting intramuscular olanzapine, lorazepam, and placebo: a double-blind, randomized study in acutely agitated patients with dementia. Neuropsychopharmacology, 26, 494–504.

Mega, M. S., Masterman, D. M., O'Connor, S. M., Barclay, T. R. & Cummings, J. L. (1999). The spectrum of behavioural responses to cholinesterase inhibitor therapy in Alzheimer disease. Archives of Neurology, 56, 1388–93.

Meythaler, J. M., Depalma, L., Devivo, M. J. et al. (2001). Sertraline to improve arousal and alertness in severe traumatic brain injury secondary to motor vehicle crashes. Brain Injury, 15, 321–31.

Meythaler, J. M., Bruner, R. C., Johnson, A. & Thomas, A. (2002). Amantadine to improve neurorecovery in traumatic brain injury-associated diffuse axonal injury: a pilot double-blind randomised trail. Journal of Head Trauma Rehabilitation, 17, 300–13.

Michals, M. L., Crismon, M. L., Roberts, S. et al. (1993). Clozapine response and adverse effects in nine brain-injured patients. Journal of Clinical Psychopharmacology, 13, 198–203.

Miller, M. D. (1989). Opportunities for psychotherapy in the management of dementia. Journal of Geriatric Psychiatry and Neurology, 2, 11–17.

Miller, S., Vermeersch, P., Bohan, K., Renbarger, K., Kruep, A. & Sacre, S. (2001). Audio presence intervention for decreasing agitation in people with dementia. Geriatric Nursing, 22, 66–70.

Mintzer, J., Faison, W., Street, J. S., Sutton, V. K. & Breier, A. (2001). Olanzapine in the treatment of anxiety symptoms due to Alzheimer's disease: a post hoc analysis. International Journal of Geriatric Psychiatry, 16 (Suppl. 1), S71–7.

Mishara, B. & Kastenbaum, R. (1973). Self-injurious behaviour and environmental change in the institutionalized elderly. International Journal of Aging and Human Development, 4, 133–45.

Molloy, D. W., McLlroy, W. E., Guyatt, G. H. & Lever, J. A. (1991). Validity and reliability of the Dysfunctional Behaviour Rating Instrument. Acta Psychiatrica Scandinavica, 84, 103–6.

Moniz-Cook, E. Stokes, G. & Agar, S. (2003). Difficult behaviour and dementia in nursing homes: Five Cases of Psychosocial Intervention. Clinical Psychology and Psychotherapy, 10, 197–208.

Montgomery, P. & Dennis, J. (2004). A systematic review of non-pharmacological therapies for sleep problems in later life. Sleep Medicine Reviews, 8, 47–62.

Mooney, G. F. & Haas, L. J. (1993). Effect of methylphenidate on brain injury related anger. Archives of Physical Medical Rehabilitation, 74, 153–60.

Moretti, R., Torre, P., Antonello, R. M., Cazzato, G. & Bava, A. (2003). Gabapentin for the treatment of behavioural alterations in dementia: preliminary 15-month investigation. Drugs and Aging, 20, 1035–40.

Morton, I. & Bleathman, C. (1991). The effectiveness of validation therapy in dementia – a pilot study. International Journal of Geriatric Psychiatry, 6, 327–30.

Mosher-Ashley, P. & Witkowski, J. (1999). Counseling older adults with dementia: a survey of therapists in Massachusetts. Journal of Clinical Geropsychology, 5, 265–79.

Muller, U., Murai, T., Bauer-Wittmund, T. et al. (1999). Paroxetine versus citalopram treatment of pathological crying after brain injury. Brain Injury, 13, 805–11.

Mulsant, B. H., Gharabawi, G. M., Bossie, C. A. et al. (2004). Correlates of anticholinergic activity in patients with dementia and psychosis treated with risperidone or olanzapine. Journal of Clinical Psychiatry, 65, 1708–14.

Nadal, M. & Allgulander, S. (1993). Normalization of sexual behaviour in a female with dementia after treatment with cyproterone. International Journal of Geriatric Psychiatry, 8, 265–7.

Nagaratnam, N., Patel, I. & Whelan, C. (2003). Screaming, shrieking and muttering: the noise-makers amongst dementia patients. Archives of Gerontology and Geriatrics, 36, 247–58.

Nagaratnam, N., Lewis-Jones M., Scott D. & Palazzi L. (1998). Behavioural and psychiatric manifestations in dementia patients in a community: caregiver burden and outcome. Alzheimer's Disease and Associated Disorders, 12, 330–4.

Negley, E. & Manley, J. (1990). Environmental interventions in assaultive behaviour. Journal of Gerontology Nursing, 16, 29–33.

Newburn, G., Edwards, R., Thomas, H. et al. (1999). Moclobemide in the treatment of major depressive disorder (DSM-III) following traumatic brain injury. Brain Injury, 13, 637–42.

Nyenhuis, D. L. & Gorelick, P. B. (1998). Vascular dementia: a contemporary review of epidemiology, diagnosis, prevention, and treatment. Journal of the American Geriatric Society, 46, 1437–48.

Nyth, A. L. & Gottfries, C. G. (1990). The clinical efficacy of citalopram in treatment of emotional disturbances in dementia disorders. A Nordic multicentre study. British Journal of Psychiatry, 157, 894–901.

Olafsson, K., Jorgensen, S., Jensen, H. V., Bille, A., Arup, P. & Andersen, J. (1992). Fluvoxamine in the treatment of demented elderly patients: a double-blind, placebo-controlled study. Acta Psychiatrica Scandinavica, 85, 453–6.

Olin, J. T., Fox, L. S., Pawluczyk, S., Taggart, N. A. & Schneider, L. S. (2001). A pilot randomized trial of carbamazepine for behavioural symptoms in treatment-resistant outpatients with Alzheimer disease. American Journal of Geriatric Psychiatry, 9, 400–5.

Onder, G., Zanetti, O., Giacbini, E. et al. (2005). Reality orientation therapy combined with cholinesterase inhibitors in Alzheimer's disease: randomised controlled trial. British Journal of Psychiatry, 187, 450–5.

Opie, J., Doyle, C. & O'Connor, D. (2002). Challenging behaviours in nursing home residents with dementia: a randomised controlled trial of multidisciplinary interventions. International Journal of Geriatric Psychiatry, 17, 6–13.

Oslin, D. W., Ten Have, T. R., Streim, J. E. et al. (2003). Probing the safety of medications in the frail elderly: evidence from a

randomized clinical trial of sertraline and venlafaxine in depressed nursing home residents. *Journal of Clinical Psychiatry*, **64**, 875–82.

Parmalee, D. X. & O'Shanick, G. J. (1998). Carbamazepine-lithium toxicity in brain-damaged adolescents. *Brain Injury*, **2**, 305–8.

Patel, V. & Hope, R. (1992). A rating scale for aggressive behaviour in the elderly – the RAGE. *Psychological Medicine*, **22**, 211–21.

Perino, C., Rago, R., Cicolin, A., Torta, R. & Monaco, F. (2001). Mood and behavioural disorders following traumatic brain injury: clinical evaluation and pharmacological management. *Brain Injury*, **15**, 139–48.

Peskind, E. R., Tsuang, D. W., Bonner, L. T. *et al.* (2005). Propranolol for disruptive behaviours in nursing home residents with probable or possible Alzheimer disease: a placebo-controlled study. *Alzheimer's Disease and Associated Disorders*, **19**, 23–8.

Petracca, G., Teson, A., Chemerinski, E., Leiguarda, R. & Starkstein, S. E. (1996). A double-blind placebo-controlled study of clomipramine in depressed patients with Alzheimer's disease. *Journal of Neuropsychiatry and Clinical Neurosciences*, **8**, 270–5.

Plenger, P. M., Dixon, C. E., Castillo, R. M. *et al.* (1996). Subacute methylphenidate treatment for moderate to moderately severe traumatic brain injury: a preliminary double blind placebo-controlled study. *Archives of Physical Medical Rehabilitation*, **77**, 536–40.

Pollock, B. G., Mulsant, B. H., Rosen, J. *et al.* (2002). Comparison of citalopram, perphenazine, and placebo for the acute treatment of psychosis and behavioural disturbances in hospitalized, demented patients. *American Journal of Psychiatry*, **159**, 460–5.

Pope, H. G., Mcelroy, S. L., Satlin, A. *et al.* (1988). Head injury, bipolar disorder and response to valproate. *Comprehensive Psychiatry*, **29**, 34–8.

Porsteinsson, A. P., Tariot, P. N., Erb, R. *et al.* (2001). Placebo-controlled study of divalproex sodium for agitation in dementia. *American Journal of Geriatric Psychiatry*, **9**, 58–66.

Proctor, R., Burns, A., Stratton-Powell, H. *et al.* (1999). Behavioural management in nursing and residential homes: a randomized controlled trial. *Lancet*, **354**, 26–9.

Pusey, H. (2000). Dementia care: interventions with people with dementia and their informal caregivers. *Mental and Health Care*, **3**, 204–7.

Rabheru, K. (2004). Special issues in the management of depression in older patients. *Canadian Journal of Psychiatry*, **49**, 41S–50S.

Rabinowitz, J., Katz, I. R., De Deyn, P. P., Brodaty, H., Greenspan, A. & Davidson, M. (2004). Behavioural and psychological symptoms in patients with dementia as a target for pharmacotherapy with risperidone. *Journal of Clinical Psychiatry*, **65**, 1329–34.

Ragneskog, H., Asplund, K., Kihlgren, M. & Norberg, A. (2001). Individualized music played for agitated patients with dementia: analysis of video-recorded sessions. *International Journal of Nursing Practice*, **7**, 146–55.

Ragneskog, J., Bräne, G., Karlsson, I. & Kihlgren, M. (1996). Influence of dinner music on food intake and symptoms common in dementia. *Scandinavian Journal of Caring Sciences*, **10**, 11–17.

Ranen, N. G., Lipsey, J. R., Treisman, G. *et al.* (1996). Sertraline in the treatment of severe aggressiveness in Huntingdon's disease. *Journal of Neuropsychiatry and Clinical Neurosciences*, **8**, 338–40.

Raskin, A. & Crook, T. (1988). Global Assessment of Psychiatric Symptoms (GAPS). *Psychopharmacology Bulletin*, **24**, 721–5.

Ratey, J. J., Leveroni, C. L., Miller, A. C. *et al.* (1992). Low-dose buspirone to treat agitation and maladaptive behaviour in brain-injured patients: two case reports (letter). *Journal of Clinical Psychopharmacology*, **12**, 362–4.

Reeve, W. & Ivison, D. (1985). Use of environmental manipulation and classroom and modified informal reality orientation with institutionalised, confused elderly patients. *Age and Aging*, **14**, 119–21.

Reifler, B. V., Teri, L., Raskind, M. *et al.* (1989). Double-blind trial of imipramine in Alzheimer's disease patients with and without depression. *American Journal of Psychiatry*, **146**, 45–9.

Reinhard, D. L., Whyte, J. & Sandel, E. (1996). Improved arousal and initiation following tricyclic antidepressant use in severe brain injury. *Archives of Physical Medical Rehabilitation*, **77**, 80–3.

Reisberg, B., Borenstein, J., Salob, S. P., Ferris, S. H., Franssen, E. & Georgotas, A. (1987). Behavioral symptoms in Alzheimer's disease: phenomenology and treatment. *Journal of Clinical Psychiatry*, **48** (Suppl.), 9–15.

Reisberg, B., Auer, S. & Monteiro, I. (1996). Behavioural pathology in Alzhemer's disease. (BEHAVE-AD) rating scale. *International Psychogeriatrics*, **8** (Suppl. 3), 301–8.

Reisberg, B., Doody, R., Stoffler, A., Schmitt, F., Ferris, S. & Mobius, H. J. (2003). Memantine in moderate-to-severe Alzheimer's disease. *New England Journal of Medicine*, **348**, 1333–41.

Remington, R. (1999). Calming music and hand massage with agitated elderly. Unpublished doctoral dissertation. University of Massachusetts: Amherst and Worcester MA.

Robichaud, L., Hebert, R. & Desrosiers, J. (1994). Efficacy of a sensory integration program on behaviours of inpatients with dementia. *American Journal of Occupational Therapy*, **48**, 355–60.

Rockwood, K., Mintzer, J., Truyen, L., Wessel, T. & Wilkinson, D. (2001). Effects of a flexible galantamine dose in Alzheimer's disease: a randomised, controlled trial. *Journal of Neurology, Neurosurgery and Psychiatry*, **71**, 589–95.

Rosberger, Z. & MacLean, J. (1983). Behavioural assessment and treatment of "organic" behaviours in an institutionalized geriatric patient. *International Journal of Behavioural Geriatrics*, **1**, 33–46.

Rosen, J., Burgio, L., Kollar, M. *et al.* (1994). The Pittsburg Agitation Scale: a user-friendly instrument for rating agitation in dementia patients. *American Journal of Geriatric Psychiatry*, **2**, 52–9.

Rosin, A. J. (1977). The physical and behavioural complex of dementia. *Gerontology*, **23**, 37–46.

Rosler, M., Retz, W., Retz-Junginger, P. & Dennler, H. J. (1998). Effects of two-year treatment with the cholinesterase inhibitor rivastigmine on behavioural symptoms in Alzheimer's disease. *Behavioral Neurology*, **11**, 211–16.

Rovner, B. W., Steele, C. D., Shmuely, Y. & Folstein, M. F. (1996). A randomised trial of dementia care in nursing homes. *Journal of the American Geriatric Society*, **44**, 7–13.

Rowland, T., Mysiw, W. J., Bogner, J. *et al.* (1992). Trazodone for post traumatic agitation. *Archives of Physical Medical Rehabilitation*, **73**, 963.

Rubin, E. H., Drevets W. C. & Burke, W. J. (1988). The nature of psychotic symptoms in senile dementia of the Alzheimer type. *Journal of Geriatric Psychiatry and Neurology*, **1**, 16–20.

Sadavoy, J. (2004). Antipsychotic agents. In *Psychotropic Drugs and the Elderly: Fast Facts*, pp. 240–1. New York: WW Norton and Co.

Sadavoy, J. (1991). Psychodynamic perspectives on dementia: Alzheimer's disease and the individual. *American Journal of Alzheimer's Care and Research*, **6**, 12–20.

Sadavoy, J. & Robinson, A. (1989). Psychotherapy with the cognitively impaired elderly. In *Psychiatric Consequences of Brain Disease in the Elderly: Focus on Management*, ed. D. Conn, A. Grek & J. Sadavoy. New York: Plenum Press.

Sanders, J. F. (1965). Evaluation of oxazepam and placebo in emotionally disturbed aged patients. *Geriatrics*, **20**, 739–46.

Satlin, A., Volicer, L., Ross, V. *et al.* (1992). Bright light treatment of behavioural and sleep disturbances in patients with Alzheimer's disease. *American Journal of Psychiatry*, **149**, 1028–32.

Schatzberg, A. F., Kremer, C., Rodrigues, H. E. & Murphy, G. M., Jr. (2002). Double-blind, randomized comparison of mirtazapine and paroxetine in elderly depressed patients. *American Journal of Geriatric Psychiatry*, **10**, 541–50.

Schiff, H. B., Sabin, T. D., Geller, A. *et al.* (1982). Lithium in aggressive behaviour. *American Journal of Psychiatry*, **139**, 1346–8.

Schneider, L. S., Pollock, V. E. & Lyness, S. A. (1990). A metaanalysis of controlled trials of neuroleptic treatment in dementia. *Journal of the American Geriatrics Society*, **38**, 553–63.

Schneider, W. N., Drew-Cates, J., Wong, T. M. *et al.* (1999). Cognitive and behavioural efficacy of amantadine in acute traumatic brain injury: an initial double-blind placebo-controlled study. *Brain Injury*, **13**, 863–72.

Scott, J. & Clare, L. (2003). Do people with dementia benefit from psychological interventions offered on a group basis? *Clinical Psychology and Psychotherapy*, **10**, 186–96.

Shaw, S. H. Curson, H. & Coquelin, J. P. (1992). A double-blind, comparative study of zolpidem and placebo in the treatment of insomnia in elderly psychiatric in-patients. *Journal of International Medical Research*, **20**, 150–61.

Shelton, P. S. & Hocking, L. B. (1997). Zolpidem for dementia-related insomnia and nighttime wandering. *Annals of Pharmacotherapy*, **31**, 319–22.

Siegler, I. C., Dawson, D. V. & Welsh, K. A. (1994). Caregiver rating of personality change in Alzheimer's disease patients: A replication. *Psychology and Aging*, **9**, 464–6.

Sinha, D., Zemlan, F. P., Nelson, S. *et al.* (1992). A new scale for assessing behavioral agitation in dementia. *Psychiatry Research*, **41**, 73–88.

Sink, K. M., Holden, K. F. & Yaffe, K. (2005). Pharmacological treatment of neuropsychiatric symptoms of dementia: a review of the evidence. *Journal of the American Medical Association*, **293**, 596–608.

Sival, R. C., Haffmans, P. M., Jansen, P. A., Duursma, S. A. & Eikelenboom, P. (2002). Sodium valproate in the treatment of aggressive behaviour in patients with dementia – a randomized placebo controlled clinical trial. *International Journal of Geriatric Psychiatry*, **17**, 579–85.

Skovdahl, K., Kihlgren, A. L. & Kihlgren, M. (2003a). Different attitudes when handling aggressive behaviour in dementia – narratives from two caregiver groups. *Aging and Mental Health*, **7**, 277–86.

Skovdahl, K., Kihlgren, A. L. & Kihlgren, M. (2003b). Dementia and aggressiveness: video recorded morning care from different care units. *Journal of Clinical Nursing*, **12**, 888–95.

Skovdahl, K., Kihlgren, A. L. & Kihlgren, M. (2004). Dementia and aggressiveness: stimulated recall interviews with caregivers after video-recorded interactions. *Journal of Clinical Nursing*, **13**, 515–25.

Slaughter, J., Bobo, W. & Childers, M. K. (1999). Selective serotonin reuptake inhibitor treatment of post-traumatic Kluver–Bucy syndrome. *Brain Injury*, **13**, 59–62.

Sloane, P., Hoeffer, B., Mitchell, C. *et al.* (2004). Effect of person-centered showering and the towel bath on bathing-associated aggression, agitation, and discomfort in nursing home residents with dementia: a randomized, controlled trial. *Journal of the American Geriatrics Society*, **52**, 1795–804.

Smallwood, J., Brown, R., Coulter, F., Irvine, E. & Copland, C. (2001). Aromatherapy and behaviour disturbances in dementia: a randomized controlled trial. *International Journal of Geriatric Psychiatry*, **16**, 1010–13.

Smith, K. R., Goulding, P. M., Wilderman, D. *et al.* (1994). Neurobehavioural effects of phenytoin and carbamazepine in patients recovering from brain trauma. *Archives of Neurology*, **51**, 653–60.

Snowden, M., Sato, K. & Roy-Byrne, P. (2003). Assessment and treatment of nursing home residents with depression or behavioural symptoms associated with dementia: a review of the literature. *Journal of the American Geriatric Society*, **51**, 1305–17.

Snyder, M., Egan, E. & Burns, K. (1995). Efficacy of hand massage in decreasing agitation behaviours associated with cure activities in persons with dementia. *Geriatric Nursing*, **16**, 60–3.

So, C. C. & Wong, K. F. (2002). Valproate-associated dysmyelopoiesis in elderly patients. *American Journal of Clinical Pathology*, **118**, 225–8.

Solms, M. & Turnbull, O. (2002). *The Brain and the Inner World: An Introduction to Neuroscience of Subjective Experience*. London: Karnac Press.

Spayd, C. S. & Smyer, M. A. (1988). Interventions with agitated, disoriented, or depressed residents. In *Mental Health Constitution in Nursing Homes*, ed. M. A. Smyer, M. D. Cohn & D. Brannon, pp. 123–41. New York: University Press.

Spector, A., Orrell, M., Davies, S. & Woods, R. (2003). Reminiscence therapy for dementia. *Cochrane Database of Systematic Reviews*, **3**. Oxford: Update Software Ltd.

Spector, A., Orrell, M., Davies, S. & Woods, R. T. (1999). Reality orientation for dementia. *Cochrane Database of Systematic Reviews*, **4**. Oxford: Update Software Ltd.

Speech, T. J., Rao, S. M., Osmon, D. C. & Sperrys, L. T. (1993). A double-blind controlled study of methylphenidate treatment in closed head injury. *Brain Injury*, **7**, 333–8.

Stanislav, S. W. (1997). Cognitive effects of antipsychotic agents in persons with traumatic brain injury. *Brain Injury*, **11**, 335–41.

Stanislav, S. W. & Childs, A. (2000). Evaluating the usage of droperidol in acutely agitated persons with brain injury. *Brain Injury*, **14**, 261–5.

Stanislav, S. W., Fabre, T., Crismon, M. L. *et al.* (1994). Buspirone's efficacy in organic-induced aggression. *Journal of Clinical Psychopharmacology*, **14**, 126–30.

Stewart, J. T. & Hemsath, R. H. (1988). Bipolar illness following traumatic brain injury: treatment with lithium and carbamazepine. *Journal of Clinical Psychiatry*, **49**, 74–5.

Stotsky, B. (1984). Multicenter study comparing thioridazine with diazepam and placebo in elderly, nonpsychotic patients with emotional and behavioural disorders. *Clinical Therapy*, **6**, 546–59.

Strauss, M. Lee, M. & DiFilippo, J. (1997). Premorbid personality and behavioural symptoms in Alzheimer's disease: some cautions. *Archives of Neurology*, **54**, 257–9.

Streams, M., Wackerbarth, S. & Maxwell, A. (2003). Diagnosis-seeking at specialty memory clinics: trigger events. *International Journal of Geriatric Psychiatry*, **18**, 915–24.

Street, J. S., Clark, W. S., Gannon, K. S. *et al.* (2000). Olanzapine treatment of psychotic and behavioural symptoms in patients with Alzheimer disease in nursing care facilities: a double-blind, randomized, placebo-controlled trial. The HGEU Study Group. *Archives of Genernal Psychiatry*, **57**, 968–76.

Street, J. S., Clark, W. S., Kadam, D. L. *et al.* (2001). Long-term efficacy of olanzapine in the control of psychotic and behavioural symptoms in nursing home patients with Alzheimer's dementia. *International Journal of Geriatric Psychiatry*, **16** (Suppl. 1), S62–70.

Sultzer, D. L., Gray, K. F., Gunay, I., Berisford, M. A. & Mahler, M. E. (1997). A double-blind comparison of trazodone and haloperidol for treatment of agitation in patients with dementia. *American Journal of Geriatric Psychiatry*, **5**, 60–9.

Sunderland, T., Weingartner, H., Cohen, R. M. *et al.* (1989). Low-dose oral lorazepam administration in Alzheimer subjects and age-matched controls. *Psychopharmacology (Berlin)*, **99**, 129–33.

Suzuki, M., Kanamori, M., Watanable, M. *et al.* (2004). Nakahara Behavioral and endocrinological evaluation of music therapy for elderly patients with dementia. *Nursing and Health Sciences*, **6**, 11–18D.

Swearer, J. M., Drachman, D. A., O'Donnell, B. F. & Mitchell, A. L. (1988). Troublesome and disruptive behaviours in dementia. Relationships to diagnosis and disease severity. *Journal of the American Geriatrics Society*, **36**, 784–90.

Tabloski, P., McKinnon-Howe, L. & Remington, R. (1995). Effects of calming music on the level of agitation in cognitively impaired nursing home patients. *American Journal of Alzheimer's Case and Related Disorders and Research*, **10**, 10–15.

Takahashi, H., Yoshida, K., Sugita, T., Higuchi, H. & Shimizu, T. (2003). Quetiapine treatment of psychotic symptoms and aggressive behaviour in patients with dementia with Lewy bodies: a case series. *Progress in Neuropsychopharmacology and Biological Psychiatry*, **27**, 549–53.

Taragano, F. E., Lyketsos, C. G., Mangone, C. A., Allegri, R. F. & Comesaña-Diaz, E. (1997). A double-blind, randomized, fixed-dose trial of fluoxetine vs. amitryiptyline in the treatment of major depression complicating Alzheimer's disease. *Psychosomatics*, **38**, 246–52.

Tariot, P. N., Erb, R., Leibovici, A. *et al.* (1994). Carbamazepine treatment of agitation in nursing home patients with dementia: a preliminary study. *Journal of the American Geriatrics Society*, **42**, 1160–6.

Tariot, P. N. (1996). CERAD behavior rating scale for dementia. *International Psychogeriatrics*, **8** (Suppl. 3), 317–20; discussion 351–4.

Tariot, P. N., Erb, R., Podgorski, C. A. *et al.* (1998). Efficacy and tolerability of carbamazepine for agitation and aggression in dementia. *American Journal of Psychiatry*, **155**, 54–61.

Tariot, P. N., Jakimovich, L. J., Erb, R. *et al.* (1999). Withdrawal from controlled carbamazepine therapy followed by further carbamazepine treatment in patients with dementia. *Journal of Clinical Psychiatry*, **60**, 684–9.

Tariot, P. N., Solomon, P. R., Morris, J. C., Kershaw, P., Lilienfeld, S. & Ding, C. (2000). A 5-month, randomized, placebo-controlled trial of galantamine in AD. The Galantamine USA-10 Study Group. *Neurology*, **54**, 2269–76.

Tariot, P. N., Cummings, J. L., Katz, I. R. *et al.* (2001a). A randomized, double-blind, placebo-controlled study of the efficacy and safety of donepezil in patients with Alzheimer's disease in the nursing home setting. *Journal of the American Geriatrics Society*, **49**, 1590–9.

Tariot, P. N., Schneider, L. S., Mintzer, J. E. & Cutler, A. J. (2001b). Safety and tolerability of divalproex sodium in the treatment of signs and symptoms of mania in elderly patients with dementia: results of a double-blind, placebo-controlled trial. *Current Therapy in Research and Clinical Experimentation*, **62**, 51–67.

Tariot, P. N., Farlow, M. R., Grossberg, G. T., Graham, S. M., McDonald, S. & Gergel, I. (2004). Memantine treatment in patients with moderate to severe Alzheimer disease already receiving donepezil: a randomized controlled trial. *Journal of the American Medical Association*, **291**, 317–24.

Taverni, J. P., Seliger, G. & Lichtman, S. W. (1997). Donepezil mediated memory improvement in traumatic brain injury during post acute rehabilitation. *Brain Injury*, **12**, 77–80.

Teri, L., Truax, P., Logsdon, R., Uomoto, J., Zarit, S. & Vitaliano, P. P. (1992). Assessment of behavioral problems in dementia: the revised memory and behavior problems checklist. *Psychology and Aging*, **7**, 622–31.

Thomas, D., Heitman, R. & Alexander, T. (1997). The effects of music on bathing cooperation for residents with dementia. *Music Therapy*, **34**, 246–59.

Thorgrimsen, L., Spector, A., Wiles, A. & Orrell, M. (2003). Aromatherapy for dementia. *Cochrane Database of Systematic Reviews*. Oxford: Update Software Ltd.

Tierney, M., Naglie, G., Jaglal, S., Kiss, A. & Fisher, R. (2004). Risk factors for harm in cognitively impaired seniors who live alone: a prospective study. *Journal of the American Geriatrics Society*, **52**, 1435–41.

Trannel, T. J., Ahmed, I. & Goebert, D. (2001). Occurrence of thrombocytopenia in psychiatric patients taking valproate. *American Journal of Psychiatry*, **158**, 128–30.

Trinh, N. H., Hoblyn, J., Mohanty, S. & Yaffe, K. (2003). Efficacy of cholinesterase inhibitors in the treatment of neuropsychiatric symptoms and functional impairment in Alzheimer disease: a meta-analysis. *Journal of the American Medical Association*, **289**, 210–16.

Vaccaro, F. J. (1988a). Successful operant conditioning procedures with an institutionalized aggressive geriatric patient. *International Journal of Aging and Human Development*, **26**, 71–9.

Vaccaro, F. J. (1988b). Application of operant procedures in a group of institutionalized aggressive geriatric patients. *Psychology and Aging*, **3**, 22–8.

Vaccaro, F. J. (1990). Application of social skills training in a group of institutionalized aggressive elderly subjects. *Psychology and Aging*, **5**, 369–78.

Whall, A., Black, M., Groh, C., Yankou, D., Kupferschmid, B. & Foster, N. (1997). The effect of natural environments upon agitation and aggression in late state dementia patients. *American Journal of Alzheimer's Disease*, **12**, 216–20.

Whelihan, W. M. Psychotherapy with elderly clients: A behavioural approach. NEED COMPLETE REFERENCE

Whyte, J., Hart, T., Schuster, K. *et al.* (1997). Effects of methylphenidate on attentional function after traumatic brain injury. A randomised, placebo-controlled trial. *American Journal of Physical Medical Rehabilitation*, **76**, 440–50.

Woods, P. & Ashley, J. (1995). Simulated presence therapy: using selected memories to manage problem behaviours in Alzheimer's disease patients. *Geriatric Nursing*, **16**, 9–14.

Woods, R. (1996). Psychosocial therapies in dementia. In *Handbook of the Clinical Psychology of Aging*, ed. R. T. Woods, pp. 575–699. Chichester: John Wiley and Sons.

Wooltorton, E. (2002). Risperidone (Risperdal): increased rate of cerebrovascular events in dementia trials. *Canadian Medical Association Journal*, **167**, 1269–70.

Wooltorton, E. (2004). Olanzapine (Zyprexa): increased incidence of cerebrovascular events in dementia trials. *Canadian Medical Association Journal*, **170**, 1395.

Wroblewski, B. A., Mccolgan, K., Smith, K. *et al.* (1990). The incidence of seizures during tricyclic antidepressant drug treatment in a brain-injured population. *Journal of Clinical Psychopharmacology*, **10**, 124–8.

Wroblewski, B. A., Leary, J. M., Phelan, A. M. *et al.* (1992). Methylphenidate and seizure frequency in brain injured patients with seizure disorders. *Journal of Clinical Psychiatry*, **53**, 86–9.

Wroblewski, B. A., Joseph, A. B., Kupfer, J. *et al.* (1997). Effectiveness of valproic acid on destructive and aggressive behaviours in patients with acquired brain injury. *Brain Injury*, **11**, 37–47.

Wystanski, M. (2000). Assaultive behaviour in psychiatrically hospitalized elderly: a response to psychosocial stimulation and changes in pharmacotherapy. *International Journal of Geriatric Psychiatry*, **15**, 582–5.

Zafonte, R. D., Watanabe, T. & Mann, N. R. (1998). Amantadine: a potential treatment for the minimally conscious state. *Brain Injury*, **12**, 617–21.

Zimmer, J., Watson, N. & Treat, A. (1984). Behavioural problems among patients in skilled nursing facilities. *American Journal of Public Health*, **74**, 1118–21.

Zisselman, M., Rovner, B., Shmuley, Y. & Ferrie, P. (1996). A pet therapy intervention with geriatric psychiatry impatients. *American Journal of Occupational Therapy*, **50**, 47–51.

11

Dementia: pharmacological and non-pharmacological treatments and guideline review

Martine Simard and Elizabeth L. Sampson

Editor's note

This is a valuable chapter and a highly topical one, which overlaps with Chapter 10. Here we have clear evidence for the value of acetylcholinesterase (AChE) inhibitors and, to a lesser extent, memantine, in all common forms of dementia, and there is also some evidence that these benefits are long-lasting. Because these studies are well-integrated and follow similar methodologies, the systematic reviews are highly informative and suggest that these drugs are effective across the range of severity of dementia, and although there are few differences between individual compounds, it is valuable to have the detailed results available for direct comparison. The current argument over who should qualify for treatment is a highly contentious one, with many arguing that all early diagnosed cases should be treated. However, in the UK, the official NICE guidelines argue that this is not cost-effective. While we realize that the chapter is long, we think that this is an exciting and fast-moving area of enquiry. No doubt much will flow from this rich seam of new therapeutic endeavour, and hopefully we may soon arrive at treatments that can significantly change the difficult path that these patients and their families follow.

Introduction

The prevalence estimates of the Canadian Study of Health and Aging (CSHA) suggested that 8% of all Canadians aged 65 and over meet the criteria for dementia. The corresponding figures for Alzheimer's disease (AD) were 5.1% overall (Canadian Study of Health and Aging Working Group, 1994). The prevalence of multi-infarct dementia in Western countries has been estimated to be 7–10% (Jellinger, 2002), whereas epidemiological data collected in Japan between 1985 and 1992 showed that 48.5% of the individuals aged 65 years and over had vascular dementia (VaD; Yanagihara, 2002). Dementia with Lewy Bodies (DLB) is reported to be the second most common cause of dementia after Alzheimer's disease, accounting for 20% of all cases of dementia in old age (McKeith et al., 1992; McKeith, 2000), and to be as common as vascular dementia in a general population aged 75 years and older (Rahkonen et al., 2003). Clearly, AD, VaD and DLB are common among the elderly population, and they significantly impact on the survival and the quality of life of the patients. The early diagnosis and, most importantly, the treatment of these disorders are becoming critical issues as the proportion of aging individuals increases dramatically in Western countries.

Various pharmacological compounds have been developed to specifically alleviate the symptoms of dementia. The acetylcholinesterase inhibitors and memantine are among treatments for dementia. Hence the emerging evidence base for vitamin E, oestrogen, gingko biloba, selegiline, and these compounds. Eventually, other agents initially developed for other diseases may also be used, such as non-steroidal anti-inflammatory drugs (NSAIDs in AD, and the use of aspirin reported for treatment of vascular dementia). Non-pharmacological approaches that encompass cognitive rehabilitation, cognitive training, reminiscence therapy and reality orientation therapy have also been studied and implemented in some clinical settings in the UK, and the USA.

The goal of the present chapter is to critically and exhaustively review the evidence reported in the literature regarding the efficacy, tolerability and safety of various cognitive-enhancing drugs and non-pharmacological interventions for treatment of Alzheimer's disease, vascular dementia, and dementia with Lewy Bodies. Specifically, a systematic review will first examine the

Cambridge Textbook of Effective Treatments in Psychiatry, ed. Peter Tyrer and Kenneth R. Silk. Published by Cambridge University Press.
© Cambridge University Press, 2008.

efficacy, tolerability and safety of donepezil, rivastigmine, galantamine and memantine in improving the cognitive and functional symptoms in AD, VaD and DLB. This systematic review will be followed by a review of the efficacy and safety of vitamin E, oestrogen, Ginkgo biloba, selegiline, non-steroidal anti-inflammatory drugs, cognitive rehabilitation, cognitive training, reminiscence therapy and reality orientation therapy in AD, as well as aspirin in VaD, using principally the results of meta-analyses and previous systematic reviews.

Cholinesterase inhibitors

The acetylcholinesterase inhibitors

The use of AChE inhibitors (AChEI) increases the concentration of acetylcholine (ACh) available for synaptic transmission by inhibiting one or more of the enzymes responsible for its hydrolysis (i.e. butyrylcholinesterase and acetylcholinesterase). Butyrylcholinesterases (BChE) are present in the brain where they originate from glial cells. There is preliminary evidence to suggest that brain butyrylcholinesterase may play a role in the initiation of the neuronal damage of Alzheimer's disease. However, it is centrally active AChE that is involved in synaptic function and which represents the current principal therapeutic target for drug intervention (Nordberg & Svensson, 1998; Krall et al., 1999).

Alzheimer's disease

Donepezil

Nine randomized, double-blind, placebo-controlled (R-DB-PC) phase II and III multicenter trials (Rogers et al., 1996, 1998a, 1998b; Homma et al., 2000; Feldman et al., 2001; Mohs et al., 2001; Tariot et al., 2001; Winblad et al., 2001; AD2000 Collaborative Group, 2004), three open-label multicenter extension studies (Rogers & Friedhoff, 1998; Rogers et al., 2000; Doody et al., 2001), four open label trials (Matthews et al., 2000; Relkin et al., 2003; Boada-Rovira et al., 2004; Fröelich et al., 2004), and one post-marketing surveillance study, have assessed the efficacy and safety of donepezil in patients meeting the National Institute of Neurological and Communicative Disorders and Stroke-Alzheimer's Disease and Related Disorders Association (NINCDS-ADRDA; McKhann et al., 1984) work group criteria for probable AD and/or the DSM–IV criteria for dementia of the Alzheimer type (American Psychiatric Association, 1994).

The initial phase II R-DB-PC trial of Rogers & Friedhoff (1996) involved 161 patients with mild to moderate AD at baseline receiving either 1, 3, or 5 mg/day of donepezil or placebo, lasted 12 weeks, and was followed by a 2-week single-blind placebo washout period. This R-DB-PC study was then followed by 98-week (Rogers & Friedhoff, 1998) and 240-week (Rogers et al., 2000) follow-up extension studies both involving 133 patients with AD at the beginning of the follow-up, and receiving 3–10 mg/day of donepezil. In these studies, the efficacy was assessed using the Alzheimer's Disease Assessment Scale-cognitive subscale score (ADAS-Cog; Rosen et al., 1984), the Mini-Mental State Examination (MMSE; Folstein et al., 1975; Rogers & Friedhoff, 1996) and the Sum of the Boxes of the Clinical Dementia Rating Scale (CDR-SB; Hughes et al., 1982) (Rogers & Friedhoff, 1998; Rogers et al., 2000). The ADAS-Cog is widely used as a primary outcome in AD trials and is a 70-point scale with higher scores indicating worse cognitive function. The results of the R-DB-PC trial indicated that the improvements in the ADAS-Cog were significantly greater with donepezil 5 mg/day than with placebo, and there was a 50% reduction in the percentage of patients showing clinical decline with donepezil 5 mg/day (11%) compared with placebo (20%) (Rogers & Friedhoff, 1996). The 98-week open label extension study of donepezil (up to 10 mg/day) showed that donepezil produced improvements on the ADAS-Cog which remained superior to baseline for 38 weeks, whereas the CDR-SB scores maintained near baseline values for 26 weeks (Rogers & Friedhoff, 1998). However, after 6–9 months of treatment, mean ADAS-Cog and CDR-SB scores gradually deteriorated (Rogers et al., 2000). The most common adverse events were related to the nervous and digestive systems, were generally mild and transient, and resolved without the need for dose modifications (Rogers & Friedhoff, 1996, 1998; Rogers et al., 2000).

The initial phase III R-DB-PC trials of Rogers et al. (1998a, 1998b) involved respectively at baseline 468 and 473 patients with mild to moderate AD receiving either 5 or 10 mg/day of donepezil or placebo, lasted 12 (Rogers et al., 1998a) and 24 weeks (Rogers et al., 1998b), and were followed by a 3-week (Rogers et al., 1998a) and a 6-week (Rogers et al., 1998b) single-blind placebo washout period. These R-DB-PC studies were then followed by a 144-week (Doody et al., 2001) follow-up extension study involving 763 patients with AD at the beginning of the follow-up, combining the patients of the two previous studies (Rogers et al., 1998a, 1998b). In these studies, the primary efficacy measures were the ADAS-Cog, the Clinician Interview-Based Impression of Change-plus information from the Caregiver (CIBIC-plus; Knopman et al., 1994; Schneider et al., 1997; Rogers et al., 1998a) and/or the CDR-SB, whereas the MMSE and the patient-rated Quality of Life

(QoL; Blau, 1977) were the secondary measures (Rogers *et al.*, 1998b; Doody *et al.*, 2001). The Intention-to-Treat (ITT) analyses showed that after 15 and 24 weeks of treatment, donepezil 5 mg/day and 10 mg/day produced significant dose-related improvement in ADAS-Cog (improvement from −0.67 in the 5 mg/day to −2.7 units in the 10 mg/day groups) and MMSE scores (improvement from 1 in the 5 mg/day to 1.36 points in the 10 mg/day groups), relative to placebo, and significant improvement (Rogers *et al.*, 1998a) or less clinical deterioration on the CIBIC-plus and CDR-SB compared with placebo (Rogers *et al.*, 1998b). Following the 3-week washout period (Rogers *et al.*, 1998a), the donepezil-associated benefits remained above original baseline values for an additional 24 weeks of open-label treatment (Doody *et al.*, 2001). However, during the longer 6-week placebo washout period (Rogers *et al.*, 1998b), donepezil-associated benefits were lost (Doody *et al.*, 2001). Thus the mean change in ADAS-Cog scores from baseline did not improve to the original baseline values of the double-blind study at any time during the open label extension trial for that particular cohort (Doody *et al.*, 2001). Benefits on the ADAS-Cog scores for patients who received 10 mg/day in the double-blind study were slight, but evident, compared with the other groups for 108 weeks of open-label treatment (Doody *et al.*, 2001).

Patients who originally received placebo in the double-blind study showed a larger decline in ADAS-Cog scores after 1, 2 and 3 years of donepezil treatment than did those who had taken donepezil from the beginning of the double-blind studies (Doody *et al.*, 2001). Regarding safety issues, the most common adverse events (AE) were associated with the nervous and digestive systems (insomnia, nausea, diarrhea), and were dose-related and generally mild and transient (Rogers *et al.*, 1998a, 1998b; Doody *et al.*, 2001); 16−17% of patients' discontinuation were associated with adverse events in the double-blind and 144-week open-label extension studies (Doody *et al.*, 2001; Rogers *et al.*, 1998b).

Two European (AD2000 Collaborative Group, 2004; Winblad *et al.*, 2001), one USA (Mohs *et al.*, 2001), and one Japanese (Homma *et al.*, 2000) multicenter R-DB-PC trials involved respectively at baseline 656, 286, 431 and 268 patients with mild to moderate AD receiving either 5 or 10 mg/day of donepezil or placebo, and lasted 1 (Homma *et al.*, 2000; Mohs *et al.*, 2001; Winblad *et al.*, 2001) and 2 years (AD2000 Collaborative Group, 2004). The donepezil-treated group received either 5 mg/day of donepezil for the first 28 days and 10 mg/day thereafter (Mohs *et al.*, 2001; Winblad *et al.*, 2001), or 5 mg/day during all the trial (Homma *et al.*, 2000). After a year of treatment, least-squares (LS) mean change from baseline in

Gottfries-Bråne-Steel (GBS; Bråne *et al.*, 2001; Gottfries *et al.*, 1982), MMSE and Progressive Deterioration Scale (PDS; DeJong *et al.*, 1989) scores showed that the group treated with donepezil 10 mg/day declined by approximately half as much as the patients receiving placebo (Winblad *et al.*, 2001), whereas Kaplan–Meier estimates of time to clinically functional decline as judged by investigators for the ITT population revealed that donepezil treatment extended the median time to functional decline compared with placebo (Mohs *et al.*, 2001). An improvement was also observed on a Japanese version of the ADAS-Cog after one year in the Japanese patients treated with 5 mg/day of donepezil (Homma *et al.*, 2000). Slightly more patients with donepezil than placebo experienced AEs mostly related to the nervous, digestive and urogenital systems; with 7−9.3% of donepezil and 5.5−6.3% of placebo-treated patients discontinuing because of adverse events during a 1-year treatment period (Mohs *et al.*, 2001; Winblad *et al.*, 2001). Following two years of treatment, no benefits were registered with donepezil 5 and 10 mg/day compared with placebo in institutionalization and progression of disability as measured by the Bristol Activities of Daily Living (BADLS; Bucks *et al.*, 1996) (AD2000 Collaborative Group, 2004). In addition, no significant differences were seen between donepezil and placebo in behavioural and psychological symptoms, carer psychopathology, formal care costs, unpaid caregiver time, adverse events or deaths, or between 5 mg and 10 mg donepezil (AD2000 Collaborative Group, 2004).

A USA (Tariot *et al.*, 2001) and a collaborative Australian–Canadian–French (Feldman *et al.*, 2001) 24-week R-DB-PC trial involved respectively at baseline 208 and 290 patients with mild to severe (Tariot *et al.*, 2001), and moderate to severe AD (Feldman *et al.*, 2001) receiving either 5 or 10 mg/day of donepezil or placebo. The primary outcome measures were the CIBIC-plus (Feldman *et al.*, 2001) and the Neuropsychiatric Inventory-Nursing Home Version (NPI-NH; Cummings *et al.*, 1994) (Tariot *et al.*, 2001). Patients receiving donepezil showed benefits on the CIBIC-plus, compared with placebo, at all visits up to week 24, and at week 24 last observation carried forward (LOCF) ($P < 0.0001$) (Feldman *et al.*, 2001), whereas there was no significant difference between the donepezil and the placebo groups on the NPI-NH (Tariot *et al.*, 2001). The performance of the donepezil-treated group compared with placebo improved significantly at week 24 on the secondary measures such as the MMSE, Severe Impairment Battery (SIB; Saxton *et al.*, 1990), Disability Assessment for Dementia (DAD; Gélinas *et al.*, 1999), and CDR-SB in the 2 studies (Feldman *et al.*, 2001; Tariot *et al.*, 2001). However, only the donepezil-treated patients of

Feldman *et al.* (2001) improved their functional level as measured by the modified Instrumental Activities of Daily Living (IADL+) and Physical Self-Maintenance Scale (PSMS+) (Lawton & Brody, 1969) at week 24 LOCF (Feldman *et al.*, 2001). Regarding safety issues, overall rates of occurrence and severity of AEs were similar between the two groups (respectively, 83–96% in the donepezil and 80–97% in the placebo groups) (Feldman *et al.*, 2001; Tariot *et al.*, 2001). The discontinuation rates because of AEs were similar between the donepezil and placebo-treated patients aged < 85 years (respectively 14% and 13%), but were greater in the placebo than in the donepezil-treated patients aged ≥ 85 years (respectively, 20% and 9%) (Tariot *et al.*, 2001). There was no difference between the discontinuation rates because of adverse events in the study of Feldman *et al.* (2001) with 8% of the donepezil- versus 6% of the placebo-treated who discontinued the trial (Feldman *et al.*, 2001).

Four open label trials were conducted in an outpatient clinic in Southampton, UK (n = 80) (Matthews *et al.*, 2000), in 37 routine clinical practice centers in Germany (Froelich *et al.*, 2004), in 255 USA sites (Relkin *et al.*, 2003), and in 246 sites located in 18 countries worldwide (n = 1113). Patients with mild to moderate AD received donepezil 5 mg/day for 28 days, after which the dosage was increased to 10 mg/day of donepezil for periods of 12 weeks (Boada-Rovira *et al.*, 2004; Relkin *et al.*, 2003), 24 weeks (Froelich *et al.*, 2004), and 18 months (Matthews *et al.*, 2000). Improvements of at least 4 points on the ADAS-Cog and the NPI were maintained for 6 (ADAS-Cog) and 18 months (NPI) in 37–39% of patients (Matthews *et al.*, 2000), whereas an improvement of 0.8–1.6 points on the MMSE was maintained for 12 months in 68% of the patients (Froelich *et al.*, 2004). The two 12-week trials showed an improvement of +1.73 ± 0.10 (Boada-Rovira *et al.*, 2004) and +1.54 ± 3.05 points (Relkin *et al.*, 2003) on the MMSE total scores at the end point in the donepezil-treated patients. Nearly all patients in these two trials presented at least one comorbid medical condition or were taking at least one concomitant medication (Relkin *et al.*, 2003; Boada-Rovira *et al.*, 2004). Five percent (Boada-Rovira *et al.*, 2004) to 12% (Froelich *et al.*, 2004; Matthews *et al.*, 2000; Relkin *et al.*, 2003) of patients prematurely discontinued the trial because of adverse events such as agitation, confusion, dizziness, headache, nausea, vomiting and diarrhea (Matthews *et al.*, 2000; Relkin *et al.*, 2003; Boada-Rovira *et al.*, 2004; Froelich *et al.*, 2004).

Finally, one post-marketing surveillance study conducted in Germany (Frölich *et al.*, 2002) included 913 patients with mild to moderate AD with (CVD+; n = 251)

and without cerebrovascular disease (CVD−; n = 595), and treated with either 5 or 10 mg/day of donepezil during a mean period of 3.4 months. After 3 months, patients had improved by a mean MMSE change from baseline of 2.2 points (CVD+: 2.4 pts, CVD−: 2.1 pts), whereas quality of life as assessed by the investigator (choice of response: improved/unchanged/worsened) was judged improved in 70.0% of patients (Frölich *et al.*, 2002).

A Cochrane meta-analysis synthesizing the evidence from 22 methodologically adequate R-DB-PC trials (total of 5205 participants) (Birks & Harvey 2006) found statistically significant improvements for both 5 mg and 10 mg per day of donepezil on the ADAS-Cog scale (−2.8 points, mean difference 95% CI −3.74 to −2.10, $P < 0.00001$, for the 10 mg dose). Benefits for treatment were also seen for activities of daily living and behavior but not on quality of life.

Rivastigmine

Three randomized, double-blind, placebo-controlled multicenter trials (Corey-Bloom *et al.*, 1998; Forette *et al.*, 1999; Rösler *et al.*, 1999), four open-label multicenter extension studies (Farlow *et al.*, 2000, 2005; Aupperle *et al.*, 2004; Grossberg *et al.*, 2004), and one open-label phase IV trial (Bilikiewicz *et al.*, 2002) were found. The study of Aupperle *et al.* (2004) is an open-label prospective extension trial of a previous 26-week open-label study (Cummings *et al.*, 2000). All the studied patients met the NINCDS-ADRDA criteria for probable AD and/or the DSM–IV criteria for dementia of the Alzheimer's type. In these studies, the ADAS-Cog, CIBIC-plus and PDS were the primary outcome measures whereas the MMSE, and Global Deterioration Scale (GDS; Reisberg *et al.*, 1982) were the disease severity measures.

The initial 26-week R-DB-PC trial of Corey-Bloom *et al.* (1998) involved 699 patients with mild to moderate AD at baseline receiving either 1–4 mg/day or 6–12 mg/day of rivastigmine or placebo. This US multicenter R-DB-PC study was then followed by a 52-week (Farlow *et al.*, 2000) and a 5-year (Farlow *et al.*, 2005) follow-up extension studies involving 532 (Farlow *et al.*, 2000) and 37 (Farlow *et al.*, 2005) patients with AD at the beginning of the follow-up, and receiving 1–12 mg/day of rivastigmine. At week 26 of the R-DB-PC trial, patients showed benefit from high doses of rivastigmine (6–12 mg/day) treatment on all outcome measures, and especially on the ADAS-Cog (4.94 points better than those who received placebo – as per the observed cases analyses). For both low- and high doses-groups, the mean changes from baseline on the ADAS-Cog and CIBIC-plus were different from those of placebo ($P < 0.05$) (Corey-Bloom *et al.*, 1998). A total of

545 out of 699 patients (78%) successfully completed the initial R-DB-PC trial. The principal cause of the 22% withdrawal rate was attributable to AEs (Corey-Bloom *et al.*, 1998). Of the 532 patients who entered the 6-month extension study, 513 completed the initial 6-month R-DB-PC, and 19 patients were from the retrieved drop-out population (Farlow *et al.*, 2000). At week 52, patients originally treated with 6–12 mg/day of rivastigmine had significantly better cognitive function, as measured by the ADAS-Cog, than patients originally treated with placebo (Farlow *et al.*, 2000). Five years later, 5/37 patients chose to not continue with the long-term extension trial, 25/37 patients had withdrawn from the study in the first 9 months of the open-label extension, and 7/37 patients were still taking rivastigmine (Farlow *et al.*, 2005). The two-thirds of the participants still enrolled at week 234 were in the original high-dose rivastigmine group, suggesting that early therapy may confer some benefit in delaying long-term progression of symptoms. For the end point defined as a 5-point drop from the baseline MMSE score, the group mean was 94 weeks. Of the 25 withdrawn patients, 7 discontinued because of AEs, and 5 died (Farlow *et al.*, 2005).

Two multinational (Forette *et al.*, 1999; Rösler *et al.*, 1999) R-DB-PC trials involved respectively at baseline 114 and 725 patients with mild to moderate AD receiving up to 12 mg/day of rivastigmine or placebo, and lasted 18 (Forette *et al.*, 1999) and 26 weeks (Rösler *et al.*, 1999). The best results in these two trials were obtained with higher doses of rivastigmine 10–12 mg/day, with the patients of Forette *et al.* (1999) best tolerating the 10 mg/day dosage. The cognitive improvement on the ADAS-Cog in the high dose-rivastigmine group compared with placebo was only statistically significant at the end of the trial in the study of Rösler *et al.* (1999). In that particular trial, 24% of the 6–12 mg/day rivastigmine group vs 16% of the placebo improved by 4 points or more on the ADAS-Cog. Improvements were also significant on the CIBIC-Plus (Forette *et al.*, 1999; Rösler *et al.*, 1999), the GDS and the PDS (Rösler *et al.*, 1999), as well as on the Nurses' Observation Scale for Geriatric Patients (NOSGER; Spiegel *et al.*, 1991), a measure of various cognitive function and behavior as related to activities of daily living (Forette *et al.*, 1999). Between 32 and 35% in the high-dose rivastigmine-treated vs 8%–13% in the placebo-treated patients discontinued the trials because of adverse events (Forette *et al.*, 1999; Rösler *et al.*, 1999).

The paper of Grossberg *et al.* (2004) reports the results of two 2-year open label extension studies from 4 R-DB-PC trials (Corey-Bloom *et al.*, 1998; Rösler *et al.*, 1999; Anand *et al.*, 2000), and involving 2010 patients with mild to moderate AD. The clinical course of AD patients treated with 2–12 mg/day of rivastigmine was compared with a prediction of their course derived by a baseline-dependent historical model of disease progression developed from data in untreated patients with AD (polynomial-regression model; Stern *et al.*, 1994). After 2 years of treatment on rivastigmine, there was less cognitive deterioration than in historical-control subjects as measured by observed cases (OC) of the rivastigmine groups and predicted (controls) on the ADAS-Cog and MMSE total scores (Grossberg *et al.*, 2004). Treatment-emergent adverse events were the commonly seen side effects of cholinesterase inhibitors, such as gastrointestinal symptoms, and were similar in frequency to those reported in patients assigned to shorter-term rivastigmine therapy (Grossberg *et al.*, 2004).

The USA 52-week open-label extension trial of Aupperle *et al.* (2004) was conducted in 13 centers, including 29 nursing homes, and involved at baseline 95 patients with moderate to severe AD receiving 3–12 mg/day of rivastigmine for an extension period of 26 weeks following the initial 26 weeks of open-label trial (Cummings *et al.*, 2000). After 52 weeks of treatment with rivastigimine, 10–12 domains of the NPI-NH significantly improved from baseline in LOCF patients with behavioral symptoms present at baseline. Over half (57.2%) of the OC and 56.9% of the LOCF analyses showed improved or stable global function as measured by the simplified CIBIC-plus (Aupperle *et al.*, 2004). Only 4/95 (4.2%) patients discontinued treatment due to adverse events (Aupperle *et al.*, 2004).

Finally, the open-label 26-week multicenter phase IV trial conducted in five clinical centers in Poland involved at baseline 62 patients (56% with concomitant disease) with mild to moderate AD receiving 3–12 mg/day of rivastigmine (Bilikiewicz *et al.*, 2002). The MMSE, ADAS-Cog and GDS scores of the patients treated for 26 weeks were not significantly different from those of baseline. Eleven percent of patients discontinued the trial because of adverse events principally related to the gastrointestinal system (Bilikiewicz *et al.*, 2002).

A Cochrane review analyzing data on 3660 participants demonstrated that rivastigmine (6–12 mg daily) was associated with a 2.1 point improvement in cognitive function on the ADAS-Cog score compared with placebo (weighted mean difference −2.09, 95% confidence interval −2.65 to −1.54, on an intention-to-treat basis) and a 2.2 point improvement in Activities of Daily Living assessed on the Progressive Deterioration Scale (weighted mean difference −2.15, 95% confidence interval −3.16 to −1.13, on an intention-to-treat basis) at 26 weeks. There were statistically significantly higher levels of nausea, vomiting, diarrhea, anorexia, headache, syncope, abdominal pain and dizziness among patients taking high-dose rivastigmine than among those taking placebo (Birks *et al.*, 2000).

Galantamine

Five randomized, double-blind, placebo-controlled multi-center trials (Raskind *et al.*, 2000; Tariot *et al.*, 2000; Wilcock *et al.*, 2000; Rockwood *et al.*, 2001; Wilkinson *et al.*, 2001), and three open-label multicenter phase III extension studies (Lyketsos *et al.*, 2004; Pirtillä *et al.*, 2004; Raskind *et al.*, 2004) were found. All the patients met the NINCDS-ADRDA criteria for probable AD. In these studies, the ADAS-Cog, and CIBIC-plus were the primary outcome measures whereas the NPI and the Alzheimer's Disease Cooperative Study Activities of Daily Living inventory (ADCS/ADL; Galasko *et al.*, 1997) or the DAD were the secondary efficacy measures.

The 5-month US multicenter R-DB-PC trial of Tariot *et al.* (2000) involved at baseline 978 patients with mild to moderate AD receiving either 8 mg/day or 16 mg/day or 24 mg/day of galantamine or placebo, and was followed by a 12-month open-label extension trial (Lyketsos *et al.*, 2004) involving 699 patients with AD. These patients had their dosage titrated up to 24 mg/day (12 mg b.i.d.) during a period of 2 weeks and were treated for 12 months. After 5 months, the ITT analyses showed that the galantamine–placebo differences on the ADAS-Cog were 3.3 points for the 16 mg/day group and 3.6 points for the 24 mg/day group ($P < 0.001$ versus placebo for both doses) (Tariot *et al.*, 2000). The galantamine-treated groups also had significantly better outcome on the CIBIC-Plus, the ADCS/ADL and NPI scores (Tariot *et al.*, 2000). Patients taking galantamine continuously throughout the double-blind and open-label studies (n = 288) demonstrated sustained cognitive benefits on the ADAS-Cog/11 scores, and did not experience further deterioration in behavior (NPI) at 18.5 months (Lyketsos *et al.*, 2004). Ten percent of galantamine-treated patients versus 7% placebo-treated patients discontinued the trial because of adverse events in the 5-month R-DB-PC trial, and 11.8%–15.3% patients treated with galantamine in the extension trial discontinued due to adverse events (Tariot *et al.*, 2000; Lyketsos *et al.*, 2004).

Two 6-month R-DB-PC trials involved respectively 636 (Raskind *et al.*, 2000) and 653 (Wilcock *et al.*, 2000) patients with mild to moderate AD at baseline recruited in 33 USA sites (Raskind *et al.*, 2000), and in multinational sites (Wilcock *et al.* 2000), and receiving either 24 mg/day or 32 mg/day of galantamine or placebo (Raskind *et al.*, 2000; Wilcock *et al.*, 2000). Six months later, the patients treated with galantamine had a significantly better outcome on the ADAS-Cog/11 (improvement of 2.9–3.9 points for the 24 mg/day group and of 3.1–3.8 points for the 32 mg/day group), the CIBIC-Plus and DAD scores than patients in the placebo group (Raskind *et al.*, 2000; Wilcock *et al.*, 2000). Apolipoprotein E genotype had no effect on therapeutic response to galantamine (Raskind *et al.*, 2000; Wilcock *et al.*, 2000). Discontinuation rates due to adverse events were 18–27% in the galantamine- versus 8–9% in the placebo-treated patients (Raskind *et al.*, 2000; Wilcock *et al.*, 2000). The R-DB-PC trial of Raskind *et al.* (2000) was followed by a 4-week single-blind placebo washout period, and a first open-label extension of 5.5 months involving 353 patients which showed that the ADAS-Cog and DAD scores did not significantly change from baseline for patients who received galantamine 24 mg/day throughout the 12 months (Raskind *et al.*, 2000). The discontinuation rate due to adverse events (predominantly gastrointestinal) was 16% (Raskind *et al.*, 2000).

The two 3-month R-DB-PC trials of Rockwood *et al.* (2001) and Wilkinson *et al.* (2001) involving respectively at baseline 386 and 285 patients with mild to moderate AD, receiving either 18–36 mg/day (Wilkinson *et al.*, 2001), or 24–32 mg/day of galantamine or placebo (Rockwood *et al.*, 2001), also reported a significantly better outcome on the ADAS-Cog (Rockwood *et al.*, 2001; Wilkinson *et al.*, 2001), CIBIC-Plus and DAD (Rockwood *et al.*, 2001) in patients treated with 24 (Wilkinson *et al.*, 2001) and 32 mg/day of galantamine compared with placebo (Rockwood *et al.*, 2001). In these two trials, 17.9–44.4% of galantamine-treated patients withdrew because of adverse events (principally gastrointestinal) compared with 4–9.2% of placebo-treated patients (Rockwood *et al.*, 2001; Wilkinson *et al.*, 2001).

The 2-year open-label trial of Raskind *et al.* (2004) was an extension study of two previous R-DB-PC trials (Raskind *et al.*, 2000; Rockwood *et al.*, 2001), and involved 194 patients with AD at the beginning of the follow-up receiving 24 mg/day of galantamine. This extension trial showed that the cognitive decline of patients treated continuously with galantamine for 36 months was approximately 50% less than that predicted for untreated patients (Raskind *et al.*, 2004). Patients discontinuing galantamine therapy before 36 months (38.7% of patients) had declined at a similar rate before discontinuation as those completing 36 months of treatment (Raskind *et al.*, 2004).

Finally, the 2-year open-label trial of Pirtillä *et al.* (2004) was the extension of two earlier galantamine double-blind studies and open-label extensions published by Janssen Research Foundation (1999a; 1999b). This study involved 491 patients with mild to moderate AD who had previously been on galantamine for 12 months (thus a total exposure up to 36 months), and received galantamine 24 mg/day

(Pirttilä *et al.*, 2004). Patients with stable and well-controlled concomitant disease were included. Initial improvement in cognitive function during the first 6 months was maintained for 12 months, but was followed by a gradual decline for the remainder of the trial, as measured by increased ADAS-Cog/11 scores of 12.4 ± 0.80 points at 36 months versus a projected 22-point increase for untreated patients (Pirttilä *et al.*, 2004).

A Cochrane synthesis of the evidence from 10 trials (6805 subjects) demonstrated that treatment with galantamine led to a significantly greater reduction in ADAS-Cog score at all dosing levels with greater effect over 6 months compared with 3 months. For example, treatment effect for 24 mg/day over 6 months was a 3.1 point reduction in ADAS-Cog (95% CI 2.6–3.7, $k=4$, intent to treat (ITT)). Functional and neuropsychiatric outcomes were reported only in a small proportion of trials; all showed significant treatment effect in some individual trials at least. Galantamine's adverse effects appeared similar to those of other cholinesterase inhibitors and to be dose related (Loy & Schneider, 2006).

Memantine

Three R-DB-PC multicenter trials (Reisberg *et al.*, 2003; Tariot *et al.*, 2004; Winblad *et al.*, 1999), and one prospective phase IV post-marketing surveillance study (Rüther *et al.*, 2000) were found, and involved patients with moderate to severe dementia.

The Swedish multicenter 12-week R-DB-PC trial of Winblad *et al.* (1999) involved 166 patients meeting the DSM–III–R criteria for severe dementia, and who were later separated clinically between AD ($n=79$) or vascular dementia (VaD)/mixed dementia ($n=87$) sub-groups using the Modified Hachinski Ischemic Scale cut-off scores of < 5 for AD and ≥ 5 for VaD (Rosen *et al.*, 1980). The patients received either memantine 5 mg/day during the first week and 10 mg/day during the next 11 weeks, or matching placebo tablets. Minimal (52% of patients) to much improvement (21% of patients) in the Clinical Global Impression of Change assessment (CGI-C; Schneider *et al.*, 1997) was observed in the ITT analyses of the memantine-treated group, versus 45% improvement in the placebo-treated patients, independent of the etiology of dementia. Regarding safety issues, 18 memantine (22%) and 18 placebo patients (21%) had AEs. Four memantine (5%) and five placebo (6%) patients had serious adverse events such as worsening of heart failure and hypostatic pneumonia, cardiac arrest, apnoea and unconsciousness.

The US R-DB-PC trials of Reisberg *et al.* (2003) and Tariot *et al.* (2004) involved respectively 252 and 404

patients with moderate to severe dementia meeting the NINCDS-ADRDA criteria for probable AD, and receiving 20 mg/day of memantine or placebo (Reisberg *et al.*, 2003), and 5–20 mg/day of memantine or placebo (Tariot *et al.*, 2004) for periods of 24 (Tariot *et al.*, 2004) and 28 weeks (Reisberg *et al.*, 2003). Interestingly, ongoing donepezil therapy for more than 6 months before entrance into the trial at a stable dose (5–10 mg/day) for at least 3 months was one of the inclusion criteria for the study of Tariot *et al.* (2004), and concomitant medications were allowed. The two trials found a significantly better outcome in the memantine-treated compared with the placebo-treated patients, as measured by the CIBIC-plus, the ADCS-ADL and the Severe Impairment Battery (SIB; Saxton *et al.*, 1990) at weeks 24 (Tariot *et al.*, 2004) and 28 (LOCF analyses; Reisberg *et al.*, 2003). Treatment discontinuations because of adverse events for memantine vs placebo were 7.4–13% vs 12.4–17% respectively (Reisberg *et al.*, 2003; Tariot *et al.*, 2004). The most frequently reported adverse events were agitation, confusion, fall, influenza-like symptoms, dizziness, headache, urinary incontinence, urinary tract infection, insomnia and diarrhea (Reisberg *et al.*, 2003; Tariot *et al.*, 2004).

Finally, the phase IV post-marketing surveillance study (Rüther *et al.*, 2000) included 531 patients with primary dementia of Global Deterioration Scale (Reisberg *et al.*, 1982) stages 5 to 7 (moderate to severe dementia), receiving 5 mg of memantine in the first week followed by a dose increase of 5 mg at weekly intervals up to 15 mg/day of memantine during 44 days. After 6 weeks of treatment, 75.5% of patients were scored as improved on the CGI-C completed by the physicians, and this improvement appeared in all three stages of dementia (GDS 5 to 7), but were more distinct at stage 5 (Rüther *et al.*, 2000).

McShane *et al.* (2006) undertook a Cochrane meta-analysis of the evidence and concluded that memantine was well tolerated in patients with Alzheimer's disease. In patients with moderate to severe AD pooled data indicated a beneficial effect at six months on cognition (2.97 points on the 100 point Severe Impairment Battery, 95% CI 1.68 to 4.26, $P < 0.00001$), activities of daily living (1.27 points on the 54 point ADCS-ADLsev, 95% CI 0.44 to 2.09, $P = 0.003$) and behaviour (2.76 points on the NPI, 95% CI 0.88 to 4.63, $P = 0.004$).

Head-to-head comparisons of cholinesterase inhibitors for Alzheimer's disease

There has been one R-DB-PC trial comparing rivastigmine (a maximum of 12 g per day) and donepezil (a maximum of 10 mg per day). Study duration was 104 weeks. In total, 994 patients received cholinesterase inhibitor treatment (rivastigmine, n = 495; donepezil, n = 499), and 57.9% of patients completed the study. Rivastigmine and donepezil had similar effects on measures of cognition and behavior as measured by the GDS. However, analysis of withdrawals before the end of the study period showed significant differences between donepezil and rivastigmine, in favour of donepezil after 2 years of treatment (182/499 vs 234/495, OR 0.64, 95% C.I. 0.5–0.83, $P < 0.0006$). Similarly, adverse events (nausea, vomiting, anorexia and weight loss at 12–16 weeks and 16 weeks to 2 years) were also greater in the donepezil-treated group. A meta-analysis that pooled data from R-DB-PC compared the effect of galantamine, rivastigmine and donepezil on safety (drop-outs due to adverse events) and selected cognitive outcomes; the ADAS-Cog and the CIBIC-plus (Ritchie *et al*, 2004). All three drugs showed benefit on ADAS-Cog scores compared with placebo, with a dose-related effect observed for donepezil and rivastigmine of approximately 3 points on the ADAS-Cog. Galantamine showed a similar effect across all dose levels. Donepezil and galantamine were associated with improvement on the CGI scale, but in this case the effect was not dose-related, possibly due to the insensitivity of the scale. There was evidence for increased drop-out rates with galantamine and rivastigmine.

Vascular dementia

Some findings in regards to ACh levels in the brains of patients with VaD suggest that AChE inhibitors (AChEIs) might be efficacious as symptomatic treatment for VaD. Neuropathological studies showed that compared with healthy controls, patients with VaD had decreased brain choline acetyltransferase (ChAT) activity located in the cortex, hippocampus and striatum (Gottfries *et al.*, 1994). Levels of ChAT are typically reduced when nicotinic acetylcholine receptor (nAChR) numbers are decreased. Reductions in nAChRs are reported in AD and DLB, as well as in other neuropsychiatric disorders, but may not be associated with reduced cortical cholinergic innervation observed in VaD (Graham *et al.*, 2002). Pimlott *et al.* (2004) showed that the reductions of nAChRs, as measured by decreased 5-[^{125}I]-A-85380 binding (a marker of the alpha4beta2 nicotinic receptor subtype) in the striatum of patients with AD, DLB and Parkinson's disease, were not apparent in VaD. These reductions of striatal 5-[^{125}I]-A-85380 binding in AD were thought to be related to reduced cortical inputs (Pimlott *et al.*, 2004). In addition, the levels of acetylcholine (ACh) and choline in the cerebrospinal fluid (CSF) of patients with VaD and of patients with AD were significantly lower than those of controls in the study of Jia *et al.* (2004). These CSF concentrations correlated positively with the MMSE scores of the three groups (Jia *et al.*, 2004). However, the CSF concentrations of choline were significantly higher in patients with VaD than in patients with AD (Jia *et al.*, 2004). These data altogether suggest that the mechanism of decreased acetylcholine activity in VaD is different and potentially less severe than that of AD.

On the other hand, excitotoxicity might justify the use of N-methyl-D-aspartate antagonists, such as memantine, in the treatment of vascular dementia. Ischemia, the sudden interruption of blood flow to the brain, may cause nerve cell death in the adult brain. Ischemic nerve cell death is thought to occur through excitotoxicity which appears to be mediated by excessive release of glutamate. This excess of glutamate over-activates the N-methyl-D-aspartate receptor/channel complex (NMDAR), allowing the influx of toxic levels of Ca^{2+} into nerve cells (Baskys & Blaabjerg, 2005, for a review).

Donepezil

Two multinational 24-week R-DB-PC trials involved 603 (Black *et al.*, 2003) and 616 (Wilkinson *et al.*, 2003) patients with mild dementia meeting the National Institute of Neurologic Disorders and Stroke-Association International pour la Recherche et l'Enseignement en Neurosciences (NINDS-AIREN; Román *et al.*, 1993) criteria for vascular dementia (VaD) who received either donepezil 5 mg/day or 10 mg/day (5 mg/day for first 28 days) or placebo. In both studies, the ADAS-Cog, the Clinician's Interview-Based Impression of Severity (CIBIS) and the CIBIC-plus were the primary outcome measures whereas the MMSE, the CDR-SB and the Alzheimer's Disease Functional Assessment and Change Scale (ADFACS; Gottfries *et al.*, 1994) were the secondary efficacy measures. Analyses were based on the intent-to-treat population. At week 24, both donepezil groups showed significant improvement in cognition versus placebo on the ADAS-Cog with mean endpoint treatment differences, as measured by the change from baseline score, of −1.90 ($P = 0.001$) (Black *et al.*, 2003) and −1.65 ($P = 0.003$) (Wilkinson *et al.*, 2003) for the groups receiving donepezil 5 mg, and of −2.33 ($P < 0.001$) (Black *et al.*, 2003) and −2.09 ($P = 0.0002$) (Wilkinson *et al.*, 2003) for the groups receiving donepezil 10 mg.

Regarding safety, the proportion of donepezil-treated patients experiencing adverse events was very high, but similar to placebo (88.4% and 86.5%; Black *et al.*, 2003; Wilkinson *et al.*, 2003) in the 5 mg/day group (88.9% and 90.4%; Black *et al.*, 2003; Wilkinson *et al.*, 2003), and similar (91.6%; Wilkinson *et al.*, 2003) or higher than placebo in the 10 mg/day group (94.7%, $P = 0.03$; Black *et al.*, 2003). In the two studies, the adverse events were generally mild to moderate in intensity. In the study of Black *et al.* (2003), stroke was the most common serious adverse event in the donepezil-treated groups, and the second most common serious adverse event after transient ischemic attack in the placebo group. However, the discontinuation rate (placebo = 11%; donepezil 5 mg/day = 11%; donepezil 10 mg/day = 23%) due to adverse events was related to dosage, and withdrawal principally due to stroke remained relatively low (Black *et al.*, 2003).

Meta-analysis has demonstrated from pooled data (n = 1219) that donepezil shows improvement compared with placebo on cognitive function, clinical global impression and activities of daily living. For example on 10 mg of donepezil per day, those who completed at 24 weeks showed an improvement of -2.21 points (95% CI -3.07 to -1.35, $P < 0.00001$) (Malouf & Birks, 2004).

Rivastigmine

The only 26-week R-DB-PC trial reported for the use of rivastigmine related to dementia and vascular problems is a secondary analysis (Kumar *et al.*, 2000) of the R-DB-PC of Corey-Bloom *et al.* (1998), involving patients with mild to moderate dementia, meeting the NINCDS-ADRDA criteria for AD and presenting vascular risk factors (VRF) as measured by a Modified Hachinski Ischemic Score of > 5 (MHIS; Rosen *et al.*, 1980). In this study, 697 patients were dichotomized as having MHIS = 0 or MHIS > 0 at baseline. All analyses were then based on the patients' MHIS dichotomization and randomized treatment group (6–12 mg/day, 1–4 mg/day and placebo), and were performed on the observed cases. At week 26, the improvement from the baseline ADAS-Cog score was significant ($P < 0.001$) for the patients in the MHIS > 0 category treated with high-dose (6–12 mg/day) rivastigmine compared with placebo controls (endpoint, mean change from baseline = -0.4 and -3.7 for respectively the 6–12 mg/day rivastigmine-treated and the placebo groups). The adverse events were mild to moderate in severity, dose related during the titration phase, and of limited duration (Kumar *et al.*, 2000).

Galantamine

One multinational 6-month R-DB-PC trial involved 592 patients with mild to moderate dementia, meeting the NINDS-AIREN criteria for probable VaD or the NINCDS-ADRDA criteria for possible AD (with CVD) who received either galantamine 24 mg/day or placebo (Erkinjuntti *et al.*, 2002). This study was followed by two open-label

trial extension studies lasting 6 (Erkinjuntti *et al.*, 2003) and 24 months (Kurz *et al.*, 2003), and including respectively 459 (Erkinjuntti *et al.*, 2003) and 326 patients (Kurz *et al.*, 2003) with either VaD or AD with CVD. In addition, the 12-month open-label extension study of Bullock *et al.* (2004) especially followed the subgroup of patients with AD and CVD. In the initial R-DB-PC trial (Erkinjuntti *et al.*, 2003), 285 patients with AD + CVD were randomized to receive either placebo (n = 97) or galantamine 24 mg/day (n = 188) for 6 months. A total of 238 patients (n = 86 from the placebo group and n = 152 from the galantamine group) continued with the open label extension and were treated with galantamine 24 mg/day (Bullock *et al.*, 2004).

In all these studies, the ADAS-Cog/11 (including 11 items), and the CIBIC-plus were the primary outcome measures whereas the DAD, the NPI and the MMSE were the secondary efficacy measures (Erkinjuntti *et al.*, 2002; 2003; Kurz *et al.*, 2003; Bullock *et al.*, 2004). The LOCF analyses performed at the end of the 6-month R-DB-PC trial revealed that galantamine had better efficacy than placebo on the ADAS-Cog/11 (respectively, improvement of 1.7 points ($P < 0.0001$) and deterioration by 1.0 points ($P = 0.045$)). After 6 months, 74% of galantamine-group patients remained stable or had improved on the CIBIC-plus compared with 59% of those assigned placebo, and Activities of Daily Living as measured by the DAD were maintained in the galantamine-treated group but deteriorated in the placebo group, whereas behavioral symptoms (especially anxiety and apathy), as measured by the NPI, significantly improved compared with placebo (Erkinjuntti *et al.*, 2002). At month 12 of the open-label extension study (Erkinjuntti *et al.*, 2003), 6 months following the end of the R-DB-PC trial, improvements from baseline (the start of the double-blind phase) in ADAS-Cog/11 scores were observed in both the group that received placebo during the double-blind phase (placebo/galantamine group: -0.3 point; 95% CI, -1.64 to 1.06), and the group that received galantamine during the double-blind phase (galantamine/galantamine group: -0.9 point; 95% CI, -1.73 to 0.03). Improvement from baseline on the DAD was also significant in both the placebo/galantamine and the galantamine/galantamine groups (Erkinjuntti *et al.*, 2003). At month 12, all patients with AD + CVD treated with galantamine remained near baseline levels, but patients treated with galantamine over the full 12-month study period appeared to have deteriorated less than those who were switched from placebo to galantamine. At month 24 of the open-label extension study (Kurz *et al.*, 2003), patients taking galantamine for the entire study (since the start of the double-blind phase) demonstrated the least cognitive decline on the

ADAS-Cog/11. The long-term benefits of galantamine were maintained for approximately 21 months in patients with VaD, and for 12 months in patients with AD and CVD (Kurz *et al.*, 2003).

Regarding safety and tolerability issues, concomitant disorders were present in 97% and 96% of patients in the galantamine and placebo groups respectively (Erkinjuntti *et al.*, 2002). Overall, 23% of patients were taking neuroleptics and 28% antidepressants at baseline of the R-DB-PC trial. More galantamine than placebo patients discontinued the R-DB-PC trial, principally as a result of AEs (19.7% vs. 8.2%). The discontinuation rates were 26.8% in the placebo/galantamine and 13.9% in the galantamine/galantamine groups involved in the 6-month extension trial (Erkinjuntti *et al.*, 2003), and 8.1% in the galantamine/galantamine/galantamine and 8.6% in the placebo/galantamine/galantamine groups in the 2-year extension trial (Kurz *et al.*, 2003). Adverse events were the most common cause of discontinuation, although they were considered mild or moderate. The adverse events were principally gastrointestinal and cholinergic in nature in the 6-month extension trial (Erkinjuntti *et al.*, 2003), whereas cerebrovascular disorder (1%), myocardial infarction (1%) and pneumonia were the adverse events most commonly associated with discontinuation in the galantamine/galantamine/galantamine group of the 24-month extension trial (Kurz *et al.*, 2003).

Memantine

One multicenter 28-week R-DB-PC trial conducted in France included 321 patients with mild to moderate dementia meeting the NINDS-AIREN criteria for probable VaD (Orgogozo *et al.*, 2002). These patients received 20 mg/day of memantine or placebo, following an initial 3-week titration period. After 28 weeks, the analyses performed on the ITT population showed that the mean ADAS-Cog total scores improved significantly (mean of 0.4) from baseline in the memantine-treated group compared with a deterioration in the placebo group (mean of 1.6; 95% confidence interval, 0.49 to 3.60). The analyses of the secondary variables were performed on the observed cases and showed an improvement of $1.8 + 3.51$ on the MMSE, and of -0.74 on the intellectual function part of the Gottfries–Brane–Steen (GBS) scale in the memantine patients, whereas the placebo group remained stable on these measures after 28 weeks. Memantine-treated patients were significantly superior to placebo in terms of the number of patients improving/stabilizing or deteriorating on the CGI-C investigator rating ($P = 0.032$). There was no significant difference between the two groups in the motor, emotional and different symptoms

subscores of the GBS, as well as in the behavioral and function symptoms measured by the NOSGER.

In terms of safety, 49 memantine (30%) and 38 placebo (24%) patients discontinued. The most common cause of early discontinuation was related to adverse events, namely, agitation, confusion and dizziness. Thirty-eight (23%) memantine patients and 40 (26%) placebo patients experienced serious adverse (cerebrovascular) events, in keeping with the pathology of VaD. There were no treatment-related deaths during the study in either group.

Dementia with Lewy Bodies

Perry and collaborators (1990a, 1990b, 1993) described reductions in the cortical cholinergic enzyme choline acetyltransferase (ChAT) greater in individuals with (80–85%) than in those without (50–55%) hallucinations. These ChAT reductions were more extensive in neo- as opposed to archi-cortical regions (Crystal *et al.*, 1990; Langlais *et al.*, 1993; Perry *et al.*, 1993), and were more marked in the parietal and temporal cortex (Perry *et al.*, 1990b) as well as in the hippocampus and entorhinal cortex than in other brain regions (Perry *et al.*, 1993). As a consequence of these ChAT reductions, there was a lack of cortical acetylcholine (ACh) in brains of patients with dementia with Lewy Bodies (DLB). Perry *et al.* (1999) suggested that the pathology of mesopontine cholinergic neurons might impair the level of conscious awareness and thus the sleeping and daytime activity cycle in DLB. Consequently, the administration of cholinergic agents should theoretically improve the level of consciousness and vigilance in subjects with DLB, and should also impact on their cognitive and behavioral functioning. Indeed, the results of a retrospective neuropathological study seem to support the view of an important role of ACh depletion in the cognitive impairment found in dementia with Lewy bodies (Levy *et al.*, 1994). In that particular study, it was found that three subjects, among those initially diagnosed with AD, and who had presented more significant improvement in cognition after receiving tacrine in a R-DB-PC trial (Eagger *et al.*, 1991), were in fact presenting with Lewy Bodies in the cingulate cortex, in addition to senile plaques and neurofibrillary tangles typical of Alzheimer's disease in the frontal, temporal, parietal and occipital lobes (Levy *et al.*, 1994). More recently, Tiraboschi *et al.* (2002) studied the timing of cholinergic deficits in 50 patients with DLB compared with 89 subjects with AD and 18 healthy controls. They found that the patients with mild DLB had significantly less ChAT activity in the superior temporal, inferior parietal and mid-frontal cerebral areas than the controls, whereas the patients with mild AD had ChAT activity comparable to that of controls. When less impaired patients underwent separate analysis, the correlations of ChAT activity with the MMSE score were significant only for the DLB group. Thus there is a biological rationale for the use of acetylcholinesterase inhibitors in dementia with Lewy Bodies.

Only articles on the use of donepezil, rivastigmine and galantamine in DLB were found. All the patients with DLB (except one case; Kaufer, 2004) included in the studies of the present review met the clinical diagnostic criteria of the Consortium on Dementia with Lewy Bodies for probable DLB (McKeith et al., 1996).

Donepezil

Thirteen studies, including eight case reports (Geizer & Ancill, 1998; Kaufer et al., 1998; Aarsland et al., 1999; Fergusson & Howard, 2000; Skjerve & Nygaard, 2000; Rojas-Fernandez, 2001; Coulson et al., 2002; Khotianov et al., 2002), two case series (Shea et al., 1998; Lanctôt & Herrmann, 2000), two open-label studies with between diagnostic group comparisons (Samuel et al., 2000; Minett et al., 2003) and one double-blind cross-over study (Beversdorf et al., 2004) described the effects of 5–10 mg/day of donepezil in a total of 46 subjects with DLB. The study of Samuel et al. (2000) compared the efficacy of 5 mg/day of donepezil in four subjects with DLB, and 12 subjects with AD over 6 months, whereas the study of Minett et al. (2003) compared the efficacy of up to 10 mg/day of donepezil in 9 subjects with DLB, and 15 subjects with Parkinson's disease and dementia (PDD) over 20 weeks followed by a 6-week withdrawal period. Beversdorf et al. (2004) studied the efficacy of 5 mg/day of donepezil in seven subjects with DLB in a double-blind, double-crossover 16-week trial, involving switches of condition after blocks of 4 weeks of treatment. The duration of the 14 studies varied from 4 weeks to one year.

According to the MMSE scores at baseline, the patients with DLB had mild (Geizer & Ancill, 1998; Kaufer et al., 1998; Aarsland et al., 1999; Fergusson & Howard, 2000; Samuel et al., 2000; Coulson et al., 2002; Khotianov et al., 2002), moderate (Shea et al., 1998; Lanctôt & Herrmann, 2000; Skjerve & Nygaard, 2000; Minett et al., 2003; Beversdorf et al., 2004), and severe dementia (Kaufer et al., 1998; Shea et al., 1998; Fergusson & Howard, 2000). Overall, the subjects with DLB were aged from 65 to 90 years (when age was mentioned).

Cognition has principally been assessed with the MMSE in 12/13 papers (Geizer & Ancill, 1998; Kaufer et al., 1998; Shea et al., 1998; Aarsland et al., 1999; Fergusson & Howard, 2000; Lanctôt & Herrmann, 2000; Samuel et al.,

2000; Skjerve & Nygaard, 2000; Coulson et al., 2002; Khotianov et al., 2002; Minett et al., 2003; Beversdorf et al., 2004), and with the ADAS-Cog in one trial (Beversdorf et al., 2004). Thirty-eight of the 46 subjects who received donepezil improved their cognitive functioning 4 weeks to 1 year post-baseline whereas 8 subjects did not register any improvement in cognition. The baseline and post-treatment MMSE scores were available in 35/38 of the 'improved' cases described in nine different anecdotal reports (Geizer & Ancill, 1998; Kaufer et al., 1998; Shea et al., 1998; Aarsland et al., 1999; Fergusson & Howard, 2000; Lanctôt & Herrmann, 2000; Skjerve & Nygaard, 2000 Coulson et al., 2002; Khotianov et al., 2002), two open-label studies (Samuel et al., 2000; Minett et al., 2003), and one double-blind cross-over study (Beversdorf et al., 2004), and revealed positive changes from 1 to 23 points. Three other cases without any MMSE or other psychometric assessment were reported to clinically improve, either by a clinician or a caregiver (Shea et al., 1998; Fergusson & Howard, 2000; Rojas-Fernandez, 2001). Only two studies utilized specific instruments to measure function, namely the Physical Self-Maintenance Scale (PSMS; Lawton & Brody, 1969), and the Instrumental Activities of Daily Living (IADL) questionnaire (Shea et al., 1998; Beversdorf et al., 2004). Improvements in function were described in 5/9 patients of Shea et al. (1998), but were not significant in the 7 subjects of Beversdorf et al. (2004).

Regarding safety issues, in the majority of these studies, there was no deterioration in extrapyramidal symptoms (EPS) as assessed by physician observation. In the two studies using the Unified Parkinson's Disease Rating Scale (UPDRS; Fahn & Elton, 1987), there was no significant change in EPS (Minett et al., 2003; Beversdorf et al., 2004). However, Shea et al. (1998) specifically reported that EPS worsened in two subjects, and fluctuated in another subject. Five subjects with DLB (moderate dementia) did not respond well or experienced adverse events (Lanctôt & Herrmann, 2000; Minett et al., 2003; Shea et al., 1998). One subject, receiving 5 mg/day, discontinued the treatment 4 weeks post-baseline because of insufficient response; two patients receiving 5 mg/day discontinued the treatment respectively after 1 and 6 weeks because of serious adverse events such as, in the first case, somnolence and exacerbation of previously stable chronic obstructive pulmonary disease, and in the second case, syncope, bradycardia and sweating (Lanctôt & Herrmann, 2000). Finally, one patient receiving 5 mg/day had a worsening of his psychotic symptoms, and then short-lived episodes of improvement after an increase of the dose to 10 mg/day (Shea et al., 1998). One subject with

DLB, and four subjects with Parkinson's disease and dementia, discontinued the 20-week open-label trial of Minett *et al.* (2003) because of gastro-intestinal side effects, increased hallucinations and EPS. Among them, one patient was also hospitalized with a gastric ulcer and empyema of the gall bladder (Minett *et al.*, 2003).

Rivastigmine
Seven papers, including one randomized double-blind placebo-controlled (R-DB-PC) trial (McKeith *et al.*, 2000a) with further cognitive analyses on this trial (McKeith *et al.*, 2004; Wesnes *et al.*, 2002), three open-label follow-up studies (McKeith *et al.*, 2000b; Grace *et al.*, 2000, 2001), and one case series (Maclean *et al.*, 2001) were found. Only the case series of Maclean *et al.* (2001) is unrelated to the trial of McKeith *et al.* (2000a). The subjects included in all the studies had mild to moderate dementia, and were aged between a mean of 74.25 and 78.5 years in the open-label trials (McKeith *et al.*, 2000b, Grace *et al.*, 2000; 2001) and in the case series (Maclean *et al.*, 2001). The treatment and placebo groups were aged 73.9 ± 6.5 and 73.9 ± 6.4 years in the studies of McKeith *et al.* (2000a, 2004) and Wesnes *et al.* (2002) respectively.

In order to measure changes in cognition, four studies utilized the MMSE (McKeith *et al.*, 2000a, 2000b; Grace *et al.*, 2000, 2001), three papers utilized the Cognitive Drug Research (CDR) computerized assessment system (McKeith *et al.*, 2000a, 2004; Wesnes *et al.*, 2002), and one study (Maclean *et al.*, 2001) utilized a modified and lengthier version of the MMSE, the Modified Mini-Mental State Examination (3MS; Teng & Chui, 1987). The CDR computerized assessment system consists of tests of attention, working memory and episodic memory, which have previously been validated in trials of acetylcholinesterase inhibitors in AD (Simpson *et al.*, 1991; Nicholl *et al.*, 1995).

Regarding the assessment of change in behavioral symptoms, four studies used either one or several versions of the Neuropsychiatric Inventory, e.g. the complete NPI, the NPI-4 or NPI-10 (nursing home version) (McKeith *et al.*, 2000a, 2000b; Grace *et al.*, 2001; Maclean *et al.*, 2001). One study (Grace *et al.*, 2000) utilized the Epworth Sleepiness Scale (ESS; Johns, 1993) and the Pittsburgh Sleep Quality Inventory (PSQI; Buysse *et al.*, 1989) to measure changes in sleep pattern.

Regarding the assessment of safety, three studies (McKeith *et al.*, 2000a, 2000b; Grace *et al.*, 2001) measured changes in EPS using the UPDRS together with a discontinuation rate. The remaining studies did not report the use of a quantifying method to record adverse events.

The R-DB-PC study included 120 subjects with DLB assigned to active treatment (n = 59) or placebo (n = 61) for 20 weeks (McKeith *et al.*, 2000a); the treatment phase was followed by a discontinuation period of 3 weeks. The 6–12 mg/day doses were reached by 44 of the 48 patients. In the paper of McKeith *et al.* (2000a), the results represented the sum of latencies measured from the CDR computerized assessment tests calculated as the unweighted sum of simple, choice, digit vigilance, numeric working memory, spatial memory, word recognition, and picture recognition reaction times. These results were given as change values in milliseconds, and were provided in three sets of data: intent to treat (ITT), last observation carried forward (LOCF), and observed cases (OC). A significant improvement in cognition occurred in the rivastigmine group, as measured by the computerized cognitive assessment system, in all three data sets at week 12 (ITT $P = 0.10$; LOCF $P = 0.005$; OC $P = 0.002$) and at week 20 (ITT $P = 0.048$; LOCF $P = 0.046$; OC $P = 0.017$), with the following mean change values from baseline: 1084 and 1318 ms at weeks 12 and 20 respectively, compared with the placebo group (mean change values: -2503 and -991 ms). The mean changes on the MMSE and the Clinical Global Change-plus were not significant. Regarding behavioral symptoms, the rivastigmine group had a significant improvement, compared with the placebo group, as measured by the NPI-4 and the NPI-10. Regarding safety issues, the rivastigmine group had a higher discontinuation rate of 30.5% (n = 18) compared with 16.4% (n = 10) in the placebo group. More patients on rivastigmine (54.92%) than placebo (46.75%) experienced adverse events, principally cholinergic in nature: nausea, vomiting, anorexia and somnolence. There was no change in the EPS of the rivastigmine and placebo groups, as measured by the UPDRS; however an emergent tremor was registered as an adverse event in four patients treated with rivastigmine (McKeith *et al.*, 2000a).

The study of Wesnes *et al.* (2002) provided further analyses on the cognitive functioning of the patients involved in the trial of McKeith *et al.* (2000a) using specific factors of the CDR computerized assessment system. In that particular study, cognitive data were available for 116 of the initial 120 patients with DLB who entered McKeith's R-DB-PC trial. The group receiving rivastigmine improved compared with the placebo group on power of attention, speed of memory processes and overall quality. Subsequent analyses performed on the R-DB-PC study revealed that among patients receiving rivastigmine, the hallucinators at baseline (74% of the patients) registered the most significant improvement at weeks 12 and 20 on the scores of power of attention and quality of memory, when compared with the non-hallucinators (26% of the patients) (McKeith *et al.*, 2004).

The open-label trial of McKeith *et al.* (2000b) was started after a 3-week washout period following the treatment period of the R-DB-PC study (McKeith *et al.*, 2000a). Eleven subjects completed 12 weeks of treatment with a mean daily dose of 9.6 ± 3.2 mg of rivastigmine at endpoint. At baseline, the patients had EPS (mean UPDRS score $= 24.5 \pm 14.1$), behavioral problems (mean NPI-4 $= 13.6 \pm 7.1$), and were all taking concomitant medications. At the end of the trial, delusions, apathy, agitation and hallucinations, as measured by the NPI-4, had significantly improved. There was no significant change in cognition on the MMSE or NPI. The authors did not mention the proportion of the 11 subjects who received rivastigmine in the R-DB-PC study. Thus some of these subjects might have been exposed to rivastigmine for the first time in the open-label trial as opposed to other subjects who may have received rivastigmine previously, in the R-DB-PC study. These latter subjects may have benefited from a longer exposure to the compound. Therefore, one does not know if the results of this open-label trial reflect a new or a continued response to the drug. Regarding safety, EPS had significantly decreased (24% on the UPDRS). Nausea and diarrhea were the most common reported side effects; no severe adverse events occurred.

The 12-week open-label trial of Grace *et al.* (2000) particularly studied the effect of rivastigmine, at maximum tolerated doses, on the sleeping profile of six subjects with DLB, as measured by the ESS (Johns, 1993), and the PSQI (Buysse *et al.*, 1989). At baseline, the subjects with DLB had a tendency to fall asleep at inappropriate times during the day. The sleeping patterns of the patients with DLB improved on the PSQI and on the ESS. Cognition also improved, as assessed by the MMSE, from a mean of 18.5/30 at baseline to 23/30 at week 12. Unfortunately, no variance analyses were performed due to the small sample size.

The study of Grace *et al.* (2001) is the continuation of the previous open-label trials of McKeith *et al.* (2000b) and Grace *et al.* (2000), and included 29 subjects with DLB. Cognition (as measured by the MMSE), behavioral disturbances (as measured by the NPI-4) and EPS (as measured by the UPDRS) significantly improved 12 and 24 weeks post-baseline, with 3–12 mg/day of rivastigmine. The scores on the NPI-4 and the UPDRS went back to those of baseline at weeks 36 and 96, whereas the scores on the MMSE went back to those of baseline at week 36, and declined below baseline scores at weeks 84 and 96. There was a high discontinuation rate of 31%.

In the case series of Maclean *et al.* (2001) involving a total of eight subjects, two subjects received 6 mg/day,

one subject received 7.5 mg/day, three subjects received 9 mg/day, and two subjects received 12 mg/day of rivastigmine. Three to 24 weeks post-baseline, cognition and behavior had improved in 7/8 subjects (their scores on the 3MS increased from a mean of 55/100 to a mean of 85/100; and their scores on the NPI-10 decreased from a mean of 46/120 to a mean of 7/120). Six cases reported better sleep; five cases reported some improvement in ADLs and two cases reported an improvement in EPS. However, the changes in sleep pattern, Activities of Daily Living and EPS were not formally assessed with psychometric instruments. Only one subject registered a lack of change in cognition and behavior after a month of receiving 9 mg/day and was thus discontinued because of the lack of efficacy (Maclean *et al.*, 2001).

Galantamine

Three studies including two case reports (Holm, 2004; Kaufer, 2004), and one open-label study (n = 25) (Edwards *et al.*, 2004) described the effects of 4 mg b.i.d. to 8 mg b.i.d. of galantamine in 28 subjects with DLB. The duration of the three studies varied from 4 weeks (Holm, 2004) to 14 months (Kaufer, 2004). The subjects included in all the studies had mild (Edwards *et al.*, 2004; Holm, 2004) to severe dementia (Kaufer, 2004). The patients of Edwards *et al.* (2004) had a mean age of 76.32 years, whereas the patients of Holm (2004) were 65 and 68 years old, and the patient of Kaufer (2004) was 89 years old.

Cognition was assessed with the MMSE in 2/3 papers (Edwards *et al.*, 2004; Holm, 2004), the CGIC and the ADAS-Cog/11score (including sub-tests of Word Recall and Word Recognition) in 1/3 papers (Edwards *et al.*, 2004), and by physician's notes in 1/3 papers (Kaufer, 2004). Twenty-six of the 28 subjects who received galantamine 8–24 mg/day improved their cognitive functioning 4 weeks to 14 months post-baseline, whereas two subjects did not register any significant improvement in cognition (Holm, 2004; Kaufer, 2004), though they improved significantly in their psychotic, mood and behavioral symptoms. The baseline and post-treatment MMSE scores were available in the two 'improved' cases described in the article of Holm (2004), and in the 25 patients of the 12-week open trial of Edwards *et al.* (2004). Only one of Holm's patients registered positive change (from 12 to 19 points on the MMSE), whereas the 25 patients in the 12-week open-label trial of Edwards *et al.* (2004) significantly improved by 1.58 points on the MMSE ($P = 0.05$), 6.63 points on the ADAS-Cog/11score ($P = 0.004$) (secondary measures) and 0.95 points ($P = 0.02$) on the CGIC (primary measure). However, the most significant improvement in this trial occurred on a behavioral measure, the NPI-4, with a change of 5.04 points ($P = 0.003$) (Edwards *et al.*, 2004).

Regarding safety issues, EPS were not systematically quantified at baseline and post-baseline in the two case reports (Holm, 2004; Kaufer, 2004), which instead used physicians' observations, but were systematically assessed using the UPDRS in the open-label trial (Edwards *et al.*, 2004). The two patients of Holm (2004) were reported to improve their posture, gait, motor abilities and tremulousness, whereas Kaufer (2004) made no comment in this regard. However, the patient of Kaufer was strongly suspected to meet the diagnostic criteria of Parkinson's disease with dementia rather than the diagnosis of DLB, given the duration of the parkinsonian symptoms (more than 1 year) before the onset of cognitive deficits. The 25 patients of Edwards registered an improvement on the UPDRS from a score of 20.1 at baseline to a score of 17.5 at week 12, thus showing some amelioration in EPS. During this trial, two patients (8%) dropped out, 48% of the patients reported adverse events, mostly gastrointestinal in nature, and only one serious adverse event occurred (this was a hospitalization for myocardial infarction, an event that was judged unrelated to the study medication).

Summary

The quality of evidence for studies in AD is generally good and abundant, whereas the quality of evidence in VaD is good, though still relatively scarce and hence somewhat preliminary at the moment. Most of the early phase II–III studies assessing the efficacy of AChEIs in Alzheimer's disease (AD) and vascular dementia (VaD) have involved only subjects with mild to moderate dementia, and have employed broad exclusion criteria (e.g. many comorbid medical conditions and psychiatric disorders as well as concurrent medications). Therefore, some caution needs to be applied before generalizing the results of these early trials to the excluded groups (e.g. to those with severe dementia, residing in institutions or having a complicating medical condition).

In patients with AD and VaD mildly to moderately demented at baseline, the efficacy of donepezil was significant, but modest, and was investigated most often solely in terms of impact on cognition. The drug is usully started at a dose of 5 mg/day, and if no dramatic improvement is seen (usually after 2 weeks to 2 months) then the dose is increased to 10 mg. The trials with donepezil obtained the best results on the ADAS-Cog, the CIBIC-plus and the MMSE with a dose of 10 mg/day, and have shown some improvement over baseline values for the first 6–9 months of treatment, and then a slowing in the cognitive decline

compared with placebo. The ADAS-Cog and the CIBIC-plus are the two clinical primary indicators of change recognized by the US Federal Food and Drug Administration (Jann, 2000). However, the effect of donepezil on behavior and function is not well known for short-term intervals, since it has been measured only with the CIBIC-plus in AD, and with the ADFACS in VaD. Trials of discontinuation (washout periods) of the drug in AD have shown that the positive effects of donepezil can be maintained over a period of 3 weeks, but not over a 6-week period. Large R-DB-PC and open-label trials over longer time periods (up to 2 years) and initiated in patients with mild-moderate dementia at baseline have demonstrated that donepezil may slow the cognitive and functional deterioration in AD for at least a year. However, over a 2-year period, no benefits were registered over placebo. In patients with moderate-severe dementia and AD, donepezil showed some benefits over placebo on cognition and on some measures of function, but not on behavior, mood and psychosis, as measured by the NPI. Donepezil was in general well tolerated in mildly to severely demented patients with AD and VaD, even with those presenting concomitant medical conditions and taking additional medications.

In the trials with rivastigmine, the best results in patients with AD and AD with vascular risk factors as measured by the Modified Hachinski Ischemic Score were obtained with higher doses of 10–12 mg/day. The cognitive improvement from baseline was minimal on the ADAS-Cog and the CIBIC-plus in the first 6 months of the treatment. Mood, behavior and function have been only preliminarily investigated (CIBIC-Plus, NOSGER, PDS), and have also shown minimal improvement over placebo. These benefits were maintained over the placebo group, in terms of slowed cognitive decline, for periods of up to 2 years in AD. The utilization of the PDS as a measure of functionality was criticized by Bentham *et al.* (1999). These authors mention that the PDS was developed to measure quality of life and not activities of daily living, and therefore contains few pertinent questions related to ADL. Although the discontinuation rates due to adverse events are higher in rivastigmine than in donepezil trials, rivastigmine can nonetheless be considered to be relatively well tolerated in mildly to severely demented patients with AD, even with those followed in clinical settings and presenting with concomitant medical conditions and taking additional medications. The most frequently reported adverse events were gastrointestinal.

In the trials studying galantamine, patients with AD and VaD were mildly to moderately demented at baseline and the results were dose-dependent up to 24 mg/day (AD and VaD) and 32 mg/day (AD). Cognition measured with the ADAS-Cog and the CIBIC-plus remained stable or minimally improved following 5 and 6 months of randomized double-blind placebo-controlled trials. Behavior (measured with the NPI) and function (measured with the DAD and the ADCS/ADL) also remained stable (NPI, DAD) or minimally improved (ADCS/ADL) after 5–6 months of treatment. These improvements were generally maintained for a year and then were followed by a gradual decline in long-term extension studies in both AD and VaD. However, the long-term benefits of galantamine tended to be maintained longer in VaD (21 months) than in AD + CVD (12 months). Thus these results suggest that galantamine is efficacious in maintaining cognition, behavior and function in AD and VaD. It appears also to be relatively safe, especially in AD. Treatment discontinuations due to adverse events in the galantamine-treated groups receiving up to 24 mg/day were generally comparable with those in the placebo group in AD, but were higher in VaD who first received placebo. Adverse events were principally cholinergic in nature, transient, and decreased in frequency during the long-term extension studies.

The memantine trials were conducted in AD patients with moderate to severe dementia and in VaD patients with mild to moderate dementia. The memantine trials were short (from 44 days to 28 weeks). Some improvements in cognition, behavior and function occurred in moderate to severe dementia in subjects with AD, with a dosage of 10 mg/day of memantine over periods of 6 months, even in patients with concomitant medications and/or already stable on donepezil. However, the cognitive measures were psychometrically poor (the CGI-C and CIBIC-plus). Only one R-DB-PC study showed that patients with mild to moderate VaD also minimally improved compared with baseline and placebo on cognition and function. Memantine has proven to be relatively safe, with discontinuation rates due to adverse events comparable in the memantine and placebo-treated groups in both AD and VaD. Thus, phase II and III randomized double-blind placebo controlled trials should take place in subjects with mild to moderate Alzheimer's disease and vascular dementia.

In regards to dementia with Lewy Bodies, despite evident methodological limitations, preliminary evidence showed some efficacy in improving principally psychotic and behavioral symptoms, and to a lesser extent, cognition, using donepezil (5–10 mg/day), rivastigmine (3–13 mg/day) and galantamine (8–24 mg/day) in patients with DLB who were mildly to moderately demented. The three AChEIs particularly improved visual hallucinations,

paranoid delusions and level of nighttime and daytime activity (hypersomnolence during the day; sleeping profile at night; apathy; aggressiveness; agitation). However, more R-DB-PC trials are required before the use of any AChEI can be clinically recommended, since the quality of evidence was generally poor, especially for the donepezil and galantamine data. The majority of the studies were case reports, case series or open label trials. There were only two R-DB-PC trials, and the data of these two trials are derived from the same sample of subjects tested with rivastigmine. The size of the samples was also very limited: the largest sample involved 59 and 61 patients in the treatment and placebo groups respectively in the R-DB-PC trial of McKeith et al. (2000a).

Another problem with some of the DLB papers included in the present review was a lack of psychometric measurement for behavioral symptoms, activities of daily living, and extrapyramidal symptoms, as well as a lack of sensitive measurement of cognitive function, especially in the studies on donepezil and galantamine. The MMSE that was generally utilized in those trials lacks sensitivity to measure the cognitive deficits characterizing early DLB, such as problems with vigilance, working memory, attention, executive functions, and episodic memory with free and cued recall paradigm (see Simard et al., 2000, for a review). Interestingly, none of the studies included in the current review commented on the effects of donepezil, rivastigmine or galantamine on cognitive fluctuations, even though these symptoms were mentioned in a large number of subjects across the three drugs' data set. This situation might partly be attributed to the fact that there is no clear definition of "cognitive or confusion fluctuations" in terms of the intensity, duration and frequency of the episodes, according to the Consortium on Dementia with Lewy Bodies Criteria (McKeith et al., 1996), and also because until very recently, there was no instrument available to measure the cognitive or confusion fluctuations.

In terms of safety, one should pay attention to the impact of the AChEI on cardiac function in DLB: often patients with DLB have a cardiac condition and take cardiac medication, and some subjects with DLB may even present with cerebrovascular lesions (Barber et al., 1999, 2000; Ballard et al., 2000). The present review, though lacking of data in many instances, has evidenced that such a condition can negatively affect the outcome of an AChEI trial (see the results of Lanctôt & Herrmann, 2000). In addition, the pro-cholinergic effect of the acetylcholinesterase inhibitors might theoretically cause a worsening of EPS in the treated patients. However, such a worsening was only reported anecdotally in a few subjects of the R-DB-PC trial with rivastigmine. In fact, in many cases, rivastigmine and galantamine improved EPS in subjects with DLB as demonstrated by significant improvements on the UPDRS. Comparatively, when treated with donepezil, three subjects from three different studies were reported to have a significant decrease in their EPS up to 6 months post-baseline. The reason for this improvement is not clear; however, modulation activity between the cortical inhibition of ChEI and levels of cortical catecholamines and between the dopaminergic and ACh-nicotinic striatal receptors reported in the literature might be responsible. Donepezil has been shown to increase levels of catecholamines, including dopamine, in the cortex of rats (Giacobini *et al.*, 1996). The activation of the nicotinic acetylcholine receptors in the dorsal striatum has been demonstrated to contribute to dopamine and activity-dependent changes in synaptic efficacy (Partridge *et al.*, 2002). These AChEI and ACh activities might affect the dopamine levels and possibly improve EPS.

The discontinuation rates of the patients with DLB in the rivastigmine studies are comparable to those described in rivastigmine trials with Alzheimer's disease. The side effects were the usual gastro-intestinal cholinergic effects, with no serious consequences. The R-DB-PC trial of rivastigmine (McKeith *et al.*, 2000a) clearly identified a number of concomitant and previous medications as well as a number of concomitant medical conditions in the subjects involved in the study; the absence of severe adverse events found in this particular study suggests that rivastigmine might potentially be administered to more severely demented subjects with DLB.

Practice guidelines

Donepezil was the first nootropic for treatment of AD to be approved by the US Federal Food and Drug Administration (FDA) in 1996, by Health Canada in 1997, and to be licensed in the UK in 1997. Rivastigmine was the second agent to receive approval from the FDA and Health Canada in 2000, and to be licensed in the UK in 1998. Galantamine was the third acetylcholinesterase inhibitor to be approved by the FDA in 2001, Health Canada in 2003, and to be licensed in the UK in 2000. The last nootropic for treatment of dementia to be approved for marketing was memantine in 2003 by the FDA, and in 2004 by Health Canada. Memantine was launched in 2002 in the UK, but is currently not recommended in National Institute for Clinical Excellence (NICE) guidelines www.nice.org.uk/cg42/niceguidance/pdf/English. The acetylcholinesterase inhibitors are currently approved only for the treatment of mild to moderately severe AD, whereas memantine is only approved for the treatment of moderately severe to severe AD.

National health advisory agencies in the UK, USA and Canada have recently adopted different positions in regards to prescribing guidelines in dementia (Kmietowicz, 2005). According to the new guidance from the NICE in the UK, donepezil, rivastigmine and galantamine should only be prescribed on the National Health Service (NHS) to treat those with moderately severe Alzheimer's disease (MMSE scores of less than or equal to 21) (http://www.nice.org.uk/page.aspx?o=324234). Memantine is no longer recommended as an effective treatment. However these decisions were based on a controversial economic analysis that concluded these drugs (around GBP 2.50 per day) were not cost-effective for the NHS (Day, 2006). As this book goes to press, the manufacturers of these drugs are seeking judicial review in the UK courts in an attempt to overturn this decision.

In an update of the American Psychiatric Association guidelines for treatment of Alzheimer's disease and other dementias of late life first issued in 1997 (APA, 1997), Rabins (2004) suggests that all the cholinesterase inhibitors and memantine, although only FDA approved for the treatment of AD, may also be beneficial for the treatment of dementia with Lewy bodies and vascular dementia. Physicians must also employ alternative strategies including ensuring general good health, avoiding sedating and anticholinergic drugs, and encouraging mental and physical activity (Rabins, 2004). Canadian psychiatrists generally follow the APA prescribing guidelines.

Conclusion

Strong evidence indicates that the cholinesterase inhibitors may successfully delay cognitive and functional decline in mild to moderate AD. The evidence is less robust in regards to memantine, due to the paucity of trials (which involve, for the most part, moderate to severe AD). In addition, preliminary evidence suggests that these agents could also provide benefit in VaD and DLB. A comparative economic analysis conducted in 2003, based on the Cochrane reviews, tends to support the present findings. The economic analysis showed that while all cholinesterase inhibitors reduced the need for full-time care, only galantamine and donepezil 10 mg reduced the overall costs of AD patients in Canada. The somewhat greater cognitive effect provided by galantamine leads to the longest delay before full-time care is required, and consequently contributes to lowering of the overall cost, with savings estimated between US $323 and $4246 (Caro *et al.*, 2003).

However, much of the research in AD and VaD employed cognitive testing as the principal outcome of interest, and the results, in terms of improvement from baseline and compared with placebo were, for the most part, modest (a few points on the ADAS-Cog or on the MMSE). Thus, clinically, it is more appropriate to describe the findings as maintaining the current level of functioning rather than significantly improving the symptoms. However, one must bear in mind the psychometric weaknesses of the instruments used to measure cognitive improvement. The ADAS-Cog, the MMSE and the GDS have notably been criticized for their lack of sensitivity (Nelson *et al.*, 1986; Eisdorfer *et al.*, 1992; Mohs *et al.*, 1997; Simard, 1998; Simard & van Reekum, 1999), whereas the CIBIC-plus and the CGIC generally have poor psychometric qualities, being dependent on the subjective judgement of the rater following a semi-structured interview that may vary in content from site to site (Knopman *et al.*, 1994; Heun *et al.*, 1998). It is thus possible that some cognitive improvements might not have been captured by the instruments. However, the ADAS-Cog and the CIBIC-plus are the two primary indicators of change recognized by the FDA (Jann, 2000).

In the past 5 years, the potential effect of these medications on functional abilities, mood and behavior have begun to be taken into account by some researchers, especially in galantamine trials. However, quality of life and cost of care still need to be investigated, using well validated instruments to properly assess these aspects.

Since relative discontinuation rates due to adverse events were often slightly to moderately higher in the drug-treated than in the placebo-treated groups, the clinician will need to consider the potential for side effects and the costs of these drugs. Given the neuronal destruction associated with progression of the disease, efficacy may well be reduced for most compounds in the moderate-severe stages of AD and in VaD.

Other treatments

Vitamin E

Vitamin E is an antioxidant and may act by protecting neurones against damage by free radicals. Vitamin E, in the form of alpha-tocopherol, is not routinely prescribed in the UK but is widely purchased as a dietary supplement over the counter at pharmacies and health food shops. In an update of the American Psychiatric Association guidelines for treatment of Alzheimer's disease and other dementias of late life first issued in 1997 (APA, 1997), Rabins (2004) mentions that the only available study (Sano *et al.*, 1997) examining the efficacy of vitamin E supports the use of 2000 international units (IU) daily in patients with moderately severe impairment for slowing disease progression.

There has been one systematic review (Tabet *et al.*, 2000) (updated February 2002). This identified one multicenter randomized controlled trial (RCT) of acceptable methodological quality (Sano *et al.*, 1997) that compared alpha-tocopherol (2000 IU daily), selegiline and a combination of both with placebo in 169 patients with moderate Alzheimer's disease over 2 years. The four primary outcomes were time to death, institutionalization, change in dementia severity and loss of Activities of Daily Living. In the alpha-tocopherol group there was a significant delay to these outcomes (risk ratio 0.47; $P = 0.001$). There was no significant effect on cognitive function as measured on the cognitive section of the Alzheimer's Disease Assessment Scale (ADAS-Cog). In the RCT there was a significant increase in the number of falls and syncopal attacks in the treatment group. At baseline, the placebo group had significantly less severe dementia (as measured on the MMSE). The positive effect of alpha-tocopherol in delaying time to adverse outcomes was found after controlling for this difference, and this adjustment may weaken the validity of these findings.

Most studies of the potential benefit of Vitamin E on prevention and treatment of Alzheimer's disease are epidemiological and further RCTs are required. There is no evidence available for Lewy Body disease or vascular dementia. Vitamin E is popular amongst Alzheimer's disease patients and their carers because it is seen as a dietary supplement and not as an "active medication". However, it is not without side effects and high dose vitamin E may be associated with abdominal cramps and diarrhea. A meta-analysis of 135 967 patients involved in clinical trials of Vitamin E (for a variety of chronic diseases) demonstrated a significant increase in all-cause mortality (Miller *et al.*, 2005) and currently there is little evidence to support its use in Alzheimer's disease.

Estrogen

Women have a higher risk of developing Alzheimer's disease and it has been postulated that this is related to the peri- and postmenopausal decrease in estrogen levels. It may act through antioxidant, antiamyloidgenic and neurotrophic mechanisms. Estrogen is a prescription-only medication and is not routinely prescribed for the treatment of cognitive impairment in the UK. In the USA and Canada, estrogen is also a prescription-only medication. The 1997 American Psychiatric Association guidelines for treatment of patients with Alzheimer's disease and other dementias of late life suggested that postmenopausal women weighing the risks and benefits of estrogen replacement might consider the preliminary evidence reporting a later onset and/or decreased risk of cognitive decline. However, since the publication of these guidelines, the efficacy of estrogen to decrease the likelihood of cognitive decline in postmenopausal women has become a controversial matter, especially after the publication of The Women's Health Initiative Memory Study (Craig *et al.*, 2005). Despite this new evidence, the recent Guideline Watch (Rabins, 2006) did not modify the 1997 APA prescription in this regard (available online at http://www.psych.org/psych_pract/treatg/pg/prac_guide.cfm).

There has been one systematic review of estrogen as a treatment for Alzheimer's disease (Hogervorst *et al.*, 2002). This examined five RCTs including a total of 210 postmenopausal women with mild to moderate Alzheimer's disease. Studies were of 8 weeks to 6 months duration and the effects of estrogen replacement alone and combined with a progestogen were assessed. The reviewers performed a large number of meta-analyses on a variety of outcomes including global cognitive function, memory, language, processing speed, concentration, clinical impression of change, dementia severity and depression. Overall there was no clinically relevant effect of preventing decline in cognitive function in Alzheimer's disease. Prolonged use of estrogen increases the risk of breast cancer, endometrial cancer (risk reduced by additional progestogen) and thrombo-embolism (Rossouw *et al.*, 2002). The studies included in the systematic review included women from a wide age range and participants were a mixed population of those with surgical and natural menopause.

Epidemiological data have suggested that the use of estrogen and hormone replacement therapy may decrease the risk of developing Alzheimer's disease (relative risk 0.56, 95% CI 0.46–0.68) (Hogervorst *et al.*, 2000). However these observational studies and the intervention trials included in the systematic review have been criticized for not controlling for important confounders such as age and education. The most recent evidence from the Women's Health Initiative Memory Study found that estrogen did not reduce the incidence of dementia and may adversely affect global cognitive function. When the data for estrogen alone and estrogen plus progestogen were pooled there was actually an increased risk for minimal cognitive impairment and Alzheimer's disease (Espeland *et al.*, 2004; Shumaker *et al.*, 2004). There are no data available for vascular dementia or Lewy Body disease.

In conclusion there is no indication for the use of estrogen to treat or prevent Alzheimer's disease in women over 65 years of age and its use may actually be harmful for cognition.

Ginkgo biloba

The most commonly used form of ginkgo biloba is the high potency extract EGb761. Ginkgo has vasodilator activity and may reduce neuronal damage by free radicals. Ginkgo is available without prescription as a food supplement in the UK and USA, therefore the strength and purity of preparations varies widely. It must be obtained on prescription in Germany where it is one of the most commonly prescribed medications. In the USA, Rabins (2004) cautiously mentions that the only study supporting use of gingko biloba as a treatment for dementia (Le Bars *et al.*, 1997) has not been replicated (Solomon *et al.*, 2002). Thus the utilization of this agent in North America for treatment of cognitive disorder is not common.

There has been one systematic review (most recent amendment August 2002) that includes 33 double-blind, placebo-controlled RCTs, few of which used intention-to-treat analysis (Birks *et al.*, 2002). Patients had a range of diagnoses including dementia of any type and "age related cognitive impairment". Significant benefits compared with placebo were found at 24–26 weeks for physician-assessed Clinical Global Improvement, cognition, activities of daily living and mood and emotion. One large study that included people with a diagnosis of Alzheimer's disease (n = 236), where intention to treat analysis was used, found significant improvement in cognition (ADAS-Cog scale, −1.7 points, 95% CI −3.1 to −0.20) (Le Bars *et al.*, 1997).

The meta-analysis found no differences between ginkgo or placebo groups in terms of adverse events. Ginkgo has few reported side effects, those occurring most commonly being bleeding, gastrointestinal disturbance and headaches (Cupp, 1999).

The meta-analysis pooled all data regardless of patients' diagnosis and it is difficult to extrapolate these results to specific dementia subtypes, although from individual trials there is evidence of efficacy for Alzheimer's disease and vascular dementia (Kanowski *et al.*, 1996; Le Bars *et al.*, 1997). Many studies of Ginkgo have not been methodologically rigorous and over the counter Ginkgo preparations vary in formulation. Despite these reservations, the available evidence suggests that Ginkgo appears to be safe and may be of benefit to patients with Alzheimer's disease and vascular dementia. However, a recently coupled large trial as yet unpublished (McCarney *et al.*) showed no evidence of any benefit for Ginkgo in dementia.

Selegiline

Selegiline (also known as L-Deprenyl) is a mono-amine oxidase β inhibitor. The enzyme is decreased in the brains of people with Alzheimer's disease. Selegiline increases dopamine synthesis by inhibiting pre-synaptic uptake and may also decrease oxidative stress. In the UK, selegiline is a prescription-only medication licensed for use in Parkinson's disease and is used very infrequently for the treatment of dementia. In 1997, the American Psychiatric Association (APA, 1997) suggested that selegiline might be used in mildly impaired patients with Alzheimer's disease. However, the APA preferred vitamin E over selegiline in the moderate stage of the disease, because of its low toxicity and lack of drug interaction. In the severe stage of the disease, the APA observed at the time that there were no available data about whether selegiline retards the process of the disease. Rabins (2004), in an update of the guidelines, did not provide further information.

There has been one systematic review that focused on the efficacy of selegiline (10 mg daily) in 17 RCTs of patients with mild to moderate Alzheimer's disease (most recent amendment October 2002) (Birks & Flicker, 2003). Using results from combined memory tests, there was a significant improvement in cognitive function at 4 months (standard mean difference 0.44, 95% CI 0.04–0.84, $P = 0.03$). There was little evidence for significant improvement in Activities of Daily Living or global assessment or emotional state.

There were a low number of patient withdrawals and adverse events in the trials. Side-effects such as nausea, dry mouth and postural hypotension were rare. Trials used a wide range of outcomes, varied greatly in size (10–41 participants) and few lasted longer than 3 months. There is little justification for further investigation of selegiline, or for its use in the treatment of Alzheimer's disease (Birks & Flicker, 2003;Wilcock et al., 2002).

Non-steroidal anti-inflammatory drugs (NSAIDs)
Laboratory evidence suggests that inflammatory pathways mediate the neuronal damage caused by β amyloid plaques. Non-steroidal anti-inflammatory drugs (NSAIDs) inhibit prostaglandin and cytokine synthesis, decreasing the inflammatory response. They are not routinely prescribed or recommended for the treatment of Alzheimer's disease in the UK. In the USA, Rabins (2004) mentions that efficacy of the NSAIDs has yet to be demonstrated in prospective trials before these compounds can be considered as interventions decreasing the likelihood of developing Alzheimer's disease.

Epidemiological evidence suggests that NSAIDs reduce the risk of developing Alzheimer's disease. A meta-analysis of prospective studies (11 902 participants) has demonstrated that use of NSAIDs for 2 years or more gives a combined risk estimate of 0.42 (95% CI = 0.26–0.66) (Szekely et al., 2004). This is supported by evidence that patients on

long-term NSAID treatment for arthritis are also less likely to develop Alzheimer's disease (McGeer et al., 1996).

Aspirin is a cyclo-oxygenase 1 (COX-1) inhibitor that acts by inhibiting platelet aggregation therefore decreasing the risk of cerebrovascular events. It is frequently prescribed to patients with vascular dementia in the UK (one survey found that 80% of patients with vascular dementia were prescribed aspirin; Dennis & Boyle 1998), probably because it is of proven benefit in stroke (Benavente et al., 2000). In 1997, the APA indicated that good control of blood pressure and perhaps low-dose aspirin may help to prevent further strokes in patients with dementia and a history of strokes (APA, 1997). However, in the 2004 update of the APA guidelines, Rabins mentions that efficacy has yet to be demonstrated in prospective trials before specific interventions (including anti-hypertensive medications) can be prescribed to decrease the likelihood of developing AD. In Canada, aspirin is indicated to reduce the risk of cerebral transient ischemic attacks and to prevent cerebral atherothrombotic infarcts by the Compendium of Pharmaceuticals and Specialities (Rabins, 2004).

There has been one systematic review of its use in vascular dementia (most recently amended November 2003) and no randomized controlled trials are available. There is currently no clear evidence that aspirin is a beneficial treatment for vascular dementia.

There has been one systematic review (most recent amendment May 2004) (Tabet & Feldman, 2003) of the effectiveness of indomethacin in Alzheimer's disease and this identified one double-blind placebo-controlled randomized trial (Rogers et al., 1993). This included 44 patients with mild to moderate Alzheimer's disease (NINCDS-ADRDA criteria) (McKhann et al., 1984) treated with 100–150 mg of indomethacin per day (adjusted for body weight). The results for cognitive tests, i.e. the MMSE (Folstein et al., 1975), ADAS-Cog (Rosen et al., 1984), Boston Naming test (Kaplan et al., 1978) and the Token test (DeRenzi & Vignolo 1962) were combined and patients in the indomethacin group showed significantly improved cognition (1.3% mean increase with indomethacin vs 8.4% mean decline with placebo, $P < 0.003$). However, when the meta-analysis examined these cognitive tests separately, only the ADAS-Cog showed significant improvement for the indomethacin group (MD 14.70, 95% CI 0.11–29.29, $P = 0.05$). The study had a high rate of patient withdrawals (42% of the active treatment group, 30% of the placebo group) and gastrointestinal side effects were common.

A subsequent 25-week study of diclofenac 50 mg plus misoprostol 200 μg per day in 41 patients with mild to moderate Alzheimer's disease found that there were no significant differences in cognitive function between the active treatment and placebo groups as measured on the ADAS-Cog and the Clinicians Interview Based Impression of Change score (Scharf *et al.*, 1999). The addition of the gastroprotective agent misoprostol did not appear to improve tolerability and 12/24 patients in the active treatment group withdrew (compared with 2/17 in the placebo group).

The largest randomized controlled trial (351 patients with mild to moderate Alzheimer's disease) compared the COX-2 inhibitor rofecoxib 25 mg daily or naproxen 225 mg daily and placebo (Aisen *et al.*, 2003). After one year there were no significant differences in cognition on the ADAS-Cog scale between either of the active treatments and placebo. Dizziness, fatigue and hypertension were more common in the rofecoxib and placebo groups. There were no significant differences in the frequency of gastrointestinal side effects between active treatment and placebo groups although gastrointestinal bleeds occurred in one patient on placebo, two of those on naproxen and four of those on rofecoxib.

The promising results of epidemiological and observational studies suggesting NSAIDs may be a treatment for Alzheimer's disease have been widely contradicted by the results of clinical trials. Sample sizes in the studies with weakly positive findings are small and the largest trial, involving rofecoxib and naproxen, did not find any significant improvements in patients on active treatments. It may be that the Alzheimer's disease of patients entering these trials has already progressed too far and that oxidative damage can only be prevented in the pre-clinical stage, the point where older people may enter an epidemiological study (Stewart *et al.*, 1997). There are also serious concerns about tolerability, particularly in elderly people where comorbid conditions are common. Recent concerns about the increase in adverse cardiovascular events in elderly people taking the COX-2 inhibitors rofecoxib (Levesque *et al.*, 2005) and the subsequent withdrawal of rofecoxib and celecoxib in the UK and the USA mean that currently NSAIDs cannot be recommended for the treatment of Alzheimer's disease.

Cognitive rehabilitation and cognitive training

These techniques are based on those developed for younger people with acquired brain injury and encompass a broad range of therapies that can be given to individual patients, in a group therapy setting or with the assistance of informal caregivers. There is considerable overlap between the two methods. Cognitive training tends to focus on practice tasks for specific domains such as memory and executive function. Cognitive rehabilitation is more individualized and may involve the patient and

carer identifying goals that are important to them such as particular activities of daily living. These therapies are not used as part of routine clinical practice in the UK but are administered at some specialist centres.

In the USA and Canada, cognitive rehabilitation and/or cognitive training are not currently used as part of routine clinical practice. The 1997 APA Practice Guidelines stated that the use of cognition-oriented treatments such as cognitive remediation and skills training was not supported by efficacy data. A recent systematic review however concluded that some of these interventions preliminarily showed some efficacy, but still required further investigation before they can be prescribed on a current basis for patients with Alzheimer's disease (Grandmaison & Simard, 2003).

There has been one systematic review (most recent amendment August 2003) (Clare *et al.*, 2003) that identified six trials, all involving cognitive training interventions. Patients were of varied diagnosis including Alzheimer's disease, vascular dementia and dementia associated with Parkinson's disease. The interventions varied widely; some were delivered to groups, others to individuals. Tools used included computers, work books and home work exercises. It was only possible to pool limited data for meta-analysis because of the range of different outcome measures used and differences in patient populations. There were no observable benefits found for cognitive retraining and the reviewers concluded that present findings do not provide strong support for cognitive training in early Alzheimer's disease.

Reminiscence therapy

Reminiscence therapy involves a structured and guided process of reflecting on a person's life. The therapy usually takes place in groups where older people discuss past events sometimes using aids such as videos or pictures. It is based on the principle that remote long-term memory is often relatively well preserved until the later stages of Alzheimer's disease. The principles of reminiscence therapy are used widely throughout specialist dementia care settings in the UK but they are often not consistently or systematically applied. The 1997 APA Practice Guidelines stated that emotion-oriented treatments such as reminiscence therapy showed modest efficacy on a wide variety of outcome measures, and thus may be helpful for some patients.

There has been one systematic review of reminiscence therapy (Woods *et al.*, 2005). The review identified five trials (total of 144 participants). At 4- or 6-week follow-up, reminiscence therapy was associated with significant improvements in cognition (SMD 0.5; 95% CI 0.07–0.92; $z = 2.31$, $P = 0.02$). There are considerable methodological difficulties in pooling data from these trials. Sample sizes, with the exception of one study by Lai *et al.* (2004) which had 101 participants, were small (15–27 patients) and every study used a different method of reminiscence therapy. Therefore data from group work and individual therapy were combined. None of the studies examined potential harms or side effects of reminiscence therapy.

Reality orientation therapy

Reality orientation therapy involves re-orientating the person with dementia in place, person and time. The intensity of the intervention varies from the use of a simple calendar board to a more intense and formal "class room" approach where patients participate in exercises. Intensive reality orientation therapy is not in widespread use in specialist dementia settings in the UK but elements such as orientation boards are used commonly. The 1997 APA practice guidelines noted that reality orientation has produced modest transient improvement in verbal orientation, as well as adverse effects such as anger, frustration, and depression in a number of studies conducted in institutionalized and non-institutionalized patients. The guidelines therefore finally concluded that this treatment was not supported by efficacy data, and also had the potential to produce adverse effects.

There has been one systematic review of reality orientation therapy (most recent amendment May 2000) (Spector *et al.*, 2000) that identified six randomized controlled trials (125 participants). Cognition was significantly better in those receiving orientation therapy (SMD −0.586, 95% CI −0.952 to −0.220). There are a number of methodological problems with these studies which recruited dementia patients with a range of etiologies. There was little use of standardized interventions or outcomes, there was a risk of contamination between control and intervention groups and most studies had small samples. The systematic review was withdrawn in February 2003.

No studies have examined potential side effects of reality orientation therapy and there have been some concerns that reality orientation does not take account of the needs of the individual and can be confrontational in its delivery (Dietch *et al.*, 1989). There is some evidence that reality orientation may be beneficial to cognition but more information on long-term benefit is required.

The level of evidence for each of the interventions discussed in this chapter is summarized in Table 11.1.

Table 11.1. Summary of evidence base for drug treatments of cognitive deficits in dementia

Treatment	Form of treatment	Type of dementia	Level of evidence for efficacy	Comments
Acetylcholin-esterase (AChE) inhibitors (Cholinesterase inhibitors)	Donepezil 5–10 mg	Mild to moderate Alzheimer's disease	Ia	Improvements in cognition demonstrated for first 9–12 months of treatment
	Rivastigmine 6–12 mg	Alzheimer's disease	Ia	Results as for donepezil but possibly longer period of efficacy in published studies
	Galantamine 16–24 mg	Ditto	Ia	As for rivastigmine
N-methyl-D-aspartate antagonists	Memantine	Mild to moderate Alzheimer's	Ia	Similar efficacy to AChEs
AChE inhibitors	Donezepil 5–10 mg	Vascular dementia	Ia	Effective at least till 24 weeks
	Rivastigmine 6–12 mg	Ditto	Ia	Effective at least till 24 weeks
	Galantamine 24 mg	Ditto	Ia	Probably effective until 1 year
N-methyl-D-aspartate antagonists	Memantine 20 mg	Vascular dementia	Ia	Effective until at least 9 months
AChE inhibitors	Donezepil 5–10 mg	Full range of severity of Lewy body dementia	Ib	Effective up to one year
	Rivastigmine 6–12 mg		Ib	Effective up to 6 months
	Galantamine 24 mg		III	May specifically improve behaviour
Vitamin E	alpha-tocopherol (2000 IU daily)	Alzheimer's disease	Ib	Little change in cognition but delay in death, severity of dementia and daily living
Estrogen	Drugs and dose?	Alzheimer's disease	Ib	No evidence of value
Gingko biloba	Leaf extract	Alzheimer's disease	Ib	No clear evidence of efficacy in large trials
Mono-amine oxidase B inhibitor	Selegiline 10 mg	Alzheimer's disease	Ib	Small but significant improvement at 4 months – needs confirmation

REFERENCES

Aarsland, D., Bronnick, K. & Karlsen, K. (1999). Donepezil for dementia with Lewy Bodies: a case study. *International Journal of Geriatric Psychiatry*, **14**, 69–74.

AD2000 Collaborative Group (2004). Long-term donepezil treatment in 565 patients with Alzheimer's disease (AD2000): randomized double-blind trial. *Lancet*, **363**, 2105–15.

Aisen, P. S., Schafer, K. A., Grundman, M. *et al.* (2003). Effects of rofecoxib or naproxen vs placebo on Alzheimer disease progression: a randomized controlled trial. *Journal of the American Medical Association*, **289**, 2819–26.

American Psychiatric Association (1994). *Diagnostic and Statistical Manual of Mental Disorders*, 4th edn. Washington, DC: APA.

American Psychiatric Association (1997). Practice Guideline for the treatment of patients with Alzheimer's disease and other dementias of late life. *American Journal of Psychiatry*, **154** (Suppl.), 1–39.

Anand, R., Messina, J. & Hartman, R. (2000). Dose-response effect of rivastigmine in the treatment of Alzheimer's disease. *International Journal of Geriatric Psychopharmacology*, **2**, 68–72.

Aupperle, P. M., Koumaras, B., Ohen, M., Rabinowicz, A. & Mirski, D. (2004). Long-term effects of rivastigmine treatment on neuropsychiatric and behavioral disturbances in nursing home residents with moderate to severe Alzheimer's disease: results of a 52-week open-label study. *Current Medical Research and Opinions*, **20**, 1605–12.

Ballard, C., O'Brien, J., Barber, B. *et al.* (2000). Neurocardiovascular instability, hypotensive episodes, and MRI lesions in neurodegenerative dementia. *Annals of New York Academy of Sciences*, **903**, 442–5.

Barber, R., Scheltens, P., Gholkar, A. *et al.* (1999). White matter lesions on magnetic resonance imaging in dementia with Lewy bodies, Alzheimer's disease, vascular dementia, and normal ageing. *Journal of Neurology, Neurosurgery and Psychiatry*, **67**, 66–72.

Barber, R., Gholkar, A., Scheltens, P., Ballard, C., McKeith, I. G. & O'Brien, J. T. (2000). MRI volumetric correlates of white matter lesions in dementia with Lewy bodies and Alzheimer's disease. *International Journal of Geriatric Psychiatry*, **15**, 911–16.

Baskys, A. & Blaabjerg, M. (2005). Understanding regulation of nerve cell death by mGluRs as a method for development of successful neuroprotective strategies. *Journal of the Neurological Sciences*, **229–30**, 201–9.

Benavente, O., Hart, R., Koudstaal, P., Laupacis, A. & McBride, R. (2000). Oral anticoagulants for preventing stroke in patients with non-valvular atrial fibrillation and no previous history of stroke or transient ischemic attacks. *Cochrane Database of Systematic Reviews*, **2**, CD001927. Oxford: Update Software Ltd.

Bentham, P., Gray, R., Sellwood, E. & Raftery J. (1999). Effectiveness of rivastigmine in Alzheimer's disease. *British Medical Journal*, **319**, 640–1.

Beversdorf, D. Q., Warner, J. L., Davis, R. A., Sharma, U. K., Nagaraja, H. N. & Scharre, D. W. (2004). Donepezil in the treatment of dementia with Lewy Bodies. *American Journal of Geriatric Psychiatry*, **12**, 542–4.

Bilikiewicz, A., Opala, G., Podemski, R. *et al.* (2002). An open-label study to evaluate the safety, tolerability and efficacy of rivastigmine in patients with mild to moderate probable Alzheimer's disease in the community setting. *Medical Science Monitor*, **8**, PI9–15.

Birks, J. & Flicker, L. (2003). Selegiline for Alzheimer's disease. *Cochrane Database of Systematic Reviews*, **1**, CD000442.

Birks, J. & Harvey, R. J. (2006). Donepezil for dementia due to Alzheimer's disease. *Cochrane Database of Systematic Reviews*, **1**, CD001190.

Birks, J., Grimley Evans, J., Iakovidou, V. & Tsolaki, M. (2000). Rivastigmine for Alzheimer's disease. *Cochrane Database of Systematic Reviews*, **4**, CD001191.

Birks, J., Grimley, E. V. & Van Dongen, M. (2002). Ginkgo biloba for cognitive impairment and dementia. *Cochrane Database of Systematic Review*, **4**, CD003120.

Black, S., Román, G. C., Geldmacher, D. S. *et al.* (2003). Efficacy and tolerability of donepezil in vascular dementia. Positive results of a 24-week, multicenter, international randomized, placebo-controlled clinical trial. *Stroke*, **34**, 2323–32.

Blau, T. H. (1977). Quality of life, social indicators and criteria of change. *Professional Psychology: Research and Practice*, **8**, 464–73.

Boada-Rovira, M., Brodaty, H., Cras, P. *et al.* (2004). Efficacy and safety of donepezil in patients with Alzheimer's disease: results of a global, multinational, clinical experience study. *Drugs and Aging*, **21**, 43–53.

Bråne, G., Gottfries, C. G. & Winblad, B. (2001). The Gottfries-Brane-Steen scale: validity, reliability and application in anti-dementia drug trials. *Dementia and Geriatric Cognitive Disorders*, **12**, 1–14.

Bucks, R. S., Ashworth, D. L., Wilcock, G. K. & Siegfried, K. (1996). Assessment of activities of daily living in dementia: development of the Bristol activities of daily living scale. *Age and Ageing*, **25**, 113–20.

Bullock, R., Erkinjuntti, T., Lilienfeld, S. & GAL-INT-6 Study Group (2004). Management of patients with Alzheimer's disease plus cerebrovascular disease: 12-month treatment with galantamine. *Dementia and Geriatric Cognitive Disorders*, **17**, 29–34.

Buysse, D. J., Reynolds, C. F. 3rd, Monk, T. H., Berman, S. R. & Kupfer, D. J. (1989). The Pittsburgh Sleep Quality Index: a new instrument for psychiatric practice and research. *Psychiatry Research*, **28**(2), 193–213.

Canadian Study of Health and Aging Working Group (1994). Canadian Study of health and aging: study methods and prevalence of dementia. *Canadian Medical Association Journal*, **150**, 899–913.

Caro, J., Getsios, D., Migliaccio-Walle, K., Ishak, J., El-Hadi, W. & the AHEAD Study Group. (2003). Rational choice of cholinesterase inhibitor for the treatment of Alzheimer's disease in Canada: a comparative economic analysis. *BioMed Central Geriatrics*, **3**, 6.

Clare, L., Woods, R. T., Moniz Cook, E. D., Orrell, M. & Spector, A. (2003). Cognitive rehabilitation and cognitive training for early-stage Alzheimer's disease and vascular dementia. *Cochrane Database of Systematic Reviews*, **4**, CD003260.

Corey-Bloom, J., Anand, R. & Veach, J. for the ENA 713 B352 Study Group (1998). A randomized trial evaluating the efficacy and safety of ENA 713 (rivastigmine tartrate), a new acetylcholinesterase inhibitor, in patients with mild to moderately severe Alzheimer's disease. *International Journal of Geriatric Psychopharmacology*, **1**, 55–65.

Coulson, B. S., Fenner, S. G. & Almeida, O. P. (2002). Successful treatment of behavioural problems in dementia using a cholinesterase inhibitor: the ethical questions. *Australian and New Zealand Journal of Psychiatry*, **36**, 259–262.

Craig, M. C., Maki, P. M. & Murphy, D. G. (2005). The Women's Health Initiative Memory Study: findings and implications for treatment. *Lancet Neurology*, **4**, 190–4.

Crystal, H. A., Dickson, D. W., Lizardi, J. E., Davies, P. & Wolfson, L. I. (1990). Antemortem diagnosis of diffuse Lewy body disease. *Neurology*, **40**, 1523–8.

Cummings, J. L., Anand, R., Koumaras, B. *et al.* (2000). Rivastigmine provides behavioural benefits to Alzheimer's disease patients residing in a nursing home: findings from a 26-week trial. *Neurology*, **54**, A468. [Abstract S79.002]

Cupp, M. J. (1999). Herbal remedies: adverse effects and drug interactions. *American Family Physician*, **59**, 1239–45.

Day, M. (2006). NICE says anti-dementia drugs should be used only for moderate Alzheimer's disease. *British Medical Journal*, **333**, 774.

DeJong, R., Osterlund, O. W. & Roy, G. W. (1989). Measurement of quality-of-life changes in patients with Alzheimer's disease. *Clinical Therapeutics*, **11**, 545–54.

Dennis, M. & Boyle, A. (1998). Management of cognitive impairment of vascular origin. *Psychiatric Bulletin: The Journal of Trends in Psychiatric Practice*, **22**, 287.

DeRenzi, E. & Vignolo, L. (1962). The token test: a sensitive test to detect receptive disturbances in aphasics. *Brain*, **85**, 665–78.

Dietch, J. T., Hewett, L. J. & Jones, S. (1989). Adverse effects of reality orientation. *Journal of the American Geriatric Society*, **37**, 974–6.

Doody, R. S., Geldmacher, D. S., Gordon, B., Perdomo, C. A., Pratt, R. D. & the Donepezil Study Group (2001). Open-label, multicenter, phase 3 extension study of the safety and efficacy of donepezil in patients with Alzheimer disease. *Archives of Neurology*, **58**, 427–33.

Eagger, S., Levy, R. & Sahakian, B. (1991). Tacrine in Alzheimer's disease. *The Lancet*, **337**, 989–92.

Edwards, K. R., Hershey, L., Wray, L. *et al.* (2004). Efficacy and safety of galantamine in patients with dementia with Lewy bodies: a 12-week interim analysis. *Dementia and Geriatric Cognitive Disorders*, **17**(Suppl. 1), 40–8.

Eisdorfer, C., Cohen, D., Paveza, G. J. *et al.* (1992). An empirical evaluation of the Global Deterioration Scale for staging Alzheimer's disease. *American Journal of Psychiatry*, **149**, 190–4.

Erkinjuntti, T., Kurz, A., Gauthier, S., Bullock, R., Lilienfeld, S. & Damaraju, C. V. (2002). Efficacy of galantamine in probable vascular dementia and Alzheimer's disease combined with cerebrovascular disease: a randomised trial. *Lancet*, **359**, 1283–90.

Erkinjuntti, T., Kurz, A., Small, G. *et al.* (2003). An open-label extension trial of galantamine in patients with vascular dementia and mixed dementia. *Clinical Therapeutics*, **25**, 1765–82.

Espeland, M. A., Rapp, S. R., Shumaker, S. A. *et al.* (2004). Conjugated equine estrogens and global cognitive function in postmenopausal women: Women's Health Initiative Memory Study. *Journal of the American Medical Association*, **291**, 2959–68.

Fahn, S. & Elton, R. L. (1987). The UPDRS Development Committee. Unified Parkinson's Disease Rating Scale. In *Recent Developments in Parkinson's Disease*, ed. S. Fahn, C. D. Marsden & M. Goldstein, pp. 153–63, 293–304. New York: Macmillan.

Farlow, M., Anand, R., Messina, J., Hartman, R. & Veach, J. (2000). A 52-week study of the efficacy of rivastigmine in patients with mild to moderately severe Alzheimer's disease. *European Neurology*, **44**, 236–41.

Farlow, M., Lilly, M. L. & the ENA 713 B352 Study Group (2005). Rivastigmine: an open-label, observational study of safety and effectiveness in treating patients with Alzheimer's disease for up to 5 years. *BioMed Central Geriatrics*, **5**, 1–7.

Feldman, H., Gauthier, S., Hecker, J. *et al.* (2001). A 24-week, randomized, double-blind study of donepezil in moderate to severe Alzheimer's disease. *Neurology*, **57**, 613–20.

Fergusson, E. & Howard, R. (2000). Donepezil for the treatment of psychosis in dementia with Lewy bodies. *International Journal of Geriatric Psychiatry*, **15**, 280–1.

Folstein, M. F., Folstein, S. E. & McHugh, P. R. (1975). "Mini-Mental State" – a practical method for grading the cognitive state of patients for the clinician. *Psychiatry Research*, **12**, 189–98.

Forette, F., Anand, R. & Gharabawi, G. (1999). A phase II study in patients with Alzheimer's disease to assess the preliminary efficacy and maximum tolerated dose of rivastigmine (Exelon). *European Journal of Neurology*, **6**, 423–9.

Fröelich, L., Gertz, H.-J., Heun, R. *et al.* (2004). Donepezil for Alzheimer's disease in clinical practice – the DONALD study. *Dementia and Geriatric Cognitive Disorders*, **18**, 37–43.

Frölich, L., Klinger, T. & Berger, F. M. (2002). Treatment with donepezil in Alzheimer patients with and without cerebrovascular disease. *Journal of the Neurological Sciences*, **203–4**, 137–9.

Galasko, D., Bennett, D., Sano, M. *et al.* (1997). An inventory to assess activities of daily living for clinical trials in Alzheimer's disease. The Alzheimer's Disease Cooperative Study. *Alzheimer Disease and Associated Disorders*, **11**(Suppl. 2), S33–9.

Geizer, M. & Ancill, R. J. (1998). Combination of risperidone and donepezil in Lewy Body dementia. *Canadian Journal of Psychiatry*, **43**, 421–2.

Gélinas, I., Gauthier, L., McIntyre, M. & Gauthier, S. (1999). Development of a functional measure for persons with Alzheimer's disease: the Disability Assessment for Dementia. *American Journal of Occupational Therapy*, **53**, 471–81.

Giacobini, E., Zhu, X. D., Williams, E. & Sherman, K. A. (1996). The effect of the selective reversible acetylcholinesterase inhibitor E2020 on extracellular acetylcholine and biogenic amine levels in rat cortex. *Neuropharmacology*, **35**, 205–11.

Gottfries, C. G., Blennow, K., Karlsson, I. & Wallin, A. (1994). The neurochemistry of vascular dementia. *Dementia*, **5**, 163–7.

Gottfries, C. G., Bråne, G., Gullberg, B. & Steen, G. (1982). A new scale for dementia syndromes. *Archives of Gerontology and Geriatrics*, **1**, 311–30.

Grace, J., Daniel, S., Stevens, T. *et al.* (2001). Long-term use of rivastigmine in patients with dementia with Lewy Bodies: an open-label trial. *International Psychogeriatrics*, **13**, 199–205.

Grace, J. B., Walker, M. P. & McKeith, I. G. (2000). A comparison of sleep profiles in patients with dementia with Lewy Bodies and Alzheimer's disease. *International Journal of Geriatric Psychiatry*, **15**, 1028–33.

Graham, A. J., Martin-Ruiz, C. M., Teaktong, T., Ray, M. A. & Court, J. A. (2002). Human brain nicotinic receptors, their distribution and participation in neuropsychiatric disorders. *Current Drug Targets – CNS & Neurological Disorders*, **1**(4), 387–97.

Grandmaison, E. & Simard, M. (2003). Critical review of memory stimulation programs in Alzheimer's disease. *Journal of Neuropsychiatry and Clinical Neurosciences*, **15**, 130–44.

Grossberg, G., Irwin, P., Satlin, A., Mesenbrink, P. & Spiegel, R. (2004). Rivastigmine in Alzheimer's disease. Efficacy over two years. *American Journal of Geriatric Psychiatry*, **12**, 420–31.

Heun, R., Papassotiropoulos, A. & Jennssen, F. (1998). The validity of psychometric instruments for detection of dementia in the elderly general population. *International Journal of Geriatric Psychiatry*, **13**, 368–80.

Hogervorst, E., Williams, J., Budge, M., Riedel, W. & Jolles, J. (2000). The nature of the effect of female gonadal hormone replacement therapy on cognitive function in post-menopausal women: a meta-analysis. *Neuroscience*, **101**, 485–512.

Hogervorst, E., Yaffe, K., Richards, M. & Huppert, F. (2002). Hormone replacement therapy to maintain cognitive function in women with dementia. *Cochrane Database of Systemetic Reviews*, **3**, CD003799.

Holm, A. C. (2004). Alleviation of multiple abnormalities by galantamine treatment in two patients with dementia with Lewy bodies. *American Journal of Alzheimer's Disease and Other Dementias*, **19**, 215–18.

Homma, A., Takeda, M., Imai, Y. *et al.* (2000). Clinical efficacy and safety of donepezil on cognitive and global function in patients with Alzheimer's disease. A 24-week, multicenter, double-blind, placebo-controlled study in Japan. E2020 Study Group. *Dementia and Geriatric Cognitive Disorders*, **11**, 299–313.

Hughes, C. P., Berg, L., Danziger, W. L., Cohen, L. A. & Martin, R. L. (1982). A new clinical scale for the staging of dementia. *British Journal of Psychiatry*, **140**, 566–72.

Jann, M. W. (2000). Rivastigmine, a new-generation cholinesterase inhibitor for the treatment of Alzheimer's disease. *Pharmacotherapy*, **20**, 1–13.

Jellinger, K. A. (2002). Vascular-ischemic dementia: an update. *Journal of Neuronal Transmission*, **62** (Suppl.), 1–23.

Jia, J. P., Jia, J. M., Zhou, W. D. *et al.* (2004). Differential acetylcholine and choline concentrations in the cerebrospinal fluid of patients with Alzheimer's disease and vascular dementia. *Chinese Medical Journal (England)*, **117**, 1161–4.

Janssen Research Foundation (1999a). Data on file, Study Report No. GAL-INT-3. Titusville, NJ.

Janssen Research Foundation (1999b). Data on file, Study Report No. GAL-INT-7. Titusville, NJ.

Johns, M. W. (1993). Sleepiness, snoring, and obstructive sleep apnea. The Epworth Sleepiness Scale. *Chest*, **103**, 30–6.

Kanowski, S., Herrmann, W. M., Stephan, K., Wierich, W. & Horr, R. (1996). Proof of efficacy of the ginkgo biloba special extract EGb 761 in outpatients suffering from mild to moderate primary degenerative dementia of the Alzheimer type or multi-infarct dementia. *Pharmacopsychiatry*, **29**, 47–56.

Kaplan, E., Goodglass, H. & Weintraub, S. (1978). *Boston Naming Test*. Philadelphia, PA: Lea and Febiger.

Kaufer, D. (2004). A case study in the treatment of dementia with Lewy bodies. *Acta Psychiatrica Scandinavica*, **110**: 73–6.

Kaufer, D. I., Catt, K. E., Lopez, O. L. & DeKosky, S. T. (1998). Dementia with Lewy bodies; Response of delirium-like features to donepezil. *Neurology*, **51**, 1512.

Khotianov, N., Singh, R. & Singh, S. (2002). Lewy Body dementia: case report and discussion. *Journal of the American Board of Family Practice*, **15**, 50–4.

Kmietowicz, Z. (2005). NICE proposes to withdraw Alzheimer's drugs from NHS. *British Medical Journal*, **330**, 495.

Knopman, D. S., Knapp, M. J., Gracon, S. I. & Davis, C. S.. (1994). The Clinician Interview Based Impression (CIBI): a clinician's global change rating scale in Alzheimer's disease. *Neurology*, **44**, 2315–21.

Krall, W. J., Sramek, J. J. & Cutler, N. R. (1999). Cholinesterase inhibitors: a therapeutic strategy for Alzheimer disease. *Annals of Pharmacotherapy*, **33**, 441–50.

Kumar, V., Anand, R., Messina, J., Hartman, R. & Veach, J. (2000). An efficacy and safety analysis of Exelon in Alzheimer's disease patients with concurrent vascular risk factors. *European Journal of Neurology*, **7**, 159–69.

Kurz, A., Erkinjuntti, T., Small, G., Lilienfeld, S. & Damaraju, C. V. (2003). Long-term safety and cognitive effects of galantamine in the treatment of probable vascular dementia or Alzheimer's disease with cerebrovascular disease. *European Journal of Neurology*, **10**, 633–40.

Lai, C. K., Chi, I. & Kayser-Jones, J. (2004). A randomized controlled trial of a specific reminiscence approach to promote the well-being of nursing home residents with dementia, *International Psychogeriatrics*, **16**, 33–49.

Lanctôt, K. L. & Herrmann, N. (2000). Donepezil for behavioural disorders associated with Lewy Bodies: a case series. *International Journal of Geriatric Psychiatry*, **15**, 338–45.

Langlais, P. J., Thal, L. J., Hansen, L., Galasko, D., Alford, M. & Masliah, E. (1993). Neurotransmitters in basal ganglia and cortex of Alzheimer's disease with and without Lewy bodies. *Neurology*, **43**, 1927–34.

Lawton, M. P. & Brody, E. M. (1969). Assessment of older people: self-maintaining and instrumental activities of daily living. *Gerontologist*, **9**, 179–86.

Le Bars, P. L., Katz, M. M., Berman, N., Itil, T. M., Freedman, A. M. & Schatzberg, A. F. (1997). A placebo-controlled, double-blind, randomized trial of an extract of ginkgo biloba for dementia. North American EGb Study Group. *Journal of the American Medical Association* **278**, 1327–32.

Levesque, L. E., Brophy, J. M. & Zhang, B. (2005). The risk for myocardial infarction with cyclooxygenase-2 inhibitors: a population study of elderly adults. *Annals of Internal Medicine*, **142**, 481–9.

Levy, R., Eagger, S., Griffiths, M. *et al.* (1994). Lewy bodies and response to tacrine in Alzheimer's disease. *Lancet*, **343**, 176.

Loy, C. & Schneider, L. (2006). Galantamine for Alzheimer's disease and mild cognitive impairment. *Cochrane Database of Systematic Reviews*, **1**. Oxford: Update Software Ltd.

Lyketsos, C. G., Reichman, W. E., Kershaw, P. & Zhu, Y. (2004). Long-term outcomes of galantamine in patients with Alzheimer's disease. *American Journal of Geriatric Psychiatry*, **12**, 473–82.

Maclean, L. E., Collins, C. C. & Byrne, E. J. (2001). Dementia with Lewy Bodies treated with rivastigmine: effects on cognition, neuropsychiatric symptoms, and sleep. *International Psychogeriatrics*, **13**, 277–88.

Malouf, R. & Birks, J. (2004). Donepezil for vascular cognitive impairment. *Cochrane Database of Systematic Reviews*, **1**, CD004395. Oxford: Update Software Ltd.

Matthews, H. P., Korbey, J., Wilkinson, D. G. & Rowden, J. (2000). Donepezil in Alzheimer's disease: eighteen month results from Southampton Memory Clinic. *International Journal of Geriatric Psychiatry*, **15**, 713–20.

McGeer, P. L., Schulzer, M., & McGeer, E. G. (1996). Arthritis and anti-inflammatory agents as possible protective factors for Alzheimer's disease: a review of 17 epidemiologic studies. *Neurology*, **47**, 425–32.

McKeith, I. G. (2000). Clinical Lewy body syndromes. *Annals of New York Academy of Sciences*, **920**, 1–8.

McKeith, I. G., Perry, R. H., Fairbairn, A. F., Jabeen, S. & Perry, E. K. (1992). Operational criteria for senile dementia of Lewy body type (SDLT). *Psychological Medicine*, **22**, 911–22.

McKeith, I. G., Galasko, D., Kosaka, K. *et al.* (1996). Consensus guidelines for the clinical and pathologic diagnosis of dementia with Lewy bodies (DLB): report of the consortium on DLB international workshop. *Neurology*, **47**, 1113–24.

McKeith, I., Del Ser, T., Spano, P. *et al.* (2000a). Efficacy of rivastigmine in dementia with Lewy bodies: a randomised, double-blind, placebo-controlled international study. *Lancet*, **356**, 2031–6.

McKeith, I. G., Grace, J. B., Walker, Z. *et al.* (2000b). Rivastigmine in the treatment of dementia with Lewy bodies: Preliminary findings from an open trial. *International Journal of Geriatric Psychiatry*, **15**, 387–92.

McKeith, I. G., Wesnes, K. A., Perry, E. & Ferrara, R. (2004). Hallucinations predict attentional improvements with rivastigmine in dementia with Lewy Bodies. *Dementia and Geriatric Cognitive Disorders*, **18**, 94–100.

McKhann, G., Drachman, D., Folstein, M., Katzman, R., Price, D. & Stadlan, E. M. (1984). Clinical diagnosis of Alzheimer's disease: report of the NINCDS-ADRDA Work Group under the auspices of Department of Health and Human Services Task Force on Alzheimer's Disease. *Neurology*, **34**, 939–44.

McShane, R., Areosa Sastre, A. & Minakaran, N. (2006). Memantine for dementia. *Cochrane Database of Systematic Reviews*, **2**, CD003154. Oxford: Update Software Ltd.

Miller, E. R., III, Pastor-Barriuso, R., Dalal, D., Riemersma, R. A., Appel, L. J. & Guallar, E. (2005). Meta-analysis: high-dosage vitamin E supplementation may increase all-cause mortality. *Annals of Internal Medicine*, **142**, 37–46.

Minett, T. S. C., Thomas, A., Wilkinson, L. M. *et al.* (2003). What happens when donepezil is suddenly withdrawn? An open label trial in dementia with Lewy bodies and Parkinson's disease with dementia. *International Journal of Geriatric Psychiatry*, **18**, 988–93.

Mohs, R. C., Doody, R. S., Morris, J. C. *et al.* (2001). A 1-year, placebo-controlled preservation of function survival study of donepezil in AD patients. *Neurology*, **57**, 481–8.

Mohs, R. C., Knopman, D., Petersen, R. C. *et al.* (1997). Development of cognitive instruments for use in clinical trials of antidementia drugs: additions to the Alzheimer's Disease Assessment Scale that broaden its scope. The Alzheimer's Disease Cooperative Study. *Alzheimer Disease and Associated Disorders*, **11** (Suppl. 2), S13–21.

Nelson, A., Fogel, B. S. & Faust, D. (1986). Bedside cognitive screening instruments, a critical assessment. *Journal of Nervous Mental Disease*, **174**, 73–83.

Nicholl, C. G., Lynch, S., Kelly, C. A. *et al.* (1995). The Cognitive Drug Research computerized assessment system in the evaluation of early dementia – is speed of the essence? *International Journal of Geriatric Psychiatry*, **10**, 199–206.

Nordberg, A. & Svensson, A.-L. (1998). Cholinesterase inhibitors in the treatment of Alzheimer's disease: a Comparison of tolerability and pharmacology. *Drug Experience*, **19**, 465–80.

Orgogozo, J. M., Rigaud, A. S., Stoffler, A., Mobius, H. J. & Forette, F. (2002). Efficacy and safety of memantine in patients with mild to moderate vascular dementia: a randomized, placebo-controlled trial (MMM 300). *Stroke*, **33**, 1834–9.

Partridge, J. G., Apparsundaram, S., Gerhardt, G. A., Ronesi, J. & Lovinger, D. M. (2002). Nicotinic acetylcholine receptors interact with dopamine in induction of striatal long-term depression. *Journal of Neurosciences*, **22**, 2541–9.

Perry, E., Walker, M., Grace, J. & Perry, R. (1999). Acetylcholine in mind: a neurotransmitter correlate of consciousness? *Trends in Neurosciences*, **22**, 273–80.

Perry, E. K., Kerwin, J., Perry, R. H, Blessed, G. & Fairbairn, A. F. (1990b). Visual hallucinations and the cholinergic system in dementia (letter). *Journal of Neurology, Neurosurgery, and Psychiatry*, **53**, 88.

Perry, E. K., Marshall, E., Perry, R. H. *et al.* (1990a). Cholinergic and dopaminergic activities in senile dementia of Lewy body type. *Alzheimer's Disease and Associated Disorders*, **4**, 87–95.

Perry, E. K., Irving, D., Kerwin, J. M. et al. (1993). Cholinergic transmitter and neuotrophic activities in Lewy body dementia: similarity to Parkinson's and distinction from Alzheimer's disease. *Alzheimer's Disease and Associated Disorders*, **7**, 69–79.

Pimlott, S. L., Piggott, M., Owens, J. et al. (2004). Nicotinic acetylcholine receptor distribution in Alzheimer's disease, dementia with Lewy Bodies, Parkinson's disease, and vascular dementia: in vitro study using 5-[^{125}I]-A-85380. *Neuropsychopharmacology*, **29**, 108–16.

Pirtillä, T., Wilcock, G., Truyen, L. & Damaraju, C. V. (2004). Long-term efficacy and safety of galantamine in patients with mild-to-moderate Alzheimer's disease: multicenter trial. *European Journal of Neurology*, **11**, 734–41.

Rabins, P. V. (2006). *Guideline Watch: Practice Guideline for the Treatment of Patients With Alzheimer's Disease and Other Dementias of Late Life*. Washington, DC: American Psychiatric Association.

Rahkonen, T., Eloniemi-Sulkava, U., Rissanen, S., Vatanen, A., Viramo, P. & Sulkava, R. (2003). Dementia with Lewy bodies according to the consensus criteria in a general population aged 75 or older. *Journal of Neurology and Neurosurgery Psychiatry*, **74**, 720–4.

Raskind, M. A., Peskind, E. R., Truyen, L., Kershaw, P. & Damaraju, C. V. (2004). The cognitive benefits of galantamine are sustained for at least 36 months. *Archives of Neurology*, **61**, 252–6.

Raskind, M. A., Peskind, E. R., Wessel, T., Yuan, W. & The Galantamine USA-1 Study Group (2000). Galantamine in AD: a 6-month randomized, placebo-controlled trial with a 6-month extension. The Galantamine USA-1 Study Group. *Neurology*, **54**, 2261–8.

Reisberg, B., Ferris, S. H., De Leon, M. J. & Crook, T. (1982). The Global Deterioration Scale for assessment of primary degenerative dementia. *American Journal of Psychiatry*, **139**, 1136–9.

Reisberg, B., Doody, R., Stöffler, A., Schmitt, F., Ferris, S. & Möbius, H. J. for the Memantine Study Group (2003). Memantine in moderate-to severe Alzheimer's disease. *New England Journal of Medicine*, **348**, 1333–41.

Relkin, N. R., Reichman, W. E., Orazem, J. & McRae, T. (2003). A large, community-based, open-label trial of donepezil in the treatment of Alzheimer's disease. *Dementia and Geriatric Cognitive Disorders*, **16**, 15–24.

Ritchie, C. W., Ames, D., Clayton, T. & Lai, R. (2004). Metaanalysis of randomized trials of the efficacy and safety of donepezil, galantamine, and rivastigmine for the treatment of Alzheimer disease. *American Journal of Geriatric Psychiatry*, **12**, 358–69.

Rockwood, K., Mintzer, J., Truyen, L., Wessel, T. & Wilkinson, D. (2001). Effects of a flexible galantamine dose in Alzheimer's disease: a randomized, controlled trial. *Journal of Neurology, Neurosurgery, and Psychiatry*, **71**, 589–95.

Rogers, S. L. & Friedhoff, L. T. (1998). Long-term efficacy and safety of donepezil in the treatment of Alzheimer's disease: an interim analysis of the results of a US multicentre open label extension study. *European Neuropsychopharmacology*, **8**, 67–75.

Rogers, J., Kirby, L. C., Hempelman, S. R. et al. (1993). Clinical trial of indomethacin in Alzheimer's disease. *Neurology*, **43**, 1609–11.

Rogers, S. L. & Friedhoff, L. T. (1996). The efficacy and safety of donepezil in patients with Alzheimer's disease: results of a US multicentre, randomized, double-blind, placebo-controlled trial. The Donepezil Study Group. *Dementia*, **7**, 293–303.

Rogers, S. L., Doody, R. S., Mohs, R. C., Friedhoff, L. T. & the Donepezil Study Group (1998a). Donepezil improves cognition and global function in Alzheimer disease. A 15-week, double-blind, placebo-controlled study. *Archives of Internal Medicine*, **158**, 1021–31.

Rogers, S. L., Farlow, M. R., Doody, R. S., Mohs, R., Friedhoff, L. T. & the Donepezil Study Group (1998b). A 24-week, double-blind, placebo-controlled trial of donepezil in patients with Alzheimer. *Neurology*, **50**, 136–45.

Rogers, S. L., Doody, R. S., Pratt, R. D. & Ieni, J. R. (2000). Long-term efficacy and safety of donepezil in the treatment of Alzheimer's disease: final analysis of a US multicentre open-label study. *European Neuropsychopharmacology*, **10**, 195–203.

Rojas-Fernandez, C. H. (2001). Successful use of donepezil for the treatment of dementia with Lewy Bodies. *Annals of Pharmacotherapy*, **35**, 202–5.

Román, G. C., Tatemichi, T. K., Erkinjuntti, T. et al. (1993). Vascular dementia: Diagnostic criteria for research studies. Report of the NINCDS-AIREN International Workshop. *Neurology*, **43**, 250–60.

Rosen, W. G., Mohs, R. C. & Davis, K. L. (1984). A new rating scale for Alzheimer's disease. *American Journal of Psychiatry*, **141**, 1356–64.

Rosen, W. G., Terry, R. D., Fuld, P. A., Katzman, R. & Peck, A. (1980). Pathological verification of ischemic score in differentiation of dementias. *Annals of Neurology*, **7**, 486–8.

Rösler, M., Anand, R., Cicin-Sain, A. et al. (1999). Efficacy and safety of rivastigmine in patients with Alzheimer's disease: international randomised controlled trial. *British Medical Journal*, **318**, 633–8.

Rossouw, J. E., Anderson, G. L., Prentice, R. L. et al. (2002). Risks and benefits of estrogen plus progestin in healthy postmenopausal women: principal results from the Women's Health Initiative randomized controlled trial. *Journal of the American Medical Association*, **288**, 321–33.

Rüther, E., Glaser, A., Bleich, S., Degner, D. & Wiltfang, J. (2000). A prospective PMS study to validate the sensitivity for change of the D-Scale in advanced stages of dementia using the NMDA-antagonist memantine. *Pharmacopsychiatry*, **33**, 103–8.

Samuel, W., Caligiuri, M., Galasko, D. et al. (2000). Better cognitive and psychopathologic response to donepezil in patients prospectively diagnosed as dementia with Lewy Bodies: a preliminary study. *International Journal of Geriatric Psychiatry*, **15**, 794–802.

Sano, M., Ernesto, C., Thomas, R. G. et al. (1997). A controlled trial of selegiline, alpha-tocopherol, or both as treatment for Alzheimer's disease. The Alzheimer's Disease Cooperative Study. *New England Journal of Medicine*, **336**, 1216–22.

Saxton, J., McGonigle-Gibson, K., Swihart, A., Miller, M. & Boller, F. (1990). Assessment of the severely impaired patient: description and validation of a new neuropsychological test battery.

Psychological Assessment: Journal of Consulting and Clinical Psychology, **2**, 298–303.

Scharf, S., Mander, A., Ugoni, A., Vajda, F. & Christophidis, N. (1999). A double-blind, placebo-controlled trial of diclofenac/misoprostol in Alzheimer's disease. *Neurology*, **53**, 197–201.

Schneider, L. S., Olin, J. T., Doody, R. S. *et al.* (1997). Validity and reliability of the Alzheimer's Disease Cooperative Study – clinical global impression of change. *Alzheimer's Disease and Associated Disorders*, **11** (Suppl. 2), S22–32.

Shea, C., MacKnight, C. & Rockwood, K. (1998). Donepezil for treatment of Dementia with Lewy Bodies: a case series of nine patients. *International Psychogeriatrics*, **10**, 229–38.

Shumaker, S. A., Legault, C., Kuller, L. *et al.* (2004). Conjugated equine estrogens and incidence of probable dementia and mild cognitive impairment in postmenopausal women: Women's Health Initiative Memory Study. *Journal of the American Medical Association*, **291**, 2947–58.

Simard, M. (1998). The MMSE: strengths and weaknesses of a clinical instrument. *The Canadian Alzheimer Disease Review*, **2**, 10–12.

Simard, M. & van Reekum, R. (1999). Memory assessment in studies of cognition-enhancing drugs for Alzheimer's disease. *Drugs and Aging*, **14**, 197–230.

Simard, M., van Reekum, R. & Cohen, T. (2000). Review of cognitive and behavioral symptoms in dementia with Lewy Bodies. *Journal of Neuropsychiatry and Clinical Neurosciences*, **12**, 425–50.

Simpson, P. M., Surmon, D. J., Wesnes, K. A. *et al.* (1991). The cognitive drug research computerized assessment system for demented patients: a validation study. *International Journal of Geriatric Psychiatry*, **6**, 95–102.

Skjerve, A. & Nygaard, H. A. (2000). Improvement in sundowning in dementia with Lewy Bodies after treatment with donepezil. *International Journal of Geriatric Psychiatry*, **15**, 1147–51.

Solomon, P. R., Adams, F., Silver, A., Zimmer, J. & DeVeaux, R. (2002). Gingko for memory enhancement: a randomized controlled trial. *Journal of the American Medical Association*, **290**, 2015–22.

Spector, A., Orrell, M., Davies, S. & Woods, R. T. (2000). Reminiscence therapy for dementia. *Cochrane Database of Systematic Reviews*, **2**, CD001120. Oxford: Update Software.

Spiegel, R., Brunner, C., Ermini-Funfschilling, D. *et al.* (1991). A new behavioral assessment scale for geriatric out- and in-patients: the NOSGER (Nurses' Observation Scale for Geriatric Patients). *Journal of the American Geriatric Society*, **39**, 339–47.

Stern, R. G., Mohs, R. C., Davidson, M. *et al.* (1994). A longitudinal study of Alzheimer's disease: measurement, rate, and predictors of cognitive deterioration. *American Journal of Psychiatry*, **151**, 390–6.

Stewart, W. F., Kawas, C., Corrada, M. & Metter, E. J. (1997). Risk of Alzheimer's disease and duration of NSAID use. *Neurology*, **48**, 626–32.

Szekely, C. A., Thorne, J. E., Zandi, P. P. *et al.* (2004). Nonsteroidal anti-inflammatory drugs for the prevention of Alzheimer's disease: a systematic review. *Neuroepidemiology*, **23**, 159–69.

Tabet, N. & Feldman, H. (2003). Indomethacin for the treatment of Alzheimer's disease patients. *Cochrane Database of Systematic Reviews*, **2**, CD003673. Oxford: Updated Software Ltd.

Tabet, N., Birks, J. & Grimley, E. J. (2000). Vitamin E for Alzheimer's disease. *Cochrane Database of Systematic Reviews*, **4**, CD002854. Oxford: Update Software Ltd.

Tariot, P. N., Cummings, J. L., Katz, I. R. *et al.* (2001). A randomized, double-blind, placebo-controlled study of the efficacy and safety of donepezil in patients with Alzheimer's disease in the nursing home setting. *Journal of the American Geriatrics Society*, **49**, 1590–9.

Tariot, P. N., Solomon, P. R., Morris, J. C. *et al.* (2000). A 5-month, randomized, placebo-controlled trial of galantamine in AD. *Neurology*, **54**, 2269–76.

Tariot, P. N., Farlow, M. R., Grossberg, G. T. *et al.* (2004). Memantine treatment in patients with moderate to severe Alzheimer's disease already receiving donepezil. A randomized controlled trial. *Journal of the American Medical Association*, **291**, 317–24.

Teng, E. L. & Chui, H. C. (1987). The Modified Mini-Mental State (3MS) examination. *Journal of Clinical Psychiatry*, **48**, 314–18.

Tiraboschi, P., Hansen, L. A., Alford, M. *et al.* (2002). Early and widespread cholinergic losses differentiate dementia with Lewy bodies from Alzheimer's disease. *Archives of General Psychiatry*, **59**, 946–51.

Wesnes, K. A., McKeith, I. G., Ferrara, R. *et al.* (2002). Effects of rivastigmine on cognitive function in dementia with Lewy Bodies: a randomised placebo-controlled international study using the cognitive drug research computerised assessment system. *Dementia and Geriatric Cognitive Disorders*, **13**, 183–92.

Wilcock, G. K., Birks, J., Whitehead, A. & Evans, S. J. (2002). The effect of selegiline in the treatment of people with Alzheimer's disease: a meta-analysis of published trials. *International Journal of Geriatric Psychiatry*, **17**, 175–83.

Wilcock, G. K., Lilienfeld, S. & Gaens, E. on behalf of the Galantamine International-1 Study Group. (2000). Efficacy and safety of galantamine in patients with mild to moderate Alzheimer's disease: multicentre randomized controlled trial. *British Medical Journal*, **321**, 1–7.

Wilkinson, D. & Murray, J. in collaboration with the Galantamine Research Group (2001). Galantamine: a randomized, double-blind, dose comparison in patients with Alzheimer's disease. *International Journal of Geriatric Psychiatry*, **16**, 852–7.

Wilkinson, D., Doody, R., Helme, R. *et al.* (2003). Donepezil in vascular dementia. A randomized, placebo-controlled study. *Neurology*, **61**, 479–86.

Winblad, B. & Poritis, N. (1999). Memantine in severe dementia: results of the 9M-Best study (Benefit and Efficacy in Severely Demented patients during treatment with memantine). *International Journal of Geriatric Psychiatry*, **14**, 135–46.

Winblad, B., Engedal, K., Soininen, H. *et al.* (2001). A 1-year, randomized, placebo-controlled study of donepezil in patients with mild to moderate AD. *Neurology*, **57**, 489–95.

Woods, B., Spector, A., Jones, C., Orrell, M. & Davies, S. (2005). Reminiscence therapy for dementia. *Cochrane Database for Systematic Reviews*, **2**, CD001120. Oxford: Update Software.

Yanagihara, T. (2002). Vascular dementia in Japan. *Annals of New York Academy of Sciences*, **977**, 24–8.

12

Pharmacological treatment of psychosis and depression in neurological disease in older adults

Mark Rapoport, Cara Brown and Craig Ritchie

Editors' note

Conventional diagnostic descriptions are not satisfactory for many late life disorders in which multiple pathology is common. This chapter examines two frequent clinical syndromes, psychotic and depressive disorders, in those who have significant neurological disorders; mainly dementia, parkinsonism, cerebrovascular disease and traumatic brain injury. It will be noted that the evidence base and recommendations for treatment are often very different in the presence of other pathologies, and that there are many important gaps in our knowledge. The reader will also be reminded that dosage of drugs is crucial in this population and often differs from the equivalent conditions in adult psychiatry.

Introduction

Many neurological diseases have an increased incidence in old age. Alzheimer's disease (AD) is present in 8% of the Canadian population over the age of 65 (Lindsay *et al.*, 2004), and this prevalence will climb as the population ages in the decades to come, since the prevalence of AD doubles every 5 years up to the age of 85 (United States General Accounting Office, 1998). Stroke is a major leading cause of death and disability for older adults. The prevalence of Parkinson's disease (PD) and Parkinsonian symptoms increase dramatically with age (Bennett *et al.*, 1996; Van Den Eeden *et al.*, 2003). Traumatic brain injury (TBI) is generally more common in younger adults, in whom it is often associated with alcohol or substance misuse. There is a second peak in TBI incidence in later life, largely due to falls and motor vehicle accidents, but little is known about the psychiatric sequelae of TBI in later life (Rapoport & Feinstein, 2000).

Psychiatric sequelae can be early or late manifestations of these diseases. While AD is the leading cause of dementia, significant cognitive impairment is also associated with PD and stroke. Traumatic brain injury is often associated with post-concussive cognitive complaints, but it may also be a risk factor for Alzheimer's disease over time. The psychiatric sequelae of these neurological diseases can either accompany the cognitive impairment (or dementia) or occur independently.

Psychosis in neurological disease

Delusions and hallucinations likely represent the most dramatic, odd, challenging and fascinating manifestations of neurological disease, as they are substantially out of keeping from the premorbid functioning of afflicted patients. Treatment is most commonly pharmacological in nature, but it must be kept in mind that drug treatment should be reserved for the treatment of psychosis that is disruptive to patients' functioning, and/or causing distress to patients and/or caregivers, not of symptoms alone. Pharmacological treatment, usually with antipsychotics, is often useful in reducing the intensity of the psychotic symptoms, allowing improvement in functioning, but often patients with neurological disease are left with residual, albeit muted psychotic symptoms. The evidence of the effectiveness of pharmacological treatment in neurological disease in older adults is rather limited. Most of the evidence is accumulated in patients with Alzheimer's and Parkinson's disease, and therefore these diseases will be the focus of the present section, followed by comments about the literature on the pharmacological treatment of psychosis in stroke and traumatic brain injury.

Cambridge Textbook of Effective Treatments in Psychiatry, ed. Peter Tyrer and Kenneth R. Silk. Published by Cambridge University Press.
© Cambridge University Press, 2008.

Treating psychosis in dementia

Delusions and hallucinations are common sequelae of Alzheimer's disease and can occur at any stage of the illness. Particularly frequent psychotic symptoms include delusions of theft, and misidentification delusions such as the phantom boarder syndrome. In this condition the patient falsely believes there are people in their home; this occurs in approximately 23% of patients with dementia (Hwang *et al.*, 2003). Schneider *et al.* (2003) have operationalized criteria for "psychosis of Alzheimer's disease" as the exhibition of paranoid or delusional ideation and/or hallucinations over a period of at least 2–4 weeks. Effective treatment for psychosis in AD is critical, as psychosis is invariably associated with impaired functioning, caregiver distress and institutionalization (Lawlor, 2004) in this population. The prevalence of psychosis in AD has been estimated at an overall median of 34% in clinic populations and a range of 7–20% in community and clinical trial populations (Schneider & Dagerman, 2004).

A recent large-scale retrospective cohort study revealed that upon admission to a nursing home, antipsychotics are dispensed to 17% of older adults within 100 days, and to 24% within the first year (Bronskill *et al.*, 2004). Dementia was associated with a 3.5 times increased likelihood of an antipsychotic prescription. Only rarely (14%) did these patients receive geriatric or psychiatric consultation. Behavioral measures should be instituted in these patients concomitant to the medication use, and in many cases may obviate the need for pharmacotherapy (Cohen-Mansfield, 2001).

Typical antipsychotics in dementia

Until the advent of the atypical antipsychotics, there was considerable agreement on the use of typical antipsychotics for the treatment of psychosis in dementia (Alessi, 1991; Devanand & Levy, 1995; Sunderland, 1996; Tariot, 1996; Borson & Raskind, 1997). A meta-analysis suggested moderate superiority of typical antipsychotics over placebo in treatment of psychosis and other disruptive behaviors in dementia, although the effect size was only 18%, and diagnostic heterogeneity and concomitant medications make some of these studies difficult to interpret (Schneider *et al.*, 1990). A randomized placebo-controlled dose-comparison study for psychotic or disruptive outpatients with AD found that a standard dose of haloperidol (2–3 mg/day) was superior to a lower dose (0.5–0.75 mg/day) (Devanand *et al.*, 1998). However, a subgroup of patients in the standard dose group developed significant neurological side effects, yielding a

recommendation of starting at 1 mg/day, with gradual upward titration.

Tardive dyskinesia (TD) is a concerning side effect of the typical antipsychotics and older patients with neurological disease including dementia are likely at the highest risk (Caligiuri *et al.*, 2000). The cumulative incidence of TD in older patients is quite high, 2.5% after 1 year, 12.1% after 2 years, and 22.9% after 3 years (Caligiuri *et al.*, 1997) with another study estimating 26%, 52% and 60% after 1, 2 and 3 years, respectively (Jeste *et al.*, 1995).

Two studies have investigated the impact of discontinuation of antipsychotics in patients with dementia on chronic typical antipsychotics whose behavioral disturbance was well-controlled. One group randomized 34 patients with dementia in long-term care to either continue with their antipsychotics or to have them discontinued, for a 6-month study (van Reekum *et al.*, 2002). Their primary finding was that the group whose antipsychotics were continued had more behavioral disturbances than those in the discontinuation group. A similar study was conducted in 82 patients with AD in long-term care (Ballard *et al.*, 2004). They found that the baseline level of behavioral disturbances predicted outcome depending on the treatment received. In particular, those with low levels of baseline neurobehavioral disturbance had a better outcome if switched to placebo, whereas patients with a higher level of disturbance at baseline had significant problems when their antipsychotics were discontinued.

Typical antipsychotics should be reserved for patients who have previously not responded to atypicals, who responded well to typicals in the past and tolerated them, or where cost, availability, or medical issues preclude the use of atypicals. They should not otherwise be regarded as a first-line treatment (Rapoport & van Reekum, 2000). When there is particular concern over the use of risperidone and olanzapine in view of their risk of cerebrovascular accidents (see below), typical antipsychotics may be preferred.

Atypical antipsychotics

The advent of atypical antipsychotics made treatment of psychosis more feasible because of more favorable side-effect profiles. Antipsychotic prescriptions have been climbing in the elderly over the last 10 years in the community (Rapoport *et al.*, 2004) and in long-term care (Liperoti *et al.*, 2003), and this changing trend is largely attributable to the atypical antipsychotics.

Risperidone

The first multicenter, double-blind, placebo-controlled 12-week randomized clinical trial (RCT) of risperidone found that fixed doses of 1 or 2 mg/day, but not 0.5 mg/day significantly improved symptoms of psychosis and aggressive behaviour in 625 institutionalized patients with severe dementia (Katz et al., 1999). A subsequent subgroup analysis of 463 patients who fulfilled operationalized criteria for psychosis of dementia confirmed this finding (Schneider & Dagerman 2004). Falls, accidental injury and peripheral edema were common side effects, and there was a dose-dependent increase in somnolence and extrapyramidal symptoms (EPS), with treatment with 2 mg/day risperidone causing a significant increase in EPS (Katz et al., 1999).

Another double-blind, placebo-controlled 13-week RCT examining flexible doses (0.5–4 mg/day) of risperidone and haloperidol found that risperidone was associated with a reduction in aggression compared with placebo in patients with AD and other dementias, but did not find statistically significant improvement in overall behavioral disturbance (De Deyn et al., 1999). Nonetheless, risperidone was well tolerated, with EPS similar to placebo and less than with haloperidol. A recent multicenter, double-blind placebo-controlled 12-week RCT similarly examined risperidone in 337 elderly nursing home patients with severe dementia (AD, vascular and mixed dementias) and aggressive behaviors, and found a significant reduction in both aggression and psychosis (Brodaty et al., 2003). Somnolence was common with risperidone, but there was no significant overall increase in EPS observed.

A post hoc exploratory analysis of the above three RCTs also concluded that risperidone was significantly more effective than placebo in treating non-paranoid delusions and other scales of aggression, but not paranoid delusions or visual hallucinations (Rabinowitz et al., 2004). Two smaller RCTs in Asian patients (Chan et al., 2001; Suh et al., 2004) confirmed the findings of reduced psychosis associated with risperidone, and lessened EPS compared with haloperidol in dementia.

The above studies therefore suggest efficacy of risperidone in a dose of 1–2 mg for reducing psychosis in dementia. However, caution must be made in interpreting these data clinically, as psychosis was not a necessary inclusion criteria for most studies, the specific dementia diagnoses were mixed, most patients were female, and all were institutionalized. Dose-dependent increases in EPS, particularly above 1 mg/day, are a matter of concern, and doses above 1 mg/day may be associated with increased falls (Katz et al., 2004). The increase in "cerebrovascular-like events" in one of the recent studies (Brodaty et al., 2003) led to a review of four placebo-controlled trials with risperidone showing that there were twice as many reported cerebrovascular adverse events with risperidone

as compared to placebo (Health Canada, 2000). However, in the risperidone RCTs, patients with vascular dementia were included and not randomly assigned to treatment groups, and cerebrovascular-like events were ill-defined. Furthermore, a recent retrospective epidemiological study found that olanzapine and risperidone were not associated with an increased risk of stroke compared with typical antipsychotics among patients 65 and over (Herrmann et al., 2004).

Olanzapine

Two recent RCTs have shown positive effects of olanzapine in the treatment of psychosis and other behavioral disturbances in patients with AD (Street et al., 2000; De Deyn et al., 2004). The first was a multicenter, double-blind, placebo-controlled, 6-week trial in 206 elderly nursing home residents with severe AD who had either psychosis and/or other behavioral disturbances (Street et al., 2000). Low fixed-dose olanzapine (5 or 10 mg/day) was found to be safe, well tolerated and superior to placebo in treating aggression, agitation and psychosis, with the 5 mg/day dose having the greatest effect. Somnolence and gait disturbances were the principal adverse events, and a group randomized to 15 mg/day showed no improvement in symptoms and significant peripheral anticholinergic effects. An 18-week, open-label, flexible dose follow-up of this trial in 105 patients found continued significant improvement in agitation/aggression and delusions (Street et al., 2001). A post hoc analysis of the acute trial also suggested that olanzapine reduced the emergence of psychosis, especially hallucinations, in 165 patients with no or minimal psychosis at baseline (Clark et al., 2001).

The second RCT was a multicenter, double-blind, placebo-controlled, 10-week trial in 652 long-term or continuing care patients with moderate AD and delusions or hallucinations of moderate severity (impairing function or posing a threat to self) lasting at least one month (De Deyn et al., 2004). Given the large sample size, the authors were able to use various fixed doses. They found a significant improvement in delusions and hallucinations in all treatment groups compared with placebo. A 2.5 mg dose showed the greatest improvement in overall clinician-rated global improvement, whereas the 7.5 mg/day dose showed the greatest improvement in delusions and hallucinations. While there was no increase in extrapyramidal symptoms, the treatment group had a higher incidence of weight gain, anorexia and incontinence.

Whereas a large retrospective study found olanzapine to be associated with greater improvement in psychotic symptoms in dementia than risperidone or haloperidol (Edell & Tunis, 2001), two smaller randomized controlled trials comparing olanzapine and risperidone showed no differences between them in efficacy against overall behavioural symptomatology in dementia (Fontaine *et al.*, 2003; Gareri *et al.*, 2004). Olanzapine at 5 or 10 mg/day was generally well tolerated in the trials reported above. None reported treatment emergent EPS, orthostatic hypotension, cognitive or cardiovascular adverse effects. Somnolence, accidental injury and weight gain were found in some studies, but clinical anticholinergic effects were not present at lower doses. It is important to note that, unlike in the risperidone studies, the large RCTs of olanzapine focused solely on AD, and several factors limit the generalizability of the findings: these included the institutional status of all patients, the preponderance of females, and in the first RCT, the absence of psychosis as an inclusion criteria.

Quetiapine

Two small open-label studies of quetiapine in patients with AD and behavioural symptoms suggested improvement in delusions and aggression without inducing adverse effects on cognition or EPS (Scharre & Chang, 2002; Fujikawa *et al.*, 2004). One study reported drowsiness or sedation in 40% of the subjects (Scharre & Chang, 2002), but the other did not assess for non-EPS adverse effects. Another open-label study in older adults with psychotic disorders including but not limited to dementia was similarly positive (Tariot *et al.*, 2000). Nonetheless, in that study, somnolence, dizziness and postural hypotension were common, and the drop-out rate was high. Whilst the data for quetiapine are promising, there is no published RCT evidence for the use of quetiapine for psychosis in dementia. Thus, information is needed on the relative benefit of quetiapine over placebo, and compared with the other atypical antipsychotics, as well as the most appropriate dose regimes.

Cholinesterase inhibitors

Acetylcholinesterase inhibitors have been established as a treatment to delay progression of cognitive impairment in AD, but preliminary evidence suggests that they may also be effective for the many non-cognitive phenomena associated with the disease (Wynn & Cummings, 2004). Some evidence of reduction in psychosis in AD is provided by open-label studies of rivastigmine (Rosler *et al.*, 1998), tacrine (Kaufer *et al.*, 1998), and a placebo-controlled trial of metrifonate (Morris *et al.*, 1998) for AD. There is also a placebo-controlled trial of rivastigmine in Lewy Body dementia (McKeith *et al.*, 2000). However, the results of the extant studies related to behavioral improvements associated with cholinesterase inhibitors have been fairly mixed, the subjects included have principally had milder forms of behavioral disturbance at baseline, and the subjects were not randomized to treatment group based on severity of behavioral disturbance (Wynn & Cummings, 2004).

Antidepressants and anticonvulsants

The specific serotonin reuptake inhibitors represent yet another potential strategy for the treatment of psychotic symptoms in AD. Antidepressants are generally used for depression in dementia (Doody *et al.*, 2001), and are commonly prescribed in long-term care facilities (Conn & Goldman, 1992), but a retrospective chart review showed improvement of both depression and psychosis in 15 of 20 patients with dementia, with a more robust response in patients with AD (Burke *et al.*, 1997). A recent randomized controlled trial for hospitalized patients with psychosis and/or behavioral disturbances in the context of dementia, showed citalopram, but not perphenazine, to be associated with significantly greater improvement in psychosis and other disturbances than placebo (Pollock *et al.*, 2002). That study suggested a potential "neuroleptic" effect of SSRIs, although it was unclear to what extent the improvement was an epiphenomenon of a reduction in agitation and anxiety. Whilst anticonvulsants are often used for treatment of behavioural disturbance in AD (Herrmann & Lanctot, 1997), there is no clear evidence that they specifically reduce psychotic symptomatology. A recent case report, however, showed a reduction of psychosis with the use of lamotrigine, a newer anticonvulsant, in a patient with AD (De Leon, 2004).

Treating psychosis in Parkinson's disease

Features of parkinsonism are found in 15% of adults aged 65–74 but are as high as 52% for adults age 85 and over (Bennett *et al.*, 1996). In this sample, parkinsonism was associated with an increased relative risk of death of 2.0 (95% confidence interval, 1.6 to 2.6) (Bennett *et al.*, 1996). Psychotic symptoms are common in PD, although rates have varied across studies, depending on the setting. For example, delusions or hallucinations were present in 16% of a community sample (Aarsland *et al.*, 1999) and 27% of a clinical sample of patients with PD (Giladi *et al.*, 2000). Psychosis carries a poor prognosis in PD and is often associated with the need for institutional care or death (Factor *et al.*, 2003). Psychotic symptoms have long been recognized as potential sequelae of available dopaminergic treatments for PD (Celesia & Barr, 1970; Knopp, 1970; Pearlman *et al.*, 1972), and conversely, traditional antipsychotics have a known propensity to induce parkinsonism.

Generally, to reduce psychotic symptoms, a reduction of the dopaminergic therapy or treatment with antipsychotics are required, but this often induces worsening of motor symptoms (Knapp *et al.*, 2002). The advent of the atypical antipsychotics with their mixed action and lower affinity for the D2 receptor, therefore, showed promise in the realm of treating the psychotic phenomena of PD. The first of these to be recognized as useful in psychosis of PD was clozapine, and subsequently other atypical antipsychotics have been assessed.

Clozapine
Clozapine has been reported in many open studies to be effective in treating psychosis in PD, even at low doses, and in some patients the treatment has been successful for years (Musser & Akil, 1996). Clozapine has also been found to be effective in at least two randomized placebo-controlled trials for the treatment of psychosis in PD without worsening of motor symptoms (Parkinson Study Group, 1999; Pollak *et al.*, 2004). These trials each had 60 patients and utilized a dose of less than 50 mg/day. Open-label extensions of these studies for 12 weeks showed that the improvement was sustained (Factor *et al.*, 2001; Pollak *et al.*, 2004). The effectiveness of treatment disappeared in one trial when the drug was discontinued (Pollak *et al.*, 2004). Somnolence is common, and while agranulocytosis is rare, these adverse effects warrant careful clinical attention especially in treating older patients with PD. Clozapine also has a tendency to lower the seizure threshold. The somnolence and necessity of frequent laboratoty work associated with clozapine often lead clinicians to consider the newer antipsychotics first. However, a careful trial of clozapine should be considered in patients with distressing symptoms of psychosis, particularly given the concerns about the newer agents discussed below.

Other atypical antipsychotics
While risperidone is a newer "atypical" antipsychotic, it still has potent D2 receptor blockade at higher doses. In vulnerable patients such as those with PD, this blockade may become clinically evident even at low doses. While two case series reported risperidone to be safe and effective in treating patients with psychosis in PD without motor worsening the sample sizes were only 9 (Workman *et al.*, 1997) and 16 (Mohr *et al.*, 2000). Another series showed substantial worsening of PD symptoms in a series of five of six Parkinsonian patients (Rich *et al.*, 1995). A randomized comparison of risperidone with clozapine in PD showed similar improvements in psychosis but a trend towards worsening of motor symptoms in the risperidone group (Ellis *et al.*, 2000). The sample size of

10 may have been too small to detect statistical differences in tolerability. The concerns about motor side effects have led some experts to recommend thinking of risperidone as a "typical" antipsychotic for patients with PD and to consider alternate options (Factor *et al.*, 2002).

Small case series have demonstrated worsening parkinsonism with the use of olanzapine in patients who were stabilized on clozapine (Friedman *et al.*, 1998), in hallucinating patients with PD (Graham *et al.*, 1998), and in patients with hallucinations and PD dementia (Marsh *et al.*, 2001). A randomized placebo-controlled trial of olanzapine in patients with L-dopa-induced psychosis showed no superiority of olanzapine and a worsening of motor symptoms (Breier *et al.*, 2002). A randomized controlled comparison of clozapine and olanzapine for hallucinating patients with PD was discontinued for safety reasons when the olanzapine group worsened in their parkinsonism (Goetz *et al.*, 2000). In contrast, a small placebo-controlled trial of olanzapine in patients with Lewy Body dementia, an entity related pathologically to PD, showed that olanzapine reduced delusions and hallucinations without worsening motor or cognitive functioning (Cummings *et al.*, 2002).

Open-label studies have shown quetiapine to be a potentially useful option in treating psychotic PD patients. A 1-year open-label follow-up in 35 patients revealed significant improvement in delusions and hallucinations (Mancini *et al.*, 2004). While 9% of patients were able to reduce their dosage of dopaminergic therapy, 43% of patients required an increased dose. Nonetheless, there were no changes in overall motor symptoms. Another open-label study revealed improvement in hallucinations in 6 out of 11 patients at 12 weeks without worsening of motor functioning (Targum & Abbott, 2000). However, delusions were less responsive to treatment, and only 5 out of 11 completed the full year of the study. Encouragingly, an open-label study of 29 elderly patients who did not respond to the other atypical antipsychotics indicated an improvement in psychosis and cognition without worsening parkinsonism with quetiapine (Juncos *et al.*, 2004). Another open-label study showed marked improvement in psychosis in 20 of 24 neuroleptic-naïve PD patients with L-dopa-induced psychosis (Fernandez *et al.*, 1999). However, 6 of 11 psychiatrically stable PD patients were unable to switch from olanzapine or clozapine, and this suggests quetiapine to be more useful as a first than second-line agent in this population. A naturalistic study of response to quetiapine in 87 patients with PD compared with 11 LBD patients showed similar effectiveness and tolerability, with 80 and 90% of patients, respectively, having at least partial resolution of psychosis

(Fernandez *et al.*, 2002). While motor worsening was seen in 32% of PD patients and 27% of LBD patients, quetiapine was generally well tolerated. There are no randomized placebo controlled trials of quetiapine in PD, but a randomized comparison with clozapine in 20 patients for 12 weeks was favorable (Morgante *et al.*, 2002). The quetiapine patients did not improve in their motor function, but they were no worse, while the patients with clozapine had improved motor function. While this study was randomized and the rater was blinded, the patients and families were aware of the treatment condition.

Given the existing evidence, it is difficult to make firm recommendations on pharmacological treatment of psychosis in PD. Informed consent and monitoring of adverse effects is clearly warranted. Typical antipsychotics almost uniformly increase extrapyramidal and related symptoms. There are no controlled data with quetiapine, there are many reports of increased symptoms with olanzapine, and there are inconsistent reports of increased symptoms with risperidone. At present, the bulk of the evidence for efficacy rests with clozapine, although careful monitoring of sedation and hematological indices is warranted. Clinicians using other atypicals should be advised to use low doses and monitor EPS carefully, while they work in close conjunction with the neurological treatment team, as doses of dopaminergic agents may need to be adjusted.

Treating psychosis in cerebrovascular disease and traumatic brain injury

Little is known about the phenomenology of psychosis in the context of cerebrovascular disease although the incidence of this seems to be exceedingly low. Rabins *et al.* (1991) screened all patients admitted post-stroke over a period of 9 years and found only five patients with post-stroke psychosis. There are no published studies about the use of antipsychotics or other pharmacological agents for the treatment of psychosis in this population. The controversies regarding risk of stroke associated with antipsychotics is described above.

The incidence of TBI has a bimodal age distribution with a second peak in later life (Fields & Coffey, 1994). Much of this is a consequence of falls, but motor vehicle accidents are common as well. There is no research on the phenomenology and epidemiology of psychosis following TBI in late life, and psychosis is generally rare following TBI in younger adults. Nonetheless, the risk of psychosis after TBI is two or three times greater than in the general population (Davison & Bagley, 1969). Whilst psychosis can develop acutely, it may often be delayed for several years, and as such may be a late manifestation of injury or related to other non-injury factors (Arciniegas *et al.*, 2003). There are no published studies investigating the effectiveness of antipsychotics for the treatment of psychosis following TBI.

Nonetheless, typical antipsychotics carry with them a risk of central anticholinergic side effects, lower the seizure threshold, and induce extrapyramidal side effects, and these are all particularly relevant for the elderly and those with acquired neurological disease (Arciniegas *et al.*, 2003). Typical antipsychotics have been shown to prolong post-traumatic amnesia (Rao *et al.*, 1985) and confusion (Stanislav, 1997) following brain injury, and to delay acute recovery post-stroke (Goldstein, 1995). The atypical antipsychotics are generally safer and better tolerated in this population (Arciniegas *et al.*, 2003), but it is also fair to add that we do not have the equivalent of the large-scale pragmatic trials such as CATIE and CutLass in old age psychiatry, so we cannot be certain if this population is qualitatively different. Clozapine has been used in an open-label study of agitated or psychotic patients with TBI, with mixed results, including induction of seizures in two of nine patients (Michals *et al.*, 1993). There are only scattered anecdotal reports of improvement of psychosis following TBI with the newer atypical antipsychotics (Arciniegas *et al.*, 2003).

Clinicians treating older patients with psychosis following TBI or stroke are usually suggested to consider cautious introduction of atypical antipsychotics at low doses for patients in whom behavioral measures do not suffice, with careful attention to informed consent and monitoring for adverse effects.

Conclusions

The treatment of psychosis in neurological disease can be as challenging in clinical practice as in the design of the studies described in this chapter. As they add substantially to the morbidity of the neurological diseases, and can hasten institutionalization or even mortality, careful clinical attention to psychotic phenomena is needed. Treatment must be individualized for each patient, particularly since the subjects included in the RCTs may not be generalizable to the multiply-comorbid patients seen in typical practice. Furthermore, in the dementia studies, patients with more severe behavioral disturbance or psychosis may have been excluded.

Although the atypical antipsychotics hold promise for the treatment of psychosis in neurological diseases in old age, most of the evidence for their use is in the treatment of psychosis in dementia. The atypicals are clearly not free of adverse effects, and more information is needed in this population. Whilst motor side effects are fewer, sedation, anticholinergic effects, EPS and TD are indeed still possible with the atypical antipsychotics, in addition to possible cardiovascular effects, weight gain, the consequences of high prolactin levels, falls, and osteoporosis. The promise of efficacy was not borne out in the studies of risperidone and olanzapine in Parkinson's disease, so added caution is needed before we extend to widespread use in other neurological diseases.

Response to atypicals may indeed be disease-specific. Further data are also required about the potential increased risk of cerebrovascular-like events associated with these agents. In the meantime, empiric trials of pharmacological agents may be warranted in patients with psychosis in neurological disease, particularly when behavioral measures fail, provided caution is taken regarding informed consent, and there is vigilant monitoring of potential drug interactions and adverse reactions. Response to antipsychotics may be incomplete, with patients continuing to harbor delusions and/or hallucinations. However, often patients respond to antipsychotic treatment with a reduction in distress and preoccupation with the psychotic material. Once patients have responded and their psychotic symptoms have been in remission, consideration should be given to reducing the dose or discontinuing the antipsychotic over time, particularly given the lack of long-term data and the risk of sedation and other common adverse effects.

Depression

Introduction

Mood disorders are frequently associated with neurological conditions in latelife and can arise as a psychological reaction to the illness itself or as a symptom of the underlying neuropathology. It is often hard to disentangle which of these two pathways predominates in the individual with depression. The three neurological conditions discussed here that are associated with depression in later life are dementia, stroke and Parkinson's disease. Neurological conditions that persevere into, though rarely have their onset in, late life such as multiple sclerosis and motor neurone disease will not be discussed in this chapter. The management of depressions as sequelae of neurological illness is similar to the standard treatment of idiopathic depression (i.e. a combination of social, psychological and pharmacological interventions). The focus here will be on pharmacological interventions.

Depression in dementia

Alzheimer's disease (AD) is the most common of the dementias. The condition is recognized as a disorder predominantly of higher cortical function with clear cognitive symptoms. It has long been known that patients with AD also exhibit behavioral and psychological symptoms, though it is only recently that these symptoms have been categorized under the classification of BPSD (Behavioural and Psychological Symptoms of Dementia). This classification arose as an attempt to understand both the etiology and management of behavioral and psychological symptoms in the context of dementia. One such symptom is depression. The array and timing of BPSD symptoms varies greatly between individuals with the same subtype of dementia, between subtypes and even within individuals during the course of their illness. There is no typical picture of BPSD symptoms in AD. Nor is there any characteristic presentation of depression. However, it is generally considered that depression developing in milder illness presents in a similar fashion to that observed in nondemented individuals, whereas in more severe dementia, the presentation of depression is characterized by predominantly behavioral problems, for example, aggression. It is important to recognize clinically that challenging behaviors may be secondary to lowered mood so that appropriate treatment can be instigated. Overall, major depression affects between 3% and 25% of patients who have AD, with consequences being felt by both patient and caregiver (Reichman & Coyne, 1995; Newman, 1999).

Pharmacological treatment of depression

There are very few high quality clinical trials specifically investigating the pharmacological management of depression in AD. Lyketos *et al.* (2003) investigated the use of sertraline in a single blind randomized trial and found that treated patients were significantly more likely to respond 20/24 (83%) than those receiving placebo 7/20 (35%) ($P = 0.007$). Concurrently, sertraline-treated patients exhibited significant improvement in the Cornell Scale for Depression in Dementia and the Hamilton Depression Rating Scale (Lysketos *et al.*, 2003). Interestingly, behavioral outcome measures also significantly improved, while there was no effect on cognition. These findings strengthened trends observed in an earlier analysis of the trial by the same group (Lysketos *et al.*, 2000). In an open-label Italian study (Moretti *et al.*, 2002), it was demonstrated that citalopram, given concurrently with donepezil hydrochloride, resulted in improved depression ratings and improved quality of life in both patient and caregiver. Most studies have involved investigation of an SSRI, as the anticholinergic effects of tricyclic antidepressants would intuitively be contraindicated in patients with AD. An earlier study compared fluoxetine and amitriptyline in 37 patients with AD and major depression (Taragano et al., 1997) and showed that both drugs were equally effective under double-blind conditions in reducing depression and improving cognition. However, the interpretation of these findings were complicated by the unequal drop-out rate between arms, with only 8/19 (42%) of amitriptyline treated patients tolerating 45 days of treatment whereas 14/18 (78%) of patients treated with fluoxetine completed the trial. The use of acetylcholinesterase inhibitors specifically in terms of changes to mood symptoms in AD has also been examined. Weiner et al. (2000) showed that donepezil had a mildly positive effect in emotional and behavioral symptoms in 25 patients with AD under open-label conditions. Cochrane reviews of acetylcholinesterase inhibitors in AD have been published and comment on the positive effects of this class of drug on behavioral symptoms in AD (Birks et al., 2000; Birks & Harvey, 2003; Olin & Schneider, 2004). However, the cited trials were not designed to specifically look at mood disorder in AD, and the measurement of these symptoms was of secondary concern to the investigators with the concurrent limits this places on interpretation.

What little evidence exists suggests that SSRIs are an effective and well-tolerated treatment for major depression in AD. Poor tolerability and the mode-of-action, especially cardiac effects, would argue against the use of tricyclic antidepressants in this population. All the studies to date with the SSRIs, however, have only treated patients with milder AD, and there is little understanding of the most effective intervention for mood disorder occurring later in the course of AD.

Depression and vascular dementia

Most investigators have shown that depression is more common in vascular dementia then it is in AD (Ballard et al., 1996; Newman, 1999). Studies have calculated the risk being between two and seven times higher in vascular dementia (Reichman & Coyne, 1995; Newman, 1999). Moreover, there is a large body of evidence associating late-onset depression with vascular risk factors such as hypertension (Van den Berg et al., 2001), carotid stenosis (Rao et al., 2001), peripheral arterial disease (Arseven et al., 2001) and global cardiovascular risk (Lyness et al., 2000). It would seem that cerebrovascular disease, whether or not leading to stroke, is associated with major depression. The course of vascular dementia is even less predictable than in AD, and the timing and features of a depressive episode in the course of the illness are poorly described (Ballard et al.,

1996). What information that does exist suggests that depression associated with vascular dementia is more pervasive than in AD (Ballard et al., 1996). Clinically, the depressions and personality change appear similar irrespective of the underlying subtype of dementia (Reichman & Coyne, 1995), and there is no difference in risk associated with different degrees of insight which is often considered greater in vascular dementia (Verhey et al., 1995).

Despite the increased risk of depression in vascular dementia, there have been no well-designed clinical trials of pharmacological interventions in this population. As is the case with AD, the trials of agents targeting cognitive symptoms in vascular dementia have identified benefit of acetylcholinesterase inhibitors in a range of behavioral symptoms associated with this condition (Erkinjuntti et al., 2004).

Depression and diffuse Lewy Body dementia

Diffuse Lewy Body dementia (DLBD) is the third most common type of dementia. Pathologically, it is characterized by cortical Lewy Bodies which are aggregations of intra-cellular α-synuclein. In the basal ganglia these lesions are the hallmark of Parkinson's disease, and there is, therefore, much overlap between the two conditions. The management of depression associated with Parkinson's disease is discussed later in this chapter. Diffuse Lewy Body dementia follows a much more aggressive course from onset to death than either AD or vascular dementia. It also differs clinically with a predominance of neuropsychiatric symptoms (in particular visual hallucinations), deficits of attention (with relative preservation of memory), parkinsonism and fluctuations in symptoms over a short period of time but sometimes over days (McKeith et al., 1996). Despite the frequency of neuropsychiatric symptoms, there has been little systematic enquiry into the association between DLBD and depression, though more recent consensus guidelines have recognized the importance clinically of this concurrent diagnosis (McKeith et al., 1999). From the available literature, it has been observed that depression is more common in DLBD than in AD (Ballard et al., 2002).

There have been no specific trials of anti-depressant treatment in patients with concurrent DLBD and major depression.

Depression following stroke

The occurrence of mood symptoms in the post-stroke period not only complicates short-term recovery and rehabilitation, but has also been associated with long-term mortality. Epidemiological evidence suggests that depression follows stroke in between 20% and 40% of patients at some time point (Vataja *et al.*, 2002).

There are different models which explain the frequently observed association between depression and stroke. Firstly, depression may precede and be a risk factor for stroke. Secondly, depression may be a symptom of stroke due to the area and extent of cortical damage. Thirdly, depression may occur as an affective response to the physical sequelae of stroke. Finally, the two conditions (both being reasonably common in late life) may co-exist in the same individual through chance (Stewart, 2002).

Early work suggested that the site of infarct is relevant to the risk of developing depression post-stroke. Robinson and colleagues demonstrated that left-sided lesions were more likely to be associated with depression, and this risk was further increased in anterior lesions with a further positive association between the risk of depression and increasing distance from the brain's frontal pole (Robinson *et al.*, 1983; Starkstein *et al.*, 1987). This work stimulated many researchers to investigate the "localization" hypothesis with conflicting and inconclusive results (Singh *et al.*, 1999; Carson *et al.*, 2000) possibly due to the differing definitions of depression and stroke types included in studies. There is continued uncertainty about whether there are any specific relationships between the site of stroke and depression (Vataja *et al.*, 2002). Intriguingly, Ballard *et al.* (2000) demonstrated that in patients with vascular dementia and similar levels of cognitive impairment, individuals with smaller infarct volumes (< 15 ml) were more likely to suffer from depression. These individuals were also more likely to demonstrate white matter lesions and perivascular changes. Therefore, in the context of more diffuse cerebrovascular disease, depression would appear to be a recognizable clinical sequela.

The pharmacological treatment of depression following stroke

The incidence and recognition of the association between stroke and depression has stimulated research to investigate the safest and most effective pharmacological intervention for depression in this population. There has been more systematic enquiry in this field than other groups of neurologically impaired patients with depression. For the most part trials have investigated the safety and efficacy of the newer antidepressants (Table 12.1) that have now superseded clinically the use of psychostimulants such as methylphenidate in this population.

Several themes emerge. Firstly, antidepressant treatment would appear to be useful as a prophylactic against depression. Secondly, SSRIs appear to have a rapid effect on pathological crying and emotionality before one would normally expect to see a classical antidepressant effect. Thirdly, antidepressant treatment appears to have a long-term effect on mortality well after the discontinuation of therapy. This would suggest that the mode of action of antidepressants may aid cerebral recovery in the immediate post-stroke period. This effect seems to be limited to antidepressants acting predominantly on the serotonergic pathways i.e. fluoxetine, sertraline and mirtazapine. Additionally, a 3-month randomized trial comparing fluoxetine, maprotiline and placebo in hemiplegic patients demonstrated that post-stroke functional recovery was greatest in the fluoxetine group and least good with maprotiline, though both active interventions were equally good at reducing depressive symptomatology (Dam *et al.*, 1996). Fourthly, augmentation of standard antidepressant treatment with calcium channel blockers may provide even greater efficacy. Finally, the clinical symptoms of depression and central serotonergic function (Morris *et al.*, 2003) post-stroke are very similar to those encountered in non-cerebrovascular related depression and hence drug treatments, diagnoses and measures of symptom progression used in general depression would be appropriate.

In conclusion, antidepressants may well have a dual role in stroke, initially to manage symptoms of depression or prevent its onset, but also and more far-reaching, they may also aid cerebral recovery and have an impact on the long-term survival from stroke. Further research in a large, multi-centre study would be welcome to elaborate on this latter observation. Table 12.1 summarizes the studies of pharmacologic treatment of post-stroke depression.

Depression in Parkinson's disease

The association between depression and Parkinson's disease (PD) is well documented (Cummings, 1992) and effects 40% of the observed variance in quality of life in PD patients (Klaassen *et al.*, 1995; Schrag *et al.*, 2000). There may also be an impact on physical symptom progression, activities of daily living and cognitive performance (Leentjens, 2004). Moreover, the impact of a depressed mood on inherent cognitive symptoms in PD may mimic dementia and the clinical picture is further clouded by the effects of antidepressants on parkinsonism and anti-parkinsonian medication on cognition and other neuropsychiatric symptoms. The high prevalence of PD and strong association with depression has led to the development of a database of clinical trials that have been subject to two systematic reviews (Klaassen *et al.*, 1995) with one published in two locations (Chung *et al.*, 2003; Ghazi-Noori *et al.*, 2003).

Table 12.1. Summary of trials of antidepressants for post-stroke depression

Drug	Author	Population	N	Design	Key findings
Mirtazapine	Neidermaier et al. (2004)	Post-stroke	70	Prophylaxis open-label RCT – investigational drug on 1st post-stroke day for up to 360 days	Risk ratio for depression; treated vs non-treated = 0.14 (5.7% in treated vs 40% in non-treated)
Sertraline	Spalletta & Caltagirone (2003)	Post-stroke cases of major depressive disorder	20	Single arm – open label for 8 weeks	At end point: 35% persistent MDD; 20% minor depression; 45% no mood disorder
	Rasmussen et al. (2003)	Post-stroke	137	Prophylaxis double-blind RCT. 12-month study	Risk ratio for depression; treated vs non-treated = 0.33 (10% in treated vs 30% in placebo)
Citalopram vs Reboxetine	Rampello et al. (2004)	Post-stroke depression (anxious or retarded subtype)	74	Double blind RCT. Active comparator. 16-week study	Citalopram superior for anxious patients, Reboxitine superior for retarded patients
Citalopram	Andersen et al. (1994)	Post-stroke depression	28	Double-blind RCT placebo-controlled. 6-week study	Citalopram significantly superior to placebo. High spontaneous recovery in early depression post-stroke compared with late (> 7 weeks post-stroke) depression.
	Andersen et al. (1993)	Pathological crying – post-stroke	16	Double-blind RCT, placebo controlled. 9 week study	50% reduction in crying observed in 100% treated versus 33% un-treated. Effect observed within several days of treatment commencement. Concomitant improvement in depression
Fluoxetine or Nortriptyline	Jorge et al. (2003)	Post-stroke	104	Random assignment to placebo or antidepressant for 12 weeks under double blind conditions in first 6 months post-stroke. Mortality survival analysis to 9 years	67.9% survival at 9 years in treated group v. 35.7 in placebo group. Conclusions maintained once post-stroke depression controlled for.
	Narushima et al. (2002)	Post-stroke euthymic patients.	48	3-arm, double-blind RCT for 3 months. Total follow-up – 21 months	Reduced incidence of depression in fluoxetine and nortriptyline during treatment. Increased risk of depression in nortriptyline group at 6 months
Fluoxetine	Fruehwald et al. (2003)	Post-stroke depression	54	Double-blind RCT, placebo controlled. Depression within 2 weeks of stroke. Review at 4, 12 and 72 weeks	High spontaneous recovery at week 4. Treatment effect significant at weeks 12 and 72 due to deterioration in placebo group and maintained improvement in treated group
	Wiart et al. (2000)	Post-stroke depression (ICD–10), hemiplegic	31	Double blind RCT, placebo-controlled. 6-weeks treatment	62.5% treated patients responded vs. 33.3% untreated. Significant difference in symptoms scores also noted
	Brown et al. (1998)	Post-stroke "emotionalism"	19	Double-blind RCT, placebo-controlled	Rapid (from Day 3) improvement in symptoms noted in treatment arm. Significant improvement in emotionality noted with fluoxetine treatment

Table 12.1. (cont.)

Drug	Author	Population	N	Design	Key findings
Milnacipran	Kimura et al. 2002	Post-stroke depression	12	Open-label pilot study. 6-week treatment	58.3% of starting patients recovered and 70% of completing (n = 10) recovered.
Nimodipine	Taragano et al. (2001)	Vascular depression	84	Double-blind RCT. Inactive comparator (Vitamin C). Up to 300 days of treatment. Augmentation study	After 60 days, nimodipine group 7.4% relapse rate vs 32% on antidepressant alone. At study end, Nimodipine augmentation led to full remission in 45% vs 25% in antidepressant alone. Also, significant improvement in symptom rating
Mianserin	Palomaki et al. (1999)	Post-stroke	100	Double-blind RCT. Placebo controlled. 1-year treatment with additional 6-month follow-up	6, 12 and 18 months risk of depression similar between the two groups
Methylphenidate	Lazarus et al. (1992)	Post-stroke depression	10	Open-label, single arm study. 3 weeks duration	8/10 (80%) full or partial response as measured by Hamilton Depression Rating Scale
	Johnson et al. (1992)	Post-stroke depression	10	Chart review	7/10 (70%) "improvement noted".
	Masand et al. (1991)	Post-stroke depression	17	Chart review of patients treated with either methylphenidate or dextroamphetamine	47% "marked or moderate improvement noted". Response rapid and usually within 1–2 days

Table 12.2. Individual trials included in Cochrane review (Ghazi-Noori *et al.*, 2003)

Author	Sample size and duration	Investigational drugs	Design	Outcome
Andersen *et al.* (1980)	N = 22; 16 weeks (crossover at week 8)	Nortryptyline 25–150 mg & placebo	Double-blind, randomized, cross-over	Significant improvement in "unique" depression rating scale with no effect on motor symptoms
Rabey *et al.* (1996)	N = 47 (length uncertain)	Fluvoxamine (mean 78 mg) and amitryptyline (mean 69 mg)	Open-label, randomized	50% of amitryptyline and 60% of fluvoxamine group achieved 50% reduction in Hamilton after 16 and 17 months respectively
Wermuth *et al.* (1998)	N = 37; 52 weeks (6 Rx weeks and 46 FU weeks)	Citalopram (20 mg < 65 and 10 mg > 65) dose doubled in non-responders.	Double-blinded, randomized, parallel group	Reduction in Hamilton and Melancholia scale in both groups, no between-group differences. No change to parkinsonian symptoms

The pharmacological treatment of depression in Parkinson's disease

The systematic review by Ghazi-Noori in early 2003 identified three RCTs of sufficient quality to be included. Since their review, one further trial that investigates the impact of citalopram on anxiety, disability and cognition, has been published (Menza *et al.*, 2004), though this trial had no control groups and was open-label so would not have been included in the Cochrane review. Forty other papers identified by the Cochrane review were rejected, though this level of academic endeavor reflects the importance of this clinical problem. The earlier review by Klaassen *et al.* (1995) identified no papers of sufficient quality to merit inclusion in their review.

The three papers included in the Cochrane review are summarized in Table 12.2 (Andersen *et al.*, 1980; Rabey *et al.*, 1996; Wermuth *et al.*, 1998). These investigators investigated the use of nortriptyline, citalopram, fluvoxamine and amitriptyline.

The results of even these trials were inconclusive and the reviewers called for larger, well-designed RCTs. This would seem particularly urgent as it would appear that mood problems have a greater impact on quality of life and carer burden than the motor symptoms (GPDS, 2000).

Conclusions

The extent of the problem of depression associated with neurological disorders in late life is not matched by the evidence level for the most effective treatments. This disappointing observation is an echo of the situation with regard to other psychiatric disorders in the elderly (Ritchie, 2005).

It is highly unlikely that the commercial benefits of large, well-designed trials in any of these conditions are such that they will persuade the pharmaceutical industry to invest in such studies. It will therefore fall upon academics to secure funding through non-commercial channels to conduct urgently needed studies. In some regard, though small, low-quality trials have their place in moving our thinking forward with regard to treatment, large, multicenter trials are needed.

The prevalence of cerebrovascular illness and Parkinson's disease and the strong relationship between these conditions and depression argue, in particular, for these two areas to be the primary focus of academic and clinicians. It is a sobering thought that depression places a greater burden on patients and their caregivers than do motor symptoms in Parkinson's disease. Yet there is no good research into the management of these depressions.

The long-term effects of acute stroke treatment with SSRIs is also noteworthy, and again large multicenter trials over a long duration are necessary to determine whether initial findings with regard to reduced overall mortality are valid. In essence, the evidence that is available would indicate that depression arising in the context of neurological conditions in late life should be treated with SSRIs. In the case of vascular dementia, augmentation with a calcium channel blocker may be useful. Larger trials are needed, however, to identify whether there are any particular safety issues, drug–drug interactions or sub-populations that exhibit differing responses to this standard recommendation.

The level of evidence for each of the interventions discussed in this chapter is summarized in Tables 12.3 and 12.4.

Table 12.3. Summary of evidence base for treatments of psychosis in dementia, Parkinson's disease and traumatic brain injury

Treatment	Form of treatment	Psychiatric disorder	Level of evidence for efficacy	Comments
Typical antipsychotic drugs (initiation)	Haloperidol or equivalent	Psychosis in dementia	Ia	Not first line, lower dosage needed initially than for younger patients
Typical antipsychotic drugs (discontinuation)	Haloperidol or equivalent	Psychosis in dementia (symptoms well controlled)	Ib	Worse outcome in those with high baseline disturbance
Atypical antipsychotic drugs	Risperidone	Psychosis in dementia, also with concomitant aggression	Ib	1–2 mg daily effective, worse EPS with 2 mg daily, dose-dependent risk of somnolence and falls
Atypical antipsychotic drugs	Olanzapine	Psychosis in dementia (Alzheimer's Disease)	Ib	2.5–10 mg daily effective, 15 mg ineffective with anticholinergic side effects
Atypical antipsychotic drugs	Quetiapine	Behavioral symptoms, including psychosis, in dementia (Alzheimer's disease)	III	Small open-label studies only
Acetylcholinesterase inhibitors (AChEI)	Rivastigmine, metrifonate	Behavioral symptoms, including psychosis, in dementia (metrifonate for Alzheimer's disease; rivastigmine in Lewy Body dementia).	Ib	Some evidence of superiority in mild to moderate cases but few trials
Selective serotonin-reuptake inhibitors (SSRIs)	Citalopram	Behavorial symptoms and psychosis in dementia (Alzheimer's disease)	Ib	Small short-term study, greater efficacy of citalopram than perphenazine or placebo but mechanism unclear
Atypical antipsychotic drugs	Clozapine	Psychosis in Parkinson's disease	Ib	Dose < 50 mg daily, good response, but risk of sedation and careful blood monitoring needed
Atypical antipsychotic drugs	Olanzapine	Psychosis in Parkinson's disease	IV	Little consistent evidence of efficacy and worsens motor symptoms
Atypical antipsychotic drugs	Risperidone	Psychosis in Parkinson's disease	Ib	Small trial, not first line, may worsen motor symptoms
Atypical antipsychotic drugs	Quetiapine	Psychosis in Parkinson's disease	III	Motor symptoms not worsened
Atypical antipsychotic drugs	Atypical antipsychotics	Psychosis in traumatic brain injury	IV	Little evidence of treatment indications, anecdotal improvement, cautious low dose use due to risk of side effects

Table 12.4. Summary of evidence base for treatments of depression in dementia, Parkinson's disease and post-stroke

Treatment	Form of treatment	Condition	Level of evidence for efficacy	Comments
Tricyclic antidepressants	Nortryptiline	Parkinson's disease	Ib	Improvement
	Amitryptyline	Parkinson's disease	IIb	Improvement
Selective – serotonin reuptake inhibitors	Fluvoxamine	Parkinson's disease	IIb	50% reduction in Hamilton, but it may take months to show this effect
	Citalopram	Parkinson's disease	Ib	Improvement in depression. No change in Parkinson's symptoms
Tri-and tetracyclic antidepressants	Nortriptyline	Post-stroke depression	Ib	Acutely effective though no better than placebo after 6 months
	Mianserin	Post-stroke depression	Ib	No evidence of efficacy from RCT
Selective-serotonin reuptake inhibitors	Sertraline (treatment)	Post-stroke depression	III	Improvement found in two-thirds of sample
	Sertraline, citalopram, fluoxetine	Post-stroke depression	Ib	Effective. Citalopram may have particular effect on crying and anxiety
	Milnacipran	Post-stroke depression	III	Small Ns but did show effectiveness
Other antidepressants	Mirtazapine	Post-stroke depression	Ib	Effective as a prophylaxis when begun on day 1 and continued for a year
	Methylphenidate	Post-stroke depression	III	Between 50% and 75% showed improvement
	Reboxitine	Post-stroke depression	Ib	For retarded depression
Other pharmacological agents	Nimodipine	Post-stroke depression	Ib	In "vascular depression", as an adjunct to antidepressant
Tricyclic antidepressants	Amitryptyline	Alzheimer's disease (mild)	Ib	Though very high drop-out rates observed from this treatment
Selective serotonin reuptake inhibitor	Sertraline, fluoxetine	Alzheimer's disease	Ib	Improvement in depression
	cipramil (with donepezil)	Alzheimer's disease	II	Questionable improvement

REFERENCES

Aarsland, D., Larsen, J. P., Cummins, J. L. & Laake, K. (1999). Prevalence and clinical correlates of psychotic symptoms in Parkinson disease: a community-based study. *Archives of Neurology*, **56**, 595–601.

Alessi, C. A. (1991). Managing the behavioral problems of dementia in the home. *Clinical Geriatric Medicine*, **7**, 787–801.

Andersen, G., Vestergaard, K. & Riis, J. O. (1993). Citalopram for post-stroke pathological crying. *Lancet*, **342**, 837–9.

Andersen, G., Vestergaard, K. & Lauritzen, L. (1994). Effective treatment of poststroke depression with the selective serotonin reuptake inhibitor citalopram. *Stroke*, **25**, 1099–104.

Andersen, J., Aabro, E., Gulmann, N. *et al.* (1980). Antidepressive treatment in Parkinson's disease. A controlled trial of the effect of nortryptiline in patients with Parkinson's disease treated with L-dopa. *Acta Neurologica Scandinavica*, **62**, 210–19.

Arciniegas, D. B., Harris, S. N. & Brousseau, K. M. (2003). Psychosis following traumatic brain injury. *International Review of Psychiatry*, **15**, 328–40.

Arseven, A., Guralnik, J. M., O'Brien, E. *et al.* (2001). Peripheral arterial disease and depressed mood in older men and women. *Vascular Medicine*, **6**, 229–34.

Ballard, C., Bannister, C., Solis, M. *et al.* (1996). The prevalence, associations and symptoms of depression amongst dementia sufferers. *Journal of Affective Disorders*, **22**, 135–44.

Ballard, C., McKeith, I., O'Brien, J. *et al.* (2000). Neuropathological substrates of dementia and depression in vascular dementia, with a particular focus on cases with small infarct volumes. *Dementia and Geriatric Cognitive Disorders*, **11**, 59–65.

Ballard, C., Johnson, M., Piggot, M. *et al.* (2002). A positive association between 5HT re-uptake binding sites and depression in dementia with Lewy bodies. *Journal of Affective Disorders*, **69**, 219–23.

Ballard, C. G., Thomas, A., Fossey, J. *et al.* (2004). A 3-month, randomized, placebo-controlled, neuroleptic discontinuation study in 100 people with dementia: the neuropsychiatric inventory median cutoff is a predictor of clinical outcome. *Journal of Clinical Psychiatry*, **65**, 114–19.

Bennett, D. A., Beckett, L. A., Murray, A. M. *et al.* (1996). Prevalence of parkinsonian signs and associated mortality in a community population of older people. *New England Journal of Medicine*, **334**, 71–6.

Birks, J. S. & Harvey, R. (2003). Donepezil for dementia due to Alzheimer's disease. *Cochrane Database of Systematic Reviews*, **3**, CD001190. Oxford: Update Software Ltd.

Birks, J., Grimley Evans, J., Iakovidou, V. & Tsolaki, M. (2000). Rivastigmine for Alzheimer's disease. *Cochrane Database of Systematic Reviews*, **4**, CD001191. Oxford: Update Software Ltd.

Borson, S. & Raskind, M. A. (1997). Clinical features and pharmacologic treatment of behavioral symptoms of Alzheimer's disease. *Neurology*, **48** (Suppl. 6), S17–24.

Breier, A., Sutton, V. K., Feldman, P. D. *et al.* (2002). Olanzapine in the treatment of dopamimetic-induced psychosis in patients with Parkinson's disease. *Biological Psychiatry*, **52**, 438–45.

Brodaty, H., Ames, D., Snowdon, J. (2003). A randomized placebo-controlled trial of risperidone for the treatment of aggression, agitation, and psychosis of dementia. *Journal of Clinical Psychiatry*, **64**, 134–43.

Bronskill, S. E., Anderson, G. M., Sykora, K. *et al.* (2004). Neuroleptic drug therapy in older adults newly admitted to nursing homes: incidence, dose, and specialist contact. *Journal of the American Geriatric Society*, **52**, 749–55.

Brown, K. W., Sloan, R. L. & Pentland, B. (1998). Fluoxetine as a treatment for post-stroke emotionalism. *Acta Psychiatrica Scandinavica*, **98**, 455–8.

Burke, W. J., Dewan, V., Wengel, S. P., Roccaforte, W. H., Nadolny, G. C. & Folks, D. G. (1997). The use of selective serotonin reuptake inhibitors for depression and psychosis complicating dementia. *International Journal of Geriatric Psychiatry*, **12**, 519–25.

Caligiuri, M. P., Lacro, J. P., Rockwell, E., McAdams, L. A. & Jeste, D. V. (1997). Incidence and risk factors for severe tardive dyskinesia in older patients. *British Journal of Psychiatry*, **171**, 148–53.

Caligiuri, M. R., Jeste, D. V. & Lacro, J. P. (2000). Antipsychotic-induced movement disorders in the elderly: epidemiology and treatment recommendations. *Drugs Aging*, **17**, 363–84.

Carson, A. J., MacHale, S., Allen, K. *et al.* (2000). Depression after stroke and lesion location: a systematic review. *Lancet*, **356**, 122–6.

Celesia, G. G. & Barr, A. N. (1970). Psychosis and other psychiatric manifestations of levodopa therapy. *Archives of Neurology*, **23**, 193–200.

Chan, W. C., Lam, L. C., Choy, C. N., Leung, V. P., Li, S. W. & Chiu, H. F. (2001). A double-blind randomised comparison of risperidone and haloperidol in the treatment of behavioural and psychological symptoms in Chinese dementia patients. *International Journal of Geriatric Psychiatry*, **16**, 1156–62.

Chung, T. H., Deane, K. H., Ghazi-Noori, S. *et al.* (2003). Systematic review of antidepressant therapies in Parkinson's disease. *Parkinsonism and Related Disorders*, **10**, 59–65.

Clark, W. S., Street, J. S., Feldman, P. D. & Breier, A. (2001). The effects of olanzapine in reducing the emergence of psychosis among nursing home patients with Alzheimer's disease. *Journal of Clinical Psychiatry*, **62**, 34–40.

Cohen-Mansfield, J. (2001). Nonpharmacologic interventions for inappropriate behaviors in dementia: a review, summary, and critique. *American Journal of Geriatric Psychiatry*, **9**, 361–81.

Conn, D. K. & Goldman, Z. (1992). Pattern of use of antidepressants in long-term care facilities for the elderly. *Journal of Geriatric Psychiatry and Neurology*, **5**, 228–32.

Cummings, J. L. (1992). Depression and Parkinson's disease: a review. *American Journal of Psychiatry*, **149**, 443–54.

Cummings, J. L., Street, J., Masterman, D. & Clark, W. S. (2002). Efficacy of olanzapine in the treatment of psychosis in dementia with lewy bodies. *Dementia and Geriatric Cognitive Disorders*, **13**, 67–73.

Dam, M., Tonin, P., De Boni, A. *et al* (1996). Effects of fluoxetine and maprotiline on functional recovery in poststroke hemiplegic patients undergoing rehabilitation therapy. *Stroke*, **27**, 1211–14.

Davison, K. & Bagley, C. R. (1969). Schizophrenia-like psychoses associated with organic disorders of the central nervous system: a review of the literature. In *Current Problems in Neuropsychiatry: Schizophrenia, Epilepsy, and the Temporal Lobe*, ed. R. N. Herrington, pp. 113–84. London: Headley.

De Deyn, P. P., Carrasco, M. M., Deberdt, W. *et al.* (2004). Olanzapine versus placebo in the treatment of psychosis with or without associated behavioral disturbances in patients with Alzheimer's disease. *International Journal of Geriatric Psychiatry*, **19**, 115–26.

De Deyn, P. P., Rabheru, K., Rasmussen, A. *et al.* (1999). A randomized trial of risperidone, placebo, and haloperidol for behavioral symptoms of dementia. *Neurology*, **53**, 946–55.

De Leon, O. A. (2004). Treatment of psychotic symptoms with lamotrigine in Alzheimer disease. *Journal of Clinical Psychopharmacology*, **24**, 232–3.

Devanand, D. P. & Levy, S. R. (1995). Neuroleptic treatment of agitation and psychosis in dementia. *Journal of Geriatric Psychiatry and Neurology*, **8** (Suppl. 1), S18–27.

Devanand, D. P., Marder, K., Michaels, K. S. *et al.* (1998). A randomized, placebo-controlled dose-comparison trial of haloperidol for psychosis and disruptive behaviors in Alzheimer's disease. *American Journal of Psychiatry*, **155**, 1512–20.

Doody, R. S., Stevens, J. C., Beck, C. *et al.* (2001). Practice parameter: management of dementia (an evidence-based review). Report of the Quality Standards Subcommittee of the American Academy of Neurology. *Neurology*, **56**, 1154–66.

Edell, W. S. & Tunis, S. L. (2001). Antipsychotic treatment of behavioral and psychological symptoms of dementia in geropsychiatric inpatients. *American Journal of Geriatric Psychiatry*, **9**, 289–97.

Ellis, T., Cudkowicz, M. E., Sexton, P. M. & Growdon, J. H. (2000). Clozapine and risperidone treatment of psychosis in Parkinson's disease. *Journal of Neuropsychiatry and Clinical Neuroscience*, **12**, 364–9.

Erkinjuntti, T., Roman, G., Gauthier, S. *et al.* (2004). Emerging therapies for vascular dementia and vascular cognitive impairment. *Stroke*, **35**, 1010–17.

Factor, S. A., Friedman, J. H., Lannon, M. C., Oakes, D. & Bourgeois, K. (2001). Clozapine for the treatment of drug-induced psychosis in

Parkinson's disease: results of the 12 week open label extension in the PSYCLOPS trial. *Movement Disorders*, **16**, 135–9.

Factor, S. A., Molho, E. S. & Friedman, J. H. (2002). Risperidone and Parkinson's disease. *Movement Disorders*, **17**, 221–2.

Factor, S. A., Feustel, P. J., Friedman, J. H. *et al.* (2003). Longitudinal outcome of Parkinson's disease patients with psychosis. *Neurology*, **60**, 1756–61.

Fernandez, H. H., Friedman, J. H., Jacques, C. & Rosenfeld, M. (1999). Quetiapine for the treatment of drug-induced psychosis in Parkinson's disease. *Movement Disorders*, **14**, 484–7.

Fernandez, H. H., Trieschmann, M. E., Burke, M. A. & Friedman, J. H. (2002). Quetiapine for psychosis in Parkinson's disease versus dementia with Lewy bodies. *Journal of Clinical Psychiatry*, **63**, 513–15.

Fields, R. B. & Coffey C. E. (1994). Traumatic brain injury. In *Textbook of Geriatric Neuropsychiatry*, ed. C. E. Coffey & J. L. Cummings, pp. 479–508. Washington, DC: American Psychiatric Press.

Fontaine, C. S., Hynan, L. S., Koch, K., Martin-Cook, K., Svetlik, D. & Weiner, M. F. (2003). A double-blind comparison of olanzapine versus risperidone in the acute treatment of dementia-related behavioral disturbances in extended care facilities. *Journal of Clinical Psychiatry*, **64**, 726–30.

Friedman, J. H., Goldstein, S. & Jacques, C. (1998). Substituting clozapine for olanzapine in psychiatrically stable Parkinson's disease patients: results of an open label pilot study. *Clinical Neuropharmacology*, **21**, 285–8.

Fruehwald, S., Gatterbauer, E., Rhak, P. & Baumhackl, U. (2003). Early fluoxetine treatment of post-stroke depression – a 3-month double blind, placebo-controlled study with an open-label long-term follow up. *Journal of Neurology*, **250**, 347–51.

Fujikawa, T., Takahashi, T., Kinoshita, A. *et al.* (2004). Quetiapine treatment for behavioral and psychological symptoms in patients with senile dementia of Alzheimer type. *Neuropsychobiology*, **49**, 201–4.

Gareri, P., Cotroneo, A., Lacava, R. *et al.* (2004). Comparison of the efficacy of new and conventional antipsychotic drugs in the treatment of behavioral and psychological symptoms of dementia (BPSD). *Archives of Gerontology Geriatric Supplement*, **9**, 207–15.

Ghazi-Noori, S., Chung, T. H., Deane, K. H. O. *et al.* (2003). Therapies for depression in Parkinson's disease. *Cochrane Database of Systematic Reviews*, **3**, CD003465. Oxford: Update Software Ltd.

Giladi, N., Treves, T. A., Paleacu, D. *et al.* (2000). Risk factors for dementia, depression and psychosis in long-standing Parkinson's disease. *Journal of Neural Transmission*, **107**, 59–71.

Goetz, C. G., Blasucci, L. M., Leurgans, S. & Pappert, E. J. (2000). Olanzapine and clozapine: comparative effects on motor function in hallucinating PD patients. *Neurology*, **55**, 789–94.

Goldstein, L. B. (1995). Common drugs may influence motor recovery after stroke. *The Sygen In Acute Stroke Study Investigators. Neurology*, **45**, 865–71.

GPDS (2000). *Global Parkinson's Disease Survey*. PDGS pamphlet.

Graham, J. M., Sussman, J. D., Ford, K. S. & Sagar, H. J. (1998). Olanzapine in the treatment of hallucinosis in idiopathic Parkinson's disease: a cautionary note. *Journal of Neurology, Neurosurgery and Psychiatry*, **65**, 774–7.

Health Canada (2000). Updated safety information for risperdal (risperidone) in elderly dementia patients. Announced in Canada by Janssen-Ortho Inc Oct 17, 2000. Available at http://www.hc-sc.gc.ca/hpfb-dgpsa/tpd-dpt/risperdal2_e.html. Accessed November 5 2004.

Herrmann, N. & Lanctot, K. L. (1997). From transmitters to treatment: the pharmacotherapy of behavioural disturbances in dementia. *Canadian Journal of Psychiatry*, **42** (Suppl. 1), 51S–64S.

Herrmann, N., Mamdani, M. & Lanctôt, K. L. (2004). Atypical antipsychotics and risk of cerebrovascular accidents. *American Journal of Psychiatry*, **161**, 1113–15.

Hwang, J. P., Yang, C. H. & Tsai, S. J. (2003). Phantom boarder symptom in dementia. *International Journal of Geriatric Psychiatry*, **18**, 417–20.

Jeste, D. V., Caligiuri, M. P., Paulsen, J. S. *et al.* (1995). Risk of tardive dyskinesia in older patients. A prospective longitudinal study of 266 outpatients. *Archives of General Psychiatry*, **52**, 756–65.

Johnson, M. L., Roberts, M. D., Ross, A. R. & Witten, C. M. (1992). Methylphenidate in stroke patients with depression. *American Journal of Physical Medical Rehabilitation*, **71**, 239–41.

Jorge, R. E., Robinson, R. G., Arndt, S. & Starkstein, S. (2003). Mortality and poststroke depression: a placebo controlled trial of antidepressants. *American Journal of Psychiatry*, **160**, 1823–9.

Juncos, J. L., Roberts, V. J., Evatt, M. L. *et al.* (2004). Quetiapine improves psychotic symptoms and cognition in Parkinson's disease. *Movement Disorders*, **19**, 29–35.

Katz, I. R., Jeste, D. V., Mintzer, J. E., Clyde, C., Napolitano, J. & Brecher, M. (1999). Comparison of risperidone and placebo for psychosis and behavioral disturbances associated with dementia: a randomized, double-blind trial. Risperidone Study Group. *Journal of Clinical Psychiatry*, **60**, 107–15.

Katz, I. R., Rupnow, M., Kozma, C. & Schneider, L. (2004). Risperidone and falls in ambulatory nursing home residents with dementia and psychosis or agitation: secondary analysis of a double-blind, placebo-controlled trial. *American Journal of Geriatric Psychiatry*, **12**, 499–508.

Kaufer, D., Cummings, J. L. & Christine, D. (1998). Differential neuropsychiatric symptom responses to tacrine in Alzheimer's disease: relationship to dementia severity. *Journal of Neuropsychiatry and Clinical Neurosciences*, **10**, 55–63.

Kimura, M., Kanetani, K., Imai, R. *et al.* (2002). Therapeutic effects of milnacipran, a serotonin and noradrenaline reuptake inhibitor, on post stroke depression. *International Clinical Psychopharmacology*, **17**, 121–5.

Klaassen, T., Verhey, F. R. J., Sneijders, G. H. J. M. *et al.* (1995). Treatment of depression in Parkinson's disease: a meta-analysis. *Journal of Neuropsychiatry and Clinical Neurosciences*, **7**, 281–6.

Knapp, M., Ilson, S. & David, A. (2002). Depot antipsychotic preparations in schizophrenia: the state of the economic evidence. *International Clinical Psychopharmacology*, **17**, 135–40.

Knopp, W. (1970). Psychiatric changes in patients treated with levodopa. I. The clinical experiment. *Neurology*, **20**, 23–30.

Lawlor, B. A. (2004). Behavioral and psychological symptoms in dementia: the role of atypical antipsychotics. *Journal of Clinical Psychiatry*, **65** (Suppl. 11), 5–10.

Lazarus, L. W., Winemiller, D. R., Lingam, V. R. *et al.* (1992). Efficacy and side effects of methylphenidate for poststroke depression. *Journal of Clinical Psychiatry*, **53**, 447–9.

Leentjens, A. F. (2004). Depression in Parkinson's disease: conceptual issues and clinical challenges. *Journal of Geriatric Psychiatry and Neurology*, **17**, 120–6.

Lindsay, J., Sykes, E., McDowell, I., Verreault, R. & Laurin, D. (2004). More than the epidemiology of Alzheimer's disease: contributions of the Canadian Study of Health and Aging. *Canadian Journal of Psychiatry*, **49**, 83–91.

Liperoti, R., Mor, V., Lapane, K. L., Pedone, C., Gambassi, G. & Bernabei, R. (2003). The use of atypical antipsychotics in nursing homes. *Journal of Clinical Psychiatry*, **64**, 1106–12.

Lyketos, C. G., DelCampo, L., Steinberg, M. *et al.* (2003). Treating depression in Alzheimer's disease: efficacy and safety of sertraline therapy, and the benefits of depression reduction: the DIADS. *Archives of General Psychiatry*, **60**, 737–46.

Lyness, J. M., King, D. A., Conwell, Y. *et al.* (2000). Cerebrovascular risk factors and 1-year depression outcome in older primary care patients. *American Journal of Geriatric Psychiatry*, **157**, 1499–501.

Lysketos, C. G., Sheppard, J. M., Steele, C. D. *et al.* (2000). Randomised, placebo-controlled, double blind clinical trial of sertraline in the treatment of depression complicating Alzheimer's disease: initial results from the Depression in Alzheimer's Disease study. *American Journal of Psychiatry*, **157**, 1686–9.

Mancini, F., Tassorelli, C., Martignoni, E. *et al.* (2004). Long-term evaluation of the effect of quetiapine on hallucinations, delusions and motor function in advanced Parkinson disease. *Clinical Neuropharmacology*, **27**, 33–7.

Marsh, L., Lyketsos, C. & Reich, S. G. (2001). Olanzapine for the treatment of psychosis in patients with Parkinson's disease and dementia. *Psychosomatics*, **42**, 477–81.

Masand, P., Murray, G. B. & Picket, P. (1991). Psychostimulants in post-stroke depression. *Journal of Neuropsychiatry and Clinical Neurosciences*, **3**, 23–7.

McKeith, I. G., Galasko, D., Kosaka, K. *et al.* (1996). Consensus guidelines for the clinical and pathological diagnosis of dementia with Lewy bodies (DLB): report of the consortium on DLB international workshop. *Neurology*, **47**, 1113–24.

McKeith, I. G., Perry, E. K. & Perry, R. H. (1999). Report of the second Dementia with Lewy body International Workshop: diagnosis and treatment. Consortium on Dementia with Lewy Bodies. *Neurology*, **53**, 902–5.

McKeith, I., Del Ser, T., Spano, P. *et al.* (2000). Efficacy of rivastigmine in dementia with Lewy bodies: a randomised, double-blind, placebo-controlled international study. *Lancet*, **356**, 2031–6.

Michals, M. L, Crismon, M. L., Roberts, S. & Childs, A. (1993). Clozapine response and adverse effects in nine brain-injured patients. *Journal of Clinical Psychopharmacology*, **13**, 198–203.

Mohr, E., Mendis, T., Hildebrand, K. & De Deyn, P. P. (2000). Risperidone in the treatment of dopamine-induced psychosis in Parkinson's disease: an open pilot trial. *Movement Disorders*, **15**, 1230–7.

Moretti, R., Torre, P., Antonello, R. M. *et al.* (2002). Depression and Alzheimer's disease: symptom or comorbidity? *American Journal of Alzheimer's Disease and Other Dementias*, **17**, 338–44.

Morgante, L., Epifanio, A., Spina, E. *et al.* (2002). Quetiapine versus clozapine: a preliminary report of comparative effects on dopaminergic psychosis in patients with Parkinson's disease. *Neurological Sciences*, **23** (Suppl. 2), S89–90.

Morris, J. C., Cyrus, P. A., Orazem, J. *et al.* (1998). Metrifonate benefits cognitive, behavioral, and global function in patients with Alzheimer's disease. *Neurology*, **50**, 1222–30.

Morris, P., Hopwood, M., Maguire, K. *et al.* (2003). Blunted prolactin response to D-fenfluramine in post-stroke major depression. *Journal of Affective Disorders*, **76**, 273–8.

Musser, W. S. & Akil, M. (1996). Clozapine as a treatment for psychosis in Parkinson's disease: a review. *Journal of Neuropsychiatry and Clinical Neurosciences*, **8**, 1–9.

Narushima, K., Kosier, J. T. & Robinson, R. G. (2002). Preventing poststroke depression: a 12-week double-blind randomized treatment trial and 21 month follow up. *Journal of Nervous and Mental Disease*, **190**, 296–303.

Neidermaier, N., Bohrer, E., Schulte, K. *et al.* (2004). Prevention and treatment of poststroke depression with mirtazapine in patients with acute stroke. *Journal of Clinical Psychiatry*, **65**, 1619–23.

Newman, S. C. (1999). The prevalence of depression in Alzheimer's disease and vascular dementia in a population sample. *Journal of Affective Disorders*, **52**, 169–76.

Olin, J. & Schneider L. (2004). Galantamine for Alzheimer's disease. *Cochrane Database of Systematic Reviews*, **4**, CD001747. Oxford: Update Software Ltd.

Palomaki, H., Kaste, M. & Berg, A. (1999). Prevention of poststroke depression: 1 year randomized placebo controlled, double blind trial of mianserin with 6-month follow up after therapy. *Journal of Neurosurgery and Psychiatry*, **66**, 490–4.

Parkinson Study Group (1999). Low-dose clozapine for the treatment of drug-induced psychosis in Parkinson's disease. *New England Journal of Medicine*, **340**, 757–63.

Pearlman, C. A., Jr., Sax, D. S. & Feldman, R. D. (1972). Psychiatric aspects of L-dopa therapy of Parkinson's disease. *Psychiatry and Medicine*, **3**, 45–50.

Pollak, P., Tison, F., Rascol, O. *et al.* (2004). Clozapine in drug induced psychosis in Parkinson's disease: a randomised, placebo controlled study with open follow up. *Journal of Neurology, Neurosurgery and Psychiatry*, **75**, 689–95.

Pollock, B. G., Mulsant, B. H., Rosen, J. *et al.* (2002). Comparison of citalopram, perphenazine, and placebo for the acute treatment of psychosis and behavioral disturbances in hospitalized, demented patients. *American Journal of Psychiatry*, **159**, 460–5.

Rabey, J. M., Orlov, E. & Korcyzn, A. D. (1996). Comparison of fluvoxamine versus amitryptiline for treatment of depression in Parkinson's disease. *Neurology*, **46**, A374.

Rabinowitz, J., Katz, I. R., De Deyn, P. P., Brodaty, H., Greenspan, A. & Davidson, M. Behavioral and psychological symptoms in patients with dementia as a target for pharmacotherapy with risperidone. *Journal of Clinical Psychiatry*, **65**, 1329–34.

Rabins, P. V., Starkstein, S. E. & Robinson, R. G. (1991). Risk factors for developing atypical (schizophreniform) psychosis following stroke. *Journal of Neuropsychiatry and Clinical Neurosciences*, **3**, 6–9.

Rampello, L., Chiechio, S., Nicoletti, G. *et al.* (2004). Prediction of the response to citalopram and reboxetine in post-stroke depressed patients. *Psychopharmacology (Berl.)*, **173**, 73–8.

Rao, N., Jellinek, H. M. & Woolston, D. C. (1985). Agitation in closed head injury: haloperidol effects on rehabilitation outcome. *Archives of Physical and Medical Rehabilitation*, **66**, 30–4.

Rao, R., Jackson, S. & Howard, R. (2001). Depression in older people with mild stroke, carotid stenosis and peripheral vascular disease: a comparison with healthy controls. *International Journal of Geriatric Psychiatry*, **16**, 175–83.

Rapoport, M. J. & Feinstein, A. (2000). Outcome following traumatic brain injury in the elderly: a critical review. *Brain Injuries*, **14**, 749–61.

Rapoport, M. J., Mamdani, M., Shulman, K. I., Herrmann, N. & Rochon, P. A. (2004). *Antipsychotic prescriptions in the elderly: Changing trends and increasing costs*. Poster presented at the American Psychiatric Association 157th Annual Meeting, May 1–6, New York, NY., 2004

Rapoport, M. J., & van Reekum, R. (2000). Treating psychosis in dementia. In *Treating Dementia: Cognition and Beyond*. ed. R. J. Ancill, S. G. Holliday, L. Thorpe & K. Rabheru. Vancouver, BC: Canadian Academic Press.

Rasmussen, A., Lunde, M., Poulsen, D. L. *et al.* (2003). A double-blind, placebo-controlled study of sertraline in the prevention of depression in stroke patients. *Psychosomatics*, **44**, 216–21.

Reichman, W. E. & Coyne, A. C. (1995). Depressive symptoms in Alzheimer's disease and multi-infarct dementia. *Journal of Geriatrics, Psychiatry and Neurology*, **8**, 96–9.

Rich, S. S., Friedman J. H. & Ott, B. R. (1995). Risperidone versus clozapine in the treatment of psychosis in six patients with Parkinson's disease and other akinetic-rigid syndromes. *Journal of Clinical Psychiatry*, **56**, 556–9.

Ritchie, C. W. (2005). The use of antipsychotic medication for schizophrenia occurring in late life. In *Psychosis in the Elderly*, ed. A. Hassett, D. Ames & E. Chiu. London: Taylor Francis Publishing.

Robinson, R. G., Kubos, K. L., Starr, L. B. *et al.* (1983). Mood changes in stroke patients: relationship to lesion location. *Comprehensive Psychiatry*, **24**, 555–66.

Rosler, M., Retz, W., Retz-Junginger, P. & Dennler, H. J. (1998). Effects of two-year treatment with the cholinestcrase inhibltor rivastigmine on behavioural symptoms in Alzheimer's disease. *Behavioral Neurology*, **11**, 211–16.

Scharre, D. W. & Chang, S. I. (2002). Cognitive and behavioral effects of quetiapine in Alzheimer disease patients. *Alzheimer Disease and Associated Disorders*, **16**, 128–30.

Schneider, L. S., Pollock, V. E. & Lyness, S. A. (1990). A meta-analysis of controlled trials of neuroleptic treatment in dementia. *Journal of the American Geriatrics Society*, **38**, 553–63.

Schneider, L. S., Katz, I. R., Park, S., Napolitano, J., Martinez, R. A., Azen, S. P. (2003). Psychosis of Alzheimer disease: validity of the construct and response to risperidone. *American Journal of Geriatric Psychiatry*, **11**, 414–25.

Schneider, L. S. & Dagerman, K. S. (2004). Psychosis of Alzheimer's disease: clinical characteristics and history. *Journal of Psychiatric Research*, **38**, 105–11.

Schrag, A., Jahanashani, M. & Quin N. (2000). What contributes to quality of life in patients with Parkinson's disease. *Journal of Neurology, Neurosurgery and Psychiatry*, **69**, 308–12.

Singh, A., Hermann, N. & Black, S. E. (1999). The importance of lesion location in post-stroke depression: a critical review. *Canadian Journal of Psychiatry*, **43**, 921–7.

Spalletta, G. & Caltagirone, C. (2003). Sertraline treatment of post-stroke major depression: an open study in patients with moderate to severe symptoms. *Functional Neurology*, **18**, 227–32.

Stanislav, S. W. (1997). Cognitive effects of antipsychotic agents in persons with traumatic brain injury. *Brain Injury*, **11**, 335–41.

Starkstein, S. E., Robinson, R. G. & Price, T. R. (1987). Comparison of cortical and subcortical lesions in the production of post-stroke mood disorders. *Brain*, **110**, 1054–9.

Stewart, R. (2002). The interface between cerebrovascular disease, depression and dementia. In *Vascular Disease and Affective Disorders*, ed. E. Chiu, D. Ames & C. Katona London: Martin Dunitz Publishing.

Street, J. S., Clark, W. S., Gannon, K. S. *et al.* (2000). Olanzapine treatment of psychotic and behavioral symptoms in patients with Alzheimer disease in nursing care facilities: a double-blind, randomized, placebo-controlled trial. The HGEU Study Group. *Archives of General Psychiatry*, **57**, 968–76.

Street, J. S., Clark, W. S., Kadam, D. L. *et al.* (2001). Long-term efficacy of olanzapine in the control of psychotic and behavioral symptoms in nursing home patients with Alzheimer's dementia. *International Journal of Geriatric Psychiatry*, **16** (Suppl. 1), S62–70.

Suh, G. H., Son, H. G., Ju, Y. S. *et al.* (2004). A randomized, double-blind, crossover comparison of risperidone and haloperidol in Korean dementia patients with behavioral disturbances. *American Journal of Geriatric Psychiatry*, **12**, 509–16.

Sunderland, T. (1996). Treatment of the elderly suffering from psychosis and dementia. *Journal of Clinical Psychiatry*, **57** (Suppl. 9), 53–6.

Taragano, F. E., Allegri, R. & Vicario, A. (2001). A double-blind, randomized clinical trial assessing the efficacy and safety of augmenting standard antidepressant therapy with nimodipine in the treatment of 'vascular depression'. *International Journal of Geriatric Psychiatry*, **16**, 254–60.

Taragano, F. E., Lysketos, C. G., Mangone, C. A. *et al.* (1997). A double-blind, randomised, fixed-dose trial of fluoxetine vs. amitryptiline in the treatment of major depression complicating Alzheimer's disease. *Psychosomatics*, **38**, 246–52.

Targum, S. D. & Abbott, J. L. (2000). Efficacy of quetiapine in Parkinson's patients with psychosis. *Journal of Clinical Psychopharmacology*, **20**, 54–60.

Tariot, P. N. (1996). Treatment strategies for agitation and psychosis in dementia. *Journal of Clinical Psychiatry*, **57** (Suppl. 14) 21–9.

Tariot, P. N., Salzman, C., Yeung, P. P., Pultz, J., Rak, I. W. (2000). Long-term use of quetiapine in elderly patients with psychotic disorders. *Clinical Therapist*, **22**, 1068–84.

United States General Accounting Office (1998). *Alzheimer's Disease: Estimates of Prevalence in the United States*. Washington, DC: United States General Accounting Office.

Van den Berg, M. D., Oldehinkel, A. J., Bouhuys, A. L. *et al.* (2001). Depression in late life: three etiologically different subgroups. *Journal of Affective Disorders*, **65**, 19–26.

Van Den Eeden, S. K., Tanner, C. M., Bernstein, A. L. (2003). Incidence of Parkinson's disease: variation by age, gender, and race/ethnicity. *American Journal of Epidemiology*, **157**, 1015–22.

van Reekum, R., Clarke, D., Conn, D. *et al.* (2002). A randomized, placebo-controlled trial of the discontinuation of long-term antipsychotics in dementia. *International Psychogeriatrics*, **14**, 197–210.

Vataja, R., Pohjasvaara, T., Leppavuori, A. & Erkinjutti, T. (2002). Post stroke depression. In *Vascular Disease and Affective Disorders*, ed. E. Chiu, D. Ames & C. Katona. London: Martin Dunitz Publishing.

Verhey, F. R., Ponds, R. W., Rozendaal, N. & Jolles, J. (1995). Depression, insight, and personality changes in Alzheimer's disease and vascular dementia. *Journal of Geriatrics, Psychiatry and Neurology*, **8**, 23–7.

Weiner, M. F., Martin-Cook, K., Foster, B. M. *et al.* (2000). Effects of donepezil on emotional/behavioural symptoms in Alzheimer's disease patients. *Journal of Clinical Psychiatry*, **61**, 487–92.

Wermuth, L., Sorensen, P. S., Timm, B. *et al.* (1998). Depression in idiopathic Parkinson's disease treated with citalopram – a placebo controlled trial. *Nordic Journal of Psychiatry*, **52**, 163–9.

Wiart, L., Petit, H., Joseph, P. A. *et al.* (2000). Fluoxetine in early post-stroke depression: a double-blind placebo-controlled study. *Stroke*, **31**, 1829–32.

Workman, R. H., Jr., Orengo, C. A., Bakey, A. A., Molinari, V. A. & Kunik, M. E. (1997). The use of risperidone for psychosis and agitation in demented patients with Parkinson's disease. *Journal of Neuropsychiatry and Clinical Neurosciences*, **9**, 594–7.

Wynn, Z. J. & Cummings, J. L. (2004). Cholinesterase inhibitor therapies and neuropsychiatric manifestations of Alzheimer's disease. *Dementia and Geriatric Cognitive Disorders*, **17**, 100–8.

Alcohol

Section editors

Kirk J. Brower and Mike Crawford

13

Psychological treatments of alcohol use disorders

Deirdre Conroy, Kirk J. Brower, Jane Marshall and Mike Crawford

Editor's note

Many interventions appear effective in the treatment of severe alcohol dependence except brief interventions and psychodynamic psychotherapy. Brief interventions are effective in alcohol users at risk to develop problems and in those whose alcohol-related problems are mild to moderate. More severe alcohol usage and subsequent dependence responds to motivational enhancement therapy or motivational interviewing, cognitive-behavioral therapy, and twelve step facilitation therapy. Other behavior therapies and couples and marital therapies are also effective here. In the USA, psychodynamic psychotherapy (for which there is very little if any evidence for effectiveness) is probably the most common form of therapy for alcohol misuse conducted outside formal alcohol treatment programs, while twelve step facilitation therapy is probably the most common form of treatment conducted within alcohol treatment programs. In the UK, motivational interviewing is the predominant mode of therapy.

Introduction

Treatment for alcohol dependence is usually composed of three phases: management of the alcohol withdrawal syndrome, motivation for and initiation of abstinence, and prevention of relapse. Both pharmacological and psychosocial interventions are used in the prevention of relapse, either separately or in combination. These interventions do not operate in a clinical vacuum, and their effectiveness is associated with a number of variables, including pre-morbid client/patient characteristics; severity of alcohol dependence; therapist characteristics and the process of treatment delivery. Treatment outcomes are likely to be different in different countries. For instance, European outcomes have historically been less favorable than outcomes in the USA. Although severe alcohol problems are chronic and intermittent, randomized studies have not been designed to study the long-term treatment perspective. Most studies assess treatment interventions between 1–3 months duration with 1-year follow-up. There is a need for long-term studies. In this chapter we focus on the psychosocial treatments. The pharmacological treatments have been addressed in another chapter.

Psychological treatments, which include psychosocial and behavioral treatments, involve a professional relationship between a therapist and a patient who work together to accomplish specific improvements in behavior, thinking, mood regulation and self-esteem. They constitute the primary professional interventions for alcohol dependence, whereas pharmacotherapy and other interventions are generally thought of as adjunctive to psychological treatment. Treatment goals that include sobriety or moderate drinking, depend on a thorough assessment of the patient's drinking history and severity of problems, drinking diagnosis (abuse vs. dependence), co-occurring medical and psychiatric disorders, readiness to change, and psychosocial stressors and supports. How to conduct these assessments is beyond the scope of this book and is reviewed elsewhere (Brower & Severin, 1997), but screening for and assessment of at-risk drinking, alcohol abuse, and alcohol dependence should be an essential part of standard healthcare in all relevant clinical settings (NIAAA, 2007).

The behavioral and psychosocial interventions are essentially "talking therapies", based on conceptual models of addiction, which can be delivered on a one-to-one basis, in a group setting, or as part of a couples/family therapy approach. Elements of effective treatments are aimed at building motivation, enabling behavioral change and modifying the social context. They are thought to enable or enhance the naturally occurring processes of recovery. It can sometimes be difficult to distinguish between some of these interventions, so it is important for definitions of treatments as well as the severity of the alcohol use disorder in the target group to be defined clearly both in systematic reviews and meta-analyses.

In this chapter, we review a range of psychological treatments for which there is an evidence base including brief intervention (BI), motivational enhancement therapy (MET), cognitive-behavioral therapy (CBT), twelve step facilitation (TSF) therapy, interactional group therapy, contingency management, cue exposure therapy, behavioral couples therapy, and family/network-based interventions, It is interesting that although psychodynamic therapies have less supporting evidence, they are commonly used in the USA so they will be discussed. Some other psychological therapies are discussed in the chapter on Complex Interventions because they are either multidimensional (e.g. community reinforcement approach) or designed to be used in combination with medication (e.g. medical management). Alcoholics Anonymous (AA) does not strictly meet the definition of a psychological therapy because it does not involve a relationship with a professional therapist. Alcoholics Anonymous is discussed in the chapter on Complex Interventions because of its multidimensional nature.

Brief interventions

Introduction

Overall the evidence indicates that screening and brief intervention (SBI) is effective in reducing excessive alcohol consumption to safer levels (Moyer *et al.*, 2002). Brief interventions (BIs) are designed to be conducted by health professionals who typically do not specialize in addiction treatment such as in general medical and other primary care settings. Brief interventions generally consist of four or fewer visits that range from a few minutes to an hour in duration. They are used for preventing alcohol-related problems in heavy drinkers at risk to develop those problems and for acute intervention for patients with established alcohol use disorders. They are not primarily used as a maintenance therapy for alcohol use disorders. For at-risk drinkers and patients with alcohol problems of low to moderate severity (i.e. alcohol abuse or mild alcohol dependence), the goals of BI include either moderate drinking or abstinence to prevent the development of more severe problems. For patients with moderate-to-

severe alcohol problems or dependence, the goals are abstinence and acceptance of an addiction specialty referral when indicated (Bien *et al.*, 1993; Graham & Fleming, 1998; O'Connor & Schottenfeld, 1998). When BIs are targeted at non-treatment-seeking populations by non-specialists, they are referred to as opportunistic (Moyer *et al.*, 2002).

Although brief interventions are sometimes discussed as a homogeneous category of interventions, they are considerably heterogeneous and vary along a number of different dimensions. The content of brief interventions for alcohol misuse varies but generally includes features incorporated in the acronym 'FRAMES': **F**eedback about the adverse effects of alcohol, an emphasis on personal **R**esponsibility for changing drinking behavior, **A**dvice about reducing or abstaining from alcohol consumption, a **M**enu of options for further help to meet treatment goals, an **E**mpathic stance towards the patient, and an emphasis on **S**elf-efficacy (Miller & Rollnick, 1991). For example, BIs may differ in intensity from a single 5-minute session of simple advice to stop drinking (World Health Organization (WHO), 1996) to multiple sessions lasting up to 60 minutes each. Brief interventions also differ in terms of the therapeutic techniques utilized. Some BIs are based on the techniques of motivational interviewing (Dunn *et al.*, 2001) and involve personalized feedback about drinking-related consequences, an emphasis on personal responsibility and self-efficacy, and negotiated goals and methods for change, in addition to direct advice (Miller & Rollnick, 1991). Other BIs involve brief cognitive-behavioral counseling techniques (Israel *et al.*, 1996) or simple advice as mentioned above.

The essential techniques or effective ingredients of BIs are not known. They may be delivered in a variety of different clinical and non-clinical settings to drinkers with varying degrees of problem severity by professionals of different disciplines. Thus, when evaluating the effectiveness of BIs or making recommendations about their use, one must consider what type of BI, to which population, in which setting, by which type of professional (Moyer *et al.*, 2002). A number of published articles and manuals on techniques have been developed to guide clinicians at providing BIs (Dunn *et al.*, 1997; Dimeff *et al.*, 1999; US Department of Health and Human Services, 2003).

While best studied for use in general practice and primary care settings, BIs have also been studied in emergency departments, trauma centers, obstetrics clinics, general hospitals, and psychiatric clinics. In the UK, these brief interventions involve a screening for alcohol misuse and are referred to as screening and brief interventions (SBI). Brief interventions have also been used in non-medical settings, particularly college campuses (Marlatt *et al.*, 1998; Larimer *et al.*, 2001; McNally *et al.*, 2005). They are not typically used in addiction-specialized settings, where the problem severity of patients usually warrants more intensive treatment strategies (Chick *et al.*, 1988; Moyer *et al.*, 2002).

A Consensus Panel of US Department of Health and Human Services recommended BI as a first line of treatment in primary health clinics (US Department of Health and Human Services, 2003). Similarly, the US Preventive Services Task Force recommended BI in primary care settings to reduce harmful alcohol use (Whitlock *et al.*, 2004). Despite their efficacy as reviewed below, BIs are underused in primary, emergency, and trauma care treatment settings in both the USA (Burman *et al.*, 2004) and the UK (Babor & Higgins-Biddle, 2000). Clinicians may lack knowledge, confidence, skills, workplace support, and time to provide them, or they may have negative attitudes towards problem drinkers and the effectiveness of BI (Danielsson *et al.*, 1999; Babor & Higgins-Biddle, 2000; Graham *et al.*, 2000; Aalto *et al.*, 2003; Anderson *et al.*, 2003, 2004; Barry *et al.*, 2004). Moreover, insurance companies in the US do not reimburse for BIs and may even deny coverage for alcohol-related injuries (Rivara *et al.*, 2000). The Scottish Intercollegiate Guidelines Network (2003) recommended that, in family practice settings, healthcare professionals should opportunistically identify hazardous and harmful drinkers and deliver a brief intervention. But in the UK, the lack of policy direction on the part of the government (Cabinet Office, 2004) means that the necessary incentives and encouragement for healthcare workers have not been put in place.

Evidence

Brief interventions are well-studied, and multiple reviews and meta-analyses of BIs have been published (Bien *et al.*, 1993; Wilk *et al.*, 1997; Poikolainen, 1999; Dunn *et al.*, 2001; D'Onofrio & Degutis, 2002; Miller & Wilbourne, 2002; Moyer *et al.*, 2002; Beich *et al.*, 2003; Daeppen 2003; Ballesteros *et al.*, 2004; Whitlock *et al.*, 2004). Brief interventions have been shown to be more effective than no treatment at all in reducing alcohol use (Bien *et al.*, 1993; US Department of Health and Human Services, 1993; Kahan *et al.*, 1995; Wilk *et al.*, 1997; Moyer *et al.*, 2002). Brief interventions are also cost-effective (Wutzke *et al.*, 2001; Fleming *et al.*, 2002; Gentilello *et al.*, 2005). A meta-analysis of 12 randomized control trials that met a set of criteria (adult subjects, sample sizes greater than 30, randomized control design, and incorporation of BI) was conducted by Wilk *et al.* (1997) to address BIs in heavy alcohol drinkers. The analysis demonstrated that those receiving

BI were two times more likely to moderate their drinking. They also calculated a combined odds ratio of close to 2 (1.91; 95% CI: 1.61–2.27) in favor of brief alcohol interventions over no interventions irrespective of gender, intensity of intervention, and type of clinical setting.

Some studies suggest that the effects of BIs are sustained over time. Randomized controlled trials have shown approximately a 10–30% reduction in the total amount of alcohol consumed and in the frequency of binge drinking by patients in the year following BI compared with the control groups (WHO, 1996; Fleming *et al.*, 1997; Wallace *et al.*, 1988; Fleming & Manwell, 1999; Gentilello *et al.*, 1999; Ockene *et al.*, 1999). Physiological changes, such as reductions in blood pressure readings (Wallace *et al.*, 1988; Maheswaran *et al.*, 1992), gamma glutamyl transferase (GGT) levels (Wallace *et al.*, 1988; Maheswaran *et al.*, 1992; Israel *et al.*, 1996), and psychosocial problems (Israel *et al.*, 1996) have also been reported at 1-year follow-up visits. Fleming *et al.* (2002) found that with the appropriate follow up, the positive effects of BI can continue for as long as 4 years after initial intervention. Without regular follow-up, however, another study found positive effects only at 9 months but not at 10 years (Wutzke *et al.*, 2002). Moreover, a meta-analysis of 34 controlled trials found that effect sizes for BIs decrease with increasing duration of follow-up (Moyer *et al.*, 2002).

Although there is general consensus about the efficacy of BI and SBI, some criticisms of the evidence should be noted. Beich *et al.* (2003) conducted a meta-analysis of eight randomized controlled trials to address the question of whether or not screening techniques in general practice settings were effective in identifying harmful users of alcohol as well as those who would benefit from BIs. Of 1000 screened patients, 90 screened positive and required further assessment. Of those 90 patients, 25 qualified for BI. In a 1-year follow-up visit, 2 patients (95% CI = 1.7–3.4) reported that they drank less than the recommended level. Although the authors agreed that BI can reduce heavy drinking, they concluded that screening for BI in general practice resulted in very few positive outcomes.

An analysis conducted by Edwards & Rollnick (1997) found that the attrition rate of eligible subjects during BI studies varied between 44% and 83% (mean 70.6%) with more heavy drinkers dropping out of the study and thereby exaggerating treatment effects compared with what might be observed in general practice. Wilk *et al.* (1997) reported that some authors provided inadequate details in their assignment of participants to intervention and control groups. According to Schulz *et al.* (1995), depending on the methodological flaws of controlled studies in general, odds ratios could be exaggerated by as much as 17–40%.

Primary care

Over 20 randomized controlled studies of BI in primary care have been conducted, and selected studies will be reviewed here. At least five large randomized controlled studies (> 500 subjects) have revealed that BIs can be successful when implemented in the primary care setting or the family practice setting. Wallace *et al.* (1988) randomly assigned 909 patients to either BI or standard care groups. After one year, the treatment group significantly reduced alcohol consumption compared to the control group. The World Health Organization (WHO, 1996) randomized 1559 heavy drinkers (81% male) to either simple advice (5 minutes), brief counseling (20-minute visit), or no intervention, and reported that both intervention groups significantly reduced alcohol consumption after nine months in men compared with the control group, but found no difference between groups in women. Fleming *et al.* (1997) randomized 774 patients after training physicians affiliated with a Health Maintenance Organization to give two 10–15 minute BI sessions to patients who scored positively on a screening survey. Nurses checked in with the patients by placing 5-minute follow-up phone calls. After one year, both patients receiving treatment and controls reduced their alcohol consumption but the group receiving BI showed a greater reduction. In a 48-month follow-up of 205 women from that study, alcohol consumption was significantly reduced in the BI compared with the control group (Manwell *et al.*, 2000). Similarly, Ockene *et al.* (1999) randomized 530 patients and examined the effects of 5–10 minutes of BI provided by a primary care physician or nurse practitioner compared with a standard care group. Weekly alcohol consumption decreased in both groups but the group receiving BI had a significantly larger reduction. Wutzke *et al.* (2002) randomized 554 heavy and problem drinkers to either a no-treatment control group or one of three BI groups that differed in duration from 5 to 60 minutes. At 9 months, all three BI groups significantly reduced their alcohol consumption compared with the control group but BI duration had no effect.

Richmond *et al.* (1995) randomized 378 patients to four groups including an assessment only, assessment + one BI visit, assessment + five BI visits, or neither assessment nor BI. At 6 months, there were no differences between groups in terms of alcohol consumption but the five-visit BI group had significantly fewer alcohol-related problems. Other studies of BI in a primary care setting have shown that BI in the form of attempted referrals (Elvy *et al.*, 1988) or general advice to reduce alcohol (Maheswaran *et al.*, 1992) is helpful in reducing the amount of alcohol consumed after treatment.

General hospitals

Emmen *et al.* (2004) reviewed the effectiveness of "opportunistic brief interventions" for problem drinking in general hospital settings in studies published between 1966 and 2001. While seven of the eight studies selected for critical analysis showed a reduction in alcohol consumption in the intervention group, only one study showed a significant reduction. Hulse & Tait (2003) recruited 120 general hospital psychiatric inpatients and randomized them to receive either an alcohol-reduction motivational interview or an information pack. Both interventions were more effective than no intervention when subjects were compared to matched controls.

Emergency departments

Few studies have examined BIs in emergency care settings such as hospital emergency departments (D'Onofrio & Degutis, 2002). An uncontrolled study of 1096 problem drinkers with a 22% follow-up rate at 60–90 days found reductions of 56% and 64%, respectively, for alcohol use and heavy drinking after a 15–20 minute BI based on motivational interviewing (MI) (Bernstein *et al.*, 1997). Among teenagers (ages 18 or 19 years old) treated in the emergency department (ED) for alcohol-related injuries, both the BI group and the control group decreased their alcohol consumption, but the BI group had fewer alcohol-related problems (i.e. drinking and driving and alcohol-related injuries) (Monti *et al.*, 1999). Another randomized controlled trial of adolescents in the ED for an alcohol-related event had better outcomes than standard care only if they screened positive for alcohol-related problems prior to the ED episode (Spirito *et al.*, 2004), but a randomized controlled trial of 655 adolescents with ED visits for minor injury revealed no significant differences in drinking outcomes at 3 and 12 months following a computer-based brief intervention (Maio *et al.*, 2005). Longabaugh *et al.* (2001) randomized 539 heavy and problem drinkers to either a motivational enhancement therapy (MET)-based BI with or without a booster session 7–10 days later or to a no-intervention control group. (See below for a fuller discussion of MET.) At 1-year, with 83% follow-up, the booster session group had significantly fewer alcohol-related injuries and other problems than the other two groups, although reduction of alcohol intake was not significantly different across the three groups. A randomized trial among 599 patients BI-plus-leaflet versus a leaflet-alone condition significantly reduced the number of weekly drinks at 6 months among the BI group, but not at 12 months, but the BI group had fewer ED visits over that year (Crawford *et al.*, 2004).

Medical and surgical clinics

Gentilello *et al.* (1999) examined alcohol intake of patients that were admitted to a trauma unit for "treatment of injuries." Patients who screened positive for alcohol problems via blood alcohol concentration, serum GGT levels and a questionnaire were randomly assigned to a control group (n = 396) or to a BI group (n = 363). Intervention groups received one motivational interview by a trained psychologist, and patients were also provided with feedback and suggestions on how to reduce alcohol consumption. After 6 months, patients in the BI group had 47% fewer new injuries and reduced their alcohol consumption by 22 drinks versus a reduction of only 7 drinks in the control group. The difference was most pronounced in patients with mild to moderate alcohol problems, and one year later, patients in the BI group continued to significantly reduce alcohol consumption compared with the control groups. Significant drinking reductions were observed over a 1-year period in a surgical clinic after a single session of BI based on motivational interviewing among 150 randomized outpatients with facial injuries (Smith *et al.*, 2003). Chang *et al.* (1999, 2005) found no difference between BI and assessment among 250 women except for the subgroup of women who entered the study abstinent who did better with BI. In another study, a single session of BI was most effective for the women with the heaviest drinking and whose partners participated in the intervention. Manwell *et al.* (2000), in a primary care clinic, found a significant effect of BI in women of childbearing age (18–40) especially among those who became pregnant during a 48-month follow-up period. Brief intervention has also proved to be a useful intervention in lowering alcohol consumption as well as blood pressure in a hypertension clinic (Maheswaran *et al.*, 1992; Fleming *et al.*, 2004).

Non-clinical settings

Randomized controlled studies of brief interventions have also been conducted on college campuses (Borsari & Carey, 2000; Ingersoll *et al.*, 2005; Larimer *et al.*, 2001; Marlatt *et al.*, 1998; Murphy *et al.*, 2001) and in the workplace (Richmond *et al.*, 2000) with promising results.

Predictors of success

Age

Fleming *et al.* (1997) found no difference in drinking reduction by age group ranging from 18 to 65 in their large-scale, primary care trial. Adolescents (Monti *et al.*, 1999), college students (Larimer *et al.*, 2001), and older adults (Fleming & Manwell, 1999) have all benefited from BI.

Gender

Some studies suggest that men may be more responsive to BIs than women (Scott & Anderson, 1990; Anderson & Scott, 1992; Babor & Grant, 1992; WHO, 1996), and other studies found that women responded better than men (Poikolainen, 1999; Richmond *et al.*, 2000), and several published meta-analyses found equal outcomes for men and women (Ballesteros *et al.*, 2004; Chang, 2002; Moyer *et al.*, 2002; Wilk *et al.*, 1997). Pregnant women (Chang et al., 2005; Manwell *et al.*, 2000) and women at risk to become pregnant (Ingersoll *et al.*, 2005) have had good outcomes with BI.

Patient motivation

Brief intervention, especially when based on motivational interviewing (Dunn *et al.*, 2001), is designed for effectiveness with patients not necessarily motivated to change their drinking behavior. As expected, higher levels of motivation predicted better outcomes in response to BI among young adults presenting to an emergency department (Leontieva *et al.*, 2005).

Duration of brief intervention

Duration of BI therapy has varied across study protocols published in the last 20 years but overall, in general, success does not depend on duration. The shortest intervention has been approximately 30 seconds with the physician simply recommending that the patient should stop drinking (Senft *et al.*, 1997) with other brief inteventions of 5–10 minutes (Wallace *et al.*, 1988; Scott & Anderson, 1990), 10–20 minutes (Aalto *et al.*, 2000, 2001; Babor & Grant 1992; Maheswaran *et al.*, 1992; Rowland & Maynard, 1993; Fleming *et al.*, 1997; Cordoba *et al.*, 1998; Watson, 1999 Manwell *et al.*, 2000), or 30 minutes (McIntosh *et al.*, 1997). Longer interventions typically range between 30 and 75 minutes (Chick *et al.*, 1985; Elvy *et al.*, 1988; Heather *et al.*, 1996). Brief interventions ranging from 5 minutes to 30 minutes have yielded similar reductions in drinking and associated negative effects of drinking. To illustrate, Maheswaran *et al.* (1992) found that 10–15 minutes of physician advice to male inpatients at a hypertension clinic was successful in significantly reducing alcohol consumption, GGT levels and diastolic blood pressure. Ten minutes of BI has been shown to significantly reduce alcohol consumption for 6 months (Ockene *et al.*, 1999) to one year

(Scott & Anderson 1990) following treatment. In a family practice setting, at 1-year follow-up, there was a general reduction of the quantity and frequency of drinking in both 5 and 30 minute intervention groups, but no statistical difference was found between the two groups (McIntosh *et al.*, 1997). Shakeshaft *et al.* (2002) found no difference in effectiveness between a 90-minute brief intervention based on the FRAMES techniques and six-weekly 45-minute sessions of cognitive-behavioral therapy in a randomized sample of 295 patients with alcohol abuse, although a low follow-up rate at 6 months (45%) limits the findings. Wutzke *et al.* (2002) found no difference between three BI groups with durations ranging from 5 to 60 minutes, and a meta-analysis of 20 studies comparing BI to extended treatment in treatment seekers found no overall differences (Moyer *et al.*, 2002).

Provider characteristics

Studies have been conducted with physicians, nurses, counselors, addiction specialists, or psychologists in order to test whether the professional discipline of the person that conducts the intervention makes a difference on patient outcome. But only one study performed a randomized comparison between two professional disciplines. McIntosh *et al.* (1997) randomized patients in a family practice setting to two 30-minute CBT informed BIs by either a nurse practitioner or a physician. There was no difference in effect between the two disciplines. Computer-based brief interventions have not been shown to be effective (Daniels *et al.*, 1992; Maio *et al.*, 2005).

Summary

Brief interventions are recommended for reduction of alcohol use for patients across age and gender who are heavy or problem drinkers who do not meet criteria for severe alcohol dependence. Although opportunistic BIs are best studied in primary care settings, evidence also supports their use in general hospitals, emergency departments, trauma centers, and some specialty clinics such as obstetrics. Brief interventions are effective when conducted by health professionals of diverse disciplines, but non-physicians may be more likely to provide them and nurses in particular should probably receive preferential training (Smith *et al.*, 2003). Brief interventions are also recommended in non-clinical settings for college students and workplace employees.

Motivational enhancement therapy (MET)

Introduction

Motivational enhancement therapy, an intervention based on motivational interviewing (Miller & Rollnick, 1991) and the stages-of-change model first proposed by Prochaska & DiClemente (1984, 1992), shares characteristics with Rogerian client-centered counseling. Motivational enhancement therapy was developed as an alternative to commonly used but comparatively ineffective directive-confrontational counseling for substance use disorders (Miller *et al.*, 1993). In MET, the clinician seeks to create a non-judgemental and respectful atmosphere while employing persuasive strategies for motivating patients to change their (drinking) behaviors. It differs from behavioral therapies which prescribe how the patient should make that change by teaching new skills and reinforcing recovery-sustaining behaviors. Instead, MET encourages patients to utilize their own skills and resources for change. Once the patient has expressed motivation for change, set an appropriate goal for change (such as abstinence), and formulated a plan for making that change, the major work of MET is completed. Motivational enhancement therapy leaves the patient with the responsibility to effect his or her own change. The style of the therapist or clinician in managing resistance to change plays a significant role in the success of MET. Confrontation is avoided. Resistance is viewed as the opposite of motivation and signals to the therapist that a change in strategy is needed. At times MET and motivational interviewing (MI) are terms used interchangeably.

Some BIs (discussed above) are based on MI techniques (Miller & Rollnick, 1991; Dunn *et al.*, 1997), but BIs may be distinguished from MET in at least two ways. First, MET was designed for patients seeking treatment for alcohol dependence (Miller *et al.*, 1995a) and is typically provided by clinicians with addiction-specialized training, whereas BIs were designed primarily for patients seen in other treatment settings to be provided by clinicians not specialized in addiction treatment. Second, MET was manualized for Project MATCH as a 4-session therapeutic intervention (Miller *et al.*, 1995b), whereas BIs based on MI are typically briefer and range from one to three sessions.

In 2004, a survey conducted on the practices of 89 clinicians from 24 public addiction treatment programs in the USA found that utilization of MET received a score of 4.11 on a scale of 1–5 with 1 = "rarely or never" and 5 = "almost always or always", suggesting a relatively high rate of use (McGovern *et al.*, 2004).

Evidence

Motivational enhancement therapy was found to be effective in 12 out of 17 studies in one review (Miller & Wilbourne, 2002). Project MATCH is one of the largest and most influential randomized trials to have examined psychosocial interventions for people with alcohol-related problems. The study involved randomizing over 1700 patients attending 10 treatment centers in North America to MET, Cognitive-behaviour therapy (CBT) or twelve step facilitation (TSF). Four sessions of MET were delivered over a 12-week period and outcomes among those randomized to MET were broadly the same as those achieved with CBT and TSF (Project MATCH Research Group, 1993, 1997a, 1997b, 1998a, 1998b). Project MATCH demonstrated that four sessions of standalone MET at the beginning of treatment or as an aftercare treatment were as effective for treating alcohol dependence as 12 sessions of CBT or TSF therapy, and that the benefits from treatment persisted for up to 3 years. Evidence also suggested that high levels of anger among outpatients at the beginning of treatment predicted better outcomes with MET than with CBT and/or TSF at both 1 and 3 years (Project MATCH Research Group, 1997b, 1998a). A subsequent evaluation of economic outcomes concluded that MET is more cost-effective than CBT or TSF for those with good prognostic factors (i.e. absence of associated mental health problems and a social network that does not support drinking; Holder et al., 2000). Cognitive-behaviour therapy and TSF will be discussed below.

Motivational enhancement therapy has also been shown to augment treatment success when combined or integrated with other treatment strategies. Sellman and colleagues (2001) randomly assigned patients with mild to moderate alcohol dependence to either MET, nondirective reflective listening (NDRL), or no further counseling (NFC) groups. All patients received an education/feedback session before randomization. Outcome was heavy drinking at 6 months following the end of treatment. Patients that underwent MET had the lowest percentage of heavy drinkers (43% MET, 63% NDRL, 65% NFC; $P = 0.04$). Lincour et al. (2002) studied 167 court-ordered patients, 80% of whom had either alcohol abuse or dependence, in a non-randomized controlled clinical trial. Patients who received six group sessions of MET prior to standard treatment attended a significantly higher proportion of their standard treatment sessions and were more likely to have completed standard treatment than patients who did not receive MET. Substance use outcomes were not reported.

Motivational enhancement therapy has also been applied with some success to specialized populations such as substance-abusing adolescents (Tevyaw & Monti, 2004) and patients comorbid for schizophrenia and alcohol use disorders (Graeber et al., 2003). Barrowclough et al. (2001) reported that integrating motivational interviewing, cognitive-behavioral therapy, and family intervention was also effective in treating substance-abusing patients with schizophrenia. Motivational enhancement therapy has been provided in both individual and group therapy formats without differences in outcome (John et al., 2003), although more studies are required to determine if selected patients do better in one format or the other.

A meta-analysis of randomized trials of motivational interviewing by Burke and colleagues (2003) identified 15 trials of MI for people with alcohol-related problems. The overall effect size of people receiving MET having short-term reductions in alcohol consumption equivalent to 20 fewer drinks per week was 0.82.

Summary

Motivational enhancement therapy as a manualized therapy developed for Project MATCH is not as well studied as BIs based on motivational interviewing techniques (Vasilaki et al., 2006). Moreover, the Project MATCH trial has been criticized for its lack of a no-treatment control group and, thus, unclear attribution of good outcomes to therapy per se (Cutler & Fishbain, 2005). Nevertheless, the existing evidence suggests that MET is effective in treatment-seeking alcohol-dependent patients with high levels of anger or resistance to treatment, and that either a group or individual format may be used.

Cognitive-behavioral therapy (CBT)

Introduction

Cognitive-behavioral therapy is a group of therapies based on social learning theory that has been given various names depending on the investigators who developed them and some differences in emphasis. These include relapse prevention strategies (Marlatt & Donovan, 2005), coping skills therapy (Monti et al., 1989), social skills training (Oei & Jackson, 1980; Monti, 2003), cognitive-behavioral coping-skills training (Longabaugh & Morgenstern, 1999), and communication skills training (Monti et al., 1990). Cognitive-behavioral therapy is employed both for abstinence-based treatment of alcohol dependence and for moderation-based treatment to reduce alcohol consumption and related problems (Marlatt & Witkiewitz, 2002). The focus of CBT is to identify and improve any deficits in skills or maladaptive thoughts that the patient may have which could lead to either a lapse to any drinking or a relapse to heavy drinking during a high-risk situation. It also teaches people who misuse alcohol to focus efforts on improving problem solving and how to avoid "alcohol cues" which lead to resumption of drinking following periods of abstinence (Morgenstern & Longabaugh, 2000). Thus, patients are encouraged to learn new behaviors and thought patterns that will help them to cope with stress and problems other than by relying on alcohol. A number of manuals are available to guide therapists in providing CBT to their patients (Monti *et al.*, 1989; Kadden *et al.*, 1994).

In 1996, there were an estimated 12 387 alcohol and drug treatment facilities in the USA. The Alcohol and Drug Services Study (SAMHSA, 2003) surveyed a nationally representative sample of 2395 of these, including the following types of programs: hospital inpatient, non-hospital residential, outpatient methadone, and outpatient non-methadone. Relapse prevention group therapy was offered at 78.8% of facilities. In a survey of leaders of 174 Department of Veterans Affairs (VA) addiction treatment programs, over 95% rated the evidence for CBT as either medium (25.6%) or high (69.8%). Ninety-three percent agreed that it should be routinely recommended, and 61.4% rated the level of implementation in their programs as high (Willenbring *et al.*, 2004). Eighty-nine clinicians from 24 public addiction treatment programs found that utilization of CBT and relapse prevention therapy received scores of 4.09 and 4.23, respectively, on a scale of 1–5 with 1 = "rarely or never" and 5 = "almost always or always" (McGovern *et al.*, 2004). Overall, the extent of use of CBT for substance use disorders in specialized treatment facilities in both the USA and the UK is high.

Evidence

Several comprehensive reviews support the efficacy of CBT for treating alcohol use disorders (Holder *et al.*, 1991; Irvin *et al.*, 1999; Kadden, 2001; McCrady, 2000). Irvin *et al.* (1999) calculated an effect size of 0.37 based on 10 studies using the weighted averaged correlation coefficient. Cognitive-behavioral therapy has been shown to be similarly effective in reducing alcohol consumption both in individual and in group formats (Oei & Jackson 1980; Irvin *et al.*, 1999; Marques & Formigoni, 2001) as well as in inpatient and outpatient settings (Irvin *et al.*, 1999). Although CBT theoretically works by

increasing coping skills, this has been difficult to prove empirically (Morgenstern & Longabaugh, 2000).

When CBT is compared with other active treatments in randomly assigned trials, it tends to produce similar outcomes with respect to main effects (Kadden *et al.*, 1989; Litt *et al.*, 2003; Project MATCH Research Group, 1997a). This may be due in part to non-specific effects of psychotherapy or to the increase in coping skills that occurs with other psychosocial therapies even if those therapies do not directly focus on coping skills (e.g., Litt *et al.*, 2003). One exception to similar outcomes was a small randomized trial of 47 outpatients that found better drinking outcomes for CBT than family systems therapy, although both therapies included the patient's spouse/partner (Karno *et al.*, 2002).

Research has aimed to determine which patients might best benefit from CBT. Analyses from the Project MATCH Research Group (1998b) where the CBT emphasized coping skills and social skills, suggested that among patients initially entering outpatient treatment, CBT more quickly reduced heavy drinking and alcohol-related consequences than MET. Thus, CBT may be best for patients that require rapid change. Other evidence from Project MATCH suggests that CBT may be most suitable for outpatients with low levels of anger and aftercare patients with low levels of dependence severity. Specifically, outpatients low in anger did better at 1 and 3 years with CBT than MET, whereas the opposite was true for outpatients high in anger (Project MATCH Research Group, 1998a). Aftercare patients with low levels of dependence did better with CBT than TSF at the 1-year follow-up, whereas the opposite was true for patients with high levels of dependence (Project MATCH Research Group, 1997b). Outpatients with low levels of psychiatric severity did worse with CBT than TSF at one year (Project MATCH Research Group, 1997a), but not at three years (Project MATCH Research Group, 1998a). No differences were seen between therapies for patients high in psychiatric severity. Complementing Project MATCH, a large (n = 3018), naturalistic comparison of VA inpatient programs using predominantly CBT, TSF, or combined CBT-TSF approaches, in general, found no differences in outcomes (Ouimette *et al.*, 1997).

Matching effects have also been used to compare CBT with interactional group therapy. Patients randomly assigned had better outcomes with CBT if they scored higher on sociopathy and global psychopathology or were classified as Type B alcoholics, whereas outcomes with interactional therapy were better for patients with cognitive impairment or classified with Type A alcoholism (Kadden *et al.*, 1989; Cooney *et al.*, 1991). Another randomized study found that antisocial personality disorder patients also responded better to CBT than to relationship enhancement treatment (Longabaugh *et al.*, 1994), but this was not found in a study by Kalman *et al.* (2000). Kadden *et al.* (2001) found mixed results when random assignment was compared to prospective matching of patients on the basis of psychopathology and sociopathy. Matching effects were not observed especially for drinking consumption; however, drinking-related adverse consequences were lower when patients with high levels of psychopathology were prospectively matched to CBT. Another study of patients randomly assigned to CBT vs. interactional therapy found no differences between treatment types but did find increases in coping skills that predicted good drinking outcomes, regardless of treatment type (Litt *et al.*, 2003).

Monti *et al.* (1990) non-randomly assigned cohorts of male VA inpatients to communication skills training (with or without family participation) or to cognitive-behavioral mood management training. Although all three therapies were CBT variants, communication skills training focused on interpersonal skills for dealing with high-risk situations while mood management training focused on coping with negative internal events such as urges to drink and anxiety. Patients who received communication skills training drank significantly less on drinking days over a 6-month follow-up period than patients who received the cognitive-behavioral mood management approach, but no differences in abstinence rates or time to relapse were noted. Rohsenow and colleagues (1991) concluded that communication skills training was (1) effective regardless of educational level, marital status, initial level of coping skills, anxiety symptoms, and urges to drink, and (2) differentially more effective than mood management training for patients with lower education, more anxiety, and greater urges to drink.

Cognitive therapy in isolation, without the behavioral aspects of treatment, has generally not been found to be as efficacious as treatment that addresses both areas (Holder *et al.*, 1991). In a review by Miller & Wilbourne in 2002, positive findings were reported in 40% of the studies reviewed that employed cognitive therapy alone whereas 49% of the studies employing self-control training (which incorporates cognitive strategies) had positive findings.

Summary

Cognitive-behavioral therapy for alcohol dependence is effective for both abstinence and harm reduction (Marlatt & Witkiewitz, 2002) especially when compared with no treatment or minimal treatment control groups.

There is little evidence that different variants of CBT are superior to one another or to other active treatments such as TSF, MET, and interactional therapy. Similarly, there is little evidence that matching patients to specific treatments on the basis of sociopathy or general psychopathology is particularly effective. On the other hand, CBT effectively increases coping skills in many studies, which are linked to better outcomes.

Twelve step facilitation (TSF) therapy

Introduction

Twelve step facilitation therapy, also tested in Project MATCH, is designed to familiarize patients with, and to encourage attendance at, twelve-step meetings, especially Alcoholics Anonymous (AA). It differs from AA in that TSF is a professionally delivered treatment designed mostly to introduce the patient to AA concepts and facilitate attendance at AA meetings, but it does not re-create the structure or strategies of AA itself. The evidence base for AA per se is reviewed in Chapter 16, but it is important to mention that patients who participate in AA or programs based on AA have better drinking outcomes (Vaillant 1983; Cross *et al.*, 1990; McCrady, 1998; Ouimette *et al.*, 1998; Project MATCH Research Group, 1998a; Humphreys *et al.*, 1999; Timko *et al.*, 2000). In contrast to AA, TSF is not viewed as a complex therapy because it does not employ multiple components and strategies to target a large number of different problem areas associated with alcoholism. The evidence for TSF efficacy, therefore, focuses both on attendance at AA as well as drinking behaviors.

The TSF psychotherapy manual which was designed for Project MATCH, specifies 12 sessions with a clinician/therapist (Nowinsky *et al.*, 1994). If the patient is in a steady relationship, two of these sessions will include the spouse/partner. Two emergency sessions are also provided. Twelve step facilitation therapy is organized into four core topics, six elective topics, and then termination. Patients are usually expected to attend AA meetings daily.

Twelve step facilitation therapy is based on a disease model of alcohol dependence. The clinician emphasizes repeatedly that they, the patients, are powerless over alcohol but that alcoholism is not their fault. Rather, patients were predisposed to develop this disease, similar to being predisposed to hypertension or diabetes. Yet, while it is not the patient's fault that they developed the disease, AA emphasizes that it is the patients' responsibility to take an active part in their recovery. And the best way to do so is to participate in twelve–step groups.

Twelve step facilitation therapy is the most common form of specialized treatment for alcoholism in the USA. Most alcohol treatment programs in the USA are based on the Minnesota Model (see Chapter 16 on complex therapies), in which TSF is a core component of treatment. The National Institute of Alcohol Abuse and Alcoholism (NIAAA 2000), reports that in 2000, participation in professional treatment therapy based on a twelve-step program such as AA was the leading treatment approach to alcoholism in the USA. A survey of 89 clinicians from 24 public addiction treatment programs found that utilization of TSF received a score of 3.86 on a scale of 1–5 with 1 = "rarely or never" and 5 = "almost always or always" (McGovern *et al.*, 2004), suggesting its relative popularity in the USA. People in the UK are often advised to seek treatment from programs such as AA, but TSF as a formal approach to treatment is much less commonly used than MI and CBT approaches.

Evidence

The Project MATCH study and smaller patient matching studies provide the support for the effectiveness of TSF programs. Patients in Project MATCH (Project MATCH 1997a, 1998b) who received outpatient TSF were most likely to abstain from alcohol during the first post-treatment year. Twelve step facilitation therapy led to a greater length of time before the patient's first relapse and to a higher percentage of abstinent patients at 1- and 3-year follow-up. Longabaugh *et al.* (1998) found that patients in Project MATCH with social networks supportive of not drinking responded better to TSF than MET, and that participation in AA was a mediator of this effect. Project MATCH (1997a) found that patients who were rated high in "meaning seeking" fared better with TSF than CBT and MET at 1-year follow-up.

In 1997, Ouimette analyzed treatment effects in 15 programs within the US VA Healthcare System that offered TSF, CBT, or a combination of TSF and CBT. Over 3000 patients were non-randomly assigned to one of these three treatments and were followed for one year. After a year, 25% of the patients participating in TSF were abstinent compared with 18% in the CBT and 20% in the mixed therapy group. Morgenstern *et al.* (1997) found that self-efficacy, commitment to abstinence, cognitive coping, behavioral coping, and primary appraisals of harm due to drinking were five patient characteristics that were related to a stronger affiliation with AA as well as a better treatment outcome.

Summary

Twelve step facilitation therapy is an effective therapy for increasing AA attendance and improving drinking outcomes in alcohol-dependent patients. Its effectiveness for problem drinkers and alcohol abuse, in the absence of a diagnosis of dependence, is not established.

Behavioral therapies

Introduction

In general, treatments that emphasize positive reinforcement for targeted behaviors have been shown to be effective in patients with alcohol use disorders (Miller & Hester, 1986; Holder *et al.*, 1991). Behavioral techniques such as behavioral contracting have been shown to be more effective and yield positive effects in 80% of studies reviewed, compared to relaxation training that yielded positive effects in only 17% of studies reviewed (Miller & Wilbourne, 2002). Two major types of behavioral treatments, contingency management (CM) and cue exposure therapy (CET) are discussed below. The community reinforcement approach (CRA), which incorporates elements of behavioral and other therapies, is briefly discussed in Chapter 16. Behavior self-control training is a well-defined treatment package, mainly aimed at promoting controlled drinking. It is probably best restricted to subjects seeking a controlled drinking outcome.

The VA facilities survey of 174 addiction treatment program leaders' opinion of evidence supporting the effectiveness of CM found that 66% rated the strength of evidence as either medium (33.3%) or high (33.3%), 43% agreed that it should be routinely recommended, but only 5.9% rated the level of implementation in their programs as high (Willenbring *et al.*, 2004). The 2004 survey of 89 clinicians from 24 public addiction treatment programs scored utilization of CM as 2.26 on a scale of 1–5 with 1 = "rarely or never" and 5 = "almost always or always" (McGovern *et al.*, 2004), and that suggested a relatively low level of use in the USA. Alternatively, CM is often incorporated into therapeutic communities, which are discussed in Chapter 16.

Use of CET for alcohol use disorders is believed to be low due to limited studies of its efficacy (Monti & Rohsenow, 1999) and the hesitancy of therapists in the USA to expose their patients to actual alcohol-related cues such as its sight, smell, or taste. In the USA, imaginary exposure in combination with CBT is more likely to be practiced than actual exposure with an expectation of simple extinction.

Evidence

Contingency management (CM)

Contingency management (CM) is based on operant conditioning theory. Substance abuse is considered an operant behavior, with the reinforcer being the substance itself and social factors, and CM provides tangible goods or services as a way to modify behavior. Few studies have been conducted for alcohol dependence in contrast to drug dependence (Kadden & Conney, 2005). In a randomized control trial of CM, Petry *et al.* (2000) provided opportunities for patients to win prizes as reinforcers by passing breathalyzer tests and by completing treatment goals. After 8 weeks, 84% of CM patients were retained in treatment compared with 22% receiving standard treatment ($P < 0.001$). One of the limitations of studies that use abstinence as a qualifier of reward in alcoholism research it is that it is difficult to verify because blood, urine, and breath analysis cannot detect alcohol for longer than 12 to 24 hours after intake.

Cue exposure treatment (CET)

Cue exposure treatment (CET) is based on the concept of extinguishing conditioned craving and drinking responses that develop after repeated pairings of urges, drinking, and the neutral stimuli that precede them (Niaura *et al.*, 1988). When patients are exposed to actual cues (e.g. the sight and smell of alcohol), a series of cognitive, emotional, and neurochemical reactions can occur which trigger drinking (Niaura *et al.*, 1988; Monti *et al.*, 1995). Repeated exposure with response prevention may result in extinction of drinking responses to cues. Alternatively, CET may be combined with CBT to teach and encourage the use of coping skills during cue exposure. Another method of exposure asks patients to imagine being in a high-risk situation involving alcohol ("imaginary exposure") (Monti & Rohsenow, 1999).

In a non-randomized, controlled trial of 35 male inpatients, CET delayed latency to heavy drinking ($P < 0.001$) and total alcohol consumption ($P < 0.01$) over a 6-month follow-up period compared with a relaxation control treatment (Drummond & Glautier, 1994). In a study among alcohol-dependent inpatients with a 2×2 design that compared two group treatments (CBT vs. education) in combination with two individual treatments (CET vs. relaxation) there were (1) main effects for CBT and CET in reducing heavy drinking days during 6 months of follow-up, (2) continued reductions after CET in heavy drinking days among patients who drank during the next 6 months of follow-up, and (3) a significant interaction between treatments such that the patients receiving both CET and CBT had the greatest reduction in drinks per drinking day during the second 6 months (Rohsenow *et al.*, 2001). In the UK, randomized trials of both cue exposure therapy (CET) and communication skills training (CST), suggest both approaches can assist people reduce their alcohol consumption (Health Technology Board for Scotland, 2002).

Cue exposure therapy has also been compared with CBT in non-dependent drinkers with alcohol abuse for which moderate drinking was the treatment goal (Sitharthan *et al.*, 1997). Subjects consumed 2–3 drinks during exposure sessions, but were required to resist an additional drink while holding it near their mouths and sniffing it. Cue exposure therapy was more effective than CBT in reducing drinking frequency and consumption over a 6-month period.

Major limitations of CET are (1) the number of cues for drinking may be too large for all of them to be readily identified and extinguished, especially if they operate outside the patient's level of awareness; (2) extinction to one set of cues may not generalize to similar cues when experienced in a different setting; and (3) up to 50% of participants may not show a response to alcohol cues (Litt *et al.*, 1990). A fourth and major limitation of CET is that patients can experience the return of previously conditioned responses when exposed to priming doses of alcohol (Drummond *et al.*, 1990). In fact, not only can drinking reverse extinction fairly rapidly, but it probably increases the difficulty of extinguishing conditioned responses with subsequent CET.

Summary

Despite evidence of its effectiveness, contingency management is underutilized and understudied as a treatment for alcohol dependence. If abstinence was simply its own reward, then CM would not be necessary. While tangible gifts in return for abstinence may seem artificial, we highly recommend helping patients to find alternative rewarding activities that can substitute for drinking alcohol (Vaillant, 1983). Patients will inevitably encounter internal and external cues that trigger urges to drink or actual drinking. We do not believe that extinguishing responses to cues by itself is an effective treatment. Successful treatment also entails utilizing coping skills to deal with those cues. Whether CET adds any additional value to CBT alone in this regard remains unclear, at least in alcohol-dependent patients embracing a goal of total abstinence.

Behavioral couples therapy/behavioral marital therapy

Introduction

Behavioral couples therapy (BCT) and behavioral marital therapy (BMT) refer to treatment approaches that include the partner or spouse of the alcoholic patient in the therapy sessions. It has its roots in both social learning theory and family systems models, and it combines efforts to develop better self-control with the spouses' support of their partners' efforts to reduce alcohol consumption. During weekly sessions, the clinician tries both to identify relationship conflicts that might trigger drinking and to develop reinforcers for abstinence (Epstein & McCrady, 1998). The clinician might also focus on different aspects of the relationship, by trying to help the couple renew their commitments to one another, by improving their communication skills, or by encouraging the couple to increase their activities together (O'Farrell & Fals-Stewart, 2000). The couple may also agree to a "Sobriety Contract," which expresses the patient's intent to stay sober and the partner's or spouse's intent to support the patient's effort. The contract also outlines the patient's commitment to attend Alcoholics Anonymous or take disulfiram if he or she elects to do so (O'Farrell & Fals-Stewart, 2000). The terms BCT and BMT are used interchangeably in this section.

Fals-Stewart and Birchler (2001) surveyed 398 randomly selected outpatient substance abuse treatment programs in the USA and reported that only 27% of the programs offered any type of couples therapy, and less than 5% offered behaviorally oriented couples therapy. In the aforementioned survey of 174 VA addiction treatment program leaders, over 68% rated the strength of evidence for behavioral marital treatment as either medium (32.4%) or high (36.5%). Fifty-three percent agreed that it should be routinely recommended, but only 7.6% rated the level of implementation in their programs as high. The 2004 survey of 89 clinicians from 24 public addiction treatment programs found that utilization of BCT received a score of only 1.6 on a scale of 1–5 with 1 = "rarely or never" and 5 = "almost always or always"(McGovern *et al.*, 2004), suggesting a very low level of use in the USA.

Evidence

A meta-analysis conducted in 2001 found a moderate effect size in 16 controlled trials of BMT (O'Farrell & Fals-Stewart, 2001), and Miller & Wilbourne (2002) found that five of eight BMT studies were effective in reducing drinking. Other marital therapy approaches such as Al-Anon facilitation and disulfiram contracting (Allen & Litten, 1992; Miller *et al.*, 1999a) have also been shown to be effective.

In addition to improved drinking outcomes, a series of studies have assessed levels of domestic violence and verbal aggression in alcoholic men before and after BCT (O'Farrell & Murphy, 1995; O'Farrell *et al.*, 1999, 2000). Couples who underwent BMT/BCT showed reduced male-to-female domestic violence and verbal aggression (O'Farrell & Murphy, 1995; O'Farrell *et al.*, 1999, 2000, 2004). The studies also showed a strong correlation between the reduction in post-treatment drinking and the reduction in the level of domestic violence, which was found to be reduced similar to the level of violence committed by non-alcoholic individuals. However, it should be noted that a large portion of the couples in the study were also participating in a trial of relapse prevention through "booster sessions" in the first year of treatment. Therefore, they received more treatment than the standard care.

O'Farrell *et al.* (2004) conducted a follow-up study which focused on violence and aggression among male alcoholic patients and their female partners in the year before and 2 years after BCT compared with a demographically matched non-alcoholic comparison sample. Results were similar to the authors' previous studies (O'Farrell & Murphy, 1995; O'Farrell *et al.*, 1999, 2000). In the year prior to treatment, 60% of 303 alcoholic men had been violent to their partner compared with 12% of 303 in the control group. After the first year of treatment, the percent of alcoholic men committing "overall violence" decreased to 24% and to 18% two years after BCT. The levels of aggression in the alcoholic men did not increase from the first to second year after BCT, which suggested that there was a stable reduction in violence. The authors attributed the decrease in violence demonstrated by the alcoholic men after treatment to enhanced relationship functioning and reduced problem drinking.

Overall, studies of BCT/BMT have found reduced alcohol consumption and partner violence, and improved marital functioning and treatment retention (McCrady *et al.*, 1999; McKay *et al.*, 1993; O'Farrell & Fals-Stewart, 2000). Behavioral marital therapy has also been shown to be more cost effective than individual therapy for reducing substance use, reducing legal, family and social problems, and for sustaining abstinence (O'Farrell *et al.*, 1985, 1993, 1996, 1998, Fals-Stewart *et al.*, 1997; O'Farrell & Fals-Stewart 2001).

Clearly further research is needed to determine if alcohol-dependent female members of a dual-gender couple benefit from BCT, since fewer cases than men have been studied (O'Farrell & Fals-Stewart, 2003).

Summary

Unfortunately, there appears to be a gap between the evidence base for BMT/BCT and its adoption by alcoholism treatment centers. According to a national survey conducted by Fals-Stewart & Birchler (2001), more than 95% of 398 addiction treatment providers had never heard of BCT. We recommend BCT when both members of a couple are motivated to participate in treatment. Although evidence indicates that BCT reduces male-to-female domestic violence when the male partner is alcohol dependent, a high potential for life-threatening violence contraindicates this type of treatment until both safety of the victim and sobriety of the abusive partner are firmly established.

Family-based intervention/concerned significant others (CSOs)

Introduction

In family-based therapy, family members and/or concerned significant others (CSOs) of the alcoholic are involved in the treatment process. The goal of the therapy is to provide a forum for the family, to exchange ideas about the treatment plan, to develop behavioral management contracts and rules for family support, and to reinforce behaviors that prevent relapse. There are several different types of family-based interventions. O'Farrell & Fals-Stewart (2003) distinguished between family-based interventions for alcohol-dependent individuals willing and not willing to be involved in treatment. The latter are referred to as unilateral family therapy approaches, and they do not require the participation of the alcohol-dependent individual. Copello et al. (2005) distinguished a third type of intervention designed to support the needs and functioning of family members themselves, independent of the alcohol-dependent patient. This type of intervention will not be discussed here. Family-based interventions designed to prevent the development of alcohol use disorders in children are outside the scope of this chapter but reviewed elsewhere (Kumpfer et al., 2003). Finally, different orientations of family therapy include systems, structural, strategic, behavioral and psychodynamic interventions. Family therapy is indicated when a maladaptive dynamic threatens a patient's abstinence (Stanton 1979).

An estimated 85.6% of US treatment facilities for substance use disorders offer some form of family counseling (SAMHSA, 2003). Especially common are education to CSOs about the nature of alcoholism and its treatment, and referrals to Al-Anon meetings in the community, a complementary twelve-step program to Alcoholics Anonymous (Al-Anon Family Groups, 1995). Similarly, it is common for CSOs to be involved in the patient's assessment, treatment planning, and discharge planning, especially at the most intensive levels of care (e.g., inpatient, residential and partial hospital treatment). Formal family psychotherapy of alcohol dependence is believed to occur less commonly because few practitioners have dual expertise or interest in both family therapy and substance use disorders. Thus, family involvement of some kind is thought to be more common than the specialized family therapies described below.

Evidence

Recent reviews have concluded that family involvement and interventions are effective treatments for alcohol use disorders (Copello et al., 2005; Liddle, 2004; Longabaugh, 2003; Steinglass & Kutch, 2004) and for engaging unwilling patients to seek treatment or reduce drinking (Barber & Gilbertson, 1997; O'Farrell & Fals-Stewart, 2003; Stanton, 2004).

In a randomized trial of 45 people who were dependent on alcohol, McCrady et al. (1991) compared the effects of minimal spouse involvement, alcohol-focused spouse involvement and spouse involvement plus BCT. While this study is small, it was unusual in having a relatively long follow-up period (18 months). While reductions in alcohol consumption were seen in all groups, those randomized to BCT showed higher levels of abstinence from alcohol and were less likely to experience marital separation.

A systematic review by the Health Technology Board for Scotland (2002) identified 22 trials involving families in the treatment of alcohol dependence. A number of different interventions were included under the term Family Therapy and studies included this with qualitatively different interventions. Although the review combined the results in a meta-analysis, the measures used in the meta-analysis were not presented. Overall this strategy was considered to be effective, and the board suggested that long-term treatment may be an important aspect of prevention of relapse.

Family interventions with unwilling alcohol-dependent patients

Several approaches have been studied in controlled trials that do not require the participation of the alcohol-dependent individual, at least initially, and are utilized when the "identified non-patient" with an alcohol use disorder refuses treatment. These approaches include the so-called Johnson Intervention (Johnson, 1986), Al-Anon Facilitation Therapy (Miller *et al.*, 1999b), Community Reinforcement and Family Training (CRAFT) (Meyers *et al.*, 1998; Miller *et al.*, 1999b), unilateral family therapy (Thomas *et al.*, 1990; Thomas & Santa, 1982), the "Pressures to Change" approach (Barber & Gilbertson, 1997) and "A Relational Intervention Sequence for Engagement" (ARISE) (Landau *et al.*, 2004). Johnson (1986) proposed that the family and other CSOs meet together with a therapist to plan a "confrontational meeting" during which they persuade the alcohol-dependent individual to enroll in a pre-selected treatment program. During the intervention, CSOs recount their direct observations of alcohol-related behaviors, their emotional responses, and the action they recommend that the patient take (i.e. treatment). One review concluded that the Johnson Intervention is ineffective at promoting treatment entry (O'Farrell & Fals-Stewart, 2003). "A Relational Intervention Sequence for Engagement" (ARISE) was developed as an alternative to the Johnson Intervention, but it is in the early stages of efficacy testing (Landau *et al.*, 2004).

Community Reinforcement and Family Training (CRAFT) is a unilateral family approach (Meyers *et al.*, 1998), and while related to the Community Reinforcement Approach to alcohol dependence, especially when used in combination with disulfiram, it is a complex behavioral treatment described in Chapter 16. CRAFT trains families or CSOs in community reinforcement techniques to help them engage the alcoholic into treatment.

As the patient proceeds through treatment, Al-Anon Facilitation Therapy suggests that the family/CSO exercise "loving detachment" and accepts its own powerlessness to change the loved one's drinking problem (Al-Anon Family Groups, 1995). Another strategy is "unilateral family therapy" in which the family or CSO group undergoes counseling without the alcoholic patient to learn how to alter a loved one's behavior and to motivate that person to change (Barber & Gilbertson 1996; Thomas & Santa, 1982; Thomas *et al.*, 1990). This technique has been shown to be effective in increasing the patient's motivation to enter therapy, increasing the level of the patient's engagement in therapy once it begins, and by reducing the patient's drinking both before and after treatment (Steinglass & Kutch, 2004).

Other family interventions

Network therapy (Galanter, 1993, 1999) is a "multimodal approach" to rehabilitating the patient that also involves the patient's family and friends in order to support and to promote attitude change. The people in the network do not receive treatment directly, but become part of the therapist's working team. To be selected as part of the team, the therapist and patient collaborate and choose people that they think will help promote abstinence. The people chosen to participate can attend therapy sessions, but the clinician should be careful to avoid focusing on the patient's family history with the other members present. Such a focus might obligate the therapist to resolve conflicts that are not necessarily associated with the addiction itself. Instead, the clinician should focus on the maintenance of abstinence, support of the network's integrity, and securing future behavior.

The effectiveness of network therapy has been studied in patients with various types of substance dependencies. Galanter (1993) followed a group of 60 patients throughout network therapy and one year after treatment. Alcohol was the primary drug of dependence for 27 patients, for 23 it was cocaine, for 3 it was marijuana, for 1 it was nicotine, and for 6 it was opiates. Of the 60 patients, 46 experienced either abstinence for at least 6 months or a marked decrease in drug use. Network therapy provided by psychiatry residents (Galanter *et al.*, 2002) and addiction counselors (Keller & Galanter, 1999) has also been effective, but randomized controlled trials of network therapy have not been conducted at this time.

In the UK a similar approach, Social Behavior and Network Therapy, involves efforts to help a person develop a positive social network that supports reductions in alcohol consumption. A single randomized trial in the UK suggested that reductions in alcohol consumption following eight 50-minute sessions of Social Behavior and Network Therapy brought about reductions of alcohol consumption equivalent to those achieved through three sessions of MET (UKATT Research Team, 2001).

Latimer *et al.* (2003) conducted a small randomized controlled trial of 43 adolescent outpatients and found superior drinking outcomes for the treatment group that integrated family therapy (16 sessions) and CBT (32 sessions) vs. a family-based psychoeducation control group (16 sessions only).

Summary

Family-based interventions are recommended for both willing and unwilling alcohol-dependent individuals. For the willing, BCT (described in the previous section), and community reinforcement therapy (described in Chapter 16) are the best-studied and have the most evidence for efficacy. Although network therapy is less well-studied, its approach is similar and can be recommended. For the unwilling, CRAFT and unilateral family therapy have the most evidence. Al-Anon Facilitation Therapy, although more commonly used, did not perform as well as CRAFT in one controlled study. Johnson-style interventions are generally not recommended.

Interactional group therapy

Introduction

Developed by Yalom and colleagues (Brown & Yalom, 1977; Matano & Yalom, 1991; Yalom et al., 1978) as a longer-term therapy of 12 months duration, interactional group therapy focuses on real-time communications and interactions between group members during the session. Group members learn about their style of relating to other people, including how they respond emotionally and to interpersonal conflicts with others, and how others respond to them. The therapy assumes that patients' maladaptive patterns of relating to others outside the group will emerge within the group as well. As patterns of interaction do emerge between group members, the therapist reinforces and helps patients to learn more effective ways of relating to others within the group. Interpersonal skills and awareness that develop during the group are expected to transfer to the patient's relationships outside of the group. To the extent that addiction is perpetuated by maladaptive interpersonal processes, interactional group therapy should help to sustain recovery from alcohol dependence after abstinence is initially established. Matano & Yalom (1991) recommend interactional group therapy as an adjunct to, not a replacement for, AA.

Group therapy is a dominant mode of treatment for alcohol dependence in the USA. Whereas other therapies, such as CBT, TSF and MET, can be delivered in either individual or group settings, interactional therapy by its nature requires a group setting. It also differs from couples, family and network therapy which involve other people who are already known to the patient. There are no good data on how frequently and extensively interactional group therapy is employed in its pure form, but it is likely that some processing of interactional events in addiction therapy groups is very common.

Evidence

A series of studies conducted by investigators from Brown University adapted interactional group therapy for short-term use (3 months) and compared it to CBT. As discussed above, effective outcomes with no overall differences between interactional group therapy and CBT were found (Kadden et al., 1989, 2001; Cooney et al., 1991; Litt et al., 2003), and this suggested that these therapies are comparable when CBT is delivered in group format.

Summary

Although less well-studied than CBT, interactional group therapy is an effective approach to treat patients with alcohol dependence, especially when combined with alcohol-focused interventions such as AA. To the extent that patients have deficits solving interpersonal problems, CBT with a focus on social skills training may be comparably beneficial.

Psychodynamic psychotherapy

Introduction

Psychodynamic psychotherapy of alcohol use disorders is generally based on a self-medication model in which patients are viewed as using alcohol to alleviate anxiety and emotional distress (Brower et al., 1989). Khantzian et al. (1990) assert that addicts compulsively self-medicate their psychological suffering because of vulnerabilities and deficits in four critical areas of psychological functioning: affect regulation, interpersonal relationships, self-care and self-esteem. These disturbances are considered to be relatively stable parts of the addict's character structure which require healing in order for recovery from addiction to occur.

Psychodynamic therapy is widely practiced in the USA by therapists of many disciplines, including those without specific training in addiction treatment. Therefore, the extent of use is likely to be high in the USA because many patients with alcohol use disorders receive treatment from generally trained psychotherapists. Addiction treatment specialists are unlikely to provide these therapies, at least as sole treatment, because of the predominance of TSF-oriented programs and because their evidence base is less convincing than for TSF and other therapies. Nevertheless, addiction therapists may sometimes explore psychodynamic issues during their individual sessions with patients, especially when those issues are interfering with recovery efforts or adherence to TSF.

Evidence

The psychodynamic approach has historically yielded little empirical support for its effectiveness in treating alcoholism (Holder *et al.*, 1991; Miller & Wilbourne, 2002). In studies reviewed between 1963 and 1981, individual psychotherapy was more effective in treating alcoholism than a control treatment in only two of eight studies, and between 1965 and 1980 group therapy with a psychodynamic focus was more effective in only two of eleven studies (Holder *et al.*, 1991). Nevertheless, controlled trials of individual or group psychotherapy based on relatively modern formulations of psychodynamic theory have not been done (Khantzian *et al.*, 1990).

Summary

There is little evidence to suggest that individual psychodynamic psychotherapy will enhance good drinking outcomes in alcohol-dependent patients. Nevertheless, psychodynamic perspectives may help some therapists to understand and empathize with their patients and, thus, establish and improve the therapeutic alliance.

Conclusions

The evidence base for psychosocial treatment in alcohol use disorders has been under increasing scrutiny in the addictions literature over the past 10–20 years, during which time relevant studies have been subjected to systematic review and meta-analysis. The Mesa Grande Project (Miller *et al.*, 1995a; Miller *et al.*, 1998; Miller & Wilbourne, 2002) is an ongoing systematic review which summarizes the current evidence of treatments for alcohol use disorders. In the most recent update, data from 361 randomized controlled trials were analyzed, and 87 treatments ranked. For psychosocial treatments, the strongest evidence of efficacy was found for brief interventions, MET and social skills training (a CBT-type intervention). See Table 13.1.

Evidence supporting the role of behavioral approaches, CBTs, BCT and case management are also reported. There are problems in interpreting the data with respect to alcohol dependence because the Mesa Grande does not separate out findings from studies among those with dependent and non-dependent drinking. But building on the data from Mesa Grande, a recent review of interventions for alcohol misuse published by the National Treatment Agency (2006), which guides delivery of substance misuse services in England, concluded that the way in which psychological treatments for alcohol use disorders are delivered may be as important as the model which is used. Nonetheless the authors state that motivational enhancement therapy provides a good starting point for treatment and that cognitive-behavioral approaches offer the best chances of success.

A systematic review of treatments for alcohol and other addictive substances by the Swedish Council on Technology Assessment in Health Care (SBU, 2001) synthesized findings from 139 randomized trials. A further 25 were added in March 2002, for the purposes of an English version of this report (Berglund *et al.*, 2003). The authors of this review concluded that "specific treatment" for alcohol-related problems is better than standard treatment. They defined specific treatment as treatment with a theoretical base, conducted by therapists with specific training and manual guided. The following treatments were considered to be effective: MET, CBT, twelve-step treatment, structured interactional therapy, marital therapy and family intervention. It was recommended that services should aim to reduce the delay between detoxification and interventions for the prevention of relapse.

The Health Technology Board for Scotland (2002) assessment of psychosocial interventions to prevent relapse in people with alcohol dependence identified four broadly defined treatments, with proven evidence of effectiveness: coping/social skills training; behavioral self control training (BSCT); marital/family therapy and motivational enhancement therapy. These interventions were not only clinically effective, but also cost-effective. However, practical limitations regarding their implementation were noted, and no one treatment was considered appropriate for every situation.

Guidelines produced by the National Drug and Alcohol Research Centre in Australia recommend that psychosocial intervention be used in an attempt to prevent relapse for all those with moderate to severe dependence on alcohol (Shand *et al.*, 2003). Motivational interviewing, problem-solving skills training and behavioural self-management are all recommended for preventing harmful and dependent use of alcohol.

Table 13.1. Effectiveness of psychological treatments of alcohol use disorders

Treatment	Form of treatment	Psychiatric disorder/ target audience	Level of evidence for efficacy	Comments
Brief interventions	Various very short psychosocial interventions	Mild to moderate alcohol misuse	Ia	Decreases alcohol consumption and alcohol related problems such as injuries and drunk driving
Motivational enhancement therapy (MET)	Specific psychosocial intervention to increase motivation and includes motivational interviewing	Alcohol dependence	Ia	Decreases alcohol consumption, days of heavy consumption. Increases attendance at treatment programs, especially in people with high levels of anger
Cognitive-behavioral therapy	Includes many different types of CBT	Alcohol dependence	Ia	Decreases alcohol consumption and increases harm avoidance. Can be delivered as individual or group treatment. There are many different types of CBT but there may be different impact with different subtypes of patients depending upon global psychopathology, sociopathy, psychiatric severity and anger.
Twelve-step facilitation therapy (TSF)	Includes but not limited to Alcoholics Anonymous (AA)	Alcohol dependence	Ia	Project MATCH. Most likely to lead to abstinence first year post treatment. Delays time to first relapse. Increased abstinence at 1 and 3 years
Behavior therapy	Includes contingency management and cue exposure therapy	Alcohol dependence	IIb	Decreases daily drinking including number of heavy drinking days, drinks per day, and overall frequency of drinking
Behavior couples/ behavior marital therapy	Various types of these treatments	Alcohol dependence	Ib	Improves drinking outcome. Decreases domestic violence and verbal abuse. Increases marital functioning. Increases retention in treatment
Family-based interventions	Various types of these treatments	Alcohol dependence	Ib	Probably need long-term treatment to be effective to prevent relapse. Increases motivation for treatment and level of engagement over time. Decreases drinking
Network therapy	Involves significant others	Alcohol dependence	Ib	Reduction in overall alcohol consumption
Interactional group therapy	Group therapy	Alcohol dependence	IIb	Comparable to CBT
Psychodynamic psychotherapy	Individual psychotherapy	Alcohol dependence	IV	No evidence for effectiveness

REFERENCES

Aalto, M., Pekuri, P. & Seppa, K. (2003). Obstacles to carrying out brief intervention for heavy drinkers in primary health care: a focus group study. *Drug and Alcohol Review*, **22**, 169–73.

Aalto, M., Saksanen, R., Laine, P. *et al.* (2000). Brief intervention for female heavy drinkers in routine general practice: a 3-year randomized, controlled study. *Alcoholism, Clinical Experimental and Research*, **24**, 1680–6.

Aalto, M., Seppa, K., Mattila, P. *et al.* (2001). Brief intervention for male heavy drinkers in routine general practice: a three year randomized controlled study. *Alcohol and Alcoholism* **36**, 224–30.

Allen, J. P., Maisto, S. A. & Connors, G. J. (1995). Self report screening tests for alcohol problems in primary care. *Archives of Internal Medicine*, **155**, 1726–30.

Allen, J. P. & Litten, R. Z. (1992). Techniques to enhance compliance with disulfiram. *Alcoholism, Clinical Experimental and Research*, **16**, 1035–41.

Al-Anon Family Groups (1995). *How Al-Anon Works for Families & Friends of Alcoholics*. Virginia Beach, VA: Al-Anon Family Group Headquarters.

Anderson, P. & Scott, E. (1992). The effect of general practitioner's advice to heavy drinking men. *British Journal of Addiction*, **87**, 891–900.

Anderson, P., Kaner, E., Wutzke, S. *et al.* (2003). Attitudes and management of alcohol problems in general practice: descriptive analysis based on findings of a World Health Organization international collaborative survey. *Alcohol and Alcoholism*, **38**, 597–601.

Anderson, P., Kaner, E., Wutzke, S. *et al.* (2004). Attitudes and managing alcohol problems in general practice: an interaction analysis based on findings from a WHO collaborative study. *Alcohol and Alcoholism*, **39**, 351–6.

Babor, T. F. & Grant, M. (ed.) (1992). *Project on Identification and Management of Alcohol Related Problems. Report on Phase II: a Randomized Clinical Trial of Brief Interventions in Primary Health Care. Program on substance abuse.* Geneva: World Health Organization.

Babor, T. F. & Higgins-Biddle, J. C. (2000). Alcohol screening and brief intervention: dissemination strategies for medical practice and public health. *Addiction* **95**, 677–86.

Ballesteros, J., Gonzalez-Pinto, A., Querejeta, I. & Arino, J. (2004). Brief interventions for hazardous drinkers delivered in primary care are equally effective in men and women. *Addiction*, **99**, 103–8.

Barber, J. G. & Gilbertson, R. (1996). An experimental study of brief unilateral intervention for the partners of heavy drinkers. *Research on Social Work Practice*, **6**, 325–36.

Barber, J. G. & Gilbertson, R. (1997). Unilateral interventions for women living with heavy drinkers. *Social Work*, **42**, 69–78.

Barrowclough, C., Haddock, G., Tarrier, N. *et al.* (2001). Randomized controlled trial of motivational interviewing, cognitive behavior therapy, and family intervention for patients with comorbid schizophrenia and substance use disorders. *American Journal of Psychiatry*, **158**, 1706–13.

Barry, K. L., Blow, F. C., Willenbring, M. L., McCormick, R., Brockmann, L. M. & Visnic, S. (2004). Use of alcohol screening and brief interventions in primary care settings: implementation and barriers. *Substance Abuse*, **25**, 27–36.

Beich, A., Thorsen, T. & Rollnick, S. (2003). Screening in brief intervention trials targeting excessive drinkers in general practice: systematic review and meta-analysis. *British Medical Journal*, **6**, 327, 536–42.

Berglund, M., Thelander, S., Francle, J., Andreasson, S. & Ojehagen, A. (2003). Treatment of alcohol and drug abuse: an evidence – based review. *Alcoholism: Clinical and Experimental Research*, **27**, 1645–1656.

Bernstein, E., Bernstein, J. & Levenson, S. (1997). Project ASSERT: an ED-based intervention to increase access to primary care, preventive services, and the substance abuse treatment system. *Annals of Emergency Medicine*, **30**, 181–9.

Bien, T. H., Miller, W. R. & Tonigan, J. S. (1993). Brief interventions for alcohol problems: a review. *Addiction*, **88**, 315–36.

Borsari, B. & Carey, K. B. (2000). Effects of a brief motivational intervention with college student drinkers. *Journal of Consulting Clinical Psychology*, **68**, 728–33.

Brown, S. & Yalom, I. D. (1977). Interational group therapy with alcoholics. *Journal of Studies on Alcoholism*, **38**, 426–56.

Brower, K. J., Blow, F. C. & Beresford, T. P. (1989). Treatment implications of chemical dependency models: an integrative approach. *Journal of Substance Abuse Treatment*, **6**, 147–57.

Brower, K. J. & Severin, J. D. (1997). Alcohol and other drug-related problems. In *Primary Care Psychiatry*, ed. D. J. Knesper, M. B. Riba & T. L. Schwenk, pp. 309–42. Philadelphia, PA: W. B. Saunders.

Burke, B. L., Arkowitz, H. & Menchola, M. (2003). The efficacy of motivational interviewing: a meta-analysis of controlled clinical trials. *Journal of Consulting and Clinical Psychology*, **71**, 843–61.

Burman, M. L., Kivlahan, D., Buchbinder, M. *et al.* (2004). Alcohol-related advice for Veterans Affairs primary care patients: who gets it? Who gives it? *Journal of Studies Alcoholism*, **65**, 621–30.

Cabinet Office, Prime Minister's Strategy Unit (2004). *Alcohol Harm Reduction Strategy for England.* London: Cabinet Office.

Chang, G. (2002). Brief interventions for problem drinking and women. *Journal of Substance Abuse Treatment*, **23**, 1–7.

Chang, G., Wilkins-Haug, L., Berman, S. & Goetz, M. A. (1999). Brief intervention for alcohol use in pregnancy: a randomized trial. *Addiction*, **94**, 1499–508.

Chang, G., McNamara, T. K., Orav, E. J. *et al.* (2005). Brief intervention for prenatal alcohol use: a randomized trial. *Obstetrics and Gynecology*, **105**, 991–8.

Chick, J., Lloyd, G. & Crombie, E. (1985). Counseling problem drinkers in medical wards: a controlled study. *British Medical Journal*, **290**, 965–7.

Chick, J., Ritson, B., Connaughton, J., Stewart, A. & Chick, J. (1988). Advice versus extended treatment for alcoholism: a controlled study. *British Journal of Addiction*, **83**, 159–70.

Cooney, N. L., Kadden, R. M., Litt, M. D. & Getter, H. (1991). Matching alcoholics to coping skills or interactional therapies: two year follow up results. *Journal of Consulting and Clinical Psychiatry*, **59**, 598–601.

Copello, A. G., Velleman, R. D. & Templeton, L. J. (2005). Family interventions in the treatment of alcohol and drug problems. *Drug and Alcohol Review*, **24**, 369–85.

Cordoba, R., Delgado, M. T., Pico, V., Altisent, R., Fores, D. & Monreal, A. (1998). Effectiveness of brief intervention on non-dependent alcohol drinkers (EBIAL): a Spanish multi-centre study. *Family Practice* **15**, 562–8.

Crawford, M. J., Patton, R., Touquet, R. *et al.* (2004). Screening and referral for brief intervention of alcohol-misusing patients in an emergency department: a pragmatic randomised controlled trial. *Lancet*, **364**, 1334–9.

Cross, G. M., Morgan, C. W., Mooney, A. J., III, Martin, C. A. & Rafter, J. A. (1990). Alcoholism treatment: a ten year follow up study. *Alcoholism Clinical and Experimental Research*, **14**, 169–73.

Cutler, R. B. & Fishbain, D. A. (2005). Are alcoholism treatments effective? The Project MATCH data. *BMC Public Health*, **5**, 75.

Daeppen, J. B. (2003). Screening and brief alcohol interventions in trauma centers. *Swiss Medical Weekly*, **133**, 495–500.

Daniels, V., Somers, M. & Orford, J. (1992). How can risk drinking amongst medical patients be modified? The effects of computer screening and advice and a self-help manual. *Behavioral Psychotherapy*, **20**, 47–60.

Danielsson, P. E., Rivara, F. P., Gentilello, L. M. & Maier, R. V. (1999). Reasons why trauma surgeons fail to screen for alcohol problems. *Archives of Surgery*, **134**, 564–8.

Dimeff, L. A., Baer, J. S., Kivlahan, D. R. & Marlatt, G. A. (1999). *Brief Alcohol Screening and Intervention for College Students: a Harm Reduction Approach.* New York, NY: Guilford Press.

D'Onofrio, G. & Degutis, L. C. (2002). Preventive care in the emergency department: screening and brief intervention for alcohol problems in the emergency department: a systematic review. *Academic Emergency Medicine*, **9**, 627–38.

Drummond, D. C. & Glautier, S. P. (1994). A controlled trial of cue exposure treatment in alcohol dependence. *Journal of Consulting and Clinical Psychology*, **62**, 809–17.

Drummond, D. C., Cooper, T. & Glautier, S. P. (1990). Conditioned learning in alcohol dependence: implications for cue exposure treatment. *British Journal of Addiction*, **85**, 725–43.

Dunn, C. W., Donovan, D. M. & Gentilello, L. M. (1997). Practical guidelines for performing alcohol interventions in trauma centers. *Journal of Trauma*, **42**, 299–304.

Dunn, C., Deroo, L. & Rivara, F. P. (2001). The use of brief interventions adapted from motivational interviewing across behavioral domains: a systematic review. *Addiction*, **96**, 1725–42.

Edwards, A. G. & Rollnick, S. (1997). Outcome studies of brief alcohol intervention in general practice: the problem of lost subjects. *Addiction*, **92**, 1699–704.

Department of Health (1993). Brief interventions and alcohol use. *Effective Health Care*, **7**, 1–13.

Elvy, G. A., Wells, J. F. & Baird, K. A. (1988). Attempted referral as intervention for problem drinking in the general hospital. *British Journal of Addiction*, **83**, 83–9.

Emmen, M. J., Schippers, G. M., Bleijenberg, G. & Wollersheim, H. (2004). Effectiveness of opportunistic brief interventions for problem drinking in a general hospital setting: systematic review. *British Medical Journal*, **328**, 318.

Epstein, E. E. & McCrady, B. S. (1998). Behavioral couples treatment of alcohol and drug use disorders: current status and innovations. *Clinical Psychology Review*, **18**, 689–711.

Fals-Stewart, W., O'Farrell, T. J. & Birchler, G. R. (1997). Behavioral couples therapy for male substance-abusing patients: a cost outcomes analysis. *Journal of Consulting and Clinical Psychology*, **65**, 789–802.

Fals-Stewart, W. & Birchler, G. R. (2001). A national survey of the use of couples therapy in substance abuse treatment. *Journal of Substance Abuse Treatment*, **20**, 277–83.

Fleming, M. F. & Manwell, L. B. (1999). Brief intervention in primary care settings: a primary treatment method for at risk problems, and dependent drinkers. *Alcohol Research and Health*, **23**, 128–37.

Fleming, M. F., Barry, K. L., Manwell, L. B., Johnson, K. & London, R. (1997). Brief physician advice for problem alcohol drinkers. A randomized controlled trial in community-based primary care practices. *Journal of the American Medical Association*, **277**, 1039–45.

Fleming, M. F., Mundt, M. P., French, M. F. *et al.* (2002). Brief physician advice for problem drinkers: long term efficacy and benefit-cost analysis. *Alcoholism, Clinical and Experimental Research*, **26**, 36–43.

Fleming, M., Brown, R. & Brown, D. (2004). The efficacy of a brief alcohol intervention combined with %CDT feedback in patients being treated for type 2 diabetes and/or hypertension. *Journal of Studies on Alcohol*, **65**, 631–7.

Galanter, M. (1993). Network therapy for substance abuse: a clinical trial. *Psychotherapy*, **30**, 251–8.

Galanter, M. (1999). *Network Therapy for Addiction: A New Approach*, Expanded Edition. New York: Guilford.

Galanter, M., Dermatis, H., Keller, D. *et al.* (2002). Network therapy for cocaine abuse: use of family and peer supports. *American Journal on Addictions*, **11**, 161–6.

Gentilello, L. M., Rivara, F. P., Donovan, D. M. *et al.* (1999). Alcohol interventions in a trauma center as a means of reducing the risk of injury recurrence. *Annals of Surgery*, **230**, 473–80.

Gentilello, L. M., Ebel, B. E., Wickizer, T. M., Salkever, D. S. & Rivara, F. P. (2005). Alcohol interventions for trauma patients treated in emergency departments and hospitals: a cost benefit analysis. *Annals of Surgery*, **241**, 541–50.

Graham, A. W. & Fleming, M. S. (1998). Brief interventions. In *Principles of Addiction Medicine*, 2nd edn, ed. A. W. Graham, T. K. Schultz & B. B. Wilfor, pp. 615–30. Chevy Chase, MD: American Society of Addiction Medicine, Inc.

Graham, D. M., Maio, R. F., Blow, F. C. & Hill, E. M. (2000). Emergency physician attitudes concerning intervention for alcohol abuse/dependence delivered in the emergency department: a brief report. *Journal of Addictive Diseases*, **19**, 45–53.

Graeber, D. A., Moyers, T. B., Grifith, G., Guajardo, E. & Tonigan, S. (2003). A pilot study comparing motivational interviewing and an educational intervention in patients with schizophrenia and alcohol use disorders. *Community and Mental Health Journal*, **39**, 189–202.

Health Technology Board for Scotland (2002). *Health Technology Assessment, Advice 3: Prevention of Relapse in Alcohol Dependence*. Norwich: The Stationery office.

Heather, N., Rollnick, S. & Bell, A. (1996). Effects of brief counseling among male heavy drinkers identified on general hospital wards. *Drug and Alcohol Review*, **15**, 29–38.

Holder, H., Longabaugh, R., Miller, W. R. & Rubonis, A. V. (1991). The cost-effectiveness of treatment for alcoholism: a first approximation. *Journal of Studies on Alcohol*, **52**, 517–40.

Holder, H. D., Cisler, R. A., Longabaugh, R., Stout, R. L., Treno, A. J. & Zweben, A. (2000). Alcoholism treatment and medical care costs from Project MATCH. *Addiction*, **95**, 999–1013.

Humphreys, K., Huebsch, P. D., Finney, J. W. & Moos, R. H. (1999). A comparative evaluation of substance abuse treatment: Substance abuse treatment can enhance the effectiveness of self-help groups. *Alcoholism, Clinical and Experimental Research*, **23**, 558–63.

Hulse, G. K. & Tait, R. J. (2003). Five-year outcomes of a brief alcohol intervention for adult in-patients with psychiatric disorders. *Addiction*, **98**, 1061–8.

Ingersoll, K. S., Ceperich, S. D., Nettleman, M. D., Karanda, K., Brocksen, S. & Johnson, B. A. (2005). Reducing alcohol-exposed pregnancy risk in college women: initial outcomes of a clinical trial of a motivational intervention. *Journal of Substance Abuse Treatment*, **29**, 173–80.

Israel, Y., Hollander, O., Sanchez-Craig, M. *et al.* (1996). Screening for problem drinking and counseling by the primary care physician – nurse team. *Alcoholism, Clinical and Experimental Research*, **20**, 1442–50.

Irvin, J. E., Bowers, C. A., Dunn, M. E. & Wang, M. C. (1999). Efficacy of relapse prevention: a meta-analytic review. *Journal of Consulting and Clinical Psychology*, **67**, 563–70.

John, U., Veltrup, C., Driessen, M., Wetterling, T. & Dilling, H. (2003). Motivational intervention: an individual counselling vs a group treatment approach for alcohol-dependent in-patients. *Alcohol and Alcoholism*, **38**, 263–9.

Johnson, V. E. (1986). *Intervention: How to Help Those Who Don't Want Help*. Minneapolis, MN: Johnson Institute.

Kadden, R. (2001). Behavioral and cognitive-behavioral treatments for alcoholism: research opportunities. *Addictive Behaviors*, **26**, 489–507.

Kadden, R. M. & Cooney, N. L. (2005). Treating alcohol problems. In *Relapse Prevention: Maintenance Strategies in the Treatment of Addictive Behaviors*, ed. G. A. Marlatt & D. M. Donovan, pp. 65–91. New York: Guilford Press.

Kadden, R. M., Cooney, N. L., Getter, H. & Litt, M. D. (1989). Matching alcoholics to coping skills or interactional therapies: post-treatment results. *Journal of Consulting and Clinical Psychology*, **57**, 698–704.

Kadden, R. M., Litt, M. D., Cooney, N. L., Kabela, E. & Getter, H. (2001). Prospective matching of alcoholic clients to cognitive-behavioral or interactional group therapy. *Journal of Studies on Alcohol*, **62**, 359–69.

Kadden, R., Carroll, K., Donovan, D. *et al.* (1994). *Cognitive-Behavioral Coping Skills Therapy Manual: A Clinical Research Guide for Therapists Treating Individuals with Alcohol Abuse and Dependence* (Project Match Monograph Series Vol. 3; NIH Publication No. 94-3724). Rockville, MD: National Institute on Alcohol Abuse and Alcoholism.

Kahan, M., Wilson, L. & Becker, L. (1995). Effectiveness of physician-based interventions with problem drinkers: a review. *Canadian Medical Association Journal*, **152**, 851–9.

Kalman, D., Longabaugh, R., Clifford, P. R., Beattie, M. & Maisto, S. A. (2000). Matching alcoholics to treatment. Failure to replicate finding of an earlier study. *Journal of Substance Abuse Treatment*, **19**, 183–7.

Karno, M. P., Beutler, L. E. & Harwood, T. M. (2002). Interactions between psychotherapy procedures and patient attributes that predict alcohol treatment effectiveness: a preliminary report. *Addictive Behaviors*, **27**, 779–97.

Keller, D. S. & Galanter, M. (1999). Technology transfer of network therapy to community based addiction counselors. *Journal of Substance Abuse Treatment*, **16**, 183–9.

Khantzian, E. J., Halliday, K. S. & McAuliffe, W. E. (1990). *Addiction and the Vulnerable Self: Modified Dynamic Group Therapy for Substance Abusers*. New York: Guilford Press.

Kumpfer, K. L., Alvarado, R. & Whiteside, H. O. (2003). Family-based interventions for substance use and misuse prevention. *Substance Use and Misuse*, **38**, 1759–87.

Larimer, M. E., Turner, A. P., Anderson, B. K. *et al.* (2001). Evaluating a brief alcohol intervention with fraternities. *Journal of Studies on Alcohol*, **62**, 370–80.

Latimer, W. W., Winters, K. C., D'Zurilla, T. & Nichols, M. (2003). Integrated family and cognitive behavioral therapy for adolescent substance abusers: a stage I efficacy study. *Drug and Alcohol Dependence*, **71**, 303–17.

Landau, J., Stanton, M. D., Brinkman-Sull, D. *et al.* (2004). Outcomes with the ARISE approach to engaging reluctant drug- and alcohol-dependent individuals in treatment. *American Journal of Drug and Alcohol Abuse*, **30**, 711–48.

Leontieva, L., Horn, K., Haque, A., Helmkamp, J., Ehrlich, P. & Williams, J. (2005). Readiness to change problematic drinking assessed in the emergency department as a predictor of change. *Journal of Critical Care*, **20**, 251–6.

Liddle, H. A. (2004). Family-based therapies for adolescent alcohol and drug use: research contributions and future research needs. *Addiction*, **99** (Suppl. 2), 76–92.

Lincour, P., Kuettel, T. J. & Bombardier, C. H. (2002). Motivational interviewing in a group setting with mandated clients: a pilot study. *Addiction Behavior*, **27**, 381–91.

Litt, M. D., Cooney, N. L. & Morse, P. (2000). Reactivity to alcohol-related stimuli in the laboratory and in the field: predictors of craving in treated alcoholics. *Addiction*, **95**, 889–900.

Litt, M. D., Kadden, R. M., Cooney, N. & Kabela, E. (2003). Coping skills and treatment outcomes in cognitive–behavioral and interactional group therapy for alcoholism. *Journal of Consulting and Clinical Psychology*, **71**, 118–28.

Litt, M. D., Cooney, N. L., Kadden, R. M. & Gaupp, L. (1990). Reactivity to alcohol cues and induced moods in alcoholics. *Addictive Behavior*, **15**, 137–46.

Longabaugh, R. (2003). Involvement of support networks in treatment. *Recent Developments in Alcoholism*, **16**, 133–47.

Longabaugh, R. & Morgenstern, J. (1999). Cognitive–behavioral coping-skills therapy for alcohol dependence: current states and future directions. *Alcohol Research and Health*, **23**, 78–85.

Longabaugh, R., Rubin, A., Malloy, P., Beattie, M., Clifford, P. R. & Noel, N. (1994). Drinking outcomes of alcohol abusers diagnosed as antisocial personality disorder. *Alcoholism, Clinical and Experimental Research*, **18**, 778–85.

Longabaugh, R., Wirtz, P., Zweben, A. & Stout, R. (1998). Network support for drinking, Alcoholics Anonymous and long term matching effects. *Addiction*, **93**, 1313–33.

Longabaugh, R., Woolard, R. E., Nirenberg, T. D. *et al.* (2001). Evaluating the effects of a brief motivational intervention for injured drinkers in the emergency department. *Journal of Studies on Alcohol*, **62**, 806–16.

Maheswaran, R., Beevers, M. & Beevers, D. G. (1992). Effectiveness of advice to reduce alcohol consumption in hypertensive patients. *Hypertension*, **19**, 79–84.

Maio, R. F., Shope, J. T., Blow, F. C. *et al.* (2005). A randomized controlled trial of an emergency department-based interactive computer program to prevent alcohol misuse among injured adolescents. *Annals of Emergency Medicine*, **45**, 420–9.

Manwell, L. B., Fleming, M. F., Mundt, M. P., Stauffacher, E. A. & Barry, K. L. (2000). Treatment of problem alcohol use in women of childbearing age: results of a brief intervention trial. *Alcoholism, Clinical and Experimental Research*, **24**, 1517–24.

Marlatt, G. A., Baer, J. S., Kivlahan, D. R. *et al.* (1998). Screening and brief intervention for high-risk college student drinkers: results from a 2-year follow-up assessment. *Journal of Consulting and Clinical Psychology*, **66**, 604–15.

Marlatt, G. A. & Donovan, D. M. (ed.) (2005). *Relapse Prevention: Maintenance Strategies in the Treatment of Addictive Behaviors*. New York: Guilford.

Marlatt, G. A. & Witkiewitz, K. (2002). Harm reduction approaches to alcohol use: health promotion, prevention, and treatment. *Addictive Behaviors*, **27**, 867–86.

Marques, A. C. & Formigoni, M. L. (2001). Comparison of individual and group cognitive-behavioral therapy for alcohol and/or drug-dependent patients. *Addiction*, **96**, 835–46.

Matano, R. A. & Yalom, I. D. (1991). Approaches to chemical dependency: chemical dependency and interactive group therapy – a synthesis. *International Journal of Group Psychotherapy*, **41**, 269–93.

McCrady, B. S. (1998). Recent research in twelve step programs. In *Principles of Addiction Medicine*, 2nd edn, ed. A. W. Graham & T. K. Schultz, pp. 707–18. Chevy Chase, MD: American Society of Addiction Medicine, Inc.

McCrady, B. (2000). Alcohol use disorders and Division 12 Task Force of the American Psychological Association. *Psychology of Addictive Behavior*, **14**, 267–76.

McCrady, B. S., Stout, R., Noel, N., Abrams, D. & Nelson, H. F. (1991). Effectiveness of three types of spouse-involved behavioral alcoholism treatment. *Addiction*, **86**, 1415–24.

McCrady, B. S., Epstein, E. E. & Hirsch, L. S. (1999). Maintaining change after conjoint behavioral alcohol treatment for men: outcomes at 6 months. *Addiction*, **94**, 1381–96.

McGovern, M., Fox, T., Xie, H. & Drake, R. (2004). A survey of clinical practices and readiness to adopt evidence-based practices: dissemination research in an addiction treatment system. *Journal of Substance Abuse Treatment*, **26**, 305–12.

McIntosh, M. C., Leigh, G., Baldwin, N. J. & Marmulak, J. (1997). Reducing alcohol consumption. Comparing three brief methods in family practice. *Canadian Family Physician*, **43**, 1959–62.

McKay, J. R., Longabaugh, R., Beattie, M. C., Maisto, S. A. & Noel, N. E. (1993). Does adding conjoint therapy to individually focused alcoholism treatment lead to better family functioning? *Journal of Substance Abuse*, **5**, 45–59.

McNally, A. M., Palfai, T. P. & Kahler, C. W. (2005). Motivational interventions for heavy drinking college students: examining

the role of discrepancy-related psychological processes. *Psychology of Addictive Behavior*, **19**, 79–87.

Meyers, R. J., Miller, W. R., Hill, D. E. & Tonigan, J. S. (1998). Community reinforcement and family training (CRAFT): engaging unmotivated drug users in treatment. *Journal of Substance Abuse*, **10**, 291–308.

Miller, W. R. & Hester, R. K. (1986). Inpatient alcoholism treatment. Who benefits? *American Psychologist*, **41**, 794–805.

Miller, W. R. & Rollnick, S. (1991). *Motivational Interviewing: Preparing People to Change Addictive Behavior*. New York: Guilford Press.

Miller, W. R. & Sanchez, V. C. (1993). Motivating young adults for treatment and lifestyle change. In *Issues in Alcohol Use and Misuse by Young Adults*, ed. G. Howard. South Bend, IN: University of Notre Dame Press.

Miller, W. R. & Wilbourne, P. L. (2002). Mesa Grande: a methodological analysis of clinical trials of treatments for alcohol use disorders. *Addiction*, **97**, 265–77.

Miller, W. R., Benefield, R. G. & Tonigan, J. S. (1993). Enhancing motivation for change in problem drinking: a controlled comparison of two therapist styles. *Journal of Consulting and Clinical Psychology*, **61**, 455–61.

Miller, W. R., Brown, J. M., Simpson, T. L. *et al.* (1995a). What works? A methodological analysis of the alcohol treatment outcome literature In *Handbook of Alcoholism Treatment Approaches: Effective Alternatives*, ed. R. K. Hester & W. R. Miller, pp. 12–44. Boston, MA: Allyn and Bacon.

Miller, W., Zweben, A., DiClemente, C. & Rychtarik, R. (1995b). *Motivational Enhancement Therapy Manual* (Project Match Monograph Series, Vol. 2). Rockville, MD: National Institute on Alcohol Abuse and Alcoholism.

Miller, W. R., Andrews, N. R., Wilbourne, P. & Bennett, M. E. (1998). A wealth of alternatives: effective treatments for alcohol problems. In *Treating Addictive Behaviours: Process of Change*, 2nd edn, ed. R. W. Miller & N. Heather, pp. 203–16. New York: Plenum Press.

Miller, W. R., Meyers., R. J. & Hiller-Sturmhofel, S. (1999a). The Community Reinforcement Approach. *Alcohol Research and Health*, **23**, 116–21.

Miller, W. R., Meyers, R. J. & Tonigan, J. S. (1999b). Engaging the unmotivated in treatment of alcohol problems: a comparison of three strategies for intervention through family members. *Journal of Consulting and Clinical Psychology*, **67**, 688–97.

Monti, P. M., Abrams, D. B., Kadden, R. M. & Cooney, N. L. (1989). *Treating Alcohol Dependence: a Coping Skills Training Guide*. New York: Guilford Press.

Monti, P. M., Abrams, D. B., Binkoff, J. A. *et al.* (1990). Communication skills training, communication skills training with family and cognitive behavioral mood management training for alcoholics. *Journal of Studies on Alcohol*, **51**, 263–70.

Monti, P. M., Colby, S. M., Barnett, N. P. *et al.* (1999). Brief intervention for harm reduction with alcohol positive older adolescents in a hospital emergency department. *Journal of Consulting and Clinical Psychology*, **67**, 989–94.

Monti, P. M. & Rohsenow, D. J. (1999). Coping skills training and cue – exposure therapy in the treatment of alcoholism. *Alcohol Research and Health*, **23**, 107–15.

Monti, P. M., Rohsenow, D. J., Colby, S. M. & Abrams, D. M. (1995). Coping and social skills training. In *Handbook of Alcoholism Treatment Approaches*, 2nd edn, ed. R. K. Hester & W. R. Miller, pp. 221–41. New York: Allyn & Bacon.

Monti, P. M. (2003). Coping and social skills training. In *Handbook of Alcoholism Treatment Approaches: Effective Alternatives*, 3rd edn, ed. R. K. Hester & W. R. Miller, pp. 213–36. Needham Heights, MA: Allyn & Bacon.

Morgenstern, J., Labouvie, E., McCrady, B. S., Kahler, C. W. & Frey, R. M. (1997). Affiliation with Alcoholics Anonymous after treatment: a study of its therapeutic effect and mechanisms of action. *Journal of Consulting and Clinical Psychology*, **65**, 768–77.

Morgenstern, J. & Longabaugh, R. (2000). Cognitive behavioral treatment for alcohol dependence: a review of evidence for its hypothesized mechanisms of action. *Addiction*, **95**, 1475–90.

Moyer, A., Finney, J. W., Swearingen, C. E. & Vergun, P. (2002). Brief interventions for alcohol problems: a meta-analytic review of controlled investigations in treatment-seeking and non-treatment-seeking populations. *Addiction*, **97**, 279–92.

Murphy, J. G., Duchnick, J. J., Vuchinich, R. E. *et al.* (2001). Relative efficacy of a brief motivational intervention for college student drinkers. *Psychology of Addictive Behavior*, **15**, 373–9.

National Treatment Agency (2006). *Review of Effectiveness of Treatment for Alcohol Problems*. London: National Treatment Agency.

National Institute on Alcohol Abuse and Alcoholism (NIAAA) (2000). New advances in alcoholism treatment. Alcohol Alert, 49. (http://pubs.niaaa.nih.gov/publications/aa49.htm), Accessed June 30, 2007.

National Institute on Alcohol Abuse and Alcoholism (NIAAA) (2007). *Helping Patients who Drink too Much: A Clinicians Guide* (Updated 2005 Edition) (NIH Publication No. 07-3769). Rockville, MD: National Institutes of Health.

Nowinski, J. Baker, S. & Carroll, K. (1994). *Twelve Step Facilitation Therapy Manual* (Project Match Monograph Series, Vol. 1; NIH Publication No. 94-3722). Rockville, MD: National Institute on Alcohol Abuse and Alcoholism.

Niaura, R. S., Rohsenow, D. J., Binkoff, J., Monti, P. M., Pedraza, M. & Abrams, D. B. (1988). Relevance of cue reactivity to understanding alcohol and smoking relapse. *Journal of Abnormal Psychology*, **97**, 133–52.

O'Connor, P. G. & Schottenfeld, R. S. (1998). Patients with alcohol problems. *New England Journal of Medicine*, **338**, 592–602.

Ockene, J. K., Adams, A., Hurley, T. G., Wheeler, E. V. & Hebert, J. R. (1999). Brief physician and nurse practioner-delivered counseling for high risk drinkers: does it work? *Archives of Internal Medicine*, **159**, 2198–205.

Oei, T. P. & Jackson, P. (1980). Long-term effects of group and individual social skills training with alcoholics. *Addictive Behaviors*, **5**, 129–36.

O'Farrell, T. J. & Murphy, C. M. (1995). Marital violence before and after alcoholism treatment. *Journal of Consulting and Clinical Psychology*, **63**, 256–62.

O'Farrell, T. J. & Fals-Steward, W. (2000). Behavioral couples therapy for alcoholism and drug abuse. *Journal of Substance Abuse Treatment*, **18**, 51–4.

O'Farrell, T. J. & Fals-Stewart, W. (2001). Family-involved alcoholism treatment. An update. *Recent Developments in Alcoholism*, **15**, 329–56.

O'Farrell, T. J. & Fals-Stewart, W. (2003). Alcohol abuse. *Journal of Marital and Family Therapy*, **29**, 121–46.

O'Farrell, T. J., Cutter, H. S. & Floyd, F. J. (1985). Evaluating behavioral therapy for male alcoholics: effects on marital adjustment and communication from before to after treatment. *Behavioral Therapy*, **16**, 147–67.

O'Farrell, T. J., Choquette, K. A., Cutter, H. S., Brown E. D. & McCourt, W. F. (1993). Behavioral marital therapy with and without additional couples relapse prevention sessions for alcoholics and their wives. *Journal of Studies on Alcohol*, **54**, 652–66.

O'Farrell, T. J., Choquette, K. A., Cutter, H. S. *et al.* (1996). Cost benefit and cost-effectiveness anlyses of behavioral marital therapy as an addition to outpatient alcoholism treatment. *Journal of Substance Abuse*, **8**, 145–66.

O'Farrell, T. J., Choquette, K. A. & Cutter, H. S. (1998). Couples relapse prevention sessions after behavioral marital therapy for male alcoholics: outcomes during the three years after starting treatment. *Journal of Studies on Alcohol*, **59**, 357–70.

O'Farrell, T. J., Van Hutton, V. & Murphy, C. M. (1999). Domestic violence before and after alcoholism treatment: a two year longitudinal study. *Journal of Studies on Alcohol*, **60**, 317–21.

O'Farrell, T. J., Murphy, C. M., Neavins, T. M. & Van Hutton, V. (2000). Verbal aggression among male alcoholic patients and their wives in the year before and two years after alcoholism treatment. *Journal of Family Violence*, **15**, 295–310.

O'Farrell, T. J., Fals-Stewart, W., Murphy, C. M., Stephan, S. H. & Murphy, M. (2004). Partner violence before and after couples-based alcoholism treatment for male alcoholic patients: the role of treatment involvement and abstinence. *Journal of Consulting and Clinical Psychology*, **72**, 202–17.

Ouimette, P. C., Finney, J. W. & Moos, R. H. (1997). Twelve step and cognitive behavioral treatment for substance abuse: a comparison of treatment effectiveness. *Journal of Consulting and Clinical Psychology* **65**(2), 220–40.

Ouimette P. C., Moos, R. H. & Finney, J. W. (1998). Influence of outpatient treatment and 12 step group involvement on one year substance abuse treatment outcomes. *Journal of Studies on Alcoholism*, **59**, 513–22.

Petry, N. M., Martin, B., Cooney, J. L. & Kranzler, H. R. (2000). Give them prizes and they will come: contingency management for treatment of alcohol dependence. *Journal of Consulting and Clinical Psychology*, **68**, 250–7.

Poikolainen, K. (1999). Effectiveness of brief interventions to reduce alcohol intake in primary health care populations: a meta analysis. *Preventive Medicine*, **28**, 503–9.

Prochaska, J. O. & DiClemente, C. C. (1984). *The Transtheoretical Approach: Crossing Traditional Boundaries of Therapy.* Homewood, IL: Dow Jones, Irwin.

Prochaska, J. O. & DiClemente, C. C. (1992). Stages of change in the modification of problem behavior. *Progress in Behavior Modification*, **28**, 183–218.

Project MATCH Research Group (1993). Project MATCH (Matching Alcoholism Treatments to Client Heterogeneity): rationale and methods for a multisite clinical trial matching patients to alcoholism treatment. *Alcoholism, Clinical and Experimental Research*, **17**, 1130–45.

Project Match Research Group (1997a). Matching alcoholism treatments to client heterogeneity: Project MATCH post-treatment drinking outcomes. *Journal of Studies on Alcoholism*, **58**, 7–29.

Project MATCH Research Group (1997b). Project MATCH secondary a priori hypotheses. *Addiction*, **98**, 1671–98.

Project MATCH Research Group (1998a). Matching alcoholism treatment to client heterogeneity: Project MATCH three-year drinking outcomes. *Alcoholism, Clinical and Experimental Research*, **22**, 1300–11.

Project MATCH Research Group (1998b). Matching alcoholism treatment to client heterogeneity: treatment main effects and matching effects on drinking during treatment. *Journal of Studies on Alcoholism*, **59**, 631–9.

Richmond, R., Heather, N., Wodak, A., Kehoe, L. & Webster, I. (1995). Controlled evaluation of a general practice-based brief intervention for excessive drinking. *Addiction*, **90**, 119–32.

Richmond, R., Kehoe, L., Heather, N. & Wodak, A. (2000). Evaluation of a workplace brief intervention for excessive alcohol consumption: the workscreen project. *Preventive Medicine*, **30**, 51–63.

Rivara, F. P., Tollefson, S., Tesh, E. & Gentilello, L. M. (2000). Screening trauma patients for alcohol problems: are insurance companies barriers? *Journal of Trauma*, **48**, 115–18.

Rohsenow, D. J., Niaura, R. S., Childress, A. R., Abrams, D. B. & Monti, P. M. (1991). Cue reactivity in addictive behaviors: theoretical and treatment implications. *International Journal of Addiction*, **25**, 957–90.

Rohsenow, D. J., Monti, P. M., Rubonis, A. V. *et al.* (2001). Cue exposure with coping skills training and communication skills training for alcohol dependence: 6- and 12-month outcomes. *Addiction*, **96**, 1161–74.

Rowland, N. & Maynard, A. K. (1993). Standardized and alcohol education: a hit or miss affair? *Health Promotion International*, **8**, 5–12.

SBU (2001). *Behandling av alcohol-och narkotikaproblem. En evidensbaserad kunskapssammanstallning.* Statens berendning for medicinsk utardering, rapport nr 156. Stockholm. ISBN: 91-87890-73-9. Also available at http://www.sbu.se/www/index.asp

Schulz, K. F., Chalmers, I., Hayes, R. J. & Altman, D. G. (1995). Empirical evidence of bias: dimensions of methodological quality associated with estimates of treatment effects in controlled trials. *Journal of the American Medical Association*, **12**, 408–12.

Scott, E. & Anderson, P. (1990). Randomized controlled trial of general practitioner intervention in women with excessive alcohol consumption. *Drug and Alcohol Review*, **10**, 313–21.

Scottish Intercollegiate Guidelines Network, (2003). *The Management of Harmful Drinking and Alcohol Dependence in Primary Care. A National Clinical Guideline.* Edinburgh: Royal College of Physicians.

Sellman, J. D., Sullivan, P. D., Dore, G. M., Adamson, S. J. & MacEwan, I. (2001). A randomized controlled trial of motivational enhancement therapy (MET) for mild to moderate alcohol dependence. *Journal of Studies on Alcoholism*, **62**, 389–96.

Senft, R. A., Polen, M. R., Freeborn, D. K. & Hollis, J. F. (1997). Brief intervention in a primary care setting for hazardous drinkers. *American Journal of Preventive Medicine*, **13**, 464–70.

Shakeshaft, A. P., Bowman, J. A., Burrows, S., Doran, C. M. & Sanson-Fisher, R. W. (2002). Community-based alcohol counselling: a randomized clinical trial. *Addiction*, **97**, 1449–63.

Shand, F., Gates, J., Fawcett, J. & Mattick, R. (2003). *Guidelines for the Treatment of Alcohol Problems.* Canberra: The Commonwealth and the National Drug and Alcohol Research Centre.

Sitharthan, T., Sitharthan, G., Hough., M. J. & Kavanagh., D. J. (1997). Cue exposure in moderation drinking: a comparison with cognitive behavior therapy. *Journal of Consulting and Clinical Psychology*, **65**, 878–82.

Smith, A. J., Hodgson, R. J., Bridgeman, K. & Shepherd, J. P. (2003). A randomized controlled trial of a brief intervention after alcohol-related facial injury. *Addiction*, **98**, 43–52.

Spirito, A., Monti, P. M., Barnett, N. P. *et al.* (2004). A randomized clinical trial of a brief motivational intervention for alcohol-positive adolescents treated in an emergency department. *Journal of Pediatrics*, **145**, 396–402.

Stanton, M. D. (2004). Getting reluctant substance abusers to engage in treatment/self-help: a review of outcomes and clinical options. *Journal of Marital and Family Therapy*, **30**, 165–82.

Stanton, M. D. (1979). Family treatment approaches to drug abuse problems: a review. *Family Process*, **18**, 251–80.

Substance Abuse and Mental Health Services Administration (SAMHSA) (2003). *Alcohol and Drug Services Study (ADSS): The National Substance Abuse Treatment System: Facilities, Clients, Services, and Staffing.* Rockville, MD: Office of Applied Studies.

Steinglass P and Kutch S (2004) Family Therapy: Alcohol, In *Textbook of Substance Abuse Treatment*, ed. Galanter and Kleber, 3rd edn. American Psychiatric Publishing, Inc.

Tevyaw, T. O. & Monti, P. M. (2004). Motivational enhancement and other brief interventions for adolescent substance abuse: foundations, applications and evaluations. *Addiction*, **99** (Suppl. 2), 63–75.

Thomas, E. & Santa, C. (1982). Unilateral family therapy for alcohol abuse: a working conception. *American Journal of Family Therapy*, **10**, 49–58.

Thomas, E. J., Adams, K. B., Yoshioka, M. R. & Ager, R. D. (1990). Unilateral relationship enhancement in the treatment of spouses for uncooperational alcohol abusers. *American Journal of Family Therapy*, **18**, 334–44.

Timko, C., Moos, R., Finney, J. W. & Lesar, M. D. (2000). Long term outcomes of alcohol use disorders: comparing untreated individuals with those in Alcoholics Anonymous and formal treatment. *Journal of Studies on Alcoholism*, **61**, 529–40.

UKATT Research Team (2001). United Kingdom Alcohol Treatment Trial: hypotheses, design and methods. *Alcohol and Alcoholism*, **36**, 11–21.

U.S. Department of Health and Human Services (2003). *Helping Patients with Alcohol Problems: A Health Practitioner's Guide.* National Institute of Health, National Institute on Alcohol Abuse and Alcoholism.

Vaillant, G. E. (1983). *The Natural History of Alcoholism: Causes, Patterns, and Paths to Recovery.* Cambridge, MA: Harvard University Press.

Vasilaki, E. I., Hosier, S. G. & Cox, W. M. (2006). The efficacy of motivational interviewing as a brief intervention for excessive drinking: a meta-analytic review. *Alcohol and Alcoholism*, **41**, 328–335.

Wallace, P., Cutler, S. & Haines, A. (1988). Randomized controlled trial of general practitioner intervention in patients with excessive alcohol consumptions. *British Medical Journal*, **297**, 663–8.

Watson, H. E. (1999). A study of minimal interventions for problem drinkers in acute care settings. *International Journal of Nursing Studies*, **36**, 425–34.

Whitlock, E. P., Polen, M. R., Green, C. A., Orleans, T. & Klein, J. (2004). Behavioral counseling interventions in primary care to reduce risky/harmful alcohol use by adults: a summary of the evidence for the U.S. Preventive Services Task Force. *Annals of Internal Medicine*, **140**, 557–68.

Wilk, A. I., Jensen, N. M. & Havighurst, T. C. (1997). Meta analysis of randomized control trials addressing brief interventions in heavy alcohol drinkers. *Journal of General Internal Medicine*, **12**, 274–83.

Willenbring, M. L., Kivlahan, D., Kenny, M., Grillo, M., Hagedorn, H. & Postier, A. (2004). Beliefs about evidence-based practices in addiction treatment: a survey of Veterans Administration program leaders. *Journal of Substance Abuse Treatment*, **26**, 79–85.

World Health Organization (WHO) Brief Intervention Study Group (1996). A cross-national trial of brief interventions with heavy drinkers. *American Journal of Public Health*, **86**, 948–55.

Wutzke, S. E., Conigrave, K. M., Saunders, J. B. & Hall, W. D. (2002). The long-term effectiveness of brief interventions for unsafe alcohol consumption: a 10-year follow-up. *Addiction*, **97**, 665–75.

Wutzke, S. E., Shiell, A., Gomel, M. K. & Conigrave, K. M. (2001). Cost effectiveness of brief interventions for reducing alcohol consumption. *Social Science and Medicine*, **52**, 863–70.

Yalom, I. D., Bloch, S., Bond, G., Zimmerman, E. & Qualls, B. (1978). Alcoholics in interactional group therapy: an outcome study. *Archives of General Psychiatry*, **35**, 419–25.

14

Pharmacotherapy of alcohol misuse, dependence and withdrawal

George A. Kenna, Kostas Agath and Robert Swift

Editor's note

While there is a large volume of research on alcohol misuse, dependence and withdrawal, the pharmacologic solutions are not as directly evident as this amount may suggest. There are widespread cultural determinants as to what constitutes alcohol misuse though the definitions for dependence are much clearer. Yet we do not have good solid pharmacologic treatments to prevent or decrease alcohol usage in the alcohol-dependent individual, though results from the recent COMBINE study suggest a more prominent and effective role for naltrexone in conjunction with medical management. Acamprosate did not fare as well in this trial even though it has been approved for alcohol dependence, and questions of heterogeneity among patient populations might explain conflicting findings. The effectiveness of disulfiram appears to rely heavily upon the patient's determination to remain abstinent. Anticonvulsants may have a role here, but more data is needed. Benzodiazepines remain the gold standard for treatment of symptoms of alcohol withdrawal, while a number of studies also support the use of some anticonvulsant drugs in assisting with withdrawal, especially in cases of mild-to-moderate severity.

Introduction

There is a large volume of research on the pharmacological treatments for alcohol misuse, dependence and withdrawal. Part of that research is marred by methodological difficulties (Moncrieff & Drummond 1997), necessitating increasingly sophisticated means of grading the available evidence to allow generalizability of findings (Mayo-Smith, 1997, Garbutt et al., 1999, Scottish Intercollegiate Guidelines Network –SIGN, 2003, Lingford-Hughes et al., 2004). This chapter summarizes the evidence base of the pharmacotherapy of alcohol misuse, dependence and withdrawal before citing examples of how that evidence has been crystallized into official guidelines shaping clinical practice. The chapter has a major limitation in that it focuses on literature available in English. It also spends some time on official guidelines issued in the United Kingdom. The relevant research findings will be presented organized under three subheadings: 'Harmful use of alcohol', 'Alcohol dependence' 'Alcohol withdrawal', reflecting the relevant diagnostic categories from the ICD-10 (World Health Organization, 1992) but also considering the DSM as well. The differences between the ICD and DSM-IV (Americans Psychiatric Association, 2000) with respect to these disorders are listed in Part I of this handbook.

Harmful use of alcohol

Harmful use refers to physical and/or mental damage due to a pattern of alcohol use in the absence of a diagnosis of another specific form of alcohol disorder (such as dependence). It is an ICD-10 diagnosis without a direct equivalent in DSM-IV, and its diagnosis depends upon the accurate reporting of alcohol-related physical or mental health problems (Babor, 1992). Harmful alcohol use (problem drinking) is believed to play a role in behavior associated with a pattern and amount of alcohol use considered hazardous such as decreased worker productivity, increased unintentional injuries, aggression and violence against others, and child and spouse abuse (Gmel & Rehm, 2003). Additionally, many individuals may periodically abuse alcohol at harmful levels, yet not be alcohol dependent. While the frequency and intensity of these markers increases with increased amounts and frequency of alcohol use, there is no firm quantitative definition for harmful alcohol use in the United States. For example, data from

Cambridge Textbook of Effective Treatments in Psychiatry, ed. Peter Tyrer and Kenneth R. Silk. Published by Cambridge University Press.

the National Health Interview Survey (Dawson, 1994), suggests that the risk of occupational injuries increases with the frequency of five or more drinks per occasion. Older workers who normally drink one or two drinks (equivalent to 1.5 ounces of 80 proof liquor) a day report the lowest risk of injuries contrasted with people who drink five or more drinks a day, who report more than a fivefold increase in risk (Zwerling et al., 1996). Heavy drinking is alcohol consumption exceeding 14 drinks per week for men (or more than four drinks per drinking occasion), more than seven drinks per week for women (or more than three drinks per occasion), and greater than seven drinks per week for all adults 65 years and older (National Institute on Alcohol Abuse and Alcoholism (NIAAA), 2000). Heavy alcohol use has also been defined (Office of Applied Studies, National Survey on Drug Use and Health (NSDUH), 2004) as drinking five or more drinks at the same time on at least five separate occasions during the previous month.

Appropriate pharmacological treatment is largely dependent on the health problem addressed (depression, anxiety, cardiovascular, endocrine, gastrointestinal abnormalities). Naltrexone has been tried but the research evidence has not supported its use in harmful use (Davidson et al., 2004, Kranzler et al., 2003, Davidson et al., 1999, Rubio et al., 2002). In the United Kingdom no official guidelines for the pharmacological treatment of harmful alcohol use exist.

Research on the use of NTX for non-dependent problem drinkers is limited. Kranzler et al. (2003) compared the effects of 50 mg of NTX or matching placebo in a sample of early problem drinkers who received NTX either daily or in targeted high-risk situations for drinking, in addition to brief coping skills therapy. Participants in the targeted group received a diminishing number of tablets (started at 1 tablet daily for week one, then 1 less tablet per week) over an 8-week treatment period. While NTX was better than placebo in reducing heavy drinking frequency, NTX did not significantly reduce the number of drinking days. Regardless of whether participants received NTX or placebo, there was a reduction in the likelihood for any drinking by participants in the targeted condition. However, as the number of tablets declined to fewer than three per week in the targeted NTX group, this group no longer exhibited a decreased risk for heavy drinking.

Davidson et al. (1999) found no differences in heavy drinkers between NTX and placebo in either drinking days or drinks per drinking day over a 7-day period in the home environment, but did find advantages of NTX for reducing craving and decreasing the reinforcing effects of alcohol. Moreover, Davidson et al. (2004) reported that placebo-treated hazardous drinkers fared better than those treated with NTX in terms of abstinence, drinks per

drinking day and craving, although the results may have been confounded by gender and family history of alcoholism. Rubio et al. (2002) in an open randomized trial with mildly dependent drinkers found delayed effects at 12 months after 12 weeks of a controlled drinking program either alone or in combination with NTX. The NTX group had fewer drinking days, heavy drinking days and less craving.

The dosing strategy for the use of naltrexone for harmful drinking in non-dependent alcoholics is unclear at present, and more details about NTX will be discussed in the other parts of this chapter. But presently, there is insufficient evidence at this time to support daily or targeted use of NTX for harmful alcohol use, and its use is best reserved for moderate-to-severe alcohol dependence (see below).

Alcohol dependence

The pharmacological treatments of alcohol dependence focus on relapse prevention once detoxification is complete. They are intended as an adjunct to psychosocial treatments (Slattery et al., 2003; Lingford-Hughes et al., 2004) and not as a monotherapy. In what follows we will review agents that research either supports their efficacy (disulfiram, acamprosate, naltrexone) or provides guidance on appropriate prescribing in common clinical scenarios (selective serotonin reuptake inhibitors – SSRIs). After a further review of non-conclusive research findings on other treatment regimes (topiramate and other anticonvulsants, antipsychotics, ondansetron, buspirone), we end the section by reporting the research findings that were crystallized into official guidelines in the United Kingdom.

Disulfiram

Despite some inconsistency in the findings, there seems to be a consensus that oral disulfiram reduces the number of drinking days (Garbutt et al., 1999). Supervision of disulfiram taking leads to a better outcome (Slattery et al., 2003), although not always in the order of a statistically significant effect (Berglund, 2003). Furthermore, for reasons that had to do with bioavailability, the therapeutic effect of disulfiram implants has not been demonstrated so far (Garbutt et al., 1999), although some authors feel positive in the light of modern formulations (Lingford-Hughes et al., 2004).

Disulfiram is an irreversible acetaldehyde dehydrogenase inhibitor that blocks alcohol metabolism creating a build-up of acetaldehyde. Disulfiram reinforces an individual's desire to stop drinking by providing a disincentive associated with the increase in acetaldehyde resulting in palpitations, hypotension, flushing, nausea and vomiting when patients consume alcohol.

In spite of the lack of evidence for its efficacy compared to placebo, some clinicians feel that disulfiram is an effective deterrent to drinking for certain individual patients. This is, in part, borne out by a survey of 1388 addiction-specialized physicians in the USA who reported that they prescribed disulfiram to only an average of 9% of their patients (Mark et al., 2003a). Another survey asked 174 addiction treatment program leaders (of which only 29% were physicians) to rate levels of disulfiram use at their Veterans Administration treatment centres in the US. The majority (58%) rated disulfiram use as low vs. 9% who rated it high (Willenbring et al., 2004). The primary issue predicting success with disulfiram is that candidates must be committed to total abstinence from alcohol. While anecdotal reports of success with this drug are common, clinical evidence suggests disulfiram appears to be most effective for alcoholics who are adherent, use which is intended for special high-risk situations (e.g. weddings, graduations, funerals) and particularly when administration is supervised (Fuller & Gordis, 2004).

Evidence

Controlled clinical trials of disulfiram have failed to consistently demonstrate a therapeutic benefit (Garbutt et al., 1999). Double-blind placebo-controlled studies using disulfiram are difficult since the psychological deterrent to use is experienced by both treatment groups and those who relapse will be unblinded when they experience the pharmacological interaction.

In the most rigorous clinical trial conducted in a population of veterans, no significant difference in abstinence rates between groups taking placebo, 1 mg or 250 mg of disulfiram was demonstrated (Fuller et al., 1986). However, patients randomized to receive 250 mg of disulfiram daily drank less frequently (significantly fewer drinking days per year). Moreover, when individuals were compliant (which was low), regardless of group, alcohol consumption was reduced. Patients who were middle-aged and had social stability were more likely to benefit from disulfiram. In another trial in which administration was supervised, patients receiving disulfiram drank less alcohol and less frequently; however upon randomization patients were unblinded to their drug (Chick et al., 1992).

Recent evidence suggests that disulfiram may provide greater benefit in treating cocaine dependence, particularly evident in those who abstained from alcohol use (Carroll et al., 2004; Gossop & Carroll, 2006). The authors suggest that differential compliance may have explained this finding. However, further studies are needed before recommendations can be made with respect to disulfiram treatment of patients with co-occurring cocaine and alcohol use disorders, and whether those recommendations should be any different than for alcoholic patients without co-occurring cocaine dependence.

The efficacy of disulfiram compared to other antidipsotropic agents such as naltrexone (De Sousa & De Sousa, 2004) is poorly studied. However, while there was no advantage for combining disulfiram with NTX in dually diagnosed alcohol-dependent patients (Petrakis et al., 2005), in another study, disulfiram combined with acamprosate (ACAM) resulted in increased days of cumulative abstinence (Besson et al., 1998).

Dosing

The recommended starting dose is 250 mg a day (Fuller & Gordis, 2004), though the manufacturer recommends 500 mg (MicroMedix, 2006a) with a range from 125–500 mg. If a patient drinks and does not experience a disulfiram–ethanol reaction, the dose can be increased to 500 mg, as a significant proportion of patients may not experience a disulfiram–alcohol reaction at the usual 250 mg daily dose (Fuller & Gordis, 2004; Brewer, 1993). However, side effects are increased at doses greater than 250 mg. Dosing starts at least 12–24 hours after abstinence initiation (when the blood or breath alcohol concentration is zero) with a maintenance dose of 250 mg daily.

Contraindications, warnings and interactions

Because of the intense cardiovascular and physical changes that occur in the disulfiram-ethanol interaction, disulfiram is contraindicated in patients with cardiac disease, coronary occlusion, cerebrovascular disease, and kidney or liver failure. Many clinicians avoid disulfiram use in elderly patients or those with any significant medical illness (e.g. diabetes). Disulfiram is teratogenic (Category C) and should not be used in pregnant women. Disulfiram can also be hepatotoxic and should be used cautiously in patients with liver disease.

Liver function tests should be monitored at baseline and periodically during treatment. Although not all clinicians agree (Chick, 1999; Dilts & Dilts, 1996), most would recommend at minimum *baseline* liver function tests (liver function tests (LFTs): ALT, AST, GGT) and withholding disulfiram when LFTs are > 3 times upper limits of normal (Saxon et al., 1998). If elevated, repeat LFTs every 1–2 weeks until normal, and then every 3–6 months if no elevations (Wright et al., 1993, 1998), with the awareness that increased LFTs may signal return to drinking rather than disulfiram toxicity. Persistently elevated LFTs may also indicate viral hepatitis (B or C), for which alcoholics are at higher risk; and thus the need to order a hepatitis profile. There are wide ranges of psychiatric adverse effects that include disorientation, agitation, depression and behavioral changes that include paranoia, withdrawal, bizarre behaviors (Daniel *et al.*, 1987; Hotson & Langston, 1976; Knee & Razani, 1974), worsening of schizophrenia especially at doses > 250 mg daily. Disulfiram should be avoided, or used very cautiously, in persons with these above conditions. On the other hand, disulfiram can be used relatively safely at a dose of 250 mg daily in alcohol-dependent patients with co-occurring psychiatric disorders, including schizophrenia (Larson *et al.*, 1992; Mueser *et al.*, 2003; Petrakis *et al.*, 2005). Common side effects of disulfiram include drowsiness, particularly in the first few weeks of treatment, a metallic or 'garlic' taste and sexual dysfunction. If drowsiness occurs, then the dose may be taken at bedtime.

Patients taking disulfiram must be informed about the dangers of consuming even small amounts of alcohol in foods, in over-the-counter medications, in mouthwashes and topical lotions and also verify that they understand the necessary precautions and the consequences of alcohol use.

Disulfiram is a potent inhibitor of the CYP2E1 oxidase, and can interact with anticoagulants (warfarin), antiepileptics (phenytoin, carbamazepine), some benzodiazepines (e.g. diazepam but not lorazepam) and tricyclic antidepressants (amitriptyline, desipramine), potentially increasing the toxicity of these medications. Delirium may result in combination with monoamine oxidase inhibitors. Other important interactions include metronidazole and omeprazole (MicroMedix, 2006a).

Summary

The social, medical and psychiatric status of a candidate is an important consideration in the use of disulfiram. Generally, clinicians do not recommend disulfiram as an initial treatment for alcohol-dependent patients because of problems with adherence, but rather reserve the medication for patients who have failed one or more episodes of psychosocial treatment. Conditions that potentially enhance the effectiveness of disulfiram include: (1) agreement by the patient to have medication administration supervized or observed by a concerned significant other; and (2) high levels of patient motivation to prove sustained abstinence, because of court-related contingencies or threatened loss of employment or licensure such as among health professionals.

Acamprosate

A series of meta-analyses and systematic reviews demonstrated that, when used as an adjunct to psychosocial interventions, acamprosate (ACAM) improves drinking outcomes such as the length and rate of abstinence (Miller & Wilbourne, 2002, Berglund, 2003, Slattery *et al.*, 2003, Mann *et al.*, 2003). This effect is doubtful if ACAM is not initiated quickly after a detoxification (Chick *et al.*, 2000; Gual & Lehert, 2001). There is evidence that the effect of ACAM on abstinence rate lasts after the treatment is stopped (Poldrugo *et al.*, 1997). The addition of NTX to ACAM compared to placebo enhances outcome even further (Kiefer *et al.*, 2003). The success of ACAM, however, seems limited to European trials as recent US trials failed to demonstrate significant results on primary outcome measures (Mason *et al.*, 2006; Anton *et al.*, 2006).

Acamprosate (ACAM) has multiple actions but is principally a glutamate and GABA modulator. *In vitro* and *in vivo* studies in animals suggest that ACAM interacts with GABA and glutamate to restore the imbalance of neuronal excitation (Zeise *et al.*, 1993) and inhibition (Daoust *et al.*, 1992) caused by chronic alcohol use. The key mechanism of action is considered to be as a weak functional antagonist of the glutamate NMDA receptor possibly mediated through indirect modulation of the receptor site via antagonism at the mGluR5 receptor (Littleton & Zieglgansberger, 2003).

ACAM appears to be especially useful in a therapeutic regimen targeted at promoting abstinence and can be used in primary care settings as well as specialized addiction treatment programs (Kiritze-Topor *et al.*, 2004). ACAM has been studied in thousands of patients, primarily in Europe, and there are few contraindications for treatment. There is little consistent information about patient characteristics that predict improvement while taking ACAM. On one hand, in a meta-analysis of all US and European studies, predictors of abstinence were motivation, readiness to change, baseline abstinence, initial first week compliance and living with a partner or child (Mason, 2005). On the other hand, a pooled analysis of seven European trials found no significant predictors of the abstinence outcome measures (Verheul *et al.*, 2005). Candidates for ACAM should be committed to abstinence and begin the medication after being abstinent from alcohol (Carmen *et al.*, 2004; Mason *et al.*, 2006).

Evidence

Evidence for the efficacy of ACAM in the treatment of alcohol dependence is a result of numerous trials involving several thousand participants. In a systematic review of the efficacy data related to ACAM, Garbutt *et al.* (1999) concluded that the proof for efficacy of ACAM was strong. Moreover, several ACAM studies have reported positive results. For example, in a study of 272 severely dependent alcoholics, patients receiving ACAM showed a significantly higher continuous abstinence rate within the first 2 months of treatment compared to patients receiving placebo (Sass *et al.*, 1996). Forty per cent of ACAM treated patients compared to 17% of those who received placebo were continuously abstinent over a 48-week period.

ACAM has also been studied for periods of up to a year. In a long-term follow-up (12 months) after trial completion, ACAM still maintained an effect on abstinence rates, but not on non-drinking days (Whitworth *et al.*, 1996). There have also been negative studies reported (e.g. Anton *et al.*, 2006; Mason *et al.*, 2006; Chick *et al.*, 2000; Namkoong *et al.*, 2003; Roussaux *et al.*, 1996), though two of the studies may have been underpowered (Namkoong *et al.*, 2003; Roussaux *et al.*, 1996). One of these studies also had a short treatment period (Namkoong *et al.*, 2003), and the other had a long delay in initiating treatment (Chick *et al.*, 2000). In sum, most studies suggest that ACAM is a safe and well-tolerated drug for the promotion of alcohol abstinence.

The question as for whether ACAM is more effective than NTX, cannot conclusively be answered at this time, but results from the COMBINE study (The Combined Pharmacotherapies and Behavioral Interventions) study suggest that it has no significant effect on drinking vs. placebo, either by itself or with any combination of the other treatments in the study. The rationale for combining these treatments was that they have different mechanisms of action (Koob & LeMoal, 2001). Despite the negative results for ACAM in the COMBINE, a prior existing randomized controlled study of 160 patients found that combining NTX and ACAM was more effective than either placebo or ACAM alone, but was not significantly more effective than NTX alone (Kiefer *et al.*, 2003). A single-blind randomized comparison of ACAM alone vs. NTX alone without a placebo comparison favored NTX in terms of abstinence rates and time to first relapse to heavy drinking (Rubio *et al.*, 2001). A final consideration is that two reviews concluded that NTX has more side effects than acamprosate (Carmen *et al.*, 2004; Mason, 2003).

The COMBINE trial randomized over 1300 individuals in a double-blind fashion to receive placebo, NTX, or ACAM alone or in combination (COMBINE Study Research Group, 2003; Anton *et al.*, 2006). In this 2 by 2 by 2 study design, there were 9 cells. The initial assignments to each cell were 153 to Medical Management (MM) + placebo, 152 to MM + ACAM, 154 to MM + NTX, 148 to MM + ACAM + NTX, 156 to MM + placebo + combined behavioural intervention (CBI), 151 to MM + ACAM + CBI, 155 to MM + NTX + CBI, 157 to MM + ACAM + NTX + CBI, and 157 to CBI alone. Reiterating the above, the COMBINE results reveal that ACAM is no better than placebo, alone or in any of the combinations where it was included in the above study design (Anton *et al.*, 2006).

Dose

ACAM is dispensed in 333 mg tablets and the usual dose is 666 mg three times daily (Forest Labs, 2004). Patients can be started on the full ACAM dose without titration. ACAM is not well absorbed into the blood from the digestive tract and it takes several days to achieve desired blood levels of the medication. The medication appears to be safe and effective in alcoholics, with minimal side effects. It does not appear to produce sedation and does not cause drug dependence. Main adverse effects of ACAM appear to be gastrointestinal, including nausea, diarrhea and bloating. Nausea or diarrhea can be usually managed with bismuth compounds, but if symptoms are severe or persistent, the dose should be reduced by one-third to one-half.

Contraindications, warnings and interactions

ACAM should not be used in patients with impaired kidney function (creatinine clearance ≤ 30 ml/min), nor in patients who previously exhibited hypersensitivity to ACAM. ACAM should only be used during pregnancy when the benefit clearly outweighs the risk as the drug has been shown to be teratogenic (Category C) in rats (Forest Labs, 2004).

Tetracyclines may be inactivated by the calcium component in acamprosate during concurrent administration (MicroMedix, 2006b). Naltrexone increases plasma levels of ACAM, although the clinical significance of this interaction is unknown (Johnson *et al.*, 2003a; Mason *et al.*, 2002).

Summary

Acamprosate was approved by the US Food and Drug Administration (FDA) in the summer of 2004 for the maintenance of abstinence in alcohol dependent individuals who are abstinent at treatment initiation. Efficacy in early studies of ACAM was demonstrated despite the lack of use of a standardised psychotherapy. A meta-analysis showed a significant effect of ACAM to improve the abstinence rate and treatment retention compared to placebo (Bouza *et al.*, 2004). Despite a strong showing in many European trials, less favorable results compared to NTX in recent studies perhaps make ACAM a good choice for heavily dependent patients coming out of detoxification with verifiable abstinence before starting the drug. We therefore suspect, that different patients will respond better to either ACAM or NTX, both drugs in combination, or neither.

Naltrexone

Evidence seems to support the use of naltrexone (NTX) as an adjunct to psychosocial interventions (Miller & Wilbourne 2002; Berglund, 2003; Slattery *et al.*, 2003, Anton *et al.*, 2006), with higher abstinence rates in short-term treatment (Srisurapanont & Jarusuraisin, 2003) and as a deterrent to progressing from a lapse to a full-blown relapse (Garbutt *et al.*, 1999). Naltrexone is as efficacious as disulfiram and probably more efficacious than ACAM (Kranzler & Van Kirk, 2001; Srisurapanont & Jarusuraisin, 2003). Addition of acamprosate to naltrexone does not enhance outcome (Kiefer *et al.*, 2003), but addition of NTX to ACAM appears to enhance outcome but probably because of the effect of the NTX (Anton *et al.*, 2006).

NTX blocks the action of endorphins when alcohol is consumed, and this results in an attenuation of dopamine release in the nucleus accumbens thought to be crucially important to positive reinforcement, reward (Koob & LaMoal, 2001) and craving, particularly in those who may be predisposed (Benjamin *et al.*, 1993).

Although NTX therapy has been recommended for all alcohol-dependent patients who do not have a medical contraindication to its use (SAMHSA, 1997), a survey of 1388 addiction-specialized physicians in the USA reported that they prescribed NTX to an average of only 13% of their patients (Mark *et al.*, 2003b). The main self-reported reasons why physicians did not prescribe NTX to more patients were that patients refused to take the medication or comply with prescribing regimes (23%), and that patients could not afford the medication (21%).

Several studies indicate that NTX is most effective in patients with strong craving (O'Malley *et al.*, 1992; Chick *et al.*, 2000; McCaul *et al.*, 2000), poor cognitive status at study entry (Jaffe *et al.*, 1996) and high compliance (Monti *et al.*, 1999; Volpicelli *et al.*, 1997). This observation is consistent with the demonstrated effect of NTX in reducing craving. There is also evidence that persons with a family history for alcoholism, early age at onset of drinking and comorbid use of other drugs are more likely to benefit from NTX (Rubio *et al.*, 2005).

Evidence

A systematic review of all data published up to 1997 concluded that NTX produced a consistent decrease in relapse rate to heavy drinking and in drinking frequency, though it did not enhance absolute abstinence rates (Garbutt *et al.*, 1999). More specifically, several studies using naltrexone report the opioid antagonist to be more effective than placebo in reducing relapse rates and increasing percent non-drinking days (Monti *et al.*, 2001; O'Malley *et al.*, 1992; Volpicelli *et al.*, 1992), or in reducing craving in heavy drinkers (Davidson *et al.*, 1999). Yet other studies fail to demonstrate a significant difference with placebo (Kranzler *et al.*, 2000; Krystal *et al.*, 2001). Several factors may explain the discrepancies in results of the different clinical trials with NTX. Many of the studies included small sample sizes and may lack the statistical power to demonstrate treatment effects (Kranzler & Van Kirk, 2001). However, several large sufficiently powered studies also reported negative results (Gastpar *et al.*, 2002; Kranzler *et al.*, 2000; Krystal *et al.*, 2001). Nonetheless, the COMBINE study clearly supports the effectiveness of NTX in that each of the groups of patients receiving NTX in conjunction with medical management had a higher percentage of days abstinent than those receiving placebo + MM without NTX or CBI (combined behavioural intervention). NTX also reduced the risk of heavy drinking.

Vivitrol 380 mg, an injectable form of NTX, was approved by the FDA and released in June 2006 to practitioners. Injectable naltrexone is safe and well tolerated in alcohol-dependent individuals (Galloway *et al.*, 2005), but has the same hepatic safety concerns as tablets. Obviously, compliance is a big advantage over tablets. In two double-blind randomized placebo-controlled trials the efficacy of once monthly long-acting injectable or depot forms of NTX was demonstrated (Garbutt *et al.*, 2005; Kranzler *et al.*, 2004); which may have the advantage of increasing compliance. In the Garbutt *et al.* trial, however, men receiving naltrexone injection had better treatment outcomes than women. Additionally, there was a robust effect for Vivitrol compared to placebo for people coming into the study abstinent. Though the sample fitting this category was only 10% of the total sample size, the FDA required the manufacturer to place a requirement for abstinence when starting the medication on its product information.

Patients receiving Vivitrol must be opioid free from 7–10 days as substantiated with a urine drug test and should be asked to wear some kind of identifier for medical emergencies. One clinical concern with long-acting injectable NTX is pain management. Any attempt to overcome the opioid blockade produced by Vivitrol using exogenous opioids may result in fatal overdose. Should a patient be in pain after receiving an injection, the first drug of choice

egelorwwhaanp

should be a non-opioid (e.g. I.M. or I.V. ketorolac or oral NSAIDs). If the patient is still in pain, an opioid can be used but will most likely have to be administered in a higher dose and more frequently. When reversal of Vivitrol blockade is required for pain management, patients should be monitored in a setting equipped and staffed for cardiopulmonary resuscitation and monitored for signs of respiratory depression.

Dose

NTX has been approved for use in the first 90 days of abstinence when the risk of relapse is highest. It has also been shown to be safe and well tolerated by patients for periods of up to a year. The usual dose of oral NTX is 50 mg daily, although doses of 25 mg to 100 mg daily have been reported to be effective, particularly those with lower blood concentrations of the drug (Rohsenow, 2004). Side effects are more common in the initial few days of therapy. Starting with a 25 mg dose (half a tablet) for the first 2 to 4 daily doses may reduce the incidence of side effects. In a year-long safety study with 570 alcohol-dependent patients, the most common side effects were nausea, headache, anxiety and sedation (Croop et al., 1997). Should such side effects occur, reducing the dosage by one-half often reduces the side effects. Nausea can be managed with bismuth compounds or antihistamines and headache with the usual over-the-counter headache remedies. Anecdotally, some practitioners suggest that, because of its long half-life, NTX may also be administered orally three times weekly in doses of 100 mg on Mondays, 100 mg on Wednesdays, and 150 mg on Fridays (or the equivalent of 50 mg daily). This method may facilitate supervised or observed administration of NTX, because only three (vs. seven) observations are required per week.

Contraindications, warnings, interactions

NTX is contraindicated in patients with a history of sensitivity to naltrexone, with acute hepatitis or liver failure, who are physically dependent on opioids, receiving opioid analgesics, or patients in acute opioid withdrawal. The benefit of using NTX during pregnancy should clearly outweigh the risk (Category C).

The concurrent administration of NTX and opioid analgesics is contraindicated. To avoid triggering an acute abstinence syndrome, patients must be opioid-free for a minimum of 7 to 10 days before initiating treatment with naltrexone, as substantiated with a urine drug test. Though rarely performed in actual practice, a naloxone challenge test can be utilized before treatment with NTX to rule out concurrent use of opioids (MicroMedix, 2006c).

Antidepressants

The SSRIs and other antidepressants seem not to be effective for the treatment of alcohol dependence (Garbutt et al., 1999; Miller & Wilburn, 2002; Berglund, 2003), although there is some evidence of a short-lived improved outcome when prescribed in higher dosages to heavy social drinkers (Lingford-Hughes et al., 2004). Additionally, in the presence of depression, SSRIs could improve mood (but not drinking outcome) when treating alcohol dependence (Berglund 2003; Lingford-Hughes et al., 2004).

Most antidepressants either block the presynaptic re-uptake of serotonin and/or norepinephrine, block their synaptic metabolism or utilize a combination of these mechanisms. Much of the research on antidepressants has focused on serotonergics. Alcohol's effects on the brain show that alcoholics and experimental animals that consume large amounts of alcohol show comparatively lower levels of serotonin than non-alcoholics (Lovinger, 1997). Considerable experimental evidence suggests that serotonin plays a crucial role in impulsivity and craving often seen in alcoholics (Ciccocioppo, 1999) and to be at least in part associated with alcohol dependence (LeMarquand et al., 1994; Myers & Martin, 1973).

There is little evidence for the use of an antidepressant for alcohol dependence, particularly as a single diagnosis or for the typical alcohol-dependent patient (Torrens et al., 2005). Even in the presence of co-occurring depression, antidepressants have only modest if any effects on drinking outcomes in randomized controlled trials (Kranzler et al., 2006; Moak et al., 2003; Nunes & Levin, 2004; Pettinati et al., 2000, 2004; Roy-Byrne et al., 2000), although some studies have reported positive effects (Cornelius et al., 1997; Hernandez-Avila et al., 2004). Nevertheless, antidepressants are commonly prescribed to patients with alcohol dependence with one study estimating a prescription rate of 46% for alcohol-dependent patients, considerably higher than prescription rates for disulfiram and naltrexone (Mark et al., 2003a). The relatively high rate of antidepressant use may be a response to high rates of co-occurring anxiety and depressive disorders among alcohol-dependent patients and some evidence that patients with untreated co-occurring mental disorders have poor outcomes. Moreover, antidepressants have small-to-medium size effects on reducing depressive symptoms among alcohol dependent patients with carefully diagnosed major depression (Nunes & Levin, 2004; Pettinati, 2004).

Evidence

Tricyclic antidepressants such as imipramine (McGrath et al., 1996) and desipramine (Mason et al., 1996) have not been effective in reducing drinking in alcohol dependent patients. One study of nortriptyline yielded mixed results depending on diagnostic subtype, but was ineffective for patients with alcohol dependence only (Powell et al., 1995). Similarly, nefazodone has not been effective in reducing drinking in most double-blind placebo-controlled trials studies (Kranzler et al., 2000; Roy-Byrne et al., 2000; Wetzel et al., 2004) with one exception (Hernandez-Avila et al., 2004). While many antidepressants have been tested for alcohol dependence, clearly SSRIs because of their mild side effect profile have produced the most trials. Conclusions of clinical trials using SSRIs are uncertain (Garbutt et al., 1999). Despite reductions in drinking in lab studies with experimental animals (Pettinati, 1996), in human drinking sessions (Pettinati, 1996; Naranjo & Bremner, 1984) and in alcoholics with major depression (Cornelius et al., 1997), most double-blind placebo-controlled studies using SSRIs including fluoxetine (Gorelick & Paredes, 1992; Kabel & Petty, 1996; Kranzler et al., 1995; Janiri et al., 1996), citalopram (Naranjo et al., 1995; Tiihonen et al, 1996), or sertraline (Pettinati et al., 2000; Kranzler et al., 2006) have not reduced any measures of alcohol consumption.

However, genotypic and phenotypic variations may differ for persons with alcohol dependence and those with comorbid alcohol dependence and depression might be an important subpopulation that could respond differently to treatment (Nellissery et al., 2003). Moreover, SSRIs do not appear to be an efficacious approach to treating heterogeneous groups of alcoholics (Johnson, 2003) though subtypes of alcoholics may respond differentially to SSRIs. Though Kranzler et al. (1995) demonstrated that using 60 mg of fluoxetine was no better than placebo in reducing alcohol consumption, two alcoholic subtypes were found to respond differentially to fluoxetine. The Type A subtype (an onset of dependence after 25 years of age, few psychopathological problems, few drinking-related problems and childhood risk factors) drank the same as the group receiving placebo. Those of the Type B subtype (an early-onset type occurring before the age of 25, with more severe psychopathology, antisocial and impulsive tendencies), drank more than those receiving placebo (Kranzler et al., 1996). As a follow-up to the Kranzler et al. study, Pettinatti and colleagues (2000) used 200 mg of sertraline and confirmed that Type B subtype alcoholics actually drank more when taking SSRIs but conflicted with the Kranzler et al. study and demonstrated that Type A subtype alcoholics drank significantly less. Moreover, the sertraline advantage for Type A alcoholics persisted for 6 months following pharmacotherapy (Dundon et al., 2004).

In addition to the Type A/Type B distinction and genotypic differences, secondary analyses of randomized controlled trial data suggest that gender (Moak et al., 2003; Pettinati et al., 2004), co-occurring cocaine use disorders (Cornelius et al., 1997; Kabel & Petty, 1996) and other psychiatric disorders (Brady et al., 2002; Powell et al., 1995) may influence antidepressant response as well. These findings support the notion that there appear to be subgroups of alcoholics who might be differentially affected by serotonin-type treatments.

Summary

Recent studies suggest a subgroup of alcohol-dependent individuals who have a later onset of the disorder and lack predisposing factors such as family history, as well as those with comorbid depression, may show some degree of success using SSRIs. At this time, however, the treatment of non-depressed alcoholics with SSRIs remains experimental and may actually worsen drinking behaviours in some individuals.

Anticonvulsants

Though more commonly used to treat alcohol withdrawal (Malcolm et al., 2001), some anticonvulsants have also been shown to reduce alcohol use. Carbamazepine, for example, is reported to reduce alcohol consumption in alcohol-dependent subjects (Malcolm et al., 1989). A double-blind study of 29 alcohol-dependent subjects receiving carbamazepine or placebo also showed reduced drinking during medication treatment (Mueller et al., 1997). Similarly, there is modest evidence from one double-blind randomized controlled trial that divalproex decreased relapse to heavy drinking in a sample of 29 subjects, although other drinking outcomes did not differ from placebo (Brady et al., 2002). Moreover, valproate significantly decreased the proportion of heavy drinking days vs. placebo when added to lithium therapy in patients with co-occurring alcohol dependence and bipolar disorder (Salloum et al., 2005). The effectiveness of another anticonvulsant agent, topiramate (TPMT), shows the most promise however. Based on the results of a preliminary study (Johnson et al., 2003b), the manufacturer has performed a large multicenter double-blind placebo-controlled trial using TPMT in alcohol dependent patients, which should yield published results by 2007.

Topiramate

Topiramate (TPMT) is a FDA approved anticonvulsant found to have multiple mechanisms of action including enhanced $GABA_A$ inhibition (White et al., 2000) that results in decreased dopamine facilitation in the midbrain thought to be of potential benefit in the treatment of addiction (Gerasimov et al., 2001). Additionally, there is antagonism of kainate to activate the kainate/AMPA glutamate receptor subtypes (Gryder & Rogawski, 2003) and inhibition of Type II and IV carbonic anhydrase isoenzymes.

Evidence

At the time of writing, the use of TPMT for alcohol dependence treatment is limited to one trial, and some anecdotal reports. Johnson and colleagues (2003b) in a randomized double-blind placebo controlled trial used an escalating dose titration from 25 mg to 300 mg per day of TPMT or matching placebo in 150 men and women non-treatment seeking alcoholics during the first 8 weeks of a 12-week period. Patients stayed at the same dose over the last 4 weeks of the study. Participants receiving TPMT reported significantly fewer drinks per day and drinks per drinking day, significantly fewer drinking days, significantly more days of abstinence and significantly less craving than placebo. The evidence suggests that since abstinence was not a goal at the start of the TPMT study, the medication may be more beneficial during the abstinence initiation phase of treatment (Swift, 2003). In the current trial, TPMT is titrated from 25 mg per day up to 200 mg a day over 5 weeks. The patient is then raised to 300 mg per day (100 mg in the am; 200 mg in the pm) or to their maximum tolerable dose. Prominent side effects include mental confusion, slowness in thinking, paresthesias, depression and somnolence which may be attenuated by titration when initiating therapy, and development of renal calculi in about 1.5% of patients (Ortho-McNeil, 2003). Adequate hydration is encouraged particularly in patients who may be at risk for developing calculi.

Contraindications, warnings, interactions

Topiramate is contraindicated in those hypersensitive to the drug. Topiramate should be used with caution in those who have a history of urolithiasis, paresthesias, secondary angle closure glaucoma, renal or hepatic impairment, and conditions or therapies that predispose to acidosis (such as renal disease, severe respiratory disorders, status epilepticus, diarrhea, surgery, ketogenic diet or drugs). Monitoring for hyperchloremic non-ionic gap metabolic acidosis is essential, and therefore baseline chemistry should be assessed. Metabolic acidosis can cause symptoms such as tiredness and loss of appetite, or more serious conditions including arrhythmia or coma. Topiramate has been found to be teratogenic in animal studies and is a pregnancy Category C medication (Ortho-McNeil, 2003).

Concomitant use of oral contraceptives, phenytoin, carbamazepine and valproic acid have been found to interact with TPMT (Ciraulo et al., 2006). Co-administration of another carbonic anhydrase inhibitor such as acetazolamide may increase the possibility of renal stone formation and should be avoided.

Summary

Much more clinical research is needed on TPMT in efficacy and effectiveness trials, as well as determining the proper dose. However, TPMT may be very useful in helping alcohol-dependent patients, who can't stop drinking at the start of treatment, initiate abstinence. Given TPMT's unique mechanism of action, co-administration with other medications such as NTX and/or ACAM, ondansetron or SSRIs may produce enhanced outcomes, particularly for various alcohol subtypes.

Antipsychotics

Reward associated with alcohol cues that influence dopamine (DA) release by the mesolimbic pathway and irrelevant stimuli interpreted as positive symptoms of schizophrenia (e.g. delusions), seem to share similar dopaminergic dysfunction (Heinz, 2002). Neuroleptics regulate dopamine occupancy at DRD2 dopamine receptors possibly causing an up-regulation of DRD2 receptors (Lidow & Rakic, 1997; Karan & Pandhi, 2000) that is associated with reduced positive symptoms of schizophrenia as well as reduced substance use (Thanos et al., 2001). Potentially this relationship influences the disproportionate prevalence of co-occurring substance abuse and schizophrenia when compared to the general population (Regier et al., 1990). The use of antipsychotics for alcoholics, therefore, may signify the correlation of an important common pathway afflicting both disorders.

Evidence

Recent reports suggest that atypical neuroleptics, such as clozapine, reduce alcohol drinking among schizophrenic and schizoaffective patients with comorbid substance abuse/dependence (Albanese et al., 1994). A naturalistic study of drinking patterns in patients receiving clozapine and typical neuroleptics showed significant reductions of alcohol use while on clozapine (Drake et al., 2000). In human laboratory studies, both typical neuroleptics (haloperidol) and atypical neuroleptics (olanzapine) reduced craving for alcohol among alcoholics and heavy social drinkers (Modell et al., 1993; Hutchison et al., 2001), though the data for olanzapine is far from conclusive. For example, Hutchinson and colleagues (2005) reported that olanzapine may be differentially effective for craving and alcohol consumption in participants who were homozygous or heterozygous for the seven or longer, repeat allele of the DRD4 variable number of tandem repeats polymorphism. Though by contrast, patients with first-episode schizophrenia and a co-occurring history of alcohol use disorder were less likely to respond to olanzapine than patients without a history of alcohol use disorder (Green *et al.*, 2004). Furthermore, a 12-week double-blind placebo-controlled trial comparing olanzapine to placebo in the treatment of 60 alcohol dependent patients demonstrated no difference in any of the drinking variables (Guardia *et al.*, 2004). Another antipsychotic, aripiprazole, a partial dopamine agonist was first proposed to be a useful treatment of alcoholism (Kenna, 2003). A case of a patient with schizophrenia and comorbid alcohol dependence receiving 20 mg daily of aripiprazole reported a reduction in alcohol use (Warsi *et al.*, 2005). Aripiprazole was tested in a Phase IV double-blind placebo-controlled clinical trial of alcohol-dependent patients by the manufacturer. The official results of that study are at this time quarantined. Quetiapine has also been reported to be useful for reducing alcohol use and craving in a bipolar patient (Longoria *et al.*, 2004) and may be useful for improving sleep and maintaining abstinence in alcohol-dependent patients (Monnelly *et al.*, 2004).

Summary

At present, there is no clinical evidence to support the prescription of antipsychotics to alcohol-dependent patients without a co-occurring diagnosis that may require the use of an antipsychotic.

Ondansetron

Ondansetron is an anti-emetic used for chemotherapy and post-operative nausea. Ondansetron has functionally opposite affects to SSRIs and blocks serotonin at 5-HT_3 post-synaptic receptors. One hypothesis states that individuals with a family history positive genetic link for alcohol dependence may be more prone to have a hyper-homozygous variant of the serotonin re-uptake transporter (5-HTTLPR) that results in more rapid serotonin removal, an up-regulation of 5-HT_3 post-synaptic receptors and attenuated dopaminergic functioning (Johnson & Ait-Doud, 2000). Yet the genotypic mechanism for this effect is far from conclusive (see Feinn *et al.*, 2005).

Evidence

While further evidence is needed, early studies suggest that ondansetron may be an important adjunctive treatment for the early onset alcoholic subgroup. Sellers *et al.* (1994) compared placebo to 1, 4 and 16 µg/kg twice a day doses of ondansetron and demonstrated that the group taking the 4 µg/kg twice a day dose drank significantly less alcohol than the other groups – suggesting a U-shaped dosing response. Following the same design, Johnson *et al.* (2000) subtyped their participants into those with a biological predisposition who were early and late onset alcoholics, consistent with previous studies (Sellers *et al.*, 1994; Pettinati *et al.*, 2000). In this study, the early onset alcoholics taking the 4 µg/kg dose of ondansetron reported less cumulative percentage drinking days than placebo (Johnson *et al.*, 2000) as well as less craving (Johnson *et al.*, 2002), again suggesting the existence of subtypes of alcoholics that have differential pharmacological responses. In sum, as demonstrated in studies with serotonergics, the variable responses based on individual variables such as onset of alcoholism, may suggest that alcoholics respond differentially based on various serotonin 5-HT subtypes.

Summary

The use of ondansetron in the treatment of alcohol dependence is still experimental, as large-scale clinical trials have yet to be conducted. The doses used in trials thus far are lower than those used to treat nausea. Additionally, at present, there is no explanation for the non-monotonic dose response. In general, future studies need to further explicate the underlying differences between alcoholic subtypes, such that reasonable predictions about treatment outcomes with serotonergics can be made (Johnson, 2003).

Buspirone

Evidence

There are seven randomised controlled studies of buspirone, a 5HT1A receptor partial agonist that is approved for the treatment of generalized anxiety disorder. In the treatment of patients with either alcohol abuse or dependence, three studies reported a positive effect on reducing drinking or craving. Bruno (1989) studied patients with 'mild to moderate alcohol abuse' and found a statistically significant reduction (buspirone vs. placebo) in both craving and the proportion of responders, with response defined as a 50% reduction in amount of drinking over the 8-week study period. Co-occurring psychiatric diagnoses were heterogeneous and included affective disorders (20%), anxiety disorders (32%), and borderline personality disorders (32%). Tollefson *et al.* (1992) studied patients after 4 weeks of abstinence that had either alcohol abuse or dependence and co-occurring generalized anxiety disorder with baseline Hamilton-Anxiety (Ham-A) scores greater than 18. Buspirone significantly decreased anxiety and craving compared to placebo, but had no overall effect on substance use. Kranzler *et al.* (1994) studied alcohol-dependent patients with depression (~25%) and/or anxiety disorders (~50%) and baseline Ham-A scores > 14. They reported differential reductions in both drinking and anxiety, but not craving. All three of these studies included both men and women with a fair proportion having anxiety disorders and mild-to-moderate alcohol problems. Of the four negative studies, only one included women and that study excluded patients with co-occurring psychiatric disorders (Malec *et al.*, 1996). Among the three negative studies that recruited men only, two included men as they were completing 4–5 weeks of inpatient treatment, indicative of high-severity alcohol dependence/problems (George *et al.*, 1999; Malcolm *et al.*, 1992). In the remaining negative study with men only, less than 5% of buspirone-treated patients had anxiety disorders (Fawcett *et al.*, 2000).

Summary

The contradictory findings across the clinical trials of buspirone may reflect between-study heterogeneity in patient characteristics. Although buspirone cannot be recommended to treat alcohol dependence in general, it may be worth trying for outpatients with either alcohol abuse or less severe forms of alcohol dependence if they also have a co-occurring anxiety disorder with high levels of anxiety.

Treatment recommendations in official national guidelines (United Kingdom)

Recommended first-line treatment in official national guidelines

General recommendations (irrespective of setting)

- Disulfiram for newly detoxified patients, preferably supervised (Department of Health, 1999) as an adjunct to psychosocial interventions in the treatment of chronic alcohol dependence (British) National Formulary ([BNF 50], 2004)
- Acamprosate for the maintenance of abstinence in alcohol dependence (BNF 50, 2004)

Primary care setting recommendations

- Acamprosate for detoxified dependent patients as an adjunct to psychosocial interventions (SIGN, 2003)
- **Recommended second-line treatment in official national guidelines**

Primary care setting recommendations

- Supervised oral disulfiram might be used to prevent relapse (SIGN, 2003)

Recommended valuable but not officially endorsed as first- or second-line treatment

General recommendations (irrespective of setting)

- Disulfiram, acamprosate and naltrexone all reported as having some effectiveness when used in alcohol dependence (National Treatment Agency (NTA), 2002)

Primary care setting recommendations

- SSRI are one of the treatment options for depressive symptoms persisting more than 2 weeks after treatment for alcohol dependence (SIGN, 2003)
- Naltrexone is not licensed for use in UK (SIGN, 2003)

Alcohol withdrawal

Introduction

For many alcohol-dependent individuals with significant physical dependence, a cluster of withdrawal symptoms known as 'alcohol withdrawal syndrome' (AWS) may occur upon cessation or reduction of alcohol consumption or reaching a level of such significant tolerance that individuals cannot consume enough alcohol to delay withdrawal. Estimates suggest that as many as 2 million Americans may experience symptoms associated with alcohol-related withdrawal annually (Abbott *et al.*, 1995). Depending directly on the degree of physical dependence, this syndrome can range from creating significant discomfort to mild tremor to alcohol withdrawal-related delirium, hallucinosis, seizures, and potentially death (Kozak *et al.*, 2000; Bayard *et al.*, 2004). Though most alcohol-dependent persons do not fit the stereotypical image of an alcoholic, individuals who are nutritionally compromised, dehydrated, or have other organ deficiencies are at more risk for withdrawal. Repeated withdrawal episodes may contribute to the development of alcohol dependence and to negative consequences associated with excessive alcohol consumption (Finn & Crabbe, 1997). Predictors for AWS complications include the duration of alcohol consumption, total number of prior detoxifications from alcohol, and previous withdrawal-related seizures and episodes of alcohol withdrawal delirium (AWD) (Asplund *et al.*, 2004).

Withdrawal-related seizure is considered a more severe manifestation of AWS, as is AWD or 'delirium tremens' as traditionally called. The incidence of seizures in alcohol dependent individuals waiting for detoxification ranges from 1% to 15% (Chan, 1985). AWD is estimated to have a mortality rate of approximately 1 in 20 patients who go into alcohol withdrawal (Trevisan *et al.*, 1998).

The pharmacological treatment of alcohol withdrawal aims at reducing the severity of non-specific features (such as elevated blood pressure, high pulse, tremor, agitation, anxiety, depression), and avoiding the occurrence of specific features (such as seizures, delirium tremens). The distinction between specific and non-specific symptoms is reflected in differential efficacy of the various pharmacological agents employed for the treatment of alcohol withdrawal.

Several reviews agree that benzodiazepines reduce both the specific and non-specific symptoms of alcohol withdrawal and are the treatment of choice for alcohol withdrawal syndrome (Mayo-Smith, 1997, Lingford-Hughes *et al.*, 2004), and the only recommended monotherapy for it (Franck, 2003). Amongst benzodiazepines there is no evidence to support one agent over another, although longer half-life seems to be better in preventing specific symptoms (Mayo-Smith, 1997) with chlordiazepoxide the most popular choice in the absence of liver failure (Lingford-Hughes *et al.*, 2004), even in the elderly (Mayo-Smith, 2004) albeit with a reduced dosage (Franck, 2003).

Apart from benzodiazepines, a few other agents were found to be superior to placebo in treating non-specific symptoms of alcohol withdrawal syndrome, although there is no consensus about their place in treatment because of either non-proven efficacy in treating specific symptoms or because of dangerous side effects. For example, chlormethiazole, a popular alternative first-line treatment of alcohol withdrawal, although superior to placebo, has no proven efficacy in the prevention of seizures and its outpatient use is marred by potentially serious side effects such as respiratory depression and increased airway secretion (Williams & McBride, 1998). Carbamazepine is also superior to placebo in treating non-specific symptoms of alcohol withdrawal (Franck, 2003), and more recent evidence shows that it is as effective as benzodiazepines in seizure prevention during withdrawal (Hilbom *et al.*, 2003), a finding that was disputed in previous reviews (Mayo-Smith, 1997, Franck, 2003).

Benzodiazepines are frequently administered in a fixed-schedule tapering regime, where clients are assigned to an initial dosage in a predetermined reduction program (Mayo-Smith, 1997). Fixed-schedule tapering regimes do not take into account the great variation of withdrawal severity apart from the onset of the regime, but their acceptability is based on the minimal need of specialist monitoring during detoxification (Mayo-Smith, 1997). Alternative benzodiazepine regimes consist of administration of a variable dose titrated against the Clinical Institute Withdrawal Assessment Alcohol revised (CIWA-Ar) scale (Sullivan *et al.*, 1989) that is administered either at set intervals during the day (such as hourly), or at the request of a client when they experience withdrawal features. Although the use of the alternative regimes is preferable in reducing the total amount of benzodiazepine administered, they need availability of trained staff and they are not suited for clients with a seizure risk (Mayo-Smith, 1997; Lingford-Hughes *et al.*, 2004).

Screening for alcohol withdrawal

Of the currently used instruments available for measuring the degree of withdrawal in an alcohol dependent patient, the most commonly used is the revised Clinical Institute Withdrawal Assessment (CIWA-Ar) (Sullivan *et al.*, 1989) with some limited use of the Sedation-Agitation Scale (SAS) (Grafenreed *et al.*, 2004). The CIWA-Ar is a validated 10-item scale used for grading severity of specific alcohol withdrawal symptoms. The assessment provides a final AWS (alcohol withdrawal syndrome) score with a maximum of 67 possible points. Generally, CIWA-Ar ratings of 8 points or less represent mild withdrawal, ratings of 9 to 15 are associated with moderate withdrawal, and ratings greater than 15 correspond to severe withdrawal, with associated increased risk of seizures and AWD with the increasing CIWA-Ar score. Pharmacotherapy of AWS can be anchored to a particular patient's CIWA score. Providers should also consider concomitant illnesses and medications when interpreting CIWA-Ar scores. Indeed, individual items in the scale are not specific to AWS, and likewise some manifestations of withdrawal may be blunted. The SAS can be used in combination with the CIWA-Ar to evaluate the level of agitation and consciousness of a patient, and be linked to administer benzodiazepines on a symptom-triggered regimen when a patient becomes agitated (for scores above 4 on a 7-point scale).

Pharmacotherapy

Benzodiazepines

Benzodiazepines modulate anxiolysis by stimulating $GABA_A$ receptors, and in doing so, substitute pharmacologically for alcohol (Schatzberg *et al.*, 2005).

Evidence

Considered the drugs of choice for alcohol withdrawal for some time (Mayo-Smith *et al.*, 1997; Lejoyeux *et al.*, 1998; Schatzberg *et al.*, 2005), long-acting benzodiazepines such as chlordiazepoxide and diazepam and short-acting agents such as lorazepam and oxazepam represent the most efficacious pharmacotherapies for the treatment

Table 14.1. Benzodiazepine comparisons

Drugs	Approximate dose equivalent (mg)	Elimination half-life (h)
Chlordiazepoxide	25	5–30
Diazepam	5	20–80
Lorazepam	0.75–1	10–20
Oxazepam	15	5–20

of acute alcohol withdrawal (Kosten & O'Connor, 2003). They are effective in preventing both first seizures and subsequent seizures during alcohol withdrawal (Hillbom *et al.*, 2003). As all benzodiazepines appear equally effective in ameliorating the signs and symptoms of alcohol withdrawal, the choice of a benzodiazepine is dependent on factors such as pharmacokinetic properties, dosage formulation, presence of liver or renal impairment, and ease of dosage titration (Mayo-Smith *et al.*, 1997). Longer-acting benzodiazepines, such as diazepam and chlordiazepoxide, may provide for easier weaning as they gradually self-taper upon metabolism and excretion; this allows for less fluctuation in plasma drug levels (Ritson & Chick, 1986). Longer-acting benzodiazepines also cause fewer rebound effects and withdrawal seizures upon discontinuation. Shorter-acting agents that do not undergo hepatic metabolism, such as lorazepam or oxazepam, require more frequent dosing but may be more appropriate for alcoholics with liver disease and the elderly (Lejoyeux *et al.*, 1998; Kraemer *et al.*, 1999). Short-acting lorazepam and long-acting diazepam also demonstrate a higher potential for abuse due to a shared rapid onset of action (Mayo-Smith *et al.*, 1997). See Table 14.1 for benzodiazepine equivalents.

Benzodiazepines are shown to be more effective than placebo in reducing the signs and symptoms of alcohol withdrawal (Adinoff, 1994). The results of a meta-analysis on treatments for alcohol withdrawal indicated a statistically significant decrease of 4.9 cases of delirium for every 100 patients treated with benzodiazepines (Mayo-Smith *et al.*, 1997). Likewise, a significant difference was shown with treatment in regard to withdrawal-related seizures, with a reduction of 7.7 cases per 100 patients treated.

In a Canadian meta-analysis, no difference was seen in adverse effects between benzodiazepines and alternative agents (Holbrook *et al.*, 1999). Even in elderly, cognitively impaired patients, benzodiazepines are recommended (Kraemer *et al.*, 1999). Notably these patients may be at an even greater risk for adverse events related to ethanol

withdrawal. Please refer to Table 14.2 for some general AWS treatment guidelines.

Dose

Two strategies for dosing benzodiazepines in AWS include 'fixed-schedule' and 'symptom-triggered' regimens. Fixed schedule regimens involve a set dose and interval for the agent chosen, which is to be tapered off at specific times, usually starting on the second day of treatment. Symptom-triggered regimens depend on the use of a rating scale of withdrawal severity, such as the CIWA-Ar previously noted, which is repeated at set intervals. Medication is only administered if the scoring from the scale is above a predetermined threshold value for treatment. In this way, the risk of under- or over-medicating patients may be minimized, as dosing is guided by the degree of withdrawal symptoms (Sullivan *et al.*, 1991). Several studies confirm that symptom-triggered regimens compared to fixed-dose regimens appear to result in a shorter duration of necessary therapy and less medication administered in total, an advantage that appears to come without any loss of efficacy.

For example, a randomized double-blind controlled trial was performed by Saitz and colleagues (1994) to determine the safety and efficacy of symptom-triggered therapy compared to a fixed-dose regimen. The study indicated a mean duration of 9 hours for treatment of withdrawal symptoms with symptom-triggered therapy compared to a duration of 68 hours with a fixed-schedule regimen. All patients in this study were assigned to receive chlordiazepoxide regardless of their respective treatment group. The symptom-triggered and fixed-dose groups had received median cumulative doses of 100 mg and 425 mg of chlordiazepoxide, respectively. Both of these outcome measures were statistically significant. No significant differences were found in the severity of withdrawal during treatment or in the incidence rates of seizures or AWD. Similar results were reported by others using oxazepam (Daeppen *et al.*, 2002). Subjects in the symptom-triggered group averaged 20 hours of treatment, while those in the fixed-dose group were treated for a mean of almost 63 hours. The mean total doses were 37.5 mg and 231.4 mg for the symptom-triggered cohort compared to the fixed-dose, respectively.

The treatment challenge associated with individuals who are in alcohol withdrawal with a comorbid medical illness is illustrated by the case of a patient with AWS who has coronary artery disease. Such a patient may be more aggressively managed for withdrawal-related hypertension and thus treated with a beta-blocker or clonidine. The result of such adjuvant treatment may be a reduced

Table 14.2. Suggested treatment strategies for alcohol withdrawal syndrome

Protocol	Special considerations	Drug	Dose range	Benefits
Symptom-triggered regimen based on CIWA-Ar score assessed as medically appropriate.	Assess patient and administer one of these drugs every hour until CIWA-Ar ≤ 8 – 10 for 24 h.	Chlordiazepoxide Diazepam	50–100 mg 10–20 mg	Less abuse potential than diazepam for outpatients. Both are low cost. long-acting
		Lorazepam	2–4 mg	Available in IM and IV form More appropriate in elderly and hepatic impairment
Fixed-schedule regimens	**Consider if:**	**Example of fixed dosing schedule using one benzodiazepine.**	**Dose, frequency and duration of treatment**	
(Provide additional medication as needed when symptoms are not controlled (i.e. CIWA-Ar ≥ 8–10.)	Mild – CIWA-Ar 8–10; SBP > 150 mmHg or DBP > 90 mmHg; HR > 100; T > 100 F. Titrate dose.	Lorazepam	1–2 mg PO every 4 to 6 hours as needed for 1 to 3 days.	Rapid onset of action
	Moderate – CIWA-Ar 8–15; SBP 150–200 mmHg or DBP 100–140 mmHg; HR 110–140; T 100–101F; Tremors, insomnia and agitation. Titrate dose	Lorazepam	Days 1 and 2 give 2 mg to 4 mg PO four times a day. On days 3 and 4 give 1 mg to 2 mg PO four times a day. On day 5 give 1 mg by mouth twice a day.	Rapid onset of action
	Severe withdrawal symptoms – CIWA-Ar > 15; SBP > 200 mmHg or DBP > 140 mmHg; HR > 140; T > 101F; Tremors, insomnia and agitation Endpoint is sedation	Lorazepam	Give 1 mg to 2 mg IV every 1 hour while awake for 3 to 5 days.	Rapid onset of action Ease of administration
Alternative therapies	Benzodiazepine class allergy or when use of a benzodiazepine is deemed medically inappropriate	Carbamazepine	Taper from 600–800 mg on Day 1 down to 200 mg over 5 days	**For both drugs:** Non-addicting
		Gabapentin	400 TID for 3 days then 400 mg BID for 1 day then 400 mg for 1 day	Few drug interactions. Causes relatively little cognitive impairment.
Adjunctive therapies	Adrenergic hyperactivity	Clonidine	0.1 mg twice daily as needed	For mild to moderate hyperactivity
	Adrenergic hyperactivity	Beta-blockers (e.g. atenolol)	50 mg daily	Shown to improve vital signs faster than oxazepam alone
	Adrenergic hyperactivity	Carbamazepine	800 mg/day tapered down to 200 mg over 5 days	Anticonvulsant activity
	Agitation, hallucinations, delirium	Neuroleptics, e.g. haloperidol	0.5–5 mg every hour; Max dose 100 mg/day	Rapid onset of action; either oral or parenteral forms

Reprinted with permission from US Pharmacist (Guirguis & Kenna, 2005).

sensitivity of the CIWA-Ar due to a masking of their autonomic manifestations of withdrawal. This could then lead to a higher likelihood of under-medicating the patient for withdrawal and may put the patient at higher risk for severe sequela from withdrawal. Because of these exclusion criteria, the symptom-triggered approach has not been tested in such populations or those with histories of severe withdrawal including seizures or delirium. Therefore, traditional fixed-dose regimens are recommended in these populations (Mayo-Smith *et al.*, 1997).

An effective approach is most likely to consider combining these two dosing strategies in developing an effective protocol rather than exclusionary for one or the other. For example, at one hospital that uses both the CIWA-Ar and the SAS, low-risk patients (no history of AWS/AWD, patient consumes low weekly amounts of alcohol and no signs or symptoms of early AWS) receive a symptom-triggered regimen (e.g. lorazepam 1 mg every hour as needed). By contrast, high risk patients (history of AWS/AWD/withdrawal seizures, consumes large daily amounts of alcohol, signs or symptoms of early AWS) receive fixed-dose lorazepam or diazepam with a tapering dose schedule and as needed benzodiazepine administration for uncontrolled alcohol withdrawal signs or symptoms.

Contraindications, warnings, interactions

Elderly patients, those with hepatic or renal insufficiency and those with medical illnesses require close observation to prevent overmedication. In patients receiving calcium channel blockers, beta-blockers, and alpha-2-adrenergic agonists, some signs of withdrawal such as hypertension, tachycardia, and tremor may be obscured.

Summary

While most clinicians have significant experience using benzodiazepines for AWS and AWD, significant questions remain to be clarified such as the most effective protocol governing drug administration and route of administration. Certainly, compared to symptom-triggered dosing, fixed dosing schedules are much easier to prescribe and carry out. Moreover, compared to anticonvulsants to be discussed next, benzodiazepines are much less expensive and afford clinical efficacy for most individuals going through alcohol withdrawal.

Anticonvulsants

Evidence

Certain anticonvulsant agents show promise for a greater role in treatment of alcohol withdrawal (Malcolm *et al.*, 2001; Book & Myrick, 2005). Some of the main reasons for interest in their use for this application include the possibility that anticonvulsants may curb the kindling phenomenon suspected in withdrawal and may therefore be neuroprotective (Zullino *et al.*, 2004). Kindling refers to long-term neuronal changes resulting from repeated detoxifications and may be associated with progressively worse AWS upon subsequent detoxifications (Bayard *et al.*, 2004). Additionally, anticonvulsants have low abuse potential and a minimal effect on cognition (Stuppaeck *et al.*, 1992).

The anticonvulsant agent carbamazepine, widely used in Europe for AWS, effectively decreases the severity of withdrawal symptoms, is comparable to the benzodiazepines in terms of adverse events, and is equally effective to oxazepam at decreasing the symptoms of alcohol withdrawal (Stuppaeck *et al.*, 1992). While limited information is available whether carbamazepine can reduce seizures or delirium associated with alcohol withdrawal in humans (Mayo-Smith, 1997), a recent study found carbamazepine to be superior to lorazepam in preventing rebound withdrawal symptoms and reducing post-treatment drinking (Malcolm *et al.*, 2002a). Also, patients treated with carbamazepine had a better success rate for subsequent rehabilitation than those managed with benzodiazepines. In that study, carbamazepine was dosed on a tapering schedule of 600–800 mg divided through day 1, down to 200 mg as a single dose on day 5. It was as equally efficacious as lorazepam in reducing most withdrawal symptoms during detoxification, and was better at reducing anxiety and promoting sleep (Malcolm *et al.*, 2002b). It should be noted that this study involved patients with mild-to-moderate AWS who were treated on an outpatient basis. An earlier study among alcohol-dependent inpatients with severe withdrawal symptoms found that carbamazepine was equally as efficacious and safe as oxazepam (Malcolm *et al.*, 1989).

The major concerns with the clinical use of carbamazepine are the risk of agranulocytosis or aplastic anemia, both potentially lethal conditions (Schatzberg *et al.*, 2005). Additionally, in the Malcolm *et al.* (2002a) study comparing carbamazepine to lorazepam, pruritus was the most frequent side effect in 18.9% of patients.

Chlormethiazole, not approved by the US Food and Drug Administration (FDA), has anticonvulsant properties and is effective in the treatment of delirium tremens (Morgan, 1995). The advantages of chlormethiazole are the low incidence of acute and chronic toxicity, rapid onset of sedation and sleep with intravenous therapy, reduction and disappearance of autonomic symptoms, and reduction of confusion. Gamma-hydroxybutyrate

(GHB), a GABA-like substance, has been reported to be as effective as chlormethiazole for the treatment of alcohol withdrawal (Nimmerrichter et al., 2002). However in the USA, GHB is a Schedule III Controlled Substance and is not recommended to treat alcohol withdrawal or dependence because of its high potential for abuse and status as a 'club drug' (Caputo et al., 2005; McDonough et al., 2004).

Although valproate sodium has been used for many years, most studies are open label (Longo et al., 2002; Myrick et al., 2000). In a small trial, valproate was reported to be equivalent to lorazepam in suppressing alcohol withdrawal symptoms (Myrick et al., 2000). One well-controlled study compared valproate and carbamazepine to placebo and reported a high rate of side effects and concluded that the initial dosages of these drugs were too high (Hillbom et al., 1989). Reoux and others (2001) performed a randomized, double-blind placebo-controlled trial evaluating the addition of divalproex to standard of care with benzodiazepines. Divalproex reduced progression of withdrawal, as measured by the CIWA-Ar, and likewise reduced benzodiazepine requirements. The investigators speculated that a loading dose of divalproex could potentially increase the magnitude of these benefits.

Gabapentin is an FDA-approved adjunctive treatment for partial seizures, and has been studied in additional trials for off-label indications including AWS. Gabapentin is not metabolized in humans, is eliminated via renal mechanisms and is therefore safe for use in those with compromised hepatic function. Additionally, as gabapentin does not induce or inhibit any liver enzymes, the impact of potential drug interactions, such as alcohol, is lessened. Its major side effects leading to discontinuance include somnolence (1.2%) and ataxia (0.8%). Gabapentin was administered to six patients in one trial (Myrick et al., 1998) and 49 patients in another (Voris et al., 2003). The 5-day dosing schedule for both of these trials was 400 mg three times a day for 3 days, 400 mg twice a day for 1 day and 400 mg for 1 day. The results of these trials suggest that gabapentin may be useful for patients with mild to moderate AWS, although another study using 400 mg four times daily showed no advantage over placebo when used adjunctively to clomethiazole (Bonnet et al., 2003). Moreover, in the Voris et al. (2003) study, those individuals who reported larger amounts of alcohol use prior to treatment required more as-needed benzodiazepines, suggesting that those with higher CIWA-Ar scores do not do as well on gabapentin. While newer anticonvulsants such as gabapentin may be useful for some patients with mild or moderate AWS, benzodiazepines are still the drugs of choice for most patients.

Summary

Anticonvulsants, particularly carbamazepine and gabapentin may offer advantages over benzodiazepines in some patients. Specifically, because they have low abuse potential, and interact minimally with alcohol, anticonvulsants may eventually be an option for outpatient treatment, and for those who are low enough risk to not necessitate hospitalization. While newer anticonvulsants such as gabapentin now in clinical trials may be useful for some patients, benzodiazepines are still the drugs of choice for most patients (Mayo-Smith et al., 2004). Finally, psychiatrists may encounter the use of intravenous ethanol for treating alcohol withdrawal in hospitalized trauma patients, however this is a practice for which there is questionable or no evidence to support its use and therefore is highly discouraged (Hodges & Mazur, 2004).

Adjunctive treatments

Alcohol-dependent clients are deficient in thiamine and have a higher risk for developing Wernicke's encephalopathy (Cook et al., 1998). Rapid correction of brain thiamine deficiency can occur with high plasma concentrations of thiamine, achieved by parenteral supplementation only, since absorption of the oral thiamine by the gastrointestinal tract is minimal, even with massive oral daily dosing (Thomson, 2000). According to the 2004 Evidence-Based Guidelines of the British Association of Psychopharmacology (Lingford-Hughes et al., 2004), to prevent the neuropsychiatric effects of thiamine deficiency, patients should receive at least 100 mg I. M. on the first day and patients should be taking 100 to 200 mg per day of thiamine for up to 30 days.

Since parenteral thiamine supplementation has been associated with anaphylactic reactions, it is only recommended as a slow intravenous injection in the presence of resuscitation facilities (BNF 50 (2004)), although some reviews site lower grade evidence in favour of oral thiamine supplementation during outpatient detoxification (Lingford-Hughes et al., 2004).

Several adjunctive medications aside from the sedative-hypnotics may serve ancillary roles in the therapy of AWS. Their selection should be based on treating specific symptoms associated with the syndrome. For instance, beta-blockers such as propranolol (Sellers et al., 1977), atenolol (Horwitz et al., 1989) or alpha-2-adrenergic agonists such as clonidine (Baumgartner & Rowen, 1987) may be used for moderate to severe hypertension or other autonomic manifestations. However, these agents can mask symptoms of severe withdrawal that may herald the onset of a seizure without providing any anti-seizure activity. Antipsychotics such as haloperidol can be used for managing hallucinations and severe agitation but care must be used as these drugs can reduce the seizure threshold (Mayo-Smith *et al.*, 2004; Schatzberg *et al.*, 2005).

Treatment recommendations in official national guidelines (United Kingdom)

Recommended first-line treatment in official national guidelines

General recommendations (irrespective of setting)
- *Agent*
  Chlordiazepoxide (Department of Health, 1999, British National Formulary 47, National Treatment Agency, 2002), or another long acting benzodiazepine (British National Formulary 47)
- *Regime*
  Chlordiazepoxide in a dose matched to the level of dependence of the client (National Treatment Agency, 2002), in a fixed schedule reducing regime (Department of Health, 1999), over 7–14 days (British National Formulary 47)
- *Vitamin supplementation*
  Thiamine 50 mg bid (twice daily) orally for three weeks, with the more severe cases receiving thiamine IV (intravenously) or IM (intramuscularly) in the presence of facilities for the treatment of anaphylaxis (Department of Health, 1999)

Primary care setting recommendations
- *Agent*
  Chlordiazepoxide (Scottish Intercollegiate Guidelines Network –SIGN, 2003)
- *Regime*
  Chlordiazepoxide in a tapered fixed dosage regime (SIGN, 2003)
- *Vitamin supplementation*
  - At-risk group (malnourished patient): 1 pair of Pabrinex (Vit B + C) amps IM daily for 3 days (SIGN, 2003)
  - Chronic alcohol problem with deficient diet: Thiamine 200–300 mg daily indefinitely (SIGN, 2003)

General hospital setting recommendations
- *Agent*
  Chlordiazepoxide (or another benzodiazepine) (The Royal College of Physicians, 2001)
- *Regime*
  Chlordiazepoxide in a fixed schedule reducing regime (The Royal College of Physicians, 2001)
- *Vitamin supplementation*
  - At risk for Wernicke's Encephalopathy: 1–2 pairs of Pabrinex (Vit B + C) amps 1–3 times daily by IV

infusion for 3–5 days or until clinical improvement ceases. (The higher the risk, the higher the prescribed dosage and the longer the period it is prescribed.) (The Royal College of Physicians, 2001)
- Low risk group (malnutrition, poor diet, weight loss): Thiamine 200 mg daily (until completion of detoxification, unless cognitive impairment persists) and Vitamin B co strong 30 mg/day (The Royal College of Physicians, 2001)
- On discharge for both groups above: Thiamine 50 mg daily (if cognitive impairment persists) and Vitamin B co strong 30 mg/day (if concerns over patient's diet) (The Royal College of Physicians, 2001)

Recommended second-line treatment in official national guidelines

Primary care setting recommendations
- Benzodiazepines (other than Chlordiazepoxide) (SIGN, 2003)

General hospital setting recommendations
- Clomethiazole (Chlormethiazole) should be used only in inpatient settings (BNF 50 (2004)) where it could be used for withdrawal fits resistant to benzodiazepines (The Royal College of Physicians, 2001)
- Lorazepam 2 mg IV in prolonged and recurrent seizures (The Royal College of Physicians, 2001)

Recommended as valuable but not officially endorsed as first- or second- line treatment

- Diazepam administered in a fixed schedule reducing regimen by experienced practitioners (Department of Health, 1999)

Used often but not endorsed or advised against

General recommendations (irrespective of setting)
- Chlormethiazole use is not recommended (Department of Health, 1999)

Primary care setting recommendations
- Clomethiazole should not be used (SIGN, 2003)
- Antiepileptics should not be used as monotherapy for alcohol detoxification (SIGN, 2003)

General hospital setting recommendations
- Conventional antiepileptics use in the treatment/prophylaxis of withdrawal seizures is not endorsed (The Royal College of Physicians, 2001)
- Beta-blocker use as a monotherapy for alcohol withdrawal is not endorsed (The Royal College of Physicians, 2001)

The level of evidence for each of the interventions discussed in this chapter is summarized in Table 14.3.

Table 14.3. Effectiveness of pharmacotherapy treatments for alcohol misuse, dependence and withdrawal

Treatment	Form of treatment	Psychiatric disorder	Level of evidence for efficacy	Comments
Pharmacotherapy	Disulfiram	Alcohol dependence	Ib	Despite widespread belief in its effectiveness, true double-blind studies are lacking. Controlled studies reveal inconsistent results. Appears to work best in those who are truly motivated to cease drinking
Pharmacotherapy	Acamprosate	Alcohol dependence	Ia	Probably is most effective when instituted shortly after completion of detoxification. It does increase length of time of abstinence
Pharmacotherapy	Naltrexone	Alcohol dependence	Ia	A decrease in relapse rate in heavy drinkers and a decrease in drinking frequency especially is addition to psychosocial interventions. No absolute improvement in abstinence rates.
Pharmacotherapy	Antidepressants	Alcohol dependence	III	Perhaps some mild impact with comorbid anxiety or depression
Pharmacotherapy	Mood stabilisers (esp. topiramate)	Alcohol dependence	Ib	Decreased drinking per day, decreased days drinking, decreased craving and increased days of abstinence but only one RCT here
Pharmacotherapy	Ondansetron	Alcohol dependence	IIa	May be useful in subtype of early age onset drinking group
Pharmacotherapy	Buspirone	Alcohol dependence	Ia	Results are contradictory. May be useful in subtypes with co-morbid anxiety disorders
Pharmacotherapy	Benzodiazepines	Alcohol withdrawal	Ia	Clearly useful in alcohol withdrawal. Dosing schedules have not been definitively determined. Longer acting may be more effective here.
Pharmacotherapy	Anticonvulsants (carbamazepine, gabapentin)	Alcohol withdrawal	Ib	May be useful in withdrawal particularly in cases of mild to moderate withdrawal.

REFERENCES

Abbott, P. J., Quinn, D. & Knox, L. (1995). Ambulatory medical detoxification for alcohol. *American Journal of Drug and Alcohol Abuse*, **21**, 549–63.

Adinoff, B. (1994). Double-blind study of alprazolam, diazepam, clonidine, and placebo in the alcohol withdrawal syndrome: preliminary findings. *Alcoholism: Clinical and Experimental Research*, **18**, 873–8.

Albanese, M. J., Khantzian, E. J. *et al.* (1994). Decreased substance use in chronically psychotic patients treated with clozapine. *American Journal of Psychiatry*, **151**, 780–1.

American Psychiatric Association (2000). *DSM-IV-TR: Diagnostic and Statistical Manual of Mental Disorders*, 4th edn. *Text Revision*. Washington DC: APA.

Anton, R. F., Moak, D. H, Latham, P. *et al.* (2005). Naltrexone combined with either cognitive behavioral or motivational enhancement therapy for alcohol dependence. *Journal of Clinical Psychopharmacology*, **25**, 349–57.

Anton, R. F., O'Malley, S. S., Ciraulo, D. A. *et al.* (2006). Combined pharmacotherapies and behavioral interventions for alcohol dependence. The COMBINE study: a randomized controlled trial. *Journal of the American Medical Association*, **295**, 2003–17.

Asplund, C. A., Aaronson, J. W. & Aaronson, H. E. (2004). 3 regimens for alcohol withdrawal and detoxification. *Journal of Family Practice*, **53**, 545–54.

Babor, T. F. (1992). Substance-related problems in the context of international classificatory systems. In *The Nature of Alcohol and Drug Related Problems*, ed. M. Lader, G. Edwards & D. C. Drummond, pp. 83–98. Oxford: Oxford University Press.

Baumgartner, G. R. & Rowen, R. C. (1987). Clonidine vs. chlordiazepoxide in the management of acute alcohol withdrawal syndrome. *Archives of Internal Medicine*, **147**, 1223–6.

Bayard, M., McIntyre, J., Hill, K. R. & Woodside J. Jr. (2004). Alcohol withdrawal syndrome. *American Family Physician*, **69**, 1443–50.

Benjamin, D., Grant, E. R. & Pohorecky, L. A. (1993). Naltrexone reverses ethanol-induced dopamine release in the nucleus accumbens in awake, freely moving rats. *Brain Research*, **621**, 137–40.

Berglund, M. (2003). Pharmacotherapy for alcohol dependence. In *Treating Alcohol and Drug Abuse: An Evidence Based Review*, ed. M. Berglund, S. Thelander & E. Jonsson. Wiley-VCH GmbH & Co.

Besson, J., Aeby, F., Kasas, A., Lehert, P. & Potgieter, A. (1998). Combined efficacy of acamprosate and disulfiram in the treatment of alcoholism: a controlled study. *Alcoholism: Clinical and Experimental Research*, **22**, 573–9.

Bonnet, M. H., Banger, M., Leweke, F. M. *et al.* (2003). Treatment of acute alcohol withdrawal with gabapentin: results from a controlled two-center trial. *Journal of Clinical Psychopharmacology*, **23**, 514–19.

Book, S. W. & Myrick, H. (2005). Novel anticonvulsants in the treatment of alcoholism. *Expert Opinion on Investigational Drugs*, **14**, 371–6.

Bouza, C., Angeles, M., Munoz, A. & Amate, J. M. (2004). Efficacy and safety of naltrexone and acamprosate in the treatment of alcohol dependence: a systematic review. *Addiction*, **99**(7), 811–28.

Brady, K. T., Myrick, H., Henderson, S. & Coffey, S. F. (2002). The use of divalproex in alcohol relapse prevention: a pilot study. *Drug and Alcohol Dependence*, **67**, 323–30.

Brewer, C. (1993). Recent developments in disulfiram treatment. *Alcohol and Alcoholism*, **28**, 383–95.

British National Formulary (BNF) (2004). British Medical Association and Royal Pharmaceutical Society of Great Britain. No. 50 (Sept 2005).

Bruno, F. (1989). Buspirone in the treatment of alcoholic patients. *Psychopathology*, **22** (Suppl. 1), 49–59.

Caputo, F., Vignoli, T., Lorenzini, F. *et al.* (2005). Suppression of craving for gamma-hydroxybutyric acid by naltrexone administration: three case reports. *Clinical Neuropharmacology*, **28**, 87–9.

Carmen, B., Angeles, M., Ana, M. & Maria, A. J. (2004). Efficacy and safety of naltrexone and acamprosate in the treatment of alcohol dependence: a systematic review. *Addiction*, **99**, 811–28.

Carroll, K. M., Fenton, L. R., Ball, S. A. *et al.* (2004). Efficacy of disulfiram and cognitive behavior therapy in cocaine-dependent outpatients: a randomized placebo-controlled trial. *Archives of General Psychiatry*, **61**, 264–72.

Chan, A. W. (1985). Alcoholism and epilepsy. *Epilepsia*, **26**, 323–33.

Chick, J. (1999). Safety issues concerning the use of disulfiram in treating alcohol dependence. *Drug Safety*, **20**, 427–35.

Chick, J., Anton R., Checinski, K. *et al.* (2000). A multicentre, randomized, double-blind, placebo-controlled trial of naltrexone in the treatment of alcohol dependence or abuse. *Alcohol and Alcoholism*, **35**, 587–93.

Chick, J., Gough K., Falkowski, W. *et al.* (1992). Disulfiram treatment of alcoholism. *British Journal of Psychiatry*, **161**, 84–9.

Chick J., Howlett, H., Morgan, M. Y. & Ritson, B. (2000). United Kingdom Multicentre Acamprosate Study (UKMAS): a 6-month prospective study of acamprosate versus placebo in preventing relapse after withdrawal from alcohol. *Alcohol and Alcoholism*, **35**, 176–87.

Ciccocioppo, R. (1999). The role of serotonin in craving: from basic research to human studies. *Alcohol*, **34**, 244–53.

Ciraulo, D. A., Shader, R. I., Greenblatt, D. J. & Creelman, W. (2006). *Drug Interactions in Psychiatry*, 3rd edn. Philadelphia PA.: Lippincott, Williams & Wilkins.

COMBINE Study Research Group (2003). Testing combined pharmacotherapies and behavioral interventions for alcohol dependence (the COMBINE) study): a pilot feasibility study. *Alcoholism: Clinical and Experimental Research*, **27**, 1123–31.

Cook, C. C. H., Hallwood, P. M., & Thomson, A. D. (1998). B-vitamin deficiency and neuro-psychiatric syndromes in alcohol misuse. *Alcohol and Alcoholism*, **33**, 317–36.

Cornelius, J. R., Salloum, I. M., Ehler, J. G. *et al.* (1997). Fluoxetine in depressed alcoholics. A double-blind placebo controlled trial. *Archives of General Psychiatry*, **23**, 193–203.

Croop, R. S., Faulkner, E. B., Labriola, D. F. *et al.* (1997). The safety profile of naltrexone in the treatment of alcoholism. Results from a multicenter usage study. *Archives of General Psychiatry*, **54**, 1130–5.

Daeppen J., Gache P., Landry, U. *et al.* (2002). Symptom-triggered vs fixed-schedule doses of benzodiazepine for alcohol withdrawal. *Archives of Internal Medicine*, **162**, 1117–21.

Daniel, D. G., Swallows, A. & Wolff, F. (1987). Capgras delusion and seizures in association with therapeutic dosages of disulfiram. *Southern Medical Journal*, **80**, 1577–9.

Daoust M., Legrand, E., Gewiss, M. *et al.* (1992). Acamprosate modulates synaptosomal GABA transmission in chronically alcoholised rats. *Pharmacology Biochemistry and Behavior*, **41**, 669–74.

Davidson D, Palfai, T., Bird, C. *et al.* (1999). Effects of naltrexone on alcohol self-administration in heavy drinkers. *Alcoholism: Clinical and Experimental Research*, **23**, 193–203.

Davidson D., Saha, C., Scifres, S., Fyffe, J., O'Connor, S. & Selzer, C. (2004). Naltrexone and brief counseling to reduce heavy drinking in hazardous drinkers. *Addictive Behaviors*, **29**, 1253–8.

Dawson, D. A. (1994). Heavy drinking and the risk of occupational injury. *Accident Analysis and Prevention*, **26**, 655–65.

De Sousa, A. & De Sousa, A. (2004). A one-year pragmatic trial of naltrexone vs disulfiram in the treatment of alcohol dependence. *Alcohol and Alcoholism*, **39**, 528–31.

Department of Health, The Scottish Office Department of Health, Welsh Office, Department of Health and Social Services, Northern Ireland (1999). *Drug Misuse and Dependence – Guidelines on Clinical Management*. London: The Stationery Office.

Dilts, S. L. & Dilts, S. L. Jr. (1996). Assessing liver function before initiating disulfiram therapy. *American Journal of Psychiatry*, **153**, 1504–5.

Drake, R. E., Xie, H., McHugo, G. J. *et al.* (2000). The effects of clozapine on alcohol and drug use disorders among patients with schizophrenia. *Schizophrenia Bulletin*, **26**, 441–9.

Dundon, W., Lynch, K. G., Pettinati, H. M. & Lipkin, C. (2004). Treatment outcomes in type A and B alcohol dependence 6 months after serotonergic pharmacotherapy. *Alcoholism: Clinical and Experimental Research*, **28**(7), 1065–73.

Fawcett, J., Kravitz, H. M., McGuire, M. *et al.* (2000). Pharmacological treatments for alcoholism: revisiting lithium and considering buspirone. *Alcoholism: Clinical and Experimental Research*, **24**, 666–74.

Feinn, R., Nellissery, M. & Kranzler, H. R. (2005). Meta-analysis of the association of a functional serotonin transporter promoter polymorphism with alcohol dependence. *American Journal of Medical Genetics, Part B Neuropsychiatric Genetics*, **133**, 79–84.

Finn, D. A. & Crabbe, J. C. (1997). Exploring alcohol withdrawal syndrome. *Alcohol Health and Research World*, **21**, 149–56.

Forest Laboratories, (2004). Acamprosate product information, Forest Pharmaceuticals, St Louis MO, April.

Franck, J. (2003). Pharmacotherapy for alcohol withdrawal syndrome. In *Treating Alcohol and Drug Abuse; Evidence Based Review*, ed. M. Berglund, S. Thelander & E. Jonsson. Wiley-VCH GmbH & Co. KgaA

Fuller, R. K., Branchey, L., Brightwell, D. R. *et al.* (1986). Disulfiram treatment of alcoholism. A Veterans Administration cooperative study. *Journal of the American Medical Association*, **256**, 1449–55.

Fuller, R. K. & Gordis, E. (2004). Does disulfiram have a role in alcoholism treatment today? *Addiction*, **99**, 21–34.

Galloway, G. P., Koch, M., Cello, R., & Smith, D. E. (2005). Pharmacokinetics, safety, and tolerability of a depot formulation of naltrexone in alcoholics: an open-label trial. *BioMed Central Psychiatry*, **5**, 18.

Garbutt, J. C., West, S. L., Carey, T. S. *et al.* (1999). Pharmacological treatment of alcohol dependence: a review of the evidence. *Journal of the American Medical Association*, **281**, 1318–25.

Garbutt, J. C., Kranzler, H. R., O'Malley, S. S. *et al.* (2005). Efficacy and tolerability of long-acting injectable naltrexone for alcohol dependence: a randomized controlled trial. *Journal of the American Medical Association*, **293**, 1617–25.

Gastpar, M., Bonnet, U., Boning, J. *et al.* (2002). Lack of efficacy of naltrexone in the prevention of alcohol relapse: results from a German multicenter study. *Journal of Clinical Psychopharmacology*, **22**, 592–8.

George, D. T., Rawlings, R., Eckardt, M. J., Phillips, M. J., Shoaf, S. E. & Linnoila, M. (1999). Buspirone treatment of alcoholism: age of onset, and cerebrospinal fluid 5-hydroxyindolacetic acid and homovanillic acid concentrations, but not medication treatment, predict return to drinking. *Alcoholism: Clinical and Experimental Research*, **23**, 272–8.

Gerasimov, M. R., Schiffer, W. K., Gardner, E. L. *et al.* (2001). GABAergic blockade of cocaine-associated cue-induced increases in nucleus accumbens dopamine. *European Journal of Pharmacology*, **414**, 205–9.

Gmel, G. & Rehm, J. (2003). Harmful Alcohol Use. http://www.niaaa.nih.gov/publications/arh 27–1/52–62.htm (accessed 8/13/04).

Gorelick, D. A. & Paredes, A. (1992). Effect of fluoxetine on alcohol consumption in male alcoholics. *Alcoholism: Clinical and Experimental Research*, **16**, 261–5.

Gossop, M. & Carroll, K. M. (2006). Disulfiram, cocaine, and alcohol: two outcomes for the price of one? *Alcohol and Alcoholism*, **41**(2), 119–20.

Grafenreed, K. M., Lobo, B., Sands, C. & Yates, M. (2004). Development of an alcohol withdrawal delirium prophylaxis protocol in a community teaching hospital. *American Journal of Health System Pharmacy*, **61**, 1151–5.

Green, A. I., Tohen, M. F., Hamer, R. M. *et al.* (2004). First episode schizophrenia-related psychosis and substance use disorders: acute response to olanzapine and haloperidol. *Schizophrenia Research*, **66**, 125–35.

Gryder, D. S. & Rogawski, M. A. (2003). Selective antagonism of GluR5 kainate-receptor-mediated synaptic currents by topiramate in rat basolateral amygdala neurons. *Journal of Neuroscience*, **23**, 7069–74.

Guardia, J., Segura, L., Gonzalvo, B. *et al.* (2004). A double-blind, placebo-controlled study of olanzapine in the treatment of alcohol-dependence disorder. *Alcoholism: Clinical and Experimental Research*, **28**, 736–45.

Gual, A. & Lehert, P. (2001). Acamprosate during and after acute alcohol withdrawal: a double-blind placebo-controlled study in Spain. *Alcohol*, **36**, 413–18.

Guirguis, A. B. & Kenna, G. A. (2005). Treatment considerations for alcohol withdrawal syndrome. *US Pharmacist*, **30**, 71–80.

Heinz, A. (2002). Dopaminergic dysfunction in alcoholism and schizophrenia-psychological and behavioral correlates. *European Psychiatry*, **17**, 9–16.

Hernandez-Avila, C. A., Modesto-Lowe, V., Feinn, R. & Kranzler, H. R. (2004). Nefazodone treatment of comorbid alcohol dependence and major depression. *Alcoholism: Clinical and Experimental Research*, **28**, 433–40.

Hillbom, M., Tokola, R., Kuusela, V. *et al.* (1989). Prevention of alcohol withdrawal seizures with carbamazepine and valproic acid. *Alcohol*, **6**, 223–6.

Hillbom, M., Pieninkeroinen, I. & Leone M. (2003). Seizures in alcohol-dependent patients: epidemiology, pathophysiology and management. *CNS Drugs*, **17**, 1013–30.

Hodges, B. & Mazur, J. E. (2004). Intravenous ethanol for the treatment of alcohol withdrawal syndrome in critically ill patients. *Pharmacotherapy*, **24**, 1578–85.

Holbrook, A. M, Crowther, R., Lotter, A., Cheng, C. & King, D. (1999). Meta-analysis of benzodiazepine use in the treatment of acute alcohol withdrawal. *Journal of the Canadian Medical Association*, **160**, 649–55.

Horwitz, R. I., Gottlieb, L. D. & Kraus, M. L. (1989). The efficacy of atenolol in the outpatient management of the alcohol withdrawal syndrome. Results of a randomized clinical trial. *Archives of Internal Medicine*, **149**, 1089–93.

Hotson, J. R. & Langston, J. W. (1976). Disulfiram-induced encephalopathy. *Archives of Neurology*, **33**, 141–2.

Hutchison, K. E., Swift, R., Rohsenow, D. J. *et al.* (2001). Olanzapine reduces urge to drink after drinking cues and a priming dose of alcohol. *Psychopharmacology*, **155**, 27–34.

Hutchison, K. E., Ray, L., Sandman, E. *et al.* (2006). The effect of olanzapine on craving and alcohol consumption. *Neuropsychopharmacology*, **31**(6), 1310–17.

Jaffe, A. J., Rounsaville, B., Chang, G. *et al.* (1996). Naltrexone, relapse prevention and supportive therapy with alcoholics: an analysis of patient-treatment matching. *Journal of Consulting and Clinical Psychology*, **64**, 1044–53.

Janiri L., Gobbi, G., Mannelli, P., Pozzi, G., Serretti, A. & Tempesta, E. (1996). Effects of fluoxetine at antidepressant doses on short-term outcome of detoxified alcoholics. *International Journal of Clinical Psychopharmacology*, **11**, 109–17.

Johnson, B. A. (2003). The role of serotonergic agents as treatments for alcoholism. *Drugs Today*, **39**, 665–72.

Johnson, B. A. & Ait-Dowd, N. (2000). Neuropharmacological treatments for alcoholism: scientific basis and clinical findings. *Psychopharmacology*, **149**, 327–44.

Johnson, B. A., Roache, J., Javors, M. A. *et al.* (2000). Ondansetron for reduction of drinking among biologically predisposed patients: a randomized controlled trial. *Journal of the American Medical Association*, **284**, 963–71.

Johnson, B. A., Roache, J. D., Ait-Daoud, N., Zanca, N. A. & Velazquez, M. (2002). Ondansetron reduces the craving of biologically predisposed alcoholics. *Psychopharmacology*, **160**, 408–13.

Johnson, B. A., O'Malley, S. S., Ciraulo, D. A. *et al.* (2003a). Dose-ranging kinetics and behavioral pharmacology of naltrexone and acamprosate, both alone and combined, in alcohol-dependent subjects. *Journal of Clinical Psychopharmacology*, **23**, 281–93.

Johnson, B. A., Ait-Doud, N., Bowden, C. L. *et al.* (2003b). Oral topiramate for treatment of alcohol dependence: a randomised controlled trial. *Lancet*, **361**, 1677–85.

Kabel, D. I. & Petty, F. (1996). A placebo-controlled, double-blind study of fluoxetine in severe alcohol dependence: adjunctive pharmacotherapy during and after inpatient treatment. *Alcoholism: Clinical and Experimental Research*, **20**, 780–4.

Karan, R. S. & Pandhi, P. (2000). D_2 and $5HT_2$ receptors: relevance to antipsychotic drugs. *Indian Journal of Pharmacology*, **32**, 187–91.

Kiefer, F., Jahn, H., Tarnaske, T. *et al.* (2003). Comparing and combining naltrexone and acamprosate in relapse prevention of alcoholism: a double-blind, placebo-controlled study. *Archives of General Psychiatry*, **60**, 92–9.

Kenna, G. A. (2003). Rationale for use of aripiprazole for alcohol dependence treatment. *Drugs of the Future*, **28**, 1227–35.

Kiritze-Topor, P., Huas, D., Rosenzweig, C., Comte, S., Paille, F. & Lehert, P. (2004). A pragmatic trial of acamprosate in the treatment of alcohol dependence in primary care. *Alcohol and Alcoholism*, **39**, 520–7.

Knee, S. T. & Razani, J. (1974). Acute organic brain syndrome: a complication of disulfiram therapy. *American Journal of Psychiatry*, **131**, 1281–2.

Koob, G. F. & Le Moal, M. (2001). Drug addiction, dysregulation of reward, and allostasis, *Neuropsychiatry*, **24**, 97–129.

Kosten, T. R. & O'Connor, P. G. (2003). Management of drug and alcohol withdrawal. *New England Journal Medicine*, **348**, 1786–95.

Kozak, L. J, Hall, M. J & Owings, M. F. (2000). National Hospital Discharge Survey: 2000 annual summary with detailed diagnosis and procedure data. *Vital Health Statistics*, **153**, 1–194.

Kraemer, K. L., Conigliaro, J. & Saitz R. (1999). Managing alcohol withdrawal in the elderly. *Drugs and Aging*, **14**, 409–25.

Kranzler, H. R. & Van Kirk, J. (2001). Efficacy of naltrexone and acamprosate for alcoholism treatment: a meta-analysis. *Alcoholism: Clinical and Experimental Research*, **25**, 1335–41.

Kranzler, H. R., Burleson, J. A., Del Boca, F. K. *et al.* (1994). Buspirone treatment of anxious alcoholics. A placebo-controlled trial. *Archives of General Psychiatry*, **51**, 720–31.

Kranzler, H. R., Burleson, J. A, Korner, P. *et al.* (1995). Placebo-controlled trial of fluoxetine as an adjunct to relapse prevention in alcoholics. *American Journal of Psychiatry*, **152**, 391–7.

Kranzler, H. R., Burleson, J. A., Brown, J. & Babor, T. F. (1996). Fluoxetine treatment seems to reduce the beneficial effects of cognitive-behavioral therapy in type B alcoholics. *Alcoholism: Clinical and Experimental Research*, **20**, 1534–41.

Kranzler, H. R., Modesto-Lowe, V. & Van Kirk, J. (2000). Naltrexone vs. nefazodone for treatment of alcohol dependence. A placebo-controlled trial. *Neuropsychiatry*, **22**, 493–503.

Kranzler, H. R., Armeli, S., Tennen, H. *et al.* (2003). Targeted naltrexone for early problem drinkers. *Journal of Clinical Psychopharmacology*, **23**, 294–304.

Kranzler, H. R., Wesson, D. R. & Billot, L. (2004). Naltrexone depot for treatment of alcohol dependence: a multicenter, randomized, placebo-controlled clinical trial. *Alcoholism: Clinical and Experimental Research*, **28**, 1051–9.

Kranzler, H. R., Mueller, T., Cornelius, J. *et al.* (2006). Sertraline treatment of co-occurring alcohol dependence and major depression. *Journal of Clinical Psychopharmacology*, **26**, 13–20.

Krystal, J. H., Cramer, J. A., Krol, W. F. *et al.* (2001). Veterans Affairs Naltrexone Cooperative Study 425 Group. Naltrexone in the treatment of alcohol dependence. *New England Journal of Medicine*, **345**, 1734–9.

Larson, E. W., Olincy, A., Rummans, T. A. & Morse, R. M. (1992). Disulfiram treatment of patients with both alcohol dependence and other psychiatric disorders: a review. *Alcoholism: Clinical and Experimental Research*, **16**, 125–30.

Lejoyeux, M., Solomon, J. & Ades, J. (1998). Benzodiazepine treatment for alcohol-dependent patients. *Alcohol and Alcoholism*, **33**, 563–75.

LeMarquand, D., Pihl, R. O. & Benkelfat, C. (1994). Serotonin and alcohol intake, abuse, and dependence: clinical evidence. *Biological Psychiatry*, **36**, 326–37.

Lidow, M. S. & Goldman-Rakic, P. S. (1997). Differential regulation of D_2 and D_4 dopamine receptors mRNAs in the primate cerebral cortex vs. neostriatum: effects of chronic treatment with typical and atypical antipsychotic drugs. *Journal of Pharmacology and Experimental Therapeutics* **283**, 939–46.

Lingford-Hughes, A. R., Welch, S. & Nutt, D. J. (2004). Evidence-based guidelines for the pharmacological management of substance misuse, addiction and comorbidity: recommendations from the British Association for Psychopharmacology. *Journal of Psychopharmacology*, **18**, 293–335.

Littleton, J. & Zieglgansberger, W. (2003). Pharmacological mechanisms of naltrexone and acamprosate in the prevention of relapse in alcohol dependence. *American Journal on Addictions*, **12** (Suppl. 1), S3–11,

Longo, L. P., Campbell, T. & Hubatch, S. (2002). Divalproex sodium (Depakote) for alcohol withdrawal and relapse prevention. *Journal of Addictive Diseases*, **21**, 55–64.

Longoria, J., Brown, E. S., Perantie, D. C., Bobadilla, L. & Nejtek, V. A. (2004). Quetiapine for alcohol use and craving in bipolar disorder. *Journal of Clinical Psychopharmacology*, **24**, 101–2.

Lovinger, D. (1997). Serotonin's role in alcohol's effects on the brain. *Alcohol Health and Research World*, **21**, 114–20.

Malcolm, R., Anton, R. F., Randall, C. L., Johnston, A., Brady, K. & Thevos, A. (1992). A placebo-controlled trial of buspirone in anxious inpatient alcoholics. *Alcoholism: Clinical and Experimental Research*, **16**, 1007–13.

Malcolm, R, Ballenger, J. C., Sturgis, E. T. & Anton, R. (1989). Double-blind controlled trial comparing carbamazepine to oxazepam treatment of alcohol withdrawal. *American Journal of Psychiatry*, **146**, 617–21.

Malcolm, R., Myrick, H., Brady, K. T. & Ballenger, J. C. (2001). Update on anticonvulsants for the treatment of alcohol withdrawal. *American Journal on Addictions*, **10** (Suppl.), 16–23.

Malcolm, R., Myrick, H., Roberts, J., Wang, W., Anton, R. F. & Ballenger, J. C. (2002a). The effects of carbamazepine and lorazepam on single versus multiple previous alcohol withdrawals in an outpatient randomized trial. *Journal of General Internal Medicine*, **17**, 349–55.

Malcolm, R., Myrick, H., Roberts, J., Wang, W. & Anton, R. F. (2002b). The differential effects of medication on mood, sleep disturbance, and work ability in outpatient alcohol detoxification. *American Journal on Addictions*, **11**, 141–50.

Malec, E., Malec, T., Gagne, M. A. & Dongier, M. (1996). Buspirone in the treatment of alcohol dependence: a placebo-controlled trial. *Alcoholism: Clinical and Experimental Research*, **20**, 307–12.

Mann, K., Lehert, P. & Morgan, M. Y. (2004). The efficacy of acamprosate in the maintenance of abstinence in alcohol-dependent individuals: results of a meta-analysis. *Alcoholism: Clinical Experimental Research*, **28**, 51–63.

Mark, T. L., Kranzler, H. R., Song, X., Bransberger, P., Poole, V. H. & Crosse, S. (2003a). Physicians' opinions about medications to treat alcoholism. *Addiction*, **98**, 617–26.

Mark, T. L., Kranzler, H. R. & Song, X. (2003b). Understanding US addiction physicians' low rate of naltrexone prescription. *Drug and Alcohol Dependence*, **71**, 219–28.

Mason, B. J. (2003). Acamprosate and naltrexone treatment for alcohol dependence: an evidence-based risk-benefits assessment. *European Neuropsychopharmacology*, **13**, 469–75.

Mason, B. (2005). *Individual patient data meta analysis of predictors of outcome including US and European studies in 'Acamprosate: New preclinical and clinical findings'*, Research Society on Alcoholism, Santa Barbara, CA. June 26.

Mason, B. J., Kocsis, J. H., Ritvo, E. C. & Cutler, R. B. (1996). A double-blind, placebo-controlled trial of desipramine for primary alcohol dependence stratified on the presence or absence of major depression. *Journal of the American Medical Association*, **275**, 761–7.

Mason, B. J., Goodman, A. M., Dixon, R. M. *et al.* (2002). A pharmacokinetic and pharmacodynamic drug interaction study of acamprosate and naltrexone. *Neuropsychopharmacology* **27**, 596–606.

Mason, B. J., Goodman, A. M., Chabac, S. & Lehert, P. (2006). Effect of oral acamprosate on abstinence in patients with alcohol dependence in a double-blind, placebo-controlled trial: the role of patient motivation. *Journal of Psychiatric Research* **40**(5), 383–93.

Mayo-Smith, M. F. (1997). Pharmacological management of alcohol withdrawal. A meta-analysis and evidence-based practice guideline. American Society of Addiction Medicine Working Group on Pharmacological Management of Alcohol Withdrawal. *Journal of the American Medical Association*, **278**, 144–151.

Mayo-Smith, M. F., Beecher, L. H., Fischer, T. L. *et al.* (2004). Management of alcohol withdrawal delirium. An evidence-based practice guideline. *Archives of Internal Medicine*, **164**, 1405–12.

McCaul, M. E., Wand, G. S., Eissenberg, T., Rohde, C. A. & Cheskin, L. J. (2000). Naltrexone alters subjective and psychomotor responses to alcohol in heavy drinking subjects. *Neuropsychopharmacology*, **22**, 480–92.

McDonough, M., Kennedy, N., Glasper, A. & Bearn, J. (2004). Clinical features and management of gamma-hydroxybutyrate (GHB) withdrawal: a review. *Drug and Alcohol Dependence*, **75**, 3–9.

McGrath, P. J., Nunes, E. V., Stewart, J. W. *et al.* (1996). Imipramine treatment of alcoholics with primary depression: a placebo-controlled clinical trial. *Archives of General Psychiatry*, **53**, 232–40.

Micromedix (2006a). Acamprosate http://healthcare.micromedex. com/mdxcgi/display.exe?CTL=/u01/mdx/mdxcgi/MEGAT.SYS& SET=80F0170C4116A485DB0D00&SYS=1&T=10&M=266655 accessed 11/18/06.

Micromedix (2006b). Disulfiram. http://healthcare.micromedex. com/mdxcgi/cgidict.exe?SRCHTERM=disulfiram&CTL=%2Fu01 %2Fmdx%2Fmdxcgi%2FMEGAT.SYS accessed 11/18/06.

Micromedix (2006c). Naltrexone. http://healthcare.micromedex. com/mdxcgi/display.exe?CTL=/u01/mdx/mdxcgi/MEGAT.SYS &SET=80F0170C411680BA5AB380&SYS=1&T=1389&D=87 accessed 11.18.06.

Miller, W. R. & Wilbourne, P. L. (2002). Mesa Grande: a methodological analysis of clinical trials of treatments for alcohol use disorders. *Addiction*, **97**, 265–77.

Moak, D. H., Anton, R. F., Latham, P. K., Voronin, K. E., Waid, R. L. & Durazo-Arvizu, R. (2003). Sertraline and cognitive behavioral therapy for depressed alcoholics: results of a placebo-controlled trial. *Journal of Clinical Psychopharmacology*, **23**, 553–62.

Modell, J. G., Mountz, J. M., Glaser, F. B. *et al.* (1993). Effect of haloperidol on measures of craving and impaired control in alcoholic subjects. *Alcoholism: Clinical and Experimental Research*, **17**, 234–40.

Moncrieff, J. & Drummond, D. C. (1997). New drug treatments for alcohol problems: a critical appraisal. *Addiction*, **92**, 939–47.

Monnelly, E. P., Ciraulo, D. A., Knapp, C., LoCastro, J. & Sepulveda, I. (2004). Quetiapine for treatment of alcohol dependence. *Journal of Clinical Psychopharmacology*, **24**, 532–5.

Monti, P. M., Rohsenow, D. J., Swift, R. M. *et al.* (2001). Naltrexone and cue exposure with coping and communication skills training for alcoholics: treatment process and 1-year outcomes. *Alcoholism: Clinical and Experimental Research*, **25**, 1634–47.

Monti, P., Rohsenow, D., Hutchison, K. E. *et al.* (1999). Naltrexone's effect on cue-elicited craving among alcoholics in treatment. *Alcoholism: Clinical and Experimental Research*, **23**, 1386–94.

Morgan, M. Y. (1995). The management of alcohol withdrawal using chlormethiazole. *Alcohol and Alcoholism*, **30**, 771–4.

Mueller, T. I., Stout, R. L., Rudden, S. *et al.* (1997). A double-blind, placebo-controlled pilot study of carbamazepine for the treatment of alcohol dependence. *Alcoholism: Clinical and Experimental Research*, **21**, 86–92.

Mueser, K. T., Noordsy, D. L., Fox, L. & Wolfe, R. (2003). Disulfiram treatment for alcoholism in severe mental illness. *American Journal on Addictions*, **12**, 242–52.

Myers, R. D. & Martin, G. E. (1973). The role of cerebral serotonin in the ethanol preference of animals. *Annals of the New York Academy of Sciences*, **215**, 135–44.

Myrick, H., Brady, K. T. & Malcolm, R (2000). Divalproex in the treatment of alcohol withdrawal. *American Journal of Drug and Alcohol Abuse*, **26**, 155–60.

Myrick, H., Malcolm, R. & Brady, K. T. (1998). Gabapentin treatment of alcohol withdrawal. *American Journal of Psychiatry*, **155**, 1632.

Namkoong, K., Lee, B. O., Lee, P. G., Choi, M. J. & Lee, E. (2003). Acamprosate in Korean alcohol-dependent patients: a multicentre, randomized, double-blind, placebo-controlled study. *Alcohol and Alcoholism*, **38**, 135–41.

Naranjo, C. A. & Bremner, K. E. (1994). Serotonin-altering medications and desire, consumption and effects of alcohol-treatment implications. *EXS*, **71**, 209–19.

Naranjo, C. A., Bremner, K. E. & Lanctot, K. L. (1995). Effects of citalopram and a brief psycho-social intervention on alcohol intake, dependence and problems. *Addiction*, **90**, 87–99.

National Institute on Alcohol Abuse and Alcoholism (2000). *Tenth Special Report to the US Congress on Alcohol and Health, 2000*, Washington, DC: US Department of Health and Human Services.

National Treatment Agency (NTA) for Substance Misuse (NTA) (2002). Models of care for treatment of adult drug misusers: framework for developing local systems of effective drug misuse treatment in England; Part 2: Full reference report. December 2002.

Nellissery, M., Feinn, R. S., Covault, J. *et al.* (2003). Alleles of a functional serotonin transporter promoter polymorphism are associated with major depression in alcoholics. *Alcoholism: Clinical and Experimental Research*, **27**, 1402–8.

Nimmerrichter, A. A., Walter, H., Gutierrez-Lobos, K. E. & Lesch, O. M. (2002). Double-blind controlled trial of gamma-hydroxybutyrate and clomethiazole in the treatment of alcohol withdrawal. *Alcohol and Alcoholism*, **37**, 67–73.

Nunes, E. V. & Levin, F. R. (2004). Treatment of depression in patients with alcohol or other drug dependence: a meta-analysis. *Journal of the American Medical Association*, **291**, 1887–96.

Office of Applied Studies (2004). Results from the 2003 National Survey on Drug Use and Health: National Findings (DHHS Publication No. SMA 04–3964, NSDUH Series H–25). Rockville, MD: Substance Abuse and Mental Health Services Administration.

O'Malley, S., Jaffe, A. J., Chang, G. *et al.* (1992). Naltrexone and coping skills therapy for alcohol dependence. *Archives of General Psychiatry*, **49**, 881–7.

Ortho-McNeil Pharmaceutical Inc. (2003). Topamax® package Insert. Raritan, NJ, Revised December.

Petrakis, I. L., Poling, J., Levinson, C., Nich, C., Carroll, K. & Rounsaville, B. (2005). Naltrexone and disulfiram in patients with alcohol dependence and comorbid psychiatric disorders. *Biological Psychiatry*, **57**, 1128–37.

Pettinati, H. M. (1996). Use of serotonin selective pharmacotherapy in the treatment of alcohol dependence. *Alcoholism: Clinical and Experimental Research*, **20** (Suppl. 7), 23A–9A.

Pettinati, H. M. (2004). Antidepressant treatment of co-occurring depression and alcohol dependence. *Biological Psychiatry*, **56**, 785–92.

Pettinati, H., Volpicelli, J., Kranzler, H. *et al.* (2000). Sertraline treatment for alcohol dependence. Interactive effects of medication and alcoholic subtype. *Alcoholism: Clinical and Experimental Research*, **24**, 1041–9.

Pettinati, H. M., Dundon, W. & Lipkin, C. (2004). Gender differences in response to sertraline pharmacotherapy in Type A alcohol dependence. *American Journal on Addictions*, **13**, 236–47.

Poldrugo, F. (1997). Acamprosate treatment in a long-term community-based alcohol rehabilitation programme. *Addiction*, **92**, 1537–46.

Powell, B. J., Campbell, J. L., Landon, J. F. *et al.* (1995). A double-blind, placebo-controlled study of nortriptyline and bromocriptine in male alcoholics subtyped by comorbid psychiatric disorders. *Alcohol Clinical and Experimental Research*, **19**(2), 462–8.

Regier, D. A, Farmer, M. E, Rae, D. S. *et al.* (1990). Comorbidity of mental disorders with alcohol and other drug abuse, *Journal of the American Medical Association*, **264**, 2511–18.

Reoux, J. P., Saxon, A. J., Malte, C. A., Baer, J. S. & Sloan, K. L. (2001). Divalproex sodium in alcohol withdrawal: a randomized double-blind placebo-controlled clinical trial. *Alcoholism: Clinical and Experimental Research*, **25**, 1324–9.

Ritson, B. & Chick, J. (1986). Comparison of two benzodiazepines in the treatment of alcohol withdrawal: effects on symptoms and cognitive recovery. *Drug and Alcohol Dependence*, **18**, 329–34.

Rohsenow, D. J. (2004). What place does naltrexone have in the treatment of alcoholism? *CNS Drugs*, **18**, 547–60.

Roy-Byrne, P. P., Pages, K. P., Russo, J. E. (2000). Nefazodone treatment of major depression in alcohol-dependent patients: a double-blind, placebo-controlled trial. *Journal of Clinical Psychopharmacology*, **20**, 129–36.

Royal College of Physicians (2001). *Alcohol – can the NHS afford it? Recommendations for a coherent alcohol strategy for hospitals.* A report of the Working Party of the Royal College of Physicians. London: Royal College of Physicians of London.

Roussaux, J. P., Hers, D. & Ferauge, M. (1996). Does acamprosate diminish the appetite for alcohol in weaned alcoholics? *Journal de Pharmacie de Belgique*, **51**, 65–8.

Rubio, G., Jimenez-Arriero, M. A., Ponce, G. & Palomo, T. (2001). Naltrexone versus acamprosate: one year follow-up of alcohol dependence treatment. *Alcohol and Alcoholism*, **36**, 419–25.

Rubio G., Manzanares, J., Lopez-Munoz, F. *et al.* (2002). Naltrexone improves outcome of a controlled drinking program. *Journal of Substance Abuse Treatment*, **23**, 361–6.

Rubio, G., Ponce, G., Rodriguez-Jimenez, R., Jimenez-Arriero, M. A., Hoenicka, J. & Palomo, T. (2005). Clinical predictors of response to naltrexone in alcoholic patients: who benefits most from treatment with naltrexone? *Alcohol and Alcoholism*, **40**, 227–33.

Saitz, R., Mayo-Smith, M. F., Roberts, M. S., Redmond, H. A., Bernard, D. R. & Calkins, D. R. (1994). Individualized treatment for alcohol withdrawal: a randomized double-blind controlled trial. *Journal of the American Medical Association*, **272**, 519–23.

Salloum, I. M., Cornelius, J. R., Daley, D. C., Kirisci, L., Himmelhoch, J. M. & Thase, M. E. (2005). Efficacy of valproate maintenance in patients with bipolar disorder and alcoholism: a double-blind placebo-controlled study. *Archives of General Psychiatry*, **62**, 37–45.

Substance Abuse and Mental Health Services Administration (SAMHSA) (1997). *National Treatment Improvement Evaluation Study*. Center for Substance Abuse Treatment.

Sass, H., Soyka, M., Mann, K. *et al.* (1996). Relapse prevention by acamprosate. Results from a placebo controlled study on alcohol dependence. *Archives of General Psychiatry*, **53**, 673–80.

Saxon, A. J., Sloan, K. L., Reoux, J. & Haver, V. M. (1998). Disulfiram use in patients with abnormal liver function test results. *Journal of Clinical Psychiatry*, **59**, 313–16.

Schatzberg, A. F., Cole, J. O. & DeBattista, C. (2005). *Manual of Clinical Psychopharmacology*, 5th edn. New York: American Psychiatric Publishing, Inc.

Scottish Intercollegiate Guidelines Network (SIGN) (2003). *The management of harmful drinking and alcohol dependence in primary care: a national clinical guideline*. Edinburgh: Scottish Intercollegiate Guidelines Network, September.

Sellers, E. M., Zilm, D. H. & Degani, N. C. (1977). Comparative efficacy of propranolol and chlordiazepoxide in alcohol withdrawal. *Journal of Studies on Alcohol*, **38**, 2096–108.

Sellers, E. M., Toneatto, T., Romach, M. K., Somer, G. R., Sobell, L. C. & Sobell, M. B. (1994). Clinical efficacy of the 5-HT3 antagonist ondansetron in alcohol abuse and dependence. *Alcoholism: Clinical Experimental Research*, **18**, 879–85.

Slattery, J., Chick, J., Cochrane, M., *et al.* (2003). *Prevention of relapse in alcohol dependence. Health Technology Assessment Report 3*. Glasgow: Health Technology Board for Scotland.

Srisurapanont, M. & Jarusuraisin, N. (2003). Opioid antagonists for alcohol dependence. In *The Cochrane Library*. Chichester: John Wiley & Sons Ltd.

Stuppaeck, C. H., Pycha, R., Miller, C., Whitworth, A. B., Oberbauer, H. & Fleischhacker, W. W. (1992). Carbamazepine versus oxazepam in the treatment of alcohol withdrawal: a double-blind study. *Alcohol and Alcoholism*, **27**, 153–8.

Sullivan, J. T., Sykora, K., Schneiderman, J., Naranjo, C. A. & Sellers, E. M. (1989). Assessment of alcohol withdrawal: the revised clinical institute withdrawal assessment for alcohol scale (CIWA-Ar). *British Journal of Addiction*, **84**, 1353–7.

Sullivan, J. T, Swift, R. M. & Lewis DC. (1991). Benzodiazepine requirements during alcohol withdrawal syndrome: clinical implications of using a standardized withdrawal scale. *Journal of Clinical Psychopharmacology*, **11**, 291–5.

Swift, R. M. (2003). Topiramate for the treatment of alcohol dependence: initiating abstinence. *Lancet*, **361**, 1666–7.

Thanos, P. K., Volkow, N. D., Freimuth, P. *et al.* (2001). Overexpression of dopamine D2 receptors reduces alcohol self-administration, *Journal of Neurochemistry*, **78**, 1094–103.

Thomson, A. D. (2000). Mechanisms of vitamin deficiency in chronic alcohol misusers and the development of the Wernicke–Korsakoff Syndrome. *Alcohol and Alcoholism*, **35** (Suppl. 1), 2–7.

Tiihonen, J., Ryynanen, O. P., Kauhanen, J., Hakola H. P. & Salaspuro, M. (1996). Citalopram in the treatment of alcoholism: a double-blind placebo-controlled study. *Pharmacopsychiatry*, **29**, 27–9.

Tollefson, G. D., Montague-Clouse, J. & Tollefson, S. L. (1992). Treatment of comorbid generalized anxiety in a recently detoxified alcoholic population with a selective serotonergic drug (buspirone). *Journal of Clinical Psychopharmacology*, **12**, 19–26.

Torrens, M., Fonseca, F., Mateu, G. & Farre, M. (2005). Efficacy of antidepressants in substance use disorders with and without comorbid depression. A systematic review and meta-analysis. *Drug and Alcohol Dependence*, **78**, 1–22.

Trevisan, L. A., Boutros, N., Petrakas, I. L. *et al.* (1998). Complications of alcohol withdrawal: pathophysiologic insights. *Alcohol Health and Research World*, **22**, 61–6.

Verheul, R., Lehert, P., Geerlings, P. J., Koeter, M. W. & van den Brink, W. (2005). Predictors of acamprosate efficacy: results from a pooled analysis of seven European trials including 1485 alcohol-dependent patients. *Psychopharmacology*, **178**, 167–73.

Volpicelli, J. R., Alterman, A. I., Hayashida, M. *et al.* (1992). Naltrexone in the treatment of alcoholism. Results from a multicenter usage study. The Naltrexone Usage Study Group. *Archives of General Psychiatry*, **49**, 876–80.

Volpicelli, J. R., Rhines, K. C., Rhines, J. S. *et al.* (1997). Naltrexone and alcohol dependence. Role of subject compliance. *Archives of General Psychiatry*, **54**, 737–42.

Voris, J., Smith, N. L., Rao, S. M., Thorne, D. L. & Flowers, Q. J. (2003). Gabapentin for the treatment of ethanol withdrawal. *Substance Abuse*, **24**, 129–32.

Warsi, M., Sattar, S. P., Bhatia, S. C. & Petty, F. (2005). Aripiprazole reduces alcohol use. *Canadian Journal of Psychiatry*, **50**, 244.

Wetzel, H., Szegedi, A., Scheurich, A. *et al.* (2004). Combination treatment with nefazodone and cognitive-behavioral therapy for relapse prevention in alcohol-dependent men: a randomized controlled study. *Journal of Clinical Psychiatry*, **65**, 1406–13.

White, H. S., Brown, S. D., Woodhead, J. H. *et al.* (2000). Topiramate modulates GABA-evoked currents in murine cortical neurons by nonbenzodiazepine mechanism. *Epilepsia*, **41**(S 1), S25–9.

Whitworth, A. B., Fischer, F., Lesch, O. M. *et al.* (1996). Comparison of acamprosate and placebo in long-term treatment of alcohol dependence. *Lancet*, **347**, 1438–42.

Willenbring, M. L., Kivlahan, D., Kenny, M., Grillo, M., Hagedorn, H. & Postier, A. (2004). Beliefs about evidence-based practices in addiction treatment: a survey of Veterans Administration program leaders. *Journal of Substance Abuse Treatment*, **26**, 79–85.

Williams, D. & McBride, A. J. (1998). The drug treatment of alcohol withdrawal symptoms: a systematic review. *Alcohol*, **33**, 103–15.

World Health Organization (1992). *The ICD-10 Classification of Mental and Behavioural Disorders*. Geneva: World Health Organization.

Wright, C., Vafier, J. A. & Lake, C. R. (1988). Disulfiram-induced fulminating hepatitis: guidelines for liver-panel monitoring. *Journal of Clinical Psychiatry*, **49**, 430–4.

Wright, C., Moore, R. D., Grodin, D. M., Spyker, D. A. & Gill, E. V. (1993). Screening for disulfiram-induced liver test dysfunction in an inpatient alcoholism program. *Alcoholism: Clinical and Experimental Research*, **17**, 184–6.

Zeise, M. L., Kasparov, S., Capogna, M. & Zieglgansberger, W. (1993). Acamprosate (calcium acetylhomotaurinate) decreases postsynaptic potentials in the rat neocortex: possible involvement of excitatory amino acid receptors. *European Journal of Pharmacology*, **26**(231), 47–52.

Zullino, D. F., Khazaal, Y., Hattenschwiler, J., Borgeat, F. & Besson, J. (2004). Anticonvulsant drugs in the treatment of substance withdrawal. *Drugs Today (Barc.)*, **40**(7), 603–19.

Zwerling, C., Sprince, N. L., Wallace, R. B., Davis, C. S., Whitten, P. S. & Heeringa, S. G. (1996). Alcohol and occupational injuries among older workers. *Accident Analysis and Prevention*, **28**, 371–6.

15

Educational interventions for alcohol use disorders

Robert Patton, Kirk J. Brower, Shannon Bellefleur and Mike Crawford

Editor's note

Educational interventions are ubiquitous in psychiatry (see Part II: Chapter 6). They are readily available, inexpensive to deliver, and can be facilitated and disseminated by non-professionals. Educational interventions have long been a staple element of treatment for problems with alcohol. They accompany many of the self-help and complex interventions used in alcohol treatment. While these interventions may be efficient from an economical point of view, they are at best only modestly effective and appear to work best among people with mild to moderate abuse. They also appear to work most effectively when combined with some additional treatment delivered by people professionally trained to deliver services. Overall didactic lectures and educational films appear to have the least benefit.

Introduction

Education is inherent in most alcohol-related treatment interventions. Physician education about medication is one essential part of pharmacotherapy. Brief interventions provide educational feedback to patients about normative patterns of drinking. Twelve-step facilitation therapy involves educating patients about the disease model of alcoholism and what to expect in meetings of Alcoholics Anonymous (Nowinski *et al.*, 1994). CBT teaches patients (1) to identify high-risk situations for relapse and (2) coping skills to prevent relapse (Kadden *et al.*, 1995).

Educational interventions are designed to increase knowledge about alcohol in such a way as to change an individual's attitude and behaviour. Providing information about health risks and brief advice emphasizing strategies to reduce consumption are the only interventions that have been recommended for both hazardous and harmful consumption of alcohol. While education may be usefully employed as part of more complex interventions, we consider it in this chapter as a 'stand-alone' treatment.

Psychoeducation, like psychotherapy, is designed to reduce drinking and improve psychological functioning. Unlike psychotherapy, however, it can be either self-administered (Mains & Scogin, 2003) or provided by para-professionals and educators who have no formal training in psychotherapy. Educational approaches may involve differing degrees of contact with an educator and as minimal as one session (Apodaca & Miller, 2003). Contact with the educator can occur in-person or by telephone, postal mail (Sobell *et al.*, 2002), or computer. Thus, it is cost-efficient and can be used in stepped care models of treatment for alcohol use disorders (Sobell & Sobell, 2000).

General advice and information

As harmful use of alcohol often persists for a long time before any help is requested, the value of educational interventions might be considered to be optimal in this group. There is some evidence that supports this. Wallace and colleagues (1988) conducted a randomised controlled trial to compare advice (a booklet combined with general advice delivered by a family practitioner) with a no-intervention control. The results showed a significantly greater reduction in the levels of gamma-glutamyl transferase in the experimental group, a valid proxy indicator of levels of alcohol consumption. In the largest randomized trial of brief interventions for alcohol misuse conducted to date, 1661 people who were misusing alcohol but were non-dependent were recruited in primary and secondary care settings across ten countries (Babor & Grant, 1992). One of the strengths of this study is that patients were recruited from study centres in Central America, Africa and Asia, in addition to centres in Europe and North America where most other trials of interventions for alcohol misuse have been conducted. The study compared the effects of screening plus 5 minutes of brief advice with screening plus 15 minutes of counseling and a 'screening alone' control arm. A follow-up rate of 73% was achieved at 9 months. The study demonstrated that 5 minutes brief advice was as effective as 15 minutes counseling. Men who received one of these two active interventions reported drinking 25% less alcohol daily compared to those who received screening alone. Among women, statistically significant differences in drinking patterns between those randomized to active and control treatments were not observed.

Findings from this and other trials involving educational intervention have subsequently been reviewed on numerous occasions (e.g. Bien *et al.*, 1993; Mullen *et al.*, 1997; Dunn *et al.*, 2001). These reviews have reached similar conclusions: that brief educational interventions directed towards those drinking excessively result in reductions in alcohol consumption and that extended interventions offer little additional benefit. In their meta-analysis of 34 trials in non-treatment seeking populations, Moyer and colleagues (2002) highlighted a trend towards brief interventions having less impact among people with more severe alcohol-related problems. Few trials have followed up people beyond 12 months and those that have suggest that benefits associated with brief educational interventions do not persist beyond this period.

Educational interventions are popular in the US. For example, they are commonly used for remediation of drunk driver offenders. Alcoholics Anonymous and other mutual help groups, such as Rational Recovery and Moderation Management, publish books and pamphlets as well as maintain websites (Finfgeld, 2000b). Indeed, most mainstream bookstores in the USA have moderately sized sections devoted to self-help and recovery books (Finfgeld, 2000a). Surveys of internet-based and mail-delivered educational interventions indicate a high degree of acceptance by users (Kypri *et al.*, 2005).

Bibliotherapy

Bibliotherapy has been defined as the use of self-help materials or "any therapeutic intervention that was presented in a written format, designed to be read and implemented by the client" (Apodaca & Miller, 2003). More simply, bibliotherapy refers to "the therapeutic use of written materials to effect behavioral change" (Walitzer &

O'Connors, 1999). Examples of bibliotherapy include the *Big Book of Alcoholics Anonymous* (A.A., 2001), which is also available on-line, and a variety of behavioural self-control training books (e.g. Sanchez-Craig, 1993). New information, however, can also be learned by listening to lectures, watching movies (Davis *et al.*, 2002), and utilizing computer-assisted formats (Hester & Delaney, 1997), including accessing websites (Cunningham *et al.*, 2005; Walters *et al.*, 2005). Obviously, psychoeducation refers to a broad category of heterogeneous interventions.

Bibliotherapy for alcohol misuse was originally developed as an adjunct to psychological treatments (Miller 1978; WHO, 1996). Cunningham and colleagues (2001) used a quasi-experimental design to evaluate the impact of supplementing routine care for people attending an alcohol treatment centre with a booklet providing advice and information aimed at people who want to reduce the amount they drink. Over a 6-month period, half of those attending the centre were provided with the booklet. Follow-up data on a subset of these patients demonstrated that people who received a booklet were drinking 1.4 fewer drinks per day than those who received standard care alone.

Apodaca & Miller (2003) conducted a meta-analysis of 22 randomized trials on the effectiveness of bibliotherapy for problem drinking. All studies involved the distribution of self-help reading materials by healthcare professionals, even when there was no direct contact with the professional. Studies involving more than one face-to-face session with a professional were excluded. Overall, the conclusion was that bibliotherapy compared to no treatment has a small beneficial effect (weighted mean effect size = 0.31). But there were other conclusions from the meta-analysis as well. First, while bibliotherapy is more effective than no treatment, it is not more effective than extensive interventions. Second, bibliotherapy is more effective for self-referred drinkers (pre/post within-group effect size of 11 studies = 0.80) than those identified through opportunistic screening in medical practice (pre/post within-group effect size of 8 studies = 0.65). The most likely explanation is that self-referred drinkers are more motivated to reduce drinking than those referred for education after opportunistic screening. Third, self-help materials that included specific behavioral strategies (such as setting drinking goals, monitoring drinking habits, and solving problems without alcohol) are more effective than those containing general information and advice to reduce drinking only. As summarized by one group of investigators, specific advice is more effective than non-specific advice (Spivak *et al.*, 1994). Finally, bibliotherapy is best studied and recommended for at-risk and problem drinkers and not for patients with severe alcohol dependence. Consistent with these conclusions, a newer study, in which emergency care patients received either screening alone or screening plus simple written advice about sensible drinking limits, showed no added effect of bibliotherapy on drinking consumption (Nordqvist *et al.*, 2005).

Other educational interventions

School-based education efforts for public and college students

Studies which have aimed to examine the impact of public education campaigns have generally reported no impact on levels of alcohol consumption (Raistrick *et al.*, 1999). Such campaigns may have modest effects on improving knowledge about alcohol but have not been demonstrated to lead to a change in behavior. Somewhat better results have been demonstrated with school-based educational programs in which information about alcohol is usually provided in the context of general information on alcohol and other drugs (White & Pitts, 1998; Botvin *et al.*, 1995). Observational studies of school-based education on alcohol have demonstrated lower levels of alcohol misuse (Dielman, 1995). More recently randomized trials of school-based educational interventions aimed at preventing alcohol and drug misuse have demonstrated changes in attitudes to alcohol but little impact on actual patterns of consumption (Palinkas *et al.*, 1996; Lindberg *et al.*, 2002). A quasi-randomized study was conducted among secondary school students in Perth, Western Australia by McBride and colleagues (2004). In this study students were provided with an intervention aimed at minimizing harm associated with excessive alcohol consumption. Teaching was combined with skills training and use of videos and workbooks and was delivered over a 2-year period. Over 1700 (76%) of the original sample were followed up over a 32-month period. In addition to changes in knowledge and attitudes to alcohol, students who received this teaching reported consuming 31% less alcohol than those who did not. Seventeen months after delivery of the intervention, students who received training continued to drink less than those who did not, but differences between groups were no longer statistically significant.

A targeted group for educational approaches has been college students for whom the goal is to reduce at-risk and problem drinking. In general, educational programs which only provide information in the absence of motivational or skills-building strategies are not effective (Larimer & Cronce, 2002). Research with college students indicates that they have a tendency to misperceive norms about drinking patterns among their peers. For example, college students typically overestimate how much other students drink. Personalized feedback comparing a student's own drinking patterns to those of age- and sex-matched peers is referred to as normative education (Walters & Neighbors, 2005). In one study of normative education, heavy-drinking college students were randomized to receive by mail either (1) a two-page information form comparing their drinking to normative drinking patterns of their peers with advice to reduce drinking, or (2) an educational brochure about alcohol use with advice to reduce drinking (Collins *et al.*, 2002). The first group had significantly fewer heavy drinking episodes at the 6-week follow-up assessment when compared to the second group, suggesting that education involving personalized feedback about drinking was more effective than general information about drinking. Similar outcomes were obtained when normative education was delivered by computer (Neighbors *et al.*, 2004).

Findings from studies among young people set outside of educational establishments have generated less positive findings. A recent systematic review concluded that there is insufficient information to support claims that they are effective (Gates *et al.*, 2006).

Other groups and other interventions

Education has long been a mainstay intervention for convicted drunk drivers. When compared to other remedial interventions for preventing repeat drunk-driver offences, education in combination with psychotherapy was more effective than education alone, which was more effective than probation alone (Wells-Parker *et al.*, 1995). The first randomized controlled trial comparing education alone to education plus exposure to a victim impact panel demonstrated no advantage of the victim impact panel (Polacsek *et al.*, 2001).

Psychoeducation for alcohol use disorders has been used as a control group in randomized controlled trials, implying that it is either an inactive or minimal intervention; yet results are mixed. For example, group psychoeducation performed as well as CBT in improving alcohol outcomes in 88 adolescents with mixed diagnoses of alcohol abuse or dependence and/or marijuana abuse or dependence (Kaminer *et al.*, 2002). On the other hand, it was inferior to standard outpatient alcoholism treatment for the outcome of abstinence in a study of male alcoholic veterans (Davis *et al.*, 2002). The latter study, however, did not control for treatment intensity and it selected for dependent drinkers.

Strengthening Families Program (SFP)

The Strengthening Families Program was designed to reduce adolescent substance misuse by increasing parenting skills and helping young people to develop their confidence and life skills (Kumpfer et al., 1996). The intervention involves parents and young people meeting separately and together in interactive groups with use of educational materials, themed discussions and role-play. In a systematic review of educational programs to prevent alcohol misuse among young people (aged 25 and under), Foxcroft et al. (2003) concluded that the SFP showed promise as an effective prevention initiative, with a number needed to treat (NNT) of 9.

Internet and computer-based education

Currently, evidence to support internet-based approaches is only beginning to accumulate (Cunningham et al., 2005; Walters et al., 2005). Although the medium is relatively novel, the educational components such as individualized and normative feedback remain similar to those delivered by other formats. The ease of accessibility may give the internet an advantage; however, the quality of information is not regulated.

Both internet and computer-based education are likely to be of value in some form as a means of reducing alcohol misuse. Joinson & Banyard (2003) present limited evidence that drinkers who are contemplating reducing their alcohol consumption are less likely to access related information of the internet compared to those who are at a pre-contemplative stage. Reis et al. (2000) presented data from an uncontrolled study of 4695 students in an evaluation of a CD-ROM aimed at preventing alcohol-related harm. Although the absence of a control group inhibits interpretation of study findings, there were suggestions of improvements in knowledge among participants.

Educational lectures and films

Miller et al. (1998) reviewed 31 studies of educational lectures and films and found that only 4 demonstrated a positive outcome. In the most recent review of alcohol treatment modalities, Miller & Wilbourne (2002) rated educational lectures, films and groups as one of the least effective approaches for reducing alcohol misuse.

Summary

There is a strong evidence base to recommend educational intervention for all patients including at-risk, problem, and dependent drinkers. Nevertheless, it is only moderately effective and appears most effective with people who have mild to moderate problems with alcohol. Education can be enhanced significantly by combining it with motivational techniques, skills training, and psychotherapy since education as a stand-alone intervention is generally less effective than when combined with other strategies.

In the UK, the importance of educational interventions is reflected in official guidelines from the World Health Organization (WHO, 2004) and in national guidelines (e.g. UK Alcohol Forum, 2001; Scottish Intercollegiate Guidelines Network, 2003), which endorse these approaches as part of first-line treatment for helping people who misuse alcohol. Self-help manuals linked to brief advice are generally recommended as second-line treatment in official guidelines (Scottish Intercollegiate Guidelines Network, 2003). The impact of other forms of educational information is less certain.

The level of evidence for each of the interventions discussed in this chapter is summarized in Table 15.1.

Table 15.1. Effectiveness of educational interventions for alcohol use disorders

Treatment	Form of treatment	Psychiatric disorder	Level of evidence for efficacy	Comments
Educational interventions	Bibliotherapy	Alcohol use disorders	Ia	Shown to have a small beneficial effect that can be enhanced by additional professional psychotherapeutic work. Works best in mild to moderate alcohol misuse
Educational interventions	Miscellaneous educational intervention including internet, formal classes, films	Alcohol use disorders	IIa	Has different impact in different populations but in general is thought to be of some help but often needs some enhancements with other more formalised treatments. Films do not appear to be effective

REFERENCES

Alcoholics Anonymous, 4th edn. (2001). *Alcoholics Anonymous*. World Services, Inc. New York, NY. Also available online at: http://www.aa.org/bigbookonline/.

Apodaca, T. R. & Miller, W. R. (2003). A meta-analysis of the effectiveness of bibliotherapy for alcohol problems. *Journal of Clinical Psychology*, **59**(3), 289–304.

Babor, T. F. & Grant, M. (1992). *Programme on substance abuse. Project on identification and management of alcohol related problems. Report on phase II: a randomised controlled trial of brief interventions in primary health care*. Geneva: World Health Organisation.

Bien, T. H., Miller, W. R. & Tonigan, J. S. (1993). Brief interventions for alcohol problems: a review. *Addiction*, **88**, 315–36.

Botvin, G. J., Baker, E., Dusenbury, L., Botvin, E. M. & Diaz, T. (1995). Long-term follow-up results of a randomized drug abuse prevention trial in a white middle-class population. *Journal of American Medical Association*, **273**, 1106–12.

Collins, S. E., Carey, K. B. & Sliwinski, M. J. (2002). Mailed personalized normative feedback as a brief intervention for at-risk college drinkers. *Journal of Studies on Alcohol*, **63**(5), 559–67.

Cunningham, J. A., Sdao-Jarvie, K., Koski-Jannes, A. & Curtis Breslin, F. (2001). Using self-help materials to motivate change at assessment for alcohol treatment. *Journal of Substance Abuse Treatment*, **20**, 301–4.

Cunningham, J. A., Humphreys, K., Koski-Jannes, A. & Cordingley, J. (2005). Internet and paper self-help materials for problem drinking: is there an additive effect? *Addictive Behaviors*, **30**(8), 1517–23.

Davis, W. T., Campbell, L., Tax, J. & Lieber, C. S. (2002). A trial of 'standard' outpatient alcoholism treatment vs. a minimal treatment control. *Journal of Substance Abuse Treatment*, **23**(1), 9–19.

Dielman, T. E. (1995). School-based research on the prevention of adolescent alcohol use and misuse: methodological issues and advances. In *Alcohol Problems Among Adolescents: Current Directions in Prevention Research*, ed. G. Boyd, J. Howard & R. A. Zucker. Hillsdale, NJ: Lawrence Erlbaum Associates.

Dunn, C., Deroo, L. & Rivara, F. P. (2001). The use of brief interventions adapted from motivational interviewing across behavioral domains: a sytematic review. *Addiction*, **96**, 1725–42.

Finfgeld, D. L. (2000a). Resolving alcohol problems using an online self-help approach: moderation management. *Journal of Psychosocial Nursing and Mental Health Services*, **38**(2), 32–8.

Finfgeld, D. L. (2000b). Use of self-help manuals to treat problem drinkers. *Journal of Psychosocial Nursing and Mental Health Services*, **38**(4), 20–7.

Foxcroft, D. R., Ireland, D., Lister-Sharp, D. J., Lowe, G., & Breen, R. (2003). Longer-term primary prevention for alcohol misuse in young people: a systematic review. *Addiction*, **98**, 397–411.

Gates, S., McCambridge, J., Smith, L. A., & Foxcroft, D. R. (2006). Interventions for prevention of drug use by young people delivered in non-school settings. *The Cochrane Database of Systematic Reviews*, **2**. Oxford: Update Software Ltd.

Hester, R. K. & Delaney, H. D. (1997). Behavioral self-control program for Windows: results of a controlled clinical trial. *Journal of Consulting and Clinical Psychology*, **65**(4), 686–93.

Joinson, A. N., & Banyard, P. (2003). Seeking alcohol information on the internet. *ASLIB Proceedings*, **55**, 313–19.

Kadden, R., Carroll, K., Donovan, D. *et al.* (1995). *Cognitive-Behavioral Coping Skills Therapy Manual*. Rockville, MD: National Institute on Alcohol Abuse and Alcoholism.

Kaminer, Y., Burleson, J. A. & Goldberger, R. (2002). Cognitive-behavioral coping skills and psychoeducation therapies for adolescent substance abuse. *Journal of Nervous and Mental Disease*, **190**(11), 737–45.

Kumpfer, K., Molgaard, V. & Spoth, R. (1996) The strengthening families programme for the prevention of delinquency and drug use. In *Preventing Childhood Disorders, Substance Abuse and Delinquency*, ed. R. Peters, & R., McMahon, pp. 241–67. Thousand Oaks, CA: Sage.

Kypri, K., Sitharthan, T., Cunningham, J. A., Kavanagh, D. J. & Dean, J. I. (2005). Innovative approaches to intervention for problem drinking. *Current Opinions in Psychiatry*, **18**(3), 229–34.

Larimer, M. E. & Cronce, J. M. (2002). Identification, prevention and treatment: a review of individual-focused strategies to reduce problematic alcohol consumption by college students. *Journal of Studies on Alcohol*, **Suppl. 14**, 148–63.

Lindberg, C. S., Solorzano, R. M., Bear, D., Strickland, O., Galvis, C., & Pittman, K. (2002). Reducing substance use and risky sexual behaviour among low-income, Mexican-American women: comparison of two interventions. *Applied Nursing Research*, **16**, 137–48.

Mains, J. A. & Scogin, F. R. (2003). The effectiveness of self-administered treatments: a practice-friendly review of the research. *Journal of Clinical Psychology*, **59**(2), 237–46.

McBride, N., Farringdon, F., Midford, R., Meuleners, L. & Phillips, M. (2004). Harm minimization in school drug education: final results of the School Health and Alcohol Harm Reduction Project (SHAHRP). *Addiction*, **99**, 278–91.

Miller, R. W. (1978). Behavioral treatment of problem drinkers: A comparative outcome study of three controlled drinking therapies. *Journal of Consulting and Clinical Psychology*, **46**, 74–86.

Miller, W. R. & Wilbourne, P. L. (2002). Mesa Grande: a methodological analysis of clinical trials of treatments for alcohol use disorders. *Addiction*, **97**, 265–77.

Miller, W. R., Andrews, N. R., Wilbourne, P. & Bennett, M. E. (1998). A wealth of alternatives: effective treatments for alcohol problems. In *Treating Addictive Behaviours: Process of Change*, ed. R. W. Miller & N. Heather, 2nd edn, pp. 203–216. New York: Plenum Press.

Moyer, A., Finney, J. W., Swearingen, C. E. & Vergun, P. (2002). Brief interventions for alcohol problems: a meta-analytic review of controlled investigations in treament-seeking and non-treatment-seeking populations. *Addiction*, **97**, 279–92.

Mullen, P. D., Simons-Morton, D. G., Ramirez, G., Frankowski, R. F., Green, L. W. & Mains, D. A. (1997). A meta-analysis of trials evaluating patient edcuation and counselling for three groups of preventive health behaviors. *Patient Educational Counselling,* **32**, 157–73.

Neighbors, C., Larimer, M. E. & Lewis, M. A. (2004). Targeting misperceptions of descriptive drinking norms: efficacy of a computer-delivered personalized normative feedback intervention. *Journal of Consulting and Clinical Psychology,* **72**(3), 434–47.

Nordqvist, C., Wilhelm, E., Lindqvist, K. & Bendtsen, P. (2005). Can screening and simple written advice reduce excessive alcohol consumption among emergency care patients? *Alcohol Alcohol,* **40**(5), 401–8.

Nowinski, J., Baker, S. & Carroll, K. (1994). *Twelve Step Facilitation Therapy Manual.* Rockville, MD: National Institute on Alcohol Abuse and Alcoholism.

Palinkas, L. A., Atkins, C. J., Miller, C. & Ferreira, D. (1996). Social skills training for drug prevention in high-risk female adolescents. *Preventative Medicine,* **25**, 692–701.

Polacsek, M., Rogers, E. M., Woodall, W. G., Delaney, H., Wheeler, D. & Rao, N. (2001). MADD victim impact panels and stages-of-change in drunk-driving prevention. *Journal of Studies on Alcohol,* **62**(3), 344–50.

Raistrick, D., Hodgson, R. & Ritson, B. (1999). *Tackling Alcohol Together.* London: Free Association Books.

Reis, J., Riley, W. & Baer, J. (2000). Interactive multimedia preventative alcohol education: an evaluation of effectiveness with college students. *Journal of Educational Computing Research,* **23**, 41–65.

Sanchez-Craig, M. (1993). *Saying When: How to Quit Drinking or Cut Down.* Toronto: Addiction Research Foundation.

Scottish Intercollegiate Guidelines Network (2003). The management of harmful drinking and alcohol dependence in primary care, a national clinical guideline. Edinburgh: Royal College of Physicians.

Sobell, L. C., Sobell, M. B., Leo, G. I., Agrawal, S., Johnson-Young, L. & Cunningham, J. A. (2002). Promoting self-change with alcohol abusers: a community-level mail intervention based on natural recovery studies. *Alcoholism: Clinical and Experimental Research,* **26**(6), 936–48.

Sobell, M. B. & Sobell, L. C. (2000). Stepped care as a heuristic approach to the treatment of alcohol problems. *Journal of Consulting and Clinical Psychology,* **68**(4), 573–9.

Spivak, K., Sanchez-Craig, M. & Davila, R. (1994). Assisting problem drinkers to change on their own: effect of specific and non-specific advice. *Addiction,* **89**(9), 1135–42.

UK Alcohol Forum (2001). *Guidelines for the Management of Alcohol Problems in Primary Care and General Psychiatry.* High Wycombe, Bucks: Tangent Medical Education.

Walitzer, K. S. & Connors, G. J. (1999). Treating problem drinking. *Alcohol Research and Health,* **23**(2), 138–43.

Wallace, P., Cutler, S. & Haines, A. (1988). Randomised controlled trial of general practitioner intervention in patients with excessive alcohol consumption. *British Medical Journal,* **297**, 663–8.

Walters, S. T., Hester, R. K., Chiauzzi, E. & Miller, E. (2005). Demon rum: high-tech solutions to an age-old problem. *Alcoholism Clinical and Experimental Research,* **29**(2), 270–7.

Walters, S. T. & Neighbors, C. (2005). Feedback interventions for college alcohol misuse: what, why and for whom? *Addictive Behavior,* **30**(6), 1168–82.

Wells-Parker, E., Bangert-Drowns, R., McMillen, R. & Williams, M. (1995). Final results from a meta-analysis of remedial interventions with drink/drive offenders. *Addiction,* **90**(7), 907–26.

White, D. & Pitts, M. (1998). Educating young people about drugs: a systematic review. *Addiction,* **93**, 1475–87.

WHO Brief Intervention Study Group (1996). A cross-national trial of brief interventions with heavy drinkers. *American Journal of Public Health,* **86**, 948–55.

WHO Collaborating Centre for Research and Training for Mental Health. (2004). *WHO Guide to Mental and Neurological Health in Primary Care.* London: RSM Press.

16

Complex interventions for alcohol use disorders

Valerie J. Slaymaker, Kirk J. Brower and Mike Crawford

Editor's note

Alcohol misuse is a complex problem and complex interventions are the norm in its management. This is illustrated well in this chapter in which all the effective treatments are not just complex, but often multi-complex, and it is not always certain what constitutes the most important elements. It is also important to note that the result of an intervention may differ at different levels of dependence. ICD-10 defines a category of 'harmful use' that is short of full dependence, and many of the simpler interventions may be more helpful in this group than when full dependence has developed.

Introduction

A complex intervention for alcohol use disorders may be defined as one that utilizes multiple therapeutic components and strategies, based on a common underlying philosophy of treatment and targeted at various facets of the disorder in a complementary and frequently simultaneous fashion. Most treatment for moderately to severely alcohol-dependent patients is complex by this definition and for good reasons. First, alcohol use disorders are heterogeneous and influenced by multiple factors in terms of their etiology, development, and course. Second, no single treatment strategy or technique is effective across all alcohol-dependent patients. Third, the active ingredients of most, if not all, psychosocial therapies for alcohol dependence are unknown.

This chapter will cover four complex interventions for which there is a base of evidence to evaluate them. They are Alcoholics Anonymous (A.A.), the Minnesota Model of treatment, Therapeutic Communities (TCs), and combined pharmacotherapy and psychotherapy. With the exception of A.A., complex interventions are generally delivered within specialized addiction treatment settings. By contrast, A.A. is a non-professional intervention available within the broader community.

Alcoholics Anonymous

Introduction

Founded in 1935 in Akron, Ohio by Dr Robert Smith and Bill Wilson, Alcoholics Anonymous (A.A.) is an extensive mutual-help organization that spans the globe. By 2002, over 100 000 groups were meeting in 150 countries (Alcoholics Anonymous World Services, 2004). As a result of A.A.'s growth and popularity, additional groups have been developed for those struggling with addiction to specific substances, including Narcotics Anonymous, Cocaine Anonymous, and Marijuana Anonymous, among others.

A.A. aims to help members with maintaining total abstinence from alcohol and drugs by living in accordance with the Twelve Steps. The Steps encompass the basic principles of the A.A. philosophy and emphasize recognition of problem drinking and alcoholism, development of hope for recovery, conducting a thorough self-inventory of personal shortcomings, implementing a behavioral plan of action to address the consequences of alcoholism, making restitution for harmful actions, engaging in regular behavior intended to maintain recovery, developing spirituality and serenity, and helping other alcoholics. Regular attendance at meetings is strongly encouraged and newcomers are advised to attend 90 meetings in 90 days whenever possible. In addition, the program philosophy encourages modification of maladaptive cognitions (referred to as "stinkin' thinkin"), behavioral changes (e.g. avoidance of drinking events, drinking friends, or relatives), and the

Cambridge Textbook of Effective Treatments in Psychiatry, ed. Peter Tyrer and Kenneth R. Silk. Published by Cambridge University Press.
© Cambridge University Press, 2008.

development of adaptive coping skills (e.g. calling a sponsor for support when needed). This multifaceted approach combines elements of cognitive and behavioral change, social support (fellowship), and spiritual growth and defines A.A. as a complex intervention.

Frequently misunderstood as a religious organization, A.A.'s spiritual principles are broad and consistent with many religious orientations. Whereas religions generally define the nature of God or some other unifying force and prescribe specific, ritualistic practices for relating to God, A.A. encourages members to define a 'Higher Power' for themselves and to find their own way of relating to that Higher Power. For example, members may choose to use the words, 'God,' 'Higher Power,' or 'Power greater than ourselves' to refer to a source of strength that assists them in maintaining recovery. The idea is that when alcoholics rely primarily on their individual selves for recovery, they are in danger of relapsing to drinking. Therefore, they need to seek a power greater than themselves for recovery. Nevertheless, some patients are unable to affiliate with A.A. because of its spiritual connotations (Walters, 2002).

A.A. is one of the most commonly sought after sources of help for alcoholism in the U.S. (Weisner *et al.*, 1995; Workgroup on Substance Abuse Self-Help Organizations, 2003), with membership estimated at over 2 000 000 people worldwide (Alcoholics Anonymous World Services, 2004). It is free, available to anyone with a desire to stop drinking, omnipresent, and compatible with professional interventions. Because A.A. participation is related to improved substance use and psychosocial outcomes, a number of national organizations recommend referral to A.A. and other Twelve Step related groups.

The most recent public policy statement written by the American Society of Addiction Medicine (ASAM, 2001) recommends the inclusion of self-help groups as an adjunct to professional treatment. Similarly, the National Institute on Alcohol Abuse and Alcoholism (NIAAA) includes A.A. in a discussion of advances in addiction treatment, noting the efficacy of A.A. in improving outcomes (NIAAA, 2000a). The Department of Veterans Affairs, perhaps one of the largest providers of substance abuse treatment in the USA, also recommends referral to self-help groups in their clinical practice guidelines, with specific strategies included for promoting meeting attendance among substance dependent patients (Veterans Health Administration Office of Quality & Performance, 2001). The American Psychiatric Association (APA) published its second edition of practice guidelines for substance use disorders in 2006, which recommend attendance and participation in meetings of A.A. or other similar self-help groups in the light of higher abstinent rates among those who participate. Acknowledging that individual patient needs and concerns must be considered when recommending A.A., the practice guideline maintains that most patients should be encouraged to attend at least some A.A. meetings on a trial basis (APA, 2006, p. 65). The Substance Abuse and Mental Health Services Administration's (SAMHSA) Center for Substance Abuse Treatment has published a series of practice guidelines in addictions treatment titled, *Treatment Improvement Protocols* (TIP). These guidelines recommend referral to A.A. and related groups for alcohol and drug addicted people including adolescents, adults, older adults, pregnant women, and those with co-occurring mental health disorders (US Department of Health and Human Services, 1993, 1994a, 1994b, 1994c, 1998, 1999). SAMHSA and the US Department of Veterans Affairs convened a group of experts to discuss mutual-help groups in the treatment of substance abuse and dependence. In a white paper outlining their clinical and policy recommendations, the resulting Workgroup on Substance Abuse Self-Help Organizations (2003) urges clinicians and program directors to implement procedures to facilitate mutual help participation, such as that offered in A.A. and related groups, among substance dependent people.

In addition to governmental agencies, groups of addiction researchers recommend referral to A.A. as part of a comprehensive treatment program. A group at the George Washington University Medical Center works to promote public knowledge, improve access to treatment, and reduce the social consequences of alcohol abuse and alcoholism through their organization, Ensuring Solutions to Alcohol Problems. To this end, the group publishes a series of primers that are summaries of research addressing specific topics related to alcohol abuse and alcoholism. In *Primer 4, The Active Ingredients of Effective Treatment for Alcohol Problems* (Ensuring Solutions to Alcohol Problems, 2003), the group identifies participation in A.A. as an important component of positive treatment outcome. Most recently, a group of nationally recognized addiction researchers published an expert consensus statement outlining policies for facilitating mutual-help group involvement (Humphreys *et al.*, 2004). Specifically, this expert panel recommended that mutual-help group attendance be viewed as an extension of professional treatment, not a substitute for it. The workgroup further specified the use of empirically validated methods to facilitate mutual-help group involvement including Twelve Step facilitation counseling, having a menu of mutual-help group options available, and encouraging clinical staff to facilitate self-help group attendance, among others.

Evidence

Several extensive and thoughtful literature reviews of A.A. effectiveness and efficacy have been recently published (Emrick & Tonigan, 2004; Humphreys, 2003; Tonigan *et al.*, 1996). The conclusion has been consistent: A.A. membership and participation is related to improved drinking and psychosocial outcomes.

At first, early research on A.A. was plagued by methodological problems. In a 1993 meta-analytic review of 107 studies available to date, Emrick and colleagues (1993) noted homogeneity of samples, potential investigator biases, pre-experimental designs, over-reliance on treatment samples, and a lack of theory-driven investigations into the interrelationships among factors related to A.A. Little attention had been paid to female members, youth, ethnic and cultural groups, and few longitudinal studies had been conducted. Despite these limitations in the published literature, the review found a positive and modest correlation between A.A. involvement and substance use outcome when professional treatment and A.A. were combined. The authors also found support for a positive, but modest, relationship between A.A. attendance and psychological health.

Tonigan *et al.* (1996) expanded upon the earlier meta-analytic review by Emrick *et al.* (1993) by considering the source of samples (whether inpatient, outpatient, or naturalistic), rating studies based on methodological rigor, and providing power estimates when possible among 74 studies reviewed. The quality rating included assessment of subject selection, subject assignment, psychometric qualities of measurement, and whether biomedical methods were undertaken to corroborate self-report. The majority of studies met only one of the five quality criteria. Researchers typically recruited from sequential admissions to either inpatient (68%) or outpatient (30%) programs. Half (51%) of the studies failed to report on the psychometric qualities of instrumentation. As a result of these problems, studies met only 'poor' or 'fair' quality ratings. Not surprisingly, power to detect differences was low among the studies, with Type II error rates ranging from 0.33 to 0.71. Overall, consistent with findings by Emrick *et al.* (1993), modest relationships in the desired direction were found between A.A. involvement and drinking and psychosocial outcome, with stronger relationships found for outpatient samples and for those studies with better methodological rigor.

As research on A.A. has progressed, increasingly sophisticated designs have included prospective measurement (e.g. McKellar *et al.*, 2003), youth samples (e.g. Kelly *et al.*, 2000), ethnic groups (e.g. Roland & Kaskutas, 2002;

Tonigan *et al.*, 1998), professionally untreated individuals in A.A. (e.g. Timko *et al.*, 2000), long-term outcomes (e.g. Moos & Moos, 2004), and a focus on the mechanisms of change within A.A. (e.g. Morgenstern *et al.*, 1997; Owen *et al.*, 2003).

Even so, as observed by Humphreys (2003) in a thoughtful review, controlled and prospective studies with random assignment to A.A. vs. no-treatment control conditions are not likely to occur. Given the extent to which A.A. is available and accessible, researchers are unable to exert the degree of control necessary to directly compare the effects of A.A. against something else. In addition, A.A. as an organization clearly states its policy against engaging in or supporting research (Alcoholics Anonymous World Services, n.d.). As a result, the majority of studies to date have had to rely on correlational and predictive analyses to understand the relationship between A.A. attendance or affiliation and drinking and psychosocial outcomes. Due to the anonymous nature of A.A., the majority of studies conducted have examined the impact of A.A. attendance following professional treatment on outcomes.

Because A.A.'s effects may be attributed to greater motivation to remain abstinent or to better overall prognosis among members, McKellar *et al.* (2003) developed a structural equation model to examine these hypothesized mediators. A sample of 2319 male alcohol-dependent veterans was contacted at 1 and 2 years following treatment. The results of the equation modeling supported the hypothesis that A.A. involvement is a cause of improved alcohol-related outcomes. Conversely, the hypothesis that reduced consumption caused greater A.A. affiliation was not supported. Furthermore, neither pretreatment motivation levels nor psychopathology explained the relationship between A.A. involvement and outcome. In summary, A.A.'s effects do not appear to be explained by increased motivation on the part of participants.

Data also suggest length of participation has a direct impact on outcomes. For example, in the study described above (McKellar *et al.*, 2003), higher levels of involvement in the first year after treatment was predictive of better outcomes at the 2-year follow-up. A prospective study conducted by Moos and Moos (2004) examined the duration and frequency of A.A. participation among 473 previously untreated men (50.3%) and women (49.7%) contacting an intake and referral alcohol treatment system. Logistic regression analyses found no outcome differences between those who attended A.A. between 1 and 16 weeks in the year following contact and those who did not attend at all. However, those who attended between 17 to 32 weeks in the first year had significantly better use outcomes, and those who attended for 33 weeks or more had better alcohol and psychosocial outcomes. Furthermore, A.A. participation frequency during the first year after contact predicted positive use and psychosocial outcomes at an 8-year follow-up.

An earlier published study of the same sample examined differences between those who attended A.A. only ($n = 66$), attended formal treatment but had no A.A. participation ($n = 74$), attended formal treatment plus A.A. ($n = 248$), and those who did not receive treatment of any type, whether formally or informally ($n = 78$) in the 8 years following initial contact (Timko et al., 2000). Those attending formal treatment plus A.A. had significantly higher rates of abstinence than those who attended formal treatment alone at the 1- and 3-year follow-ups. By 8 years, this difference dissipated.

Given the benefits of A.A. participation with regard to outcomes, researchers have begun to study the change mechanisms by which A.A. exerts its effect. Thus far, data from several well-conducted studies suggest A.A. involvement works to improve outcomes by increasing self-efficacy or the confidence to resist drinking, which in turn positively impacts abstinence. Morgenstern and colleagues (1997), for example, conducted a prospective, controlled study of 100 patients in a Twelve Step treatment program. Because problem severity, pretreatment use frequencies, baseline commitment to abstinence, and self-efficacy levels at discharge were correlated with outcome, these factors were controlled for in the analyses. Overall, affiliation with A.A. after treatment was found to promote ongoing motivation and commitment to abstinence, increased use of active coping skills, and the maintenance of self-efficacy which each, in turn, independently predicted positive substance use outcomes.

Self-efficacy as a mediator of A.A.'s effects was further supported by an analysis of Project MATCH data by Connors et al. (2001). In their examination of 914 participants, A.A. participation predicted the percentage of abstinent days in the 7–12 months after treatment. Self-efficacy was a mediator of this effect; that is, A.A. participation predicted self-efficacy levels which, in turn, predicted percentage of days abstinent at 1 year. Later analyses found this effect to persist at the 3-year follow-up (Owen et al., 2003).

Humphreys et al. (1999) found support for the role of active coping and changes in social support networks. In a study of 2337 male VA patients seeking treatment who had no involvement with A.A. or other self-help groups prior to intake, involvement after treatment was found to have a direct effect upon reduced substance abuse in the year following discharge. This effect was mediated by the use of active coping responses, the quality of friendships and support from friends to remain abstinent. These three mediators, in turn, predicted reductions in substance use.

Additional evidence suggests the role of social support within A.A. is important in understanding its impact on outcome. Bond et al. (2003) assessed 1- and 3-year outcomes among a sample of 655 people in public and private treatment facilities. A.A.'s impact on outcome was mediated by the number of A.A. contacts with people who encouraged a reduction in drinking. In a study of 112 patients in a residential treatment setting, Owen et al. (2003) found that A.A. participation in the year after treatment positively impacted lifestyle changes, which included ending relationships with using friends and making new friends in recovery. Lifestyle changes, in turn, positively impacted abstinence rates at 1-year.

A.A. participation has also been found to reduce the utilization of additional treatment services. Humphreys and Moos (1996) compared 135 individuals initially choosing to attend A.A. to 66 initially choosing outpatient treatment for alcohol problems. While the two groups were similar in terms of sex, race, marital status, employment, and alcohol dependence and depression symptoms as measured at baseline, the group choosing A.A. had lower incomes, less education, and experienced more use-related consequences than did the outpatient group. Over the course of 3 years, the A.A.-choosing group incurred an average of $1826 of subsequent professional treatment costs per person – 45% less than the outpatient group. A later study by Humphreys and Moos (2001) examined substance-dependent individuals in residential treatment programs. Those who attended programs that emphasized A.A. and related group attendance were not only more likely to be abstinent at the 1-year follow-up, they had significantly lower health care costs compared to those in cognitive-behavioral (CB) programs. Specifically, CB participants had 64% higher annual health care costs, averaging $4700.00 per patient.

Summary

While there is inherent difficulty in subjecting A.A. attendance to randomized clinical trials, increasingly sophisticated designs have been utilized in an effort to understand its impact. The available evidence to date strongly suggests that A.A. is effective for many alcohol-dependent persons. Given the strength of the evidence, the ubiquity of meeting times and places, the importance of social support for recovery, its cost-free nature, and compatibility with professional treatment, we recommend that A.A. be considered as a treatment option for all alcohol-dependent patients. We do this with the understanding that not everyone will affiliate with it long enough to benefit from its fellowship.

When patients do affiliate with A.A., however, the benefits are positive. We suggest to patients that not all A.A. meetings are created equal and that they 'shop around' or sample a variety of meetings before deciding not to attend. We also recommend that patients attend their first meeting with an A.A. member. Some meetings are specialized, such as gender-specific meetings and meetings that are closed to non-alcoholic friends of the patient. We recommend that family members be encouraged to attend Al-Anon, a Twelve Step mutual-help group for people close to the patient, who may also have suffered from the impact of the patient's alcoholism.

To facilitate A.A. attendance, professionals should ask about what the patient liked and did not like about the first meeting attended. Objections to its religious overtones, for example, may surface at this point and can be addressed. The wise clinician will explore such objections non-judgmentally in order to differentiate between patients that resist alcoholism treatment in general or A.A. specifically. Patients who conscientiously object to A.A. specifically will nevertheless manifest motivation to participate in and use other treatment strategies. Further encouragement and/or coercion to attend A.A. are contraindicated and counterproductive in such patients. Among those patients who affiliate with A.A., efforts made at facilitating ongoing participation (e.g. addressing barriers to attendance, utilizing Twelve Step facilitation techniques) should be undertaken throughout the course of treatment for substance dependence.

The Minnesota model of care

Introduction

Several interesting and informative publications document the historical development of the Minnesota Model of treatment. Interested readers are referred to Anderson (1981), Anderson *et al.* (1999), McElrath (1987), Spicer (1993), and White (1998) for thorough descriptions from which the following early historical material was gleaned.

The Minnesota Model's beginnings can be traced to a state psychiatric hospital in Willmar, Minnesota in the early 1950s where Nelson Bradley, a Canadian physician, and Dan Anderson, a psychologist, began to revolutionize addiction treatment. At the time, alcoholics (or 'inebriates' as they were known) were detoxified and institutionalized with the chronically mentally ill. Many languished. In an

effort to learn more about alcoholism, Bradley and Anderson began to attend local A.A. meetings that were springing up around the state. They quickly developed personal relationships with A.A. attendees who urged the pair to examine two new and innovative treatment programs in Minnesota that were based on the A.A. philosophy: Pioneer House and Hazelden.

Pioneer House was founded in 1948 in an effort to treat alcoholic men with families and thereby reduce the cost of welfare payments. The program was based entirely on the A.A. philosophy, involved lectures and informal discussions, and residents were required to complete the first five of the Twelve Steps before leaving. Almost simultaneously, Hazelden was founded in 1949 as an alcoholism treatment center for professionals. Following on the A.A. philosophy, the program included lectures, groups, informal discussions and recreational activities.

Based on what they learned from these programs, Bradley and Anderson developed a comprehensive philosophy of alcoholism treatment. They shunned the traditional psychoanalytic approach and instead conceptualized alcoholism as a biological, psychological, social, and spiritual disease that was a primary, progressive, and chronic illness. To best address these multiple dimensions, Bradley and Anderson convened a group of professionals into a multidisciplinary team of physicians, psychologists, nurses, social workers, and spiritual care providers. They turned traditional treatment on its head by separating alcoholics from the mentally ill, unlocking the doors, and bringing in recovering alcoholics to interact with the patients. For the first time, recovering people obtained paid positions as counselors and participated fully on the treatment team of professionals.

In the 1960s, Bradley and colleagues left Willmar State Hospital while Anderson accepted a position at Hazelden where he later became President. It was at Hazelden that the Minnesota Model continued to take shape and grow. Eventually, a cohesive model of alcoholism treatment emerged and is known even today as the 'Minnesota Model.'

The Minnesota Model has developed into a comprehensive, evidence-based, integrated treatment strategy that recognizes addiction as a chronic biopsychosocial and spiritual disease oftentimes complicated by other medical and psychiatric disorders. Treatment is approached in a holistic way, working with mind, body and spirit as components of a healthy life. Consistent with the model's origins at Willmar State Hospital, treatment is delivered by a team of professionals including substance abuse/addiction counselors, nurses, physicians, psychologists and psychiatrists, spiritual care professionals, and fitness and recreation specialists.

Abstinence from alcohol and drugs is the goal for ongoing recovery from substance dependence. Consistent with early Hazelden programming, the Twelve Steps are a foundation and guideline for living and are fully integrated into the treatment process and care plan. The steps are an integrated core of the program, applied systematically, that provide a framework to examine substance dependence, mental health, physical health, emotional well-being, relationships, spirituality, and more. Cognitive-behavioral strategies are consistently employed to identify and restructure the "stinkin' thinkin" associated with substance use. Contrary to its image as a "confrontational" approach, the model emphasizes treating all patients with dignity and respect. To this end, "hot seat" or other confrontational methods are not implemented. Instead, motivational enhancement approaches are used to facilitate problem recognition and subsequent engagement in treatment.

Programming consists of structured activities including thorough clinical assessment and evaluation, individual counseling, group therapy, and peer interaction. Care is tailored to the individual and may involve specialty groups such as relapse prevention, anger, eating issues, dual disorders, women's issues, men's issues, assertiveness, Twelve Step group study, trauma survivors, and other topics. To address co-occurring disorders, integrated mental health care is provided and may involve specialized assessments (e.g. gambling, post-traumatic stress disorder, ADHD), therapy, and medication management. Motivational lectures by clinical staff and alumni educate clients on a broad range of topics including psychological, medical, social, spiritual issues, and Twelve-Step work. Family and parent programs are also available. Treatment is provided in residential, outpatient, extended care and halfway house settings.

As the model developed at Hazelden in the 1960s, word quickly spread about the new approach to addiction treatment. Anderson, Hazelden alumni, visiting professionals and Hazelden's own publishing activities facilitated the spread of information. As a result, Hazelden expanded and community and hospital based treatment programs emulating the Minnesota Model sprang up around the country. As the years progressed, treatment centers across the country adopted a Minnesota Model approach to treatment, basing programming on the principles of the Twelve-Steps of A.A. Due to a lack of nationwide best practices or governance, the quality and type of treatment provided from one center to another varied greatly. Boundaries between Minnesota Model care and what became known as 'milieu therapy' were sometimes blurred. Because use of the descriptor 'Minnesota Model'

is widespread and unregulated, the Hazelden Foundation has recently begun to refer to its model and philosophy of treatment as the 'Hazelden Model,' nomenclature originally used in the 1960s (Anderson *et al.*, 1999).

Within the research arena, programs offering Minnesota Model care are sometimes referred to as Twelve-Step-based programs. Unfortunately, this tends to confuse comprehensive, professionally delivered, integrated treatment with the mutual- and self-help provided in A.A. Twelve-Step-based professional treatment is not A.A.; conversely, A.A. is not Twelve-Step-based treatment. Care must be made to distinguish the two when searching and reviewing literature related to outcomes.

To confuse the matter even further, Twelve-Step-based treatment (a.k.a. Minnesota or Hazelden Model) was manualized in the early-1990s in order to be subjected to a multi-site, highly controlled study called Project MATCH. The resulting manualized program was titled, '*Twelve-Step Facilitation*' (TSF; Nowinski *et al.*, 1992). The authors sought the assistance of several Hazelden employees, including Dan Anderson himself, who provided their expertise, suggestions and feedback during the development of the TSF manual. While the manualization of Twelve-Step-based professional treatment helped to address fidelity and issues of variation from one center to another in the course of a clinical trial, Twelve-Step Facilitation is sometimes mistaken as an entirely different treatment approach than the Minnesota or Hazelden Model. Addressing this issue, Nowinski & Baker (2003), authors of the TSF manual for Project MATCH, note that TSF is "... informed by and consistent with what is more generally known as the Minnesota Model..." (p. xxviii) and add "... TSF, as well as the treatment program offered at Hazelden, are well-developed, structured approaches, with specific goals and objectives" (p. xxix). When reviewing literature, it is helpful to keep in mind that the phrases "Twelve-Step-based treatment" and "Twelve-Step Facilitation" are used interchangeably with "Minnesota" or "Hazelden Model" treatment programming.

The Minnesota Model of care is historically one of the most commonly used treatment approaches in the United States (Fuller, 1989; Institute of Medicine, 1990), and its use has spread to other parts of the world (Cook, 1988; Keso & Salaspuro, 1990). Because this complex model is composed of multiple components, the extent to which it has been *fully* incorporated into treatment programs around the world has not been measured. However, data from the National Treatment Improvement Evaluation Study (Center for Substance Abuse Treatment, 1997) provide information on the utilization of several of its components. In a survey of 519 outpatient, residential, and specialty care facilities receiving grant funding from the Centers for Substance Abuse Treatment in the early 1990s, 71% of programs indicated they placed 'moderate' to 'great' therapeutic emphasis on the Twelve Steps. Other components included supportive individual counseling (89%), supportive group counseling (86%), and spirituality (51%), among others.

Due to advances in research on this model, its position as an effective treatment for alcohol dependence is recognized at the national level. Perhaps the strongest commendatory statement has come from the National Institutes of Health. In the 10th special report to the U.S. Congress in 2000, the National Institute on Alcohol Abuse and Alcoholism (2000b) recognized the empirical support for Twelve-Step-based professional treatment and concluded, "Professional treatments based on 12-step approaches can be as effective as other therapeutic approaches and may actually achieve more sustained abstinence" (p. 448). The Department of Veterans Affairs, in their detailed clinical practice guidelines for the management of substance use disorders, specifies, "Consider addiction-focused psychosocial interventions with the most consistent empirical support," and includes Twelve-Step-based professional treatment in the list of equally acceptable interventions for the treatment of substance dependence (Veterans Health Administration Office of Quality & Performance, 2001).

The Minnesota Model's efficacy as a treatment approach for youth is also recognized. The Substance Abuse and Mental Health Services Administration's Center for Substance Abuse Treatment provides direction on delivering Twelve-Step based treatment to adolescents in *Treatment Improvement Protocol #32: Treatment of adolescents with substance use disorders* (U.S. Department of Health and Human Services, 1999).

Evidence

Research on the efficacy of the Minnesota Model dates back to its beginnings. The earliest reports of the model's effectiveness were unpublished evaluation studies conducted by the staff of treatment agencies. The very first published outcome study was conducted at the Willmar State Hospital in the early 1960s where the Minnesota Model had its origins (Rossi *et al.*, 1963). Hazelden, where the model fully developed, has systematically evaluated and reported its outcomes for over 30 years, first via in-house reports and books, and later via published articles.

Methodological problems (e.g. sampling, response rates, lack of control conditions) limit the conclusions that can be drawn from the early reports. Even so, the

data provided valuable information and a starting point for more rigorous evaluations that came later. Laundergan (1982), for example, examined outcomes of a sample of 3638 patients discharged from Hazelden from mid-1973 through 1975. The sample was composed of those who remained in treatment for a period of at least 5 days. Self-report questionnaires were initially mailed with attempts made to reach non-respondents by phone. Of the sample, 12-month outcome data were obtained from 1899 patients, a response rate of only 52%. Among respondents, 50% reported having maintained abstinence in the year following treatment, an additional 17.6% were 'improved,' and 32.4% were 'not improved.' A similar study was conducted by Gilmore (1985) who reported outcomes obtained from a sample of 1531 patients discharged from Hazelden during 1978, 1980, and 1983. Response rates were improved compared to the earlier study, with 75% accounted for at one-year following discharge. Overall, 89% were reported to have attained either abstinence or reduced alcohol use after treatment. Another evaluation by Higgins and colleagues (1991) of 1655 patients discharged from Hazelden in 1985 and 1986 found 66% abstinent at both the 6-month and 1-year follow-ups. However, patients who were unavailable for follow-up, who stayed at Hazelden less than 5 days, returned to treatment, or were incarcerated were excluded from the study, and these methodological issues inflated abstinence rates.

Early studies such as these, while providing useful information about Minnesota Model outcomes, were limited by either treatment-completion samples, low response rates, and/or the reliance on self-report to assess outcomes. In an effort to expand upon earlier work, Stinchfield and Owen (1998) prospectively assessed 1, 6, and 12-month outcomes among an intent-to-treat sample of 1083 patients at Hazelden. To corroborate self-report, collaterals were contacted at 1-year. The 1-year follow-up response rate was 71% among patients and 55% among collaterals (or 83% among collaterals for the 713 patients who identified a contact person). At 1-year follow-up, 53% of the sample reported continuous abstinence since discharge from treatment, with an additional 35% reporting reduced alcohol and drug use. Perfect agreement between patient and collateral report was 78% with the remainder divided between those who reported more substance use than collaterals (10%) and collaterals who reported more patient use than patients (12%).

Evaluations of Minnesota Model outcomes are not limited to Hazelden samples. The outcomes of Minnesota Model programs participating in the Chemical Abuse Treatment Outcome Registry (CATOR) were assessed by

Hoffman and Harrison (1991) who examined the data of 3304 patients entering Minnesota Model programs across the country between 1983 and 1986. Although approximately two-thirds reported abstinence in the year following treatment, response rates were low leading the authors to estimate corrected 1-year abstinence rates at 40%.

McLellan and colleagues (1993) compared outcomes among two inpatient and two outpatient programs in the Philadelphia area that emphasized A.A. and the Twelve-Steps. The sample was composed of 198 alcohol and/or cocaine dependent males referred to treatment by an Employee Assistance Program. A 6-month follow-up included urine and breath tests in addition to self-report. A 94% response rate was achieved. Overall, 59% were abstinent from alcohol and 84% were abstinent from drugs at the time of the follow-up. Psychosocial functioning was also improved from pre- to post-testing. However, the types and quantities of services offered differed among programs, differential outcomes were found, and the degree to which the programs were Minnesota Model based was unclear.

In addition to descriptive designs, quasi-experimental studies have been conducted to compare outcomes among those treated in Minnesota Model programs to those treated with other approaches. Ouimette and colleagues (1997), for example, compared outcomes among 3018 patients in Twelve Step, cognitive-behavioral, or mixed treatment programs. Patients in Twelve-Step-based programming were more likely to be abstinent at one year (25%) than patients from the mixed (20%) or cognitive-behavioral groups (18%).

The earliest randomized trial to test the Minnesota Model was conducted in the late 1980s in Finland. Keso and Salaspuro (1990) randomized 141 alcohol dependent patients into either a 28-day program emulating the Minnesota/Hazelden Model ($n = 74$) or a 6-week traditional psychiatric facility ($n = 67$). Follow-ups were conducted bimonthly for 1 year after treatment and included biological measures of alcohol consumption in addition to self-report. Groups did not differ on pretreatment demographic, substance use, or prior treatment characteristics. On the Ward Atmosphere Scale (Moos, 1996), the Minnesota/Hazelden model program exhibited significantly greater performance on dimensions of Involvement, Support, Spontaneity, Personal Problem Orientation, and Order and Organization. Significantly more patients treated in the Minnesota/Hazelden model program attended A.A. meetings (59.5%) in the year after treatment than those randomized to the psychiatric rehabilitation facility (19.4%). More patients in the psychiatric facility made subsequent outpatient clinic visits (31.3%) than those assigned to the Minnesota/Hazelden model program

(16.3%). While groups did not differ in terms of alcohol use quantity in the year after treatment, significantly more Minnesota/Hazelden model patients were abstinent during the 8–12 month follow-up period (26.3%) than those treated in the psychiatric facility (9.8%). Overall, 14.0% of Minnesota/Hazelden model patients maintained continuous abstinence during the entire follow-up year compared to 1.9% of the psychiatric facility patients, a difference that was statistically significant.

As discussed earlier, Twelve Step Facilitation (TSF) is a manualized version of Minnesota Model treatment. As such, discussion of Project MATCH outcomes is relevant here in that the study provides empirical support for this model of care. Project MATCH was the first large-scale, randomized, multi-site study to examine whether patients could be "matched" to one of three treatment approaches: TSF, Cognitive-Behavioral Therapy (CBT), and Motivational Enhancement Therapy (MET; Project MATCH Research Group, 1993). Over 1700 participants were enrolled and randomized. The TSF was as effective in promoting abstinence and reducing drinking at one year as CBT and MET approaches (Project MATCH Research Group, 1997). At the 3-year follow-up, a significantly higher abstinence rate was found for TSF participants compared to the other two conditions (Project MATCH Research Group, 1998). Furthermore, alcohol-dependent patients who had networks supportive of drinking (i.e. a high percentage of family members and friends were drinkers and less supportive of abstinence), fared significantly better in the TSF condition than those in MET condition at three years (Longabaugh *et al.*, 1998).

In a more recent, prospective and quasi-experimental design, Humphreys and Moos (2001) examined outcomes among 1774 veterans admitted to a sample of 10 inpatient treatment programs. The programs were chosen on the extent to which the program philosophy and treatment emphasis was Twelve-Step based ($n = 5$) or cognitive-behaviorally oriented ($n = 5$). Although patients were not randomly assigned to conditions, they were matched on pre-treatment mental health care utilization costs. Groups did not differ at intake in terms of marital status, employment, presence of a co-occurring psychiatric condition, psychological distress, self-help group meeting attendance, or frequency of contact with an A.A. or other Twelve Step mutual-help group sponsor. Significantly more patients in Twelve-Step-based programming attended mutual-help groups (59.4%) than did those in cognitive-behavioral programs (48%) in the year following treatment. In addition, patients in cognitive-behavioral programs exhibited a 70% higher inpatient and outpatient mental health care utilization rate in the year following treatment, incurring

$12 129 of costs, on average, compared to expenses of $7400 among patients treated in Twelve-Step-based programs. Patient groups were also compared on the basis of abstinence in the 3 months prior to the 12-month follow-up. Patients treated in Twelve-Step programs had significantly higher abstinence rates (45.7%) compared to those treated in cognitive-behavioral programs (36.2%).

The Minnesota Model of care has also been found helpful with youth. Several evaluation studies have demonstrated favorable use and psychosocial outcomes following treatment (Brown *et al.*, 1989; Harrison & Hoffman, 1989; Knapp *et al.*, 1991; Richter *et al.*, 1991). Harrison & Hoffman (1989), for example, utilized the national CATOR outcomes database and evaluated the 6- and 12-month outcomes of 942 youth who completed treatment in Minnesota Model programs. Among respondents, 42% reported continuous abstinence during the follow-up period and 23% reported a brief relapse. However, response rates were low with only 52% contacted at follow-up. Alford *et al.* (1991) evaluated 157 youth 6, 12, and 24-months after treatment in a facility based on the Minnesota Model. Follow-up rates were high at 96%, 93%, and 89% at each follow-up period, respectively. Overall, 71% of male and 79% of female treatment completers were either abstinent or had experienced one or two slips of less than 1 week's duration at the 6-month mark. At 1 year, these numbers fell to 48% and 70% for males and females, respectively. By 2 years, 40% of males and 61% of females were classified in this category of outcomes. Winters *et al.* (2000) conducted a quasi-experimental study of 245 youth referred for treatment by comparing those who entered either a residential or outpatient Twelve-Step Minnesota Model program to those placed on a waiting list. Both urinalysis and parental report of functioning were collected at follow-up to verify self-report. Response rates were high with only 13 participants lost to follow-up or who had withdrawn from the study. At 12 months after treatment, 53% of those who completed treatment were either abstinent or experienced a minor lapse, defined as one to two instances of substance use. In contrast, treatment non-completers and wait-list participants fared significantly worse with only 15% and 27% either abstinent or having experienced a minor lapse by 12 months, respectively. No differences were found between residential or outpatient groups.

Summary

Early descriptive reports of Minnesota Model programs provided valuable information and set the stage for more rigorous evaluations of the model. Later studies, including empirically sound randomized and quasi-experimental designs, demonstrate the effectiveness of the Minnesota Model in improving both substance use and psychosocial outcomes among substance dependent individuals.

The Minnesota Model was the first comprehensive and cohesive model of care developed for alcoholism. It revolutionized treatment by abandoning custodial, psychiatric hospitalization approaches for an active program of care delivered by a multidisciplinary team of professionals. Though the model expanded and became the most common form of treatment in the USA, relatively little research attention was given to it, with most studies limited to descriptive evaluations of outcomes. The Minnesota Model was commonly delegated to "treatment as usual" status, if included in studies at all. More recently, increasingly sophisticated designs have been used to evaluate the model. The advent of Project MATCH, a multi-site, randomized trial that illustrated the efficacy of Twelve-Step-based professional treatment, led national agencies to recognize its effectiveness as a model of care. Given the positive impact of Minnesota Model treatment upon substance use and psychosocial functioning, it is recommended this effective model of care be considered when referral to treatment for alcohol dependence is deemed necessary.

Therapeutic communities

Introduction

"Therapeutic community" (TC) is a term that was first applied in the United Kingdom in the early 1950s to describe a newly developed treatment method for psychiatric inpatients. As a form of substance abuse treatment, therapeutic communities (TCs) were developed independently by recovering individuals with substance use disorders as a mutual self-help alternative to traditional medical and psychiatric treatment approaches (De Leon, 2004). TCs are highly structured hierarchical settings in which members of the community progress through a series of stages characterized by their length in treatment, motivation and commitment, status in the TC, and achievement of specific goals. Individuals in TCs are viewed as community members or residents, rather than patients or clients. The TC is a self-operating, working environment in which cooking, cleaning, and repairs within its expertise are performed by member residents. Community status such as junior, intermediate, or senior peer resident is assigned according to length and progress in treatment. Junior members perform the most basic or menial tasks and advance through the ranks over time to become senior members who serve as role models, conduct house meetings and lead peer encounter groups, and provide support and confrontation to more junior members. Community rules and expected conduct are clearly defined. Contingency management is utilized such that adherence to rules and treatment expectations are rewarded with an increase in privileges and community status, whereas rule violations are sanctioned by loss of privileges and status which can be regained with appropriate behavior and therapeutic progress. Early in treatment, motivation may be mostly external in origin, and members comply with the rules primarily to avoid sanctions or discharge. Later in treatment, members may conform to community rules because they actively seek affiliation with the community. In the final stages of treatment, members are ideally motivated by their commitment to enhance the community and provide leadership.

TCs are widely used in the USA over 500 member treatment programs belong to Therapeutic Communities of America (TCA), a non-profit association established in 1975 to represent therapeutic communities in the United States and Canada (TCA, 2005).

The American Psychiatric Association's *Practice Guideline for the Treatment of Patients with Substance Use Disorders*, 2nd edn (APA, 2006, p. 15) notes the utility of TCs when patients with opioid, cocaine or multiple substance use disorders do not benefit from less intensive treatment settings, but does not specifically recommend TCs for patients with only alcohol use disorders.

The VA/DOD (2001) *Clinical Practice Guideline Summary for the Management of Substance Use Disorders* does not mention therapeutic communities specifically, although it does specify '24-Hour Supervision' as a housing option in which supervision is provided by other patients, volunteers, and paraprofessionals. It also specifies homelessness, lack of social supports and an inability to maintain abstinence without supervision as indications for this level of care.

Evidence

Therapeutic Communities for substance use disorders can be broadly categorized by chronology into 'traditional' and 'modified' TCs. The evidence for their efficacy will be discussed in sequence.

Traditional TCs
Traditional TCs emerged in the 1960s and refer to abstinence-based residential treatment programs of 15–24 months in duration (De Leon, 2004). The traditional TCs served mostly male heroin-dependent individuals without serious Axis I psychiatric disorders. As such, study findings of the effectiveness of traditional TCs may not generalize well to alcohol-dependent patients, but are included here for background information and because traditional TCs are better studied than modified TCs.

The evidence for the effectiveness of traditional TCs comes primarily from naturalistic treatment outcome studies (DeLeon, 2004). As is generally consistent with such studies, time in treatment is positively correlated with good outcomes. DeLeon (2004) cites 'success rates' (defined as a composite index of neither substance use nor criminal activity) as 90% for patients who complete treatment, 50% for those who remain in treatment for at least 1 year, and 25% for those who stay less than 1 year. Unfortunately, retention rates at 1 year are about 20–35%. Therefore, using an intent-to-treat computation, 10–18% of patients are successful. Nevertheless, traditional TCs typically accept patients with high-severity substance use disorders that are characterized by criminality and Axis II psychopathology, all of which portend poor outcomes.

Modified TCs
Beginning in the 1980s with the emergence of the crack cocaine epidemic in the USA, the addicted population shifted and included more individuals with cocaine dependence and polysubstance dependence, both of which are frequently associated with heavy alcohol consumption and alcohol-related problems. As programs became more integrated, individuals with severe, chronic, and treatment-resistant forms of alcohol dependence, who required global lifestyle changes, were also accepted into TCs even in the absence of other drug use disorders.

Around the same time, TCs were modified to make them more widely available by reducing costs and accommodating special populations. Costs were reduced by introducing TC concepts and treatment methods into shorter stay residential programs (3–12 months) and non-residential outpatient programs (e.g. partial hospital and other abstinence-based outpatient programs as well as methadone maintenance programs). Recommended lengths of treatment in abstinence-based outpatient TCs range from 6 to 12 months (De Leon, 2004). Special populations have included incarcerated individuals, addicted mothers and their children, individuals with co-occurring psychiatric disorders, and adolescents. Outcomes of modified TCs were first published in the late 1990s and also demonstrate effectiveness (Hubbard *et al.*, 1997; Simpson *et al.*, 1997), especially for patients with lower problem severity in shorter stay programs (Melnick *et al.*, 2000).

Summary

Therapeutic Communities are effective for some patients and effectiveness is associated with length of treatment but retention rates are low. They are especially recommended with patients who have a primary substance problem with opioids or cocaine, with or without alcohol use disorders, who are at high risk for relapse and unlikely to respond to less structured treatments because they have a high severity of dependence, lack of social resources (e.g. unemployment, few social supports, no safe place to stay), and they need help developing prosocial behaviors. Although some TCs have been adapted for incarcerated individuals and those with severe and persistent mental illness, less evidence is available to recommend them for these specialized populations. Moreover, the quality of such programs varies considerably which requires consideration when making a referral. Nevertheless, the evidence is strong enough to recommend modified and adapted TCs for selected patients who have not fared well with other forms of treatment.

Combined pharmacotherapy and psychotherapy

Introduction

Combining pharmacotherapy and psychotherapy for alcohol use disorders has the potential for achieving greater efficacy than either one alone. Psychotherapy here includes all forms of therapy: dynamic, milieu and cognitive-behavioural. Theoretically, the two types of treatment could operate synergistically through different mechanisms. For example, naltrexone might reduce both urges to drink and the reinforcing effects of drinking, while cognitive-behavioral therapy (CBT) might increase a patient's skills and confidence at managing high-risk situations that had previously triggered drinking. Similarly, patients that take disulfiram abstain from drinking to avoid aversive medical complications, while behavioral therapies can be used to enhance compliance with disulfiram and reinforce other recovery activities. These two examples also illustrate that different medications might be optimized by different types of psychotherapy (i.e. CBT and behavioral therapy for naltrexone and disulfiram, respectively).

Current consensus recommends against the use of medication to treat alcohol dependence without also using addiction-focused psychotherapy. Nevertheless, knowledge about which particular psychotherapy (e.g. CBT, MET or TSF) should be combined with a given medication is limited. Conversely, psychotherapy for alcohol dependence is commonly provided in the absence of addiction-specific medication. Therefore, knowledge about the added value of a particular medication when combined with a specific psychotherapy will be a fruitful area for future research to guide treatment options.

The use of alcohol-specific medications to prevent relapse is uncommon in the USA despite the growing evidence in support of these medications. (See Part III: Chapter 4). The latest National Survey of Substance Abuse Treatment Services from 2003, for example, found that only 20% of treatment centers were using pharmacotherapies (17% using disulfiram; 12% using naltrexone; 5% using buprenorphine; Substance Abuse and Mental Health Service Administration, 2004). Moreover, relapse prevention medications are viewed as adjunctive to psychosocial treatment in the USA, and simple medication monitoring by itself is not considered sufficient treatment. This guideline is reflected in the FDA labeling for disulfiram and acamprosate, and in the US Department of Health and Human Services practice guideline for naltrexone (O'Malley, 1998). The guideline implies that combination therapy will usually be administered in specialized addiction treatment settings because this is where addiction-focused psychosocial therapy is predominantly available. Further studies are needed to determine the efficacy of simple medical management approaches (Johnson et al., 2003; Pettinati et al., 2004; Volpicelli et al., 2001). It is emphasized, however, that even 'simple' medical management approaches require highly trained healthcare professionals who help patients set goals and solve problems in addition to simply writing prescriptions (Pettinati et al., 2004). Nevertheless, if medical management approaches prove effective, then pharmacotherapy could favorably be administered in primary care settings, and the use of relapse prevention medications could potentially increase. As discussed below, preliminary evidence supports this approach.

Evidence

The optimal research design to evaluate if the combination of psychosocial therapy and medication works better than either therapy alone randomizes patients to at least four conditions using a two-by-two (2×2) factorial (or cell) design: double-blind administered active drug vs. placebo crossed with two different psychotherapy conditions. This design allows interactions between medication and psychotherapy to be analyzed. In addition, the design ideally includes as a control a minimal psychotherapy condition, analogous to a placebo medication condition.

Examples include supportive therapy, medical management, or compliance enhancement treatment (Johnson et al., 2003; Pettinati et al., 2004). Unlike medication groups, however, psychotherapy conditions cannot be blinded from the patient or therapist, but they can, and should, be blinded from the outcomes evaluator. Typically, minimal psychotherapies consist of several individual sessions with the prescribing medical professional and focus mostly on providing education and instruction about the medication, monitoring for side effects and medication adherence, making dose adjustments, and giving encouragement about the potential effectiveness of medication. They do not, however, focus specifically on how to manage any urges to drink, negative emotional states, and/or interpersonal conflicts that may trigger drinking. Nor do they facilitate social support outside of the treatment relationship such as attendance at Twelve-Step meetings. Consequently, the minimal psychotherapy condition could be delivered by a primary care provider, and it is an excellent comparison to evaluate any added value that a more specialized addiction-focused psychosocial therapy may provide. Few combination studies have employed all of these gold-standard design features. Studies employing the 2×2 design are noted below.

A note on the COMBINE study

The first results from the COMBINE (2003) trial (The Combined Pharmacotherapies and Behavioral Interventions (COMBINE 2003; Anton et al., 2006)) appeared as this book was going to press. The COMBINE Study was a 16-week randomized controlled trial of 1383 alcohol-dependent individuals that aimed to determine which treatment or combination of treatments for alcohol dependence, including both medications and psychosocial interventions, would be most efficacious. Two medications, naltrexone (NTX) 100 mg po daily and acamprosate (ACAM) 1 gm po TID, were tested alone and in combination vs. placebo, both with and without a Combined Behavioral Intervention (CBI). CBI consisted of up to 20 50-minute sessions of psychosocial therapy by specialists trained in alcohol counseling, and it combined elements from three other evidence-based psychosocial treatments for alcohol dependence, i.e. motivational enhancement therapy, cognitive-behavioral therapy, and twelve-step facilitation therapy (Miller, 2004). In addition, all subjects assigned to get either active or placebo medication received Medical Management (MM), a supportive therapy designed to monitor a patient's drinking and related consequences, educate the patient about the medications used in the study, and promote medication

adherence. Medical Management was delivered by a physician, a nurse, a physician's assistant, or a clinical pharmacist as might occur in a primary care practice, and consisted of nine sessions, including a first session averaging 45 minutes and eight sessions averaging 20 minutes each (Pettinati et al., 2004).

The primary analyses of the COMBINE Study investigated the main and interactive effects of the three interventions: NTX, ACAM, and CBI. The primary analyses were based on randomization of subjects to eight cells or treatment conditions (i.e. a $2 \times 2 \times 2$ study design): NTX or placebo vs. ACAM or placebo vs. CBI or no CBI. All eight of these treatment groups received MM. The two primary outcome variables that measured efficacy were percentage of days abstinent and time to relapse to first heavy drinking day during the 16-week trial.

Briefly the primary analyses of the COMBINE Study revealed a main effect for NTX in delaying the time to relapse when compared to placebo; however ACAM was no better than placebo in terms of delaying time to relapse or increasing the percentage of days abstinent. In addition, the combination of ACAM and NTX was no more effective than NTX alone, and the combination of ACAM and CBI was no more effective than placebo plus CBI. Finally, a significant interaction between NTX and CBI was found such that any combination which included either NTX or CBI (i.e. NTX + CBI, NTX + no CBI, and placebo + CBI) performed better than placebo plus no CBI. In the context of medical management (MM), therefore, NTX or CBI significantly increased the odds of a good clinical outcome above that achieved with MM and placebo without CBI.

A secondary analysis was conducted to determine the effect of MM and placebo when compared to CBI alone without any pills or MM (a ninth cell of the study). The question to be answered was whether or not CBI, a specialized addiction-focused psychotherapy, performed better than supportive MM plus placebo pill taking (i.e. MM even without active medication). Surprisingly, MM combined with placebo increased the percentage of abstinent days significantly more than CBI alone. The result suggests that alcohol dependence can be managed successfully in non-specialized settings, as long as frequent interactions between the patient and a medication-knowledgeable licensed healthcare professional occur over a sustained period of several months and some medication is utilized. It is emphasized, however, that MM with its nine visits (each at least 20-minutes in duration) over a 16-week period is more intensive than usual treatment provided in the ordinary primary care setting.

Also, at 1 year after the treatments ended most of the effects noted during the treatment period faded although the relative pattern of results observed across the treatments were still evident.

Overall, the COMBINE Study reported negative results for CBI alone (without pills and MM) and for ACAM both alone and in combination. While NTX was effective, there was no advantage to combining it with either ACAM or CBI. The negative findings, however, need to be interpreted with the following caveats. First, a higher dose of NTX (100 mg daily) than approved by the FDA (50 mg daily) was used in this study. Thus, no conclusions about the effect of a 50-mg dose, which is ordinarily used in clinical practice, can be made. Two, although the 9-session MM with placebo seemed to work as well if not better than the up to 20-session CBI alone, the median number of actual sessions received during the trial was 9 and 10 for MM and CBI, respectively. Third, attendance at meetings of A.A. has been associated with good drinking outcomes. While no formal analysis of A.A. attendance appeared in this first publication of results, the investigators noted that A.A. attendance rates across treatment groups were similar.

Naltrexone

At least five 2 × 2 randomized studies have examined NTX vs. PLA when combined with either CBT or a minimal psychotherapy. In the first of these, O'Malley et al. (1992) randomized 97 subjects to treatment with NTX vs. PLA and CBT vs. supportive therapy. The investigators distinguished between abstinence (defined as no drinking) and relapse (defined as heavy drinking and requiring > 4 drinks in a day for women and > 5 drinks per day for men). After 12 weeks, the naltrexone group did not relapse to heavy drinking as quickly and had significantly fewer drinking days and fewer drinks than the placebo group. Although no difference between NTX and PLA was found in the initial duration of abstinence (i.e. time to first drink), a significant interaction occurred with the NTX + supportive therapy group having the longest duration of initial abstinence. Among those patients who did drink during the study ($n = 58$), the NTX + CBT group had the longest time to first heavy drinking day (i.e., the longest duration before relapsing). A good response to NTX was predicted by increased craving and decreased cognitive functioning at baseline, whereas a good response to CBT was predicted by increased verbal learning skills (Jaffe et al., 1996). When 80 of the original 97 subjects were followed to 6 months after completing the treatment phase, the group that had received NTX still showed a significant advantage vs. PLA at preventing any heavy drinking, but no difference between the four groups was observed for complete abstinence across the 6 months, and no interactions with psychotherapy were found

(O'Malley et al., 1996). These are complicated results but suggest that interactions between medication and psychotherapy vary according to both the particular outcome variable selected and the duration of the outcome period assessed. Specifically, during 12 weeks of combination treatment, a significant advantage for NTX + supportive therapy was observed for delaying any episode of drinking, whereas a significant advantage for NTX + CBT was observed for delaying any heavy drinking among patients who drank at all. This interaction was no longer evident after 6 months of completing treatment.

In a second American study, Monti et al. (2001) randomized 128 alcohol-dependent outpatients to four treatment groups defined by crossing NTX vs. PLA and CBT + cue exposure treatment (CBT/CET) vs. education + relaxation (Ed/Relax). Twelve weeks of treatment was followed by outcomes reassessments at 6 and 12 months. No treatment interactions were observed, but treatment effects were time-dependent. At the end of treatment (3 months), patients receiving NTX did significantly better than those getting PLA whereas no psychotherapy effects were observed. By contrast, no differences between NTX and PLA were found at the 6- and 12-month follow-up periods; however, the CBT/CET groups did significantly better than the Ed/Relax groups.

Heinala et al. (2001) conducted a 2 × 2 randomized placebo-controlled trial of NTX that contrasted CBT to supportive therapy among 121 alcohol-dependent patients. A positive interaction was found in which the best outcomes occurred in patients receiving both CBT and NTX, whereas the worst outcomes occurred with CBT and PLA. For patients receiving supportive therapy, there were no differences between the NTX and PLA groups. Balldin et al. (2003) randomized 118 patients to receive either NTX or PLA and CBT vs. treatment as usual. After 6 months of treatment a positive interaction was found with CBT + NTX group having the best outcomes.

In a fifth study, Anton et al. (2006) randomized 160 alcoholic outpatients to either NTX vs. PLA for 12 weeks and either 12 sessions of CBT or 4 sessions of motivational enhancement therapy (MET, see Part III: Chapter 21). An advantage for the CBT + NTX combination was demonstrated. For two primary outcome variables, percent of patients relapsing to heavy drinking and percent days abstinent during the 12-week study, the CBT + NTX group did better than the CBT + PLA group whereas the MET + NTX group did no better than the MET + PLA. For time to first relapse, NTX did better than placebo; for time to third and fourth relapses, the CBT + NTX group had the longest intervals.

In addition to these five 2 × 2 studies, O'Malley et al. (2003) published a study of naltrexone treatment in primary vs. specialty care. Outpatients ($n = 197$) received 10 weeks of open-label NTX following randomization to either primary care management or CBT. Over the course of 10 weeks, there were no differences between the two groups except that during the last 4 weeks the CBT group had a greater percentage of abstinent days than the primary care group. Patients who responded to treatment in the first 10 weeks were then randomized in a 24-week maintenance trial to either NTX or PLA while continuing with an additional seven sessions of their initial psychotherapy. For those who had responded initially in the first 10 weeks to primary care management + open-label NTX ($n = 53$), NTX produced better outcomes than placebo (81% vs. 52% response rate) in the 24-week double-blind phase. For those who had responded initially to CBT + open-label NTX ($n = 60$), there were no differences between NTX and PLA (83% vs. 70% response rate) in the 24-week double-blind phase. In other words, those who had initially received the CBT + NTX combination maintained their gains with CBT even in the absence of maintenance NTX; whereas those who had initially received primary care management + NTX required maintenance NTX to maintain their gains with primary care management.

Overall, these studies provide a mixture of complicated results, but nevertheless suggest that NTX + CBT may produce better drinking-related outcomes than NTX in combination with other psychosocial therapies such as MET or supportive therapy. Primary care management and medical management (as operationalized in the COMBINE study) also show promise in combination with NTX.

Acamprosate

As reviewed above, Project COMBINE is a recently completed US study for which results have just been published (Combine Study Research Group, 2003; Anton et al., 2006). It is arguably the most sophisticated and ambitious combination study conducted to date. This study showed that ACAM was no better than PLA, either by itself or in combination with any of the psychosocial treatments in the COMBINE study (i.e. MM, CBI or both). It also did not improve on the outcomes that NTX achieved even when added to NTX (Anton et al., 2006).

Published results of other ACAM-related comparative psychotherapy trials administered acamprosate in open label fashion without a PLA control group (De Wildt et al., 2002; Feeney et al., 2002; Soyka et al., 2002). In the absence of other evidence, they will be reviewed here. De Wildt et al. (2002) randomized 241 intention-to-treat patients to one of three groups, all of which received ACAM for 28 weeks: MM alone (6 sessions), MM + MET

(3 extra sessions), and MM + CBT (7 extra sessions). No differences between the three groups were noted at either the end of treatment or 6 months later. The authors concluded that intensive psychosocial intervention was not always necessary when prescribing ACAM. Soyka et al. (2002) found a similar result after assigning 753 patients in a multicenter trial to one of five therapies (individual counseling, group counseling, behavioral treatment, brief intervention, or family therapy). However, this was not an intention-to-treat study and patients were withdrawn if they relapsed during the first 14 days of treatment. Finally, Feeney et al. (2002) compared 50 patients who received 8 sessions of CBT + 12 weeks of ACAM to 50 matched historical controls that received CBT only. The combination group did better than the CBT only group, but the lack of randomization as well as a lack of a PLA group limits any firm conclusions.

Before leaving this topic, a word must be added as to why ACAM did not appear to be effective in the COMBINE study. The authors of that study gave two explanations. First, they stated that, in previous studies, the number of days of abstinence before prescribing ACAM was longer than the 4 days needed for the COMBINE trial. Perhaps, then, there was some patient selection bias occurring in these other studies. Second, others studies used less frequent assessments and the other studies did not have PLA controls, and in COMBINE, ACAM did not better than placebo.

Disulfiram

In general, disulfiram (DSF) is minimally effective because compliance rates are low (Fuller et al., 1986; Fuller & Gordis, 2004). There is general consensus, however, that supervised DSF administration in which someone observes the alcoholic patient taking DSF increases both compliance and effectiveness (Brewer, 1993; Chick et al., 1992; Fuller & Gordis, 2004). This may be particularly true when taking DSF under observation is linked to receiving particular incentives, a characteristic of behavioral therapies such as the community reinforcement approach (CRA), behavioral couple's therapy (BCT), and contingency management techniques. Contingency management techniques involve the use of tangible incentives such as money (Bigelow et al., 1976) or methadone privileges for methadone-maintained opioid-dependent alcoholics (Bickel et al., 1987). Both BCT and CRA utilize the intangible incentive of social reinforcement (O'Farrell et al., 1995). In BCT, the therapist insures that a specific DSF contract is agreed to and signed by both the patient and the concerned significant other (O'Farrell et al., 1995, p. 69). The contract specifies that the alcoholic will voluntarily take DSF daily while the partner observes and then records the observation on a calendar. Social reinforcement is immediately given and takes the form of thanking the patient and showing appreciation for taking the medication. In the BCT approach, the couple also agrees in the contract not to discuss past drinking episodes or fears of future drinking episodes. The purpose of this latter agreement is to reduce potentially negative social interactions between them. In CRA, the patient and partner agree to DSF monitoring but discussions about drinking are not prohibited (O'Farrell *et al.*, 1995; Miller *et al.*, 2001).

There is moderate evidence that DSF therapy is enhanced when combined with the CRA (Berglund, 2005; O'Farrell & Fals-Stewart, 2003; Roozen *et al.*, 2004). This was first suggested in a randomized study by Azrin (1976) in which treatment as usual plus ordinarily prescribed DSF was compared to CRA plus a DSF contract. The CRA group drank less than the control group at the 6-month follow-up and it continued to fare well for up to two years, but the study was limited by a small sample size of 18 patients. Also, it was not possible to discern the active ingredient of the more improved group: CRA vs. the DSF contract. Subsequently, Azrin *et al.* (1982) replicated their results using a randomized three-group design with 43 outpatients. The best drinking-related outcomes at 6 months occurred in the group receiving CRA plus a DSF contract, whereas the worst outcomes were seen with the group receiving traditional individual counseling plus DSF without a contract. An intermediate and mixed result was seen in a third group receiving traditional individual counseling and a DSF contract involving a significant other, which worked well for married/cohabiting patients but not for single ones. A third study by Miller *et al.* (2001) analyzed 157 DSF-eligible outpatients using intent-to-treat analyses after randomization to one of four groups based on DSF monitoring or not and CRA vs. treatment as usual (TAU = traditional disease model counseling). The four groups were CRA + DSF monitoring, CRA without DSF, TAU + DSF monitoring, and TAU + DSF option. With the DSF option, patients were encouraged but not required to take DSF, and DSF monitoring was not offered. In the CRA without DSF, DSF was neither encouraged nor prescribed. Although complex, the key results will be summarized briefly. CRA was similarly effective with or without DSF monitoring; TAU with DSF monitoring was generally better than TAU without DSF monitoring; and TAU did not differ significantly from CRA when both were combined with DSF monitoring. In contrast to the study by Azrin *et al.* (1982), marital status did not affect the efficacy of TAU + DSF monitoring, but the investigators concede that the power to analyze that interaction was low. Considering all three studies together, combining DSF monitoring with TAU is a reasonable practice, especially for married or cohabiting couples. Combining DSF monitoring with CRA does not appear to confer any advantage to CRA alone with the possible exception of patients without a partner.

Nefazodone

Although negative, this study is presented for completeness. A 2×2 study involving nefazodone vs. PLA and CBT vs. group counseling showed no advantage of nefazodone regardless of therapy (Wetzel *et al.*, 2004). This result is consistent with another study that failed to find any advantage of nefazodone vs. PLA when combined with CBT for the treatment of non-depressed alcoholics (Kranzler *et al.*, 2000).

Summary

Medications to reduce drinking and prevent relapse are adjunctive to addiction-focused psychosocial therapy. The question of which psychotherapy is optimal in combination with particular medications appears to vary by medication. Current evidence suggests that CBT adds benefit when combined with NTX. Current evidence also suggests that supervised DSF monitoring is superior to unsupervised administration of DSF when combined with traditional disease-model psychosocial therapy. If an intimate partner cannot be involved with DSF monitoring, then combining DSF with CRA may confer an advantage compared to disease-model psychosocial therapy, although this recommendation is based on one small study. The results from the COMBINE Study (Anton *et al.*, 2006) do not provide us with evidence to support any particular psychotherapy over another. Although some authors have suggested that addiction-focused psychosocial therapies may be no more effective than simple MM or brief intervention when combined with NTX or ACAM (and COMBINE seems to suggest that that may, in some respects be true for NTX), these other studies were not placebo-controlled (DeWildt *et al.*, 2002; Latt *et al.*, 2002; Soyka *et al.*, 2002). Nevertheless, they provide encouragement that some alcohol-specific medications, especially naltrexone, can be prescribed effectively in primary care settings with short-term psychosocial interventions.

The level of evidence for each of the interventions discussed in this chapter is summarized in Table 16.1.

Table 16.1. Effectiveness of complex interventions for alcohol use disorders

Treatment	Form of treatment	Psychiatric disorder	Level of evidence for efficacy	Comments
Complex intervention	Alcoholics Anonymous	Alcohol dependence	Ib	A.A. attendance is difficult to study in clinical trials. Evidence suggests modest but consistent improvements in days of sobriety, improved social skills, and increased self-efficacy. Length of participation as well as concurrent professional treatment also leads to improved outcomes
Complex intervention	The Minnesota Model including Twelve-Step Facilitation (TSF)	Alcohol dependence	Ia	Substantial evidence supports that these programs significantly improve sobriety and social functioning. A number of studies show that in many the gains are maintained
Complex intervention	Therapeutic Community	Alcohol dependence	III	Despite the complexity of the treatment and the low rate of retention until completion of the program, there is some evidence that in certain populations, it is an effective treatment
Complex intervention	Combined pharmacotherapy and psychotherapy	Alcohol dependence	Ib	The COMBINE study and other open label studies suggest that the combination of psychotherapy and medication can be useful. Most evidence supports NTX as the pharmacologic agent with weaker support for ACAM and little for DSF

REFERENCES

Alcoholics Anonymous World Services (n.d.). *A.A. at a glance.* Retrieved September 7, 2004, from the Alcoholics Anonymous website: www.alcoholics-anonymous.org.

Alcoholics Anonymous World Services (1976). *Alcoholics Anonymous*, 3rd edn. New York: Author.

Alford, G. S., Koehler, R. A. & Leonard, J. (1991). Alcoholics Anonymous–Narcotics Anonymous model inpatient treatment of chemically dependent adolescents: a 2-year outcome study. *Journal of Studies on Alcohol*, **52**, 118–26.

American Psychiatric Association (2005). Web page citation. http://www.psych.org/psych_pract/treatg/pg/prac_guide.cfm.

American Psychiatric Association (2006). Practice guideline for the treatment of patients with substance use disorders, second edition. *American Journal of Psychiatry*, **163**(8 Suppl), 1–82.

American Society of Addiction Medicine (2001). *ASAM public policy statement*. Retrieved August 30, 2004, from the American Society of Addiction Medicine Web site: www.asam.org/ppol/treatment.htm.

Anderson, D. (1981). *Perspectives on Treatment: The Minnesota Experience*. Center City, MN: Hazelden.

Anderson, D. J, McGovern, J. P. & DuPont, R. L. (1999). The origins of the Minnesota Model of addiction treatment – a first person account. *Journal of Addictive Diseases*, **18**, 107–14.

Anton, R. F., Moak, D. H., Waid, L. R., Latham, P. K., Malcolm, R. J. & Dias, J. K. (1999). Naltrexone and cognitive behavioral therapy for the treatment of outpatient alcoholics: results of a placebo-controlled trial. *American Journal of Psychiatry*, **156**, 1758–64.

Anton, R. F., O'Malley, S. O., Ciraulo, D. A. *et al.* (2006). Combined pharmacotherapies and behavioral; interventions for alcohol dependence. The COMBINE study: a randomized controlled trial. *Journal of the American Medical Association*, **295**, 2003–17.

Azrin, N. H. (1976). Improvements in the community-reinforcement approach to alcoholism. *Behavior Research Therapy*, **14**, 339–48.

Azrin, N. H., Sisson, R. W., Meyers, R. & Godley, M. (1982). Alcoholism treatment by disulfiram and community reinforcement therapy. *Journal of Behaviour Therapy and Experimental Psychiatry*, **13**(2), 105–12.

Balldin, J., Berglund, M., Borg, S. *et al.* (2003). A 6-month controlled naltrexone study: combined effect with cognitive behavioral therapy in outpatient treatment of alcohol dependence. *Alcoholism: Clinical and Experimental Research*, **27**, 1142–9.

Berglund, M. (2005). A better widget? Three lessons for improving addiction treatment from a meta-analytical study. *Addiction*, **100**, 742–50.

Bickel, W. K., Marion, I. & Lowinson, J. H. (1987). The treatment of alcoholic methadone patients: a review. *Journal of Substance Abuse Treatment*, **4**, 15–19.

Bigelow, G., Strickler, D., Liebson, I. & Griffiths, R. (1976). Maintaining disulfiram ingestion among outpatient alcoholics: a security-deposit contingency contracting procedure. *Behavior Research Therapy*, **14**, 378–81.

Bond, J., Kaskutas, L. A. & Weisner, C. (2003). The persistent influence of social networks and Alcoholics Anonymous on abstinence. *Journal of Studies on Alcohol*, **64**, 579–88.

Brewer, C. (1993). Recent developments in disulfiram treatment. *Alcohol and Alcoholism*, **28**, 383–95.

Brown, S. A., Vik, P. W. & Creamer, V. A. (1989). Characteristics of relapse following adolescent substance abuse treatment. *Addictive Behaviors*, **14**, 291–300.

Center for Substance Abuse Treatment. (1997). *NTIES: The National Treatment Improvement Evaluation Study final report, March 1977*. Rockville, MD: U.S. Department of Health and Human Services.

Chick, J., Gough, K., Falkowski, W. *et al.* (1992.) Disulfiram treatment of alcoholism. *British Journal of Psychiatry*, **161**, 84–9.

Christo, G. & Franey, C. (1995). Drug users' spiritual beliefs, locus of control, and the disease concept in relation to Narcotics Anonymous attendance and six-month outcomes. *Drug and Alcohol Dependence*, **38**, 51–6.

Cocaine Anonymous World Service (n.d.). *Welcome to Cocaine Anonymous*. Retrieved September 7, 2004, from the Cocaine Anonymous Web site: www.ca.org.

COMBINE Study Research Group (2003). Testing combined pharmacotherapies and behavioral interventions in alcohol dependence: rationale and methods. *Alcoholism: Clinical and Experimental Research*, **27**, 1107–22.

Connors, G. J., Tonigan, J. S. & Miller, W. R. (2001). A longitudinal model of A.A. affiliation, participation, and outcome: retrospective study of the Project MATCH outpatient and aftercare samples. *Journal of Studies on Alcohol*, **62**, 817–25.

Cook, C. C. H. (1988). The Minnesota Model in the management of drug and alcohol dependency: miracle, method or myth? Part I. The philosophy and the programme. *British Journal of Addiction*, **83**, 625–34.

De Leon, G. (2000). *The Therapeutic Community: Theory, Model, and Method*. New York: Springer.

De Leon, G (2004). Therapeutic communities. In *Textbook of Substance Abuse Treatment*, ed. M. Galanter & H. D. Kleber, 3rd edn., pp. 485–501. Washington, DC: American Psychiatric Press.

De Wildt, W. A., Schippers, G. M., Van Den Brink, W., Potgieter, A. S., Deckers, F. & Bets, D. (2002). Does psychosocial treatment enhance the efficacy of acamprosate in patients with alcohol problems? *Alcohol and Alcoholism*, **37**, 375–82.

Emrick, C. D. & Tonigan, J. S. (2004). Alcoholics Anonymous and other 12-Step groups. In *The American Psychiatric Publishing Textbook of Substance Abuse Treatment*, ed. M. Galanter & H. D. Kleber, 3rd edn, pp. 433–43. Washington, DC: American Psychiatric Press.

Emrick, C. D., Tonigan, J. S., Montgomery, H. & Little, L. (1993). Alcoholics Anonymous: what is currently known? In *Research on Alcoholics Anonymous: Opportunities and alternatives*, ed. B. S. McCrady & W. R. Miller, pp. 41–76. New Brunswick, NJ: Rutgers Center for Alcohol Studies.

Ensuring Solutions to Alcohol Problems (2003). *Primer 4: The Active Ingredients of Effective Treatment for Alcohol Problems*. Available online http://www.ensuringsolutions.org/images/primers/prim4.pdf.

Feeney, G. F., Young, R. M., Connor, J. P., Tucker, J. & McPherson, A. (2002). Cognitive behavioural therapy combined with the relapse-prevention medication acamprosate: are short-term treatment outcomes for alcohol dependence improved? *Australian and New Zealand Journal of Psychiatry*, **36**, 622–8.

Fuller, R. (1989). Current status of alcoholism treatment outcome research. In *Problems of drug dependence 1989: Proceedings of the 51st Annual Scientific Meeting* (NIDA Research Monograph 95, ed. L. S. Harris), pp. 85–91. Rockville, MD: National Institute on Drug Abuse.

Fuller, R. K. & Gordis, E. (2004). Does disulfiram have a role in alcoholism treatment today? *Addiction*, **99**, 21–4.

Fuller, R. K., Branchey, L., Brightwell, D. R. *et al.* (1986). Disulfiram treatment of alcoholism. *Journal of the American Medical Association*, **11**, 1449–55.

Gilmore, K. (1985). Hazelden primary treatment program: 1985 profile and patient outcome. Unpublished research report. Center City, MN: Hazelden.

Harrison, P. A. & Hoffmann, N. G. (1989). *CATOR report: Adolescent treatment completers one year later*. St. Paul, MN: CATOR.

Heinala, P., Alho, H., Kiianmaa, K., Lonnqvist, J., Kuoppasalmi, K. & Sinclair, J. D. (2001). Targeted use of naltrexone without prior detoxification in the treatment of alcohol dependence: a factorial double-blind, placebo-controlled trial. *Journal of Clinical Psychopharmacology*, **21**, 287–92.

Higgins, P., Baeumler, R., Fisher, J. & Johnson, V. (1991). Treatment outcomes for Minnesota Model programs. In *Does Your Program Measure Up? An Addiction Professional's Guide to Evaluating Treatment Effectiveness*, ed. J. Spicer, pp. 93–114. Center City, MN: Hazelden.

Hoffman, N. & Harrison, P. (1991). The Chemical Abuse Treatment Outcome Registry (CATOR): Treatment outcome from private programs. In *Does Your Program Measure Up? An Addiction Professional's Guide to Evaluating Treatment Effectiveness*, ed. J. Spicer, pp. 115–33. Center City, MN: Hazelden.

Humphreys, K. (2003). Alcoholics Anonymous and 12-Step alcoholism treatment programs. In *Recent Developments in Alcoholism, Vol 16: Research on Alcoholism Treatment*, ed. M. Galanter, pp. 149–64. New York: Kluwer Academic/Plenum.

Humphreys, K. & Moos, R. H. (1996). Reduced substance abuse-related health care costs among voluntary participants in Alcoholics Anonymous. *Psychiatric Services*, **47**, 709–13.

Humphreys, K. & Moos, R. H. (2001). Can encouraging substance abuse patients to participate in self-help groups reduce demand for health care? A quasi-experimental study. *Alcoholism: Clinical and Experimental Research*, **25**, 711–16.

Humphreys, K., Mankowski, E. S., Moos, R. H. & Finney, J. W. (1999). Do enhanced friendship networks and active coping mediate the effect of self-help groups on substance abuse? *Annals of Behavioral Medicine*, **21**, 54–60.

Humphreys, K., Wing, S., McCarty, D. *et al.* (2004). Self-help organizations for alcohol and drug problems: Toward evidence-based practice and policy. *Journal of Substance Abuse Treatment*, **26**, 151–8.

Institute of Medicine (1990). *Broadening the base of treatment for alcohol problems*. Washington, DC: National Academy Press. Retrieved June 1, 2005 from http://www.nap.edu/openbook/0309040388/html/.

Jaffe, A. J., Rounsaville, B., Chang, G., Schottenfeld, R. S., Meyer, R. E. & O'Ma Weiss, R. (2004). Self-help organizations for alcohol and drug problems: Toward evidence-based practice and policy. *Journal of Substance Abuse Treatment*, **26**, 151–8.

lley, S. S. (1996). Naltrexone, relapse prevention, and supportive therapy with alcoholics: an analysis of patient treatment matching. *Journal of Consulting and Clinical Psychology*, **64**, 1044–53.

Johnson, B. A., DiClemente, C. C., Ait-Daoud, N. & Stoks, S. S. (2003). Brief behavioral compliance enhancement treatment (BBCET) manual. In *Handbook of Clinical Alcoholism Treatment*, ed. B. Johnson, P. Ruiz & M. Galanter, pp. 282–301. Philadelphia: Lippincott, Williams & Williams.

Kelly, J. F., Myers, M. G. & Brown, S. A. (2000). A multivariate process model of adolescent 12-Step attendance and substance use outcome following inpatient treatment. *Psychology of Addictive Behaviors*, **14**, 376–89.

Keso, L. & Salaspuro, M. (1990). Inpatient treatment of employed alcoholics: a randomized clinical trial of Hazelden-type and traditional treatment. *Alcoholism: Clinical and Experimental Research*, **14**, 584–9.

Kessler, R. C., Mickelson, K. D. & Zhao, S. (1997). Patterns and correlates of self-help group membership in the United States. *Social Policy*, **27**, 27–46.

Knapp, J., Templer, D., Cannon, W. G. & Dobson, S. (1991). Variables associated with success in an adolescent drug treatment program. *Adolescence*, **26**, 305–17.

Kranzler, H. R., Modesto-Lowe, V. & Van Kirk, J. (2000). Naltrexone vs. nefazodone for treatment of alcohol dependence. A placebo-controlled trial. *Neuropsychopharmacology*, **22**(5), 493–503.

Latt, N. C., Jurd, S., Houseman, J. & Wutzke, S. E. (2002). Naltrexone in alcohol dependence: a randomised controlled trial of effectiveness in a standard clinical setting. *Medical Journal of Australia*, **176**, 530–4.

Laundergan, J. C. (1982). *Easy Does It: Alcoholism Treatment Outcomes, Hazelden, and the Minnesota Model*. Center City, MN: Hazelden.

Longabaugh, J. C., Wirtz, P., Zweben, A. & Stout, R. (1998). Network support for drinking: Alcoholics Anonymous and long-term matching effects. *Addiction*, **93**, 1313–33.

McElrath, D. (1987). *Hazelden: A Spiritual Odyssey*. Center City, MN: Hazelden.

McKellar, J., Stewart, E. & Humphreys, K. (2003). Alcoholics Anonymous involvement and positive alcohol-related outcomes: cause, consequence, or just a correlate? A prospective 2-year study of 2,319 alcohol-dependent men. *Journal of Consulting and Clinical Psychology*, **71**, 302–8.

McLellan, A. T., Grissom, G. R., Brill, P., Durell, J., Metzger, D. S. & O'Brien, C. P. (1993). Private substance abuse treatments: are some programs more effective than others? *Journal of Substance Abuse Treatment*, **10**, 243–54.

Meyers, R. J. & Smith, J. E. (1995). *Clinical Guide to Alcohol Treatment: The Community Reinforcement approach*. New York: Guilford.

Miller, W. R. (2004). *Combined behavioral intervention manual: a clinical research guide for therapists treating people with alcohol abuse and alcohol dependence*. (NIAAA COMBINE Monograph Series, Volume 1). Bethesda, MD: DHHS Publication No. (NIH) 04-5288.

Monti, P. M., Rohsenow, D. J., Swift, R. M. *et al.* (2001). Naltrexone and cue exposure with coping and communication skills training for alcoholics: treatment process and 1-year outcomes. *Alcohol Clinical and Experimental Research*, **25**, 1634–47.

Moos, R. H. (1996). *Ward Atmosphere Scale*. Redwood City, CA: Mind Garden.

Moos, R. H. & Moos, B. S. (2004). Long-term influence of duration and frequency of participation in Alcoholics Anonymous on individuals with alcohol use disorders. *Journal of Consulting and Clinical Psychology*, **72**, 81–90.

Morgenstern, J., Labouvie, E., McCrady, B. S., Kahler, C. W. & Frey, R. M. (1997). Affiliation with Alcoholics Anonymous after treatment: a study of its therapeutic effects and mechanism of action. *Journal of Consulting and Clinical Psychology*, **65**, 768–77.

Narcotics Anonymous World Services (n.d.). *Facts about Narcotics Anonymous*. Retrieved September 7, 2004, from the Narcotics Anonymous Web site: www.na.org.

National Institute on Alcohol Abuse and Alcoholism (2000a). *Alcohol Alert No. 49: New Advances in Alcoholism Treatment*. Rockville, MD: Author.

National Institute on Alcohol Abuse and Alcoholism (2000b). *10th special report to the US Congress on alcohol and health: Highlights from current research*. Rockville, MD: Author. Also available on-line: http://www.niaaa.nih.gov/publications/publications.htm.

Nowinski, J. & Baker, S. (2003). *The Twelve-Step Facilitation Handbook: A Systematic Approach to Recovery From Substance Dependence*. Center City, MN: Hazelden.

Nowinski, J., Baker, S. & Carroll, K. (1992). *Twelve Step Facilitation therapy manual: A clinical research guide for therapists treating individuals with alcohol abuse and dependence* (DHHS Publication No. ADM 92–1893). Rockville, MD: US Department of Health and Human Services.

O'Farrell, T. J. & Fals-Stewart, W. (2003). Alcohol abuse. *Journal of Marital and Family Therapy*, **29**, 121–46.

O'Farrell, T. J., Allen, J. P. & Litten, R. Z. (1995). Disulfiram (Antabuse) contracts in treatment of alcoholism. *NIDA Research Monograph Series*, **150**, 65–91.

O'Malley, S. (1998). *Naltrexone and alcoholism treatment. Treatment Improvement Protocol (TIP) Series 28.* (DHHS Publication No. [SMA] 98–3206). Rockville, MD: US Department of Health and Human Services.

O'Malley, S. S., Jaffe, A. J., Chang, G., Schottenfeld, R. S., Meyer, R. E. & Rounsaville, B. (1992). Naltrexone and coping skills therapy for alcohol dependence. A controlled study. *Archives of General Psychiatry*, **49**, 881–7.

O'Malley, S. S., Jaffe, A. J., Chang, G. *et al.* (1996). Six-month follow-up of naltrexone and psychotherapy for alcohol dependence. *Archives of General Psychiatry*, **53**, 217–24.

O'Malley, S. S., Rounsaville, B. J., Farren, C. *et al.* (2003). Initial and maintenance naltrexone treatment for alcohol dependence using primary care vs specialty care: a nested sequence of 3 randomized trials. *Archives of Internal Medicine*, **163**, 1695–704.

Ouimette, P. C., Finney, J. W. & Moos, R. H. (1997). Twelve-step and cognitive-behavioral treatment for substance abuse: a comparison of treatment effectiveness. *Journal of Consulting and Clinical Psychology*, **65**, 230–40.

Owen, P. L., Slaymaker, V., Tonigan, J. S. *et al.* (2003). Participation in Alcoholics Anonymous: intended and unintended change mechanisms. *Alcoholism: Clinical and Experimental Research*, **27**, 524–32.

Pettinati, H. M., Weiss, R. D., Miller, W. R., Donovan, D., Ernst, D. B. & Rounsaville, B. J. (2004). *Medical management treatment manual: a clinical research guide for medically trained clinicians providing pharmacotherapy as part of the treatment for alcohol dependence.* (NIAAA COMBINE Monograph Series, Volume 2). Bethesda, MD: DHHS Publication No. (NIH) 04-5289.

Project MATCH Research Group (1998). Matching alcoholism treatments to client heterogeneity: Project MATCH three year drinking outcomes. *Alcoholism: Clinical and Experimental Research*, **22**, 1300–11.

Project MATCH Research Group (1997). Matching alcoholism treatments to client heterogeneity: Project MATCH post-treatment drinking outcomes. *Journal of Studies on Alcohol*, **58**, 7–29.

Project MATCH Research Group (1993). Project MATCH: Rationale and methods for a multisite clinical trial matching patients to alcoholism treatment. *Alcoholism: Clinical and Experimental Research*, **17**, 1130–45.

Richter, S. S., Brown, S. A. & Mott, M. A. (1991). The impact of social support and self-esteem on adolescent substance abuse treatment outcome. *Journal of Substance Abuse*, **3** (4), 371–85.

Roland, E. J. & Kaskutas, L. A. (2002). Alcoholics Anonymous and church involvement as predictors of sobriety among three ethnic treatment populations. *Alcoholism Treatment Quarterly*, **20**, 61–77.

Roozen, H. G., Boulogne, J. J., van Tulder, M. W., van den Brink, W., De Jong, C. A. & Kerkhof, A. J. (2004). A systematic review of the effectiveness of the community reinforcement approach in alcohol, cocaine and opioid addiction. *Drug and Alcohol Dependence*, **74**, 1–13.

Rossi, J. J., Stach, A. & Bradley, N. J. (1963). Effects of treatment of male alcoholics in a mental hospital. *Quarterly Journal of Studies on Alcohol*, **24**, 91–8.

Smith, J. W., Frawley, P. J. & Polissar, L. (1991). Six- and twelve-month abstinence rates in inpatient alcoholics treated with aversion therapy compared with matched inpatients from a treatment registry. *Alcoholism: Clinical and Experimental Research*, **15**, 862–70.

Soyka, M., Preuss, U. & Schuetz, C. (2002). Use of acamprosate and different kinds of psychosocial support in relapse prevention of alcoholism. Results from a non-blind, multicentre study. *Drugs in R & D*, **3**, 1–12.

Spicer, J. (1993). *The Minnesota Model: The Evolution of the Multidisciplinary Approach to Addiction Recovery.* Center City, MN: Hazelden.

Stinchfield, R. & Owen, P. (1998). Hazelden's model of treatment and its outcome. *Addictive Behaviors*, **23**, 669–83.

Therapeutic Communities of America – TCA (2005). Web page citation. http://www.therapeuticcommunitiesofamerica.org.

Timko, C., Moos, R. H., Finney, J. W. & Lesar, M. D. (2000). Long-term outcomes of alcohol use disorders: comparing untreated individuals with those in Alcoholics Anonymous and formal treatment. *Journal of Studies on Alcohol*, **61**, 529–40.

Tonigan, J. S., Connors, G. J. & Miller, W. R. (1998). Special populations in Alcoholics Anonymous. *Alcohol Health and Research World*, **22**, 281–5.

Tonigan, J. S., Miller, W. R. & Schermer, C. (2002). Atheists, agnostics and Alcoholics Anonymous. *Journal of Studies on Alcohol*, **63**, 534–41.

Tonigan, J. S., Toscova, R. & Miller, W. R. (1996). Meta-analysis of the literature on Alcoholics Anonymous: Sample and study characteristics moderate findings. *Journal of Studies on Alcohol*, **57**, 65–72.

US Department of Health and Human Services (1993). *TIP 2: Pregnant, substance-using women* (DHHS Publication No. SMA 95-3056). Rockville, MD: Author.

US Department of Health and Human Services (1994a). *TIP 8: Intensive outpatient treatment for alcohol and other drug abuse* (DHHS Publication No. SMA 94B2077). Rockville, MD: Author.

US Department of Health and Human Services (1994b). *TIP 9: Assessment and treatment of patients with coexisting mental illness and alcohol and other drug abuse* (DHHS Publication No. SMA 95-3061). Rockville, MD: Author.

US Department of Health and Human Services (1994c). *TIP 10: Assessment and treatment planning for cocaine-abusing methadone-maintained patients* (DHHS Publication No. SMA 94–3003). Rockville, MD: Author.

US Department of Health and Human Services (1998). *TIP 26: Substance abuse among older adults* (DHHS Publication No. SMA 98-3179). Rockville, MD: Author.

US Department of Health and Human Services (1999). *TIP 32: Treatment of adolescents with substance use disorders* (DHHS Publication No. SMA 99-3283). Rockville, MD: Author.

Veterans Health Administration Office of Quality & Performance VA(DOD) (2001). *Management of substance use disorders in the primary care setting.* Washington, DC: Author. Also available: Office of Quality and Performance publication 10Q-CPG/SUD-01. Retrieved from the VA Office of Quality & Performance Web site: http://209.42.214.199/cpg/cpg.htm.

Walters, G. D. (2002). Twelve reasons why we need to find alternatives to Alcoholics Anonymous. *Addiction Disorders and Their Treatment,* **1**, 53–9.

Weisner, C., Greenfield, T. & Room, R. (1995). Trends in the treatment of alcohol problems in the U.S. general population, 1979 through 1990. *American Journal of Public Health,* **85**, 55–60.

Wetzel, H., Szegedi, A., Scheurich, A. *et al.* (2004). Combination treatment with nefazodone and cognitive-behavioral therapy for relapse prevention in alcohol-dependent men: a randomized controlled study. *Journal of Clinical Psychiatry,* **65**, 1406–13.

White, W. L. (1998). *Slaying the Dragon: The History of Addiction Treatment and Recovery in America.* Bloomington, IL: Chestnut Health Systems.

Winters, K. C., Stinchfield, R. D., Opland, E., Weller, C. & Latimer, W. W. (2000). The effectiveness of the Minnesota Model approach in the treatment of adolescent drug abusers. *Addiction,* **95**, 601–12.

Workgroup on Substance Abuse Self-Help Organizations (2003). Self-help organizations for alcohol and drug problems: Towards evidence-based practice and policy. Retrieved from the Center for Healthcare Evaluation Website: http://www.chce.research.med.va.gov/chce/pdfs/VAsma_feb1103.pdf

17

Complementary and alternative medicine for alcohol misuse

Elizabeth A. R. Robinson, Stephen Strobbe and Kirk J. Brower

Editor's note

As described in Part II of this text, complementary and alternative medicines and therapies are widespread. They have certainly been applied to the treatment of conditions related to alcohol misuse. While they may be popular in the treatment of these disorders, there is little hard evidence for their effectiveness. Part of the lack of evidence has to do with the methodological issues related to treatments such as acupuncture, biofeedback, and meditation. For example, it is difficult to create true 'blind' or 'placebo' conditions, given the nature of these interventions. There may be, however, some effectiveness for these treatments, particularly in helping the individual assume greater control over their behavior and teach the individual that they may be able to alter difficult affective and psychological states by learning strategies for better managing one's body and lifestyle.

Introduction

This chapter reviews the existing evidence of the effectiveness of a range of complementary and alternative medicine (CAM) treatment modalities for alcoholism that have been investigated, focusing in particular on acupuncture, biofeedback, and meditation. To date, rigorous empirical evidence of their effectiveness in treating alcohol problems is lacking. While many CAM approaches are used and have been advocated, support for their use has primarily been case studies, anecdotes, or conceptual arguments.

The National Health Interview Survey (NHIS; Barnes *et al.*, 2004) of the Center for Disease Control (CDC) classifies CAM modalities into four basic types: (a) alternative medical systems, (b) mind–body therapies, (c) biologically-based therapies, and (d) manipulative body-based therapies. This chapter reviews one type of alternative medical system, acupuncture, as there is some empirical literature published on its use with alcohol use disorders. The mind–body therapies are a broad category that includes biofeedback, meditation, guided imagery, progressive relaxation, deep breathing exercises, hypnosis, yoga, tai chi and qi gong. We will present the empirical literature on biofeedback and meditation. We will not review the other CAM therapies, as the scientific literature on these therapies is sparse.

The NHIS has documented the widespread use of complementary and alternative medicine (CAM) for health problems in the United States in its survey of over 31 000 adults (NHIS, Barnes *et al.*, 2004). (See Chapter 7.) They estimated that 75% of the US population has used some form of CAM therapy at some time in their lives. This estimate included the use of prayer for health reasons. When such prayer was excluded and the time span limited to the last 12 months, 36% or more than one-third of US adults have used CAM therapies recently. The most commonly used therapies, besides prayer, are: natural products (used by 19%), deep breathing exercises (12%), meditation (8%), chiropractic care (8%), yoga (5%), and massage (5%). The most common conditions for which CAM therapies were used were pain (in the back, neck, or joints), head or chest colds, anxiety, and depression.

The NHIS provides data on CAM use by lifetime alcohol drinking status (Table 17.1).

These data indicate that drinkers at all levels, including former drinkers (such as those in recovery), are interested in and likely to use alternative approaches. These data do not indicate whether CAM is used specifically to address alcohol problems.

Cambridge Textbook of Effective Treatments in Psychiatry, ed. Peter Tyrer and Kenneth R. Silk. Published by Cambridge University Press.
© Cambridge University Press, 2008.

Table 17.1. Age-adjusted percent of adults who used any CAM in the last 12 months by lifetime alcohol drinking status (from Barnes *et al.*, 2004)

Lifetime alcohol use status	All CAM use including prayer and megavitamin therapy	Mind–body therapies including prayer	Mind–body therapies excluding prayer	Prayer only**	Alternative medical systems	All other CAM use*
Lifetime abstainer	61.6	56.9	10.8	46.1	1.5	21.2
Former drinker	69.2	62.3	16.6	45.7	2.3	30.4
Current infrequent/ light drinker	62.2	51.6	19.6	32.0	3.1	28.3
Current moderate/ heavier drinker	57.0	43.5	18.4	25.1	3.4	38.2

*Includes: biologically-based therapies including megavitamin therapy, energy therapies, and manipulative and body-based therapies.
**Estimate based on difference between columns 2 and 3.

Acupuncture

Description

Acupuncture as an alternative medical system based on Traditional Chinese Medicine is described in Chapter 7. It has been defined as "stimulation, primarily by the use of solid needles, of traditionally and clinically defined points on or beneath the skin, in an organized fashion for therapeutic and/or preventative purposes" (Klein & Trachtenberg, 1997; cited in Han *et al.*, 2004, p. 743).

In Traditional Chinese Medicine, acupuncture is thought to promote health through the stimulation of specific anatomical points which, in turn, facilitates the natural flow of qi, or vital energy. These points, including those used in auricular acupuncture, correspond to certain organs and systems in the body, along with their attendant physical, emotional, and spiritual responses. The experience of properly administered acupuncture has been described as a subjective state of well-being, and represents the recruitment of natural, internal resources directed toward healing. Benefits are thought to be additive and cumulative over time. In contrast, Western medicine has conceptualized acupuncture in terms of its effect on endogenous endorphins (Pomeranz, 1989; Ulett, 1989). It has been posited that the stimulation of endorphin production has the capacity to reduce symptoms of withdrawal and craving, not only for exogenous opioids, but for other drugs of abuse as well, including alcohol (Scott & Scott, 1997).

The most commonly used and researched acupuncture protocol in alcoholism treatment is a 5-point technique, often referred to as the "NADA protocol," or "acudetox." Developed by Lincoln Hospital in the South Bronx of New York City, it has been adopted by the National Acupuncture Detoxification Association (NADA, 1995) and is the standard in the education and training of those seeking certification as Acupuncture Detoxification Specialists (ADSs). It was developed by Smith (1999) and is based on the work of Wen & Cheung (1973) and Wen & Teo (1975). From the outset, this acupuncture protocol was designed to serve as "a foundation for psycho-social rehabilitation" (Smith, 1999, p. 11). Much of the subsequent research on acupuncture and addiction has been based on some variation of this protocol.

Acupuncture is one of the more frequently used CAM modalities for the treatment of addictions in the United States (Boucher *et al.*, 2003). Results from the National Survey of Substance Abuse Treatment Services (N-SSATS) in 2003 showed that 5% (or approximately 700) of all known substance abuse treatment facilities in the United States, both public and private, listed acupuncture as one of the services offered (Substance Abuse and Mental Health Services Administration, SAMHSA, 2004). These figures do not indicate the extent to which acupuncture is used specifically for alcohol use disorders.

Evidence

Studies on acupuncture have been criticized for a number of limitations in methodology. Perhaps foremost among these is an inherent inability to provide double-blind, placebo-controlled treatment conditions. Researchers have attempted to compensate for this through the use of "sham" or "non-specific" acupuncture. Under these circumstances, subjects in a given control group, who are known to the acupuncturists but not to the evaluators, receive acupuncture at localized points adjacent to, but a few millimeters away from, what are considered to be true and active sites. Critics contend that this makes for an inadequate control condition, since acupuncture could still be producing an effect, even at non-specific sites. As a result, differences between an active treatment and a placebo condition may be rendered indiscernible. Other limitations and criticisms have included small sample sizes, high drop-out rates, and potentially insufficient doses of acupuncture.

It has been difficult to make comparisons or to draw conclusions across studies. Populations have differed on inpatient or outpatient status, the number and types of substances being used, the stage of the addictive disorder, and the symptoms being treated. Different techniques have been employed, including the use of standard acupuncture needles, either with or without electrical stimulation. More recently, "low level laser stimulation," also known as "laser acupuncture," has been tried (Trumpler et al., 2003), but this raises questions about what qualifies as acupuncture. Doses of acupuncture have varied greatly across studies, both in terms of quantity and frequency, from a single episode to multiple treatments over a period of days, weeks, or months. Numbers and locations of acupuncture points have also differed, using single or multiple sites, auricular acupuncture, body acupuncture or a combination of these techniques. Some protocols have been standardized while others were individualized, based on presenting symptoms. The qualifications and skills of those administering acupuncture can also vary. Finally, an inconsistent and wide array of outcomes have been measured, including craving, withdrawal, participation in other aspects of substance abuse treatment, psychiatric symptoms, reductions in alcohol and other drug use, abstinence and relapse rates, and readmissions to hospitals or treatment programs.

In an extensive and systematic review of the literature, the British Columbia Office of Health Technology Assessment published a report entitled, "Acupuncture in the management of alcohol and drug dependence" (Kazanjian & Rothon, 2002). From a total of 234 relevant documents retrieved, the authors identified 24 randomized controlled trials, with 5 specifically addressing "the effect of acupuncture in alcohol-dependent patients" (Kazanjian & Rothon, 2002, p. 27). Of these, three studies (Worner et al., 1992; Toteva & Milanov, 1996; Rampes et al., 1997) were given less weight for failing to meet "empirically-supported quality criteria" (p. ix), based on a

modified version of the Jadad scale (Jadad et al., 1996). In brief, Worner et al. (1992, US) randomized 56 outpatient alcoholics (49 male, 7 female) to one of three treatment groups who received: (1) a combination of fixed-point body and auricular acupuncture administered 3 times a week for 3 months, (2) sham transdermal stimulation, or (3) standard care. The authors reported "no significant differences in attendance at Alcoholics Anonymous meetings, number of outpatient sessions attended, number of weeks in either the study or in the outpatient program, number of persons completing treatment or in the number of relapses," and cautioned against "the routine use of this treatment until more randomized controlled trials demonstrate a beneficial effect" (p. 169).

Toteva & Milanov (1996, Bulgaria) compared "the treatment efficacy of body acupuncture with conventional (outpatient) medical detoxification for [118] subjects with alcohol dependence and withdrawal syndrome" (p. 19). Results included significantly better outcomes in the acupuncture group, including a lower drop-out rate, decreased desire for alcohol use, decreased depressive symptoms, increased participation in psychotherapeutic programs, reduction of tremor, and a higher remission rate 6 months post-treatment. The authors concluded that "acupuncture is useful for treatment of alcohol dependence, and particularly for the alleviation of withdrawal symptoms" (p. 24).

Rampes et al. (1997, UK) randomized a total of 59 patients, who were receiving care in the context of a community alcohol team (CAT) approach, to one of three groups to determine whether auricular electroacupuncture reduced craving for alcohol. Participants received (1) specific electroacupuncture plus treatment as usual, (2) non-specific electroacupuncture plus treatment as usual, or (3) treatment as usual. The authors "did not find any major advantage in treating auricular acupuncture points regarded as specific for addiction" (p. 19).

Kazanjian & Rothon (2002) identified two studies that met their "minimum quality criteria" (p. 27) for randomized controlled trials. In the first of these, Bullock et al. (1987) reported significant and positive findings among a population of "54 hardcore alcoholic recidivists" (p. 292), half of whom received an extended course of auricular acupuncture, supplemented with wrist points, following medical detoxification. In comparison, members of the control group received non-specific acupuncture. In terms of retention, only 2 control patients completed the study (7%), compared with 10 of the treatment patients (37%). During a 6-month follow-up period, patients in the treatment group reported less need for alcohol, had fewer drinking episodes, and had fewer readmissions to the detoxification center. Using similar study procedures, Sapir-Weise *et al.* (1999, Sweden) were unable to replicate these findings, and indicated that "the effects of acupuncture were less pronounced than those previously reported" (p. 629). In an executive summary, Kazanjian & Rothon (2002) concluded that, "The trials that scored highly in methodological quality did not conclusively demonstrate the effectiveness of acupuncture for the management of alcohol and drug dependence" (p. ix).

Two other randomized controlled trials were published after the release of the British Columbia report. Bullock *et al.* (2002) set out to design a study "that would provide sufficient power and clarity to answer definitively the question of whether auricular acupuncture is effective in the treatment of alcohol dependence," using analytic approaches that would "address the needs of skeptics and advocates alike" (p. 76). Toward that end, 503 patients were randomized to one of four conditions for a study period of three weeks, with follow-up at 3 months, 6 months, and 12 months. The study conditions were: (1) specific 4-point auricular acupuncture, (2) non-specific auricular acupuncture, (3) symptom based acupuncture, or (4) conventional treatment alone. While subjects who received both acupuncture and conventional treatment reported a reduction in the desire for alcohol, this finding did not translate into improved drinking outcomes. "In summary," the authors stated, "our findings do not support the addition of acupuncture to conventional treatment in the treatment of alcoholism" (p. 77).

Finally, Trumpler *et al.* (2003, Switzerland) randomized 48 inpatients undergoing medical detoxification for alcohol withdrawal to one of three conditions: (1) laser acupuncture, (2) needle acupuncture, or (3) sham laser stimulation. The primary outcome measure was duration of withdrawal symptoms. The researchers did not detect a difference in outcomes between those receiving laser acupuncture and those who received sham laser stimulation. The authors further noted an absence of any sham condition for needle acupuncture, which appeared to preclude blinding for this treatment condition even among study participants themselves. While those who received needle acupuncture had a shorter duration of detoxification, and a shorter duration of prescribed sedative use, these findings were no longer significant when adjusted for baseline differences. In conclusion, the authors found "no evidence to suggest a beneficial effect of auricular acupuncture in alcohol withdrawal" (p. 372).

Summary

Based on a handful of randomized controlled trials, most of which have reported negative findings, there is currently insufficient evidence to recommend the routine use of acupuncture in the treatment of alcohol use disorders, and alcohol withdrawal. Nonetheless, acupuncture may still become useful in the treatment of select populations. Included among these are pregnant women requiring detoxification from alcohol, since traditional pharmacotherapy for withdrawal is contraindicated as potentially harmful to the fetus. In an uncontrolled study, Sanders *et al.* (1998) reported that satisfaction with services among pregnant and postpartum women was positively correlated with the use of acupuncture and subsequent retention in a peer counseling substance abuse treatment program. Randomized controlled trials are needed to substantiate these findings.

The inability to conduct true double-blind placebo-controlled trials has remained a source of frustration and limitation to researchers and reviewers alike. It will be interesting to see to what degree, if any, the advent of a "newly designed placebo needle for clinical trials" (Fink *et al.*, 2001) affects future studies of acupuncture and alcohol use disorders.

Mind–body therapies: biofeedback and meditation

Mind–body therapies include a wide range of approaches, including biofeedback and meditation, that are intended to enhance the mind's capacity to affect bodily function and symptoms. First, however, we should mention research on prayer, the most common CAM intervention that individuals use outside of professional treatment. The NHIS-CDC study of CAM use found that about 36% of the US population has used prayer and *only* prayer to address a health problem. To date, the only published research has been on intercessory prayer, in which an individual with a health problem is prayed for by others. In a double-blind study with treated alcoholics, Walker *et al.* (1997) found no differences in subsequent alcohol consumption between the experimental groups. Interestingly, the investigators found that frequency of clients' prayer at intake was significantly and negatively associated with amount of alcohol used at 2–3-month follow-up.

Biofeedback

Biofeedback is a technique used to induce relaxation by training individuals to voluntarily control selected physiological parameters (e.g. blood pressure, muscle tone, or brainwaves). By monitoring and providing real-time information or feedback about those measured parameters during the treatment session, individuals can learn to control them. At least three different techniques of feedback have been studied in alcohol-dependent patients. Brainwave biofeedback (Graap & Freides, 1998; Peniston & Kulkosky, 1989; Saxby & Peniston, 1995) utilizes electroencephalography (EEG) to train patients to increase the quantity of their alpha (8–11 Hz) and/or theta (4–7 Hz) frequency waveforms. Electromyography (EMG) biofeedback trains patients to relax selected muscle groups such as the frontalis facial muscle (Tarbox, 1983ab; Weingarten et al., 1980). A third type of biofeedback training monitors physiological signs such as heart rate, blood pressure and finger temperature (Sharp et al., 1997).

Biofeedback is not commonly used in addiction treatment settings in the USA to induce states of physiological relaxation or to prevent relapse in alcohol-dependent patients.

Evidence

Watson et al. (1978) conducted an 18-month follow-up of 46 alcoholic men who had been assigned to either alpha EEG biofeedback therapy or a matched control group during an inpatient treatment episode and reported that the biofeedback group had significantly more consecutive days of abstinence ($P < .05$). The finding was attributed to chance because no significant differences between the two groups were found for five other consumption-related outcome variables, including total number of abstinent days, number of excessive-consumption days, and drinking parameters during the two weeks prior to follow-up. Peniston & Kulkosky (1989) randomly assigned 20 alcohol-dependent males to either alpha-theta brainwave biofeedback training or treatment as usual. After 13 months of follow-up, significantly more biofeedback patients completely abstained from alcohol than patients that received treatment as usual. Saxby & Peniston (1995) reported on 14 alcohol-dependent outpatients that received alpha-theta brainwave biofeedback training, and only one relapsed after 21 months of follow-up. Small sample sizes, no control group in the latter study, and other methodological issues (Graap & Freides, 1998) severely limit the evidence provided by these reports.

Using EMG biofeedback, Weingarten et al. (1980) did not find a relationship between reduction in muscle tension and completion of treatment. Both completers and drop-outs were able to significantly decrease their muscle tension with biofeedback. Denney et al. (1991) conducted a retrospective, naturalistic outcomes study among 233 male inpatients and found a relationship between the number of thermal and EMG biofeedback training

sessions completed and continuous abstinence for 3–12 months post-treatment. Among 82 male inpatients that completed at least six thermal/EMG biofeedback sessions, reduction of anxiety symptoms following treatment was correlated with abstinence at 3 and 6 months post-discharge, but a control group was not included (Denney & Baugh, 1992). Sharp et al. (1997) conducted a randomized controlled trial of fingertip temperature feedback to facilitate autogenic relaxation training; however, neither alcohol consumption nor drinking-related consequences were studied as outcomes.

Summary

The methodological quality of biofeedback studies does not permit any conclusions about efficacy. Therefore, the use of biofeedback-induced relaxation states to promote abstinence or prevent relapse to heavy drinking cannot be recommended.

Meditation

Over 30 years of published research indicate that meditation may help with a variety of presenting psychiatric problems, including depression, anxiety, stress disorders, and possibly substance misuse (Grossman et al., 2004; Baer, 2003; Alexander et al., 1994). A primary rationale for using meditation training in alcoholism treatment is the evidence that stress plays a role in substance use disorders (Adinoff et al., 1998; Brady & Sonne, 1999; Brown et al., 1995; Kreek & Koob, 1998; Lamon & Alonzo, 1997), and psychophysiological evidence that meditation may alter stress reactions (e.g. Harte et al., 1995; Carlson et al., 2004).

However, a review of this research is murky, as the meditation technique is often not clearly defined. In particular, meditation is often confused with relaxation, in part because this is a noticeable benefit or side effect of meditating. Some studies of relaxation focus on meditation; others do not. The secular offshoot of Transcendental Meditation (TM) developed by Herbert Benson (Meditation Training, 1975) is often called relaxation training. Unfortunately Jacobson's Progressive Relaxation (1938, 1987) is also sometimes referred to as relaxation training. In addition, biofeedback, music therapy, and some other alternative mind–body interventions often include a relaxation training component. Another complication in reviewing this literature is that a number of investigators have used 'relaxation training' as a control condition, assuming that it has no effect on outcomes. The assumption that meditation and relaxation are synonymous is incorrect, but the prevalence of this assumption complicates a thorough review of meditation's use in alcohol treatment, as the term 'relaxation' is used with various degrees of empirical precision, historical source, and relationship to meditation. Further confusing an understanding of the potential benefit of meditation is that a number of researchers have tested interventions that combine meditation with other components, some of which may be traditional treatment components (such as CBT) as well as other types of CAM. In this review we will limit ourselves to empirical studies of meditation's particular contribution to treatment of alcoholism.

The subsequent discussion presents studies by type of meditation: transcendental meditation, secular concentration approaches (including Benson's), and mindfulness techniques. Only studies that include alcohol use as an outcome are covered, although we recognize that other benefits of meditation are also possible (see Grossman *et al.*, 2004; Walsh & Shapiro, 2006; Baer, 2003; Alexander *et al.*, 1994).

The definition of meditation applied in this review follows that recently provided by Walsh and Shapiro: "The term meditation refers to a family of self-regulation practices that focus on training attention and awareness in order to bring mental processes under greater voluntary control and thereby foster general mental well-being and development and/or specific capacities such as calm, clarity, and concentration." (Walsh & Shapiro 2006, pp. 228–9).

Note that this differentiates meditation from strategies that focus primarily on changing mental content, such as psychotherapies, self-hypnosis, and visualization, and from strategies that may involve controlling the breath, body movements or postures, or energy manipulation (e.g. yoga).

Meditation practices differ in many ways, including the focus of the attention one cultivates, the extent one intends to alter or manipulate internal experience, and the goal. Attention can be concentrated, that is focused on a specific object, such as the breath, a sound, or a concept (e.g. loving kindness, a deity, etc.). Alternatively, one can cultivate developing moment-to-moment awareness, attending to and observing whatever internal experience is dominant (e.g. physical sensations, thoughts, even emotions). Both TM and Benson's approach are generally considered examples of concentration approaches, whereas mindfulness approaches emphasize awareness of the current moment. Although many religions have meditative traditions, the two most researched practices are TM and mindfulness, based, respectively, in Hindu and Buddhist practices. Secularized versions of both types of approaches also exist.

The degree that treatment programs are using meditation-based approaches is unknown. Unlike acupuncture, the use of meditation is not tabulated in SAMHSA's annual report on treatment program approaches (2004).

Evidence

Transcendental meditation (TM)

Transcendental meditation was introduced to the West in the 1970s by a minor Indian adept, now known as Maharishi, and became very popular. It is taught in a standard seven-step course which includes group and individual instruction. Unlike the other forms of meditation training presented here, the training itself is secret and is not manualized in a form accessible to researchers. The claims made for TM's positive effects are passionate and enthusiastic, but they beg for corroboration by independent researchers and more rigorous designs and measures.

Since the early 1970s, many studies have investigated the impact of TM on drinking behaviors, although only one study has recruited a sample of individuals with alcohol problems and used a control group with random assignment (Taub *et al.*, 1994). All of these less rigorous studies describe decreases in consumption of alcohol (see review by Alexander *et al.*, 1994). However, all but the Taub study have serious methodological weaknesses in their design and samples. They are either retrospective (e.g. Benson, 1975) or use a pre-test–post-test design without follow-up. A few used matched comparison groups. The samples are students or community members who took a TM course, not individuals with alcohol problems or individuals in treatment for alcohol use disorders. Measures of alcohol use, alcohol diagnoses, and related variables are inadequate. There are few, if any, studies of TM and substance use that are recent.

The study by Taub *et al.* (1994) is the most relevant to treatment of those with alcohol and drug use disorders. Subjects were randomly assigned to four treatment conditions: treatment as usual (TAU; $n = 31$), TAU with transcendental meditation (TM; $n = 35$), TAU with EMG biofeedback (BF; $n = 24$), and TAU with electronic neurotherapy (NT; $n = 26$). Increases in percent days abstinent were significantly higher in the TM and BF groups than the TAU and NT groups, ranging from 24%–39% fewer drinking days. Also, the percent of subjects who were abstinent was 1.5 to 2.5 times higher in the TM and BF groups, than in the NT and TAU groups, although this did not reach significance. When the TM and BF group data were combined and compared to the combined TAU and NT group, differences were statistically significant. The authors also report that, in the TM group pre–post-mood improved significantly as reflected by higher scores on 5 of 6 POMS (Profile of Mood States) scales. For the BF group, increases occurred in 2 of the 6 scales.

Secular mantra-based techniques

Benson's meditation training. Benson, a physician impressed by the results he saw and experienced with Transcendental Meditation, developed a secularized version of TM (manualized in Benson, 1975). He is also credited with describing the hypometabolic state often experienced in meditation which is thought to reduce tension and mitigate reaction to stress, as reflected in the title of his book, *The Relaxation Response.* The Benson meditation technique uses concentration, instructing users of this technique to silently say the word 'one' in time with one's breath. When distractions occur, users are instructed to ignore them and continue to repeat the word 'one.' Two 20-minute practice sessions a day are recommended.

There is one study of Benson's approach relevant to this review, which is unfortunately more than 20 years old. Marlatt *et al.* (1984) described a well-designed randomized controlled trial of 4 conditions with 41 heavy drinking college students. The conditions were the Benson model, Jacobson's progressive relaxation, an attention-placebo control (bibliotherapy), and a no-treatment control. Data on alcohol consumption were obtained during a 2-week baseline period, the 6-week treatment period, and a 7-week follow-up. Significant decreases in alcohol consumption occurred in all three active conditions from baseline to post-treatment and significant differences were found between each active treatment condition and the no-treatment control. Unfortunately, these gains were not maintained at follow-up. Almost all subjects in the active treatment conditions discontinued their practice, and there appeared to be a temporal association between discontinuation of practice and increased alcohol consumption. The authors conclude that the common characteristic of the active conditions, i.e., daily 'time-out' periods for one's self, contributed to an increased sense of personal control which in turn resulted in a decrease in alcohol consumption. In their discussion, they note that the subjects in the meditation control were more invested and involved in the intervention, as they were slower to decrease their practice. In addition, in the meditation group, there was a linear relationship between reported relaxation over time and decreased alcohol consumption.

Carrington's standardized meditation. Another study, also by Marlatt and colleagues (Murphy *et al.*, 1986), investigated the impact on alcohol consumption of meditation, exercise (i.e. running), and a no-treatment control of 43 heavy social drinkers randomly assigned to the three conditions. They taught a meditation technique, standardized by Carrington (1978), which is also a mantra-based concentration technique. Pre–post-alcohol consumption dropped significantly

for all treatment conditions. The only significant difference at post-treatment between the three groups was between the exercise group and the control group; the alcohol consumption of the meditation group fell between the other two groups. Follow-up data at 11–16 weeks post-baseline on 72% of the subjects found no significant differences between the 3 groups, although subjects in all 3 conditions increased their alcohol intake during follow-up. Subject adherence appeared to be a significant contributor to reduced alcohol intake; subjects in the meditation condition who practiced more than 5 times/week had a reduced ethanol consumption of 60%, which is similar to that of the subjects in the exercise group.

Mindfulness/Vipassana

A promising set of meditation interventions that are currently being investigated by a number of researchers are mindfulness-based approaches. This form of meditation is based primarily on Vipassana, a Buddhist form from Southeast Asia, sometimes called insight meditation. It emphasizes the development of moment-to-moment awareness, unlike the mantra-based approaches discussed above. Mindfulness is the non-judgmental observation of our current experience of internal and external stimuli, as they arise and pass away. Jon Kabat-Zinn (1990) developed a secularized version, Mindfulness-Based Stress Reduction (MBSR), which he and his colleagues used with some success for chronic pain patients (1985, 1987), anxiety disorders (1992), and psoriasis (1998). Other investigators report positive results investigating the use of mindfulness interventions with a number of other conditions (for reviews, see Grossman *et al.*, 2004; Reibel *et al.*, 2001; and Baer, 2003), including eating disorders (Kristeller & Hallett, 1999), anxiety disorders (Kabat-Zinn *et al.*, 1992), and depression (Mindfulness-Based Cognitive Therapy or MBCT; Teasdale *et al.*, 1999; Teasdale *et al.*, 1995; Teasdale *et al.*, 2000; Segal *et al.*, 2002). In addition to mental health, mindfulness meditation has been studied for its potential impact on the physiology of stress reactions (e.g., Carlson *et al.*, 2004). Both MBSR and MBCT are manualized interventions, accessible to patients, psychotherapists and researchers. Vipassana is not manualized as a mental health intervention, although many books are available describing it (e.g., Goldstein & Kornfield, 1987; Gunaratana, 1991; Braza, 1997). Buddhist teachers of Vipassana can be found on the web (e.g., http://www.dharma.org/teachers/index.htm). Also of interest is that several empirically-supported clinical interventions incorporate mindfulness concepts or practices into their approaches, including Linehan's Dialectical Behavior Therapy (1993a, b), Hayes' acceptance and commitment therapy (ACT; Hayes *et al.*, 1999) and, most relevant to alcoholism treatment, Marlatt's relapse prevention (Marlatt & Gordon, 1985; Marlatt & Donovan, 2005).

However, published studies of the impact of mindfulness-based interventions on individuals with alcohol dependence are rare. Marlatt and colleagues (Bowen *et al.*, 2006; Marlatt *et al.*, 2004; Parks *et al.*, 2003) presented results from a quasi-experimental study of incarcerated individuals in a minimum security correctional and rehabilitation facility who were offered a Vipassana meditation course compared to a matched control group. Although formal alcohol diagnoses were not presented, high quality drinking and drug use data was described which indicated that this population had a history of heavy use of alcohol and other substances. In addition, half of the incarcerated population at this facility participated in substance abuse treatment. Twenty-nine inmates participated in a 10-day silent Vipassana retreat; 50 inmates who did not participate provided comparison data. Data was obtained before and 3 months after the course. Significant main effects at follow-up were found within the Vipassana group in number of alcoholic drinks, marijuana and crack use in the last week. Although there was a trend for the control group to also decrease their use of alcohol and drugs, it was only significant for marijuana use. In addition, the Vipassana group showed significant decreases on measures of the consequences of alcohol and drug use and drug abuse severity. However, the treatment-by-time analysis of the decrease in alcohol use did not reach statistical significance, probably as a consequence of the low power in this study.

A related study of individuals in a therapeutic community for substance abuse treatment investigated changes in stress levels after a Mindfulness-Based Stress Reduction intervention (Marcus *et al.*, 2003). This pre–post-design found significant changes in salivary cortisol levels after the intervention. Self-reported stress decreased, but not scores on the Perceived Stress Scale. Unfortunately, the authors did not follow up with participants after they left the community to see if these changes in cortisol and self-reported stress were maintained, nor did they provide any data on alcohol use.

Summary

There is insufficient empirical evidence of a suitably rigorous quality at this time to suggest that teaching alcoholics meditation techniques will support their sobriety. Nevertheless, there is reason to suspect from theory, neurophysiological effects, and their efficacy with comorbid disorders, that mindfulness approaches may, in time, be shown to have an impact on alcohol treatment and recovery.

Conclusions

There is very little data to support the use of alternative medicine techniques in either alcohol dependence or withdrawal, largely because adequate studies have not been carried out. However, all is not lost. CAM techniques, especially biofeedback and meditation, can help patients feel more in control over their bodies, minds and behavior and may be able to temper some of the anxiety and other physiologic states involved in both alcohol use, as well as withdrawal from alcohol.

The level of evidence for each of the interventions discussed in this chapter is summarized in Table 17.2.

Table 17.2. Effectiveness of complementary and alternative medicine for alcohol misuse

Treatment	Form of treatment	Psychiatric disorder	Level of evidence for efficacy	Comments
Alternative medicine	Acupuncture	Alcohol use disorders	III	Because of the nature of acupuncture, difficult to do placebo-controlled trials. Evidence is contradictory and plagued by methodological issues
Alternative medicine	Biofeedback	Alcohol use disorders	III	Methodological issues prevent us from making any recommendations
Meditation	Transcendental meditation and other mantra-based approaches (TM)	Alcohol use disorders	Ib	One study revealed increases in days abstinent and greater total abstinence in TM group and In biofeedback group as well. Improvement was not maintained after meditation ended
Meditation	Mindfulness/ Vipassana	Alcohol use disorders	IIb	While there appeared to be some benefit for meditation, treatment group-by-time analysis was not

REFERENCES

Adinoff, B., Iranmanesh, A., Feldhuis, J. & Fisher, L. (1998). Disturbances of the stress response: the role of the HPA Axis during alcohol withdrawal and abstinence. *Alcohol, Health and Research World*, **22** (1), 67–72.

Alexander, C. N., Robinson, P. & Rainforth, M. (1994). Treating and preventing alcohol, nicotine, and drug abuse through Transcendental Meditation: a review and statistical meta-analysis. *Alcoholism Treatment Quarterly*, **11** (1/2), 13–87.

Baer, R. A. (2003). Mindfulness training as a clinical intervention: a conceptual and empirical review. *Clinical Psychology: Science and Practice*, **10** (2), 125–43.

Barnes, P. M., Powell-Griner, E., McFann, K. & Nahin, R. L. (2004). Complementary and alternative medicine use among adults: United States, 2002. *Advance Data from Vital and Health Statistics*, No. 343, May 27. Center for Disease Control and Prevention, US Dept. Health & Human Services.

Benson, H. (1975). *The Relaxation Response*. New York: William Morrow & Co.

Boucher, T. A., Kiresuk, T. J. & Trachtenberg, A. I. (2003). Complementary and alternative therapies. In *Principles of Addiction Medicine*, ed. A. W. Graham, T. K. Schultz, M. F. Mayo-Smith, R. K. Ries & R. B. Wilford, 3rd edn. pp. 509–32. Chevy Chase, MD: American Society of Addiction Medicine, Inc.

Bowen, S., Witkiewitz, K., Dillworth, T. M. *et al.* (2006). Mindfulness meditation and substance use in an incarcerated population. *Psychology of Addictive Behaviors*, **20** (3), 343–7.

Brady, K. T. & Sonne, S. C. (1999). The role of stress in alcohol use, alcoholism treatment, and relapse. *Alcohol Research and Health*, **23** (4), 263–71.

Braza, J. (1997). *Moment by Moment: The Art and Practice of Mindfulness*. Boston, MA: Charles E. Tuttle, Co.

Brown, S. A., Vik, P. W., Patterson, T. L., Grant, I. & Schuckit, M. A. (1995). Stress, vulnerability and adult alcohol relapse. *Journal of Studies on Alcohol*, **56**, 538–45.

Bullock, M. L., Umen, A. J., Culliton, P. D. & Olander, R. T. (1987). Acupuncture treatment of alcoholic recidivism: a pilot study. *Alcoholism: Clinical and Experimental Research*, **11**(3), 292–5.

Bullock, M. L., Kiresuk, T. J., Sherman, R. E. *et al.* (2002). A large randomized placebo controlled study of auricular acupuncture for alcohol dependence. *Journal of Substance Abuse Treatment*, **22**, 71–7.

Carrington, P. (1978). *Freedom in Meditation*. New York: Crown.

Carlson, L. E., Speca, M., Patel, K. D. & Goodey, E. (2004). Mindfulness-based stress reduction in relation to quality of life, mood, symptoms of stress and levels of cortisol, dehydroepiandrosterone sulfate (DHEAS) and melatonin in breast and prostate cancer outpatients. *Psychoneuroendocrinology*, **29**, 448–74.

Denney, M. R. & Baugh, J. L. (1992). Symptom reduction and sobriety in the male alcoholic. *International Journal of Addictions*, **27**(11), 1293–300.

Denney, M. R., Baugh, J. L. & Hardt, H. D. (1991). Sobriety outcome after alcoholism treatment with biofeedback participation: a pilot inpatient study. *International Journal of Addictions*, **26**(3), 335–41.

Fink, M., Gutenbrunner, C., Rollnik, J. & Karst, M. (2001). Credibility of a newly designed placebo needle for clinical trials in acupuncture research. *Forsch Komplementarmed Klass Naturheilkd*, **8**(6), 368–72.

Goldstein, J. & Kornfield, J. (1987). *Seeking the Heart of Wisdom: The Path of Insight Meditation*. Boston, MA: Shambhala

Graap, K. & Freides, D. (1998). Regarding the database for the Peniston alpha-theta EEG biofeedback protocol. *Applied Psychophysiological Biofeedback*, **23**(4), 265–72; 273–5.

Grossman, P., Niemann, L., Schmidt, S. & Walach, H. (2004). Mindfulness-based stress reduction and health benefits: a meta-analysis. *Journal of Psychosomatic Research*, **57**, 35–43.

Gunaratana, H. (1991). *Mindfulness in Plain English*. Boston, MA: Wisdom Publications.

Han, J. S., Trachtenberg, A. I. & Lowinson, J. H. (2004). Acupuncture. In *Substance Abuse: A Comprehensive Textbook*, ed. J. H. Lowinson, P. Ruiz, R. B. Millman & J. G. Langrod, 4th edn. Philadelphia, PA: Lippincott Williams & Wilkins.

Harte, J. L., Eifert, G. H. & Smith, R. (1995). The effect of running and meditation on beta-endorphin, corticotropin-releasing hormone and cortisol in plasma, and on mood. *Biological Psychiatry*, **40**, 251–65.

Hayes, S. C., Strosahl, K. D. & Wilson, K. G. (1999). *Acceptance and Commitment Therapy: An Experiential Approach to Behavior Change*. New York: Guilford Press.

Jacobson, E. (1938). *Progressive Relaxation*. Chicago: University of Chicago Press.

Jacobson, E. (1987). Progressive relaxation. *American Journal of Psychology*, **100** (3–4), 522–37.

Jadad, A. R., Moore, R. A., Carroll, D. *et al.* (1996). Assessing the quality of reports of randomized clinical trials: Is blinding necessary? *Clinical Controlled Trials*, **17**(1), 1–12.

Kabat-Zinn, J. (1990). *Full Catastrophe Living: Using the Wisdom of Your Body and Mind to Face Stress, Pain, and Illness*. New York: Delacorte.

Kabat-Zinn, J., Lipworth, L. & Burney, R. (1985). The clinical use of mindfulness meditation for the self-regulation of chronic pain. *Journal of Behavioral Medicine*, **8**, 163–90.

Kabat-Zinn, J., Lipworth, L., Burney, R. & Sellers, W. (1987). Four-year follow-up of a meditation-based program for the self-regulation of chronic pain: treatment outcomes and compliance. *Clinical Journal of Pain*, **2**, 159–73.

Kabat-Zinn, J., Massion, M. D., Kristeller, J. *et al.* (1992). Effectiveness of a meditation-based stress reduction program in the treatment of anxiety disorders. *American Journal of Psychiatry*, **149**, 936–43.

Kabat-Zinn, J., Wheeler, E., Light, T. *et al.* (1998). Influence of a mindfulness meditation-based stress reduction intervention on rates of skin clearing in patients with moderate to severe psoriasis undergoing phototherapy (UVB) and photochemotherapy (PUVA). *Psychosomatic Medicine*, **50**, 625–32.

Kazanjian, A. & Rothon, D. A. (2002). *Acupuncture in the Management of Alcohol and Drug Dependence*. Vancouver, BC: British Columbia Office of Health Technology Assessment, University of British Columbia.

Kreek, M. J. & Koob, G. F. (1998). Drug dependence: stress and dysregulation of brain reward pathways. *Drug and Alcohol Dependence*, **51**, 23–47.

Kristeller, J. L. & Hallett, C. B. (1999). An exploratory study of a meditation-based intervention for binge eating disorder. *Journal of Health Psychology*, **4**, 357–63.

Lamon, B. C. & Alonzo, A. (1997). Stress among males recovering from substance abuse. *Addictive Behaviors*, **22** (2), 195–205.

Linehan, M. M. (1993a). *Cognitive Behavioral Treatment of Borderline Personality Disorder*. New York, NY: Guilford Press.

Linehan, M. M. (1993b). *Skills Training Manual for Treating Borderline Personality Disorder*. New York, NY: Guilford Press.

Manheimer, E., Anderson, B. J. & Stein, M. D. (2003). Use and assessment of complementary and alternative therapies by intravenous drug users. *American Journal of Drug and Alcohol Abuse*, **29** (2), 401–13.

Marcus, M. T., Fine, M., Moeller, G. *et al.* (2003). Change in stress levels following mindfulness-based stress reduction in a therapeutic community. *Addictive Disorders and their Treatment*, **2**(3), 63–68.

Marlatt, G. A. & Donovan, D. M. (2005). *Relapse Prevention: Maintenance Strategies in the Treatment of Addictive Behaviors*, 2nd edn. New York, NY: Guilford Press.

Marlatt, G. A. & Gordon, J. R. (1985). *Relapse Prevention: Maintenance Strategies in the Treatment of Addictive Behaviors*. New York, NY: Guilford Press.

Marlatt, G. A., Pagano, R., Rose, D. & Marques, J. (1984). Effect of meditation and relaxation training upon alcohol use in male social drinkers. In *Meditation: Classic and Contemporary Perspectives*, ed. D. Shapiro & R. Walsh, pp. 105–20. New York: Aldine.

Marlatt, G. A., Witkiewitz, K., Dillworth, T. M. *et al.* (2004). Vipassana meditation as a treatment for alcohol and drug use disorders. In *Mindfulness and Acceptance: Expanding the Cognitive Behavioral Tradition*, ed. S. C. Hayes, V. M. Follette & M. M. Linehan. New York: Guilford Press.

Murphy, T. J., Pagano, R. R. & Marlatt, G. A. (1986). Lifestyle modification with heavy alcohol drinkers: Effects of aerobic exercise and meditation. *Addictive Behaviors*, **11**, 175–86.

National Acupuncture Detoxification Association (NADA) (1995). NADA FAQs: How did NADA originate? Retrieved May 30, 2005 from http://www.acudetox.com/index.htm.

Parks, G. A., Marlatt, G. A., Bowen, S. W. *et al.* (2003). The University of Washington vipassana meditation research project at the North Rehabilitation Facility. *American Jails*, **17**, 13–17.

Peniston, E. G. & Kulkosky, P. J. (1989). Alpha-theta brainwave training and beta-endorphin levels in alcoholics. *Alcoholism; Clinical and Experimental Research*, **13**(2), 271–9.

Pomeranz, B. (1989). Acupuncture research related to pain, drug addiction and nerve regeneration. In *Scientific Bases of Acupuncture*, ed. B. Pomeranz, G. Stux, pp. 35–52. Berlin, Germany: Springer-Verlag.

Rampes, H., Pereira, S., Mortimer, A., Manoharan, S. & Knowles, M. (1997). Does electroacupuncture reduce craving for alcohol? A randomized controlled study. *Complementary Therapies in Medicine*, **5**, 19–26.

Reibel, D. K., Greeson, J. M., Brainard, G. C. & Rosenzweig, S. (2001). Mindfulness-based stress reduction and health-related quality of life in a heterogeneous patient population. *General Hospital Psychiatry*, **23**, 183–92.

Sanders, L. M., Trinh, C., Sherman, B. R. & Banks, S. M. (1998). Assessment of client satisfaction in a peer counseling substance abuse treatment program for pregnant and postpartum women. *Evaluation and Program Planning*, **21**(3), 287–96.

Sapir-Weise, R., Berglund, M., Frank, A. & Kristenson, H. (1999). Acupuncture in alcoholism treatment: a randomized outpatient study. *Alcohol and Alcoholism*, **34**(4), 629–35.

Saxby, E. & Peniston, E. G. (1995). Alpha-theta brainwave neurofeedback training: an effective treatment for male and female alcoholics with depressive symptoms. *Journal of Clinical Psychology*, **51**(5), 685–93.

Segal, Z. V., Williams, J. M. G. & Teasdale, J. D. (2002). *Mindfulness-based Cognitive Therapy for Depression: A New Approach to Preventing Relapse*. New York: Guilford Press.

Scott, S. & Scott, W. N. (1997). A biochemical hypothesis for the effectiveness of acupuncture in the treatment of substance abuse: acupuncture and the reward cascade. *American Journal of Acupuncture*, **25**(1), 33–8.

Sharp, C., Hurford, D. P., Allison, J., Sparks, R. & Cameron, B. P. (1997). Facilitation of internal locus of control in adolescent alcoholics through a brief biofeedback-assisted autogenic relaxation training procedure. *Journal of Substance Abuse Treatment*, **14**(1), 55–60.

Smith, M. O. (1999). *Acupuncture For Addiction Treatment*. Vancouver, WA: J. & M. Reports.

Substance Abuse and Mental Health Services Administration (SAMHSA), Office of Applied Studies (2004). *National Survey of Substance Abuse Treatment Services (N-SSATS): 2003. Data on substance abuse treatment facilities*, DASIS Series: S-24, DHHS Publication no. (SMA) 04-3966. Rockville, MD: Author.

Tarbox, A. R. (1983a). Alcoholism, biofeedback and internal scanning. *Journal of Studies on Alcohol*, **44** (2), 246–61.

Tarbox, A. R. (1983b). Neuromuscular learning in middle-stage male alcoholics. *Alcoholism: Clinical & Experimental Research*, **7**(1), 38–41.

Taub, E., Steiner, S. S., Weingarten, E & Walton, K. G. (1994). Effectiveness of broad spectrum approaches to relapse prevention in severe alcoholism: a long-term, randomized, controlled trial of Transcendental Meditation, EMG biofeedback and electronic neurotherapy. *Alcoholism Treatment Quarterly*, **11**(1/2), 187–220.

Teasdale, J. D. (1999). Metacognition, mindfulness, and the modification of mood disorders. *Clinical Psychology and Psychotherapy*, **6**, 146–55.

Teasdale, J. D., Segal, Z. V. & Williams, M. G. (1995). How does cognitive therapy prevent depressive relapse and why should attentional control (mindfulness training) help? *Behavior Research and Therapy*, **33**, 25–39.

Teasdale, J. D., Williams, J. M., Soulsby, J. M., Segal, Z. V., Ridgeway, V. A. & Lau, M. A. (2000). Prevention of relapse/recurrence in major depression by mindfulness-based cognitive therapy. *Journal of Consulting and Clinical Psychology*, **68**, 615–23.

Toteva, S. & Milanov, I. (1996). The use of acupuncture for treatment of alcohol dependence and withdrawal syndrome: a controlled study. *American Journal of Acupuncture*, **24**(1), 19–26.

Trumpler, F., Oez, S., Stahli, P., Brenner, H. D. & Juni, P. (2003). Acupuncture for alcohol withdrawal: a randomized, controlled trial. *Alcohol and Alcoholism*, **38**, 369–75.

Ulett, G. A. (1989). Studies supporting the concept of physiological acupuncture. In *Scientific Bases of Acupuncture*, ed. B. Pomeranz & G. Stux, pp. 177–96. Berlin, Germany: Springer-Verlag.

Walker, S. R., Tonigan, J. S., Miller, W. R., Comer, S. & Kahlich, L. (1997). Intercessory prayer in the treatment of alcohol abuse and dependence: a pilot investigation. *Alternative Therapies in Health & Medicine*, **3**(6), 79–86.

Walsh, R. & Shapiro, S. L. (2006). The meeting of meditative disciplines and Western psychology: a mutually enriching dialogue. *American Psychologist*, **61**(3), 227–39.

Watson, C. G., Herder, J. & Passini, F. T. (1978). Alpha biofeedback therapy in alcoholics: an 18-month follow-up. *Journal of Clinical Psychology*, **34**(3), 765–9.

Weingarten, E., Hartman, L. & Holcomb, Z. (1980). Frontalis EMG of dropouts from inpatient treatment for alcoholism. *International Journal of the Addictions*, **15**(7), 1113–17.

Wen, H. L. & Cheung, S. Y. C. (1973). Treatment of drug addiction by acupuncture and electrical stimulation. *Asian Journal of Medicine*, **9**, 138–41.

Wen, H. L. & Teo, S. W. (1975). Experience in the treatment of drug addiction by electro-acupuncture. *Modern Medicine of Asia*, **11**(6), 23–7.

Worner, T. M., Zeller, B., Schwarz, H., Zwas, F. & Lyon, D. (1992). Acupuncture fails to improve treatment outcome in alcoholics. *Drug and Alcohol Dependence*, **30**, 169–73.

Drug misuse

Section editors

Owen Bowden-Jones and Tony P. George

18

Empirically validated psychological therapies for drug dependence

Tara M. Neavins, Caroline J. Easton, Janet Brotchie and Kathleen M. Carroll

Editors' note

This chapter reviews empirically validated psychological therapies for adults with substance use problems. There is not a corresponding chapter in this section for psychopharmacologic treatment for substance dependence because psychopharmacology in these disorders is much more limited and may be substance class specific. Psychopharmacologic approaches are covered in the chapters on the specific disorders, while the psychological therapies, almost all of which fall into the broader psychological therapy categories, can extend across the classes of substances that are frequently misused. CBT, especially when accompanied by contingency management, is effective in cocaine and opioid dependence, while CBT alone is effective in cocaine and cannabis abuse. Contingency management with vouchers may also, by itself, be effective in cocaine and opioid abuse as well. Behavioral couples therapy appears to be effective in reducing opioid and cocaine use. Motivational interviewing appears effective in alcohol or cannabis misuse in adults. Other forms of psychological/psychosocial therapy may be effective for other types of substance misuse, but the empirical evidence is not as strong. Often these interventions are combined with some psychopharmacologic intervention that has been shown to reduce, in some instances, craving for the particular substance. Sections of this chapter are adapted from Carroll, 2000; Carroll & Onken, 2005, McGovern & Carroll, 2003, and Rounsaville & Carroll, 1997, and are used here with permission.

Introduction

During the past 10–15 years, tremendous gains have been made in the development of effective psychological therapies for drug abuse and dependence for adults. An increasing number of well-conducted randomized controlled trials have shown the effectiveness of many psychological therapies in treating drug dependence. Whereas there are highly effective pharmacotherapies for some classes of drug dependence (e.g. opioids), treatment outcomes often dramatically improve with the addition of psychological therapies in areas such as patient motivation, medication compliance, self-efficacy, and overall reduced treatment cost. For other classes of drugs (e.g. cocaine) where pharmacological interventions do not yet exist, psychological approaches are the state-of-the-art treatments. Today, many psychological approaches have been evaluated in rigorous controlled clinical trials. Treatment manuals and training materials are available, which facilitate the use of these psychological approaches by a wider variety of clinicians and within and across a multidisciplinary approach. Thus, the medical treatment of patients who are dependent on illicit drugs likely will be improved with a basic understanding of these therapies and their underlying principles.

This chapter begins with a general explanation of the guiding principles of psychological therapies in treating drug dependence. Next, the available evidence regarding treatment effectiveness of psychological therapies for the following drugs will be considered: opioids, cocaine, amphetamines and methamphetamines, and cannabis. For each drug category, availability of empirical validation of psychological therapies, through randomized trials, will be considered. Although this review will focus primarily on adult drug dependence, young adult drug dependence also will be included.

To provide a context for this chapter, three issues deserve emphasis. First, "talk" therapies remain the most common form of drug dependence treatment in the United States, excluding treatment facilities that focus on detoxification or methadone maintenance services (Simpson et al., 1997). Second, there tends to be limited interaction between

Cambridge Textbook of Effective Treatments in Psychiatry, ed. Peter Tyrer and Kenneth R. Silk. Published by Cambridge University Press.
© Cambridge University Press, 2008.

clinical researchers and clinicians (Institute of Medicine, 1998). so that, on the one hand, psychological treatments found to be effective in clinical trials often are not incorporated into mainstream clinical practice, and, on the other hand, many widely utilized clinical treatments have not been subjected to randomized trials. Third, for the majority of illicit drugs, no generally effective pharmacotherapies have been developed. Classes of drug use for which no effective pharmacotherapies yet exist include cocaine, amphetamines, methamphetamines, sedative/hypnotic/anxiolytics, cannabis, phencyclidine (PCP), hallucinogens, club drugs (e.g. MDMA), and inhalants. Although strides have been made in discovering the physiological mechanisms of action for many of these illicit substances, behavioral approaches remain the only available treatment for most types of drug dependence (O'Brien, 1996).

Within the UK treatment context there has been a focus on two approaches to the treatment of problematic drug use that have resulted in different developments in relation to the use of psychological approaches within the drug treatment system. First, UK statutory treatment providers have focused largely on the provision of pharmacological interventions to primary heroin-using clients. This pharmacological orientation has led to the position that treatment often equates to the provision of methadone for heroin-dependent clients, while clients who use other substances receive minimal interventions. It is rare in the UK for non-opioid using clients to be the focus of treatment provision, or indeed for non-opioid use in opioid-using clients to be targeted. As poly-drug use grows and the numbers of clients who use other illicit drugs increases, the UK is addressing the need to implement more evidence-based psychological interventions. However, at this time there is a paucity of provision of evidence-based psychological interventions within the drug treatment system as a whole. The second approach to treatment that has influenced the provision of psychological interventions has been the focus on harm reduction as a primary intervention for opioid and non-opioid-using clients. Here harm reduction has often meant that clients receive psychoeducational interventions, with the focus being on changing risk-related behaviors rather than changing drug use per se.

Goals of psychological therapies in treating drug dependence

Overview

Psychological therapies encompass a variety of roles in the treatment of drug abuse. These roles differ from those of

pharmacotherapy in their time to effect, durability of action, and target symptoms. Unlike psychological therapies that tend to require more time to reveal their effects, pharmacotherapies often exert their effects very soon after their initiation. However, psychological therapies often have more long-lasting effects after completion of treatment and broader applicability than do most pharmacotherapies now in existence. Specifically, most cognitive-behavioral and behavioral therapies can be used across various treatment settings (e.g. inpatient, outpatient, residential), modalities (e.g. group, individual, and family) and a myriad of substance users. Psychological therapies often rely on teaching coping skills or on employing a motivational approach and are applicable to a large extent to patients who are opiate, cocaine, barbiturate, or cannabis users. In contrast, most pharmacotherapies are warranted only for a single class of substance use and target a relatively narrow band of symptoms. Methadone, for instance, creates cross-tolerance for opioids but would not be expected to (and indeed does not) have an effect on concurrent cocaine dependence; similarly, disulfiram produces nausea after alcohol ingestion but not after intake of other substances (Carroll, 2000).

Although theoretical and technical differences are apparent, cognitive-behavioral and behavioral therapies for drug dependence generally have many similarities. The following discussion highlights the issues that are present, to varying degrees, in most psychological therapies. Moreover, currently available pharmacotherapies for drug dependence would be expected to have little or no effect in these areas commonly addressed by cognitive-behavioral and behavioral treatments (Rounsaville & Carroll, 1997).

Cessation of drug use

Ambivalence regarding cessation of drug use is common for individuals who present with drug dependence. Even after negative consequences of drug use have become so overwhelming that treatment may be sought, drug users typically can state several benefits of drug use, express a strong desire or perceived need for drugs, and struggle to imagine what life might be like without drug use (Rounsaville & Carroll, 1997). On the other hand, many drug users may be even more uncertain about treatment given that they have presented for counseling due to the external demands of the legal system, family, friends and relationship partners. Treatments rooted in motivational psychology, including Motivational Interviewing (Miller & Rollnick, 1991; Rollnick *et al.*, 1999) and Motivation Enhancement Therapy (Miller *et al.*, 1992), concentrate almost exclusively on strategies intended to bolster the patient's own motivational resources. Specifically, clients may first need to see reasons for changing their behavior before they can benefit from treatment. Motivational therapies are client-centered and understand the ambivalence that many individuals face when considering reducing or eliminating their drug use. However, the majority of psychological therapies elect to explore the pros and cons of continued substance use in an attempt to increase motivation for treatment and abstinence. In addition to exploring the pros and cons of drug use, motivational strategies general provide clients with feedback derived from an initial assessment session. This feedback often serves to increase motivation to change drug patterns (Carroll, 2000; Rounsaville & Carroll, 1997).

Teaching coping skills and relapse prevention
Social learning theory posits that substance use may represent a means of coping with such things as difficult situations, positive and negative emotional states, and invitations by peers to engage in substance use (Bandura, 1977a, 1977b). By the time that substance use has evolved to the point of drug dependence and treatment-seeking, substance use may represent the individual's single, over-generalized pattern of coping with a variety of situations, settings, and states. In order to maximize the probability of achieving and maintaining abstinence, patients would be best-served by understanding high-risk situations that might increase their temptation to use substances and learning more effective means of coping with these risky circumstances. Relapse prevention (Marlatt & Gordon, 1985), a means of increasing self-control and learning to cope with cravings to use substances, has been found to be particularly effective with cocaine-dependent individuals (Carroll *et al.*, 1991a; National Institute on Drug Abuse, 2004). Although cognitive-behavioral therapies are focused primarily on skills training in order to prevent relapse to substances (Carroll, 1998; Marlatt & Gordon, 1985; Monte *et al.*, 1989), many other behavioral therapies devote at least some time to addressing high-risk situations. Childress *et al.*'s (1984, 1993) work, for instance, has addressed relapse-prevention by examining cue exposure and reactivity, which may enhance patients' capacity to cope effectively with craving for drugs (Carroll, 2000).

Changing reinforcement contingencies
At the point of entry into drug dependence treatment, many individuals may spend the vast majority of their time acquiring, using, and recovering from substance use to the exclusion of other endeavors and rewards (Rounsaville & Carroll, 1997). Frequently, the drug abuser

is isolated from friends and family. The drug addict's world tends to consist of individuals who use drugs. If the individual happens to be employed, work may have lost any value except for serving as a means of earning enough money to buy more drugs. Hobbies, sports, community and religious group involvement, and other leisure pursuits have probably faded to the background to be replaced by the active demands of drug dependence. Frequently, daily rewards are narrowed progressively to those derived from drug use, and other diversions may no longer be available or may simply fail to be perceived as pleasurable. When abstinence from substance use is achieved, addicts may be at a loss as to how to structure their time that previously was consumed with acquiring, using, and recovering from drugs. Similarly, newly abstinent addicts may struggle to find rewards that can replace those derived from drug use. In light of these factors, behavioral therapies, such as the Community Reinforcement Approach (CRA (Azrin, 1976)) and voucher-based contingency management (Budney & Higgins, 1998; Budney *et al.*, 2000), assist patients with identifying and creating fulfilling and reinforcing alternatives to drug use (Carroll, 2000).

Fostering management of painful affects
Negative emotions and affects appear to be strong catalysts for relapse to substance use (Marlatt & Gordon, 1985). Some clinicians have asserted that inability to regulate affect is a salient factor underlying the development of compulsive drug use (Khantzian, 1975). Moreover, it is commonly believed that substances enable addicts to 'numb' their feelings of anger, sadness, loss, betrayal, guilt and other difficult emotions. Empirical investigations have demonstrated that substance abusers have compromised ability to identify and explicate their affect states (Keller *et al.*, 1995; Taylor *et al.*, 1990). Consequently, an important component of cognitive-behavioral and behavioral therapies' abilities to treat drug dependence is to help addicts create ways of coping with strong negative affects and to learn to recognize the source of these disturbing emotions (Rounsaville & Carroll, 1997). While many psychodynamically oriented treatments, such as Supportive-Expressive Therapy (Luborsky, 1984), emphasize the role of affect in the treatment of cocaine abuse, for instance, many types of psychological therapies give attention to a myriad of ways to cope with strong emotions (Carroll, 2000).

Improving interpersonal functioning and enhancing social support
Studies have repeatedly shown that the presence of an adequate network of social support is protective in

preventing relapse to drug dependence (Longabaugh *et al.*, 1993; Marlatt & Gordon, 1985). Three issues are particularly relevant to the social networks of many drug addicts. First, even prior to onset of drug use, these individuals often have failed to develop meaningful relationships with peers, intimate partners and family members. Second, if they have been able to achieve satisfactory relationships, these relationships tend to erode under the weight of the drug use. Third, drug misusers tend to have few individuals in their social circles that do not abuse substances (Rounsaville & Carroll, 1997). Given these facts, many cognitive-behavioral and behavioral therapies, including family therapy (McCrady & Epstein, 1995), twelve-step approaches (Nowinski *et al.*, 1992), interpersonal therapy (Rounsaville, 1995), and network therapy (Galanter, 1993), place a premium on teaching addicts how to create and maintain a social network devoid of substance users (Carroll, 2000).

Another advantage of twelve-step and network therapy approaches is that once a drug-dependent individual has acquired various skills and knowledge with a particular therapist in a given service, the client can go on to develop contact with a broader network of supportive non-using peers such as that provided by Alcoholics Anonymous (AA). As a consequence, the client can successfully terminate treatment at a service because he/she has not become dependent on one therapist or agency.

Fostering compliance with pharmacotherapy
Substance users often struggle to be compliant with treatment, particularly with pharmacotherapies. Psychological treatments may help serve as vital adjuncts to pharmacotherapies by increasing client levels of compliance. The vast majority of techniques to improve compliance are psychosocial (Carroll, 1997). Examples of these strategies include regular monitoring of medication compliance with feedback; encouraging patients to engage in self-monitoring (e.g. through medication logs or diaries); clear communication between patient and staff about the study medication, its anticipated effects, side effects, and benefits; clearly describing the benefits of adherence and the risks of non-compliance; contracting with the patients for adherence; directly reinforcing adherence through incentives or rewards; providing telephone reminders or other cues for taking medication; frequent contact and the provision of support (Haynes *et al.*, 1979; Meichenbaum & Turk, 1987). Given the success of these strategies, it comes as no surprise that research consistently has demonstrated the benefit of adding cognitive-behavioral and behavioral treatments to pharmacological treatments for substance use (Carroll, 1997;

McLellan & McKay, 1998). Several of the landmark investigations illustrating the merit of appealing to psychological treatments to enhance outcome for pharmacotherapeutic treatment of drug dependence will be highlighted in the sections that follow.

Evidence-based cognitive-behavioral and behavioral treatments for drug dependence

Overview

The purpose of empirical validation of psychological therapies is to identify effective treatments that assist clinicians in delivering appropriate therapies (Chambless *et al.*, 1996; Chambless *et al.*, 1998). In general, this review focuses on interventions classified as 'empirically validated' or 'likely to be efficacious'. To be considered empirically validated, it is necessary that a given treatment demonstrate efficacy in at least two randomized controlled trials (RCTs (McGovern & Carroll, 2003)). Included studies should be methodologically sound and incorporate features such as treatment manuals, random assignment to targeted and appropriate control and treatment conditions, and use validated measures. Moreover, a treatment's efficacy should be confirmed by at least two independent investigation teams. In contrast, to be considered 'probably efficacious', a treatment's efficacy must be confirmed by at least two positive randomized clinical trials with a waiting list control group, a small series of single case experiments, or one or more experiments meeting criteria for empirical validation but not by independent teams. Although this framework has generated considerable controversy, this model afforded a standard by which to compare treatments (McGovern & Carroll, 2003).

Psychological therapies and opioid dependence

Behavioral therapies in the context of methadone maintenance
The development of methadone maintenance treatment revolutionized the treatment of opioid addiction by producing outcomes far surpassing those produced by the use of non-pharmacologic treatments (Carroll, 2000; Rounsaville & Carroll, 1997). Specifically, methadone maintenance treatment allowed addicts to remain in treatment and to reduce their illicit opioid use (Brill, 1977; Nyswander *et al.*, 1958; O'Malley *et al.*, 1972). In addition, methadone maintenance is associated with less risk of HIV infection and other medical complications by decreasing intravenous drug use (Ball *et al.*, 1988; Metzger *et al.*, 1993; Sorenson & Copeland, 2000).

Methadone maintenance, particularly when given at therapeutic doses and combined with drug counseling, substantially reduces illicit opioid use, injection drug use, criminal activity, and morbidity as well as mortality risk (Institute of Medicine, 1998). Another advantage to methadone maintenance is that by stabilizing patients and retaining them in treatment it creates an opportunity to address concurrent disorders, including medical problems, family issues, and psychiatric conditions (Lowinson *et al.*, 1992).

Despite the enormous success of methadone maintenance treatments, several problems with this approach are evident. First, different methadone maintenance programs vary widely in their success rates, which may in part be attributed to variability in delivery of therapeutic dosing of methadone as well as variability in provision and quality of psychosocial services (Ball & Ross, 1991). Second, it is not uncommon for methadone maintenance clients to sell their take-home methadone doses or to use other substances, especially alcohol, benzodiazepines, and cocaine, while on methadone (Kosten & McCance, 1996).

Before describing specific behavioral therapies useful in enhancing the effectiveness of methadone maintenance treatment, a landmark study will first be summarized to clarify the importance of psychosocial treatments even within the framework of a pharmacotherapy as potent as methadone. In their 24-week trial, McLellan *et al.* (1993) randomly assigned 92 opiate-dependent individuals to one of three conditions: (1) methadone maintenance alone, without psychosocial services, (2) methadone maintenance with standard services, which included regular meetings with a counselor, and (3) enhanced methadone maintenance, which included regular counseling plus on-site medical, employment and family therapy services. Although some patients did reasonably well in the methadone alone condition, 69% of this group had to be removed from this condition within the first 3 months of the study protocol as their substance use did not improve or had worsened, or they experienced significant medical or psychiatric difficulties which necessitated a higher level of care. With regard to substance use and psychosocial functioning, success rates were highest in the enhanced methadone maintenance condition followed by the standard methadone maintenance condition. Comparatively, individuals in the methadone alone condition fared most poorly. Thus, although basic methadone maintenance treatment aids in treatment retention and reduces continued illicit opioid abuse as well as associated illegal and dangerous behavior, a purely pharmacologic approach may not be sufficient for the vast majority of opioid

addicts. Outcomes can be improved with higher levels of behavioral treatment (McLellan *et al.*, 1993).

Contingency management approaches and opioid dependence

The effectiveness of decreasing opioid use via contingency management as an adjunct to methadone maintenance treatment has received wide empirical attention (Carroll, 2000; Rounsaville & Carroll, 1997). In these studies, patients who meet delineated target behaviors, such as providing drug-free urine specimens, attaining certain treatment goals, or attending treatment session, receive a reinforcer (reward). An example of an inexpensive, readily-available reinforcer is having methadone take-home privileges be conditional upon a demonstration of a decrease in drug use. Stitzer and her colleagues (1992, 1993) have devoted considerable attention to evaluating methadone take-home privileges as a reward for reduced illicit drug use. In a series of well-controlled trials, these investigators have documented several findings: (1) the relative benefits of positive contingencies (e.g. rewarding desired behaviors such as abstinence) compared with negative contingencies (e.g. punishing undesired behaviors such as continued drug use through discharges or dose reductions; (Stitzer *et al.*, 1986)), (2) the desirability of take-home privileges over other incentives available within methadone maintenance clinics (Stitzer & Bigelow, 1978), and (3) the relative effectiveness of rewarding drug-free urines compared with other target behaviors (Iguchi *et al.*, 1996).

Drawing upon the compelling work of Higgins and colleagues (2000) (outlined in later discussion), Silverman and his colleagues (1996a) evaluated a voucher-based contingency management system to reduce concurrent illicit drug use (generally cocaine) among methadone-maintained opioid addicts. This approach requires urine specimens thrice weekly in order to reliably detect drug use. Abstinence, verified through drug-free urine screens, is reinforced through a voucher system through which patients receive points redeemable for items consistent with an abstinence-based (drug-free) lifestyle. In other words, these vouchers are intended to help patients create alternate reinforcers to drug use (e.g. movie tickets, sporting events). Using this voucher system, Silverman and colleagues (Robles *et al.*, 2002; Silverman *et al.*, 1996a, 1996b, 1998, 2001) demonstrated less opioid and cocaine use amongst individuals participating in methadone-maintenance treatment.

In a very elegant series of studies, Silverman and his colleagues (1996a, 1996b, 1998) built upon the voucher method. These investigators (Silverman *et al.*, 2001) created the 'therapeutic workplace' in which methadone-maintained study participants are paid to work in a job but only are allowed to work and get financial compensation on the days on which they provide drug-free urines. These jobs follow an initial employment training program during which time individuals' participation in this orientation program is considered their job. Similar to their findings with their previous voucher system, their 'therapeutic workplace' treatment models resulted in less opioid and cocaine use as well as produced additional treatment benefits among methadone-maintained opioid addicts (Silverman *et al.*, 2001; Wong *et al.*, 2003, 2004).

Other psychological approaches and opioid dependence

Relatively few studies have evaluated the efficacy of formal psychotherapy in enhancing outcomes achieved by methadone maintenance treatment. Woody and colleagues (1983) randomly assigned 110 opiate addicts who were starting a methadone maintenance program to one of three conditions: (1) drug counseling alone, (2) drug counseling plus supportive-expressive psychotherapy (SE), or (3) drug counseling plus cognitive psychotherapy (CT). After 6 months of treatment, there was little difference between the SE and CT groups on the majority of outcome measures. However, opiate addicts who received either of the two types of professional psychotherapy demonstrated greater strides in more outcome domains than opiate addicts who simply received drug counseling (Woody *et al.*, 1983). In addition, treatment gains made by the subjects in the professional psychotherapy conditions were sustained over a 1-year follow-up. In contrast, treatment advances made by subjects in the drug counseling condition tended to dissipate over time (Woody *et al.*, 1995). Furthermore, this study showed that methadone-maintained opiate addicts with higher levels of psychopathology, as contrasted with those having lower levels of psychopathology, tended to improve only if they received professional psychotherapy. This finding indicates a differential response to psychotherapy based on patient characteristics, which may suggest the best use of psychotherapy (relative to drug counseling) when resources are scarce.

Behavioral couples therapy and opioid dependence

One form of psychotherapy that has received increasing empirical validation for individuals with opioid dependence is behavioral couples therapy (O'Farrell & Fals-Stewart, 2000). Behavioral couples therapy has several critical components. First, the patient develops a 'sobriety contract' such that the patient promises to their partner that the patient will not use drugs that day. The partner then reciprocates by indicating that they know the patient can succeed. Second, there is effort to 'catch your partner doing something nice' and offering compliments. Third, partners set up a 'caring day' for each other so that partners can take turns making the other one feel special. Fourth, 'shared rewarding activities' provide an opportunity for partners to engage in mutually satisfying endeavors, which are substance-free. Finally, time is devoted to 'communication skills' and relapse-prevention skills in order to best cope with daily stressors without returning to drug use.

The first randomized clinical trial to examine behavioral couples therapy was conducted with married (or co-habitating), male, substance treatment, outpatients who were struggling primarily with opioid or cocaine dependence (Fals-Stewart *et al.*, 1996). These investigators randomly assigned 80 participants to: (1) behavioral couples therapy (BCT; one weekly couples session with their female partner and one weekly individual session) or (2) individual treatment (IT; two weekly individual sessions). Although both groups similarly had few urine samples positive for substances during the 12-week comparison, men in the BCT condition self-reported significantly fewer days of using drugs, fewer drug-related consequences and greater lengths of abstinence than did men in the IT condition. These self-reported findings were noted through the 12-month follow-up assessment. In addition, men (and their female partners) had better couple functioning and were less apt to abuse each other than was true for men (and their female partners) assigned to the IT condition. These results have been replicated with female, substance-abusing, patients who have participated in BCT with their male, non-drug-abusing, male, partners (Winters *et al.*, 2002). Furthermore, Fals-Stewart *et al.* (1997) showed that BCT was a better value treatment economically than individual behavioral therapy.

Fals-Stewart *et al.* (2001) randomly assigned 36 married (or co-habitating) men, who were beginning methadone maintenance (MM) treatment, to: (1) individual-based MM treatment (IBMM; two individual, weekly, counseling sessions in addition to methadone maintenance) or (2) behavioral couples therapy (BCT; a weekly couples session with female partner, a weekly individual session, and MM). During treatment, men in the BCT condition produced fewer opioid- and cocaine-positive urine specimens than did men in the IBMM condition. In addition, the BCT condition was associated with greater relationship satisfaction during the study and better dyadic functioning at the end of the study. Finally, BCT participants noted fewer family and social problems post-treatment than did IBMM participants.

Psychological therapies and cocaine dependence

In contrast to the treatment of opioid dependence, where behavioral therapies have been most effective when combined with pharmacotherapies (especially agonist interventions, such as methadone maintenance), the cocaine literature is marked by strong evidence suggesting the effectiveness of purely behavioral treatments. Despite many clinical trials examining several pharmacologic agents, no pharmacotherapy currently is available for the general population of cocaine users (Carroll *et al.*, 2000). In contrast, several investigations have shown that comparatively brief, purely behavioral approaches can be both sufficient and effective for the majority of patients.

Behavioral therapies in the context of cocaine dependence

Voucher-based contingency management and cocaine dependence Higgins *et al.*'s (1991, 1993, 2000; Budney & Higgins, 1998) Community Reinforcement Approach (Azrin, 1976) has paved the way toward the success of psychosocial treatments for cocaine dependence. Their treatment regime consists of the following elements: positive incentives for abstinence from cocaine, reciprocal relationship counseling, and disulfiram. This treatment has four essential guiding principles rooted in behavioral pharmacology: (1) drug use and abstinence must be detected both quickly and accurately, (2) abstinence is positively reinforced, (3) drug use results in loss of reinforcement, and (4) the development of competing reinforcers to drug use is emphasized (Higgins *et al.*, 1993).

There are several other important features of the treatment program established by Higgins and colleagues (1991, 1993). In this program, urine samples are obtained thrice weekly. Abstinence, assessed through drug-free urine screens, is reinforced using a voucher system in which patients receive points redeemable for items consistent with a drug-free lifestyle, such as movie tickets, sporting events and similar items. In order to encourage longer periods of drug abstinence, the points earned by patients increase in value with each successive clean urine specimen. Moreover, the value of the points is reset back to its original level when patients produce a drug-positive urine screen or when patients fail to provide a urine screen.

In a series of well-controlled clinical trials, Higgins and colleagues reliably have demonstrated the following: (1) high acceptance, retention, and rates of abstinence for patients involved with this approach (i.e. 85% completing 12 weeks of treatment and 65% achieving 6 or more weeks of abstinence) relative to standard substance abuse counseling (Higgins *et al.*, 1991, 1993); (2) rates of abstinence not declining substantially when less valuable incentives are substituted for the voucher system (Higgins *et al.*, 1993); (3) the value of the voucher system itself (as opposed to other program elements) in yielding good outcomes by comparing the behavioral system with and without the vouchers (Higgins *et al.*, 1994); and, (4) durable effects of the voucher system (Higgins *et al.*, 2000). The initial work with voucher-based contingency management conducted by Higgins and associated investigators now has been widely-replicated in a diverse array of settings and populations, including homeless substance abusers (Milby *et al.*, 1996), freebase cocaine users (Kirby *et al.*, 1998), alcohol-dependent individuals (Petry, 2000a), and cocaine-dependent individuals within methadone maintenance treatment programs (Peirce *et al.*, 2006; Silverman *et al.*, 1996a, 1996b; Rawson *et al.*, 2002).

Low-cost contingency management of cocaine dependence One of the more innovative, state-of-the-art, approaches to treatment of cocaine dependence, derived from work with alcohol-dependent patients, involves providing clients with prizes at variable intervals using the 'fishbowl' methodology (Petry, 2000a). This methodology is an inherently 'low-cost' alternative to traditional, fixed participant, financial reimbursement and is based on extensive demonstrations of the empirical validity of contingency management approaches (Higgins *et al.*, 2000; Petry, 2000b; Petry & Martin, 2002; Petry *et al.*, 2000, 2001, 2005). This technique affords clients the opportunity to choose a prize card from a bowl. Typically, prizes range from $1 to $100 (Petry *et al.*, 2000). The success of this approach is rooted in utilizing this variable schedule of reinforcement, which has been associated with sustained behavioral change (Skinner, 1984). In addition, as only a small percentage of clients win the largest monetary amounts, researchers can minimize their study costs to a greater extent than they could were they to pay each participant the same, fixed amount (Petry *et al.*, 2000).

Petry & Martin (2002) randomly assigned 42 methadone-maintenance patients to 12 weeks of standard treatment or to 12 weeks of standard treatment plus contingency management (CM; fishbowl technique). In the CM condition, drawing from the fishbowl was contingent upon producing cocaine- and opioid-free urines. Individuals in the CM condition had significantly longer episodes of sustained abstinence from cocaine and opioids than individuals in the standard condition. Furthermore, these treatment gains were maintained over a 6-month interval.

Petry *et al.* (2004) expanded the fishbowl technique by randomly assigning cocaine-using individuals to one of three conditions: (1) standard care, (2) standard care plus CM ($80), or (3) standard care plus CM ($240). Both CM conditions yielded similar rates of abstinence from cocaine for individuals whose urines were negative for drugs at intake. However, individuals who produced intake urines positive for drugs had significantly greater abstinence from cocaine when placed in the larger ($240) CM condition than those who only received standard care.

In their study of 120 cocaine-dependent individuals who participated in a methadone maintenance program, Rawson *et al.* (2002) directly compared CM and CBT. Participants were randomly assigned to one of four cells for the 16-week study period: (1) CM (based on providing cocaine-negative urine samples), (2) CBT, (3) CM/CBT, or (4) methadone maintenance treatment program alone (3 weekly clinic visits; MMTP). Three prominent findings emerged. First, during treatment, the CM condition yielded the best outcome in terms of within-treatment, cocaine-free, urine specimens. In contrast, the CBT and MMTP conditions had similar, cocaine-positive, within-treatment urine specimens. Second, the CM, CBT, and CM/CBT conditions all revealed fewer self-reported days of cocaine use by the end of the study period than did the MMTP condition. Third, at both 26- and 52-week follow-up, the CBT condition showed a successful outcome and was indistinguishable from the CM and CM/CBT conditions when considering both cocaine-free urine specimens and self-reported cocaine use. Thus, although CM produced quicker results than were seen within treatment, CBT produced similar success at post-treatment and 6-month follow-up. Furthermore, combining CM and CBT did not lead to a more successful outcome than either condition alone. However, given the more immediate effects of CM and the more delayed effects of CBT in this study, the researchers wondered whether it might be useful to deliver CM initially and CBT later in the treatment process.

Like Rawson *et al.* (2002), Epstein *et al.* (2003) wished to examine whether a combination of CM and CBT might produce superior results for 193 cocaine-using patients (41% were cocaine-dependent) in a methadone maintenance treatment program who were randomized to 12 weeks of group treatment (CBT or a social support control group) and CM (based on providing cocaine-negative urines or based on being yoked to CM participants' urine sample results). In all conditions, individuals received methadone maintenance. For the control condition, participants were unknowingly yoked to an individual in the CM condition, such that they would receive vouchers whenever this other individual received them regardless of their own behavior. Participants in the control condition were told that they would receive vouchers on "a totally unpredictable schedule" as long as they gave a urine sample (Epstein *et al.*, 2003). These investigators discovered that initially, CBT hampered the very strong

effects of CM on reducing cocaine use. However, when comparing the 12-month and 3-month post-treatment results, significant reductions in cocaine use were seen for the CBT/CM condition at 12 months post-treatment.

Other cognitive-behavioral therapies and cocaine dependence Based on social learning theories pertaining to the acquisition and maintenance of substance use disorders (Marlatt & Gordon, 1985), cognitive-behavioral treatment (CBT) has demonstrated effectiveness in the treatment of cocaine-dependent individuals (Carroll, 1998). The goal of CBT (also frequently called relapse prevention or coping skills therapy) is to foster abstinence by teaching patients a set of individualized coping strategies as effective alternatives to substance use. Among the skills typically taught are the following: (1) exploring the positive and negative outcomes of continued use as a means to promote motivation to stop cocaine and other substances; (2) creating a functional analysis of substance use (i.e. understanding substance use in relation to its antecedents and consequences); (3) developing strategies for coping with high-risk situations, including cocaine craving; (4) preparing for emergencies and coping with a relapse to substance use; and (5) identifying and confronting thoughts about substance use (Carroll, 1998).

A number of randomized clinical trials among several diverse cocaine-dependent populations have yielded several salient conclusions. First, compared with other popular psychological therapies for cocaine dependence, CBT appears to be especially more effective with individuals who have more severe cocaine problems or who also have comorbid disorders (Carroll *et al.*, 1991a, 1994a, b; Maude-Griffin *et al.*, 1998; McKay *et al.*, 1997). Second, CBT is significantly more effective than less intensive approaches that have been considered control conditions (Carroll *et al.*, 1998; Monti *et al.*, 1997). Third, CBT is equivalent to or more effective than manualized disease-model approaches (Carroll *et al.*, 1998; Maude-Griffin *et al.*, 1998). Fourth, CBT appears to be a particularly durable treatment with several studies suggesting that patients who participated in CBT may continue to reduce their cocaine use even 1–2 years after leaving treatment (Carroll *et al.*, 1994b, 2000; McKay *et al.*, 1999). Finally, for individuals who have non-drug-abusing partners who are willing to participate in treatment, behavioral couples therapy has been shown to be more effective than individual therapy in terms of reducing within-treatment, cocaine-positive urine samples, for men in methadone maintenance treatment (Fals-Stewart *et al.*, 2001) and for reducing self-reported cocaine use for both male and female outpatients enrolled in substance use treatment (Fals-Stewart *et al.*, 1996; Winters *et al.*, 2002).

Disease model approaches to cocaine dependence and other substances of abuse

The NIDA Collaborative Cocaine Treatment Study (CCTS), a multi-site randomized trial of psychotherapeutic treatments for cocaine dependence (Crits-Christoph *et al.*, 1999), offered strong evidence of the effectiveness of a manualized treatment approach known as Individual Drug Counseling (Carroll, 2000; Mercer & Woody, 1992). In this study, 487 cocaine-dependents were randomized to one of four manual-guided treatment conditions: (1) Cognitive Therapy (Beck *et al.*, 1993) plus Group Drug Counseling (Mercer *et al.*, 1994); (2) Supportive Expressive Therapy, a short-term psychodynamically oriented approach, which helps people feel comfortable discussing personal problems while learning ways to identify and work through interpersonal problems (Luborsky, 1984; Mark & Luborsky, 1992) plus Group Drug Counseling; (3) Individual Drug Counseling, focused on abstinence from drugs and solving areas of impaired functioning (e.g. illegal activity, family issues, and unemployment), plus Group Drug Counseling; or, (4) Group Drug Counseling alone. The treatments offered were intensive (36 individual and 24 group sessions over 24 weeks – a total of 60 sessions) and were met with comparatively poor retention, with patients on average completing less than one-half of sessions offered, with higher rates of retention for subjects assigned to Cognitive Therapy or Supportive-Expressive Therapy (Crits-Christoph *et al.*, 1999). Outcomes on the whole were good, with all groups significantly reducing their cocaine use from baseline; however, the best cocaine outcomes were seen for subjects who received Individual Drug Counseling (Carroll *et al.*, 2000).

The findings from these studies offer compelling support for the efficacy of manual-guided disease-model approaches (Carroll, 2000). This result has important clinical implications, as these approaches are similar to the dominant model applied in most community treatment programs (Horgan and Levine, 1998), and thus may be more easily mastered by "real world" clinicians than approaches such as CM or CBT, treatments whose theoretical underpinnings may not be seen as highly compatible with disease model approaches (Carroll, 2000).

Psychological therapies and amphetamine and methamphetamine dependence

Given the relative ease with which amphetamines and methamphetamines can be manufactured and the minimal cost involved in doing so, it is not surprising that amphetamine and methamphetamine dependence are commonplace (World Health Organization, 2001). Despite the prevalence of amphetamine and methamphetamine dependence, no empirically validated pharmacological and only one empirically validated behavioral treatment of methamphetamine dependence currently exists (Rawson *et al.*, 2004; World Health Organization, 2001).

Baker *et al.* (2001) conducted a randomized controlled trial of brief psychological treatments for regular amphetamine users (individuals who used one or more times per month). Amphetamine users were assigned to one of three conditions: (1) four sessions of CBT (including Motivational Interviewing [MI], relapse-prevention, skills training, coping with cravings) plus a self-help booklet, (2) two sessions of CBT (including a motivational interview and skills training) plus a self-help booklet, or (3) an assessment and a self-help booklet. Overall, all participants, irrespective of treatment assignment, reduced their amphetamine use throughout the course of the study. Participants in either of the CBT conditions reported more than two times less daily amphetamine use than participants in the self-help booklet (control) condition. In addition, at 6-month follow-up, a significantly greater number of individuals in the CBT conditions were abstinent from amphetamine use as compared with the control condition.

Although efficacious behavioral treatments for amphetamine dependence need considerable investigation, the Matrix Model (a manualized, intensive, 16-session treatment which broadens CBT by supplementing it with family education, drug education, and Alcoholics or Narcotics Anonymous meetings) offers some promise for methamphetamine abuse and dependence (Huber *et al.*, 1997; Rawson *et al.*, 2004) after successful use with cocaine addicts (Rawson *et al.*, 1991, 1995). In the biggest randomized clinical trial in existence for methamphetamine dependence, Rawson *et al.* (2004) randomized 978 methamphetamine users at eight sites to one of two outpatient treatment conditions: (1) the Matrix Model or (2) a control condition (standard treatment). The superiority of the Matrix Model, as evidenced by a higher percentage of treatment sessions attended, longer involvement in treatment, greater number of methamphetamine-negative urines, and more days of methamphetamine abstinence, was observed during the treatment phase. However, patients showed less drug use and greater functioning in both conditions when the treatment ended and at 6-month follow-up. That is, the Matrix Model was not significantly better than standard treatment at the end of treatment or at 6-month follow-up.

Low-cost contingency management of amphetamine and methamphetamine dependence Petry *et al.* (2005) randomly assigned 415, outpatient substance abuse treatment, methamphetamine (or cocaine) users to either standard treatment or contingency management (CM; based on providing substance-free urine specimens) and standard treatment. This study was unique in that it was run across eight community-based agencies. Participants in the CM plus standard treatment condition stayed in treatment longer, attended more counseling sessions, produced more substance-free urine specimens (in terms of alcohol, cocaine, and methamphetamines), and achieved abstinence for longer periods of the 12-week study. Surprisingly, the two groups did not differ in terms of the percentage of urine specimens which were positive for substances. These researchers found this treatment to be very cost-effective and noted that the average amount spent on incentives per individual was only $203.

Building upon the earlier work of Petry *et al.* (2005), Peirce *et al.* (2006) conducted a multi-site investigation at six methadone maintenance treatment programmes in various community settings. A total of 388 participants, over 80% of whom were abusing or dependent upon cocaine, methamphetamines, and/or amphetamines (as well as heroin) were randomized either to CM (based on submitting alcohol-free breathalyzer readings and urine samples free of cocaine, methamphetamines, or amphetamines) or a non-CM (standard treatment) condition during the 12-week study. Among the most significant study findings, Peirce *et al.* observed that the CM group was two times more apt as the standard treatment condition to produce alcohol-free and stimulant-free (cocaine, methamphetamines, and amphetamines) urine specimens. Overall, CM participants had 11 times greater chance of remaining abstinent from stimulants than standard treatment participants. No differences were found between the two groups with regard to remaining in the study or attending sessions. Furthermore, the average cost per participant (i.e. $120/day) was approximately 40% less than that found by Petry *et al.* (2005).

Psychological therapies and cannabis dependence

Although it is the most commonly used illicit substance, treatment of cannabis dependence is a comparatively understudied area to date, in part, because relatively few individuals present for treatment with a primary complaint of cannabis dependence. No effective pharmacotherapies for cannabis dependence exist (see Chapter 22), and only a few controlled trials of psychosocial approaches have been completed for adults (Budney *et al.*, 1997; Stephens *et al.*, 1994). In their innovative study using vouchers, Budney *et al.* (2000) randomly assigned outpatients to one of three interventions: (1) motivational enhancement (MET), (2) MET plus behavioral coping skills therapy (MBT), or (3) a combination of the first two approaches plus

voucher-based incentives (MBTV). Overall, the MBTV intervention was the most successful approach as noted by greater marijuana abstinence both during and after treatment. There were no significant differences in patient outcomes between the MET and MBT conditions.

Stephens *et al.* (2000) compared a delayed treatment control, a two-session motivational approach, and a more intensive (14-session) relapse prevention approach. These investigators found better cannabis outcomes for the two active treatments compared with the delayed-treatment control group but no significant differences between the brief and the more intensive treatment. More recently, a replication and extension of the Stephens study (Stephens *et al.*, 2000) involving a multisite trial of 450 adult cannabis-dependent patients, compared three approaches: (1) a delayed treatment control, (2) a 2-session motivational approach, and (3) a 9-session combined motivational/coping skills (case management)/CBT approach (The Marijuana Treatment Research Project Group, 2004). There were four assessment periods: baseline, 4-month, 9-month, and 15-months. Results suggested that both active treatments were associated with significantly greater reductions in marijuana use than the delayed treatment control through the 15-month follow-up. In addition, the 9-session intervention was significantly more effective than the 2-session intervention. Moreover, this effect also was sustained through the 15-month follow-up.

Psychotherapy approaches and cannabis dependence amongst Young adults (ages 18–25 years old)

Drug dependence amongst young adults has begun to receive greater attention in recent years with the vast majority of clinical trials aimed at addressing marijuana use. Sinha *et al.* (2003), for example, compared a three-session motivational enhancement therapy (MET only) with a three-session MET and contingency management therapy (MET/CM). In the CM condition, individuals were given vouchers as a reward for attending treatment. Sixty-five, primarily cannabis-dependent, probation-referred patients, between the ages of 18 to 25 years, were randomly assigned to one of the two conditions. These investigators found that treatment completion was significantly higher in the MET/CM condition than in the MET only condition. Participants in both conditions had significantly less cannabis usage and fewer legal problems than they did before this brief treatment.

Carroll *et al.* (2006) recently studied 136 marijuana-dependent 18- to 25-year-olds who were all referred by the Office of Adult Probation. Individuals were randomly assigned to one of four treatment modalities: (1) motivational enhancement therapy/cognitive-behavioral therapy

Table 18.1. A summary of selected empirically validated cognitive-behavioral and behavioral therapies by drug dependence category

Selected empirically validated treatments	References	Evidence rating
Cognitive-behavioral therapy (CBT); relapse-prevention; coping skills therapy	Cocaine (Carroll, 1998; Carroll *et al.*, 1991b, 1994a, 1994b, 1998, 2000; Epstein *et al.*, 2003; Maude-Griffin *et al.*, 1998; McKay *et al.*, 1997, 1999; Monti *et al.*, 1997; Rawson *et al.*, 2002)	1
	Amphetamines/Methamphetamines (Baker *et al.*, 2001; Huber *et al.*, 1997; Rawson *et al.*, 2004)	2
	Cannabis (Adults: Budney *et al.*, 1997, 2000; The Marijuana Treatment Project Research Group, 2004; Stephens *et al.*, 1994, 2000)	1
	Cannabis (Young Adults: Carroll *et al.*, in press)	2
Motivational enhancement Therapy (MET); Motivational interviewing	Amphetamines/Methamphetamines (Baker *et al.*, 2001)	2
	Cannabis (Adults: Budney *et al.*, 2000; The Marijuana Treatment Project Research Group, 2004)	1
	Cannabis (Young Adults: Carroll *et al.*, in press; Sinha *et al.*, 2003)	2
Twelve-step facilitation therapy (TSF)	Cocaine (Carroll *et al.*, 1998; Maude-Griffin *et al.*, 1998)	2
Drug counseling treatment (group; individual)	Opioids (Institute of Medicine, 1998; McLellan *et al.*, 1993)	2
	Cocaine (Mercer & Woody, 1992)	2
	Amphetamines/Methamphetamines (Institute of Medicine, 1998)	2
Contingency management approaches (CM; including low-cost strategies and vouchers)	Opioids (Iguchi *et al.*, 1996; Petry & Martin, 2002; Robles *et al.*, 2002; Silverman *et al.*, 1996a, 1996b, 2001; Stitzer *et al.*, 1986, 1992, 1993; Stitzer & Bigelow, 1978; Wong *et al.*, 2003, 2004)	1
	Cocaine (Budney & Higgins, 1998; Epstein *et al.*, 2003; Higgins *et al.*, 1991, 1993, 1994, 2000; Kirby *et al.*, 1998; Petry, 2000a; Petry *et al.*, 2004; Petry & Martin, 2002; Peirce *et al.*, 2006; Petry *et al.*, 2005; Rawson *et al.*, 2002; Robles *et al.*, 2002; Silverman *et al.*, 1996a, 1996b, 1998, 2001)	1
	Amphetamines/Methamphetamines (Peirce *et al.*, 2006; Petry *et al.*, 2005)	2
	Cannabis (Adults: Budney *et al.*, 2000)	2
	Cannabis (Young Adults: Carroll *et al.*, in press; Sinha *et al.*, 2003)	2
Behavioral couples therapy; family therapy; family education	Opioids (Fals-Stewart *et al.*, 1996, 2001; McLellan *et al*, 1993; Winters *et al.*, 2002)	2
	Cocaine (Fals-Stewart *et al.*, 1996, 2001; Rawson *et al.*, 1991, 1995; Winters *et al.*, 2002)	2
	Amphetamines/Methamphetamines (Huber *et al.*, 1997; Rawson *et al.*, 2004)	2
Cognitive therapy	Opioids (Woody *et al.*, 1983)	2
	Cocaine (Crits-Christoph *et al.*, 1999)	2
Supportive-Expressive Therapy	Opioids (Woody *et al.*, 1983)	2
	Cocaine (Crits-Christoph *et al.*, 1999)	2

Effectiveness ratings:

1 = Strong Evidence for Efficacy, 2 = Modest Evidence for Efficacy, 3 = No evidence of efficacy.

(MET/CBT) in addition to voucher-based contingency management (CM) based either on attending therapy sessions or providing urine samples free of marijuana, (2) MET/CBT alone, (3) individual drug counseling (DC) in addition to CM, and (4) DC alone. Four primary findings emerged. First, individuals assigned to CM stayed in the study longer and were more apt to provide cannabis-free urine samples than were individuals who were not assigned to CM.

Second, the MET/CBT plus CM condition was superior to all other study treatment modalities in terms of promoting greater study session attendance, consecutive urine samples free of cannabis, and likelihood of having at least one cannabis-free urine sample during the study. Third, these same outcome measures were significantly worse for individuals in the DC alone condition. Finally, individuals in either MET/CBT condition were able to maintain their treatment gains by continuing to use cannabis less frequently at 6-month follow-up than they did pre-treatment.

Summary and conclusions

In conclusion, a variety of effective psychological treatments for drug dependence disorders have been identified in recent years for adult opioid-, cocaine-, amphetamine-, methamphetamine-, and cannabis-dependent populations (Table 18.1). Less work has focused on individuals with sedatives (other than alcohol), phencyclidine (PCP), ecstasy (MDMA) dependence, or inhalants. For drug use disorders, such as cocaine dependence, where no overall effective pharmacotherapies exist, a number of brief psychological approaches have been demonstrated to yield robust and durable effects. For classes of drug dependence for which powerfully effective pharmacotherapies exist, such as opioid dependence, psychological treatments have been found with some consistency to extend, strengthen and augment treatment effects.

Despite these advances, the identification of empirically valid psychological therapies has not been met with their rapid integration into general clinical practice (Carroll, 2000; Carroll & Onken, 2005). A number of barriers exist which impede the broader use of effective therapies (Simpson *et al.*, 1997). Among the frequently cited barriers are the lack of an organized system for disseminating effective psychological treatments to the clinical community and failure of researchers to design their studies with critical clinical questions in mind and as well as consideration for cost-effectiveness. Yet, encouraging signs continue to emerge. As an example, several rigorous trials evaluating psychological treatments have taken seriously the need to report cost-effectiveness data (Avants *et al.*, 1999; Kraft *et al.*, 1997). Similar to cost evaluations of psychotherapeutic approaches for other psychiatric conditions (Gabbard, 2000), these novel studies have highlighted how psychological therapies for treating drug dependence are associated with a number of significant cost savings (Carroll, 2000; Klostermann *et al.*, 2004; Fals-Stewart *et al.*, 1997; Petry *et al.*, 2005; Peirce, *et al.*, 2006).

The level of evidence for each of the interventions discussed in this chapter is summarized in Table 18.2.

Table 18.2. Effectiveness of empirically validated psychological therapies for drug dependence

Treatment	Form of treatment	Psychiatric disorder/ target audience	Level of evidence for efficacy	Comments
Behavioral Therapy	Contingency Management	Opioid dependence	Ia	Multiple studies including community-based programs support the effectiveness in reducing opiate usage
Behavioral Therapy	Voucher-based contingency management	Cocaine dependence	Ia	High acceptance, retention and rates of abstinence
Psychological Therapy/ Psychotherapy	Supportive-expressive or cognitive	Opioid dependence	Ib	Both types of psychological therapy more effective than drug counseling alone
Psychological Therapy/ Psychotherapy	Cognitive- behavioral therapy	Cocaine dependence	Ia	Very effective in severe cocaine abuse and in people with co-morbidities and effects appear to be durable
Psychological Therapy/ Psychotherapy	Individual Drug Counseling (A Manualized Treatment)	Cocaine dependence	Ia	As effective as CBT and Supportive-Expressive therapy with best outcomes for Individual Drug Counseling and cocaine
Psychological Therapy/ Psychotherapy	Cognitive- behavioral therapy	Amphetamine dependence	Ib	CBT groups reported two times less daily amphetamine usage
Psychological Therapy/ Psychotherapy	Motivational enhancement plus vouchers	Cannabis dependence	Ib	Both types of psychological therapy more effective than drug counseling alone
Psychological Therapy/ Psychotherapy	Behavioral Couples Therapy	Opioid and Cocaine Dependence	Ib	Shown to be more effective than individual counseling

REFERENCES

Avants, S. K., Margolin, A., Sindelar, J. L. *et al.* (1999). Day treatment versus enhanced standard methadone services for opioid-dependent patients: a comparison of clinical efficacy and cost. *American Journal of Psychiatry*, **156**, 27–33.

Azrin, N. H. (1976). Improvements in the community-reinforcement approach to alcoholism. *Behavior Research and Therapy*, **14**, 339–48.

Baker, A., Boggs, T. G. & Lewin, T. J. (2001). Randomized controlled brief cognitive-behavioural interventions among regular users of amphetamine. *Addiction*, **96**, 1279–87.

Ball, J. C. & Ross, A. (1991). *The Effectiveness of Methadone Maintenance Treatment*. New York: Springer-Verlag.

Ball, J., Lange, W. R., Myers, C. P. & Friedman, S. R. (1988). Reducing the risk of AIDS through methadone maintenance treatment. *Journal of Health and Social Behavior*, **29**, 214–16.

Bandura, A. (1977a). *Social Learning Theory*. Englewood Cliffs, NJ: Prentice-Hall.

Bandura, A. (1977b). Self-efficacy: Towards a unifying theory of behavior change. *Psychological Review*, **84**, 191–215.

Beck, A. T., Wright, F. D., Newman, C. F. & Liese, B. S. (1993). *Cognitive Therapy of Substance Abuse*. New York: Guilford Press.

Brill, L. (1977). The treatment of drug abuse: evolution of a perspective. *American Journal of Psychiatry*, **134**, 157–160.

Budney, A. J. & Higgins, S. T. (1998). *A Community Reinforcement Plus Vouchers Approach: Treating Cocaine Addiction*. Rockville, MD: NIDA.

Budney, A. J., Kandel, D. B., Cherek, D. R., Martin, B. R., Stephens, R. S. & Roffman, R. (1997). Marijuana use and dependence. *Drug and Alcohol Dependence*, **45**, 1–11.

Budney, A. J., Higgins, S. T., Radonovich, K. J. & Novy, P. L. (2000). Adding voucher-based incentives to coping skills and motivational enhancement improves outcomes during treatment for marijuana dependence. *Journal of Consulting and Clinical Psychology*, **68**, 1051–61.

Carroll, K. C. (2000). Science-based therapies for drug dependence. *The Economics of Neuroscience*, **2**, 41–7.

Carroll, K. M. (1997). Integrating psychotherapy and pharmacotherapy to improve drug abuse outcomes. *Journal of Addictive Behaviors*, **22**, p. 233–45.

Carroll, K. M. (1998). *A Cognitive-Behavioural Approach: Treating Cocaine Addiction*. Rockville, MD: National Institute on Drug Abuse.

Carroll, K. M. & Onken, L. S. (2005). Behavioral therapies for drug abuse. *American Journal of Psychiatry*, **162**, 1452–60.

Carroll, K., Rounsaville, B. & Keller, D. (1991a). Relapse prevention strategies for the treatment of cocaine abuse. *American Journal of Drug and Alcohol Abuse*, **17**(3), 249–65.

Carroll, K. M., Rounsaville, B. J. & Gawin, F. H. (1991b). A comparative trial of psychotherapies for ambulatory cocaine abusers: Relapse Prevention and Interpersonal Psychotherapy. *American Journal of Drug and Alcohol Abuse*, **17**, 229–47.

Carroll, K. M., Rounsaville, B. J., Gordon, L. T. *et al.* (1994a). Psychotherapy and pharmacotherapy for ambulatory cocaine abusers. *Archives of General Psychiatry*, **51**, 177–87.

Carroll, K. M., Rounsaville, B. J., Nich, C., Gordon, L. T., Wirtz, P. W. & Gawin, F. H. (1994b). One year follow-up of psychotherapy and pharmacotherapy for cocaine dependence: delayed emergence of psychotherapy effects. *Archives of General Psychiatry*, **51**, 989–97.

Carroll, K. M., Nich, C., Ball, S. A., McCance-Katz, E. F., Frankforter, T. & Rounsaville, B. J. (2000). One year follow-up of disulfiram and psychotherapy for cocaine-alcohol abusers: sustained effects of treatment. *Addiction*, **95**(9), 1335–49.

Carroll, K. M., Easton, C. J., Nich, C. *et al.* (2006). The use of contingency management and motivational/skills-building therapy to treat young adults with marijuana dependence. *Journal of Consulting and Clinical Psychology*, **74**, 955–66.

Carroll, K. M., Nich, C., Ball, S. A., McCance, E. & Rounsaville, B. J. (1998). Treatment of cocaine and alcohol dependence with psychotherapy and disulfiram. *Addiction*, **93**, 713–28.

Chambless, D. L., Sanderson, W. C., Shoham, V. *et al.* (1996). An update on empirically validated therapies. *The Clinical Psychologist*, **49**, 5–18.

Chambless, D. L., Baker, M. J., Baucom, D. H. *et al.* (1998). Update on empirically validated therapies, II. *The Clinical Psychologist*, **51**, 3–16.

Childress, A. R., McLellan, A. T. & O'Brien, C. P. (1984). Assessment and extinction of conditioned withdrawal-like responses in an integrated treatment for opiate dependence. In *Problems of Drug Dependence*, ed. L. S. Harris, pp. 202–10. National Institute on Drug Abuse: Rockville, MD.

Childress, A. R., Hole, A. V., Ehrman, R. N., Robbins, S. J., McLellan, A. T. & O'Brien, C. P. (1993). Cue reactivity and cue reactivity interventions in drug dependence. In *Behavioural Treatments for Drug Abuse and Dependence*, ed. L. S. Onken, J. D. Blaine, & J. J. Boren, pp. 73–95. Rockville, MD: National Institute on Drug Abuse.

Crits-Christoph, P., Siqueland, L., Blaine, J. *et al.* (1999). Psychosocial treatments for cocaine dependence: results of the National Institute on Drug Abuse Collaborative Cocaine Study. *Archives of General Psychiatry*, **56**, 495–502.

Epstein, D. H., Hawkins, W. E., Covi, L., Umbricht, A. & Preston, K. L. (2003). Cognitive-behavioral therapy plus contingency management for cocaine use: Findings during treatment and across 12-month follow-up. *Psychology of Addictive Behaviors*, **17**, 73–82.

Fals-Stewart, W., Birchler, G. R. & O'Farrell, T. J. (1996). Behavioral couples therapy for male substance-abusing patients: effects on relationship adjustment and drug-using behavior. *Journal of Consulting and Clinical Psychology*, **64**, 959–72.

Fals-Stewart, W., O'Farrell, T. J. & Birchler, G. R., (1997). Behavioral couples therapy for male substance abusing patients: a cost outcomes analysis. *Journal of Consulting and Clinical Psychology*, **65**, 789–802.

Fals-Stewart, W., O'Farrell, T. J. & Birchler, G. R., (2001). Behavioral couples therapy for male methadone maintenance patients:

effects on drug-using behavior and relationship adjustment. *Behavior Therapy*, **32**, 391–411.

Gabbard, G. O. (2000). Is psychotherapy cost-effective? *The Economics of Neuroscience*, **2**, 40–3.

Galanter, M. (1993). *Network Therapy for Alcohol and Drug Abuse: A New Approach in Practice*. New York: Basic Books.

Haynes, R. B., Taylor, D. W. & Sackett, D. L. (1979). *Compliance in Health Care*. Baltimore, MD: Johns Hopkins University Press.

Higgins, S. T., Delaney, D. D., Budney, A. J. *et al.* (1991). A behavioural approach to achieving initial cocaine abstinence. *American Journal of Psychiatry*, **148**, 1218–24.

Higgins, S. T., Budney, A. J., Bickel, W. K. & Hughes, J. R. (1993). Achieving cocaine abstinence with a behavioural approach. *American Journal of Psychiatry*, **150**, 763–9.

Higgins, S. T., Budney, A. J., Bickel, W. K., Foerg, F. E., Donham, R. & Badger, G. J. (1994). Incentives improve outcome in outpatient behavioural treatment of cocaine dependence. *Archives of General Psychiatry*, **51**, 568–76.

Higgins, S. T., Wong, C. J., Badger, G. J., Haug-Ogden, D. E. & Dantona, R. L. (2000). Contingent reinforcement increases cocaine abstinence during outpatient treatment and one year follow-up. *Journal of Consulting and Clinical Psychology*, **68**, 64–72.

Horgan, C. M. & Levine, H. J. (1998). The substance abuse treatment system: What does it look like and whom does it serve? Preliminary findings from the Alcohol and Drug Services Study. In *Bridging the Gap Between Practice and Research: Forging Partnerships with Community-Based Drug and Alcohol Treatment*, ed. S. Lamb, M. R. Greenlick, & D. McCarty, pp. 186–97. Washington, DC: National Academy Press.

Huber, A., Ling, W., Shoptaw, S., Gulati, V., Brethen, P. & Rawson, R. (1997). Integrating treatments for methamphetamine abuse: a psychosocial perspective. *Journal of Addictive Diseases*, **16**, 41–50.

Iguchi, M. Y., Lamb, R. J., Belding, M. A., Platt, J. J., Husband, S. D. & Morral, A. R. (1996). Contingent reinforcement of group participation versus abstinence in a methadone maintenance program. *Experimental and Clinical Psychopharmacology*, **4**, 1–7.

Institute of Medicine (1998). *Bridging the Gap Between Practice and Research: Forging Partnerships with Community-based Drug and Alcohol Treatment*. Washington, DC: National Academy Press.

Keller, D. S., Carroll, K. M., Nich, C. & Rounsaville, B. J. (1995). Differential treatment response in alexithymic cocaine abusers: findings from a randomized clinical trial of psychotherapy and pharmacotherapy. *American Journal on Addictions*, **4**, 234–44.

Khantzian, E. J. (1975). Self-selection and progression in drug dependence. *Psychiatry Digest*, **10**, 19–22.

Kirby, K. C., Marlowe, D. B., Festinger, D. S., Lamb, R. J. & Platt, J. J. (1998). Schedule of voucher deliver influences initiation of cocaine abstinence. *Journal of Consulting and Clinical Psychology*, **66**, 761–7.

Klostermann, K., Fals-Stewart, W. & Yates, B. T. (2004). Behavioral couples therapy for substance abuse: a cost analysis. *Alcoholism, Clinical, and Experimental Research*, **28**, 164A.

Kosten, T. R. & McCance, E. F. (1996). A review of pharmacotherapies for substance abuse. *American Journal on Addictions*, **5**, 58–64.

Kraft, M. K., Rothbard, A. B., Hadlye, T. R., McLellan, A. T. & Asch, D. A. (1997). Are supplementary services provided during methadone maintenance really cost-effective? *American Journal of Psychiatry*, **154**, 1214–19.

Longabaugh, R., Beattie, M., Noel, R., Stout, R. & Malloy, P. (1993). The effect of social support on treatment outcome. *Journal of Studies on Alcohol*, **54**, 465–78.

Lowinson, J. H., Marion, I. J., Joseph, H. & Dole, V. P. (1992). Methadone maintenance. In *Comprehensive Textbook of Substance Abuse*, 2nd edn, ed. J. H. Lowinsohn, P. Ruiz, & R. B. Millman. New York: Williams and Wilkins.

Luborsky, L. (1984). *Principles of Psychoanalytic Psychotherapy: A Manual for Supportive-Expressive (SE) Treatment*. New York: Basic Books.

Mark, D. & Luborsky, L. (1992). *A Manual for the Use of Supportive-Expressive Psychotherapy in the Treatment of Cocaine Abuse*. Philadelphia, PA: Department of Psychiatry, University of Pennsylvania.

Marlatt, G. A. & Gordon, J. R. (1985). *Relapse Prevention: Maintenance Strategies in the Treatment of Addictive Behaviors*. New York: Guilford Press.

Maude-Griffin, P. M., Hohenstein, J. M., Humfleet, G. L., Reilly, P. M., Tusel, D. J. & Hall, S. M. (1998). Superior efficacy of cognitive-behavioural therapy for crack cocaine abusers: main and matching effects. *Journal of Consulting and Clinical Psychology*, **66**, 832–7.

McCrady, B. S. & Epstein, E. E. (1995). Marital therapy in the treatment of alcohol problems. In *Clinical Handbook of Couple Therapy*, ed. N. S. Jacobson & A. S. Gurman, pp. 369–93.

McGovern, M. P. & Carroll, K. M. (2003). Evidence-based practices for substance use disorders. *Psychiatric Clinics of North America*, **26**, 991–1010.

McKay, J. R., Alterman, A. I., Cacciola, J. S., Rutherford, M. J., O'Brien, C. P. & Koppenhaver, J. (1997). Group counseling versus individualized relapse prevention aftercare following intensive outpatient treatment for cocaine dependence. *Journal of Consulting and Clinical Psychology*, **65**, 778–88.

McKay, J. R., Alterman, A. I., Cacciola, J. S., O'Brien, C. P., Koppenhave, J. M. & Shepard, D. S. (1999). Continuing care for cocaine dependence: Comprehensive 2-year outcomes. *Journal of Consulting and Clinical Psychology*, **67**, 420–7.

McLellan, A. T. & McKay, J. R. (1998). The treatment of addiction: what can research offer practice? In *Bridging the Gap Between Practice and Research: Forging Partnerships with Community Based Drug and Alcohol Treatment*, ed. S. Lamb, M. R. Greenlick & D. McCarty, pp. 147–85. Washington, DC: National Academy Press.

McLellan, A. T., Arndt, I. O., Metzger, D. S., Woody, G. E. & O'Brien, C. P. (1993). The effects of psychosocial services in substance abuse treatment. *Journal of the American Medical Association*, **269**, 1953–9.

Meichenbaum, D. & Turk, D. C. (1987). *Facilitating Treatment Adherence*. New York: Plenum.

Mercer, D. & Woody, G. (1992). *Addiction Counseling*. Philadelphia, PA: Center for Studies of Addiction, University of Pennsylvania/Philadelphia VAMC.

Mercer, D., Carpenter, G., Daley, D., Patterson, C. & Volpicelli, J. (1992). *Addiction Recovery Manual* (Vol 2). Philadelphia, PA: Treatment Research Unit, University of Pennsylvania.

Metzger, D.S.W., McLellan, A.T., O'Brien, C.P., Druley, P., Navaline, H., Dephilippis, D. *et al.* Human immunodeficiency virus seroconversion along in and out-of-treatment drug users: An 18-month prospective follow-up. *Journal of AIDS*, 1993. **6**, 1049–56.

Milby, J.B., Schumacher, J.E., Raczynski, J.M. *et al.* (1996). Sufficient conditions for effective treatment of substance abusing homeless persons. *Drug and Alcohol Dependence* **43**, 23–8.

Miller, W.R. & Rollnick, S. (1991). *Motivational Interviewing: Preparing People to Change Addictive Behavior*. New York: Guilford Press.

Miller, W.R., Zweben, A., DiClemente, C.C. & Rychtarik, R.G. (1992). *Motivational enhancement therapy manual: A clinical research guide for therapists treating individuals with alcohol abuse and dependence*. NIAAA Project MATCH Monograph Series. Vol. 2. Rockville, MD: National Institute on Alcohol Abuse and Alcoholism.

Monti, P.M., Abrams, D.B., Kadden, R.M. & Cooney, N.L. (1989). *Treating Alcohol Dependence: A Coping skills training guide in the treatment of alcoholism*. 1989, New York: Guilford.

Monti, P.M., Rohsenow, D.J., Michalec, E., Martin, R.A. & Abrams, D.B. (1997). Brief coping skills treatment for cocaine abuse: substance abuse outcomes at three months. *Addiction*, **92**, 1717–28.

National Institute on Drug Abuse (2004). Scientifically based approaches to drug addiction treatment. *Principle of Drug Addiction Treatment: A Research Based Guide*, pp. 1–7. Rockville, MD: National Institute on Drug Abuse.

Nowinski, J., Baker, S. & Carroll, K.M., (1992). *Twelve-step Facilitation Therapy Manual: A Clinical Research Guide for Therapists Treating Individuals with Alcohol Abuse and Dependence*. NIDA Research Monograph Series. Vol. 1. Rockville, MD: National Institute on Alcohol Abuse and Alcoholism.

Nyswander, M., Winick, C., Bernstein, A., Brill, I., & Kaufer, G. (1958). The treatment of drug addicts as voluntary outpatients: a progress report. *American Journal of Orthopsychiatry*, **28**, 714–27.

O'Brien, C.P. (1996). Recent developments in the pharmacotherapy of substance abuse. *Journal of Consulting and Clinical Psychology*, **64**, 677–86.

O'Farrell, T.J. & Fals-Stewart, W. (2000). Behavioral couples therapy for alcoholism and drug abuse. *Journal of Substance Abuse Treatment*, **18**, 51–4.

O'Malley, J.E., Anderson, W.H. & Lazare, A. (1972). Failure of outpatient treatment of drug abuse. I. Heroin. *American Journal of Psychiatry*, **128**, 865–8.

Peirce, J.M., Petry, N.M., Stitzer, M.L. *et al.* (2006). Effects of lower-cost incentives on stimulant abstinence in methadone maintenance treatment: A National Drug Abuse Treatment Clinical Trials Network study. *Archives of General Psychiatry*, **63**, 201–8.

Petry, N.M. (2000a). Given them prizes and they will come: Contingency management for the treatment of alcohol dependence. *Journal of Consulting and Clinical Psychology*, **68**, 250–7.

Petry, N.M. (2000b). A comprehensive guide for the application of contingency management procedures in standard clinic settings. *Drug and Alcohol Dependence*, **58**, 9–25.

Petry, N.M. & Martin, B. (2002). Low-cost contingency management for treating cocaine- and opioid-abusing methadone patients. *Journal of Consulting and Clinical Psychology*, **70**(2), 398–402.

Petry, N.M., Martin, B., Cooney, J.L. & Kranzler, H.R. (2000). Give them prizes, and they will come: contingency management for treatment of alcohol dependence. *Journal of Consulting and Clinical Psychology*, **68**(2), 250–7.

Petry, N.M., Tedford, J. & Martin, B. (2001). Reinforcing compliance with non-drug related activities. *Journal of Substance Abuse Treatment*, **158**, 694–702.

Petry, N., Tedford, J., Austin, M., Nich, C., Carroll, K.C. & Rounsaville, B.J. (2004). Prize reinforcement contingency management for treating cocaine users: How long can we go, and with whom. *Addiction*, **99**(3), 349–60.

Petry, N.M., Peirce, J.M., Stitzer, M.L. *et al.* (2005). Effect of prize-based incentives on outcomes in stimulant abusers in outpatient psychosocial treatment programs: A National Drug Abuse Treatment Clinical Trials Network study. *Archives of General Psychiatry*, **62**, 1148–56.

Rawson, R.A., Obert, J.L., McCann, M.J. & Ling, W. (1991). Psychological approaches for the treatment of cocaine dependence – A neurobehavioral approach. *Journal of Addictive Diseases*, **11**, 97–119.

Rawson, R., Shoptaw, S., Obert, J.L. *et al.* (1995). An intensive outpatient approach for cocaine abuse: the matrix model. *Journal of Substance Abuse Treatment*, **12**(2), 117–27.

Rawson, R.A., Huber, A., McCann, M.J. *et al.* (2002). A comparison of contingency management and cognitive-behavioral approaches during methadone maintenance for cocaine dependence. *Archives of General Psychiatry*, **59**, 817–24.

Rawson, R.A., Marinelli-Casey, P., Anglin, M.D. *et al.* (2004). (Methamphetamine Treatment Project Corporate Authors) A multi-site comparison of psychosocial approaches for the treatment of methamphetamine dependence. *Addiction*, **99**(6), 708–17.

Robles, E., Stitzer, M.L., Strain, E.C., Bigelow, G.E. & Silverman, K. (2002). Voucher-based reinforcement of opiate abstinence during methadone detoxification. *Drug and Alcohol Dependence*, **65**(2), 179–89.

Rollnick, S., Mason, P. & Butler, C. (1999). *Health Behavior Change: A Guide for Practitioners*. London, UK: Harcourt Brace and Company Limited.

Rounsaville, B.J. (1995). Can psychotherapy rescue naltrexone treatment of opioid addiction? In *Potentiating the Efficacy of Medications: Integrating Psychosocial Therapies with*

Pharmacotherapies in the Treatment of Drug Dependence, ed. L. S. Onken & J. D., Blaine, pp. 37–52. Rockville, MD: National Institute on Drug Abuse.

Rounsaville, B. J. & Carroll, K. M. (1997). Individual psychotherapy. In *Comprehensive Textbook of Substance Abuse*, 3rd edn, ed. J. H. Lowinsohn, P. Ruiz & R. B. Millman, pp. 430–9. New York: Williams and Wilkins.

Silverman, K., Higgins, S. T., Brooner, R. K. *et al.* (1996a). Sustained cocaine abstinence in methadone maintenance patients through voucher-based reinforcement therapy. *Archives of General Psychiatry*, **53**, 409–15.

Silverman, K., Wong, C. J., Higgins, S. T. *et al.* (1996b). Increasing opiate abstinence through voucher-based reinforcement therapy. *Drug and Alcohol Dependence*, **41**, 157–65.

Silverman, K., Wong, C. J., Umbricht-Schneiter, A., Montoya, I. D., Schuster, C. R. & Preston, K. L. (1998). Broad beneficial effects of cocaine abstinence reinforcement among methadone patients. *Journal of Consulting and Clinical Psychology*, **66**, 811–24.

Silverman, K., Svikis, D., Robles, E., Stitzer, M. L. & Bigelow, G. E. (2001). A reinforcement-based Therapeutic Workplace for the treatment of drug abuse: six-month abstinence outcomes. *Experimental and Clinical Psychopharmacology*, **9**, 14–23.

Simpson, D. D., Joe, G. W., Broome, K. M., Hiller, M. L., Knight, K. & Rowan-Szal, G. A. (1997). Program diversity and treatment retention rates in the Drug Abuse Treatment Outcome Study (DATOS). *Psychology of Addictive Behaviors*, **11**, 279–93.

Sinha, R., Easton, C., Renee-Aubin, L. & Carroll, K. M. (2003). Engaging young probation-referred marijuana-abusing individuals in treatment: A pilot trial. *The American Journal on Addictions*, **12**, 314–23.

Skinner, B. F. (1984). *About Behaviorism*. New York: Random House, Inc.

Sorenson, J. L. & Copeland, A. L. (2000). Drug abuse treatment as an HIV prevention strategy: a review. *Drug and Alcohol Dependence*, **59**, 17–31.

Stephens, R. S., Roffman, R. A. & Simpson, E. E. (1994). Treating adult marijuana dependence: a test of the relapse prevention model. *Journal of Consulting and Clinical Psychology*, **62**, 92–9.

Stephens, R. S., Roffman, R. A. & Curtin, L. (2000). Comparison of extended versus brief treatments for marijuana use. *Journal of Consulting and Clinical Psychology*, **68**(5), 898–908.

Stitzer, M. L. & Bigelow, G. E. (1978). Contingency management in a methadone maintenance program: availability of reinforcers. *International Journal of the Addictions*, **13**, 737–46.

Stitzer, M. L., Bickel, W. K., Bigelow, G. E & Liebson, I. A. (1986). Effect of methadone dose contingencies on urinalysis test results of polydrug-abusing methadone maintenance patients. *Drug and Alcohol Dependence*, **18**, 341–8.

Stitzer, M. L., Iguchi, M. Y. & Felch, L. J. (1992). Contingent take-home incentive: effects on drug use of methadone maintenance patients. *Journal of Consulting and Clinical Psychology*, **60**, 927–34.

Stitzer, M. L., Iguchi, M. Y., Kidorf, M. & Bigelow, G. E. (1993). Contingency management in methadone treatment: the case for positive incentives. In *Behavioural Treatments for Drug Abuse and Dependence*, ed. L. S. Onken, J. D. Blaine, J. J., Boren, pp. 19–36. Rockville, MD: National Institute on Drug Abuse.

Taylor, G. J., Parker, J. D. & Bagby, R. M. (1990). A preliminary investigation of alexithymia in men with psychoactive substance dependence. *American Journal of Psychiatry*, **147**, 1228–30.

The Marijuana Treatment Project Research Group (2004). Brief treatments for cannabis dependence: Findings from a randomized multisite trial. *Journal of Consulting and Clinical Psychology*, **72**(3), 455–66.

Winters, J., Fals-Stewart, W., O'Farrell, T. J., Birchler, G. R. & Kelley, M. L. (2002). Behavioral couples therapy for female substance-abusing patients: effects on substance use and relationship adjustment. *Journal of Consulting and Clinical Psychology*, **70**, 344–55.

Wong, C. J., Dillon, E. M., Sylvest, C. E. & Silverman, K. (2004). Contingency management of reliable attendance of chronically unemployed substance abusers in a therapeutic workplace. *Experimental and Clinical Psychopharmacology*, **12**(1), 39–46.

Wong, C. J., Sheppard, J-M., Dallery, J. *et al.* (2003). Effects of reinforcer magnitude on data-entry productivity in chronically unemployed drug abusers participating in a therapeutic workplace. *Experimental and Clinical Psychopharmacology*, **11**(1), 46–55.

Woody, G. E., Luborsky, L., McLellan, A. T. *et al.* (1983). Psychotherapy for opiate addicts: does it help? *Archives of General Psychiatry*, **40**, 639–45.

Woody, G. E., McLellan, A. T., Luborsky, L. & O'Brien, C. P. (1995). Psychotherapy in community methadone programs: a validation study. *American Journal of Psychiatry*, **152**, 1302–8.

World Health Organization (2001). *Systematic Review of Treatment for Amphetamine-related Disorders*. Management of substance dependence review series. Geneva, Switzerland: WHO.

19

Treatment of stimulant dependence

Mehmet Sofuoglu, Kostas Agath and Thomas R. Kosten

Editor's note

Cocaine, amphetamine and methamphetamine are the stimulants considered in this chapter. Yet most of the treatments discussed primarily deal with issues related to cocaine. Despite a growing knowledge base as to the underlying action of stimulants, we have not found psychopharmacologic treatments that consistently can be counted upon to be effective in the treatment of the misuse of substances within this class. There are single randomized control trials that show effectiveness for fluoxetine, imipramine, disulfiram, some dopamine agents and adrenergic blocking agents, but there are few RCT replications of the effectiveness of these agents. The treatment of stimulant abuse remains primarily psychosocial, especially treatments that use a cognitive-behavioral approach, an approach whose effectiveness can be further enhanced with contingency management and the use of vouchers. There is some growing interest and studies of combined cognitive behavioral approaches with pharmacotherapy, but even here no single pharmacotherapeutic agent or class of agents stands out. The measures of effectiveness are usually (a) the presence of drug-free urines and (b) the continued involvement in the treatment program which is referred to as treatment retention.

Introduction

Cocaine and amphetamine addictions have become major public health concerns for over 20 years worldwide. The estimated annual prevalence of cocaine abusers in the population over 15 years of age is 0.3% globally, 0.4% in Europe and 1.7% in the Americas, while the relevant figures for amphetamine abusers are 0.6% globally, 0.7% in Europe and 0.7% in the Americas (United Nations Office for Drug Control and Crime Prevention, 2000). Of all treatment cases (excluding alcohol), cocaine abuse represents 29% in USA and 5% in the European Union (United Nations Office for Drug Control and Crime Prevention, 2000). Over the last decade there was a decrease in cocaine consumption in USA and an increase of consumption of both cocaine and amphetamine-type stimulants in Europe (United Nations Office for Drug Control and Crime Prevention, 2000). Methamphetamine abuse is an international public health problem, with two-thirds of the world's 33 million amphetamine abusers living in Asia (Ahmad, 2003).

In the US, there are an estimated 2 million dependent cocaine and amphetamine users (National Institute on Drug Abuse, 1998; SAMHSA, 2000). In the UK the misuse of cocaine is higher than the use of amphetamines. Of the treatment services users in the UK, 6% report cocaine and 4% report amphetamine as a primary drug (National Treatment Agency, 2002), although misuse within a multi-substance misuse pattern seems to be more frequent, with 50% of heroin users reporting use of stimulants in the last 3 months (Gossop et al., 1998), 60% of problematic crack misusers being opiate users (Greater London Alcohol and Drug Alliance, 2004) and 34% of stimulant users being problem drinkers (Farrell et al., 1998). Crack cocaine misuse is twice as frequent as cocaine powder misuse (Greater London Alcohol and Drug Alliance, 2004).

The risks associated with stimulant use are enormous and include increased risk of HIV, hepatitis C and B infection, increased crime and violence, as well as medical, financial, and psychosocial problems. Thus developing effective treatments for stimulant addiction is an essential goal. In this chapter, we will provide a brief overview of current treatment approaches for stimulant use disorders.

For cocaine, smoking free base cocaine (crack) is the preferred method of use. Intranasal and intravenous routes are also commonly used. The effects of snorted

Cambridge Textbook of Effective Treatments in Psychiatry, ed. Peter Tyrer and Kenneth R. Silk. Published by Cambridge University Press.
© Cambridge University Press, 2008.

cocaine generally occur within 15 to 20 minutes, whereas the peak effects from intravenous or smoked cocaine are reached within 3–5 minutes (Benowitz, 1993). Amphetamines are usually taken orally or intravenously and produce actions similar to those of cocaine. Similar to crack-cocaine, a smoked version of methamphetamine (Ice, Crank) is also available (Cho & Melega, 2002). Due to its long duration of action, methamphetamine can produce euphoria lasting 12 to 24 hours.

Clinical aspects of stimulant use

As defined by DSM-IV, stimulant dependence is characterized by compulsive use of stimulants at the expense of important activities and responsibilities. Stimulant use is continued in spite of the physical or psychological problems caused by drug use and the individual has a chronic desire or makes unsuccessful attempts to cut down or quit stimulant use. Dependence may have a physiological component characterized by tolerance or withdrawal. Stimulant abuse, on the other hand, is a maladaptive drug use with associated social, and medical consequences but without the typical compulsive drug use pattern of drug dependence (American Psychiatric Association, 1994).

Stimulant intoxication is characterized by euphoria, hyperalertness, grandiosity, anxiety, restlessness, stereotypical behavior, psychomotor agitation, and impaired judgment (American Psychiatric Association, 1994). Physical signs and symptoms include tachycardia, bradycardia, dilated pupils, elevated or lowered blood pressure, perspiration or chills, nausea or vomiting, weight loss, chest pain, cardiac arrhythmia, confusion, seizures, dyskinesia or dystonias. Treatment of stimulant intoxication includes close monitoring of the symptoms in a safe environment until the symptoms subside. In most cases, benzodiazepines are sufficient to alleviate the symptoms of intoxication. Judicious use of antipsychotics should be reserved for more severe cases when psychosis is present (Kosten, 2002).

Stimulant-induced psychotic disorder is seen in high-dose, chronic stimulant users, often during binge episodes or during withdrawal (Brady *et al.*, 1991; Manschreck *et al.*, 1998; Satel & Edell, 1991; Satel *et al.*, 1991). The clinical presentation includes delusions, hallucinations, paranoid thinking, and stereotyped compulsive behavior. Amphetamines are more likely to induce paranoia than cocaine, perhaps due to their longer elimination half-life (Ujike, 2002). Treatment of stimulant intoxication paranoia involves close clinical monitoring and short-term treatment with antipsychotics.

Following heavy use, stimulants can also produce a state of mental confusion and excitement, known as stimulant delirium (Nakatani & Hara, 1998; Ruttenber *et al.*, 1997). Delirium is characterized with disturbances in consciousness, disorientation and perceptual disturbances such as visual and auditory hallucinations (American Psychiatric Association, 1994). Since delirium indicates stimulant overdose, patients need intensive monitoring for medical complications associated with stimulant overdose including seizures, cardiac arrhythmias, vascular and pulmonary complications (Shanti & Lucas, 2003). Benzodiazepines are preferred over antipsychotics for control of agitation since antipsychotics may decrease seizure threshold and worsen the hyperthermia associated with stimulant overdose. Acutely, benzodiazepines can also help minimize the need for physical restraints.

Stimulant withdrawal is characterized by depressed mood; fatigue; vivid, unpleasant dreams; insomnia or hypersomnia; increased appetite; and psychomotor retardation or agitation following cessation of stimulant use (American Psychiatric Association, 1994). Greater amounts and more sustained duration of use are associated with more severe withdrawal symptoms and more severe withdrawal symptoms seem to be associated with poor treatment outcome (Kampman *et al.*, 2001a; Sofuoglu *et al.*, 2003). Clinically, stimulant withdrawal is generally self-limited and does not require specific treatment.

Treatment for stimulant use disorder

In the UK, the contact of a stimulant user with the treatment delivery system usually follows a crisis relating to the psychiatric and physical comorbidity and increased social problems the stimulant misuse is associated with (Department of Health, 1996; Farrell *et al.*, 1998; Karch, 2002), and this is also true in the USA. Yet treatment for the stimulant user is still not well-established. Though there is a growing knowledge base about the neurobiological actions of stimulants, unfortunately this has not yet led to the development of effective pharmacotherapies.

Most of the clinical trials for the pharmacological and behavioral treatments for stimulant dependence have focused on cocaine. However, the treatment approaches used for cocaine addiction are now also being tested for the treatment of amphetamine use. And while strides are being made in trying to study systematically the effectiveness of treatments for stimulant abusers, the research on the treatment of stimulant misuse is characterized by heterogeneity of study populations and large variations in

Table 19.1. Potential pharmacological treatments for stimulant dependence

Antidepressants
- Serotonin reuptake blockers: Fluoxetine, Sertraline, Paroxetine
- Serotonin/Norepinephrine Reuptake Blockers: Bupropion, Desipramine, Imipramine, Venlafaxine
- 5-HT$_{2A}$ antagonists: Mirtazapine, Nefazodone

Dopaminergic medications
- Dopamine agonists: Bromocriptine, Amantadine
- Monoamine oxidase inhibitors: Phenelzine, Selegiline
- Inhibitor of dopamine-beta-hydroxylase: Disulfiram
- Other stimulants: Methylphenidate, Amphetamine, Pemoline, Modafinil

GABA medications
- GABA$_B$ agonist: Baclofen
- GABA Transporter inhibitor: Tiagabine
- GABA Transaminase inhibitor: Vigabatrin
- GABA$_A$ agonist: Progesterone

Glutamate release inhibitors
- Lamotrigine, Riluzole

Glutamate receptor antagonist
- Topiramate

Adrenergic inhibitors
- Propranolol, carvedilol, clonidine

Pharmacokinetic mechanisms
- Cocaine vaccine

Cerebral blood flow enhancers
- Piracetam, Hydergine

Herbal products and nutritional supplements
Ginkgo biloba, Amino acid mixtures, L-carnitine/coenzyme Q10, Hypericum (St John's wort), Ibogaine

drop out rates (Lima *et al.*, 2002a, 2002b; Soares *et al.*, 2002). These factors may account for some of the reasons why findings often cannot be replicated. In outcome studies, the most frequently used outcome measures are cocaine urine testing and treatment retention. There are a variety of secondary outcome measures employed such as craving, depressive symptoms and various other self-reported measures (Johansson, 2003; Lima *et al.*, 2002a).

Pharmacotherapy of cocaine dependence or misuse

Table 19.1 summarizes the large number of medications that have been investigated in randomized clinical trials but none have shown consistent efficacy. These trials have mainly focused on abstinence initiation rather than on relapse prevention and have been relatively brief, covering a 3 to 6 months follow-up or outcome period. We will briefly review findings from these clinical trials.

Antidepressants

The rationale to use antidepressants as a treatment for stimulant addiction is the proposed downregulation of synaptic monoamine receptors. The downregulation is opposite to the upregulation of monoamine receptors caused by chronic stimulant use (Gawin & Ellenwood, 1988). A number of antidepressants including imipramine, desipramine, bupropion and SSRIs have been studied as a treatment for cocaine dependence. A recent review concluded that there was no evidence supporting the clinical use of antidepressants in the treatment of cocaine dependence (de Lima *et al.*, 2002). There is no difference from placebo when urine testing and treatment retention are the outcome measures (Johansson, 2003; Lima *et al.*, 2002a). This lack of efficacy is found when employing tricyclic antidepressants, selective serotonin reuptake inhibitors, lithium, or bupropion (Johansson, 2003), and it is irrespective of treatment setting, co-existing opioid dependence (Lima *et al.*, 2002a) or co-morbid depression (Carroll *et al.*, 1995). If there are any exceptions to this conclusion, it is found in a small study by Batki *et al.* (1996) that found better retention in those treated with fluoxetine and improvement on self-ratings of clinical response in a study by Nunes *et al.* (1995). Other studies that revealed more improvement with desipramine (Gawin *et al.*, 1989; Levin & Lehman, 1991) have been challenged by the meta-analysis of Lima *et al.* (2002a).

These studies had high drop-out rates, and the idea of adding psychotherapy to medication treatment was recommended to improve patient retention. In a recent randomized clinical trial of desipramine and contingency management (CM), neither treatment alone significantly reduced cocaine abuse in buprenorphine maintained cocaine abusers (Kosten *et al.*, 2003). However, the combination of desipramine and CM showed efficacy in increasing cocaine free urines. These promising findings using desipramine and contingency management need to be replicated in future studies.

Dopamine agonists (amantadine, bromocriptine)

Reviews and meta-analyses conclude that dopamine agonists are not superior to placebo in reducing cocaine abuse or in improving retention (Johansson, 2003; Soares *et al.*, 2002), and this lack of effectiveness was irrespective of treatment setting, co-morbid opioid dependence or alcohol abuse (Malcolm *et al.*, 2000; Soares *et al.*, 2002).

Amantadine is an antiviral agent mainly used for the treatment of Parkinson's disease and drug-induced extrapyramidal reactions (Blanchet et al., 2003; Crosby et al., 2003). Amantadine increases dopaminergic transmission and may also affect cholinergic and NMDA receptors (Nastuk et al., 1976; Stoof et al., 1992). In a randomized clinical study, amantadine (100 mg twice daily) treatment showed some efficacy (Alterman et al., 1992). However, in other randomized clinical studies amantadine was no more effective than placebo (Handelsman et al., 1995; Kampman et al., 1996; Shoptaw et al., 2003). Interestingly, reanalysis of one of the negative studies suggested that amantadine was more effective than placebo in reducing cocaine use among subjects with severe cocaine withdrawal symptoms at the start of treatment (Kampman et al., 2000). Additional controlled studies are needed to determine whether amantadine is more effective in cocaine users with high withdrawal severity.

Bromocriptine is a D_2-like receptor agonist and a partial D_1-like receptor agonist. It is used mainly for Parkinson's disease and hyperprolactinemic states (Ho & Thorner, 1988; Jackson et al., 1988). In a randomized clinical trial with cocaine users, the bromocriptine group had more urine toxicology screens negative for cocaine than those randomized to placebo, 67% vs. 31%, (Moscovitz et al., 1993) These initial positive findings could not be replicated in a randomized clinical trial with methadone maintained cocaine users (Handelsmann et al., 1997).

In comparing bromocriptine to amantadine, amandatine showed a positive effect on cocaine use in a two-week treatment (Alterman et al., 1992; Johansson, 2003). But amantadine, in looking at some non-significant trends, is poorer than bromocriptine in decreasing craving but better in retention than bromocriptine (Giannini et al., 1989; Tennant & Saghera, 1987).

Disulfiram

Disulfiram is used as a deterrent agent for alcohol dependence due to its aldehyde dehydrogenase inhibitor effects, which mediate the alcohol-disulfiram reaction (Hughes & Cook, 1997). Disulfiram also inhibits dopamine-β-hydroxylase (DBH). DBH converts dopamine to norepinephrine, and leads to increased dopamine and decreased norepinephrine levels in the brain yielding some dopamine agonist-like effects of this medication. A number of randomized controlled trials found disulfiram, at 250 mg/day, effective for the treatment of cocaine dependence. The beneficial effects of disulfiram for cocaine dependence does not seem to be mediated through a decrease in alcohol use. Initially disulfiram showed efficacy in cocaine users with concurrent alcohol abuse or dependence (Carroll et al.,

1998), both in increased retention and decreased cocaine use. It has also shown efficacy in opioid and cocaine dependent subjects maintained on methadone (Petrakis et al., 2000) or buprenorphine (George et al., 2000) and in cocaine users without concomitant dependence on other drugs (Carroll et al., 2004). Altogether, these results suggest that disulfiram may be an effective medication in reducing cocaine use. Further studies are needed to develop guidelines for disulfiram treatment in clinical settings.

Antiepileptics

Tiagabine

Tiagabine, an antiseizure medication, increases the synaptic levels of GABA by inhibiting a GABA transporter (Schachter, 2001). In a recent randomized clinical study, the efficacy of tiagabine for cocaine use was investigated in opioid dependent patients maintained on methadone (González et al., 2003a, 2003b). In that study, tiagabine at 24 mg/day (in twice daily dosing) was more effective than placebo in reducing cocaine use, suggesting that tiagabine may be a promising medication for cocaine dependence pharmacotherapy. These findings are currently being replicated in a larger clinical trial.

Topiramate

Topiramate is an antiseizure medication with multiple pharmacological effects in the brain including blockage of glutamate receptors and potentiation of GABAnergic transmission (Shank et al., 2000). In a recent randomized controlled study with cocaine users, topiramate at 200 mg/day decreased cocaine use behavior (Kampman et al., 2003). A recent randomized controlled study suggested that topiramate may also have efficacy for the treatment of alcohol dependence (Johnson et al., 2003). Whether topiramate will have clinical utility in cocaine or mixed cocaine and alcohol use disorders needs to be further investigated.

Carbamazepine and phenytoin each has been reported in a single methodologically flawed study, to decrease use of cocaine (Crosby et al., 1996; Halikas et al., 1997).

Baclofen

Baclofen is a non-selective $GABA_B$ receptor agonist that is used for muscle spasticity and acts through both presynaptic and post-synapatic $GABA_B$ receptors (Misgeld et al., 1995). In a recent randomized controlled study, baclofen at 60 mg/day reduced cocaine use more than placebo (Shoptaw et al., 2003). Interestingly, baclofen was more effective in the subgroup of patients with greater cocaine use at baseline.

Adrenergic blockers

Cocaine activates the adrenergic system which mediates the physiological responses to cocaine including an increase in heart rate, blood pressure and arousal (Robbins *et al.*, 1998; Schindler *et al.*, 1995). Two human laboratory studies showed that alpha and beta-adrenergic blockers, labetalol and carvedilol, effectively attenuated smoked-cocaine induced heart rate and blood pressure changes (Sofuoglu *et al.*, 2000a, b). In a randomized clinical trial, propranolol, a non-selective beta-adrenergic blocker, led to better retention and greater drug-free urines than placebo in a subgroup of cocaine dependent subjects (Kampman *et al.*, 2001b). Propranolol, 100 mg/day, was more effective than placebo only in the group with severe cocaine withdrawal symptoms at baseline. These studies suggest that adrenergic blockers may be effective in attenuating some of the physiological effects of cocaine and may be effective in the subgroup with high cocaine withdrawal severity.

Other pharmacologic data

Dexamphetamine was found to be better than placebo in increasing retention (Grabowski *et al.*, 2001), though the results were not always consistent and positive (Shearer *et al.*, 2003). Naltrexone, when used in conjunction with relapse prevention, was associated with decreased cocaine use (Schmitz *et al.*, 2001). Buspirone helped with the symptoms of withdrawal (but not treatment retention) from day 5 onwards in a 4-week study (Giannini *et al.*, 1993).

Immunotherapies: cocaine vaccine

More than 25 years ago, the concept of treating drug dependence with immunotherapy was first demonstrated by vaccination of primates against heroin (Bonese *et al.*, 1974). The heroin dose needed to re-instate drug taking by the primate was increased by 16-fold suggesting that vaccination may be an effective strategy in decreasing the reinforcing effects of drugs of abuse and maintaining abstinence. The proposed mechanism of action for immunotherapies is that as a result of binding of the drug peripherally, the entry of drug into the brain is prevented or at least delayed (Kosten *et al.*, 2002). Currently, there is a cocaine vaccine undergoing clinical trial for safety and efficacy in cocaine users. This vaccine has used cholera toxin B subunit as the carrier protein and is linked to a norcocaine derivative at the methyl ester group as an immunogen. Ongoing studies with cocaine users are examining whether this vaccine will attenuate the effects of cocaine and be effective in preventing relapse (Kosten *et al.*, 2002).

Pharmacotherapy of amphetamine dependence or misuse

A recent meta-analysis of relevant studies with fluoxetine, imipramine, desipramine and amlodipine concluded that none was demonstrated to be effective in the treatment of amphetamine misuse and dependence (Srisurapanont *et al.*, 2002). The only significant results observed were that fluoxetine decreased craving at the start of the treatment. Imipramine increased adherence to treatment in the medium term.

The lack of efficacy of pharmacotherapy to amphetamine dependence, seems to also hold true of dexamphetamine, for which, despite the contrary evidence of descriptive studies (Lingford-Hughes *et al.*, 2004), the only randomized controlled trial failed to show that it is better than weekly counseling (Shearer *et al.*, 2001).

Psychosocial treatments

Summarizing the role of psychosocial treatment in stimulant misuse is difficult given the large number of treatments and diversity of treatment populations, settings and protocols. A recent meta-analysis grouped psychosocial treatments in three groups: supportive (counseling, relaxation, acupuncture, etc.), re-educative (CBT, drug counseling, Twelve-Step approach, cue exposure, contingency management, community reinforcement approach, etc.) and re-constructive (dynamic therapy, family therapy, interpersonal psychotherapy, supportive-expressive therapy etc. (Fridel, 2003)) and showed that (a) re-educative therapies marginally but significantly reduce cocaine use especially during the first 6 months of the intervention, and (b) re-constructive therapies increase treatment retention up to 1 year.

Behavioral therapies

Behavioral therapies are an important component of stimulant treatment, and they are reviewed in detail in Chapter 18. A wide range of behavioral treatments have been used for the treatment of stimulant use disorders (Hennessy *et al.*, 2003; McGovern & Carroll, 2003). In contrast to pharmacotherapies, behavioral therapies are not specific for a given addiction and can be used for a range of substance use disorders. Among behavioral treatments, cognitive-behavioral therapy (CBT) and contingency management (CM) have been studied in randomized clinical trials for stimulant use disorders, and it may be useful to add promising pharmacotherapies as adjuncts to these empirically validated behavioral interventions for the treatment of stimulant dependence (e.g. Carroll *et al.*, 2004).

Cognitive behavioral therapy (CBT)

CBT is extensively discussed in Chapter 18, and we will not go into great detail here. The goal of CBT is to teach new cognitive and coping skills for substance use behavior. Social and coping skills training and relapse prevention are also successfully added to CBT of cocaine use disorders.

CBT has been studied with manual assisted delivery in cocaine misuse and dependence. CBT has been shown to decrease cocaine use behavior in randomized controlled trials (Siqueland & Crits-Christoph, 1999). In comparing CBT vs a Twelve-step treatment, CBT was found better than (Maude-Griffin *et al.*, 1998), equal to (Wells *et al.*, 1994), or worse than (Crits-Christoph *et al.*, 1999) a Twelve-step facilitation treatment in reducing cocaine use. Differences in findings are probably because of differences in the study participants' features especially with respect to co-morbidities: alcohol misuse in Wells *et al.* alcohol/cannabis dependence in Crits-Cristoph *et al.* and homelessness and psychiatric comorbidity in Maude-Griffin *et al.* In the latter study, there was some evidence in favour of treatment matching with CBT being better than 12-step facilitation for patients with a history of depression, and 12-step being a better choice for clients with low levels of abstract reasoning or strong religious beliefs (Maude-Griffin *et al.*, 1998).

Contingency management (CM)

CM is a specific behavioral approach which systematically reinforces abstinence in exchange for treatment compliance or drug-free urines. Most often the client is offered a reward such as a voucher, usually for providing negative urine tests. The goal of CM is to decrease behavior maintained by drug reinforcers and increase behavior maintained by non-drug reinforcers. There are two critical steps for successful implementation of CM. First, the target behavior (e.g. drug-free urines) has to be reliably detected with frequent monitoring such as three times weekly drug screening. Second, whenever the target behavior is observed (e.g. clean urine), a tangible reinforcer such as a token, a clinic privilege, or a voucher exchangeable for retail goods is provided (Petry & Simcic, 2002).

Contingency management with voucher rewards have been used successfully to initiate abstinence and prevent relapse in cocaine use disorders (Higgins *et al.*, 2000a, 2000b, 2003). It was also found to increase cocaine abstinence in methadone patients (Kirby *et al.*, 1998; Silverman *et al.*, 1998), although in the Kirby *et al.* study (1998) the effect on cocaine dependent clients was not replicated. Contingency management in methadone maintenance cocaine dependent clients was found to be more effective

than CBT during treatment, but the effect disappeared at the 6-month and 1-year follow-up (Rawson *et al.*, 2002).

In contingency management with vouchers, the type of the voucher schedule is important, with the reward after each negative urine testing being more powerful than weekly vouchers (Kirby *et al.*, 1998). A start-up bonus voucher made no difference in initiating abstinence (Silverman *et al.*, 1998). Reward with vouchers is not the only effective means of CM. Housing reinforcement improves cocaine abstinence amongst homeless cocaine or multi-substance misusers (Milby *et al.*, 2000).

Most of the studies evaluating the efficacy of the CM approach have been conducted in research settings. Further studies need to be conducted in order to provide guidelines to implement CM in community settings. Preliminary studies are evaluating the combinations of behavioral therapies such as CBT and CM with promising pharmacotherapies, and this appears to have become standard clinical practice in both the USA and UK.

Drug counseling

Individual Twelve-step-based drug counseling was better than CBT or supportive – expressive therapy when each was combined with Twelve-step-based group counseling for the treatment of cocaine dependence (Crits-Christoph *et al.*, 1999). The results could be due to the simple unequivocal message of counseling (do not use drugs) or to the structured nature of counseling employed in the study.

Community reinforcement approach (CRA)

The community reinforcement approach (CRA) is multimodal treatment comprising a mixture of relapse prevention, skills training, Twelve-step approach and other interventions. The CRA as a structured behavior intervention was effective in cocaine dependence but not in methadone maintenance (Roozen *et al.*, 2004). When compared with drug counseling in opioid/cocaine dependence, CRA was not different from drug counseling (Scottenfeld *et al.*, 2000). When combined with vouchers, CRA was more efficacious in cocaine dependent outpatients (Higgins *et al.*, 2003).

Acupuncture

There is no consensus on the efficacy of acupuncture in cocaine dependence. Two RCT trials have shown acupuncture to be associated with decreased cocaine use in cocaine dependent clients with (Avants *et al.*, 2000) and without (Lipton *et al.*, 1994) opioid dependence, while two further RCTs with blind study design have failed to show any efficacy (Bullock *et al.*, 1999; Otto *et al.*, 1998). This is not surprising considering that both real and 'sham' acupuncture needle sites were found to be effective in the treatment of cocaine dependence (Margolin *et al.*, 2002). In stimulant misuse, acupuncture is probably not useful as a stand alone intervention but only as an integrated part of a broader treatment plan (Margolin *et al.*, 2002).

Psychiatric comorbidity

In treatment-seeking cocaine users, major depression, bipolar disorder, PTSD and phobias, ADHD, and antisocial personality are common psychiatric disorders co-morbid with stimulant dependence (Rounsaville *et al.*, 1991). Co-morbid psychiatric disorders may increase the risk for drug use by multiple mechanisms including self-medication by patients to ease psychiatric symptoms. Treatment adherence can also be more difficult in stimulant users with psychiatric comorbidity than in those without comorbidity (Daley *et al.*, 1998). Thus, an effective treatment plan needs to address both the stimulant addiction and the comorbid disorder.

Although, guidelines for the pharmacotherapy of stimulant addiction and psychiatric comorbidity have not been developed, certain pharmacotherapies may be particularly useful for stimulant abusers with psychiatric comorbidity. For instance, in a clinical trial with depressed cocaine users, treatment with antidepressant medications such as imipramine (150–300 mg), desipramine (150 mg/day) and bupropion (300 mg/day) have reduced depressive symptoms, cocaine use and craving (Margolin *et al.*, 1995; Nunes *et al.*, 1995; Ziedonis & Kosten, 1991). In depressed cocaine users the combination of CBT with desipramine treatment improved treatment retention and abstinence, underscoring the importance of the combination of pharmacotherapy and psychotherapy as an effective treatment of depressed stimulant users (Carroll *et al.*, 1995). In cocaine users with comorbid ADHD, a randomized controlled trial with methylphenidate showed attenuation of ADHD symptoms without affecting cocaine use (Schubiner *et al.*, 2002).

Concomitant addictions

Opioid addiction

Cocaine use is especially common in individuals who are addicted to other drugs of abuse. In opioid users who are engaged in methadone maintenance, treatment rates of cocaine use range from 30 to 80 percent (DesJarlais *et al.*, 1992; Grella *et al.*, 1997). Cocaine use has devastating consequences in this population including poor treatment outcome and relapse to IV drug use. In opioid- and cocaine-dependent patients, treatment with methadone or buprenorphine alone does not reduce cocaine use (Schottenfeld *et al.*, 1997; Strain *et al.*, 1994). While there are no proven pharmacotherapies for concomitant opioid and stimulant addiction, some medications showed promising findings. In opioid dependent cocaine users, a combination of buprenorphine and desipramine reduced both opioid and cocaine use (Oliveto *et al.*, 1999). As mentioned previously, in a recent study, the anticonvulsant tiagabine, in combination with methadone, reduced cocaine and opioid use (González *et al.*, 2003a, 2003b).

Alcohol addiction

Thirty percent of treatment-seeking cocaine users report alcoholism (Carroll *et al.*, 1993). Concomitant alcohol use is a poor prognostic factor in stimulant users and clearly deserves attention for a successful treatment outcome (Heil *et al.*, 2002). As mentioned before, disulfiram at 250 mg/day has been shown to decrease both alcohol and cocaine use in these dual abusers (Carroll *et al.*, 1998).

Tobacco addiction

In a community sample, 85% of cocaine users were current cigarette smokers (Richter *et al.*, 2002). In drug-addicted individuals, smoking is a significant cause of mortality (Hser *et al.*, 1994; Hurt *et al.*, 1996), emphasizing the need for smoking cessation in stimulant users. Specific treatment approaches for stimulant and tobacco addiction have not been developed. Following the guidelines published by the US Public Health Service, every smoker, including stimulant users, should be asked about their tobacco use. Those attempting to quit smoking should be prescribed at least one of the first-line pharmacotherapies, nicotine replacement treatments or bupropion, in the absence of contraindications for these medications (Fiore, 2000). For the depressed patient dependent on tobacco and stimulants, bupropion might be a particularly apt pharmacotherapy.

Summary and conclusions

Before treatment initiation, stimulant users require a comprehensive psychiatric, medical, and laboratory examination. Psychiatric comorbidity is common in stimulant users and needs to be addressed together with stimulant addiction. The clinician also needs to be aware that stimulant users commonly use other drugs of abuse including alcohol and heroin, which may result in serious overdose and death. Pharmacological intervention may be necessary during stimulant-induced drug states. For instance, benzodiazepines may be useful in controlling stimulant-induced intoxication and antipsychotics may be useful in stimulant induced- psychosis or delirium.

To date, no effective medications are available for stimulant dependence, although progress has been made in the development of pharmacotherapies. Behavioral treatments aimed at maintaining drug abstinence and

preventing relapse have shown favorable results and are essential components to provide effective adherence to any pharmacotherapy. Further research is needed to develop effective pharmacotherapies for stimulant addiction.

The level of evidence for each of the interventious discussed in this chapter is summarized in Table 19.2.

Table 19.2. Effectiveness of treatments for stimulant dependence

Treatment	Form of treatment	Psychiatric Disorder/ target audience	Level of evidence for efficacy	Comments
Pharmacotherapy	Antidepressant	Cocaine dependence	Ib	Score is lower here because most studies that have shown improvement have been difficult to replicate. Some evidence in small study for fluoxetine and imipramine but the evidence is very weak
Pharmacotherapy	Disulfiram	Cocaine dependence	Ia	Better retention in program and better impact on decreasing cocaine usage
Pharmacotherapy	Dopamine agonists Amantadine, Bromcriptine	Cocaine dependence	Ib	Amantadine may be better at retaining people in a treatment program, especially in the short-term while bromcriptine may be better at reducing craving
Pharmacotherapy	Tiagabine Topiramate	Cocaine dependence	Ib	Appears to reduce cocaine usage and cocaine use behavior
Pharmacotherapy	Baclofen	Cocaine dependence	Ib	Better than placebo
Pharmacotherapy	Adrenergic blockers	Cocaine dependence	Ib	Better than placebo (and may have some efficacy in cocaine + alcohol abuse)
Pharmacotherapy	Antidepressant (tricyclics, bupropion)	Cocaine dependence plus depression	IIa	Reduction of depressive symptoms and cocaine craving
Psychosocial treatment	Cognitive Behavioral Therapy	Cocaine dependence	Ia	Has been shown to be effective especially for reducing cocaine usage for the first 6 months, and better than a 12-step program in achieving that goal. It may also be better than a 12-step approach in patients with comorbid depression.
Psychosocial treatment	Contingency Management	Cocaine dependence	Ib	Has been shown to be effective in initiating abstinence and to prevent relapse. It may be more effective than CBT in the initiation of abstinence phase of treatment.
Psychosocial treatment	Individual 12-step counseling	Cocaine dependence	III	Probably has some impact when joined with group 12-step approach
Psychosocial treatment	Community Reinforcement Approach	Cocaine dependence	III	Effective in cocaine dependence but not in methadone maintenance. May be more effective when combined with CM
Combined treatment	Psychotherapy (Contingency management) and pharmacotherapy [desipramine])	Cocaine dependence	IIa	Only the combination showed significant improvement
Combined treatment	CBT and desipramine	Cocaine dependence and depression	III	Improved treatment retention and abstinence
Alternative treatment	Acupuncture	Cocaine dependence	IIa	Results are inconsistent. Probably may be good in a multimodal treatment but not as a stand alone treatment

ACKNOWLEDGMENT

Supported by the National Institute on Drug Abuse grants P50-DA12762 K05-DA0454 (TRK), R01-DA 14537, and K12 00167 (MS).

REFERENCES

Ahmad, K. (2003). Asia grapples with spreading amphetamine abuse. *Lancet*, **361**, 1878–9.

Alterman, A. I., Droba, M., Antelo, R. E. *et al.* (1992). Amantadine may facilitate detoxification of cocaine addicts. *Drug Alcohol Dependence*, **31**, 19–29.

American Psychiatric Association (1994). *Diagnostic and Statistical Manual of Mental Disorders*, 4th edn: DSM-IV. Washington, DC: American Psychiatric Association.

Avants, S. K., Margolin, A., Holford, R. & Kosten, T. R. (2000). A randomised controlled trial of auricular acupuncture for cocaine dependence. *Archives of Internal Medicine*, **160**, 2305–12.

Batki, S. L., Washburn, A. M., Delucchi, K. & Jones, R. T. (1996). A controlled trial of fluoxetine in crack cocaine dependence. *Drug and Alcohol Dependence*, **41**, 137–42.

Benowitz, N. L. (1993). Clinical pharmacology and toxicology of cocaine. *Pharmacol Toxiccol*, **72**, 3–12.

Blanchet, P. J., Metman, L. V. & Chase, T. N. (2003). Renaissance of amantadine in the treatment of Parkinson's disease. *Advances in Neurology*, 251–7.

Bonese, K. F., Wainer, B. H., Fitch, F. W., Rothberg, R. M. & Schuster, C. R. (1974). Changes in heroin self-administration by a rhesus monkey after morphine immunization. *Nature*, **252**, 708–10.

Brady, K. T., Lydiard, R. B., Malcolm, R. & Ballenger, J. C. (1991). Cocaine-induced psychosis. *Journal of Clinical Psychiatry*, **52**, 509–12.

Bullock, M. L., Kiresuk, T. J., Pheley, A. M., Culliton, R. D. & Lenz, S. K. (1999). Auricular acupuncture in the treatment of cocaine abuse. A study of efficacy and dosing. *Journal of Substance Abuse Treatment*, **16**(1), 31–8.

Carroll, K. M., Rounsaville, B. J. & Bryant, K. J. (1993). Alcoholism in treatment-seeking cocaine abusers: clinical and prognostic significance. *Journal of Studies in Alcoholism*, **54**, 199–208.

Carroll, K. M., Nich, C. & Rounsaville, B. J. (1995). Differential symptom reduction in depressed cocaine abusers treated with psychotherapy and pharmacotherapy. *Journal of Nervous and Mental Disease*, **183**, 251–9.

Carroll, K. M., Nich, C., Ball, S. A., McCance, E. & Rounsaville, B. J. (1998). Treatment of cocaine and alcohol dependence with psychotherapy and disulfiram. *Addiction*, **93**, 713–27.

Carroll, K. M., Fenton, L. R., Ball, S. A. *et al.* (2004). Efficacy of disulfiram and cognitive behavior therapy in cocaine-dependent outpatient: a randomised placebo-controlled trial. *Archives of General Psychiatry*, **61**, 264–72.

Cho, A. K. & Melega, W. P. (2002). Patterns of methamphetamine abuse and their consequences. *Journal of Addictive Diseases*, **21**, 21–34.

Crits-Christoph, P., Siqueland, L., Blaine, J. *et al.* (1999). Psychosocial treatments for cocaine dependence: National Institute on Drug Abuse Collaborative Cocaine Treatment Study. *Archives of General Psychiatry*, **56**, 493–502.

Crosby, R. D., Pearson, V. L., Eller, C., Winegarden, T. & Graves, N. L. (1996). Phenytoin in the treatment of cocaine abuse: a double–blind study. *Clinical and Pharmacological Therapy*, **59**, 458–68.

Crosby, N., Deane, K. H. & Clarke, C. E. (2003). Amantadine in Parkinson's disease. *Cochrane Database Systematic Reviews*, CD003468. Oxford: Update Software Ltd.

Daley, D. C., Salloum, I. M., Zuckoff, A., Kirisci, L. & Thase, M. E. (1998). Increasing treatment adherence among outpatients with depression and cocaine dependence: results of a pilot study. *American Journal of Psychiatry*, **155**, 1611–13.

de Lima, M. S., de Oliveira Soares, B. G., Reisser, A. A. & Farrell, M. (2002). Pharmacological treatment of cocaine dependence: a systematic review. *Addiction*, 931–49.

Department of Health (1996). The Task Force to Review Services for Drug Misusers: report of an Independent Review of Drug Treatment Services in England.

Des Jarlais, D. C., Wenston, J., Friedman, S. R., Sotheran, J. L., Maslansky, R. & Marmor, M. (1992). Crack cocaine use in a cohort of methadone maintenance patients. *Journal of Substance Abuse Treatment*, **9**, 319–25.

Farrell, M., Howes, S., Griffiths, P., Williamson, S. & Taylor, C. (1998). *Stimulant Needs Assessment Project*. London: Department of Health.

Fiore, M. and United States. Tobacco Use and Dependence Guideline Panel. (2000). *Treating Tobacco Use and Dependence*. Rockville, MD: US Department of Health and Human Services, Public Health Service.

Fridell, M. (2003). Psychosocial treatment for drug dependence. In *Treating Alcohol and Drug Abuse: An Evidence Based Review*, ed. M. Berglund, S. Thelander & E. Jonsson. Berlin: Wiley-VCH GmbH & Co. KgaA.

Gawin, F. H. & Ellinwood, E. H. (1988). Cocaine and other stimulants: actions, abuse and treatment. *New England Journal of Medicine*, 1173–82.

Gawin, F. H., Kleber, H. D., Byck, R. *et al.* (1989). Desipramine facilitation of initial cocaine abstinence. *Archives in General Psychiatry*, **46**, 117–21.

George, T. P., Chawarski, M. C., Pakes, J., Carroll, K. M., Kosten, T. R. & Schottenfeld, R. S. (2000). Disulfiram versus placebo for cocaine dependence in buprenorphine-maintained subjects: a preliminary trial. *Biological Psychiatry*, **47**, 1080–6.

Giannini, A. J., Folts, D. J., Feather, J. N. & Sullivan, B. S. (1989). Bromocriptine and Amantadine in Cocaine Detoxification. *Psychiatry Research*, **29**, 11–16.

Giannini, A. J., Loiselle, R. H., Graham, B. H. & Folts, D. J. (1993). Behavioural response to buspirone in cocaine and phencyclidine withdrawal. *Journal of Substance Abuse Treatment*, **10**, 523–7.

González, G., Sevarino, K., Sofuoglu, M. *et al.* (2003a). Tiagabine increases cocaine-free urines in cocaine-dependent methadone-treated patients: results of a randomized pilot study. *Addiction*, **98**, 1625–32.

González, G., Sofuoglu, M., Gonsai, K., Poling, J., Oliveto, A. & Kosten, T. R. (2003b). Efficacy of tiagabine or gabapentin in reducing cocaine use in methadone-stabilized cocaine abusers [abstract]. College on Problems of Drug Dependence. 65th Annual Scientific Meeting; 2003 June 14–19; Bal Harbour.

Gossop, M., Marsden, J., Steward, D. *et al.* (1998). Substance use, health and social problems of service users at 54 drug treatment agencies: intake data form the National Treatment Outcome Research Study (NTORS). *British Journal of Psychiatry*, **173**, 166–71.

Grabowski, J., Rhodes, H., Schmitz, J. M. *et al.* (2001). Dextroamphetamine for cocaine – dependence treatment: a double blind randomised clinical trial. *Journal of Clinical Psychopharmacology*, **31**, 522–6.

Greater London Alcohol and Drug Alliance (2004). An evidence base for the London crack cocaine strategy: a consultation document prepared for the Greater London Alcohol and Drug Alliance. Greater London Authority.

Grella, C. E., Anglin, M. D. & Wugalter, S. E. (1997). Patterns and predictors of cocaine and crack use by clients in standard and enhanced methadone maintenance treatment. *American Journal of Drug and Alcohol Abuse*, **23**, 15–42.

Halikas, J. A., Crosby, R. D., Pearson, V. L. & Graves, N. L. (1997). A randomized double-blind study of carbamazepine in the treatment of cocaine abuse. *Clinical and Pharmacological Therapy*, **62**, 89–105.

Handelsman, L., Rosenblum, A., Palij, M. *et al.* (1997). Bromocriptine for cocaine dependence. A controlled clinical trial. *American Journal of Addiction*, **6**, 54–64.

Handelsman, L., Limpitlaw, L., Williams, D., Schmeidler, J., Paris, P. & Stimmel, B. (1995). Amantadine does not reduce cocaine use or craving in cocaine-dependent methadone maintenance patients. *Drug and Alcohol Dependence*, **39**, 173–80.

Heil, S. H., Holmes, H. W., Bickel, W. K. *et al.* (2002). Comparison of the subjective, physiological, and psychomotor effects of atomoxetine and methylphenidate in light drug users. *Drug and Alcohol Dependence*, **67**, 149–56.

Hennessy, G. O., De Menil, V. & Weiss, R. D. (2003). Psychosocial treatments for cocaine dependence. *Current Psychiatry Reports*, **5**, 362–4.

Higgins, S. T., Badger, G. J. & Budney, A. J. (2000a). Initial abstinence and success in achieving longer term cocaine abstinence. *Experimental and Clinical Psychopharmacology*, **8**, 377–86.

Higgins, S. T., Wong, C. J., Badger, G. J., Ogden, D. E. & Dantona, R. L. (2000b). Contingent reinforcement increases cocaine abstinence during outpatient treatment and 1 year of follow-up. *Journal of Consulting and Clinical Psychology*, **68**, 64–72.

Higgins, S. T., Sigmon, S. C., Wong, C. J. *et al.* (2003). Community reinforcement therapy for cocaine-dependent outpatients. *Archives of General Psychiatry*, **60**, 1043–52.

Ho, K. Y. & Thorner, M. O. (1988). Therapeutic applications of bromocriptine in endocrine and neurological diseases *Drugs*, 67–82.

Hser, Y. I., McCarthy, W. J. & Anglin, M. D. (1994). Tobacco use as a distal predictor of mortality among long-term narcotics addicts. *Preventative Medicine*, **23**, 61–9.

Hughes, J. C. & Cook, C. C. (1997). The efficacy of disulfiram: a review of outcome studies. *Addiction*, **92**, 381–95.

Hurt, R. D., Offord, K. P., Croghan, I. T. *et al.* (1996). Mortality following inpatient addictions treatment. Role of tobacco use in a community-based cohort. *Journal of the American Medical Association*, **275**, 1097–103.

Jackson, D. M., Jenkins, O. F. & Ross, S. B. (1988). The motor effects of bromocriptine – a review. *Psychopharmacology (Berlin)*, 433–46.

Johansson, B. A. (2003). Pharmacotherapy for cocaine dependence. *Treating Alcohol and Drug Abuse: An Evidence Based Review*, ed. M. Berglund, S. Thelander & E. Jonsson. Berlin: Wiley-VCH GmbH & Co.

Johnson, B. A., Ait-Daoud, N., Bowden, C. L. *et al.* (2003). Oral topiramate for treatment of alcohol dependence: a randomised controlled trial. *Lancet*, **361**, 1677–85.

Kampman, K., Volpicelli, J. R., Alterman, A. I. *et al.* (1996). Amantadine in the early treatment of cocaine dependence: a double-blind, placebo-controlled trial. *Drug and Alcohol Dependence*, 25–33.

Kampman, K. M., Volpicelli, J. R., Alterman, A. I., Cormish, J. & O'Brien, C. P. (2000). Amantadine in the treatment of cocaine-dependent patients with severe withdrawal symptoms. *American Journal of Psychiatry*, 2052–4.

Kampman, K. M., Alterman, A. I., Volpicelli, J. R. *et al.* (2001a). Cocaine withdrawal symptoms and initial urine toxicology results predict treatment attrition in outpatient cocaine dependence treatment. *Psychology of Addictive Behavior*, **15**, 52–9.

Kampman, K. M., Volpicelli, J. R., Mulvaney, F. *et al.* (2001b). Effectiveness of propranolol for cocaine dependence treatment may depend on cocaine withdrawal symptom severity. *Drug and Alcohol Dependence*, **63**, 69–78.

Kampman, K. M., Pettinati, H., Lynch, K. *et al.* (2003). A pilot trial of topiramate for cocaine dependence [abstract]. College on Problems of Drug Dependence. 65th Annual Scientific Meeting, June 14–19; Bal Harbour.

Karch, S. B. (2002). *Pathology of Drug Abuse*, 3rd edn. USA: CRC Press.

Kirby, K. C., Marlowe, D. B., Festinger, D. S., Lamb, R. J. & Platt, J. J. (1998). Schedule of voucher delivery influences initiation of cocaine abstinence. *Journal of Consulting and Clinical Psychology*, **66**(5), 761–7.

Kosten, T. R. (2002). Pathophysiology and treatment of cocaine dependence. In *Neuropsychopharmacology: The Fifth Generation of Progress*, ed. C. Nemeroff, pp. 1461–73. Baltimore, MD: Lippincott Williams & Wilkins.

Kosten, T., Oliveto, A., Feingold, A. *et al.* (2003). Desipramine and contingency management for cocaine and opiate dependence in buprenorphine maintained patients. *Drug and Alcohol Dependency*, **70**, 315–25.

Kosten, T. R., Rosen, M., Bond, J. *et al.* (2002). Human therapeutic cocaine vaccine: safety and immunogenicity. *Vaccine*, **20**, 1196–204.

Levin, R. L. & Lehman, A. F. (1991). Meta-analysis of desipramine as an adjunct in the treatment of cocaine addiction. *Journal of Clinical Psychopharmacology*, **11**(6), 374–8.

Lima, A. R., Lima, M. S., Soares, B. G. O. & Farrell, M. (2002a). Carbamazepine for cocaine dependence (Cochrane Review). In *The Cochrane Library*, **2**. Oxford: Update Software.

Lima, M. S., Reisser, A. A. P., Soares, B. G. O. & Farrell, M. (2002b). Antidepressants for Cocaine Dependence (Cochrane Review). In *The Cochrane Library*, **2**. Oxford: Update Software.

Lingford-Hughes, A. R., Welch, S. & Nutt, D. J. (2004). Evidence-based guidelines fro the pharmacological management of substance misuse, addiction and comorbidity: recommendation form the British Association for Psychopharmacology. *Journal of Psychopharmacology*, **18**(3), 293–355.

Lipton, D. S., Brewington, V. & Smith, M. (1994). Acupuncture for crack-cocaine detoxification: experimental evaluation of efficacy. *Journal of Substance Abuse Treatment*, **11**(3), 205–15.

Malcolm, R., Kajdasz, K., Herron, J., Anton, R. F. & Brady, K. T. (2000). A double–blind placebo-controlled outpatient trial of pergolide for cocaine dependence. *Drug and Alcohol Dependence*, **60**, 161–8.

Manschreck, T. C., Laughery, J. A., Weisstein, C. C. *et al.* (1988). Characteristics of freebase cocaine psychosis. *Yale Journal of Biological Medicine*, **61**, 115–22.

Margolin, A., Kosten, T. R., Avants, S. K. *et al.* (1995). A multi-center trial of bupropion for cocaine dependence in methadone-maintained patients. *Drug and Alcohol Dependence*, **40**, 125–31.

Margolin, A., Kleber, H. D., Avants, S. K. *et al.* (2002). Acupuncture for the treatment of cocaine addiction: a randomised controlled trial. *Journal of the American Medical Association*, **287**(1), 55–63.

Maude-Griffin, P. M., Hohenstein, G. L., Hamfleet, G. L., Reilly, P. M., Tusel, D. J., & Hall, S M. (1998). Superior efficacy of cognitive-behavioural therapy for urban crack-cocaine abusers: main and matching effects. *Journal of Consulting and Clinical Psychology*, **66**(5), 832–7.

McGovern, M. P. & Carroll, K. M. (2003). Evidence-based practices for substance use disorders. *Psychiatric Clinics of North America*, **26**, 991–1010.

Milby, J. B., Schumacher, J. E., McNamara, C. *et al.* (2000). Initiating abstinence in cocaine abusing dually diagnosed homeless persons. *Drug and Alcohol Dependence*, **60**, 55–67.

Misgeld, U., Bijak, M. & Jarolimek, W. (1995). A physiological role for GABAB receptors and the effects of baclofen in the mammalian central nervous system. *Progress in Neurobiology*, **46**, 423–62.

Moscovitz, H., Brookoff, D. & Nelson, L. (1993). A randomized trial of bromocriptine for cocaine users presenting to the emergency department. *Journal of General Internal Medicine*, 1–4.

Nakatani, Y. & Hara, T. (1998). Disturbance of consciousness due to methamphetamine abuse. A study of 2 patients. *Psychopathology*, **31**, 131–7.

Nastuk, W. L., Su, P. & Doubilet, P. (1976). Anticholinergic and membrane activities of amantadine in neuromuscular transmission. *Nature*, 76–9.

National Institute on Drug Abuse (1998). National Survey Results on Drug Use from Monitoring the Future Survey.

National Treatment Agency for Substance Misuse (2002). *Models of care for treatment of adult drug misusers: framework for developing local systems of effective drug misuse treatment in England*. London.

Nunes, E. V., McGrath, P. J., Quitkin, F. M. *et al.* (1995). Imipramine treatment of cocaine abuse: possible boundaries of efficacy. *Drug and Alcohol Dependence*, **39**, 185–95.

Oliveto, A. H., Feingold, A., Schottenfeld, R., Jatlow, P. & Kosten, T. R. (1999). Desipramine in opioid-dependent cocaine abusers maintained on buprenorphine vs methadone. *Archives of General Psychiatry*, **56**, 812–20.

Otto, K., Quinn, C. & Sung, Y. F. (1998). Auricular acupuncture as an adjunctive treatment for cocaine addiction. *American Journal of Addiction*, **7**, 164–70.

Petrakis, I., Carroll, K., Nich, C. *et al.* (2000). Disulfiram treatment for cocaine dependence in methadone-maintained opioid addicts. *Addiction*, **95**, 219–28.

Petry, N. M. & Simcic, F., Jr (2002). Recent advances in the dissemination of contingency management techniques: clinical and research perspectives. *Journal of Substance Abuse Treatment*, **23**, 81–6.

Rawson, R. A., Huber, A., McCann, M. *et al.* (2002). A comparison of contingency management and cognitive-behavioral approaches during methadone maintenance treatment for cocaine dependence. *Archives of General Psychiatry*, **59**, 817–24.

Richter, K. P., Ahluwalia, H. K., Mosier, M. C., Nazir, N. & Ahluwalia, J. S. (2002). A population-based study of cigarette smoking among illicit drug users in the United States. *Addiction*, **97**, 861–9.

Robbins, T. W., Granon, S., Muir, J. L., Durantou, F., Harrison, A. & Everitt, B. J. (1998). Neural systems underlying arousal and attention. Implications for drug abuse. *Annals of New York Academy of Sciences*, **846**, 222–37.

Roozen, H., Boulogne, J., Tulder, M., van den Brink, W., De Jong, C. A., & Kerkhof, A. J. (2004). A systematic review of the effectiveness of the community reinforcement approach in alcohol, cocaine and opioid addiction. *Drug and Alcohol Dependence*, **74**, 1–13.

Rounsaville, B. J., Anton, S. F., Carroll, K. M. *et al.* (1991). Psychiatric diagnosis of treatment seeking cocaine abusers. *Archives of General Psychiatry*, **18**, 43–51.

Ruttenber, A. J., Lawler-Heavner, J., Yin, M., Wetli, C. V., Hearn, W. L. & Mash, D. C. (1997). Fatal excited delirium following cocaine use: epidemiologic findings provide new evidence for mechanisms of cocaine toxicity. *Journal of Forensic Science*, **42**, 25–31.

Satel, S. L. & Edell, W. S. (1991). Cocaine-induced paranoia and psychosis proneness. *American Journal of Psychiatry*, **148**, 1708–11.

Satel, S. L., Southwick, S. M. & Gawin, F. H. (1991). Clinical features of cocaine-induced paranoia. *American Journal of Psychiatry*, **148**, 495–8.

Schachter, S. C. (2001). Pharmacology and clinical experience with tiagabine. *Expert Opinions in Pharmacotherapy*, **2**, 179–87.

Schindler, C. W., Tella, S. R., Erzouki, H. K. & Goldberg, S. R. (1995). Pharmacological mechanisms in cocaine's cardiovascular effects. *Drug and Alcohol Dependence*, **37**, 183–91.

Schmitz, J. M., Stotts, A. L., Rhoades, J. M., & Grabowski, J. (2001). Naltrexone and relapse prevention treatment for cocaine dependent patients. *Addictive Behaviours*, **26**, 167–80.

Schottenfeld, R. S., Pakes, J. R., Oliveto, A., Ziedonis, D. & Kosten, T. R. (1997). Buprenorphine vs methadone maintenance treatment for concurrent opioid dependence and cocaine abuse. *Archives in General Psychiatry*, **54**, 713–20.

Schottenfeld, R. S., Pantalon, M. V., Chawarski, M. C. & Paker, J. (2000). Community reinforcement approach for combined opioid and cocaine dependence: patterns of engagement in alternative activities. *Journal of Substance Abuse Treatment*, **18**, 255–61.

Schubiner, H., Saules, K. K., Arfken, C. L. *et al.* (2002). Double-blind placebo-controlled trial of methylphenidate in the treatment of adult ADHD patients with comorbid cocaine dependence. *Experimental and Clinical Psychopharmacology*, **10**, 286–94.

Shank, R. P., Gardocki, J. F., Streeter, A. J. & Maryanoff, B. E. (2000). An overview of the preclinical aspects of topiramate: pharmacology, pharmacokinetics, and mechanism of action. *Epilepsia*, **41**, S3–9.

Shanti, C. M. & Lucas, C. E. (2003). Cocaine and the critical care challenge. *Critical Care Medicine*, **31**, 1851–9.

Shearer, J., Wodak, A., Mattick, R. P. *et al.* (2001). Pilot randomised controlled study of dexamphetamine substitution for amphetamine dependence. *Addiction*, **96**, 1289–96.

Shearer, J., Wodak, A., van Beek I., Mattick, R. P. & Lewis, J. (2003). Pilot randomised double blind placebo-controlled study of dexamphetamine for cocaine dependence. *Addiction*, **98**, 1137–41.

Shoptaw, S., Yang, X., Rotheram-Fuller, E. J. *et al.* (2003). Randomized placebo-controlled trial of baclofen for cocaine dependence: preliminary effects for individuals with chronic patterns of cocaine use. *Journal of Clinical Psychiatry*, **64**, 1440–8.

Silverman, K., Wong, C. M., Umbricht-Schneiter, A., Montoya, I. D., Schuster, C. R. & Preston, K. L. (1998). Broad beneficial effects of cocaine abstinence reinforcement among methadone patients. *Journal of Consulting and Clinical Psychology*, **66**(5), 811–24.

Siqueland, L. & Crits-Christoph, P. (1999). Current developments in psychosocial treatments of alcohol and substance abuse. *Current Psychiatry Reports*, **1**, 179–84.

Soares, B. F. O., Lima, M. S., Reisser, A. A. P. & Farrell, M. (2002). Dopamine agonists for cocaine dependence (Cochrane Review). In *The Cochrane Library*, **2**. Oxford: Update Software (Meta-analysis).

Sofuoglu, M., Brown, S., Babb, D. A., Pentel, P. R. & Hatsukami, D. K. (2000a). Carvedilol affects the physiological and behavioral response to smoked cocaine in humans. *Drug and Alcohol Dependence*, **60**, 69–76.

Sofuoglu, M., Brown, S., Babb, D. A., Pentel, P. R., & Hatsukami, D. K. (2000b). Effects of labetalol treatment on the physiological and subjective response to smoked cocaine. *Pharmacological and Biochemical Behavior*, **65**, 255–9.

Sofuoglu, M., Dudish-Poulsen, S., Brown, S. B. & Hatsukami, D. K. (2003). Association of cocaine withdrawal symptoms with more severe dependence and enhanced subjective response to cocaine. *Drug and Alcohol Dependence*, **69**, 273–82.

Srisurapanont, M., Jarusuraisin, N. & Kittirattanapaiboon, P. (2002). Treatment for amphetamine dependence and abuse (Cochrane Review). In *The Cochrane Library*, **2**. Oxford: Update Software.

Stoof, J. C., Booij, J., Drukarch, B. & Wolters, E. C. (1992). The anti-parkinsonian drug amantadine inhibits the N-methyl-D-aspartic acid-evoked release of acetylcholine from rat neostriatum in a non-competitive way. *European Journal of Pharmacology*, **213**, 439–43.

Strain, E. C., Stitzer, M. L., Liebson, I. A. & Bigelow, G. E. (1994). Buprenorphine versus methadone in the treatment of opioid-dependent cocaine users. *Psychopharmacology (Berl.)*, **116**, 401–6.

Substance Abuse and Mental Health Services Administration (SAMHSA) (2000). Department of Health and Human Services, Substance Abuse and Mental Health Administration, Rockville, M.D.

Tennant, F. S. Jr, & Sagherian, A. A. (1987). Double-blind comparison of amantadine and bromocriptine for ambulatory withdrawal from cocaine dependence. *Archives of Internal Medicine*, **147**(1), 109–12.

Ujike, H. (2002). Stimulant-induced psychosis and schizophrenia: the role of sensitization. *Current Psychiatry Reports*, **4**, 177–84.

United Nations Office for Drug Control and Crime Prevention (2000). *World Drug Report 2000*. Oxford: Oxford University Press.

Wells, E. A., Peterson, P. L., Gainey, R. R., Hawlins, J. D. & Catalano, R. F. (1994). Outpatient treatment for cocaine abuse: a controlled comparison of relapse prevention and twelve step approaches. *American Journal of Drug and Alcohol Abuse*, **20**(1), 1–17.

Ziedonis, D. M. & Kosten, T. R. (1991). Depression as a prognostic for pharmacological treatment of cocaine dependence. *Psychopharmacology Bulletin*, **27**, 337–43.

Substance Abuse and Mental Health Services Administration (SAMHSA) (2000). Department of Health and Human Services, Substance Abuse and Mental Health Services Administration Rockville, MD.

20

Treatment of opioid dependence

Leslie L. Buckley, Nicholas Seivewright, Mark Parry, Abhijeetha Salvaji and Richard Schottenfeld

Editor's note

Opiate addiction is one misuse and dependence disorder for which we have good pharmacological treatments. Both methadone and buprenorphine are effective in withdrawing individuals from opiates via substitution, and their use in maintenance treatment has an excellent track record. Naltrexone may also be efficacious for selected patients. Psychosocial and behavioral treatments play a role too, most often in combination with pharmacological treatments or for patients who do not want pharmacological treatments. This is one subject in which practice varies enormously in different parts of the world. Readers who look at the text closely will notice considerable geographical variation in treatment polices, and it is a tribute to our authors that they have kept this to a minimum in this combined chapter.

Introduction

Opioid dependence is a chronic disorder characterized by relapse, increased mortality, significant medical morbidity, psychiatric sequelae and impaired social function in the individual. Accompanying these detrimental effects to the dependent individual are costs to their families and society secondary to impaired social and occupational functioning and increased criminal behavior or violence. In recent years there have been considerable gains in our understanding of the neurobiology of opioid dependence and in the development of new pharmacological and behavioral treatments for opioid dependence.

Epidemiology

In 1999 there were estimated to be 1 million chronic users of heroin in the United States, or 0.4% (4 per 1000) of the population (Rhodes et al., 2000). The amount of money approximated to have been spent by heroin users to purchase heroin in the United States in 2000 was $10 billion (Rhodes et al., 2000). In recent years there have been changes in the pattern of heroin use among North Americans. The availability of more pure forms of heroin since the 1980s and concerns about HIV transmission have led to decreased injection drug use and increased intranasal use, a route of administration that is perceived as more palatable and less dangerous than injection use (US Department of Justice, Drug Enforcement Administration (DEA), 2003). During the same time, the relative cost of heroin has decreased (DEA, 2003). Survey data demonstrates that the annual number of new users of heroin escalated during the latter half of the 1990s. While the years 1988 to 1994 saw between 28 000 and 80 000 new heroin initiators per year, each year between 1995 and 2001 saw over 100 000 new heroin users per year. Such levels of initiation of heroin use had not been seen since the late 1970s (SAMSHA, 2004). In past surveys, an increased incidence of new use was usually followed by increased numbers of users in future years. The US Monitoring the Future study, which surveys high school students regarding substance use, found that 0.5% of twelfth grade students reported heroin use within the last month and 0.9% reported using heroin within the last year (Johnston et al., 2004).

In an official European Union report on opioid dependence treatment, the European Monitoring Center for Drugs and Drug Addiction (2000) estimated that, in the 15 member countries, the prevalence of opioid dependence was somewhere between 2 and 6+ per 1000 in people aged 16–64. Kraus et al. (2003) carefully reviewed comparable data from the same European countries plus Norway with the main multipliers being from contacts with treatment services and police, capture–recapture data, and multivariate indicators. The highest prevalence

Cambridge Textbook of Effective Treatments in Psychiatry, ed. Peter Tyrer and Kenneth R. Silk. Published by Cambridge University Press.
© Cambridge University Press, 2008.

rates of opioid use were in Italy, Luxembourg, and the UK and Spain, at 6.3–9.2 per 1000, rates 1.5 to 2 times higher than reported in the USA. Italy, Luxembourg and the UK have notably high rates of IV heroin usage.

Also of importance is the finding that there has been a recent steep escalation in the number of Americans using opioid pain medications for non-medical purposes. In 2002 there were 2 500 000 million new users of non-medically prescribed opioids compared to 92 000 new users in 1963 and 573 000 new users in 1990. It is noteworthy that the number of new users of non-medically prescribed painkillers is nearly equal to the 2.6 million new users of marijuana and greater than the 1.1 million new users of cocaine and the 1.1 million new users of ecstasy (SAMSHA, 2004). It is also important to note that dependence on non-medical painkillers can lead to dependence on heroin, especially when supply or cost favors the switch. With respect to gender, whereas illicit drug use is generally more common in males than in females, in 2002, 55% of the new initiators of non-medically prescribed painkillers were females (SAMSHA, 2004). There are similar patterns of increasing use of illicit painkillers in youth with a steady increase in the number of senior high school students reporting use. Between 1991 and 2004 there was a nearly three-fold increase in annual use of non-medically prescribed painkillers with reports of use in the past year increasing from 3.5% to 9.5% of students (Johnston *et al.*, 2004).

In Europe there is much less data on the prevalence of minor opioid abuse than on that of illicit drug use (Akram, 2000). One large survey of prescriptions dispensed in Norway found that about 8% of the population had obtained controlled analgesics (Eggen & Andrew, 1994), with the highest rates in older women. In a more recent study in Wales two-thirds of community pharmacists viewed some requests for over-the-counter medications (mostly opioids) as suspicious, from features such as frequent request from the same person, behavioral aspects and refusal to consider alternative products (Pates *et al.*, 2002).

Clinical features of opioid dependence

Opioids have long been recognized for their pain relieving and euphoric effects. Opioids produce their effects through their agonist effects at the opioid receptors in the CNS. Opioids vary in their receptor affinity and activity. Activation of the μ receptor in the central nervous system results in the classic features of opioid intoxication. Some compounds (e.g. morphine, heroin and methadone)

function as full agonists. Others (e.g. buprenorphine) are partial agonists at the μ receptor, while compounds with high affinity but no efficacy for the receptor (e.g., naltrexone) function as antagonists. Opioids also vary in their duration of action; heroin and morphine have a relatively short duration of action. Medications used for maintenance treatment, including methadone, buprenorphine or naltrexone, have significantly longer half-lives, thus facilitating increased stability and daily (or less frequent) dosing.

As with other substance-related disorders within the DSM IV, the disorders related to opioids are divided into two main groupings: substance use disorders and substance-induced disorders. Substance-induced disorders include opioid intoxication, opioid withdrawal and other clinical manifestations of acute opioid intake or withdrawal. Opioid use is followed by an initial euphoria or 'a rush' in the user which is associated with a warm flushing of the skin and heaviness in the extremities; nausea is also a common immediate effect, especially among first-time users. The acute euphoric effects may be followed by a longer but less intense period of tranquility; however, the initial euphoria may also be followed by apathy or dysphoria. Chronic use leads to the development of tolerance, and many chronic users report experiencing little or no euphoric effects from repeated use. Signs of recent opioid use include pupillary constriction, drowsiness or coma, respiratory depression, slurred speech, analgesia, delayed gastrointestinal motility, decreased spinal reflexes, decreased sympathetic activity, impairment in memory and impaired attention. Other signs and symptoms include psychomotor slowing or psychomotor agitation, impaired judgment, and impaired social/occupational function. Signs of injection use include needle marks, track marks, thrombophlebitis or abscesses near veins used for injection.

Opioid overdose is a medical emergency. The opioid antagonist, naloxone, should be administered to treat overdose and may be useful in diagnosing opioid overdose. In some cases psychosis, mood disorders or delirium can occur with intoxication or withdrawal from opioids.

The characteristic opioid withdrawal syndrome includes dysphoric or anxious mood; nausea, vomiting, diarrhea or stomach cramps; muscle aches; lacrimation, rhinorrhea, pupillary dilation, piloerection, mild tachycardia and hypertension, sweating, yawning, fever, chills and insomnia. This is accompanied by strong cravings to use opioids. The appearance or duration of intoxication and the length of time to emergence of withdrawal symptoms varies according to the half-life and duration of activity of different opioids used by the individual. Typically, withdrawal from shorter-acting opioids (e.g. heroin) begins 6 to 8 hours after last dose, reaches a peak within 2 to 3 days, and usually subsides within 5 to 10 days. Some symptoms such as insomnia, restlessness and dysphoria may be present for weeks to months. Onset of withdrawal symptoms may be delayed for several days in individuals dependent on longer-acting opioids (e.g. methadone).

Opioid dependence and opioid abuse are substance use disorders as classified and described in the DSM IV-TR (American Psychiatric Association, 2000). Opioid abuse involves a pattern of recurrent or continued use which results in one of the following: the individual fails to fulfill role obligations because of opioid use, uses the opioid in hazardous situations, incurs substance-related legal problems or continues to use despite significant interpersonal problems related to the opioid use. Opioid dependence refers to a pattern of use which is more akin to the more common term addiction. The dependent individual displays a constellation of behaviors and symptoms which must include three of seven criteria over a period of a year. These criteria include tolerance to opioids, opioid withdrawal, spending excessive amounts of time involved in procuring or using opioids, decreased participation in activities or relationships, a loss of control of the amount of opioids used or the amount of time spent taking opioids, a desire to cut down on use or unsuccessful attempts to cut down, and continuing use despite adverse psychological or physical consequences. According to the DSM-IV-TR criteria for dependence, it is not necessary to experience physiological adaptation to opioid evidenced by tolerance or withdrawal symptoms.

The psychological and physical effects of opioids will vary depending on the opioid used because of the different pharmacological properties of the opioids. Substances with a more rapid onset and higher intensity of effect are more likely to become substances that are abused (Roset et al., 2001). The route of administration will also affect the intensity of the effects of the drug, and those routes producing higher levels of drug to the brain faster (i.e. intravascular versus intranasal) will be preferred (Hatsukami & Fischman, 1996). Also important in considering the effect of opioids on the individual is the individual's history of use. As tolerance develops over time, the opioid user tends to experience less pleasure associated with the drug than experienced in earlier phases of their course of use. Opioid-dependent individuals may report that they continue to use, not in order to experience positive effects (positive reinforcer) but to avoid the extremely aversive opioid withdrawal syndrome (negative reinforcer). It is of utmost importance to remember that, after a period of withdrawal, tolerance to the opioid is decreased, and

there is a significant risk of overdose if high doses used by the individual before withdrawal are resumed.

Evidence-based treatments for opioid dependence

There are a variety of strategies used to treat those who are dependent on opioids. Pharmacological interventions include medically assisted withdrawal (MAW), using medications to minimize the symptoms of withdrawal; antagonist treatment, using naltrexone to block the acute effects of opioid use; and opioid agonist maintenance treatment, using long-acting opioid agonists (methadone) or partial agonists (buprenorphine) to prevent withdrawal and, at higher doses, decrease craving and, as a result of cross-tolerance, reduce or block the acute effects of illicit opioid use. Psychotherapeutic treatments, Twelve-step approaches and psychosocial interventions are important components of comprehensive treatment for opioid dependence.

How do we judge treatment success? In considering treatment strategies for opioid dependence, it is important to define successful treatment and clearly prioritize short and long-term treatment goals. In making these decisions, one must be mindful of the pervasive, chronic nature of opioid dependence which is characterized by frequent relapse (Hser et al., 2001). It is only through the consideration of long-term outcomes that we can adequately judge and compare treatment outcomes for a disorder often punctuated with periods of abstinence and relapse. For instance, a course of ultra-rapid withdrawal, if it is followed by a relapse one week later, may be associated with greater risk (e.g. drug overdose) than benefit, despite a successful course of withdrawal. By considering the various treatments on the merits of their long-term benefits, we increase our ability to make treatment decisions which maximize the long-term benefit to the patient. This may also help us to reduce unnecessary costs of ineffective treatments which could be reallocated to treatments with more positive outcomes.

In making decisions about care it is also important to prioritize the desired outcomes of treatment. With extremely high rates of mortality associated with opioid dependence, interventions that are associated with a decreased risk of mortality should be prioritized. The second priority of treatment is to prevent the transmission of chronic infectious diseases and other medical complications affecting the health and quality of life of the individual. Other important goals of treatment are sustained remission from opioids and improved psychosocial functioning, including employment and decreased criminal behavior. Some short-term outcomes (e.g. abstinence, reductions in illicit opioid use, or discontinuation of injection drug use) may serve as intermediate markers for other, long-term outcomes (e.g., decreased mortality or HIV risk).

Medically assisted withdrawal

Through medically assisted withdrawal (MAW), the opioid dependent patient is provided pharmacological relief of withdrawal symptoms. MAW may be accomplished through substitution of a longer-acting opioid agonist (e.g. methadone) or partial agonist (e.g. buprenorphine) followed by gradual tapering, or through pharmacological treatment of withdrawal symptoms (e.g. clonidine or its analogue lofexidine to reduce autonomic symptoms and other pharmacological treatments to reduce nausea, gastrointestinal symptoms, muscle pains, and sleep disturbance) following opioid discontinuation. Antagonist-precipitated withdrawal, with withdrawal symptoms treated by clonidine and other medications, may shorten the time period of withdrawal and facilitate induction onto antagonist maintenance treatment. The process is complete after all opioids have been discontinued for a sufficient period and the patient no longer experiences symptoms or shows signs of withdrawal in the absence of medications used to treat withdrawal symptoms. Completion of medical withdrawal may be documented by a lack of precipitated withdrawal in response to intramuscular naloxone and oral naltrexone. The time from opioid discontinuation to the ability to tolerate oral naltrexone without symptoms depends on the opioid being discontinued – longer acting opioids (e.g. methadone) require more prolonged periods (e.g. in the case of methadone, up to 14 days or longer). Although in otherwise healthy adults untreated withdrawal is not life-threatening, opioid withdrawal is extremely unpleasant and may lead to premature treatment termination and relapse.

Medically assisted withdrawal treatment begins with an initial evaluation. As with the evaluation of any substance dependent individual, a complete drug use history (including past treatment for opioid dependence), medical history, and information regarding psychosocial function should be obtained, in addition to necessary laboratory testing and mental status examination. Important complications to consider in MAW are suicide secondary to withdrawal induced anxiety and dysphoria; spontaneous abortion in pregnant women; medical complications in medically compromised patients (e.g. those with acute endocarditis); and post-withdrawal overdose upon relapsing. The interview should elicit stressors such as legal problems and interpersonal conflicts, the current support system available to the patient as well as information about coping strategies and cues affecting drug use and past relapses in the individual. Patients should be informed about the risks and benefits of MAW and alternative treatments. Because of the chronic course of opioid addiction, there is a high rate of relapse following successful withdrawal. MAW should be accompanied by support and counseling re: relapse prevention and ongoing drug abuse treatment (including, for example, drug counseling, family therapy, and naltrexone maintenance treatment) following completion of MAW.

Methadone in medically assisted withdrawal

Methadone is a long-acting, full agonist acting at the μ opioid receptor and, when used in progressively decreasing doses, reduces symptoms of withdrawal during MAW from opioids. A dose of 10 to 20 mg can be given once withdrawal symptoms are present (or before if adequate proof of dependence is available) and should relieve the symptoms within 30 to 60 minutes. A second dose can be given 2–4 hours later, if symptoms are not adequately relieved or recur, and the following day's dose should equal that given on the first day unless signs of sedation or withdrawal symptoms necessitate 5–10 mg increases or decreases. After stabilization, methadone doses may be tapered slowly. The rate of tapering may depend on setting (e.g. tapering may be more rapid in an inpatient setting) and patient comfort. During tapering and following methadone discontinuation, withdrawal symptoms may be treated using similar protocols to those described below in the section describing pharmacological treatments for relief of withdrawal symptoms.

In response to high relapse rates following rapid methadone tapering or other approaches to medically assisted withdrawal, extended withdrawal programs have been developed with the goal of reducing relapse by tapering methadone over a period of months. A randomized controlled trial by Sees *et al.* (2000) compared the efficacy of an enriched 180-day methadone detoxification to a standard methadone maintenance program. Findings showed the maintenance program was superior in reducing rates of illicit drug use and drug-related HIV risk behaviors. A cost/benefit analysis of these results showed that although the direct cost of the detoxification program was less expensive, the participants utilized significantly more medical and substance treatment resources than the maintenance group. The authors concluded that their results did not support the allocation of funds from methadone maintenance to detoxification programs and that the cost-effectiveness ratio of maintenance treatment was well within the accepted range for many other accepted medical interventions (Masson *et al.*, 2004).

Buprenorphine in medically assisted withdrawal

Buprenorphine is an opioid with unique pharmacological properties. It is a partial agonist at the μ receptor, has a very high affinity for occupying the μ receptor and also acts as an antagonist at the opioid receptor. As a high affinity, partial agonist, buprenorphine may displace μ receptor full agonists and result in withdrawal symptoms. Consequently, to reduce the risk of precipitated withdrawal, generally it should not be administered to patients with high levels of physical dependence (e.g. patients who have been maintained at methadone doses of 40 to 50 mg daily or higher) and should only be given to patients when withdrawal symptoms are already present. Because of its very slow dissociation from the μ receptor, buprenorphine discontinuation provides a self-tapering effect which results in a milder (but sometimes more prolonged) withdrawal syndrome. Because it is a partial agonist, there is a ceiling effect to buprenorphine's activation at the cellular level, and consequently a reduced risk for abuse (especially when provided in a tablet formulation combining buprenorphine and naloxone).

Pharmacological treatments for relief of withdrawal symptoms

Clonidine

Originally marketed for reducing hypertension, clonidine, an α-2 adrenergic agonist is also used to treat symptoms of opioid withdrawal. Clonidine, like opioids, reduces the activity of the locus coeruleus (LC) and thus is helpful in alleviating autonomic symptoms of withdrawal associated with hyperactivity of the LC following discontinuation of opioids after prolonged opioid use. Although successful at reducing the autonomic symptoms of withdrawal, when used alone for management of symptoms during withdrawal, α-2 adrenergic agonists are not effective in reducing the insomnia, restlessness, nausea, lacrimation, rhinorrhea and muscle cramps seen in withdrawal (Walsh *et al.*, 2003). Consequently, in MAW, clonidine is often combined with medications to reduce muscle pains and cramps, diarrhea, anxiety and insomnia, and nausea. Monitoring blood pressure and heart rate is important in the administration of clonidine, which is dosed at 0.1 to 0.3 mg tid to qid up to a maximum of 1.2 mg per day. Patients should be warned to be careful ambulating because of the potential fall in blood pressure. Clonidine (alone or in combination with other symptomatic medications) may be used for symptomatic treatment following

opioid tapering or abrupt opioid discontinuation, and it may also be used for symptomatic treatment in antagonist-precipitated withdrawal (see below). The duration of clonidine treatment depends on the anticipated duration of withdrawal symptoms (e.g. 5–7 days following heroin discontinuation or 5–14 days or longer following methadone discontinuation).

Lofexidine

Although not FDA approved in the US, lofexidine is currently used for MAW in Europe. Studies have shown this alpha 2-adrenergic agonist to be similar to clonidine in its success in reducing withdrawal symptoms. It has fewer side effects than clonidine, especially having little or no impact on blood pressure and less sedation. It is preferentially used over clonidine in outpatient settings. A number of randomized control trials using lofexidine support that it is essentially as effective as clonidine with less hypotension (Bearn *et al.*, 1996; Beswick *et al.*, 2003; Carnwath & Hardman, 1998; Howells *et al.*, 2002; Kahn *et al.*, 1997).

Antagonists in medically assisted withdrawal

Naltrexone in medically assisted withdrawal

The use of naltrexone in medically assisted withdrawal (Riordan & Kleber, 1980) functions to decrease the time of MAW to a 3-day course before initiation of a full blocking dose of the opioid antagonist, naltrexone. Naltrexone has high binding affinity for the μ opioid receptor and dissociates slowly from the receptor, leading to a prolonged duration of its binding. Because it is inactive at the receptor, it functions as a long-acting antagonist. With a high binding affinity, it competitively displaces active opioids from the receptor. In individuals who are physiologically dependent on opioids, naltrexone precipitates severe and prolonged withdrawal symptoms. In naltrexone-precipitated medically assisted withdrawal, withdrawal symptoms are aggressively treated with α-2 adrenergic agonists such as clonidine or lofexidine, and other adjunctive medications such as benzodiazepines for sleep difficulties, anxiety, muscle spasms, and other adjunctive medications for some of the symptoms of withdrawal described above. The major benefits of this method are that it decreases the time experiencing withdrawal symptoms and shortens the period before initiating blocking doses of naltrexone that may be useful in preventing relapse. The intensity of symptoms is a limitation for its use because adequate management of symptoms requires close medical supervision and support for up to 8 hours on the first day of induction. There is little evidence that the use of naltrexone in medically assisted withdrawal results in superior rates of abstinence or retention in post-withdrawal naltrexone treatment (O'Connor & Kosten, 1998). Buprenorphine substitution for up to 3 days prior to initiating naltrexone precipitated withdrawal has been found to decrease the severity of withdrawal symptoms compared to standard naltrexone precipitated withdrawal. Both approaches to naltrexone precipitated withdrawal are associated with a higher proportion of patients receiving a full blocking dose of naltrexone compared to protocols using clonidine and other medications in the absence of naltrexone precipitated withdrawal.

Ultrarapid medically assisted withdrawal

Ultrarapid medically assisted withdrawal using naltrexone precipitated withdrawal under general anesthesia or conscious sedation has been touted as faster, more comfortable and more effective than other approaches to naltrexone precipitated withdrawal or symptomatic treatment of withdrawal without administering naltrexone to precipitate withdrawal. Despite extravagant claims about its short-term and long-term effectiveness, there is at best limited scientific evidence supporting the claims, and the procedure is associated with a significant risk of medical complications, including pulmonary edema, aspiration pneumonia, delirium, and death (Hamilton *et al.*, 2002; Kleber, 1998; O'Connor & Kosten, 1998). A study by McGregor *et al.* (2002) found no advantage in 3-month outcomes of the anesthetic approach over non-anesthetic approaches, and a recent meta-analysis concluded that ultrarapid withdrawal should continue to be deemed experimental, as there is not currently proof of benefit over other methods and the costs and risks are greater (Gowing *et al.*, 2001). Because of the risk of respiratory depression and vomiting under anesthetic, the procedure should only be delivered in locations with adequate staffing and resources for intubation and assisted ventilation if required.

Opioid antagonist treatment (treatment of dependence)

Opioid antagonists are used in the treatment of opioid dependence in three ways: (1) to reverse an opioid overdose, (2) to prevent relapse by blocking opioids from producing their effect at opioid receptors, and (3) to identify those with opioid dependence by inducing withdrawal symptoms to provide evidence of opioid dependence.

Naloxone

Naloxone, a short-acting opioid antagonist, has a number of important uses in opioid treatment. The rapid metabolism of the naloxone makes it an ideal antagonist for the reversal of opioid overdose effects in emergency situations. Naloxone is also combined with buprenorphine in a special combination tablet to prevent misuse of buprenorphine. Because naloxone is minimally absorbed sublingually or orally, when combined with buprenorphine in a sublingual tablet (Suboxone) and taken sublingually, as directed, it has negligible effect. However, if the tablet is dissolved and injected, the naloxone may induce opioid withdrawal in opioid dependent individuals. Naloxone (e.g. 0.8 mg IM) may also be used to confirm physiological opioid dependence in individuals seeking maintenance treatment or MAW and may be used to verify completion of MAW prior to initiating naltrexone treatment.

Naltrexone maintenance treatment

As described above, in the medically assisted withdrawal section, naltrexone is a long-acting opioid antagonist which functions to block the effects of opioids by competitively occupying but not activating opioid receptors. Regular dosing of naltrexone prevents patients from experiencing the effects of opioids, thereby preventing relapse. Naltrexone is taken in daily doses of 50 mg or three weekly doses (e.g. 100 mg on Mondays and Wednesdays and 150 mg on Fridays). Naltrexone has good bioavailability by the oral route of administration and has a half-life of approximately four hours. An active metabolite has a half-life of 12 hours. Side effects of naltrexone have been implicated as one cause of drop-out rates in treatment. A large multi-center study which followed 570 patients taking naltrexone in its separate indication for alcohol dependence examined the rate of various side effects. The most common new onset side effects were nausea (9.8%) and headache (6.6%), with dizziness (4.4%), nervousness (3.8%), fatigue (3.6%), anxiety (2.0%) and depression (1.4%) being less common (Croop *et al.*, 1997). High doses of naltrexone (300 mg daily) used in a study of obese patients and a study of patients with Huntington's disease were associated with hepatotoxicity which was reversible on discontinuation of naltrexone. At lower doses (50 mg per day) however, a number of studies examining liver function in naltrexone treated alcohol dependent individuals have found that liver function was equivalent or improved in those receiving naltrexone compared to placebo (Croop *et al.*, 1997; O'Malley *et al.*, 1992; Volpicelli *et al.*, 1992). Liver function should be monitored during naltrexone treatment.

Abstinence-based treatment with naltrexone can be initiated only after a patient has withdrawn completely from opioids. If even minimal residual physical dependence exists, treatment with naltrexone may induce persistent and severe withdrawal symptoms, resulting in termination of treatment. A naloxone challenge can assist in determining whether physical dependence is present in an individual requesting naltrexone treatment.

An important adjunct to medically assisted withdrawal, initiation or continuation of naltrexone immediately post-MAW assists in reducing the extremely high relapse rates of MAW alone. The goal of naltrexone treatment is to avoid the positive reinforcement of opioid use thereby reducing use and interrupting the patterns of learning and conditioning that have occurred through this reinforcement. Despite initial optimism for this treatment, the effectiveness of naltrexone in practice has been very limited secondary to high drop-out rates and low patient interest in initiating antagonist treatment (Garcia Alonso et al., 1989; Gutierrez et al., 1995; Hulse & Basso, 1999; Kirchmayer et al., 2002; San et al., 1991). A lack of pharmacological positive reinforcement related to naltrexone and patients not wanting to lose the ability to get high are examples of reasons given for rates of compliance ranging as low as 0 to 10% at 6 months for naltrexone treatment alone (Rounsaville, 1995). Studies combining naltrexone treatment with psychotherapeutic interventions such as behavioral naltrexone therapy, behavioral family counseling combined with individual therapy, significant other involvement, individual counseling or contingency management have been shown to produce some improvement in outcomes (Carroll et al., 2001, 2002; Fals-Stewart & O'Farrell, 2003, Preston et al., 1999; Rothenberg et al., 2002; Stella et al., 1999). Outside of academic research centers, formal naltrexone treatment programs are rare and even when available, patients tend to show more affinity for, and better retention within, agonist treatment programs (Rounsaville, 1995). Select groups of opioid dependent individuals with high negative reinforcement for opioid use, such as healthcare professionals at risk of losing their license or business executives, tend to do better than other patients in naltrexone treatment with some rates of abstinence being as high as 80% and 95% at 1 year post-treatment (Roth et al., 1997; Washton et al., 1984). Other groups showing higher success rates in naltrexone treatment are federal probationers (Cornish et al., 1997) and populations in countries where methadone is not available and patients appear to have increased levels of family support (Krupitsky et al., 2004).

Long-acting preparations of naltrexone have been developed to avoid the problem of loss of antagonistic effect through non-compliance with a daily tablet and perhaps to improve retention. The general safety and efficacy of blockade effect of a depot were demonstrated in the USA by Comer et al. (2002), while a Spanish study found 80% retention at 6 months and 65% at one year using a subcutaneous naltrexone implant (Carreno et al., 2003).

To summarize, it appears that, although some heavily dependent opioid users with complex problems wish to receive naltrexone if they become drug free, the most frequent indication is in milder cases that detoxify easily, have a real motivation to remain opioid drug-free, have social support, and thus have a generally good prognosis. In practice, the medication clearly has a role in preventing impulsive relapses during abstinence attempts.

Opioid agonist maintenance treatment

In opioid agonist maintenance treatment, the patient is stabilized on a long-acting, orally available, medically prescribed opioid agonist or partial agonist. The goals of opioid agonist maintenance treatment are to prevent withdrawal symptoms and, with sufficient doses, to reduce craving and block or reduce the acute rewarding effects of illicit opioid use by inducing cross-tolerance to usual street doses of opioids. Maintenance treatment with opioid agonists provides a pharmacological platform that also facilitates behavioral monitoring (for illicit opioid or other drug use) and psychosocial and behavioral treatments and life-style change necessary for longer-term abstinence and recovery. Provision of drug counseling during opioid agonist maintenance treatment significantly reduces illicit opioid and other drug use and improves treatment outcome (McLellan et al., 1993). Clear and consistent program expectations, greater involvement of the methadone program director in treatment planning and provision of services, and greater program stability are also associated with improved outcomes across methadone treatment programs (Bell et al., 1997; Magura et al., 1999) The results of clinical trials, meta-analyses of clinical trials, and observational studies of treatment consistently support the effectiveness of opioid agonist maintenance treatment for reducing illicit opioid use, the mortality and medical morbidity (including HIV) and criminal activity associated with opioid dependence, and improving psychosocial functioning (Bates & Pemberton, 1996; Bertschy, 1995; Caplehorn et al., 1996; Dole et al., 1969; Farre et al., 2002; Ling & Wesson, 2003; Marsch, 1998; Mattick et al., 2002a, 2002b; Merrill, 1999; Metzger et al., 1993; Newman & Whitehall, 1979).

Methadone was the first medication used for maintenance treatment in the USA and remains the most commonly used medication currently not only in the USA, but in the UK and Europe as well. Two other medications, buprenorphine and LAAM (L-α-acetylmethadol) are currently approved by the FDA for maintenance treatment in the USA. LAAM is a methadone derivative which acts as a full agonist at the μ opioid receptor and, along with its active metabolites, has a longer half-life than methadone, allowing for three times weekly dosing. Because of a risk of cardiac conduction abnormalities (prolonged QT interval and torsades de pointes) LAAM is no longer marketed in the USA. The efficacy of buprenorphine, the most recently approved opioid agonist for treating opioid dependence, is generally comparable to methadone (Johnson *et al.*, 2000; Ling & Wesson, 2003; Strain *et al.*, 1994; West *et al.*, 2000).

Methadone maintenance treatment

Methadone maintenance treatment has been in use since the mid-1960s and is the most thoroughly studied and documented effective treatments for opioid dependence. Because the substantial evidence regarding its effectiveness derived from randomized, placebo controlled clinical trials and observational studies has been reviewed elsewhere, we do not review the evidence regarding its effectiveness in this chapter and instead briefly review some of the basic pharmacology of methadone and issues regarding methadone dose, duration of treatment, and treatment setting.

Methadone is a full agonist at the μ opioid receptor. It has an average half-life of approximately 24 hours allowing for once daily dosing in maintenance treatment. Methadone is primarily metabolized by the enzyme cytochrome P450 3A4 in the liver, although other P450 enzymes are also involved in metabolism (Iribarne *et al.*, 1997) To ensure safety, it is essential to consider drug interactions when prescribing methadone. There are numerous medications (e.g. antiretrovirals, antidepressants, anticonvulsants, and antibiotics) which interact with methadone metabolism and can decreasing methadone levels inducing withdrawal symptoms or increase methadone levels putting patients at risk of side effects or death. Common side effects of methadone include sexual dysfunction, constipation, excessive sweating, and drowsiness (Langrod *et al.*, 1981). There is a risk of overdose death associated with methadone treatment, most significantly during the first 1 to 2 weeks of treatment. Overdose risk is related to excessive initial methadone doses or too rapid and excessive dose increases and is exacerbated by the use of illicit substances, by concomitant use of medications which may interact with methadone metabolism or act synergistically as a CNS depressant, and by liver disease. Methadone overdose may cause respiratory depression, aspiration of vomit, pulmonary edema, cardiac problems, bronchopneumonia, and renal failure (Corkery *et al.*, 2004). There have been recent reports of associations between prolonged QTc interval and high dose methadone (Kornick *et al.*, 2003; Krantz *et al.*, 2003). This is an important finding that will require further study. A fine review of the possible cardiac side effects is provided by Justo *et al.* (2006).

After the initial very positive effects of methadone versus placebo (Gunne & Gronbaldh, 1981), it soon was considered unethical to conduct placebo-controlled trials because of the disadvantages of denying people methadone who needed it. There remains some controversy as to dosing, because some feel that even the current dosing may be too low. Methadone maintenance treatment is initiated at a relatively low dose (up to a maximum of 30 mg daily), which is generally sufficient to prevent or ameliorate withdrawal symptoms, and then gradually increased over a period of several weeks or more to a dose that is sufficient to reduce craving and illicit opioid use. Higher doses of methadone (60–100 mg daily) are associated with better treatment retention rates and decreased illicit drug use than lower doses (Faggiano *et al.*, 2003; Gerra *et al.*, 2003; Johnson *et al.*, 2000; Strain *et al.*, 1999). High-dose treatment has the most impact, and maintenance is more effective than short-term detoxification, though Curran *et al.* (1999) found, in a double-blind cross-over design, that in some patients a one-third increase in daily dosage increased some aspects of craving for heroin.

A prominent cohort study in the UK comparing four treatment modalities has been the National Treatment Outcome Research Study (NTORS) (Gossop *et al.*, 2003). Alongside residential programs the two pharmacological modalities are methadone maintenance and methadone reduction with staff in participating agencies initially indicating into which of these categories patients fitted. The very slow rate of dose reduction in some flexible prescribing schemes was illustrated by the finding at one year that there was no significant difference in methadone dosage between the supposed maintenance and reduction groups (Gossop *et al.*, 2000). A similar lack of distinction between treatments was present at two years (Gossop *et al.*, 2001), with those individuals who had reduced quickly having worse outcomes and higher drop-out rates. At 4 to 5 years, the 418 patients followed up in all modalities showed overall reductions in use of heroin, benzodiazepines and non-prescribed methadone as well as injecting and sharing of equipment, but measures of cocaine and alcohol use were not significantly different from intake (Gossop *et al.*, 2003). Thus one can appreciate that there is still discussion as to what is the best and proper dose to be used. Much treatment in Europe falls somewhere between these two models in slow withdrawal schemes (Seivewright & Lagundoye, 2003).

In the past two decades methadone has been the main opioid substitute treatment used in both US and European drug services. Maintenance in particular was increasingly promoted as the need to reduce HIV risk behaviours and transmission was recognized, and taking the UK as an example, successive national guidelines up to the latest version have recommended the treatment as first-line in established opiate dependence (Department of Health, 1999). Because of its potential lethality and its high risk of abuse (there is a street value), methadone treatment in the USA is tightly controlled and delivered in specialized clinics which provide counseling, medical services and may offer social work, legal services or vocational services.

Some of the more recent trials of methadone provide information as to its success and to the limits of its success. Strang et al. (1997) randomized 119 opiate-dependent subjects to methadone maintenance or reduction regimens and found most benefits occurring in the early stages before low doses had been reached. They also found equivalent rates of positive outcome when comparing oral methadone with the injectable form (Strang et al., 2000), though the prescribing of the injectable form of methadone, at least in the UK, is usually reserved for individuals who had demonstrably failed to progress on oral methadone over long periods (Battersby et al, 1992; Metrebian et al., 1998; Sell et al., 2001). In these individuals, the injectable form did lead to harm reduction benefits which included good retention, reduced illicit usage, and improved psychological well-being. Completion rates of methadone detoxification in the community are known to be low, with one trial finding 17% in outpatients as against 81% in inpatients (Gossop et al., 1986). "Flexible" prescribing, in which users have a say in their rates of reduction is often advocated, but in a study by Dawe et al. (1991), patients randomly assigned to that method progressed no better then fixed-regime subjects, with generally high rates of additional drug use. Amato et al. (2004) examined five Cochrane reviews of detoxification involving methadone, adrenergic agonists and buprenorphine and concluded that methadone had some advantages in relation to retention in treatment, relapse rates and side effects. Methadone treatment in primary care has mainly been investigated in open studies, with Keen et al. (2003) measuring one-year outcomes in Sheffield, UK, in patients receiving maintenance based on national guidelines (Department of Health, 1999). Sixty-five out of 96 recruits completed the study, showing highly significant reductions in heroin use and criminal activity as well as improvements in HIV risk behaviors, social functioning, and physical and psychological health.

The superiority of methadone maintenance over detoxification in terms of outcomes within treatment has been repeatedly shown. There is the possibility, however, that subgroups who do successfully complete withdrawal and avoid relapse into substance misuse go on to have the best quality of life, and this was demonstrated in a study in Sweden by Eklund et al. (1994). Differences between patients trying to quit their methadone and those wishing to continue on maintenance were studied by Hiltunen & Eklund (2002), while an increased mortality in the early stages of re-entering methadone treatment was among the findings in a substantial study in Amsterdam (Buster et al., 2002).

In sum, there is much consistency in the findings of studies supporting the effectiveness of methadone maintenance, for reducing illicit opioid use and improving the various medical and social outcomes. Methadone maintenance is the most established, evidence-based approach for reducing an opioid-dependent individual's drug use and associated problems. Such effectiveness is broadly proportional to dosage and length of treatment. Nevertheless, the optimal methadone dose and optimal duration of treatment needs to be determined on an individual basis for patients, since some opioid dependent patients may respond to lower methadone doses, and some patients may be able to achieve sustained benefits after discontinuing methadone maintenance treatment.

Buprenorphine maintenance treatment
Buprenorphine has been licensed in Europe and in the United States for drug dependence treatment only relatively recently. Much of the usage in the UK where it is a category B substance, has been since the latest version of national guidelines. France is somewhat exceptional in not having had widespread methadone prescribing before buprenorphine was introduced, and the latter is an especially prominent treatment there.

Treatment with buprenorphine, a partial μ receptor agonist, is slightly more complicated than with full agonist opioids such as methadone. But its partial opioid agonist/antagonist activity makes it a suitable substitution treatment in opioid dependence, and its primary effect is usually milder than that of methadone. The mixed property potentially confers some advantages over methadone, including greater safety in overdosage, less interaction with other euphoriant drugs and quicker transfer to naltrexone after detoxification (Davids & Gastpar, 2004; Kosten, 2003; Walsh & Eissenberg, 2003). The partial agonist profile makes it theoretically more attractive for detoxification than methadone, and relatively low rates of problematic withdrawal effects have been reported from clinical settings (Diamant et al., 1998; Williams et al., 2002).

Following the pivotal studies in the USA (Johnson et al., 1995), further randomized controlled trials have taken place in Europe, including in Sweden (Kakko *et al.*, 2003), Switzerland (Uehlinger *et al.*, 1998, Petitjean *et al.*, 2001), and Austria (Fischer *et al.*, 1999). The Swedish study was described as placebo-controlled with that group actually receiving just a 6-day medication reduction course. Stark differences were indeed found with buprenorphine maintenance having a 75% 12-month retention rate and no deaths, compared with 0% retention at 2 months in the placebo group and four deaths by 12 months.

In France buprenorphine is widely prescribed in primary care, with methadone reserved for use in specialist centres. There have been attempts to compare the use and effectiveness of methadone versus buprenorphine, but Barrau *et al.* (2001) considered that some differences in outcomes probably reflected features of the populations rather than true differences in effectiveness between the two medications. A cross-sectional study in the same country (Guichard *et al.*, 2003) found approximately one-third of both buprenorphine and methadone patients to be using illicit drugs, with social situation exerting some influence. Injection of buprenorphine has emerged as a substantial problem in France and several other countries. Buprenorphine and methadone outpatients in Austria were compared by Giacomuzzi *et al.* (2003), with the buprenorphine-maintained group showing less additional opioid and cocaine use over six months, and both groups having similar improvements in quality of life. Other studies comparing buprenorphine and methadone found satisfactory overall reductions in illicit drug use with both. Retention tended to be less good with buprenorphine but the Swiss investigators (Uehlinger *et al.*, 1998, Petitjean *et al.*, 2001) considered that that might be due to inadequate dosing. Clinical practice now involves higher daily dosages then were used in some early trials.

The clinical profiles of buprenorphine patients in French cities were studied by Poirier *et al.* (2004). Factors predicting a good treatment response included lack of alcohol dependence and family history of addictions, and duration of opioid dependence less then 10 years.

The relatively unique pharmacological properties of buprenorphine, including its long lasting effects on the μ opioid receptor and possible association with lower degree of physiological dependence, may offer an advantage with regard to causing neonatal withdrawal. Evidence is accumulating on the safe use of buprenorphine maintenance during pregnancy (Lacroix *et al.*, 2004), and neonatal signs which appear less marked than after methadone maintenance (Schindler *et al.*, 2003).

When initiating treatment with buprenorphine it is important to wait until there are signs of withdrawal before initiating treatment. Due to its partial activation at the opioid receptor, buprenorphine may precipitate withdrawal symptoms if it displaces opioids in the system occupying opioid receptors. Buprenorphine is a generally well-tolerated medication. Side effects include constipation, nausea, drowsiness, headache, and vomiting. There have been case reports in the literature of hepatotoxicity that is reversible on discontinuation of the medication (Herve *et al.*, 2004). It is important to monitor liver function in patients on buprenorphine. Due to its partial agonist activity there is a ceiling effect or plateau with respect to dose-dependent effects of buprenorphine and this results in a decreased risk of adverse events such as respiratory depression (Walsh *et al.*, 1994) Buprenorphine overdose, including severe respiratory depression, has been reported, however, in young children and in individuals abusing buprenorphine along with benzodiazepines. As with methadone, the efficacy of buprenorphine is dose-dependent, and higher daily doses of 12–16 mg are more effective than lower doses of 4 or 8 mg (Ling *et al.*, 1996; Montoya *et al.*, 2004; Schottenfeld *et al.*, 1997). At present, buprenorphine is mainly prescribed in tablet form and there is a significant risk of abuse by injection. To deter this a combination preparation of buprenorphine and naloxone has been developed, with the naloxone only being active parenterally. If injected, the combination product may cause severe withdrawal symptoms in heroin-dependent individuals, but its effects in individuals dependent on buprenorphine has not been systematically evaluated (Walsh & Eissenberg, 2003).

In sum, as with methadone, the general benefits of buprenorphine maintenance appear very clear in terms of reduced illicit drug use, injecting and associated problems. Meta-analyses of comparisons with methadone (Barnett *et al.*, 2001; West *et al.*, 2000) find broadly equivalent overall results. The particular impact which buprenorphine has had in France in greatly increasing the availability of substitution treatment has been emphasized by Auriacombe *et al.* (1999).

Thus, buprenorphine is an extremely important alternative to methadone, and may be preferable where a treatment plan includes possible slow reduction or detoxification. Buprenorphine appears indicated for individuals with moderate degrees of opioid dependence, but individuals with severe dependence may require a more potent opioid, usually methadone.

Diamorphine

Diamorphine is essentially heroin. Where diamorphine is able to be prescribed, as it is in the UK where this has long been part of the so-called 'British system' of drug treatment (Spear, 2002), recommendations are for use in a small minority of treatment-resistant patients. Providing diamorphine has also been advocated as a way of enrolling into treatment heroin-dependent individuals who would not enroll in methadone or buprenorphine maintenance treatment, but there have been no systematic evaluations of this approach (compared to approaches emphasizing improving the availability and accessibility of methadone or buprenorphine maintenance) regarding this goal. Programs providing diamorphine by injection may be considerably more costly and resource intensive, requiring longer hours and greater levels of staffing and more frequent program attendance for patients, compared to methadone or buprenorphine maintenance treatment. One additional disadvantage of maintenance treatment with diamorphine is the difficulty obtaining objective verification of heroin abstinence in patients; urine toxicology testing is routinely used during buprenorphine or methadone maintenance treatment to evaluate recent illicit opioid use, which patients may be hesitant to report, despite the importance of being able to adjust treatment to address ongoing heroin use.

The most systematic research regarding diamorphine has taken place in Switzerland and the Netherlands. One part of a large Swiss cohort study was a randomized trial of intravenous diamorphine prescribing plus psychological interventions versus standard treatment, usually methadone (Rehm *et al.*, 2001). At 6 months only one of 25 diamorphine subjects still used street heroin as opposed to 10 control subjects, and the diamorphine group showed better psychological health and social functioning. Two studies in the Netherlands were undertaken by van den Brink *et al.* (2003). They randomized 549 individuals who had not progressed well in methadone maintenance to injectable or smokable diamorphine plus methadone or to methadone alone. Both combination treatments appeared superior to methadone alone as measured by a combined index covering physical health, mental status and social functioning over 12 months.

In a London drug clinic 58 long-term opiate injectors who had been unsuccessful in oral methadone treatment were offered the choice of receiving injectable diamorphine or injectable methadone, and then they were followed up for 12 months (Metrebian *et al.*, 2001). Two-thirds opted for diamorphine, and that group had better retention in treatment. There were no other significant differences in outcomes that occurred. Two subjects progressed to oral methadone and one became abstinent. Sell *et al.* (2001) studied 125 patients on injectable opioid treatment in Manchester, UK with most receiving injectable methadone or diamorphine. Many of the patients on methadone ampoules stated that they would rather have

been on diamorphine. Previous high levels of risk behaviours in relation to health and blood-borne virus infection were characteristic of the population, but current self-reported risks were low. Overall, 25% continued to use some street heroin, although daily usage was rare.

Much of the Swiss research program was composed of investigations of effectiveness of diamorphine without direct comparison groups. Over 1000 individuals with severe heroin dependence and a high degree of social complications were treated with diamorphine at various stages, with much clinical information being contained in the studies by Uchtenhagen *et al.* (1996, 1997). Overall, retention rates were about 70% and the mortality rate low at 1%. There were demonstrable reductions in illicit drug use and improvements in health and social functioning apparent at 18-months follow-up. The dosage of prescribed diamorphine was around 500 mg per day, which is similar to that used in the Netherlands, but the Swiss group did not find smokable heroin as satisfactory, with very high doses required to achieve adequate effects. Long-term follow-up of police records of the Swiss participants showed marked reductions in criminal activity in most patients (Ribeaud, 2004).

The European studies have often been criticized as not being significantly rigorous, although the trials from the Netherlands appear to demonstrate benefits relating strongly to treatment medication rather than confounding factors. One of the best-known aspects of diamorphine prescribing is that it has been available as a clinical option for decades in the UK, and Metrebian *et al.* (2002) investigated the practice by surveying the 164 doctors recorded as holding the relevant license. Only 70 were definitely established to have a current license with 46 actually prescribing diamorphine, and the reasons the clinicians gave for not issuing diamorphine were the concern that the medication might be diverted, the treatment involves perpetuating the process of injection, it is costly, and many doubt it is a necessary drug beyond oral methadone. Prescribers of diamorphine describe its ability to reduce drug-related harm and improve health and stability, it is a good option when all else has failed, it is effective in detoxification, it keeps people in treatment, and it allows people continuity of care who have already been prescribed diamorphine in other settings.

Thus some countries may consider it useful to have diamorphine as an option for some treatment-resistant patients who prove unable to stop injecting with other treatments. It would be preferable to also have a non-injectable preparation with satisfactory bioavailability, to broaden usage where necessary and to enable some diamorphine patients to move on from injecting.

Other opiate agonists

Morphine Some morphine treatment was included in the Swiss diamorphine research (Uchtenhagen *et al.*, 1996), but low acceptability by patients led to two of the morphine groups being curtailed. A different patient experience with oral morphine was reported by Fischer *et al.* (1999). Patients in this trial had low rates of adverse effects. Kraigher *et al.* (2002) reported good results of oral slow-release morphine prescribing in 64 patients with improvements in well-being and highly significant reductions in craving for drugs. In this preliminary investigation over just a three-week period, a reduction in use of additional benzodiazepines was particularly noted. Morphine may ultimately have fewer adverse effects than methadone, and it may, in some individuals, be an effective oral treatment.

Dihydrocodeine and codeine In drug regulations dihydrocodeine is typically set at a lower level of control than methadone, and in the UK much dihydrocodeine prescribing takes place in primary care by doctors not necessarily involved with methadone treatment (Matheson *et al.*, 2003). In Germany there have been recent attempts to limit dihydrocodeine and codeine prescribing, linked with encouragement to use more methadone for opioid-dependent individuals. Some clinical investigators, however, consider it as a legitimate milder alternative. Banbery *et al.* (2000) used it to successfully detoxify 13 out of 20 patients from methadone maintenance. A particularly favorable report of dihydrocodeine prescribing to drug misusers was by MacLeod *et al.* (1998), who audited 200 patients in a primary care practice in Edinburgh, Scotland. Retention rates and measures of health and behavior change were good, appearing equivalent to those achieved with methadone. Thus dihydrocodeine has a place in some treatment, though is not used as a treatment in the USA, at least not formally.

Office-based care Until recently, in the USA opioid maintenance treatment has been delivered through specially licensed narcotic treatment programs resourced with an administrative framework to ensure clinic procedures which decrease the likelihood of diversion of agonists for illicit use and ensures adherence to patient eligibility criteria. Problems associated with this approach, however, include the difficulty expanding treatment accessibility, capacity and attractiveness to reach the estimated 75%–80% opioid-dependent individuals not in treatment (200 000 out of the estimated 800 000 to one million opioid dependent individuals are currently enrolled in methadone maintenance), and the lack of flexibility in dispensing procedures, the high exposure to drug users and the lack of anonymity associated with attending a methadone clinic. As an alternative to providing opioid agonist maintenance treatment in specialized narcotic treatment programs, several approaches for opioid agonist maintenance provided by physicians in office-based or primary care clinics have been evaluated. One approach, referred to as medical maintenance for stable methadone maintained patients (i.e. patients who have been abstinent from illicit drug use and have good psychosocial functioning), has been implemented in physician offices in several geographic areas of the USA. Recent evaluations indicate that medical maintenance is feasible and has comparable efficacy as continued maintenance in specialized narcotic treatment programs (Fiellin *et al.*, 2001; King *et al.*, 2002; Salsitz *et al.*, 2000).

With recent changes in federal legislation authorizing office-based prescription by specially certified physicians of Schedule III or IV medications approved for opioid agonist maintenance treatment (Drug Addiction Treatment Act of 2000) and the recent FDA approval of buprenorphine for this indication, office-based prescription of buprenorphine maintenance is now available in the USA. An early pilot study found better retention and a significantly lower proportion of opiate-positive urine tests in patients randomly assigned to three times weekly buprenorphine maintenance in a primary care clinic compared to a specialized drug treatment program (O'Connor *et al.*, 1998). Another more recent study found that, in comparison with an historical control, treatment retention and reductions of illicit drug use were similar for office-based buprenorphine and maintenance in narcotic treatment programs (Fiellin *et al.*, 2002) The optimal intensity of drug counseling, frequency of clinic attendance, and frequency of medication pick-up during buprenorphine maintenance in primary care or office-based practices are currently under investigation.

Psychosocial treatment in agonist maintenance

The management of opioid dependence involves pharmacological treatments to an extent not seen in some other forms of drug misuse where psychosocial interventions may be the only strategies. In opioid dependence the various forms of counseling tend to be viewed as additional treatments (Nyswander *et al.*, 1958; O'Malley *et al.*, 1972), but there are dangers of prescribing in isolation and drug services are increasingly recommended to provide pharmacological and psychological assistance as a combined package. There are many studies which show that outcomes are optimized in opioid dependence by combining psychosocial interventions with opioid agonist maintenance.

Stanton & Todd (1982) demonstrated that a Structured Family Therapy intervention, which involved bringing families of methadone maintained patients into a family therapy treatment, showed superior outcomes at one year follow-up in comparison to patients receiving standard treatment. In the UK, a randomized trial of family therapy and two control treatments was undertaken in 119 opioid users in a methadone reduction program (Yandoli et al., 2002). In terms of reduced drug use over 12 months, patients receiving family therapy or minimal interventions fared better than those having supportive psychotherapy, with gender and drug use in partners also exerting effects.

Cognitive-behavioral therapy (CBT) and supportive expressive therapy (SE) have also shown to be superior to standard drug counseling (DC) in methadone patients. A controlled study with three treatment groups compared DC, CBT and SE, and demonstrated increased improvement in patients in the latter two groups (Woody et al., 1983) Patients with psychiatric co-morbidity showed the most dramatic gains in SE and CBT compared to DC. An important negative finding for psychotherapy was demonstrated in a study comparing short-term Interpersonal Psychotherapy (IPT) with standard treatment (Rounsaville et al., 1983). A significant psychotherapy effect was not found; however, certain organizational elements in the study such as a low completion rate and off-site therapy rather than on-site therapy may have affected the outcome.

Motivational interviewing, an approach to drug treatment developed by Miller & Rollnick (1991), involves brief interventions with a non-judgmental style, empathic listening and the absence of confrontation. A randomized controlled trial comparing brief motivational intervention to a control group in methadone maintained patients demonstrated reduced opioid related problems, better compliance with treatment and improved retention in the experimental group (Saunders et al., 1995) Network therapy, a treatment which employs family members and/or friends to assist through supporting compliance with treatment, has been shown to increase the number of negative urine toxicology screens in patients treated with short-term office-based buprenorphine maintenance (Galanter et al., 2004).

Contingency management, a behavioral intervention which is based on the principle that behaviors that are reinforced are more likely to be exhibited, has shown success in treating substance abuse. When standard procedures of a narcotic treatment program involve providing privileges for not using illicit substances (such as take-home bottles) or costs for positive toxicology screens (increased time in counseling, losing bottle privileges or being discharged from treatment), contingency is established which helps to positively

shape the substance use behavior of the individual in treatment (Stitzer et al., 1992). Randomized controlled trials of the specific behavioral approach of community reinforcement, which can involve incentives for abstinence from drugs, were considered by Roozen et al. (2004). In a review of 11 trials there was some evidence of effectiveness within opioid maintenance and detoxification programs, although this efficacy appeared less than in cocaine or alcohol dependence. Twelve-step programs, well studied and effective for other substances of abuse, are also available for opioid dependent individuals as Narcotics Anonymous or Methadone Anonymous (Gilman et al., 2001).

Other studies have investigated the impact of alternatively structured programs and enhanced psychosocial interventions in methadone maintained patients. More intense treatments such as day programs (Ravndal, 2001; Ravndal & Valum, 1991), provided at program entry, have been investigated but have not proven to be more effective than the less intensive once weekly standard counseling (Avants et al., 1998). In addition, in this latter study, those who were socially anxious did more poorly if randomized to intensive treatment than if randomized to once weekly standard counseling (Avants et al., 1999). The UK NTORS cohort research involves the non-pharmacological modalities of inpatient care and longer-term residential rehabilitation (Gossop et al., 2003). Patients in all treatments showed marked reductions in opioid and benzodiazepine use and injecting at the various review stages, with the results of methadone prescribing and residential rehabilitation being remarkably similar at one and 4- to 5-year follow-up. The most conclusive evidence supporting the effectiveness of intensity of counseling and programming provided in treatment in opioid maintenance was drawn from a randomized controlled trial involving three different levels of psychosocial support in methadone maintenance treatment. One of the three groups received minimal treatment (methadone with no counseling), a second group received methadone with standard drug counseling, and the third received methadone and standard drug counseling plus additional services including vocation, legal and medical services. Before completion of the 6 month trial, 69% of the participants had to be protectively transferred from the minimal treatment (methadone only) group because of unremitting cocaine or opioid use or medical/psychiatric emergencies. Only 41% and 19% of the standard counseling and additional services groups, respectively, met similar criteria. Study outcomes showed significant improvement in outcome with each increased level of intervention (McLellan et al., 1993). Cost–benefit analysis of the interventions in this study revealed that, although the best outcomes at 12 months were seen in the enhanced services group, when costs of treatment were evaluated, the standard counseling group showed the best cost/benefit ratio of the three groups (Kraft *et al.*, 1997).

Alternative treatments

Geerlings *et al.* (1985) detoxified 93 opiate addicts with either electrostimulation or graded methadone withdrawal, finding more early drop-outs in the electrostimulation group. In Hamburg, Germany, acupuncture was offered to drug addiction outpatients with 96% of 159 patients participating but many dropping out in the first two weeks (Verthein *et al.*, 2002). There were some improvements in reduced withdrawal symptoms and drug usage in individuals who persisted with the treatment. A meta-analysis of studies of acupuncture in addictions was undertaken by a Dutch group (Ter-Riet *et al.*, 1990), concluding that the data in opioid dependence was of poor quality and there was little to support the treatment. The herbal treatment ibogaine was used in seven subjects with variable results by Sheppard (1994), and has since received additional study in the USA. Animal studies focusing on identifying the mechanism of action for ibogaine have increased understanding of its effects but, given the poor clinical evidence base for ibogaine, further study is necessary.

Treatment in pregnancy

The use of illicit opioids during pregnancy is associated with numerous risks to the mother and developing fetus and upon delivery, to the neonate who may experience withdrawal. Untreated, neonatal withdrawal is associated with significant mortality and morbidity. In heroin-exposed infants, withdrawal generally occurs 1 to 3 days after birth. Characteristic features include yawning, sneezing, respiratory and gastrointestinal dysfunction, tearing, frantic sucking of fists, an inconsolable high-pitch cry, irritability and difficulty feeding. Opioid dependence and withdrawal during pregnancy are associated with increased risk of spontaneous abortion, premature birth, decreased birth weight, decreased head circumference size, fetal demise and withdrawal symptoms in the neonate (Archie, 1998). Medical complications of opioid dependence (e.g. HIV, hepatitis, endocarditis) and other complications of addiction (e.g. poor nutrition, inconsistent or inadequate medical care, or violence exposure) may also complicate pregnancy, labor and delivery, and adversely affect the fetal health and development. Comprehensive methadone maintenance treatment, including co-ordinated medical and psychosocial services,

reduces episodic withdrawal and improves the health status and well-being of the pregnant woman and developing fetus. Providing the appropriate dose of methadone during pregnancy is important in order to reduce illicit drug use, minimize cravings for illicit drugs and avoid withdrawal syndromes. Although there have been concerns that higher doses of methadone during pregnancy result in an increased likelihood of neonatal abstinence syndrome, this has not been observed in two recent studies comparing mothers' doses with neonatal outcomes. A retrospective review of 100 births did not find a difference between high versus low maternal dose (above 80 mg vs. below 80 mg) in measures of neonatal abstinence scores, need for treatment of withdrawal, and duration of withdrawal (Berghella *et al.*, 2003). The study also found a trend in patterns of illicit drug use, with mothers on doses less than 80 mg being more likely to use illicit opioids during their pregnancy than those on doses above 80 mg. Another study which repeated the finding that maternal methadone dose did not predict need for neonatal treatment also showed a significant association, independent of mother's methadone dose, between a lower methadone concentration in cord blood at the time of birth, lower levels of methadone in the neonate at 48 hours, and an increased likelihood of neonatal abstinence syndrome (Kuschel *et al.*, 2004). As stated above, recent evidence appears to support the safety of buprenorphine in pregnancy (Lacroix *et al.*, 2004), and neonatal signs appear less marked than after methadone maintenance (Schindler *et al.*, 2003).

Conclusions

In the last 50 years, there have been tremendous gains in the treatment of opioid dependent individuals. Methadone maintenance was the first and remains the most thoroughly studied and documented effective treatment. Encouraging results in studies of buprenorphine treatment and office-based care indicate the potential for enhanced safety and increased access to opioid agonist maintenance. Treatment with opioid antagonists has demonstrated excellent results for select groups despite low uptake and poor efficacy in general public populations. Combined antagonist maintenance and psychotherapeutic approaches show promise and deserve further study. Medically assisted withdrawal provides a less uncomfortable withdrawal experience for patients and an opportunity to encourage ongoing substance treatment and involvement in antagonist treatment for a group of patients at high risk of relapse. New effective psychotherapeutic approaches have increased the psychosocial armamentarium of treatment providers. Ongoing creative methods of combining these approaches with pharmacological treatment where appropriate are exciting. Improved integration of these effective treatments for opioid dependence into practice in the community remains an important challenge.

The level of evidence for each of the interventions discussed in this chapter is discussed in Table 20.1.

Table 20.1. Effectiveness of treatments for opioid dependence

Treatment	Form of treatment	Psychiatric disorder/target audience	Level of evidence for efficacy	Comments
Psychopharmacology	Alpha-2 adrenergic agonists	Medically assisted opiate withdrawl	1b	Clonidine and lofexidine can both help relieve some of the more unpleasant autonomic side effects. Lofexidine has less hypotension and sedation than clonidine. They do not relieve symptoms of insomnia, restlessness, nausea, lacrimation, rhinorrhea, nausea
Psychopharmacology	Naltrexone	Opioid antagonist (maintenance) treatment	IIb	Little effect as measured by retention rates in people with little motivation to cease use. Those with high motivation (executive, professionals, probationers) have much higher retention and success rates. Improvement in retention can occur when accompanied by psychosocial interventions
Psychopharmacology	Methadone	Opioid agonist (maintenance) treatment	Ia	Effective in reducing drug usage, decreasing morbidity and mortality from the drug usage, decreases criminal activity and increases social functioning
Psychopharmacology	Buprenorphine	Opioid agonist (maintenance) treatment	Ia	Effective as is methadone in reducing drug usage, decreasing morbidity and mortality from the drug usage, decreases criminal activity and increases social functioning. It may be easier to dose than methadone and may have a greater early retention rate
Psychopharmacology	Diamorphine	Opioid agonist (maintenance) treatment	Ia	Not available in USA. Major problem is that it perpetuates the idea of injecting something rather than changing the person to an oral form of maintenance
Psychosocial and maintenance	Standard treatment versus standard treatment plus CBT versus standard treatment plus Supportive Expressive Therapy	Opioid dependence maintenance treatment	IIb	Psychosocial treatments by themselves are ineffective, but with psychopharmacological treatment, the addition of other psychosocial interventions to standard treatment, enhances outcome. Supportive Expressive and CBT did equally well
Psychosocial and maintenance	Motivational interviewing plus methadone maintenance	Opioid dependence maintenance treatment	Ib	Motivational intervention revealed reduced opioid related problems, better compliance with treatment, and improved retention
Psychosocial and maintenance	Enhanced services plus methadone maintenance	Opioid dependence maintenance treatment	Ib	Comparing methadone alone, methadone plus standard drug counselling, and methadone plus standard drug counselling plus enhanced services (vocational, medical, legal), the methadone maintenance alone did most poorly with the enhanced services doing the best
Psychosocial and maintenance	Contingency management or community reinforecement plus methadone maintenance	Opioid dependence maintenance treatment	IIa	Some evidence for effectiveness, but evidence not as strong as it is for alcohol or cocaine dependence

REFERENCES

Akram, G. (2000). Over-the-counter medcines: and emerging and neglected drug abuse?. *Journal of Substance Use*, 5, 136–42.

Amato, L., Davoli, M., Ferri, M., Gowing, L. & Perucci, C. A. (2004). Effectiveness of interventions on opiate withdrawal treatment: an overview of systematic reviews. *Drug and Alcohol Dependence*, 73, 219–26.

American Psychiatric Association (2000). *Diagnostic and Statistical Manual of Mental Disorders* (DSM-IV), 4th edn. Washington, DC: American Psychiatric Association.

Archie, C. (1998). Methadone in the management of narcotic addiction in pregnancy. *Obstetrics and Gynecology*, 10, 435–40.

Auriacombe, M., Franques, P., Daulouede, J. P. & Tignol, J. (1999). The French experience: results from extensive delimited research studies and nation-wide sample surveys. *Research and Clinical Forums*, 21, 9–15.

Avants, S. K., Margolin, A., Kosten, T. R., Rounsaville, B. J. & Schottenfeld, R. S. (1998). When is less treatment better? The role of social anxiety in matching methadone patients to psychosocial treatments. *Journal of Consulting Clinical Psychology*, 66(6), 924–31.

Avants, S. K., Margolin, A., Sindelar, J. L. *et al.* (1999). Day treatment versus enhanced standard methadone services for opioid-dependent patients: a comparison of clinical efficacy and cost. *American Journal of Psychiatry*, 156(1), 27–33.

Banbery, J., Wolff, K. & Raistrick, D. (2000). Dilhydrocodeine: a useful tool in the detoxification of methadone-maintained patients. *Journal of Substance Abuse Treatment*, 19, 301–5.

Barnett, P. G., Rodgers, J. H. & Bloch, D. A. (2001). A meta-analysis comparing buprenorphine to methadone for treatment of opiate dependence. *Addiction*, 96, 683–90.

Barrau, K., Thirion, X., Micallef, J., Chuniaud, L. C., Bellemin, B. & San-Marco, J. L. (2001). Comparison of methadone and high dosage buprenorphine users in French care centres. *Addiction*, 96, 1433–41.

Bates, M. & Pemberton, D. A. (1996). The effect of methadone prescribing in a clinic setting on the criminal activity of drug users. *Scottish Medical Journal*, 41, 173–5.

Battersby, M., Farrell, M., Gossop, M., Robson, P. & Strang, J. (1992). 'Horse trading': prescribing injectable opiates to opiates addicts. A descriptive study. *Drug and Alcohol Review*, 11, 35–42.

Bearn, J., Gossop, M. & Strang, J. (1996). Randomised double-blind comparison of lofexidine and methadone in the inpatient treatment of opiate withdrawal. *Drug and Alcohol Dependence*, 43, 87–91.

Bell, J., Mattick, R., Hay, A., Chan, J. & Hall, W. (1997). Methadone maintenance and drug-related crime. *Journal of Substance Abuse*, 9, 15–25.

Berghella, V., Lim, P. J., Hill, M. K., Cherpes, J., Chennat, J. & Kaltenbach, K. (2003). Maternal methadone dose and neonatal withdrawal. *American Journal of Obstetrics and Gynecology*, 189(2), 312–17.

Bertschy, G. (1995). Methadone maintenance treatment: an update. *European Archives of Psychiatry and Clinical Neuroscience*, 245, 114–24.

Beswick, T., Best, D., Bearn, J., Gossop, M., Rees, S. & Strang, J. (2003). The effectiveness of combined naloxone/lofexidine in opiate detoxification: results from a double-blind randomised and placebo-controlled trial. *American Journal on Addictions*, 12, 295–305.

Buster, M. C. A., van Brussel, G. H. A. & van den Brink, W. (2002). An increase in overdose mortality during the first 2 weeks after entering or re-entering methadone treatment in Amsterdam. *Addiction*, 97, 993–1001.

Caplehorn, J. R., Dalton, M. S., Haldar, F., Petrenas, A. M. & Nisbet, J. G. (1996). Methadone maintenance and addicts' risk of fatal heroin overdose. *Substance Use and Misuse*, 31(2), 177–96.

Carnwath, T. & Hardman, J. (1998). Randomised double-blind comparison of lofexdine and clonidine in the out-patient treatment of opiate withdrawal. *Drug and Alcohol Dependence*, 50, 251–4.

Carreno, J. E., Alvarez, C. E., San Narciso, G. I., Bascaran, M. T., Diaz, M. & Bobes, J. (2003). Maintenance treatment with depot opioid antagonists in subcutaneous implants: an alternative in the treatment of opioid dependence. *Addiction Biology*, 8, 429–38.

Carroll, K. M., Ball, S. A., Nich, C. *et al.* (2001). Targeting behavioral therapies to enhance naltrexone treatment of opioid dependence: efficacy of contingency management and significant other involvement. *Archives of General Psychiatry*, 58(8), 755–61.

Carroll, K. M., Sinha, R., Nich, C., Babuscio, T. & Rounsaville, B. J. (2002). Contingency management to enhance naltrexone treatment of opioid dependence: a randomized clinical trial of reinforcement magnitude. *Experimental Clinical Psychopharmacology*, 10(1), 54–63.

Comer, S. D., Collins, E. D., Kleber, H. D., Nuwayser, E. S., Kerrigan, J. H. & Fischman, M. W. (2002). Depot naltrexone: long-lasting antagonism of the effects of heroin in humans. *Psychopharmacology*, 159, 351–60.

Corkery, J. M., Schifano, F., Ghodse, A. H. & Oyefeso, A.. (2004) The effects of methadone and its role in fatalities. *Human Psychopharmacology*, 19(8), 565–76.

Cornish, J. W., Metzger, D., Woody, G. E., *et al.* (1997). Naltrexone pharmacotherapy for opioid dependent federal probationers. *Journal of Substance Abuse Treatment*, 14(6), 529–34.

Croop, R. S., Faulkner, E. B. & Labriola, D. F. (1997). The safety profile of naltrexone in the treatment of alcoholism. Results from a multicenter usage study. The Naltrexone Usage Study Group in *Archives of General Psychiatry*, 54(12), 1130–5.

Curran, H. V., Bolton, J., Wanigaratne, S. & Smyth, C. (1999). Additional methadone increases craving for heroin: a double blind, placebo-controlled study of chronic opiate users receiving methadone substitution treatment. *Addiction*, 94, 665–74.

Davids, E. & Gastpar, M. (2004). Buprenorphine in the treatment of opioid dependence. *European Neuropsychopharmacology*, 14, 209–16.

Dawe, S., Griffiths, P., Gossop, M. & Strang, J. (1991). Should opiate addicts be involved in controlling their own detoxification? A comparison of fixed versus negotiable schedules. *British Journal of Addiction*, **86**, 977–82.

Department of Health (1999). *Drug Misuse and Dependence – Guidelines on Clinical Management*. London: The Stationery Office.

Diamant, K., Fischer, G., Schneider, C. et al. (1998). Outpatient opiate detoxification treatment with *buprenorphine*. Preliminary investigation. *European Addiction Research*, **4**, 198–202.

Dole, V. P., Robinson, J. W., Orraca, J., Towns, E., Searcy, P. & Caine, E. (1969). Methadone treatment of randomly selected criminal addicts. *New England Journal of Medicine*, **280**, 1372–5.

Drug Addiction Treatment Act of 2000, Pub. L. No. 106–310 (October 17, 2000).

Eggen, A. E. & Andrew, M. (1994). Use of codeine analgesics in a general population. A Norwegian study of moderately strong analgesics. *European Journal of Clinical Pharmacology*, **46**, 491–6.

Eklund, C., Melin, L., Hiltunen, A. J. & Borg, S. (1994). Detoxification from methadone maintenance treatment in Sweden: long-term outcome and effects on quality of life and life situation. *The International Journal of the Addictions*, **29**, 627–45.

European Monitoring Centre for Drugs and Drug Addiction (EMCDDA) (2000). *Insights: reviewing current practice in drug-substitution treatment*. Luxembourg: The European Union Office for Official Publications of the European Communities.

Faggiano, F., Vigna-Taglianti, F., Versino, E. & Lemma, P. (2003). Methadone maintenance at different dosages for opioid dependence. In *Cochrane Database Systematic Review*, **3**, CD002208. Oxford: Update Software Ltd.

Fals-Stewart, W. & O'Farrell, T. J. (2003). Behavioral family counseling and naltrexone for male opioid-dependent patients. *Journal of Consulting Clinical Psychology*, **71**(3), 432–42.

Farre, M., Mas, A., Torrens, M., Moreno, V. & Cami, J. (2002). Retention rate and illicit opioid use during methadone maintenance interventions: a meta-analysis. *Drug and Alcohol Dependence*, **65**, 283–90.

Fiellin, D. A., O'Connor, P. G., Chawarski, M., Pakes, J. P., Pantalon, M. V. & Schottenfeld, R. S. (2001). Methadone maintenance in primary care: a randomized controlled trial. *Journal of the American Medical Association*, **286**(14), 1724–31.

Fiellin, D. A., Pantalon, M. V., Pakes, J. P., O'Connor, P. G., Chawarski, M. & Schottenfeld, R. S. (2002). Treatment of heroin dependence with buprenorphine in primary care. *American Journal of Drug and Alcohol Abuse*, **28**(2), 231–41.

Fischer, G., Gombas, W., Eder, H. et al. (1999). Buprenorphine versus methadone maintenance for the treatment of opioid dependence. *Addiction*, **94**, 1337–47.

Galanter, M., Dermatis, H., Glickman, L. et al. (2004). Network therapy: decreased secondary opioid use during buprenorphine maintenance. *Journal of Substance Abuse Treatment*, **26**(4), 313–18.

Garcia Alonso, F., Gutierrez, M., San, L. et al. (1989). A multicentre study to introduce naltrexone for opiate dependence in Spain. *Drug and Alcohol Dependence*, **23**, 117–21.

Geerlings, P. J., Bos, T. W., Schalken, H. F. A. & Wouters, L. F. J. M. (1985). Detoxification of heroin addicts with electrostimulation or methadone. *Tijdschrift voor Alcohol, Drugs en Andere Psychotrope Stoffen*, **11**, 80–5.

Gerra, G., Ferri, M., Polidori, E., Santoro, G., Zaimovic, A. & Sternieri, E. (2003). Long-term methadone maintenance effectiveness: psychosocial and pharmacological variables. *Journal of Substance Abuse Treatment*, **25**, 1–8.

Giacomuzzi, S. M., Riemer, Y., Ertl, M. et al. (2003). Buprenorphine versus methadone maintenance treatment in an ambulant setting: a health-related quality of life assessment. *Addiction*, **98**, 693–702.

Gilman, S. M., Galanter, M. & Dermatis, H. (2001). Methadone anonymous: a 12-step program for methadone maintained heroin addicts. *Substance Abuse*, **22**(4), 247–56.

Gossop, M., Johns, A. & Green, L. (1986). Opiate withdrawal: inpatient versus outpatient programmes and preferred versus random assignment to treatment. *British Medical Journal*, **293**, 103–4.

Gossop, M., Marsden, J., Stewart, D. & Rolfe, A. (2000). Patterns of improvement after methadone treatment: one year follow-up results from the National Treatment Outcome Research Study (NTORS). *Drug and Alcohol Dependence*, **60**, 275–86.

Gossop, M., Marsden, J., Stewart, D. & Treacy, S. (2001). Outcomes after methadone maintenance and methadone reduction treatments: two-year follow-up results from the National Treatment Outcome Research Study. *Drug and Alcohol Dependence*, **62**, 255–64.

Gossop, M., Marsden, J., Stewart, D. & Kidd, T. (2003) The National Treatment Outcome Research Study (NTORS): 4–5 year follow-up results. *Addiction*, **98**, 291–303.

Gowing, L., Ali, R. & White, J. (2001). Opioid antagonists under sedation or anaesthesia for opioid withdrawal. *Cochrane Database Systematic Reviews*, **1**, CD002022. Oxford: Update Software Ltd.

Guichard, A., Lert, F., Calderon, C. et al. (2003). Illicit drug use and injection practices among drug users on methadone and buprenorphine maintenance treatment in France. *Addiction*, **98**, 1585–97.

Gunne, L. M. & Gronbaldh, L. (1981). The Swedish methadone maintenance program: a controlled study. *Drug and Alcohol Dependence*, **7**, 249–56.

Gutierrez, M., Ballesteros, J., Gonzalez-Oliveros, R. & de Apodaka, J. R. (1995). Retention rates in to naltrexone programmes for heroin addicts in Vitoria, Spain. *European Psychiatry*, **10**, 183–8.

Hamilton, R. J., Olmedo, R. E., Shah, S. et al. (2002). Complications of ultrarapid opioid detoxification with subcutaneous naltrexone pellets. *Academic Emergency Medicine*, **9**, 63–8.

Hatsukami, D. K. & Fischman, M. W. (1996). Crack cocaine and cocaine hydrochloride: are the differences myth or reality?. *Journal of the American Medical Association*, **276**, 1580–8.

Herve, S., Riachi, G., Noblet, C. et al. (2004). Acute hepatitis due to buprenorphine administration. *European Journal of Gastroenterology and Hepatology*, **16**(10), 1033–7.

Hiltunen, A. J. & Eklund, C. (2002). Withdrawal from methadone maintenance treatment. Reasons for not trying to quit methadone. *European Addiction Research*, **8**, 38–44.

Howells, C., Allen, S., Gupta, J., Stillwell, G., Marsden, J. & Farrell, M. (2002). Prison based detoxification for opioid dependence: a randomised double blind controlled trial of lofexidine and methadone. *Drug and Alcohol Dependence*, **67**, 169–76.

Hser, Y. I., Hoffman, V., Grella, C. E. *et al.* (2001). A 33-year follow-up of narcotic addicts. *Archives of General Psychiatry*, **58**, 503–8.

Hulse, G. K. & Basso, M. R. (1999). Reassessing naltrexone maintenance as a treatment for illicit heroin users. *Drug and Alcohol Review*, **18**, 263–9.

Iribarne, C., Dreano, Y., Bardou, L. G., Menez, J. F. & Berthou, F. (1997). Interaction of methadone with substrates of human hepatic cytochrome P450 3A4. *Toxicology*, **117**(1), 13–23.

Johnson, R. E., Eissenberg, T., Stitzer, M. L., Strain, E. C., Liebson, I. A. & Bigelow, G. E. (1995). A placebo controlled clinical trial of buprenorphine as a treatment for opioid dependence. *Drug and Alcohol Dependence*, **40**, 17–25.

Johnson, R. E., Chutuape, M. A., Strain, E. C., Walsh, S. L., Stitzer, M. L. & Bigelow, G. E. (2000). A comparison of levomethadyl acetate, buprenorphine, and methadone for opioid dependence. *New England Journal of Medcine*, **343**(18), 1290–7.

Johnston, L. D., O'Malley, P. M., Bachman, J. G. & Schulenberg, J. E. (2004). *Monitoring the Future National Results on Adolescent Drug Use: Overview of Key Findings*, 2003 (NIH Publication No. 04–5506). Bethesda, MD: National Institute on Drug Abuse, 59 pp.

Justo, D., Gal-Oz, A., Paran, Y. *et al.* (2006). Methadone-associated Torsades de Pointes (polymorphic ventricular tachycardia) in opioid-dependent patients. *Addiction*, **101**, 1333–8.

Kahn, A., Mumford, J. P., Ash-Rogers, G. & Beckford, H. (1997). Double-blind study of lofexidine and clonidine in the detoxification of opiate addicts. *Drug and Alcohol Dependence*, **44**, 57–61.

Kakko, J., Svanborg, K. D., Kreek, M. J. & Heilig, M. (2003). 1-year retention and social function after buprenorphine-assisted relapse prevention treatment for heroin dependence in Sweden: a randomised, placebo-controlled trial. *Lancet*, **361**, 662–8.

Keen, J., Oliver, P., Rowse, G. & Mathers, N. (2003). Does methadone maintenance treatment based on the new national guidelines work in a primary care setting?. *British Journal of General Practice*, **53**, 461–7.

King, V. L., Stoller, K. B., Hayes, M. *et al.* (2002). A multicenter randomized evaluation of methadone medical maintenance. *Drug and Alcohol Dependence*, **65**(2), 137–48.

Kirchmayer, U., Davoli, M., Verster, A. D., Amato, L., Ferri, M. & Perucci, C. A. (2002). A systematic review on the efficacy of naltrexone maintenance treatment in opioid dependence. *Addiction*, **97**, 1241–9.

Kleber, H. D. (1998). Ultrarapid opiate detoxification. *Addiction*, **92**, 1929–33.

Kornick, C. A., Kilborn, M. J., Santiago-Palma, J. *et al.* (2003). QTc interval prolongation associated with intravenous methadone. *Pain*, **105**(3), 499–506.

Kosten, T. R. (2003). Buprenorphine for opioid detoxification: a brief review. *Addictive Disorders and Their Treatment*, **2**, 107–12.

Kraft, M. K., Rothbard, A. B., Hadley, T. R., McLellan, A. T. & Asch, D. A. (1997). Are supplementary services provided during methadone maintenance really cost-effective?. *American Journal of Psychiatry*, **154**(9), 1214–19.

Kraigher, D., Ortner, R., Eder, H., Schindler, S. & Fischer, G. (2002). Slow-release morphine hydrochloride for maintenance therapy of opioid dependence. *Wiener Klinische Wochenschrift*, **114**, 904–10.

Krantz, M. J., Kutinsky, I. B., Robertson, A. D. & Mehler, P. S. (2003). Dose-related effects of methadone on QT prolongation in a series of patients with torsade de pointes. *Pharmacotherapy*, **23**(6), 802–5.

Kraus, L., Augustin, R., Frischer, M., Kummler, P., Uhl, A. & Wiessing, L. (2003). Estimating prevalence of problem drug use at national level in countries of the European Union and Norway. *Addiction*, **98**, 471–85.

Krupitsky, E. M., Zvartau, E. E., Masalov, D. V. *et al.* (2004). Naltrexone for heroin dependence treatment in St. Petersburg, Russia. *Journal of Substance Abuse Treatment*, **26**(4), 285–94.

Kuschel, C. A., Austerberry, L., Cornwell, M., Couch, R. & Rowley, R. S. (2004). Can methadone concentrations predict the severity of withdrawal in infants at risk of neonatal abstinence syndrome?. *Archives of Diseases Child and Fetal Neonatal Education*, **89**(5), F390–3.

Lacroix, I., Berrebi, A., Chaumerliac, C., Lapeyre-Mestre, M., Montastruc, J. L. & Damase-Michel, C. (2004). Buprenorphine in pregnant opioid-dependent women: first results of a prospective study. *Addiction*, **99**, 209–14.

Langrod, J., Lowinson, J. & Ruiz, P. (1981). Methadone treatment and physical complaints: a clinical analysis. *International Journal of Addiction*, **16**(5), 947–52.

Ling, W. & Wesson, D. R.. (2003). Clinical efficacy of buprenorphine: comparisons to methadone and placebo. *Drug and Alcohol Dependence*, **70**(2 Suppl), S49–57.

Ling, W., Wesson, D. R., Charuvastra, C. & Klett, C. J. (1996). A controlled trial comparing buprenorphine and methadone maintenance in opioid dependence. *Archives of General Psychiatry*, **53**, 401–7.

MacLeod, J., Whittaker, A. & Robertson, J. R. (1998). Changes in opiate treatment during attendance at a community drug service: findings from a clinical audit. *Drug and Alcohol Review*, **17**, 19–25.

Magura, S., Nwakeze, P. C., Kang, S. Y., & Demsky, S. (1999). Program quality effects on patient outcomes during methadone maintenance: a study of 17 clinics. *Substance Use and Misuse*, **34**(9), 1299–324.

Marsch, L. A. (1998). The efficacy of methadone maintenance interventions in reducing illicit opiate use, HIV risk behaviour and criminality: a meta-analysis. *Addiction*, **93**, 515–32.

Masson, C. L., Barnett, P. G., Sees, K. L. *et al.* (2004). Cost and cost-effectiveness of standard methadone maintenance treatment compared to enriched 180-day methadone detoxification. *Addiction*, **99**(6), 718–26.

Matheson, C., Pitcairn, J., Bond, C. M., van Teijlingen, E. & Ryan, M. (2003). General practice management of illicit drug users in Scotland: a national survey. *Addiction*, **98**, 119–26.

Mattick, R. P., Breen, C., Kimber, J. & Davoli, M. (2002a). Methadone maintenance therapy versus no opioid replacement therapy for opioid dependence. *Cochrane Database Systematic Reviews*, **4**, CD002209. Oxford: Update Software Ltd.

Mattick, R. P., Kimber, J., Breen, C. & Davoli, M. (2002b). Buprenorphine maintenance versus placebo or methadone maintenance for opioid dependence. *Cochrane Database Systematic Reviews*, **4**. Oxford: Update Software Ltd.

McGregor, C., Ali, R., White, J. M. *et al.* (2002). A comparison of antagonist-precipitated withdrawal under anesthesia to standard inpatient withdrawal as a precursor to maintenance naltrexone treatment in heroin users: outcomes at 6 and 12 months. *Drug and Alcohol Dependence*, **68**, 5–14.

McLellan, A. T., Arndt, I. O., Metzger, D. S., Woody, G. E. & O'Brien, C. P. (1993). The effects of psychosocial services in substance abuse treatment. *Journal of the American Medical Association*, **269**(15), 1953–9.

Merrill, J., Alterman, A., Cacciola, J. & Rutherford, M. (1999). Prior treatment history and its impact on criminal recidivism. *Journal of Substance Abuse Treatment*, **17**, 313–19.

Metrebian, N., Shanahan, W., Wells, B. & Stimson, G. V. (1998). Feasibility of prescribing injectable heroin and methadone to opiate dependent drug users: associated health gains and harm reductions. *Medical Journal of Australia*, **168**, 596–600.

Metrebian, N., Shanahan, W., Stimson, G. V. *et al.* (2001). Prescribing drug of choice to opiate dependent drug users: a comparison of clients receiving heroin with those receiving injectable methadone at a West London drug clinic. *Drug and Alcohol Review*, **20**, 267–76.

Metrebian, N., Carnwath, T., Stimson, G. V. & Storz, T. (2002). Survey of doctors prescribing diamorphine (heroin) to opiate-dependent drug users in the United Kingdom. *Addiction*, **97**, 1155–61.

Metzger, D. S., Woody, G. E., McLellan, A. T. *et al.* (1993). Human immunodeficiency virus seroconversion among intravenous drug users in- and out-of-treatment: an 18 month prospective follow-up. *Journal of Acquired Immune Deficiency Syndrome*, **6**, 1049–56.

Miller, W. R. & Rollnick, S. (1991). *Motivational Interviewing: Preparing People for Change*, 2nd edn. New York: Guilford Press.

Montoya, I. D., Gorelick, D. A., Preston, K. L. *et al.* (2004). Randomized trial of buprenorphine for treatment of concurrent opiate and cocaine dependence. *Clinical and Pharmacological Therapy*, **75**(1), 34–48.

Newman, R. G. & Whitehill, W. B. (1979). Double-blind comparison of methadone and placebo maintenance treatments of narcotic addicts in Hong Kong. *Lancet*, **2**, 485–8

Nyswander, M., Winick, C., Bernstein, A., Brill, L. & Kaufer, G.. (1958). Treatment of the narcotic addict: workshop, 1957. 1. The treatment of drug addicts as voluntary outpatients; a progress report. *American Journal of Orthopsychiatry*, **28**(4), 714–27; discussion 727–9.

O'Connor, P. G. & Kosten, T. R. (1998). Rapid and ultrarapid opioid detoxification techniques. *Journal of the American Medical Association*, **279**, 229–234.

O'Connor, P. G., Oliveto, A. H., Shi, J. M. *et al.* (1998). A randomized trial of buprenorphine maintenance for heroin dependence in a primary care clinic for substance users versus a methadone clinic. *American Journal of Medicine*, **105**(2), 100–5.

O'Malley, J. E., Anderson, W. H. & Lazare, A. (1972). Failure of outpatient treatment of drug abuse. I. Heroin. *American Journal of Psychiatry*, **128**(7), 865–8.

O'Malley, S. S., Jaffe, A. J., Chang, G., Schottenfeld, R. S., Meyer, R. E. & Rounsaville, B. (1992). Naltrexone and coping skills therapy for alcohol dependence: a controlled study. *Archives of General Psychiatry*, **49**, 881–7.

Pates, R., McBride, A., Li, S. & Ramadan, R. (2002). Misuse of over-the-counter medicines: a survey of community pharmacies in a South Wales health authority. *The Pharmaceutical Journal*, **268**, 179–82.

Petitjean, S., Stohler, R., D-glon, J. *et al.* (2001). Double-blind randomised trial of buprenorphine and methadone in opiate dependence. *Drug and Alcohol Dependence*, **62**, 97–104.

Poirier, M. F., Laqueille, X., Jalfre, V. *et al.* (2004). Clinical profile of responders to buprenorphine as a substitution treatment in heroin addicts: results of a multicentre study of 73 patients. *Progress in Neuro-Psychopharmacology and Biological Psychiatry*, **28**, 267–72.

Preston, K. L., Silverman, K., Umbricht, A., DeJesus, A., Montoya, I. D., & Schuster, C. R. (1999). Improvement in naltrexone treatment compliance with contingency management. *Drug Alcohol Dependence*, **54**(2), 127–35.

Ravndal, E. (2001). An outcome study of a therapeutic community based in the community: a five-year prospective study of drug abusers in Norway In *Therapeutic Communities*, 4th edn. B. Rawlings & R. Yates, pp. 224–240. Philadelphia: Jessica Kingsley Publishers.

Ravndal, E. & Vaglum, P. (1991). Psychopathology and substance abuse as predictors of program completion in a therapeutic community for drug abusers: a prospective study. *Acta Psychiatrica Scandinavica*, **83**, 217–22.

Rehm, J., Gschwend, P., Steffen, T., Gutzwiller, F., Dobler-Mikola, A. & Uchtenhagen, A. (2001). Feasibility, safety and efficacy of injectable heroin prescription for refractory opioid addicts: a follow-up study. *Lancet*, **358**, 1417–20.

Rhodes, W., Layne, M., Johnston, P., & Hozik, L. (2000). *What America's Users Spend on Illegal Drugs, 1988–1998*. Office of National Drug Control Policy.

Ribeaud, D. (2004). Long-term impacts of the Swiss heroin prescription trials on crime of treated heroin users. *Journal of Drug Issues*, **34**, 163–94.

Riordan, C. E. & Kleber, H. D. (1980). Rapid opiate detoxification with clonidine and naloxone (letter). *Lancet*, **1**(8177), 1079–80.

Roozen, H. G., Boulogne, J. J., Van Tulder, M. W., van den Brink, W. & De Jong, C. A. J. (2004). A systematic review of the effectiveness of the community reinforcement approach in alcohol, cocaine and opioid addiction. *Drug and Alcohol Dependence*, **74**, 1–13.

Roset, P., Farre, M., de la Torre, R. *et al.* (2001). Modulation of rate of onset and intensity of drug effects reduces abuse potential in healthy males. *Drug Alcohol Dependence*, **64**, 285–98.

Roth, A., Hogan, I. & Farren, C. (1997). Naltrexone plus group therapy for the treatment of opiate-abusing health-care professionals. *Journal of Substance Abuse Treatment*, **14**(1), 19–22.

Rounsaville, B. J. (1995). Can psychotherapy rescue naltrexone treatment of opioid addiction?. *NIDA Research Monograph*, **150**, 37–52.

Rounsaville, B. J., Glazer, W., Wilber, C. H., Weissman, M. M. & Kleber, H. D. (1983). Short-term interpersonal psychotherapy in methadone-maintained opiate addicts. *Archives of General Psychiatry*, **40**, 629–36.

Rothenberg, J. L., Sullivan, M. A., Church, S. H. *et al.* (2002). Behavioral naltrexone therapy: an integrated treatment for opiate dependence. *Journal of Substance Abuse Treatment*, **23**(4), 351–60.

Salsitz, E. A., Joseph, H., Frank, B. *et al.* (2000). Methadone medical maintenance (MMM): treating chronic opioid dependence in private medical practice – a summary report (1983–1998). *Mount Sinai Journal of Medicine*, **67**(5–6), 388–97.

San, L., Pomarol, G., Peri, J. M., Olle, J. M. & Cami, J. (1991). Follow-up after a 6-month maintenance period on naltrexone versus placebo in heroin addicts. *British Journal of Addiction*, **86**, 983–90.

Saunders, B., Wilkinson, C. & Phillips, M. (1995). The impact of a brief motivational intervention with opiate users attending a methadone programme. *Addiction*, **90**(3), 415–24.

Schindler, S. D., Eder, H., Ortner, K. R., Rohrmeister, K., Langer, M. & Fischer, G. (2003). Neonatal outcome following buprenorphine maintenance during conception and throughout pregnancy. *Addiction*, **98**, 103–10.

Schottenfeld, R. S., Pakes, J. R., Oliveto, A., Ziedonis, D. & Kosten, T. R. (1997). Buprenorphine vs methadone maintenance treatment for concurrent opioid dependence and cocaine abuse. *Archives in General Psychiatry*, **54**(8), 713–20.

Sees, K. L., Delucchi, K. L., Masson, C. *et al.* (2000). Methadone maintenance vs 180-day psychosocially enriched detoxification for treatment of opioid dependence: a randomized controlled trial. *Journal of the American Medical Association*, **283**(10), 1303–10.

Seivewright, N. & Lagundoye, O. (2003). Withdrawal from methadone and methadone for withdrawal. In *Methadone Matters: Evolving Community Methadone Treatment of Opioid Addiction*, ed. J. Strang & G. Tober, pp. 79–87. London: Martin Dunitz.

Sell, L., Segar, G. & Merrill, J. (2001). One hundred and twenty-five prescriptions for injectable opiates in the North West of England. *Drug and Alcohol Review*, **20**, 57–66.

Sheppard, S. G. (1994). A preliminary investigation of ibogaine: Case reports and recommendations for further study. *Journal of Substance Abuse Treatment*, **11**, 379–85.

Spear, H. B. (2002). *Heroin Addiction Care and Control: The British System, 1916–1974*, ed. J. Mott. London: DrugScope.

Stanton, M. D., Todd, T. C. (1982). *The Family Therapy of Drug Abuse and Addiction*. New York: Guilford Press.

Stella, L., Cassese, F., Barone, S. *et al.* (1999). Naltrexone to keep a drug-free condition. *Research Communications in Alcohol and Substance of Abuse*, **20**, 91–8.

Stitzer, M. L., Iguchi, M. Y. & Felch, L. J. (1992). Contingent take-home incentive: effects on drug use of methadone maintenance patients. *Journal of Consulting Clinical Psychology*, **60**(6), 927–34.

Strain, E. C., Stitzer, M. L., Liebson, I. A. & Bigelow, G. E. (1994). Comparison of buprenorphine and methadone in the treatment of opioid dependence. *American Journal of Psychiatry*, **151**, 1025–30.

Strain, E. C., Bigelow, G. E., Liebson, I. A. & Stitzer, M. L. (1999). Moderate- vs high-dose methadone in the treatment of opioid dependence: a randomized trial. *Journal of the American Medical Association*, **281**, 1000–5.

Strang, J., Finch, E., Hankinson, L., Farrell, M., Taylor, C. & Gossop, M. (1997). Methadone treatment for opiate addiction: benefits in the first month. *Addiction Research*, **5**, 71–6.

Strang, J., Marsden, J., Cummins, M. *et al.* (2000). Randomised trial of supervised injectable versus oral methadone maintenance: report of feasibility and 6-month outcome. *Addiction*, **95**, 1631–45.

Substance Abuse and Mental Health Services Administration (SAMSHA). (2004). *Overview of Findings from the 2003 National Survey on Drug Use and Health*. Rockville, MD: NSDUH Series. Office of Applied Studies.

Ter-Riet, G., Kleijnen, J. & Knipschild, P. (1990). A meta-analysis of studies into the effect of acupuncture on addiction. *British Journal of General Practice*, **40**, 379–82.

US Department of Justice, Drug Enforcement Administration: (2003). *2002 Domestic Monitor Program, Drug Intelligence Report*. June, DEA-03057.

Uchtenhagen, A., Dobler-Mikola, A. & Gutzwiller, F. (1996). Medical prescription of narcotics: background and intermediate results of a Swiss national project. *European Research Journal*, **2**, 201–7.

Uchtenhagen, A., Gutzweiller, F., Dobler-Mikola, A. & Steffen, A. (1997). A programme for a medical prescription of narcotics. A synthesis of results. *European Addiction Research*, **3**, 160–16.

Uehlinger, C., Deglon, J. J., Livoti, S., Petitjean, S., Waldvogel, D. & Ladewig, D. (1998). Comparison of buprenorphine and methadone in the treatment of opioid dependence. Swiss multicentre study. *European Addiction Research*, **4**, 13–18.

van den Brink, W., Hendriks, V. M., Blanken, P., Koeter, M. W. J., van Zwieten, B. J. & van Ree, J. M. (2003). Medial prescription of heroin to treatment resistant heroin addicts: two randomised controlled trials. *British Medical Journal*, **327**, 310–12.

Verthein, U., Haasen, C. & Krausz, M. (2002). Auricular acupuncture as a treatment of cocaine, heroin and alcohol addiction: a pilot study. *Addictive Disorders and Their Treatment*, **1**, 11–16.

Volpicelli, J. R. Alterman, A. I. Hayashida, M. & O'Brien, C. P. (1992). Naltrexone in the treatment of alcohol dependence. *Archives of General Psychiatry*, **49**, 876–80.

Walsh, S. L. & Eissenberg, T. (2003). The clinical pharmacology of buprenorphine: extrapolating from the laboratory to the clinic. *Drug and Alcohol Dependence*, **70**, S13–27.

Walsh, S. L., Strain, E. C. & Bigelow, G. E. (2003). Evaluation of the effects of lofexidine and clonidine on naloxone-precipitated withdrawal in opioid-dependent humans. *Addiction*, **98**(4), 427–39.

Walsh, S. L., Preston, K. L., Stitzer, M. L., Cone, E. J. & Bigelow, G. E. (1994). Clinical pharmacology of buprenorphine: ceiling effects at high doses. *Clinical and Pharmacological Therapy*, **55**(5), 569–80.

Washton, A. M., Gold, M. S. & Pottash, A. C. (1984). Successful use of naltrexone in addicted physicians and business executives. *Advances in Alcohol Substance Abuse*, **4**(2), 89–96.

West, S. L., O' Neal, K. K. & Graham, C. W. (2000). A meta-analysis comparing the effectiveness of buprenorphine and methadone. *Journal of Substance Abuse*, **12**, 405–14.

Williams, H., Remedios, A., Oyefeso, A. & Bennett, J. (2002). Buprenorphine detoxification treatment for heroin dependence: a preliminary experience in an outpatient setting. *Irish Journal of Psychological Medicine*, **19**, 80–3.

Woody, G. E., Luborsky, L., McLellan, A. T. *et al.* (1983). Psychotherapy for opiate addicts. Does it help?. *Archives in General Psychiatry*, **40**(6), 639–45.

Yandoli, D., Eisler, I., Robbins, C., Mulleady, G. & Dare, C. (2002). A comparative study of family therapy in the treatment of opiate users in a London drug clinic. *Journal of Familiy Therapy*, **24**, 402–22.

21

Treatment of sedative-hypnotic dependence

Karim Dar and Manoj Kumar

Editor's note

Misuse and dependence upon benzodiazepines, despite much greater awareness of the dangers of these drugs, still appear to be growing problems. Misuse occurs because of dependency upon these drugs that have been prescribed for extended periods with some increasing tolerance on the part of the patient. Misuse also occurs by people who purchase or obtain these drugs by means other than prescription. The growing emphasis on insomnia and the increasing competition among various drug companies to capture the prescription sleeping pill market appears to exacerbate this problem. At the moment, a gradual tapering of the prescribed or illegally used drug, especially by substituting a longer-acting drug for a shorter-acting drug, appears to have the most supporting evidence. Little research has been done on hypnotics compared with the benzodiazepines, and this is a bit of a puzzle.

Introduction

Sedative hypnotic drugs are central nervous system depressants traditionally used to reduce anxiety and induce sleep. The sedatives under consideration in this chapter are benzodiazepines, the Z-drugs (zopiclone, zolpidem and zaleplon) and barbiturates. After their introduction in 1903, barbiturates were supplanted by the benzodiazepines which were introduced in the early 1960s. This was primarily due to concerns about the obvious toxicity of barbiturates, particularly in overdose, and knowledge of their propensity for dependence. After reaching a peak in the early 1980s, prescriptions for benzodiazepines in the UK have shown a substantial reduction; however, while annual prescriptions for benzodiazepines in England fell from 10 million to around

6 million between 1993–2003, those for the Z-drugs rose from 0.3 million to over 4 million over the same time period, mainly in older people (DoH, 2003), and this is a worldwide phenomenon. Expert bodies have long advised that use of all these group of drugs be limited to short periods and should be generally avoided in elderly people (BNF, 2004; CSM, 1988; Priest & Moutgomery, 1988)(but see Chapter 31 for a fuller discussion). Around 80% of all such prescriptions in England are for those aged 65 years or over (Curran *et al.*, 2003), and many patients remain on the drugs for months or years (Taylor *et al.*, 1998). This prescribing is likely to lead to development of dependence and many other adverse effects on health (Ashton 1995). All currently marketed hypnotics have been associated with at least some features of dependence and have demonstrated a potential for misuse and dose escalation in at least a minority of patients (Ashton, 1995; Hajak *et al.*, 2003; Lader, 1999). In this chapter we will discuss the treatment of sedative-hypnotic dependence with the primary focus on benzodiazepines (but this is partly a consequence of much less literature being available on the Z-drugs, particularly in the field of dependence, where fundamental differences from the benzodiazepines remain to be established.

Manifestations of anxiety and of sedative-hypnotic abstinence syndromes

It is important to note that the symptoms of anxiety and withdrawal syndromes from benzodiazepines overlap greatly. The psychological manifestations of anxiety include irritability, restlessness, insomnia, agitation, nightmares and difficulty in concentration. Physiological symptoms include tremors, shakiness, profuse sweating, palpitations and lethargy. In addition, in withdrawal

Cambridge Textbook of Effective Treatments in Psychiatry, ed. Peter Tyrer and Kenneth R. Silk. Published by Cambridge University Press.
© Cambridge University Press, 2008.

syndromes in particular, there is hyperexcitability of voluntary musculature and hyperacuity of sensation leading to muscle twitching, aches and pains, hypersensitivity to light, smell and sounds, a metallic taste in one's mouth and, very rarely, convulsions (Tyrer *et al.*, 1990). Other physical reactions include nausea, loss of appetite, weight loss and feeling like one has a 'flu-like' illness. Other mental status changes can involve dysphoria, impaired memory and possibly confusion, depersonalisation and derealisation, psychotic reactions, and hallucinations (APA Task Force, 1990).

Benzodiazepines

The safety of benzodiazepines was questioned when evidence of their dependence inducing properties and withdrawal effects started to be recognised in the form of case reports in the 1970s (Hall & Joffe, 1972; Woody *et al.*, 1975). However, clinical dependence on benzodiazepines was not reported in the medical literature until almost a decade later (Tyrer, 1980; Hallstrom & Lader, 1981; Tyrer *et al.*, 1981; Mackinnon & Parker, 1982; Petursson & Lader, 1981). There are two distinct groups of patients who may be abusing or dependent on benzodiazepines:

(1) Those who have taken benzodiazepines long term for a disorder such as anxiety or insomnia prescribed by a doctor but who do not abuse their prescription;

(2) Those who either abuse their prescription or have polydrug and alcohol dependence and use non-prescribed benzodiazepines. Dependence on these drugs can develop within a few weeks of regular use (Busto *et al.*, 1986a, 1986b; Hallstrom & Lader, 1981; Noyes *et al.*, 1988).

Despite the differences in origin, the basic syndrome of drug dependence is the same in each group (Seivewright & Dougal, 1993). A brief review of the kinetic properties of benzodiazepines (which applies to the barbiturate and barbiturate-like drugs as well) makes the abuse liability of these drugs understandable. There are a number of properties that increases the potency of benzodiazepines as a reinforcer of continued consumption. There is the high intrinsic pharmacological activity of drugs, their rapid absorption and rapid entry into specific brain regions. They have high oral bioavailability, low protein binding, a short half-life, a small volume of distribution and high clearance. The factors that promote physical dependence on benzodiazepines include their high intrinsic pharmacological activity, the cumulative drug load which involves dose, frequency, and duration of treatment, their small volume of distribution with a long half-life, and

their low clearance. These issues relating to physical dependence then lead to other factors that promote appearance of the withdrawal syndrome (Coppell *et al.*, 1986).

Epidemiology

The clinical descriptive data regarding benzodiazepine dependence is surprisingly sparse. There are case reports of benzodiazepine dependence (Cole & Chiarello, 1990) and reports documenting groups of benzodiazepine-dependent patients largely from addiction treatment centres (Busto *et al.*, 1986b). About 1%–3% of the population of the Western world has received continuous benzodiazepine therapy for more than 1 year. The rates of use are substantially higher among women than men and among older than younger populations (Balter *et al.*, 1984; Woods *et al.*, 1992). Previous studies have estimated the population of prescribed long-term benzodiazepine users in the UK to be about 1.2 million people (Ashton & Golding 1989; Taylor, 1987). There is some evidence that long-term prescription is higher in those who have anxiety and comorbid personality disorder (Seivewright *et al.*, 1991, Romach *et al.*, 1995).

It has been estimated that 30%–45% of patients taking regular therapeutic doses of benzodiazepines long term have withdrawal symptoms (Ashton, 1995). Among illicit drug users, the use of benzodiazepines is common. In the NTORS (National Treatment Outcome Research Study), 33%–43% were regular users of benzodiazepines (Gossop *et al.*, 2003). In a survey of drug users from clinics in seven British cities, Strang *et al.* (1994) found that temazepam and diazepam were the most frequently used benzodiazepines, and that 49% of the people misusing them had injected them. In one European study triazolam and lorazepam were found to feature more highly among individuals dependent on high doses of benzodiazepines than among those dependent on low or 'therapeutic' doses (Martinez-Cano *et al.*, 1996). Drugs such as temazepam and flunitrazepam are more frequently reported to be injected (Strang *et al.*, 1992). However, more recently the rate of physical dependence on benzodiazepines among illicit drug misusers has been found to be relatively low (Ross & Darke, 2000; Williams *et al.*, 1996). There have been suggestions that benzodiazepines of high potency and short elimination half-life (e.g. triazolam, lorazepam, alprazolam), are associated with greater dependence risk than those of low potency and long elimination half-life, (e.g. chlordiazepoxide, nitrazepam), but there have been insufficient large-scale studies to support this notion and only one randomised trial giving partial support (Murphy & Tyrer, 1991).

Treatment of benzodiazepine dependence

Pharmacological treatments

Gossop (2003) has identified four strategies that are often used to treat benzodiazepine dependent patients. The choice of treatment method would depend upon the particular benzodiazepine, the dose, the co-occurrence of other dependent drug use and the clinical setting in which treatment is provided. These four strategies are as follows:

(1) Gradual tapering doses of the drug of dependence.
(2) Substitution of short acting benzodiazepines with a long acting benzodiazepine such as diazepam which is then reduced over a period of weeks.
(3) Substitution and gradual reduction of phenobarbitone or some other long acting barbiturate.
(4) Treatment of withdrawal symptoms with carbamazepine or valproate.

Gradual reduction with benzodiazepines
There is abundant literature that highlights the elements of assessment and preparation of patients with sedative drug dependence. In most patients, particularly those prescribed long-term licit prescription of benzodiazepines, switching to a long acting compound, followed by graded reduction, is recommended. This practice is based on the belief that long acting benzodiazepines, because of their long elimination half lives, produce a gradual reduction in drug concentration and are associated with less pronounced withdrawal symptoms (Rhodes *et al.*, 1984; Tyrer *et al.*, 1981, 1983). In case of non-prescribed severe benzodiazepine abuse, the initial prescribed dose should generally be substantially less than the amount the patient claims to be taking (Harrison *et al.*, 1984; Williams *et al.*, 1996). National guidelines in the UK have recommended this treatment as first-line in established benzodiazepine dependence (DoH, 1999).

Gradual reduction of benzodiazepines, with or without cognitive-behavioural therapy, has been shown to increase successful withdrawal rates in several studies (Tyrer *et al.*, 1983; Murphy & Tyrer, 1991; Oude-Voshaar *et al.*, 2003), and a recent systematic review found that only gradual reduction (tapering) was an unequivocally effective strategy (Oude-Voshaar *et al.*, 2006b). There are a number of studies of discontinuation schedules lasting several weeks (Murphy & Tyrer, 1991; Oude-Voshaar *et al.*, 2003; Tyrer *et al.*, 1983). However a widely varying range has been used, from a 7-day schedule (Petrovic *et al.*, 1999) to discontinuation over many years (Ashton, 1987); a shorter period of 1 to 3 months is a reasonable compromise. Short-term withdrawal over 7 days or less has been reported to be successful in some studies (Cantopher *et al.*, 1990; Rickels *et al.*, 1990), and this short-term

withdrawal strategy was achieved over a week in a group of elderly inpatients in Belgium (Petrovic *et al.*, 1999). In a recent study, 81/104 patients (mean age 77 years) who wished to stop benzodiazepines after many years of use were able to withdraw successfully with blinded tapering of dose and then with gradual substitution of placebo, plus psychological support, over 8–9 weeks (Curran *et al.*, 2003). Although there is little evidence for choosing the inpatient over the outpatient setting for most patients, inpatients are more likely to complete the detoxification regimen (Gossop *et al.*, 1986) and reduction in dosage may be more rapid when the person is an inpatient (Ashton, 1987). A gradual reduction/withdrawal strategy can be employed equally successfully with phenobarbital as well as with benzodiazepines, in sedative-hypnotic tolerant patients (Perry *et al.*, 1981). However, it is thought that a type II error compromised the conclusions of this study.

Gradual discontinuation programs are successful in two-thirds of patients and can be combined with additional pharmacological or psychological treatment (Oude-Voshaar *et al.*, 2001; Oude-Voshaar *et al.*, 2006a), although a systematic review shows no strong support for any of the adjunctive therapies (Oude-Voshaar *et al.*, 2006b). Most of the studies show methodological problems including small numbers of subjects (Nathan *et al.*, 1986; Tyrer *et al.*, 1985) and lack of randomisation and blinding. There is limited data on long-term outcome of benzodiazepine withdrawal, but some degree of relapse is commonly reported (Zitman & Couvée, 2001). Nonetheless, benzodiazepine discontinuation over a period of several weeks is the most commonly used detoxification method for benzodiazepine dependence. Success rates vary and there is no clear optimal rate or duration of reduction. Discontinuation may be particularly difficult in patients with personality disorder, comorbid mental or physical illness and multiple drug use. It may be useful to arrange inpatient detoxification for complex dependence. Patients should also be given additional support throughout and after the withdrawal period.

Substitution and tapering with barbiturates
Another method to treat benzodiazepine dependence is substitution with phenobarbitone and instituting a gradual stepwise reduction in dose. Smith & Wesson (1985) developed this technique. The pharmacological rationale suggests that long acting barbiturates permit a more stable blood level (Smith *et al.*, 1989), thus allowing the safe use of gradually reducing daily doses. Moreover, signs of toxicity are easily observed and lethal doses are many times higher than toxic doses of phenobarbitone. It is also said to be rarely abused (Sees, 1991). This method is rarely used in the UK and Europe though it is still, somewhat, being recommended for

complex high dose benzodiazepine dependent patients in the United States (Dupont & Saylor, 1991).

There is no peer reviewed scientific literature originating from the UK or Europe to support this treatment method. Phenobarbitone substitution, even though fairly commonly used in the United States, has as yet not led to randomised controlled trials looking at efficacy and outcomes, and at present it cannot be recommended as routine treatment and should be restricted to those on high doses of benzodiazepines in an inpatient setting.

Substitution and tapering with carbamazepine

Even though carbamazepine was initially reported to be of value in the treatment in benzodiazepine withdrawal both in an anecdotal report (Klein *et al.*, 1986) and an open study (Ries *et al.*, 1989), carbamazepine is seldom if ever used to treat benzodiazepine dependence in Europe. In a randomised, placebo-controlled trial in which carbamazepine was administered for 2–4 weeks before benzodiazepine tapering over 4 weeks in 40 patients who had previous difficulties in withdrawing from long-term therapeutic doses of benzodiazepines, there were no significant differences from placebo in severity of withdrawal symptoms or outcomes at 12 weeks post-withdrawal (Schweizer *et al.*, 1991). Yet patients taking more than 20 mg diazepam equivalent appeared to derive benefit, and the authors suggested that carbamazepine may have some utility in patients withdrawing from high dose benzodiazepines. It may also offer some anticonvulsant cover for those with a history of epilepsy (Lader, 1991), and recent guidelines issued in the UK have suggested that carbamazepine may be used instead of benzodiazepines to control withdrawal symptoms from high doses of benzodiazepines (BAP Guidelines (Lingford-Hughes *et al.*, 2004). Carbamazepine should probably only be used in a few carefully selected cases who are on very high doses of benzodiazepines and who have had a history of epilepsy.

Additional pharmacological treatment

Medications such as antidepressants, beta-blockers and buspirone have been studied for the management of benzodiazepine withdrawal. The rationale stems from the desire to remove the patient from the reinforcing pharmacological effects of benzodiazepines. Antidepressants have been reported to be effective in assisting withdrawal from benzodiazepines (Rickels *et al.*, 1989; Tyrer, 1985). Most authors have used tricyclic antidepressants in their studies. In a double-blind placebo-controlled study using dothiepin, Tyrer *et al.* (1996) concluded that dothiepin had no value in the treatment of benzodiazepine withdrawal symptoms. However in another double-blind placebo-controlled trial using imipramine and buspirone, Rickels *et al.* (2000) found that the success rate of benzodiazepine taper was significantly higher for patients who received imipramine (82.6%) compared to patients who received buspirone (67.9%) or placebo (37.5%).

There is as yet no clear evidence from published studies for the routine use of tricyclic antidepressants in withdrawal. To date, there is little experience with SSRIs or other new antidepressants in this context. Beta-blockers such as propranolol have little effect on subjective states of anxiety and do not have clear benefit in reducing the incidence of withdrawal symptoms or drop out rates in controlled trials (Abernethy *et al.*, 1981; Ashton, 1984, 1987; Cantopher *et al.*, 1990; Lader & Higgitt, 1986; Tyrer *et al.*, 1981). A number of studies have shown buspirone to be of no value in the treatment of benzodiazepine withdrawal (Ashton *et al.*, 1990; Olajide & Lader, 1987; Rickels *et al.*, 2000; Schweizer & Rickels, 1986).

Thus there have been variable results from studies when using the pharmacological treatments mentioned above in reducing withdrawal symptom severity and discontinuation rates, but no drug has been clearly established as effective in repeated RCTs (Couvée *et al.*, 2003; Schweizer and Rickels, 1998). Antidepressants, beta-blockers and buspirone should not be used in the routine management of benzodiazepine withdrawal (Oude-Voshaar *et al.*, 2006a, 2006b).

Maintenance treatments

Maintenance prescribing of benzodiazepines occurs mostly in specialist methadone maintenance clinics in the UK. It has been suggested that this may occur more frequently in practice than is advisable (Best *et al.*, 2002; Greenwood, 1996; Seivewright & Dougal, 1993). Although a number of preliminary open studies have found that maintenance prescribing reduced other benzodiazepine use (Weizman *et al.*, 2003 Wicks *et al.*, 2000), there are as yet no controlled trials published to support this form of treatment. Current expert opinion (DoH, 1999; BAP Guidelines 2004) does not support maintenance prescribing on the basis of existing evidence. The risks of overdose, injecting and diversion in this group of misusers is well recognised, and such maintenance prescribing is best avoided.

Z-drugs

Annual prescriptions for the Z-drugs, zaleplon, zolpidem and zopiclone in England between 1993 and 2003 are rising (DoH, 2003). This suggests that prescribers may believe that changing to a Z-drug can avoid problems associated with regular hypnotic use. In reality the precautions needed are just as stringent as those for benzodiazepines (DTB 2004). Also, given the surge in direct-to-consumer advertising in the USA on drugs for insomnia, the number of prescriptions for these drugs might be expected to increase at a greater rate.

Dependence on Z-drugs is a recognised risk for some patients and its incidence may be increasing (NICE, 2004). The misuse of zopiclone and zolpidem, characterised by significant dose escalation and withdrawal symptoms, has been reported in a systematic review of case reports, particularly in patients with a history of drug or alcohol misuse or other psychiatric disorder (Hajak et al., 2003). Recently, misuse of zolpidem for its stimulant and anxiolytic actions has also been reported in patients without these characteristics (Liappas et al., 2003, Vartzopoulos et al., 2000), (Dundar et al., 2004). This omission is a matter for concern as we enter an age of greater transparency over adverse effects of treatments. Since there are as yet no published studies on the treatment of Z-drug dependence, at present prevention is probably the best form of treatment.

Based on a limited number of case reports, it is advised that normal criteria for the prescription of benzodiazepines also be used when prescribing non-benzodiazepine sedatives and hypnotics, as they act upon the same receptor, the benzodiazepine-GABA-chloride complex (Bruun, 1993; Jones & Sullivan, 1998). Patients with a history of drug abuse or dependence and those with psychiatric diseases are at increased risk of abuse of these drugs. Therefore the same caution as with benzodiazepines should be taken when considering the prescription of zolpidem and zopiclone to these special populations (Hajak et al., 2003). Overall, Z-drugs should be used cautiously and for short-term treatment of insomnia. There is a definite potential risk of dependence. Studies designed to test the comparative risks of dependence with benzodiazepines and Z-drugs have as yet not been conducted. There is also an urgent need to examine the range of treatment options for dependent patients but it would be expected that gradual withdrawal would be as prominent as with the benzodiazepines.

Barbiturates

Over recent years use and abuse of barbiturates is seen only infrequently (Fountain et al., 1999). Barbiturate withdrawal was first described in 1905, two years after they were introduced into medical practice. There have been no randomised controlled trials in the last decade evaluating treatment methods for barbiturate dependence.

Most published literature is from the early 1970s and has serious methodological problems. Treatment of withdrawal with barbiturate substitution was reported as early as 1953 (Isbell & White 1953). In 1970 and 1971, Smith & Wesson (1971) reported on a protocol that used a phenobarbital substitution, stabilisation and tapering technique to treat barbiturate dependence. Their technique is still considered to be the 'gold standard' (Eickelberg & Mayo-Smith, 1998). More recently Robinson et al. (1981) successfully used repeated oral loading doses of phenobarbital, with the doses being titrated against symptoms, for barbiturate withdrawal. Substitution of barbiturates with diazepam was successful in another study (Perry et al., 1981). Ghodse (1995) has suggested that outpatient detoxification is seldom appropriate for these patients. The greatest clinical concern with barbiturate withdrawal is to prevent grand mal seizures and toxic confusional states. Thus even though there is very limited published literature, a gradual withdrawal, preferably as an inpatient, with substitution and tapering with a long-acting barbiturate such as phenobarbitone, appears the safest option.

Psychological treatments

Certain psychological interventions, particularly cognitive behavioural strategies focusing on anxiety management, have long been thought to be useful in the treatment of benzodiazepine dependence and withdrawal (Sanchez-Craig et al., 1987; Tyrer et al., 1985). No studies looking at psychological interventions for barbiturate or Z-drug dependence could be found despite a detailed review of the literature.

The two randomised controlled trials without major methodological problems in this area were restricted to participants who met the criteria for panic disorder. Otto et al. (1993) demonstrated the superior efficacy of CBT approach in combination with slow tapering of benzodiazepines (13/17; 76% successfully discontinued) over similar tapering regimen with supportive medical management (4/16; 25% discontinued). At 3-month follow-up 77% of the patients on the cognitive-behavioural programme remained benzodiazepine free. Spiegel et al. (1994) found no difference between taper only and cognitive-behavioural treatment in the rate of discontinuation (80% and 90%), but half of the subjects who discontinued without cognitive-behavioural therapy relapsed during the 6-month follow-up period. Results are, however, difficult to generalise as the prevalence of panic disorder among those who are long-term benzodiazepine users has been estimated to be at most 27% (Rickels et al., 1986).

Oude-Voshaar *et al.* (2003) more recently conducted a 3-month randomised controlled trial in a general practice setting in which 180 people attempting to discontinue long-term benzodiazepine use were assigned to tapering off plus CBT, tapering off alone and usual care. Although tapering off led to a significantly higher proportion of successful discontinuations (62% vs. 21%), adding CBT did not increase the success rate (58% vs. 62%). The authors concluded that the addition of group CBT was of limited value. Boyce (2003) has done a useful commentary on this paper. Vorma *et al.* (2002) in a controlled trial, which included 76 patients in two nearly equal groups, compared gradual benzodiazepine taper combined with CBT with standard treatment in benzodiazepine patients. They included patients on high doses and with alcohol use disorders in the study. They did not find any significant differences in the outcomes between the two groups.

Sanchez-Craig *et al.* (1987) carried out a randomised comparison of cognitive-behavioural treatment with a rapid 4–5 week drug taper and abrupt cessation by substituting placebo tablets for benzodiazepines in 42 subjects. By the end of the treatment, a total of 39% of the subjects in the benzodiazepine group and 58% in the placebo group were abstinent. No differences in treatment outcomes between the groups were observed.

Higgitt *et al.* (1987) compared group CBT with individual telephone contact in 16 chronic benzodiazepine users over a 28-week period. The sample size was too small to find any significant differences between the groups; however, when the groups were combined, 25% of the subjects discontinued their benzodiazepines during the study period. Elsesser *et al.* (1996) evaluated the efficacy of complaints management training (CMT) compared to that of anxiety management training (AMT) in patients undergoing benzodiazepine withdrawal. Nineteen patients were randomly allocated either to CMT or AMT. Both groups received 9 weekly treatment sessions. The CMT was more successful than the AMT in terms of abstinence rate, reported number of severe withdrawal symptoms, depression and anxiety. At 6 months, there was no difference between groups in terms of abstinence rate.

Baillargeon *et al.* (2003) in a study involving participants aged over 65 years, carried out a randomised comparison of a combination of group CBT and benzodiazepine tapering to gradual tapering only over an 8-week period. Immediately after treatment a greater number (26/34; 77%) in the combined treatment group had withdrawn from benzodiazepine use completely versus (11/29; 38%) in the gradual taper only group. At the 12-month follow-up, the favourable outcome persisted (23/33; 70% v. 7/29; 24%) in the combined treatment group.

There is no reliable evidence on psychological treatment as a stand-alone method of treatment. Cognitive-behavioural therapy, anxiety management training, psycho-education and supportive therapy have been used in combination with gradual tapering. However, even the studies mentioned above have considerable methodological problems. Two studies did not compare the efficacy of additional CBT with tapering alone (Elsesser *et al.*, 1996; Sanchez-Craig *et al.*, 1987). Other studies did not randomise participants over the conditions (Higgit *et al.*, 1987) or studied a sample of fewer than 10 participants (Tyrer *et al.*, 1985). Most of these studies recruited highly selected subject groups and excluded patients with high dosage benzodiazepine dependence and comorbid alcohol or opiate misuse. Drop out rates in these studies were relatively high (Oude-Voshaar *et al.*, 2003). The recent BAP guidelines (Lingford-Hughes *et al.*, 2004) and a systematic review (Oude-Voshaar *et al.*, 2006) conclude that additional psychological therapies do not appear to increase effectiveness of graded discontinuation from benzodiazepines but should be considered on their own merits.

Minimal interventions

Minimal interventions include advisory letters, provision of other information, single consultation with a GP and short courses of relaxation. Books written for patients are also available (Trickett, 1986; Tyrer, 1986).

Cormack *et al.* (1994) in a randomised controlled trial found that a letter from the GP suggesting a reduction in the use of benzodiazepines resulted in up to a 50% reduction in dose and in about 20% of patients to total cessation. In a recent trial involving 284 patients on long-term benzodiazepines, 39% of those receiving either of two brief interventions (a short consultation or a letter from their GP advising gradual reduction in benzodiazepine intake) achieved at least a 25% reduction in their use of benzodiazepines (Heather *et al.*, 2004). In the study, 24% of a control group who completed the assessment and were randomised to 'usual GP care' also reduced their benzodiazepine use by at least 25%.

In a controlled study, Bashir *et al.* (1994) described the effectiveness of a minimal intervention in the form of brief advice from the GP supplemented by a self-help booklet compared with a control group who received 'routine' care. Eighteen percent (9/50) in the intervention group reduced benzodiazepine prescribing compared to 5% (3/55) in the control group. At six months follow up 43% reported reduction in their benzodiazepine use in the intervention group compared to 20% in the control group. The authors found that more subjects (20% vs. 7%) in the intervention group stopped benzodiazepine use completely. Furthermore, the authors concluded that this intervention did not lead to psychological distress or increased consultation.

The studies described above excluded several categories of patients such as psychiatric illness, poly-substance misusers, etc. Nevertheless, the cumulative findings demonstrate that in selected patients, an appreciable rate of success can be achieved even after many years of benzodiazepine use by using fairly simple interventions. Minimal intervention approaches have been calculated to achieve cessation of benzodiazepine use in approximately 20% of cases (Couvée *et al.*, 2003), and they are a reasonable and cost effective approach in primary care settings.

Alternative treatments

There is a general lack of research in the literature on the role and efficacy of alternative treatments in addictive disorders, and most research has focused on alcohol, nicotine, opiate and cocaine problems. There are some reports of phytotherapy and hypnotherapy being helpful for patients with benzodiazepine dependence (Rasmussen, 1997). Poyares *et al.* (2002) in a recent double blind placebo-controlled study described the effects of Valerian in patients using benzodiazepines chronically. Valerian is a naturally occurring root used in many countries by patients with insomnia and may be a useful treatment in benzodiazepine withdrawal. The authors concluded that valerian had some positive effect on benzodiazepine

withdrawal but suggested that, due to small sample size, further larger studies were needed. Thus, due to the complete lack of research in this area, alternative therapies at present cannot be recommended in the treatment of sedative-hypnotic dependence (see also Chapter 7).

Summary and Conclusions

The treatment of tranquilliser dependence is not especially satisfactory, with only gradual withdrawal, often using a different benzodiazepine, over a variable time scale, showing satisfactory levels of efficacy in almost all studies. Other forms of pharmacological substitution are of limited value, with only carbamazepine showing some hint of real benefit, and psychological treatments such as cognitive-behaviour therapy are disappointing. The best evidence for a psychological intervention is for brief self-help packages and other forms of bibliotherapy, which also have the advantage of being accessible for booster purposes at all times. However, the evidence for efficacy is better in those who are in primary care and with less intractable dependence. Interestingly, these approaches do not seem to differ in effectiveness for those who are dependent through prolonged therapeutic prescription or though deliberate misuse. The lack of information about the dependence problems of the Z-drugs (zopiclone, zolpidem and zaleplon) is troubling.

The level of evidence for each of the interentions discussed in this chapter is summarised in Table 21.1.

Table 21.1. Effectiveness of treatments for sedative-hypnotic dependence

Treatment	Form of treatment	Psychiatric disorder/ target audience	Level of evidence for efficacy	Comments
Gradual withdrawal (with or without switching to a longer-acting benzodiazepine)	Gradual reduction with longer-acting benzodiazepines NB. In practice diazepam is often used for this purpose as in chronic doses its major long-acting metabolite (nordiazepam) is the active ingredient and the range of doses (10 mg, 5 mg, 2 mg) for this drug are a practical advantage	Benzodiazepine dependence	Ia	A number of studies support the idea that about 2 out of 3 patients are able to stop benzodiazepines completely using this method. Little is known about the long-term impact of this type of intervention but recourse to brief prescriptions of benzodiazepines is common (Holton & Tyrer, 1990)
Phenobarbitone substitution	Gradual reduction after phenobarbitone substitution	Benzodiazepine dependence	III	Limited to occasional use with inpatients on high doses of benzodiazepines
Carbamazepine substitution	Carbamazepine	Benzodiazepine dependence	II	Despite some shortcomings, this is a frequently recommended form of treatment, though little is known about its long-term impact

Table 21.1. (cont.)

Treatment	Form of treatment	Psychiatric disorder/ target audience	Level of evidence for efficacy	Comments
Psychological treatment	CBT and other forms of behavioural therapy	Benzodiazepine dependence	III	There is really no evidence for the effectiveness of this treatment as a stand alone intervention and little gain when used in combination
Antidepressant substitution	Tricyclic antidepressant substitution	Benzodiazepine dependence	III	Minimal evidence of efficacy and acceptability
Brief psychological interventions and bibliotherapy	Non-specialised interventions using small resources	All tranquilliser dependence	II	Is probably more valuable than formal CBT and similar approaches and appears to have a small but significant benefit

REFERENCES

Abernethy, D. R., Greenblatt, D. J. & Shader, R. I. (1981). Treatment of diazepam withdrawal syndrome with propranolol. *Annals of Internal Medicine*, **94**, 354–5.

APA Task Force (1990). Benzodiazepine dependence, toxicity and abuse: a Task Force Report of the American Psychiatric Association. Washington DC: APA.

Ashton, C. H. (1984). Benzodiazepine withdrawal: unfinished story. *British Medical Journal*, **288**, 1135–40.

Ashton, C. H. (1987). Benzodiazepine withdrawal: outcome in 50 patients. *British Journal of Addiction*, **82**, 665–671.

Ashton, C. H. (1995). Toxicity and adverse consequences of benzodiazepine use. *Psychiatric Annales*, **25**, 158–65.

Ashton, C. H. & Golding, J. F. (1989). Tranquillisers: prevalence, predictions and possible consequences, data from a large United Kingdom survey. *British Journal of Addiction*, **84**, 541–6.

Ashton, C., Rawlins, M. & Tyrer, S. (1990). A double blind placebo-controlled study of buspirone in diazepam withdrawal in chronic benzodiazepine users. *British Journal of Psychiatry*, **157**, 232–8.

Baillargeon, L., Landreville, P., Verreault, R., Beauchemin, J. P., Gregoire, J. P. & Morin, C. M. (2003). Discontinuation of benzodiazepines among older insomniac adults treated with cognitive-behavioural therapy combined with gradual tapering: a randomized trial. *Canadian Medical Association Journal*, **169**, 1015–20.

Balter, M. B., Manheimer, D. I., Mellinger, G. D. & Uhlenhuth, E. H. (1984). A cross national comparison of antianxiety/sedative use. *Current Medical Research Opinion*, **8**, 5–20.

Bashir, K., King, M. & Ashworth, M. (1994). Controlled evaluation of brief intervention by general practitioners to reduce chronic use of benzodiazepines. *British Journal of General Practice*, **44**, 408–12.

Best, D., Noble, A., Man, L., Gossop, M., Finch, E. & Strang, J. (2002). Factors surrounding long-term benzodiazepine prescribing in methadone maintenance clients. *Journal of Substance Abuse Treatment*, **7**, 175–9.

Boyce, P. (2003). Commentary on, Gradual reduction of benzodiazepines, with or without cognitive behavioural therapy, increases successful withdrawal rates compared with no support in long-term users. *Evidence Based Mental Health*, **6**(4), 119.

Bruun, T. G. (1993). Abuse potential during use and withdrawal psychosis after treatment with the hypnotic zolpidem (Stilnoct). *Ugeskr Laeger*, **155**(51), 4194–5.

Busto, U., Sellers, E. M., Naranjo, C. A., Cappell, H., Sanchez-Craig, M. & Sykora, K. (1986a). Withdrawal reaction after long-term therapeutic use of benzodiazepines. *New England Journal of Medicine*, **315**, 854–9.

Busto, U., Sellers, E. M., Naranjo, C. A., Cappell, H. D., Sanchez-Craig, M. & Simpkins, J. (1986b). Patterns of benzodiazepine abuse and dependence. *British Journal of Addiction*, **81**, 87–94.

Cantopher, T., Olivieri, S., Cleave, N. & Edwards, G. (1990). Chronic benzodiazepine dependence: a comparative study of abrupt withdrawal under propranolol cover versus gradual withdrawal. *British Journal of Psychiatry*, **156**, 406–11.

Cole, J. O. & Chiarello, R. J. (1990). The benzodiazepines as drugs of abuse. *Journal of Psychiatric Research*, **24**, 135–44.

Committee on Safety of Medicines (CSM) (1988). Benzodiazepines, dependence and withdrawal symptoms. *Current Problems*, **21**, 1–2.

Coppell, H. D., Sellers, E. M. & Busto, U. (1986). Benzodiazepines as drugs of abuse and dependence. *Recent Advances in Alcohol and Drug Problems*, ed. H. D. Coppell, F. H. Glaser, Y. Israel *et al.*, vol. 9, p. 63. New York: Plenum Press.

Cormack, M. A., Sweeney, K. G., Hughes-Jones, H. & Foot, G. A. (1994). Evaluation of an easy, cost-effective strategy for cutting benzodiazepine use in general practice. *British Journal of Genearl Practice*, **44**(378), 5–8.

Couvée, J., Oude-Voshaar, R., van Balkom, A., & Zitman, F. (2003). Strategies to discontinue long term benzodiazepine use: a systematic review. In *Towards a Treatment of Chronic Benzodiazepine Users Suffering from Depression*, ed. J. Couvée. The Netherlands: Glaxo SmithKline BV.

Curran, H. V., Collins, R., Fletcher, S., Kee, S. C., Woods, B. & Iliffe, S. (2003). Older adults and withdrawal from benzodiazepine

410   K. Dar & M. Kumar

hypnotics in general practice: effects on cognitive function, sleep, mood and quality of life. *Psychological Medicine*, **33**, 1223–37.

Department of Health (DoH 2003). Prescription costs analysis (PCA 2003 online). Available: www.publications.doh.gov.uk/stats/pca2003.pdf.

Department of Health, Scottish Office Department of Health, Welsh Office, Department of Health and Social Services, Northern Ireland (1999). *Drug Misuse and Dependence – Guidelines on Clinical Management.*

Drug and Therapeutic Bulletin (DTB) (2004). What's wrong with prescribing hypnotics? **42**(12), 89–93.

Dundar, Y., Boland, A., Strobl, J. *et al.* (2004). Newer hypnotic drugs for the short term management of insomnia: a systematic review and economic evaluation. *Health Technology Assessment*, **8**(24), iii–x, 1–125.

DuPont, R. L. & Saylor, K. E. (1991). Sedatives/hypnotics and benzodiazepines. In *Clinical Textbook of Addictive Disorders*, ed. R. J. Frances & S. I. Miller, pp. 69–102. New York & London: Guilford Press.

Eickelberg, S. J. & Mayo-Smith, M. F. (1998). Management of sedative-hypnotic intoxication and withdrawal. In *Principles of Addiction Medicine*, ed. A. W. Graham & T. K. Schultz, pp. 441–55. ASAM Press.

Elsesser, K., Sartory, G. & Maurer, J. (1996). The efficacy of complaints management training in facilitating benzodiazepine withdrawal. *Behaviour Research and Therapy*, **34**, 149–56.

Fountain, J., Griffiths, P., Farrell, M., Gossop, M. & Strang, J. (1999). Benzodiazepines in polydrug-using repertoires: the impact of the decreased availability of temazepam gel-filled capsules. *Drugs: Education, Prevention and Policy*, **6**(1), 61–9.

Ghodse, A. H. (1995). *Drugs and Addictive Behaviour: A Guide to Treatment*, 2nd edn, pp. 268–75. Oxford: Blackwell Science.

Gossop, M. (2003). Detoxification from benzodiazepines and sedatives. In *Drug Addiction and its Treatment*, pp. 127–9. Oxford, UK: Oxford University Press.

Gossop, M., Johns, A. & Green, L. (1986). Opiate withdrawal: inpatient versus outpatient programmes and preferred versus random assignment to treatment. *British Medical Journal*, **293**, 103–4.

Gossop, M., Marsden, J., Stewart, D. & Kidd, T. (2003). The National Treatment Outcome Research Study (NTORS): 4–5 year follow-up results. *Addiction*, **98**(3), 291–303.

Greenwood, J. (1996). Six years experience of sharing the care of Edinburgh's drug users. *Psychiatric Bulletin*, **20**, 8–11.

Hajak, G., Muller, W. E., Wittchen, H. U., Pittrow, D. & Kirch, W. (2003). Abuse and dependence potential for the non-benzodiazepine hypnotics zolpidem and zopiclone: a review of case reports and epidemiological data. *Addiction*, **98**, 1371–8.

Hall, R. C. W. & Joffe, J. R. (1972). Aberrant response to diazepam: a new syndrome. *American Journal of Psychiatry*, **129**, 738–42.

Hallstrom, C. & Lader, M. (1981). Benzodiazepine withdrawal phenomena. *International Pharmacopsychiatry*, **16**, 235–44.

Harrison, M., Busto, U., Naranjo, C. A., Kaplan, H. L. & Sellers, E. M. (1984). Diazepam tapering in detoxification for high-dose benzodiazepine abuse. *Clinical Pharmacology and Therapeutics*, **36**, 527–33.

Heather, N., Bowie, A., Ashton, H. *et al.* (2004). Randomised controlled trial of two brief interventions against long-term benzodiazepine use: outcome of intervention. *Addiction Research Theory*, **12**, 141–54.

Higgitt, A., Golombok, S., Fonagy, P. & Lader, M. (1987). Group treatment of benzodiazepine dependence. *British Journal of Addiction*, **82**, 517–32.

Holton, A. & Tyrer, P. (1990). Five year outcome of patients withdrawn from long-term treatment with diazepam. *British Medical Journal*, **300**, 1241–2.

Isbell, H. & White, W. M. (1953). Clinical characteristics of addictions. *American Journal of Medicine*, **14**, 558–65.

Joint Formulary Committee (2004). *British National Formulary*. Edition 48. London: Royal Pharmaceutical Society of Great Britain and British Medical Association. Sept. 2004

Jones, I. R. & Sullivan, G. (1998). Physical dependence on zopiclone: case reports. *British Medical Journal*, **316**, 117.

Klein, E., Uhde, T. W. & Post, R. M. (1986). Preliminary evidence for the utility of carbamazepine in alprazolam withdrawal. *American Journal of Psychiatry*, **143**, 336–8.

Lader, M. H. (1999). Limitations on the use of benzodiazepines in anxiety and insomnia: are they justified? *European Neuropsychopharmacology*, **9** (Suppl. 6), S399–405.

Lader, M. H. (1991). Avoiding long-term use of benzodiazepine drugs. *Prescriber*. March, pp. 79–83.

Lader, M. H. & Higgitt, A. C. (1986). Management of benzodiazepine dependence – Update 1986. *British Journal of Addiction*, **81**, 7–9.

Liappas, I. A., Malitas, P. N., Dimopoulos, N. P. *et al.* (2003). Zolpidem dependence case series; possible neurobiological mechanisms and clinical management. *Journal of Psychopharmacology*, **17**, 131–5.

Lingford-Hughes, A. R., Welch, S. & Nutt, D. J. (BAP Guidelines) (2004). Evidence-based guidelines for the pharmacological management of substance misuse, addiction and comorbidity: recommendations from the British Association for Psychopharmacology. *Journal of Psychopharmacology*, **18**(3), 305–7.

Mackinnon, G. L. & Parker, W. A. (1982). Benzodiazepine withdrawal syndrome: a literature review and evaluation. *American Journal of Drug and Alcohol Abuse*, **9**, 19–33.

Martinez-Cano, H., Vela-Bueno, A., De Iceta, M., Pomalima, R., Martinez-Gras, I. & Sobrino, M. P.(1996). Benzodiazepine types in high versus therapeutic dose dependence. *Addiction*, **91**, 1179–86.

Murphy, S. & Tyrer, P. (1991). A double-blind comparison of the effects of gradual withdrawal of lorazepam, diazepam and bromazepam in benzodiazepine dependence. *British Journal of Psychiatry*, **158**, 511–16.

Nathan, R. G., Robinson, D., Cherek, D. R., Sebastian, C. S., Hack, M. & Davison, S. (1986). Alternative treatments for withdrawing the long-term benzodiazepine user: a pilot study. *International Journal of Addictions*, **21**(2), 195–211.

National Institute for Clinical Excellence (NICE) (2004). Guidance on the use of zaleplon, zolpidem and zopiclone for short term management of insomnia. London: NICE (Technology Appraisal 77).

Noyes, R., Garvey, M. J., Cook, B. L. & Perry, D. J. (1988). Benzodiazepine withdrawal: a review of the evidence. *Journal of Clinical Psychiatry*, **49**, 382–9.

Olajide, D. & Lader, M. H. (1987). A comparitive study of the efficacy of buspirone in relieving benzodiazepine withdrawal symptoms. *Journal of Clinical Psychopharmacology*, **7**, 11–15.

Otto, M. W., Pollack, M. H., Sachs, G. S., Reiter, S. R., Meltzer-Brody, S. & Rosenbaum, J. F. (1993). Discontinuation of benzodiazepine treatment: efficacy of cognitive behavioural therapy for patients with panic disorder. *American Journal of Psychiatry*, **150**, 1485–90.

Oude-Voshaar, R. C., Gorgels, W. J. & Mol, A. J. J. (2001). Behandelmethoden om langdurig benzodiazepinegebruik te staken [Treatment methods for discontinuation of long-term benzodiazepine use]. *Nederlands Tijdschrift voor Geneeskunde*, **145**, 1347–50.

Oude-Voshaar, R. C., Gorgels, W. J. & Mol, A. J. J. (2003). Tapering off long-term benzodiazepine use with or without group cognitive-behavioural therapy: three-condition, randomised controlled trial. *British Journal of Psychiatry*, **182**, 498–504.

Oude-Voshaar, R. C., Couvée, J. E., van Balkom, A. J. L. M., Mulder, P. G. H. & Zitman, F. G. (2006a). Strategies for discontinuing long-term benzodiazepine use: meta-analysis. *British Journal of Psychiatry*, **189**, 213–20.

Oude-Voshaar, R. C., Gorgels, W. J., Mol, A. J. *et al.* (2006b). Long-term outcome of two forms of randomised benzodiazepine discontinuation. *British Journal of Psychiatry*, **188**, 188–9.

Perry, P. J., Stambaugh, R. L., Tsuang, M. T. & Smith R. E., (1981). Sedative-hypnotic tolerance testing and withdrawal comparing diazepam to barbiturates. *Journal of Clinical Psychopharmacology*, **1**(5), 289–96.

Petrovic, M., Pevernagie, D., van den Noortgate, N. Mariman, A., Michielsen, W. & Afschrift, M. (1999). A programme for short-term withdrawal from benzodiazepines in geriatric hospital inpatients: Success rate and effect on subjective sleep quality. *International Journal of Geriatric Psychiatry*, **14**(9), 754–60.

Petursson, H. & Lader, M. (1981). Benzodiazepine dependence. *British Journal of Addiction*, **76**, 133–45.

Poyares, D. R., Guilleminault, C., Ohayon, M. M. & Tufik, S. (2002). Can valerian improve the sleep of insomniacs after benzodiazepine withdrawal?. *Progress in Neuropsychopharmacology and Biological Psychiatry*, **26**(3), 539–45.

Priest, R. G. & Montgomery, S. A. (1988). Benzodiazepines and dependence: a College statement. *Bulletin Royal College of Psychiatrists*, **12**, 107–8.

Rasmussen, P. (1997). A role for phytotherapy in the treatment of benzodiazepine and opiate drug withdrawal. *European Journal of Herbal Medicines* **3**(1), 11–21.

Rhodes, P. J., Rhodes, R. S. & McCurdy, J. H. (1984). Elimination kinetics and symptomatology of diazepam withdrawal in abusers. *Clinical Toxicology*, **22**, 371–4.

Rickels, K., Case, W. G., Schweizer, E. E., Swenson, C. & Fridman, R. (1986). Low dose dependence in chronic benzodiazepine users: a preliminary report on 119 patients. *Psychopharmacological Bulletin*, **22**, 407–15.

Rickels, K., Case, W. G., Schweizer, E., Garcia-Espana, F. & Fridman, R. (1989). Benzodiazepine dependence: management of discontinuation. *Psychopharmacology Bulletin*, **26**, 63–8.

Rickels, K., DeMartinis, N., Rynn, M. & Mandos, L. (1999). Pharmacologic strategies for discontinuing benzodiazepine treatment. *Journal of Clinical Psychopharmacology*, **19**(6) Suppl. 2, 12S–16S.

Rickels, K., Schweizer, E., Case, W. G. & Greenblatt, D. J. (1990). Long-term therapeutic use of benzodiazepines. I. Effects of abrupt discontinuation. *Archives of General Psychiatry*, **47**, 899–907.

Rickels, K., DeMartinis, N., García-España, F., Greenblatt, D. J., Mandos, L. A. & Rynn, M. (2000). Imipramine and buspirone in treatment of patients with generalized anxiety disorder who are discontinuing long-term benzodiazepine therapy. *American Journal of Psychiatry*, **157**, 1973–9.

Ries, R. K., Roy-Byrne, P. P., Ward, N. G., Neppe, V. & Cullison, S. (1989). Carbamazepine treatment for benzodiazepine withdrawal. *American Journal of Psychiatry*, **146**, 536–7.

Robinson, G. M., Sellers, E. M. & Janacek, E. (1981). Barbiturate and hypnosedative withdrawal by a multiple oral Phenobarbital loading dose technique. *Clinical and Pharmacological Therapy*, **30**(1), 71–6.

Romach, M., Busto, U., Somer, G., Kaplan, H. I. & Sellers, E. (1995). Clinical aspects of chronic use of alprazolam and lorazepam. *American Journal of Psychiatry*, **152**, 1161–7.

Ross, J. & Darke, S. (2000). The nature of benzodiazepine dependence among heroin users in Sydney, Australia. *Addiction*, **95**, 1785–93.

Sanchez-Craig, M., Cappell, H., Busto, U. & Kay, G. (1987). Cognitive-behavioural treatment for benzodiazepine dependence: a comparison of gradual versus abrupt cessation of drug intake. *British Journal of Addiction*, **82**, 1317–27.

Schweizer, E. & Rickels, K. (1986). Failure of buspirone to manage benzodiazepine withdrawal. *American Journal of Psychiatry*, **143**, 1590–2.

Schweizer, E. & Rickels, K. (1998). Benzodiazepine dependence and withdrawal: a review of the syndrome and its clinical management. *Acta Psychiatrica Scandinavica*, **98** (Suppl. 393), 95–101.

Schweizer, E., Rickels, K., Case, W. G. & Greenblatt, D. J. (1991). Carbamazepine treatment in patients discontinuing long-term benzodiazepine therapy: effects on withdrawal severity and outcome. *Archives of General Psychiatry*, **48**, 448–52.

Sees, K. L. (1991). Pharmacological adjuncts for the treatment of withdrawal syndromes. *Journal of Psychoactive Drugs*, **23**, 179–93.

Scivewright, N. & Dougal W. (1993). Withdrawal symptoms from high dose benzodiazepines in polydrug users. *Drug & Alcohol Dependence*, **32**, 15–23.

Seivewright, H., Tyrer, P., Casey, P. & Seivewright, N. (1991). A three-year follow-up of psychiatric morbidity in urban and rural primary care. *Psychological Medicine*, **21**, 495–503.

Smith, D. E. & Wesson, D. R. (1970). A new method for treatment of barbiturate dependence. *Journal of the American Medical Association*, **23**, 294–5.

Smith, D. E. & Wesson, D. R. (1971). A phenobarbital technique for the withdrawal of barbiturate abuse. *Archives of General Psychiatry*, **24**, 56–60.

Smith, D. E. & Wesson, D. R. (1985). Benzodiazepine dependence syndromes. In *The Benzodiazepines: Current Standards for Medical Practice*, ed. D. E. Smith & D. R. Wesson, pp. 235–48. Lancaster, UK: MTP Press.

Smith, D. E., Landry, M. J. & Wesson, D. R. (1989). Barbiturate, sedative, hypnotic agents. In *APA Task Force on Treatment of Psychiatric Disorders*, pp. 1294–308. Washington DC: APA.

Spiegel, D. A., Bruce, T. J., Gregg, S. F. & Nuzzarello, A. (1994). Does cognitive behaviour therapy assist slow-taper alprazolam discontinuation in panic disorder? *American Journal of Psychiatry*, **151**, 876–81.

Strang, J., Seivewright, N. & Farrell, M. (1992). Intravenous and other novel abuses of benzodiazepines; the opening of Pandora's box?. *British Journal of Addiction*, **87**(10), 1373–5.

Strang, J., Griffiths, P., Abbey, J. & Gossop, M. (1994). Survey of use of injected benzodiazepines among drug users in Britain. *British Medical Journal*, **308**, 1082.

Taylor, D. (1987). Current usage of benzodiazepines in Britain. In *Current Clinical Practice*, ed. H. Freeman & Y. Rue, pp. 13–18. London: Royal Society of Medicine.

Taylor, S., McCracken, C. F., Wilson, K. C. & Copeland, J. R. (1998). Extent and appropriateness of benzodiazepine use. Results from an elderly urban community. *British Journal of Psychiatry*, **173**, 433–8.

Trickett, S. (1986). *Coming off Tranquillisers and Sleeping Pills.* Wellingborough, Northamptonshire: Thorsons Publishing Group.

Tyrer, P. (1980). Dependence on benzodiazepines. *British Journal of Psychiatry*, **137**, 576–7.

Tyrer, P. (1985). Clinical management of benzodiazepine dependence. *British Medical Journal*, **291**, 1507.

Tyrer, P. (1986). *How to Stop Taking Tranquillisers.* London: Sheldon Press.

Tyrer, P., Rutherford, D. & Huggett, T. (1981). Benzodiazepine withdrawal symptoms and propranolol. *Lancet*, **i**, 520–2.

Tyrer, P., Owen, R. & Dawling, S. (1983). Gradual withdrawal of diazepam after long-term therapy. *Lancet*, **1**, 1402–6.

Tyrer, P., Murphy, S., Oates, G. & Kingdon, D. (1985). Psychological treatment for benzodiazepine dependence. *Lancet*, **1**, 1042–3.

Tyrer, P., Murphy, S. & Riley, P. (1990). The benzodiazepine withdrawal symptom questionnaire. *Journal of Affective Disorders*, **19**, 53–61.

Tyrer, P., Ferguson, B., Hallstrom, C. *et al.* (1996). A controlled trial of dothiepin and placebo in treating benzodiazepine withdrawal symptoms. *British Journal of Psychiatry*, **168**, 457–61.

Vartzopoulos, D., Bozikas, V., Phocas, C., Karavatos, A. & Kaprinis, G. (2000). Dependence on zolpidem in high dose. *International Clinical Psychopharmacology*, **15**, 181–2.

Vorma, H., Naukkarinen, H., Sarna, S. & Kuoppasalmi, K. (2002). Treatment of outpatients with complicated benzodiazepine dependence: comparison of two approaches. *Addiction*, **97**, 851–9.

Weizman, T., Gelkopf, M., Melamed, Y., Adelson, M. & Bleich, A. (2003). Treatment of benzodiazepine dependence in methadone maintenance treatment patients: a comparison of two therapeutic modalities and the role of psychiatric comorbidity. *Australian and New Zealand Journal of Psychiatry*, **37**, 458–63.

Wicks, W., Darke, S. & Ross, J. (2000). Clobazam maintenance among methadone maintenance patients with problematic benzodiazepine use; five case studies. *Drug and Alcohol Reviews*, **19**, 401–5.

Williams, H., Oyefeso, A. & Ghodse, A. (1996). Benzodiazepine misuse and dependence among opiate addiction treatment. *Irish Journal of Psychological Medicine*, **13**, 62–4.

Woods, J. H., Katz, J. L. & Winger, G. (1992). Benzodiazepines: use, abuse and consequences. *Pharmacological Reviews*, **44**, 151–338.

Woody, G. E., O'Brien, C. P. & Greestein, R. (1975). Misuse and abuse of diazepam: an increasingly common medical problem. *International Journal of Addiction*, **10**, 843–8.

Zitman, F. G. & Couvée, J. E. (2001). Chronic benzodiazepine use in general practice patients with depression: an evaluation of controlled treatment and taper-off. Report on behalf of the Dutch Chronic Benzodiazepine Working Group. *British Journal of Psychiatry*, **178**, 317–24.

22

Treatment of cannabis dependence

Brent A. Moore, Henrietta Bowden-Jones, Alan J. Budney and Ryan Vandrey

Editor's note

Cannabis usage is often thought not to be a problem, and recent reclassifications of the drug in the UK and groups pushing for the legalization of marijuana encourage usage. This is unfortunate because cannabis usage is often problematic. A dependency syndrome can develop, and then withdrawal symptoms can complicate the efforts to stop using the substance. There are many medical and mental health problems that occur with chronic cannabis usage, and these include, most seriously, psychoses (see Chapter 26) problems with memory, motivation, psycho-motor coordination, irritability, anxiety, and a host of other psychological difficulties. Pulmonary problems can occur because of the smoking of the substance. Yet, despite the problems inherent in chronic usage and despite the large number of people who probably have developed dependency on the substance, there remains very little in the way of effective interventions. There are not enough trials to even attempt a meta-analysis of interventions. There are really no good pharmacologic interventions. Cognitive-behavioural therapy, enhanced by contingency management techniques such as the use of vouchers, seems most effective. There is some evidence that the longer the length of exposure to these behavioural interventions, the greater the chance of success in being able to stop using the substance.

Introduction

Cannabis use remains the most prevalent form of illicit drug use in English speaking countries and the European Union, and its use is believed to be high in other countries where epidemiological data are not available (European Monitoring Centers for Drugs and Drug

Addiction, 2003; Hall et al., 1999; SAMSHA, 2002). Recent population rates of cannabis use during the past year have been found to be highest in New Zealand (20%) and Australia (17%), lower in the USA (11%) and Canada (7%), and ranges from 2% (Finland) to 11% (United Kingdom) across the European Union, with rates higher among young adult populations (European Monitoring Center for Drugs and Drug Addiction, 2003; Gledhill-Hoyt et al., 2000; SAMSHA, 2002; Swift et al., 2001). In the UK 21% of adults have tried it at least once and 16% had used it in the last year. Amongst boys aged 16–19, 32% had used it in the last year whereas amongst girls aged 16–19, 40% had done so (Caan and de Belleroche, 2002). The World Health Organization has estimated that 2.45% of the world uses cannabis on a regular basis or, to put this in perspective, 141 million people (WHO, 1997). The Conference Report from UK Dept of Environment and Transport reports that cannabis is second only to alcohol as a factor in fatal road accidents (10% of UK road deaths) because cannabis impairs psychomotor performance.

Smoking is the primary method for use of cannabis, and almost all users smoke either marijuana cigarettes ('joints') or use pipes to smoke marijuana or hashish. A range of problems have been associated with regular cannabis use including difficulty in recalling previously learned items, concentration, motivation, health, interpersonal relationships, and employment, as well as lower participation in conventional roles of adulthood, history of psychiatric symptoms and hospitalizations, and participation in deviant activities (Budney et al., 2003a; Kalant et al., 1999). One must not overlook respiratory complications and pulmonary damage secondary to chronic smoking. Yet there has been little empirical research into cannabis dependency, and there are very few randomized control trials looking at either psychological or pharmacological interventions.

Cambridge Textbook of Effective Treatments in Psychiatry, ed. Peter Tyrer and Kenneth R. Silk. Published by Cambridge University Press.

In fact, there are so few randomized trials that no meta-analyses are found in the Cochrane database, although the database now includes a systematic review of the few trials conducted.

In the UK, the reclassification of cannabis into a class C drug has worried some that the reclassification would have people believe that it is less harmful than it was previously thought to be. This possible misconception is unfortunate because research has shown that an increased perception of the risks of cannabis is strongly correlated with decreased rates of use over time (Johnston *et al.*, 2003).

Cannabis dependence

Although cannabis was previously not thought to be addictive, over the past 20 years strong evidence from epidemiology, basic neurobiology, animal research, and human laboratory and clinical studies indicates that cannabis can and does lead to a dependence syndrome similar to that seen with other drugs of abuse (Budney & Moore, 2002; Swift *et al.*, 1998). Rates of cannabis dependence (based on the *Diagnostic and Statistical Manual of Mental Disorders* or the IDC) have been examined in the United States, Australia, and Germany. In the United States approximately 12 million individuals have, at some point in their lives, met diagnostic criteria for cannabis dependence (Anthony *et al.*, 1994; Kandel *et al.*, 1997; SAMHSA, 2004). When limited to only those who have ever used cannabis, the rate of dependence, either current or past, was 9% in the national US study and 8% in a study of German youth (Anthony *et al.*, 1994; von Sydow *et al.*, 2001). Similarly, 10% of individuals who admitted using cannabis in the year prior to being interviewed met current dependence criteria (Compton *et al.*, 2004). While these conditional probabilities are lower than other common drugs of abuse such as alcohol (15%), cocaine (17%), and heroin (23%), rates are similar to anxiolytics (9%) and other stimulants (11%) (Anthony *et al.*, 1994). In addition, dependence rates increase substantially with more frequent use from approximately 20% for individuals who report using cannabis at least five times in the past year (Swift *et al.*, 2001), to more than 70% for almost daily users (Coffey *et al.*, 2002). The percentage of people reporting chronic use and rates of initiation of use among youth and young adults have increased over the last decade (Gfroerer *et al.*, 2002), accompanied by a decreased perception of the risk of regular cannabis use by youth has decreased over this same time period (Johnston *et al.*, 2003).

Cannabis withdrawal

Although early studies of cannabis tetrahydrocannabinol (THC) withdrawal suggested that some symptoms were present (Compton *et al.*, 1990; Jones, Benowitz & Bachman, 1976), compared to the dramatic medical and physiological symptoms associated with severe opioid, sedative or alcohol withdrawal, cannabis withdrawal was considered to most likely have little clinical significance. However, during the 1980s, research on tobacco identified a reliable and clinically meaningful withdrawal syndrome with symptoms less dramatic than other drugs of abuse. In addition, the discovery of the endogenous cannabinoid system indicated that a neurobiological basis for cannabis dependence existed. As a result, research interest in examining the characteristics of cannabinoid withdrawal increased. During the past 10 years, a valid and reliable cannabinoid withdrawal syndrome has been documented.

Cannabinoid withdrawal is characterized by symptoms of anger or aggression, decreased appetite or weight loss, irritability, nervousness, restlessness, sleep difficulty, and less common symptoms of chills, depressed mood, stomach pain, shakiness, and sweating (Budney *et al.*, 2004; Haney *et al.*, 1999; Kouri & Pope, 2000). The nature and severity of the symptoms characteristic of cannabinoid withdrawal appear similar to those of nicotine withdrawal (Vandrey *et al.*, 2005). Of importance, cannabinoid withdrawal has been directly linked to the endogenous cannabinoid system, specifically the CB1 receptor, since withdrawal has been reliably precipitated using the selective CB1 receptor antagonist SR141716A in a variety of non-human species (Lichtman & Martin, 2002). In addition, recent inpatient and outpatient studies suggest that withdrawal is pharmacologically specific to the active component THC found in cannabis since oral THC has been shown to alleviate cannabis withdrawal symptoms (Haney *et al.*, 2004; Budney *et al.*, in press).

The reduction in dopamine (DA) activity in brain reward systems appears to be associated with similar characteristics of withdrawal for cannabis as it is with other drugs of abuse. Withdrawal from cocaine, opiates, amphetamines, nicotine, and alcohol results in reduction of DA activity in the same reward system and this reduction of DA activation appears to be a possible explanation of the chronic and persistent dysphoric symptoms of protracted withdrawal (Fung *et al.*, 1996; Gardner, 2002; George *et al.*, 1998; Hildebrand *et al.*, 1999; Parsons *et al.*, 1991; Rossetti *et al.*, 1992; Schaefer & Michael, 1986). Similarly, THC abstinence following chronic administration results in a reduction of DA activity in the ventral tegmental area (VTA; Diana *et al.*, 1998). Since cannabis withdrawal is predominately associated with mood changes such as irritability, nervousness, anger, and restlessness, these mood characteristics may be most associated with relapse (Koob *et al.*, 1997), possibly due to the importance of the role of DA in drug reinforcement.

Clinical studies

Cannabis dependence

Human studies indicate that cannabis dependence is associated with a number of consequences such as respiratory and other physical problems, cognitive impairments in memory, concentration, and motivation, as well as psychiatric comorbidity such as depression and social and interpersonal problems (Budney *et al.*, 2003a; Kalant *et al.*, 1999). Substance dependence is characterized by feelings of loss of control of substance use and continued use despite physiological, behavioural, and interpersonal consequences of use (American Psychiatric Association, 2000).

The severity and specificity of cannabis dependence has been documented in several studies. Clinical studies of cannabis dependent individuals seeking treatment have indicated that these patients generally have long histories of regular use (average more than 10 years), use cannabis on a daily basis, and have a range of psychosocial problems related to use (Budney *et al.*, 1998; Copeland *et al.*, 2001; Stephens *et al.*, 1993). The most commonly reported problems are feeling bad/guilty about their use, procrastination, low productivity, low self-confidence, interpersonal/family problems, memory problems, and financial difficulties. Importantly, cannabis-dependent individuals report repeated unsuccessful attempts to stop using and the perception that they are unable to quit. Further, approximately 50% to 70% of cannabis dependent users also use tobacco (Moore & Budney, 2001). Tobacco use is associated with additional risk of respiratory and other health problems (see also Chapter 23 and Moore *et al.*, 2005; Taylor *et al.*, 2000). In addition, among individuals seeking treatment for cannabis dependence, tobacco use is associated with increased psychosocial problems and poorer treatment response (Moore & Budney, 2001).

A study directly comparing cannabis dependent with cocaine-dependent outpatients demonstrated that the two groups exhibited similar types of problems, but the cannabis abusers generally showed a less severe dependence

syndrome (Budney *et al.*, 1998). Both groups met multiple DSM-III-R dependence criteria, although the cocaine group reported a significantly greater number. The groups did not differ on the Medical, Legal, Family/Social, or Psychiatric severity scales of the Addiction Severity Index, but the cocaine group scored higher on the Employment Severity Scale. The cocaine group also scored higher on the ASI Drug and Alcohol severity scales; this higher score reflects greater polydrug abuse in the cocaine treatment population. Both groups showed clinically significant elevations on standardized psychiatric symptom scales, but few between-group differences were observed. Demographic variables between the groups such as marital status, income and employment status also did not differ.

Although cannabis-dependent outpatients do not typically experience the acute crises or dramatic consequences that many times drive alcohol-, cocaine- or heroin-dependent individuals into treatment, they clearly show psychosocial impairment that warrants clinical attention. In summary, evidence for a cannabis dependence disorder is strong and indicative of a disorder of substantial severity.

Treatment for cannabis dependence

Given the consequences of cannabis dependence and recent increase in initiation and use in the United States, it is perhaps not surprising that the number of individuals who seek treatment for cannabis abuse at registered treatment agencies has doubled since the early 1990s (SAMSHA, 2002). Presentation for treatment where cannabis is the primary drug of abuse represents approximately 15% of all admissions in the USA, which is a similar proportion to that for heroin (18%) and cocaine (13%). Australia and Europe have also seen similar increases in individuals seeking treatment for cannabis abuse, with the rate doubling in Australia in a single year to 21% of all substance abuse admissions. This rate is second only to alcohol (Australian Institute of Health and Welfare, 2003; European Monitoring Centres for Drugs and Drug Addiction, 2003).

Behavioural interventions (see also Chapter 18)
Many of these are reviewed in the chapter on psychotherapies in this section. Behavioural interventions have demonstrated efficacy with cannabis abusing populations (Copeland, 2004; McRae *et al.*, 2003) (see Table 22.1). To date, only a small number of studies have been published with the first randomized controlled trial evaluating treatment for adult cannabis dependence not appearing until 1994 (Stephens *et al.*, 1994). In this initial trial, 212 individuals were randomly assigned to one of two programmes:

10-week group therapy, social support or cognitive-behavioural therapy (CBT) and relapse prevention (RP). The authors predicted that the CBT and RP would reduce cannabis use to a greater extent than the social support therapy. Although both conditions were associated with significant improvement in cannabis use over the course of treatment, no significant differences were observed between the treatments.

A second study by Stephens *et al.* (2000) was designed to enhance the CBT therapy by increasing the number of sessions as well as to evaluate a brief Motivational Interviewing intervention. Importantly, this study included a delayed treatment control (DTC) to verify whether either treatment was efficacious. Individuals seeking treatment for cannabis abuse ($n = 291$) were randomly assigned to an extended 14-session cognitive behavioural and relapse prevention group therapy, a brief two session motivational assessment and intervention conducted individually, or a 4-month DTC. Again, no differences were indicated between the two active treatments; however both treatments were found to be efficacious compared to the DTC.

McCambridge and Strang (2004) found that a single session of motivational interviewing decreased the frequency of cannabis use by 66% (from 15.4 times to 5.4 times per week), while the control group had a 27% increase in frequency. At 3 months, 16% of the intervention group, but only 5% of the controls, had discontinued cannabis use. The authors found that 'intention to stop' was a strong predictor of ultimate success. Those receiving the motivational interviewing intervention were 3.5 times more likely to make the decision to stop than controls.

Additional studies of cannabis dependence have compared brief interventions to longer treatments. In the first randomized clinical trial from Australia (Copeland *et al.*, 2001), 229 individuals seeking treatment for cannabis problems were randomized to a single-session CBT, a six-session CBT, or a DTC. Both treatments were found to be more effective than the DTC, and differences were observed between the two treatment conditions. Participants in the six-session treatment had greater reductions in cannabis use than those in the single session. This was the first study to indicate that more treatment led to decreased cannabis use.

Contingency Management (CM) interventions are designed to increase motivation to change substance use and to maintain abstinence. In one study, CM was examined as an addition to a three-session individual Motivational Enhancement Therapy (MET) (Sinha *et al.*, 2003). Sixty-five participants were randomly assigned to either MET alone or MET plus CM. A total of $120 USD in vouchers was contingent on therapy session attendance. Although MET-CM participants were more likely to attend all sessions compared to MET clients, there were no differences indicated in cannabis use or other drug use outcomes. However, the effectiveness of CM is dependent on the selection of therapeutic goal (Budney *et al.*, 2006). Although treatment attendance may improve by providing vouchers contingent upon coming to sessions, drug use might not change which was supported by this study (Iguchi *et al.*, 1997).

Budney *et al.* (2000) examined the addition of CM based in the context of individual cognitive-behavioural therapy. An important difference between this study and that by Sinha *et al.* (2003) was that vouchers were contingent on cannabis negative urine screens rather than session participation. Sixty participants were randomly assigned to one of three behaviourally based treatments: a 4-session MET, a 14-session CBT, and the 14-week CBT with the addition of the voucher-based CM. The findings indicated that the addition of a voucher-based incentive programme to behaviourally based therapies leads to substantially greater level of continuous documented abstinence (as indicated by twice weekly cannabis screens) than the behavioural therapies alone. No significant differences were indicated between the MET and CBT alone conditions, although all findings were in the direction of CBT. This study extends the efficacy of CM approaches with individuals who abuse drugs such as cocaine and heroin (Bickel *et al.*, 1997; Higgins *et al.*, 1994) to cannabis dependent individuals. Although the study had low power due to the small total number of participants ($n = 60$) and did not include post-treatment assessments, the findings were consistent with prior studies that found no significant differences between a brief motivational enhancement treatment and a more costly cognitive-behavioral treatment (Stephens *et al.*, 2000).

Results from a large multi-site trial comparing a 2-session MET therapy to a 9-session cognitive-behavioural treatment (CBT + MET) and a DTC were published (Babor *et al.*, 2004). Participants ($n = 450$) were randomly assigned to a treatment condition and were assessed during treatment and at 4, 9, and 15 months post-randomization. Similar to the findings by Copeland *et al.* (2001), the longer treatment was associated with reduced use and negative consequences compared to a 2-session MET, and MET was more effective than a delayed treatment control. An important issue with this study is that its size and multi-site nature substantially generalize findings across different ethnicities, geographic areas, and clinic types that cannabis-dependence can be effectively treated with psychosocial interventions.

Recently, a larger trial extended these findings (Budney *et al.*, 2006). Ninety cannabis dependent individuals were randomly assigned to CBT alone, CBT with voucher based CM, or voucher based CM alone in a similar 14-week treatment. Abstinence-based vouchers led to greater levels of continuous documented abstinence during treatment. CBT did not increase abstinence during treatment, but led to greater maintenance of abstinence following treatment compared to voucher based CM alone. While brief treatments are effective, more extensive and costly treatments can increase treatment response.

Overall, the findings indicate that the types of effective treatments are similar to those observed with other substances of abuse and the magnitude of effects compared to delayed treatment controls also appear similar (20%–40% abstinence during treatment vs. 5%–10% for delayed treatment controls). Similar types of interventions have demonstrated efficacy in clinical trials for alcohol, cocaine, and opiate dependence (Bickel *et al.*, 1997; Higgins *et al.*, 2000; Project Match Research Group, 1997). In particular, short interventions such as brief MET and CBT have demonstrated effectiveness with cannabis-dependence. While more extensive treatments (e.g. 12 and 14 week CBT or CM combined with CBT) have been shown to be more effective than these brief treatments, the optimal duration of such interventions to maximize cost effectiveness has not been determined.

Unfortunately, as with psychosocial treatments for other drugs of abuse, many individuals do not initiate abstinence during treatment, and many who do relapse to use either during or after treatment. Relapse rates associated with treatment of cannabis dependence also appear similar to other drugs of abuse (Moore & Budney, 2003). This indicates that cannabis dependence is not easily treated with the currently available psychosocial treatments alone and that there is substantial societal need for additional treatments to improve treatment outcome such as CM or pharmacological interventions. In addition, since cannabis-dependent individuals may be particularly unwilling to seek treatment at regular substance abuse clinics (Stephens & Roffman, 1994; Stephens *et al.*, 1993), efficacious pharmacological treatments for cannabis might greatly expand access and availability of treatment for cannabis dependence since pharmacological treatments could be provided by primary care medical practitioners outside of substance abuse treatment programmes.

Psychopharmacology
Because cannabis withdrawal may contribute to cannabis dependence and relapse, decreasing cannabis withdrawal

severity may aid cessation. Several studies have examined pharmacological interventions with agents such as nefazadone, naltrexone, bupropion, divalproex, and oral THC, in an attempt to reduce cannabis withdrawal symptoms among cannabis dependent participants who were not seeking treatment or planning to quit (Haney *et al.*, 2001a, 2001b, 2003a, 2003b, 2004). Nefazadone, a serotonin reuptake inhibitor and $5HT_2$ receptor antagonist used to treat depression and anxiety was predicted to decrease cannabis withdrawal (Haney *et al.*, 2003b). Withdrawal symptoms were studied in seven non-treatment seeking, heavy cannabis users in an inpatient setting. While nefazadone decreased ratings of anxiety and muscle pain, all other ratings of withdrawal symptoms (e.g. 'Irritable', 'Miserable' and 'Trouble Sleeping') remained high.

Similarly, Haney *et al.* (2001a) hypothesized that the dopamine reuptake blocking properties of bupropion would reduce cannabis-withdrawal severity in a 58-day double-blind placebo controlled trial with cannabis abusing individuals. Ten participants received placebo or active medication in their usual environment for 11 days to allow the medication to attain steady state. Then participants transferred to an inpatient setting where they smoked active cannabis for 4 days, followed by placebo cannabis for 13 days. Participants were then crossed over to the other dose of the active medication and the procedure was replicated. Rather than decreasing withdrawal symptoms, bupropion was found to increase ratings of irritability, depression, restlessness, and trouble sleeping. This may have been due to the stimulant properties of bupropion (West, 2003) or the influence of buproprion on other systems rather than its effect on DA activity in the mesolimbic pathways (Dong & Blier, 2001).

Because cannabis withdrawal includes symptoms of irritability and aggression it was hypothesized that divalproex sodium, an anticonvulsant which has been used to treat irritability, anger, and mood lability, would decrease withdrawal symptoms. In an inpatient laboratory study examining cannabis withdrawal, divalproex was found to decrease craving for cannabis, but ratings of anxiety, irritability, and tiredness, increased (Haney *et al.*, 2004). And recently, Haney *et al.* (2004) sought to determine if a THC agonist would be effective in reducing cannabis withdrawal similar to the role of methadone and buprenorphine in opiate dependence and nicotine for cigarette cessation. They examined the effect of 10 mg oral THC taken 5 times per day, again using a double-blind, cross-over design, inpatient study. Seven participants were followed for 15 days in two inpatient segments which included 4 baseline days of no use, 4 days of active smoked marijuana use, and 5 days of either oral THC or placebo. Oral THC was effective in reducing craving and suppressed ratings of anxiety, feeling miserable, trouble sleeping, and chills. In addition, participants could not distinguish active THC from placebo. Although these findings offer promise, all of these studies involved non-treatment seekers, included single doses, and followed individuals for only a brief period in an inpatient setting rather than the individual's home environment. A recently completed trial of oral THC in an outpatient setting showed similar promising findings (Budney *et al.*, 2007). Eight daily marijuana users received daily doses of either placebo or low dose (30 mg/tid) or high dose (90 mg/tid) THC alternating with 7–9 day periods of smoking cannabis as usual. Both doses of THC reduced withdrawal discomfort, with greater suppression of symptoms noted for the higher doses. These findings indicate that oral THC may be an effective pharmacological treatment for individuals seeking to quit using cannabis. However, additional outpatient clinical trials with individuals seeking treatment are needed.

Only one preliminary study in the published literature has examined a medication, divalproex, for reducing cannabis use in a 12-week outpatient placebo-controlled trial of 19 cannabis-dependent individuals (Levin *et al.*, 2004). Findings indicated no difference between active and placebo conditions in the double-blind, crossover design. Both conditions showed reductions in cannabis use over the course of treatment that also included weekly manualized relapse prevention therapy. Although two different studies (from the same group) have suggested that divalproex was ineffective in treating cannabis dependence, there are a number of other potentially effective medications. In addition to oral THC, such promising medications include other partial agonists, cannabinoid antagonists, medications that target protracted withdrawal and decreases in DA activity in the mesolimbic dopamine pathway, and medications that target comorbid disorders such as depression or anxiety. Future research and clinical findings will need to address issues such as appropriate doses, dose changes, length of medication treatment, tapering and withdrawal, and what type and what level of psychosocial treatments are need to maximize treatment response.

Alternative and other treatments
There is no evidence that acupuncture or hypnosis works in helping people cease use of cannabis. While psychodynamic psychotherapy and family therapy have been used

to treat cannabis dependence, there is little data available as to their effectiveness.

Summary and conclusions

Cannabis dependence is a substantial worldwide problem. Although consequences associated with cannabis dependence may not be as severe as consequences with some other drugs of abuse, there are more similarities than differences between cannabis dependence and dependence for other drugs of abuse. Demand for treatment services has continued to rise in the past decade, and increased rates of cannabis use in younger populations suggests that such demand will remain high. Of particular concern is the finding that the total number of individuals seeking treatment for cannabis dependence is still a small proportion of the estimated number of dependent individuals. This indicates a vastly underserved population. Unfortunately, there is little information on how and why cannabis-dependent individuals seek or do not seek treatment and the contexts in which treatment would be best served. Some research suggests that cannabis dependent individuals may be particularly unwilling to seek treatment at regular substance abuse clinics but may be more interested in either cannabis-specific programmes or settings where cannabis dependence is addressed individually and not included with all other drugs of abuse (Stephens & Roffman, 1994; Stephens *et al.*, 1993). Additionally, since many prominent organizations promote the use of cannabis (e.g. NORML) and argue that it is non-addictive, cannabis-dependent individuals may avoid treatment or may disregard the necessity of treatment.

Research suggests that psychosocial interventions such as cognitive-behavioural, motivational enhancement, relapse prevention, and contingency management, are effective in treating cannabis dependence and should be considered as first-line treatments. However, rates of abstinence initiation and relapse appear similar to other drugs of abuse, with few differences indicated between treatments indicating that there is substantial room for improvement. Where differences have been indicated, cognitive-behavioural therapy (nine sessions), and cognitive-behaviour therapy with contingency management have been shown to be most effective. Medications may help improve cannabis-dependence treatment, but there is no empirical data to support this contention as yet, and they should be considered second-line adjuncts to behavioural treatments, especially in cases of comorbid psychiatric disorders.

The level of evidence for each of the interventions discussed in this chapter is summarized in Table 22.1.

Table 22.1. Effectiveness of treatments for cannabis dependence

Treatment	Form of treatment	Psychiatric disorder/ target audience	Level of evidence for efficacy	Comments
Psychotherapy	Cognitive-behavioural therapy	Cannabis dependence	Ia	With or without motivational interviewing, treatment group improved to a greater degree than no treatment group. Longer treatment may lead to greater effectiveness
Psychotherapy	Motivational interviewing	Cannabis dependence	IIa	Subjects receiving motivational interviewing were 3.5 times more likely to make the decision to stop than controls
Psychotherapy	Cognitive-behavioural therapy with contingency management	Cannabis dependence	Ib	Voucher based incentive programme added to a behavioural treatment led to greater levels of increased abstinence
Psychotherapy	Motivation enhancement therapy	Cannabis dependence	Ib	Found to be more effective than waiting list controls. The longer the exposure to this treatment, the better the results
Psychopharmacology	THC	Cannabis dependence	IIb	THC effective in reducing craving and in lowering withdrawal symptoms
Psychopharmacology	Divalproex	Cannabis dependence	IIb	Evidence is conflicting. Can decrease craving, but anxiety, irritability, and fatigue increased

REFERENCES

American Psychiatric Association (2000). *Diagnostic and Statistical Manual of Mental Disorders.* IV-TR edn. Washington, DC: American Psychiatric Association.

Anthony, J. C., Warner, L. A. & Kessler, R. C. (1994). Comparative epidemiology of dependence on tobacco, alcohol, controlled substances and inhalants: basic findings from the National Comorbidity Survey. *Experimental and Clinical Psychopharmacology*, **2**, 244–68.

Australian Institute of Health and Welfare (2003). Alcohol and other drug treatment services in Australia: findings from the National Minimal Data Set 2001–02. Vol. 16 Bulletin No. 10, AIHW cat. no. AUS 40. 2003, Canberra: Australian Institure of Health and Welfare.

Babor, T., Carroll, K. M., Christiansen, K. *et al.* (2004). Brief treatments for cannabis dependence: findings from a randomized multi-site trial. *Journal of Consulting and Clinical Psychology*, **72**, 455–66.

Bickel, W. K., Amass, L., Higgins, S. T., Badger, G. J. & Esch, R. A. (1997). Effects of adding a behavioral treatment to opioid detoxification with buprenorphine. *Journal of Consulting and Clinical Psychology*, **65**, 803–10.

Budney, A. J. & Moore, B. A. (2002). Development and consequences of cannabis dependence. *Journal of Clinical Pharmacology*, **42**, 28S–33S.

Budney, A. J., Radonovich, K. J., Higgins, S. T. & Wong, C. J. (1998). Adults seeking treatment for marijuana dependence: a comparison to cocaine-dependent treatment seekers. *Experimental and Clinical Psychopharmacology*, **6**(4), 419–26.

Budney, A. J., Higgins, S. T., Radonovich, K. J. & Novy, P. L. (2000). Adding voucher-based incentives to coping-skills and motivational enhancement improves outcomes during treatment for marijuana dependence. *Journal of Consulting and Clinical Psychology*, **68**, 1051–61.

Budney, A. J., Moore, B. A. & Vandrey, R. (2003a). Health consequences of marijuana use. In *Medical Consequences of Drug Abuse*, ed. J. Brick, pp. 171–218. Haworth Press.

Budney, A. J., Moore, B. A., Vandrey, R. & Hughes, J. R. (2003b). The time course and significance of cannabis withdrawal. *Journal of Abnormal Psychology*, **112**(3), 393–402.

Budney, A. J., Moore, B. A., Rocha, H. & Higgins, S. T. (2006). Voucher-based incentives and behavior therapy for adult marijuana dependence. *Journal of Consulting and Clinical Psychology*, **74**, 307–16.

Budney, A. J., Sigmon, S. C. & Moore, B. A. (2006). Contingency-management interventions for cannabis dependence. In *Cannabis Dependence: Its Nature, Consequences, and Treatment*, ed. R. A. Roffman and R. S. Stephens. Cambridge, UK: Cambridge University Press.

Budney, A. J., Vandrey, R. G., Hughes, J. R., Moore, B. A. & Bahrenburg, (2007). Oral delta-9-tetrahydrocannabinol suppresses withdrawal symptoms. *Drug and Alcohol Dependence*, **86**, 22–9.

Budney, A. J., Hughes, J. R., Moore, B. A. & Vandrey, R. (2004). Review of the validity and significance of cannabis withdrawal syndrome. *American Journal of Psychiatry*, **161**(11), 1967–77.

Caan, W. & de Belleroche, J. (2002). *Drink, Drugs and Dependence.* Routledge.

Coffey, C. E., Carlin, J. B., Degenhardt, L. Lynskey, M. T., Sanci, L. & Patton, G. C. (2002). Cannabis dependence in young adults: an Australian population study. *Addiction*, **97**, 187–94.

Compton, D. R., Dewey, W. L. & Martin, B. R. (1990). Cannabis dependence and tolerance production. *Advances in Alcohol and Substance Abuse*, **9**, 129–47.

Compton, W. M., Grant, B. F., Colliver, J. D., Glantz, M. D. & Stinson, F. S. (2004). Prevalence of marijuana use disorders in the United States; 1991–1992 and 2001–2002. *Journal of the American Medical Association*, **291**, 2114–21.

Copeland, J. (2004). Developments in the treatment of cannabis use disorder. *Current Opinion in Psychiatry*, **17**(3), 161–8.

Copeland, J., Swift, W., Roffman, R. & Stephens, R. S. (2001). A randomized controlled trial of brief cognitive-behavioral interventions for cannabis use disorder. *Journal of Substance Abuse Treatment*, **21**, 55–64.

Diana, M., Melis, M., Muntoni, A. L. & Gessa, G. L. (1998). Mesolimbic dopaminergic decline after cannabinoid withdrawal. *Proceedings of the National Academy of Sciences, USA*, **95**, 10269–73.

Dong, J. & Blier, P. (2001). Modification of norepinephrine and serotonin, but not dopamine, neuron firing by sustained bupropion treatment. *Psychopharmacology*, **155**(1), 52–7.

European Monitoring Center for Drugs and Drug Addiction (2003). Annual report 2003: the state of the drugs problem in the acceding and candidate countries to the European Union. Luxembourg: Office of the Official Publications of the European Communities.

Fung, Y. K., Schmid, M. J., Anderson, T. M. & Lau, Y.-S. (1996). Effects of nicotine withdrawal on central dopaminergic systems. *Pharmacology Biochemistry and Behavior*, **53**, 635–40.

Gardner, E. L. (2002). Addictive potential of cannabinoids: The underlying neurobiology. *Chemistry and Physics of Lipids*, **121**, 267–90.

George, T. P., Verrico, C. D. & Roth, R. H. (1998). Effects of repeated nicotine pre-treatment on mesoprefontal dopaminergic and behavioral responses to acute footshock stress. *Brain Research*, **801**, 36–49.

Gfroerer, J. C., Wu, L.-T. & Penne, M. A. (2002). *Initiation of marijuana use: trends, patterns, and implications.* Analytic Series: A-17, DHHS Publication No. SMA 02-3711. Rockville, MD: SAMHSA.

Gledhill-Hoyt, J., Lee, H., Strote, J. & Wechsler, H. (2000). Increased use of marijuana and other illicit drugs at US colleges in the 1990s: results of three national surveys. *Addiction*, **95**, 1655–67.

Hall, W., Johnston, L. & Donnelly, N. (1999). Epidemiology of cannabis use and its consequences. In *The Health Effects of Cannabis*, ed. H. Kalant *et al.*, pp. 69–126. Toronto: Centre for Addiction and Mental Health.

Haney, M., Ward, A. S., Comer, S. D., Foltin, R. W. & Fischman, M. W. (1999). Abstinence symptoms following smoked marijuana in humans. *Psychopharmacology*, **14**, 395–404.

Haney, M., Ward, A. S., Comer, S. D., Hart, C. L., Foltin, R. W. & Fischman, M. W. (2001a). Bupropion SR worsens mood during marijuana withdrawal in humans. *Psychopharmacology*, **155**, 171–9.

Haney, M., Ward, A. S., Hart, C. L., Nasser, R. W., Foltin, R. W. & Fischman, M. W. (2001b). Effects of nefazadone on marijuana withdrawal in humans. *Drug and Alcohol Dependence*, **63**, S62.

Haney, M., Bisaga, A. & Foltin, R. W. (2003a). Interaction between naltrexone and oral THC in heavy marijuana smokers. *Psychopharmacology*, **166**, 77–85.

Haney, M., Hart, C. L., Ward, A. S. & Foltin, R. W. (2003b). Nefazodone decreases anxiety during marijuana withdrawal in humans. *Psychopharmacology*, **165**, 157–65.

Haney, M., Hart, C. L., Vosburg, S. K. *et al.*, (2004). Marijuana withdrawal in humans: effects of oral THC or Divalproex. *Neuropsychopharmacology*, **29**, 158–70.

Higgins, S. T., Badger, G. J. & Budney, A. J. (2000). Predictors of abstinence and relapse in behavioral treatments for cocaine dependence. *Experimental and Clinical Psychopharmacology*, **8**, 377–86.

Higgins, S. T., Budney, A. J., Bickel, W. K., Foerg, F., Donham, R. & Badger, G. (1994). Incentives improve outcome in outpatient behavioral treatment of cocaine dependence. *Archives of General Psychiatry*, **51**, 568–76.

Hildebrand, B. E., Panagis, G., Svennson, T. H. & Nomikos, G. G., (1999). Behavioral and biochemical manifestations of mecamylamine-precipitated nicotine withdrawal in the rat: role of nicotinic receptors in the ventral tegmental area. *Neuropsychopharmacology*, **21**, 560–74.

Iguchi, M. Y., Belding, M. A., Morral, A. R., Lamb, R. J. & Husband, S. D. (1997). Reinforcement operants other than abstinence in drug abuse treatment: an effective alternative for reducing drug use. *Journal of Consulting and Clinical Psychology*, **65**(3), 421–8.

Johnston, L. D., O'Malley, P. M. & Bachman, J. G. (2002). *Monitoring the future national survey results on adolescent drug use: overview of key findings*, (NIH Publication No. 03-5374). 2003, Bethesda, MD: National Institute on Drug Abuse. 56.

Jones, R. T., Benowitz, N. & Bachman, J. (1976). Clinical studies of cannabis tolerance and dependence. *Annals New York Academy of Sciences*, **282**, 221–39.

Kalant, H., Corrigall, W. A., Hall, W. & Smart, R. G. (eds.). (1999). *The Health Effects of Cannabis*. Toronto: Centre for Addiction and Mental Health.

Kandel, D., Chen, K., Warner, L. A., Kessler, R. C. & Grant, B. (1997). Prevalence and demographic correlates of last year dependence on alcohol, nicotine, marijuana and cocaine in the U.S. population. *Drug Alcohol Dependency*, **44**, 11–29.

Koob, G. F., Caine, S. B., Parsons, L., Markou, A. & Weiss, F. (1997). Opponent process model and psychostimulant addiction. *Pharmacology, Biochemistry, and Behavior*, **57**, 513–21.

Kouri, E. M. & Pope H. G. (2000). Abstinence symptoms during withdrawal from chronic marijuana use. *Experimental and Clinical Psychopharmacology*, **8**(4), 483–92.

Levin, F. R., McDowell, D., Evans, S. M. *et al.* (2004). Pharmacotherapy for marijuana dependence: a double-blind, placebo-controlled pilot study of divalproex sodium. *American Journal on Addictions*, **13**, 21–32.

Lichtman, A. H. & Martin, B. R. (2002). Marijuana withdrawal syndrome in the animal model. *Journal of Clinical Pharmacology*, **42**, 20S–27S.

McCambridge, J. & Strang, J. (2004). The efficacy of single-session motivational interviewing in reducing drug consumption and perceptions of drug-related risk and harm among young people: results from a multi-site cluster randomized trial. *Addiction*, **99**(1), 39–52.

McRae, A. L., Budney, A. J. & Brady, K. T. (2003). Treatment of marijuana dependence: a review of the literature. *Journal of Substance Abuse Treatment*, **24**, 369–76.

Moore, B. A. & Budney, A. J. (2001), Tobacco smoking in marijuana dependent outpatients. *Journal of Substance Abuse*, **13**, 585–98.

Moore, B. A. & Budney, A. J. (2003). Relapse in outpatient treatment for marijuana dependence. *Journal of Substance Abuse Treatment*, **25**, 85–9.

Moore, B. A., Augustson, E. M., Moser, R. P. & Budney, A. J. (2005). Respiratory effects of marijuana and tobacco use in a U.S. sample. *Journal of General Internal Medicine*, **20**(1), 33–7.

Parsons, L. H., Smith, A. D. & Justice, J. B. Jr (1991). Basal extracellular dopamine is decreased in the rat nucleus accumbens during abstinence from chronic cocaine. *Synapse*, **9**, 60–5.

Project Match Research Group (1997). Matching alcoholism treatments to client heterogeneity: project MATCH posttreatment drinking outcomes. *Journal of Studies on Alcohol*, **22**, 7–29.

Rossetti, Z. L., Hmaidan, Y. & Gessa, G. L. (1992). Marked inhibition of mesolimbic dopamine release: a common feature of ethanol, morphine, cocaine, and amphetamine abstinence in rats. *European Journal of Pharmacology*, **221**, 227–34.

SAMHSA, National Survey On Drug Use And Health (2002). [Computer file]. 2nd ICPSR version. 2004, Research Triangle Institute [producer]. Ann Arbor, MI: Inter-university Consortium for Political and Social Research [distributor]: Research Triangle Park, NC.

Schaefer, G. J. & Michael, R. P. (1986). Changes in response rates and reinforcement thresholds for intracranial self-stimulation during morphine withdrawal. *Pharmacology, Biochemistry and Behavior*, **25**, 1263–9.

Sinha, R., Easton, C., Renee-Aubin, L. & Carroll, K. M. (2003). Engaging young probation-referred marijuana-abusing individuals in treatment: a pilot trial. *American Journal on Addictions*, **12**, 314–23.

Stephens, R. S. & Roffman, R. A. (1994). Adult marijuana dependence. In *Addictive Behaviors Across the Lifespan: Prevention, Treatment, and Policy Issues*, ed. J. S. Baer & R. J. McMahon, pp. 243–73. Newbury Park, CA: Sage Publications.

Stephens, R. S., Roffman, R. A. & Simpson, E. E. (1993). Adult marijuana users seeking treatment. *Journal of Consulting and Clinical Psychology*, **61**, 1100–4.

Stephens, R. S., Roffman, R. A. & Simpson, E. E. (1994). Treating adult marijuana dependence: a test of the relapse prevention model. *Journal of Consulting and Clinical Psychology*, **62**, 92–9.

Stephens, R. S., Roffman, R. A. & Curtin, L. (2000). Comparison of extended versus brief treatments for marijuana use. *Journal of Consulting and Clinical Psychology*, **68**, 898–908.

Swift, W., Hall, W., Didcott, P. & Reilly, D. (1998). Patterns and correlates of cannabis dependence among long-term users in an Australian rural area. *Addiction*, **93**(8), 1149–60.

Swift, W., Hall, W. & Teesson, M. (2001). Cannabis use and dependence among Australian adults: results from the National Survey of Mental Health and Wellbeing. *Addiction*, **96**, 737–48.

Taylor, D. R., Poulton, R., Moffitt, T. E., Ramankutty, P. & Sears, M. R. (2000). The respiratory effects of cannabis dependence in young adults. *Addiction*, **95**(11), 1669–77.

World Health Organization (1997). *Cannabis: A Health Perspective and Research Agenda*. Geneva: WHO.

Vandrey, R. G., Budney, A. J., Moore, B. A. & Hughes, J. R. (2005). A cross-study comparison of cannabis and tobacco withdrawal. *American Journal on Addictions*, **14**(1), 54–63.

von Sydow, K., Lieb, R., Pfister, H., Hofler, M., Sonntag, H. & Wittchen, H. (2001). The natural course of cannabis use, abuse and dependence over four years: a longitudinal community study of adolescents and young adults. *Drug and Alcohol Dependence*, **64**, 347–61.

West, R. (2003). Bupropion SR for smoking cessation. *Expert Opinion on Pharmacotherapy*, **4**, 533–40.

23

Treatment of nicotine dependence

Andrea H. Weinberger, Pamela Walters, Taryn M. Allen, Melissa
M. Dudas, Kristi A. Sacco and Tony P. George

Editor's note

Nicotine dependence is found in at least a billion people worldwide and in millions in the United States and Great Britain. It is a major cause of morbidity and mortality in all countries, and both active smoking and exposure to passive smoke has significant health care consequences. There currently are public health campaigns in both the UK and USA to combat smoking, and laws against smoking in public places are just one, if not one of the most visible, of the various public and community campaigns against smoking. While these campaigns are effective, most smokers wishing to quit will utilize pharmacological treatments which involve primarily nicotine replacement therapy (NRT) or the use of bupropion. Both have substantial evidence as to effectiveness, though there are other secondary pharmacological treatments that also are beginning to find some support such as vareniciline, clonidine and nortriptyline. The NRTs come in various forms from patches to nasal sprays to gum, inhalers, and lozenges. All have substantial support for their effectiveness. Cognitive-behavioural therapies, especially multimodal interventions that are tailored to the specific patient, have a good deal of success and support for that success as well. Despite these effective interventions, smoking remains a major public health problem.

Introduction

Cigarette smoking is the single largest preventable cause of substantial morbidity and mortality in developed countries. In the United States, approximately 23% of the general population reports cigarette smoking, which is the most common (> 98%) method of tobacco use (Center for Disease Control (CDC), 2002; Giovino, 2002). Approximately 430 000 people

in the USA die each year as a result of smoking-attributable medical illnesses such as lung cancer, chronic obstructive pulmonary disease, cardiovascular disease and stroke (Giovino, 2002). It is estimated that 29% of adults in the United Kingdom smoke (Lader & Meltzer, 2000). This equates to approximately 16 million British smokers. Worldwide, it is estimated that approximately 1.1 billion people use tobacco on a regular basis (CDC, 2002).

In the UK, the proportions of men and women who currently smoke are similar. Over the past 5 years the overall proportion of smokers in the UK population has stabilized, although in some groups, such as adolescents, there has been an increase. It is thought around 25% of 15-year-olds are regular smokers (NICE, 2002; Lader & Meltzer, 2000). As a result of the implementation of tobacco control policies in the USA (e.g. tobacco excise taxes, advertising health dangers), the prevalence of cigarette smoking was reduced from 45% in the 1960s to about 22.9% in 2002 (CDC, 2002). However, it appears that many of these remaining smokers have more difficulty quitting smoking, and today's smoker has often failed multiple quit attempts despite using behavioural therapies combined with pharmacological interventions such as nicotine replacement therapies (NRTs) and sustained-release bupropion. In fact, quit rates with NRTs over the past 15 years in controlled clinical trials appear to be declining (Irvin et al., 2003). The remaining population of smokers has characteristics associated with smoking persistence and quit attempt failures such as lower education attainment, less interest in behavioural treatments to assist with cessation, and medical, substance abuse and psychiatric co-morbidities (Hughes, 1996b). In addition, women are smoking at higher rates than in the past, may have more intense nicotine withdrawal and depressed mood during quit attempts than men (Gritz et al., 1996), and may be less responsive to quitting with NRTs (Perkins et al., 1999).

Cambridge Textbook of Effective Treatments in Psychiatry, ed. Peter Tyrer and Kenneth R. Silk. Published by Cambridge University Press.
© Cambridge University Press, 2008.

Smokers who have failed initial quit attempts generally embrace pharmacotherapies, and given that a large proportion of remaining smokers do not respond to conventional pharmacotherapies, the development of novel and more effective medication treatment for smoking cessation is critical in our efforts to treat nicotine dependence. Recent advances in our understanding of nicotine's effects on central neurotransmitter systems are guiding basic and clinical pharmacologists to develop medications for new pharmacological targets to treat nicotine dependence.

The hazards of smoking are important and well established. Smokers have a larger number of chronic respiratory diseases and have a substantially higher risk of cancers and cardiovascular disease. They are twice as likely as non-smokers to suffer from fatal ischemic heart disease and four times as likely to suffer a fatal aortic aneurysm (Parrott *et al.*, 1998). The National Institute for Clinical Excellence (NICE) has estimated that treatment for smoking related disease cost the National Health Service (UK) around £1.5 billion (Edwards, 2004).

Nicotine addiction is closely linked to socio-economic disadvantage. Smoking prevalence is higher and nicotine use heavier amongst poorer smokers. The socio-economic gradient in smoking behaviour accounts for about two-thirds of the excess premature mortality associated with deprivation.

Smoking is now increasing rapidly throughout the developing world, and it is estimated that current cigarette smoking will cause about 450 million deaths worldwide in the next 50 years. Reducing current smoking by 50% would prevent 20–30 million premature deaths in the first quarter of this century and 150 million in the second quarter (Doll *et al.*, 1994). For most smokers, quitting is the single most important thing they can do to improve their health.

Clinical features of nicotine dependence

Most tobacco users (> 98%) are smokers of cigarettes, and while there are a subset of cigarette smokers who do not smoke every day, most cigarette smokers are daily users and have some degree of physiological dependence on nicotine (Rigotti, 2002). Determination of nicotine dependence is typically accomplished clinically by historical documentation of daily smoking (typically 10–40 cigarettes per day) for several weeks, evidence of tolerance (e.g. lack of aversive effects of nicotine such as nausea and excessive stimulation) and the presence of symptoms of nicotine withdrawal upon smoking cessation. These withdrawal symptoms include dysphoria, anxiety, irritability, decreased heart rate, insomnia (waking in the middle of the night), increased appetite and craving for cigarettes (American Psychiatric Association, 2006). In addition, most dependent smokers state that they smoke their first cigarette of the day within thirty minutes of awakening. Scales such as the Fagerstrom Test for Nicotine Dependence (FTND) allow assessment of the level of nicotine dependence with scores of ≥ 4 on a scale of 0–10 consistent with physiological dependence to nicotine. These scales have been empirically validated (Heatherton *et al.*, 1991).

Interestingly, the positive effects of cigarette smoking (e.g. taste, satisfaction) appear to be mediated by non-nicotine components of tobacco such as tar (Dallery *et al.*, 2003). Besides positive reinforcement, withdrawal and craving, there are several secondary effects of nicotine and tobacco use that may contribute to both maintenance of smoking and to smoking relapse including mood modulation (e.g. reduction of negative affect), stress reduction, and weight control. In addition, conditioned cues can elicit the urge to smoke even after prolonged periods of abstinence. Specific effects might be most relevant to individuals high on dietary restraint (weight reduction), and psychiatric disorders (mood modulation, stress reduction) (Fig. 23.1). These secondary effects may present additional targets for pharmacological intervention in certain subgroups of smokers (e.g. schizophrenic, depressed, or overweight smokers).

National guidelines

There are clinical practice guidelines available in both the USA and UK. The US Public Health Service published the monograph *Treating Tobacco Use and Dependence* in 2000 (Fiore *et al.*, 2000), and the American Psychiatric Association recently updated its Practice Guidelines for the treatment of nicotine dependence (APA, 2006). In the UK, a series of guidelines and key documents were published in the late nineties. The paper 'Smoking kills' (DOH 98) outlined the government's plan of action to stop people from smoking. This plan included proposals for abolishing tobacco advertising and promotion. It also looked at ways of altering public attitudes, preventing tobacco smuggling and supporting further research into this important area of public health. Partnerships with other agencies such as businesses were pivotal in order to start the restriction of smoking in public places.

The Royal College of Physicians published smoking cessation guidelines in 1998 which were updated in 2000 (West *et al.*, 2000). Expert committees such as the Cochrane

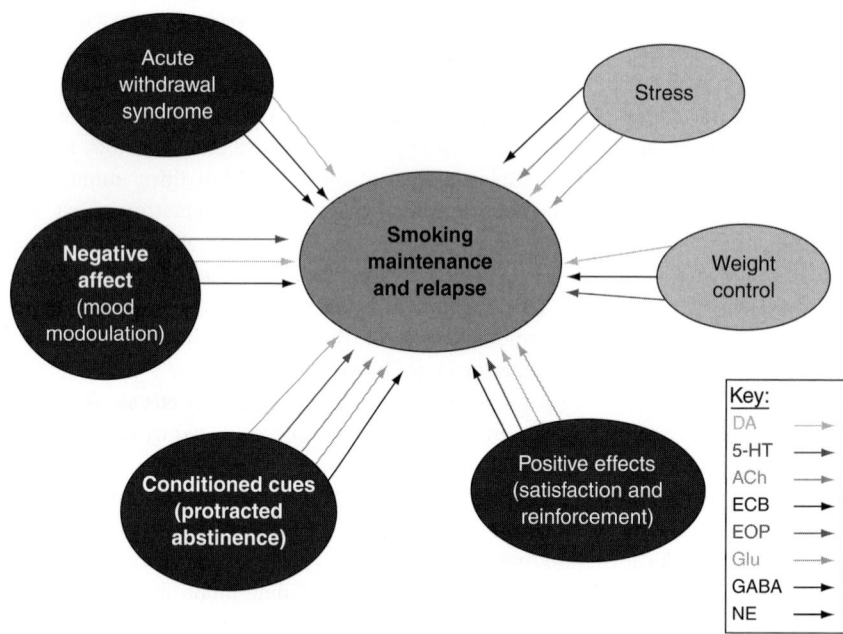

Fig. 23.1. Environmental, state, and trait factors and neurotransmitter systems that mediate smoking maintenance and relapse. The dark blue circles indicate primary contributors while the light blue circles indicate secondary contributors to smoking maintenance and relapse. Abbreviations: DA = dopamine; 5-HT = 5-hydroxytryptamine; Ach = acetylcholine (nitoinic Ach receptor); ECB = endocannabinoid (CB₁ receptor); EOP = endogenous opioid peptide; Glu = glutamate; NE = noradrenaline.

Tobacco Addiction review group were set up to operate in much the same manner as its American equivalent, The Agency for Health Care Policy Research.

As a direct result of the change in priority given to the management of smoking, smoking cessation services were launched in a variety of health action zones throughout England and Wales in 1999–2000. In the 3 years up to and including 2001–2002, £53 million was made available for these services with further substantial amounts earmarked for the years 2003–2006, £41 million, £46 million and £51 million, respectively. Quarterly reports are fed back to the government by these services so that progress towards specified targets can be audited. The government's guidance on management of smoking cessation is implemented through The National Institute for Health and Clinical Excellence (NICE). This organization is part of The National Health Service (NHS) and its role is to provide guidance for both the NHS and patients on medicines, medical equipment, and diagnostic tests. It was specifically asked to review the available evidence on nicotine replacement therapy (NRT) and bupropion and provide guidance that would inform the NHS about effective evidence-based treatments for smoking cessation.

Before we proceed to examine the treatments for smoking, a quick glance at these official guidelines suggests the manner and context in which, in the UK, smoking cessation treatment should take place. Nicotine replacement therapy or bupropion should normally only be prescribed as part of an abstinent contingent treatment (ACT) programme in which the smoker makes a commitment to stop smoking. Smokers should be offered advice and encouragement to aid their attempt to quit. Ideally, initial prescription of NRT or bupropion should be sufficient to last only until 2 weeks after the target stop date. Normally, this will be after 2 weeks of NRT and 3–4 weeks for bupropion to allow for the different methods of administration and mode of action. Second prescriptions should be given only to people who have demonstrated that their quit attempt is continuing on reassessment. If a smoker's attempt to quit is unsuccessful with treatment using either NRT or bupropion, the NHS should normally fund no further attempts within 6 months. It is thought that there is insufficient evidence to recommend a combination of bupropion and NRT (see below).

It is recommended that smokers who are under the age of 18 years, who are pregnant or breastfeeding, or who have unstable cardiovascular disorders should consult a health care professional before either treatment is prescribed. Bupropion is not recommended for smokers under the age of 18 years as its safety and efficacy have not been evaluated for this group. Women who are pregnant or breastfeeding should not use bupropion.

Evidence-based treatments for nicotine dependence

Stepped care approaches

Since the majority of smokers quit on their own or with minimal treatment (Fiore *et al.*, 1990), most existing algorithms/guidelines rely on a stepped care approach with minimal interventions early on and more intensive interventions for those who are not able to stop with minimal interventions (Fiore *et al.*, 2002; Hughes, 1994b; Rigotti, 2002). There are three issues to consider with this approach: (a) most smokers who quit on their own require several attempts before they succeed (Rigotti, 2002); thus, any success later in the algorithm cannot be attributed to the specific treatment being given at that point; (b) early cessation of smoking can prevent much of the devastating medical consequences of smoking (Bartecchi *et al.*, 1994); thus, delaying delivering a treatment known to be effective could allow a serious, irreversible consequence of smoking (e.g., an acute myocardial infarction, lung cancer) to occur; (c) the notion that most smokers can quit on their own or will need only minimal treatment is based on research on smokers without a history of psychiatric problems (Rigotti, 2002). Smokers with psychiatric problems appear to be 2–3 times less likely to successfully stop smoking than smokers without psychiatric problems (Glassman, 1993; Lasser *et al.*, 2000; McChargue *et al.*, 2001). Thus, psychiatric patients require more intensive interventions earlier on and there is some evidence that such higher intensity interventions can lead to better cessation outcomes (Addington *et al.*, 1998; Evins *et al.*, 2001; George *et al.*, 2000, 2002; Hughes & Francis, 1995).

In considering smoking cessation treatment, a number of variables should be taken into consideration. The motivation and intention to quit should be assessed. The availability of support and counseling should be considered, though there is little data to support that the presence of these significantly impact success rates. The previous attempts to stop smoker and the method(s) used in those attempts should be considered. Then the preferences of the smoker as to the type of quit aid as well as the possible side effects of the particular method and, of course, any contraindications of that method for the smoker, should be taken into account.

Medication treatments

Pharmacotherapies for nicotine dependence can be divided into nicotine replacement therapy and non-nicotine medications that mimic or antagonize nicotine/smoking effects. Non-medication somatic therapies include acupuncture and devices. The following are brief descriptions of these therapies in terms of goals of treatment, efficacy in smoking cessation, side effects and implementation issues.

Nicotine replacement therapies (NRTs)

The goal of nicotine replacement therapy is to relieve withdrawal. Relief of withdrawal will allow the patient to focus on habit and conditioning factors when attempting to stop smoking. After the acute withdrawal period, nicotine replacement therapy is gradually reduced so that little withdrawal should occur. NRTs rely on systemic venous absorption and so do not produce the rapid high levels of arterial nicotine achieved when cigarette smoke is inhaled. Thus individuals are less likely to become addicted to NRTs. Nicotine replacement therapies should be discontinued if the person restarts smoking.

Nicotine gum

Nicotine ingested through the gastrointestinal tract is extensively metabolized on first pass through the liver (Benowitz, 1988). Nicotine gum (nicotine polacrilex) avoids this problem via buccal absorption (Benowitz, 1988). The gum contains 2 or 4 mg of nicotine that can be released from a resin by chewing (Hughes, 1996b). The original recommendation was to use one piece of 2-mg gum every 15–30 minutes as needed for craving. More recent work suggests scheduled dosing (e.g. 1 piece of 2 mg gum/ hour), and use of 4 mg gum for highly nicotine-dependent smokers is more effective (Sachs, 1991). The original recommended duration of treatment was 3 months, though many experts believe longer treatment is more effective. However, the two trials of longer duration produced contradictory results (Hughes, 1991).

Nicotine absorption from the gum peaks 30 minutes after beginning to use the gum. Venous nicotine levels from 2- and 4-mg gum are about one-third and two-thirds, respectively, of the steady-state (i.e. between cigarettes) levels of nicotine achieved with cigarette smoking (Benowitz, 1988). Nicotine via cigarettes is absorbed directly into the arterial circulation; thus arterial levels from smoking are 5–10 times higher than those from the 2- and 4-mg gums (Henningfield *et al.*, 1993). Absorption of nicotine in the buccal mucosa is decreased by an acidic environment, and patients should not use beverages (e.g. coffee, soda, juice) immediately before, during, or after nicotine gum use (Henningfield *et al.*, 1993). Nicotine gum (2- and 4-mg doses) was approved as an over-the-counter (OTC) medication in the UK in 1991 and in the USA in 1996.

Significant side effects from nicotine gum are rare, and seldom deter use (Hughes, 1993). Minor side effects are of mechanical origin (e.g. difficulty chewing, sore jaw) or of local pharmacological origin (e.g. burning in mouth, throat irritation). Tolerance develops to most side effects over the first week, and education about proper use of the gum (e.g. do not chew too vigorously) decreases side effects (Hughes, 1993). Originally, some disorders were listed as contraindications to use of nicotine gum (e.g. cardiovascular disease, pregnancy, hypertension), but given that nicotine blood levels are much lower with nicotine gum than with cigarettes, these contraindications have been dropped (Benowitz, 1988; Hughes, 1993).

One potential long-term concern with the chronic use of nicotine gum is the continuance of nicotine dependence (Hughes, 1989). While abrupt cessation of nicotine gum can produce withdrawal symptoms similar to, but less intensive than, those from cigarettes, gradual reduction in the use of nicotine gum usually produces no or very minor symptoms (Hughes, 1989). About 5–20% of those who stop smoking with the help of nicotine gum continue to use nicotine gum for 9 months or more, but few use the gum longer than 2 years (Hughes, 1991). In fact, West *et al.* (2000) have conducted a study on continued use of nicotine gum and other forms of NRTs after cessation, and only 7% of smokers continued to use nicotine gum after a cessation attempt compared to 2% with patch and 10% for both nasal spray and inhaler. Thus, the abuse liability of nicotine gum appears to be minimal.

Several placebo-controlled trials established the safety and efficacy of nicotine gum for smoking cessation, and these are reviewed by Balfour and Fagerstrom (1996). There appears to be some evidence from randomized controlled trials to support using higher doses of nicotine gum (4 mg pieces) in more highly dependent cigarette smokers (Garvey *et al.*, 2000; Glover *et al.*, 1996; Herrera *et al.*, 1995; Sachs, 1995), which upholds the idea of matching nicotine gum dose to dependence level of the smoker. This appears to be independent of the intensity of behavioural therapy support, though this needs further study.

The combination of nicotine gum with nicotine patch is often used clinically to manage the treatment-resistant heavy smoker. A trial by Kornitzer *et al.* (1995) in 374 nicotine dependent cigarette smokers suggested that the combination of nicotine gum (2 mg) with patch (15 mg/day) was superior to patch alone with placebo gum, and to placebo gum and placebo at both the end of the 12-week trial (34.2 vs. 22.7 vs. 17.3%) and at the one-year follow-up (18.1 vs. 12.7 vs. 13.3%). There is some preliminary evidence that nicotine gum may have comparable efficacy for smoking cessation in smokers with a positive history of Major depressive disorder (MDD) vs.

those without such a history when combined with various levels of behavioural support (Hall *et al.*, 1996).

Transdermal nicotine patch

The four transdermal formulations take advantage of ready absorption of nicotine across the skin (Palmer & Faulds, 1992; Silagy *et al.*, 1994). Three of the patches are for 24-hour use and one is for 16-hour (waking) use. Starting doses are 21–22 mg/24-hour patch and 15 mg/16-hour patch. Patches are applied daily each morning beginning upon cessation of smoking. Nicotine via patches is slowly absorbed so that on the first day venous nicotine levels peak 6–10 hours after administration. Thereafter, nicotine levels remain fairly steady with a decline from peak to trough of 25% to 40% with 24-hour patches. Nicotine levels obtained with the use of patches are typically half those obtained by smoking (Palmer & Faulds, 1992). After 4–6 weeks patients are usually tapered to a middle dose (e.g. 14 mg/24 hours or 10 mg/16 hours) and then to the lowest dose after 2–4 more weeks (7 mg/24 hours or 5 mg/16 hours). Most, but not all, studies indicate abrupt cessation of the use of patches often causes no significant withdrawal; thus, tapering may not be necessary (Fiore *et al.*, 1994). The recommended total duration of treatment is usually 6–12 weeks (Fiore *et al.*, 1994; Silagy *et al.*, 1994). Two nicotine patches are now available over the counter with one brand at 21, 14 and 7 mg strength over 24-hour application and the other brand at 22 and 11 mg strength for a 16 hour application.

Significant adverse events with nicotine patches have not been found (Benowitz, 1988; Fiore *et al.*, 1992; Hughes, 1993; Silagy *et al.*, 1994). The most common minor side effects are skin reactions (50%), insomnia and increased or vivid dreams (15% with 24-hour patches), and nausea (5–10%) (Fiore *et al.*, 1992; Hughes, 1993; Silagy *et al.*, 1994). Tolerance to these side effects usually develops within a week. Rotation of patch sites decreases skin irritation. Although debatable, insomnia reported in the first week post-cessation appears to be mostly due to nicotine withdrawal rather than the nicotine patch itself (Wetter *et al.*, 1995). A 24-hour patch can be removed before bedtime to determine if the insomnia is due to the nicotine patch. Without treatment, insomnia usually abates after 4–7 days. Although one series of case reports suggested concomitant use of cigarettes and nicotine patches caused myocardial infarction, later analyses and prospective empirical studies in smokers with active heart disease indicated this prior report was incorrect. Abrupt cessation of the nicotine patch does not produce significant withdrawal symptoms, and long-term use has not been a problem (Fiore *et al.*, 1992). There appears to be little dependence liability associated with patch use as only 2% of patch users continue to use this product for extended period after a cessation trial (West *et al.*, 2000).

The overall efficacy of the nicotine transdermal patch (NTP) for smoking cessation has been well documented. A meta-analysis of 17 RCTs in 1994 (Fiore *et al.*, 1994) reported end of treatment abstinence rates for NTP of 27% vs. 13% for placebo patch (OR 2.6) and 22% vs. 9% at 6-month follow-up (OR 3.0). The effects of active NTP were independent of patch type, treatment duration, tapering procedures and behavioural therapy format or intensity, though it should be noted that behavioural treatment enhanced outcomes with patch compared to patch alone. NTP continued to show much more effectiveness than placebo when measured by continuous or prolonged abstinence at 1 year (Richmond, 1997).

Nicotine nasal spray

Nicotine nasal spray is a nicotine solution in a nasal spray bottle similar to those used with saline sprays and antihistamines (Fiore *et al.*, 1994; Perkins *et al.*, 1992; Schneider *et al.*, 1995). This treatment was approved by the FDA for treatment of nicotine dependence in the United States in 1996. Nasal sprays produce droplets that average about 1 mg nicotine per administration, and the patient administers the spray to each nostril every 4–6 hours (spray solutions are dispensed at 10 mg/ml). This formulation produces a more rapid rise in nicotine levels than does nicotine gum, and the rise in nicotine levels produced by nicotine spray falls between the levels produced by nicotine gum and cigarettes. Peak nicotine levels occur within 10 minutes, and venous nicotine levels are about two-thirds those of between-cigarette levels (Sutherland *et al.*, 1992). Smokers are instructed to use the nasal spray ad lib up to 30 times/day for 12 weeks, including a tapering period.

The major side effects from nicotine nasal spray are nasal and throat irritation, rhinitis, sneezing, coughing, and watering eyes (Hjalmarson *et al.*, 1994; Schneider *et al.*, 1995; Sutherland *et al.*, 1992). One or more of these side effects occur in over three-quarters of the patients. Long-term nasal problems from use of nicotine nasal spray is usually not a problem (Sutherland *et al.*, 1992). Nicotine nasal spray may have some dependence liability as indicated by the fact that in some studies several patients who quit smoking with nicotine nasal spray continued to use it for long periods (Perkins *et al.*, 1992; Sutherland *et al.*, 1992). In a controlled study by West *et al.* (2000), this prolonged use of nasal spray was determined to be the case in 10% of smokers using the nasal spray. A human laboratory study (Perkins *et al.*, 1997) suggested that nicotine nasal spray has modest reinforcing effects, so follow-up of smokers using nasal spray is recommended. Whether abrupt cessation of nasal spray produces withdrawal has not been studied.

Two randomized, double-blind, placebo-controlled trials of nasal spray versus placebo spray (Blondal *et al.*, 1997; Schneider *et al.*, 1995) have established the safety and efficacy of the nasal spray for smoking cessation. Both trials employed treatment for 3–6 months, and active nasal spray lead to a doubling of quit rates during active use. Differences were reduced or absent with extended follow-up suggesting the need for maintenance use of this agent. However, such long-term studies to date have not been published. The usefulness of combining nasal spray with patch, gum and bupropion has not been studied.

Nicotine vapour inhalers (NVI)

NVI are cartridges (plugs) of nicotine (containing about 1 mg of nicotine each) placed inside hollow cigarette-like plastic rods. The cartridges produce a nicotine vapour when warm air is passed through them (Rose & Behm, 1987; Tonnesen *et al.*, 1993). Absorption from nicotine inhaler is primarily buccal rather than respiratory (Russell *et al.*, 1987). More recent versions of inhalers produce a rise in venous nicotine levels more quickly than with nicotine gum but less quickly than with nicotine nasal spray, with nicotine blood levels of about one-third that of between-cigarette levels (Sutherland *et al.*, 1993). Smokers are instructed to puff continuously on the inhaler (0.013 mg/puff) during the day, and recommended dosing is 6–16 cartridges daily. The inhaler is to be used ad lib for about 12 weeks.

No serious medical side effects have been reported with nicotine inhalers (Leischow, 1994). About half of subjects report throat irritation or coughing (Tonnesen *et al.*, 1993). The controlled study by West *et al.* (2000) suggested that about 10% of smokers quitting smoking with nicotine inhaler continued to use it for extended periods, and thus follow-up of inhaler users is recommended.

Two 4–6 month double-blind, placebo-controlled RCTs (Bolliger *et al.*, 2000; Schneider *et al.*, 1996) have demonstrated the superiority of NVI to placebo inhalers for smoking cessation. Results revealed a 2–3 fold increases in quit rates (17–26%) at trial endpoint compared to placebo inhalers, and smaller differences at follow-up periods of 1 year or longer. These data support the short-term efficacy of NVI in cigarette smokers, but longer-term trials with the inhaler are needed. The combination of NVI with other forms of NRT (e.g. gum and patch) has not been studied.

Nicotine polacrilex lozenges

Nicotine lozenges that deliver nicotine (2 and 4 mg preparations) by buccal absorption (not swallowed, as nicotine is a gastrointestinal irritant) are now available for use in the USA as of 2002, and these lozenges offer further flexibility for nicotine replacement options for smokers, and are known to allow great absorption of nicotine as compared to nicotine gum. Mild throat and mouth irritation have been reported in preliminary trials (Shiffman *et al.*, 2002; Wallstrom *et al.*, 2000).

A 6-week double-blind, placebo-controlled RCT of 2 and 4 mg nicotine lozenges has shown their superiority to placebo lozenge (Shiffman *et al.*, 2002), with significant reduction in nicotine craving and withdrawal. Furthermore, high doses of lozenge may be more efficacious in more highly dependent smokers suggesting that lozenge dose can be matched with dependence level. The nicotine sublingual tablet (2 mg) has also been shown to be superior to placebo tablets when used for up to 6-months, nearly doubling quit rates at 6-weeks (50 vs. 29%) and 6-months (33 vs. 18%), while effects lessened at 1-year follow-up (Wallstrom *et al.*, 2000).

Summary of NRTs All commercially available forms of NRT are effective and increase quit rates by approximately 1.5 to 2-fold regardless of the setting. A meta-analysis of all 5 NRT products containing 97 RCTs involving 38 000 smokers followed for 6 months after commencing treatment found odds ratio of smoking cessation of any NRT versus placebo was 1.74 (95% CI 1.64–1.86). At 12 months, NRT versus placebo was 1.69 (95% CI 1.57–1.82). Facilitation of an intense level of support, although beneficial in facilitating the likelihood of quitting, was not essential to the success of the NRT. There was weak evidence that combination forms of NRT are more effective, and higher doses of nicotine patch may produce small increases in quit rates (Silagy *et al.*, 2002). In a review of 8 nicotine gum studies, 3 inhaler studies, and one microtab study, involving 774 subjects, the evidence for oral nicotine forms to reduce total withdrawal discomfort, irritability and anxiety was very high. There was some evidence for an effect on depressed mood and craving, though there was less evidence for nicotine gum than for other forms of oral nicotine replacement (West *et al.*, 2001).

Sustained release bupropion

The phenylaminoketone, atypical antidepressant agent bupropion, in the sustained-release (SR) formulation (Zyban®), is now considered a first-line pharmacological treatment for nicotine dependent smokers who want to quit smoking. The mechanism of action of this antidepressant agent in the treatment of nicotine dependence likely involves blockade of DA and norepinephrine reuptake (Ascher *et al.*, 1995), as well as antagonism of high-affinity

nicotinic acetylcholine receptors (Slemmer *et al.*, 2000). Yet the exact mechanism by which bupropion aids in smoking cessation is unclear (Roddy, 2004).

The goals of bupropion therapy are: (1) smoking cessation, (2) reduction of nicotine craving and withdrawal symptoms, and (3) prevention of cessation-induced weight gain. While bupropion is indicated both for the treatment of depression as well as for the treatment of smoking cessation in the USA, in the UK it is licensed only for use in smoking cessation.

The target dose of this agent in nicotine dependence is 300 mg daily (150 mg bid), and it is started 7 days prior to the target quit date (TQD) at 150 mg daily. Dosing is increased to 150 mg bid after 3–4 days. Unlike the NRTs, there is no absolute requirement that smokers completely cease smoking by the TQD, though many smokers report a significant reduction in urges to smoke and craving which facilitates cessation at the time of the TQD. Some smokers gradually reduce their cigarette smoking over several weeks prior to quitting. At the present time, there is little data as to which subgroups of smokers bupropion may have the most utility, though smokers with depressive symptoms may benefit from its antidepressant properties (Chengappa *et al.*, 2001).

The primary side effects reported with bupropion administration in cigarette smokers are headache, nausea and vomiting, dry mouth, insomnia and activation, most of which occur during the first week of treatment, though insomnia can persist. The main contraindication for the use of bupropion is a past history of seizures of any etiology. The rates of *de novo* seizures are low with this agent ($< 0.5\%$) at doses of 300 mg daily or less and have been predominantly observed when daily dosing exceeds 450 mg/day. The risk of hypertension is $< 1\%$ in smokers, but may be higher in combination with NRTs (Jorenby *et al.*, 1999).

A pivotal multi-centre study by Hurt *et al.* (1997) established the efficacy and safety of sustained-release (SR) bupropion for treatment of nicotine dependence which led to its FDA approval in the USA in 1998 and approval in the UK in 2000. In a 7-week double-blind, placebo-controlled multi-centre trial, three doses of bupropion SR (100, 150 and 300 mg/day in BID divided doses) in combination with weekly individual cessation counselling, were given to 615 cigarette smokers using at least 15 cigarettes per day. The end of trial 7-day point prevalence cessation rates were 19.0%, 28.8%, 38.6% and 44.2% for placebo, 100 mg/day, 150 mg/day and 300 mg/day bupropion doses, respectively. At 1-year follow-up, cessation rates were 12.4%, 19.6%, 22.9% and 23.1%, respectively. Bupropion treatment dose-dependently reduced weight gain associated with smoking cessation and significantly reduced nicotine withdrawal symptoms at the 150 and 300 mg/day doses.

The combination of bupropion SR with nicotine transdermal patch (NTP) was evaluated in a double-blind, double placebo-controlled, randomized multi-centre trial (Jorenby *et al.*, 1999). A total of 893 cigarette smokers, using at least 15 cigarettes per day (cpd), were randomized to one of four experimental groups: (1) placebo bupropion (0 mg/day) + placebo patch; (2) bupropion (300 mg/day) + placebo patch; (3) placebo bupropion + nicotine patch (21 mg/day for 4 weeks, with 2 weeks of 14 mg/day and 2 weeks of 7 mg/day); (4) bupropion + patch. Bupropion was administered 1 week prior to the target quit date (Day 15) at which time patch treatment was initiated for a total of 8 weeks. All subjects received weekly individual smoking cessation counselling. Cessation rates at the 1-year follow-up assessment were 15.6% for placebo; 16.4% for active NTP alone; 30.3% for bupropion alone; and 35.5% for the combination of patch and bupropion. Both bupropion + patch and bupropion alone groups were significantly better than the placebo and patch alone conditions, but the combination was not significantly better than bupropion alone. Weight suppression after cessation was most robust in the combination therapy group. Side effects were consistent with the profiles of patch and bupropion, and the combination was well-tolerated. However, a higher than expected rate of treatment-emergent hypertension (4–5%) was noted with the combination of bupropion and patch (Jorenby *et al.*, 1999). Of note, patch alone treatment was significantly different from placebo at the end of the trial, but not at the follow-up assessments.

Several recent studies have extended the use of bupropion for smoking cessation. Hays *et al.* (2001) examined the effects of bupropion versus placebo on the prevention of smoking relapse in 784 cigarette smokers who achieved smoking abstinence after a 7-week open-label trial of bupropion (300 mg/day). Abstinent smokers were then randomized to bupropion (300 mg/day) or placebo for a total of 45 weeks. Fifty-nine per cent of smokers enrolled in the open-label phase of the trial quit smoking. Significantly more smokers were abstinent at the end of the 52-week treatment period in bupropion vs. placebo groups (55.1 vs. 42.3%, $P < 0.01$), but not at the 1-year follow-up assessment. In addition, days to smoking relapse was higher in the bupropion vs. placebo group (156 vs. 65 days, $P < 0.05$). Weight gain was significantly less in the bupropion group at both the end of treatment and 1-year follow-up. The results of this study suggest the efficacy of bupropion in preventing smoking relapse. Data

regarding the effective duration of bupropion therapy as a maintenance treatment requires further study.

Other studies have suggested the efficacy of bupropion for smoking cessation in African-Americans (Ahluwalia *et al.*, 2002), as a treatment for smokers who have failed initial bupropion therapy (Gonzales *et al.*, 2001), and as a treatment for smokers with chronic obstructive pulmonary disease (Tashkin *et al.*, 2001). In an interesting study by Sampablo *et al.* (2002), patients who had higher anxiety scores on the Hamilton at outset of the effort to stop smoking did better on smoking cessation, while those with higher depression scores at outset did more poorly.

Varenicline tartarate
Varenicline tartarate (Chantix® in USA, Champix® in Europe), an $\alpha_4\beta_2$ nicotinic receptor partial agonist, was approved as a first-line smoking cessation agent by the USA FDA in the summer of 2006, and subsequently was in Canada and Europe. The results of two independent but identical phase III trials comparing varenicline (1 mg bid) to bupropion SR (150 mg bid) and placebo have recently been published (Study 1: Gonzales *et al.*, 2006; Study 2: Jorenby *et al.*, 2006). The quit rate for both studies were similar for continuous abstinence over the last 4 weeks (Weeks 9–12) of the study: Study 1: varenicline: 44.4%, bupropion SR, 29.5%, and placebo, 17.7%; Study 2: varenicline: 44.4%, bupropion SR, 29.5%, and placebo, 17.7%. Quit rates were significantly higher for participants taking varenicline compared to bupropion SR ($Ps < 0.0001$) and both drugs resulted in significantly higher quit rates than placebo. Continuous abstinence over the follow up period (week 9 to 52) were lower and participants taking varenicline continued to show a higher rate of abstinence (Study 1: 22.1%, Study 2: 23.0%) than participants taking bupropion (Study 1: 16.4%, $P < 0.001$ compared to varenicline; Study 2: 15.0%, $P = 0.064$ compared to varenicline) and placebo (Study 1: 8.4%, Study 2: 10.3%). A third study examining the efficacy of the drug on smoking relapse-prevention used a 12-week open label varenicline phase followed by randomization to 12 weeks of varenicline or placebo (Tonstad *et al.*, 2006). These investigators found that participants taking varenicline versus placebo were more likely to be continuously abstinent during weeks 13 to 24 (70.5% vs. 49.6%, $P < 0.001$) and weeks 13 to 52 (43.6% vs 36.9%, $P = 0.02$). Varenicline was found to reduce cravings and smoking satisfaction and well tolerated. There were similar discontinuous rates for varenicline and bupropion and the most common adverse event reported by the varenicline group was nausea (Study 1: 28.1%, Study 2: 29.4%).

Other non-nicotine pharmacotherapies

A number of non-nicotine pharmacotherapies have been tested for utility for treating nicotine dependence but are not currently FDA-approved for the treatment of nicotine dependence.

Nortriptyline

Nortriptyline is a tricyclic antidepressant which has been shown in several double-blind, placebo-controlled trials to be superior to placebo (Hall *et al.*, 1998; Prochazka *et al.*, 1998) and to have comparable efficacy to bupropion (Hall *et al.*, 2002). Its efficacy may be improved with higher vs. lower intensity behavioural therapies. Its mechanism of action is thought to relate to norepinephrine and serotonin reuptake blockade, two neurotransmitters which have been implicated in the biology of nicotine dependence. Side effects include dry mouth, blurred vision, constipation and orthostatic hypotension. It appears to have some utility in smokers with past histories of major depression and it can be recommended as a second line agent after nicotine replacement therapies and bupropion, though more study of this agent is necessary. SSRIs do not appear to be helpful in directly assisting in smoking cessation (Hughes *et al.*, 2003).

Clonidine

Clonidine is a pre-synaptic alpha-2 agonist that dampens sympathetic activity originating at the locus ceruleus. It appears to have some efficacy for alcohol and opioid withdrawal and thus was tested with nicotine withdrawal as well (Covey & Glassman, 1991; Hughes, 1994a). The most common side effects of clonidine are dry mouth, sedation, and constipation. Postural hypotension, rebound hypertension, and depression are rare with smoking cessation treatment (Gourlay & Benowitz, 1995).

Several clinical trials tested oral or transdermal clonidine in doses of 0.1–0.4 mg/day for 2–6 weeks with and without behaviour therapy. Three meta-analytic reviews reported that clonidine doubles quit rates (Covey & Glassman, 1991; Gorley & Benowitz, 1995; Law & Tang, 1995), but a fourth disagreed. Several studies have suggested clonidine is more effective in women than in men; however, other studies have failed to find this association (Gourlay & Benowitz, 1995). In general, the effects of clonidine have not proven to be as robust as NRTs. An initial study in $n = 71$ heavy smokers by Glassman *et al.* (1988) showed that at doses up to 0.4 mg/day, cessation rates were doubled in comparison to placebo, and in a follow-up study by this group in $n = 300$ smokers this initial finding was replicated (Glassman *et al.*, 1993). In fact, a meta-analysis by Covey and Glassman (1991) of 9 placebo-controlled studies and 813 patients found short-term quit rates of 39% on clonidine vs. 21% on placebo (OR 2.4, 1.7–32.8), and suggested that clonidine was effective in the transdermal preparation and more helpful in female smokers. A subsequent meta-analysis by Gourlay and Benowitz (1995) found long-term follow-up quit rates in 4 subsequent studies of 31% on clonidine and 17% on placebo (OR 2.0, 1.3–3.0). It appears to be useful in reducing nicotine withdrawal symptoms acutely and may have a role in smokers who have high levels of anxiety during early cessation (Gourlay *et al.*, 2001; Niaura *et al.*, 1996). Recent trials of the transdermal clonidine preparation (Niaura *et al.*, 1996) and oral clonidine (Nana & Praditsuwan, 1998) have found less impressive support for clonidine's efficacy for smoking cessation, but this agent should be considered as a second line therapy for smokers failing initial treatment with NRTs or bupropion.

Mecamylamine

Mecamylamine is a non-competitive blocker at the ion channel site of both high-affinity central nervous system and peripheral nicotinic receptors that decreases the positive subjective effects from cigarettes (Cepeda-Benito, 1993; Clarke, 1991; Stolerman, *et al.*, 1973). When mecamylamine is given to smokers who are not trying to stop smoking, they initially increase their smoking in an attempt to overcome the blockade produced by mecamylamine (Cepeda-Benito, 1993; Clarke, 1991). Mecamylamine does not precipitate withdrawal in humans perhaps because it is an indirect blocker. Early studies suggested some short-term efficacy with mecamylamine, but the high doses used produced significant dropout rates because of side effects (Cepeda-Benito, 1993; Clarke, 1991). Side effects included abdominal cramps, constipation, dry mouth, and headaches. Based on a theory that combined blockade and agonist therapy might be beneficial (Rose & Levin, 1991), similar to the nicotinic receptor partial agonist profile of varenicline, two randomized trials comparing mecamylamine (MEC) in combination with nicotine patch to placebo and nicotine patch, with the rationale that MEC would reduce the rewarding effects of nicotine, and patch would reduce nicotine withdrawal symptoms. In the first trial (Rose *et al.*, 1994), mecamylamine (up to 10 mg/day; 5 mg bid for 5 weeks) or placebo was given in combination with nicotine patch (21 mg/day) for up to 8 weeks, and cessation rates were significantly higher in the combination group than the patch alone group (12/24 [50.0%] vs. 4/24 [16.7%] respectively). Mecamylamine was reported to reduce cigarette craving and negative affect and appetite increases associated with tobacco withdrawal. Constipation was the major side effect at the MEC doses used, and there was little orthostatic hypotension noted. In the second study of 80 cigarette smokers (Rose *et al.*, 1998), MEC at doses of up to 10 mg/day was given as a pre-treatment for 4 weeks prior to nicotine patch initiation at the TQD, and the combination of MEC and patch was continued for 6 weeks. Similar to the first study, the combination of MEC with NTP increased continuous abstinence rates after the TQD compared to NTP alone (19/40 [47.5%] vs. 11/40 [27.5%], $P < 0.05$). These data suggest the efficacy of the combination of MEC with NTP. In summary, mecamylamine lacks sufficient evidence to be recommended but is considered promising (Lancaster & Stead, 2002).

Naltrexone

Naltrexone is a long-acting form of the opioid antagonist naloxone. The rationale for using naltrexone for smoking cessation is that the performance-enhancing and other positive effects of nicotine may be opioid mediated (Pomerleau & Pomerleau, 1984). Most, but not all, studies have found that naltrexone increases smoking (interpreted again as an attempt to overcome blockade (Hughes & Francis, 1995; Sutherland *et al.*, 1995)). The few side effects from naltrexone include elevated liver enzymes, nausea and blockade of analgesia from narcotic pain relievers (Hughes & Francis, 1995). There is little evidence to indicate the efficacy of naltrexone hydrochloride alone for smoking cessation (Sutherland *et al.*, 1995). A recent trial by Covey *et al.* (1999) in 68 cigarette smokers using at least 20 cigarettes per day and highly motivated to quit compared naltrexone (up to 75 mg/day) initiated 3 days prior to the TQD to placebo for a total of 4 weeks. Cessation rates in the naltrexone group were non-significantly higher than placebo (46.7% vs. 26.3%, $P < 0.10$) and at 6-month follow-up there were no group differences (27 vs. 15%). Female subjects and those with a history of major depression appeared to respond better, but a lack of power to detect significant group differences because of the small sample size studied is a major shortcoming of this study.

Another study compared naltrexone (50 mg/day) in combination with NTP (21 mg/day) to naltrexone alone, patch alone and placebo (there being no placebo patch condition) in 100 cigarette smokers for a total of 12 weeks. Cessation rates for placebo alone and naltrexone alone groups were 19 and 22%, and for patch alone and patch + naltrexone, 48% and 46%, respectively, suggesting only a main effect of nicotine patch treatment, and no effects of naltrexone on smoking cessation, either alone or in combination. The main effect of nicotine patch was lost at the 6-month follow-up assessment. In addition, there was no effect of naltrexone on amount smoked or cigarette craving. However, a preliminary study by Krishnan-Sarin *et al.* (2003) suggests that the combination of naltrexone and NTP is superior to NTP alone especially if NTP administration precedes that of naltrexone. In a larger trial of the combination of nicotine patch (21 mg/day) with four active doses of naltrexone (0, 25, 50 and 100 mg/day), it was shown that the highest dose of naltrexone with patch could significantly improve continuous smoking abstinence rates (O'Malley *et al.*, 2006). Further studies of naltrexone either alone or in combination with the patch are needed, including in patients with concurrent alcohol misuse. At this time, naltrexone lacks sufficient evidence to be recommended.

Monoamine oxidase (MAO) inhibitors

Inhibition of MAO-A and MAO-B theoretically could be helpful for smoking cessation since blockade of the metabolism of neurotransmitters involved in the biology of nicotine dependence, such as DA (MAO-B), and serotonin and norepinephrine (MAO-A) occurs, leading to increases in their synaptic levels, which are reduced during acute withdrawal. A single trial of the MAO-A inhibitor mocloclobemide (Berlin *et al.*, 1995) was conducted suggesting short-term increases in smoking cessation in $n = 88$ smokers. Furthermore, a small trial by George *et al.* (2003) in 40 smokers suggested the short-term efficacy of the MAO-B inhibitor selegiline hydrochloride for smoking cessation. Larger controlled trials of these agents are warranted before firm recommendations for the use of these agents for smoking cessation can be made.

Summary of recommendations on pharmacotherapies for nicotine dependence Nicotine patches, nicotine gum, sustained-release bupropion and varenicline are recommended initial pharmacotherapies for smoking cessation. Nicotine nasal spray and vapour inhaler are also recommended but because the studies here have a smaller empirical base and appear to have significant side effects, it is recommended primarily as a treatment for those who have failed to stop smoking using the nicotine patch or gum. Nortriptyline is a promising second-line non-nicotine pharmacotherapy than should be considered especially in smokers with co-morbid depressive symptoms, major depression or past history of major depression. Clonidine may also have some merit as a second line agents, possibly in female smokers, but side effects limit its use and probably compliance. Other consideration as third-line agents can be given to naltrexone, mecamylamine and monoamine oxidase inhibitors but their efficacy for smoking cessation has not been established.

Psychosocial treatments

Behavioural therapy

Behavioural therapy is based on the theory that learning processes operate in the development, maintenance and cessation of smoking. Many of the recommendations described under psychiatric management are actually based on the principles of behavioural therapy. The following sections briefly describe formal behavioural techniques for cessation. For more information, the reader is referred to several descriptive (Brown *et al.*, 1993; Curry, 1993; Fisher *et al.*, 1993; Glasgow, 1987; Hughes & Francis, 1994; Mermelstein *et al.*, 1992; Sachs, 1991; Schwartz, 1992; US Department of Health and Human Services (HHS), 1988) and meta-analytic reviews (Baille *et al.*, 1994) of behavioural therapy. The goals of behavioural therapies in treatment of nicotine dependence include: (1) Providing necessary skills to smokers to aid them in quitting smoking; (2) Teaching skills to avoid smoking in high risk situations; (3) Supporting and extending the effects of proven pharmacotherapies for nicotine dependence.

There are over 100 controlled prospective studies verifying the efficacy of behaviour therapy (Baille *et al.*, 1994; Lancaster & Stead, 1999a; Schwartz, 1992; Viswesvaran & Schmidt, 1992). Typically, behavioural therapies are a multimodal package of several of the specific treatments. In most reviews/meta-analyses, 6-month quit rates with behaviour therapy packages are 20%–25%, and behaviour therapy typically increases quit rates twofold over control groups (Baille *et al.*, 1994; Glasgow, 1987; Law & Tang, 1995; Schwartz, 1992; Viswesvaran & Schmidt, 1992). Given this large database of efficacy, multimodal behaviour therapy is a recommended first-line therapy.

Below follows a description of specific behavioural interventions that have been evaluated for the treatment of nicotine dependence.

Self-help materials and other brief interventions

The major goals of self-help materials and procedures are to increase motivation to quit and impart cessation skills. Several recent studies have documented that minimal behavioural interventions such as community support groups (Bakkevig *et al.*, 2000), call-back telephone counselling (Borland *et al.*, 2001; Curry *et al.*, 1995; Platt *et al.*, 1997) (but see the study by Reid *et al.* (1999) which was negative), and computer generated tailored self-help materials (Dijkstra *et al.*, 1999; Etter & Perneger, 2001) can augment smoking cessation rates in controlled settings. Materials tailored more to the specific person seemed to have greater effectiveness, but overall they do not seem to add power to other interventions

(Lancaster & Stead, 1999b). Fiore *et al.* (2000) suggest that written materials may be more effective when combined with other more intensive therapies.

Training programmes for physicians in basic behavioural supportive cessation counselling may lead to enhanced cessation rates simply because physicians are more likely to engage patients in a discussion about smoking cessation (Cornuz *et al.*, 2002). Such brief interventions also seem to have efficacy in promoting smoking cessation in hospitalized medical inpatients (Dornelas *et al.*, 2000; Rigotti *et al.*, 1997), though this is not true of all studies (Hajek *et al.*, 2002). Thus, there is good evidence to recommend their use in smokers making initial attempts at cessation, especially in light smokers (Jackson *et al.*, 1986), and in people without histories of treatment-failure. Pharmacists and other health care people may also be able to use these brief interventions with some success (Lancaster *et al.*, 2000). Community interventions, mass media campaigns and posters, etc., appear to impact, if at all, on the lighter smoker (Foulds, 1996), and provide little information as to the cost and effectiveness of workplace interventions (Moher *et al.*, 2003).

Community interventions that target adolescents appear to have very limited impact on deterring adolescents from beginning to smoke (Sowden *et al.*, 2002). There are correlations between adolescents being exposed to pro-tobacco advertising and eventually at least experimenting with tobacco (Lovato *et al.*, 2003).

Cognitive-behavioural interventions (skills training/ relapse-prevention therapies)

For the smoker who has failed initial treatments, use of more specialized and higher intensity behavioural treatments such as cognitive-behavioural therapy (CBT), in combination with NRT or bupropion, is recommended. In CBT, patients anticipate situations or processes where they are likely to smoke, and then plan strategies to cope with these situations. Behavioural coping includes removing oneself from the situation, substituting other behaviours (walking, exercising), or using skills to manage triggers (assertiveness, refusal skills, time management). Cognitive coping includes identifying maladaptive thoughts, challenging them, and substituting more effective thought patterns in order to prevent a slip from becoming a relapse (e.g. not viewing the slip as a catastrophe). Some degree of efficacy of cognitive-behavioural therapies in smokers with a history of depression, alcoholism and substance abuse (Alterman *et al.*, 2001; Brown *et al.*, 2001; Burling *et al.*, 2001; Garcia, 2000; Hall *et al.*, 1998; Patten *et al.*, 1998) and weight concerns associated with smoking cessation (Perkins *et al.*, 2001) has been demonstrated, though differences in design and control groups making comparisons amongst the studies difficult.

Motivational interventions

The goal of motivational interviewing (MI) interventions is to elicit change through examining and resolving ambivalence, increasing intrinsic motivation for change, and creating an atmosphere of acceptance in which patients take responsibility for making changes happen (Miller, 2004; Miller & Rollnick, 2002). MI has been applied to many areas of health behaviour (e.g. weight loss, HIV risk behaviours, medical adherence). The majority of research and strongest positive results have come from interventions with alcohol and illicit drug use (Burke *et al.*, 2003; Dunn *et al.*, 2001; Noonan & Moyers, 1997). Fewer studies have examined the specific area of smoking cessation. In addition, these studies have utilized a wide range of smoking populations (e.g. adolescents, adults, pregnant women) and yielded mixed results (Dunn *et al.*, 2001; Resnicow *et al.*, 2002). Burke *et al.* (2003) conducted a meta-analysis of the efficacy of MI with smoking cessation, substance abuse, HIV-risk reduction, and diet and exercise. Only two of the analysed studies examined smoking cessation: a study of adolescent smokers and a study of adult smokers. Burke *et al.* (2003) reported just one significant effect size: a small but significant effect (Cohen's $d = 0.23$) for 24-hour abstinence in Butler *et al.*'s (1999) adolescent study. Although MI has shown no effect in a number of studies (Colby *et al.*, 1998; Ershoff *et al.*, 1999; Tappin *et al.*, 2000), more recent research has shown promising results for increased smoking cessation at 6-week follow-up (Glasgow *et al.*, 2000; Stotts *et al.*, 2002), 6-month follow-up (Carpenter *et al.*, 2004), and for adolescents with low initial intention to quit (Brown *et al.*, 2003). Thus, while few studies have rigorously evaluated the efficacy of MI for smoking cessation, these preliminary positive findings suggest that the technique may be a useful intervention for smoking cessation either alone or as an adjunct to other pharmacological and psychosocial interventions. Additional research is needed to clarify the utility of MI for smoking cessation.

Summary: implementation of nicotine dependence behavioural therapies As discussed earlier in this chapter, a stepped-care approach is desirable in implementing behavioural treatments for smoking cessation. That is, minimal interventions should be tried first, and failing these minimal interventions, more intense levels of behavioural treatment should then be considered in combination with pharmacotherapies. However, as mentioned previously, initial interventions for some groups

(e.g. psychiatric populations) should consider higher intensities of behavioural therapy, given the frequent treatment failure in smoking cessation by these patients. Both group and individual formats have been used for behavioural therapies for smoking cessation, with groups being used to increase social support and individual treatment to address individual problems of the smoker. Patient preference should be considered in recommending group versus individual treatment.

Since nearly two-thirds of patients relapse in the first week after a smoking cessation attempt, most treatment is timed to occur before or just after cessation occurs. The most common providers of behavioural therapy are voluntary organizations (e.g. American Cancer Society, American Lung Association), wellness programmes, or health educators/psychologists in health care organizations (Hughes, 1996a). A major problem is that behavioural therapy is not often available to patients or available only intermittently, is costly, and is not integrated into the health care system. Consequently, many of those motivated to quit forego behavioural therapy (Hughes, 1996b).

Alternative treatments

In a study of 22 trials of acupuncture, there was a failure to detect an effect on smoking cessation (White *et al.*, 2002). Hypnotherapy has also been studied as a smoking cessation tool. There is currently no evidence that hypnotherapy has any greater effect on 6-month quit rates than any other intervention or no intervention at all (Abbot *et al.*, 1998).

Special considerations in subpopulations of smokers

Alcohol and drug abuse

There is strong evidence that rates of smoking in substance abusers are much higher than the general population (60%–90%), and that the presence of the alcohol and/or illicit drug use is a negative predictor of smoking cessation treatment outcomes (Hughes, 1996a). Conditioned effects of substance use with smoking may be one important factor in determining both the high rates of co-morbidity and treatment failure, as these behaviours are often concurrent. Nonetheless, many alcoholics and substance abusers express an interest in smoking cessation, and motivational interventions should be used in patients who do not express a current interest in quitting. There is little evidence to suggest that smoking cessation can increase the risk of relapse for alcohol and substance abuse disorders. There is little evidence to guide when cessation should be attempted in a substance abuser insofar as whether this should be attempted concurrently with drug abuse abstinence or after abstinence from drugs is completed. Perhaps the timing of the intervention might be guided by patient preference. In addition, studies of pharmacotherapies in substance abusers are few (Kalman *et al.*, 2001), but there is some evidence for the utility of nicotine replacement and behavioural approaches. Use of alcohol pharmacotherapies such as disulfiram or naltrexone might be considered in alcoholic smokers, but there are no empirical studies to suggest their efficacy in smoking cessation. In any case, such smoking cessation treatment should be made available in substance abuse treatment programmes.

Depression

Persons with depressive symptoms or major depression have high rates of smoking (40%–60% prevalence), and depression appears to be a negative predictor of treatment outcome during smoking cessation (Covey *et al.*, 2000; Niaura *et al.*, 2001). Pharmacotherapies for smoking cessation have not been carefully tested in patients with major depression, but antidepressants such as bupropion and nortriptyline should be strongly considered. Behavioural therapies such as CBT should also be strongly considered for the depressed smokers, as they are likely to fail with more minimal interventions. After smoking cessation, plasma levels of some antidepressants (e.g. tricyclic antidepressants) which are metabolized by CYP 1A2 may increase, necessitating close monitoring of levels and antidepressant side effects.

Schizophrenia

As with depression and substance abuse disorders, rates of smoking in schizophrenic patients are much higher (58%–88%) when compared to the general population (Kalman *et al.*, 2005). Motivation to quit smoking is often poor in these patients, and thus motivational interventions as initial treatments are strongly suggested. Quit rates for these patients are very low (Lasser *et al.*, 2000), suggesting that more intense interventions are needed, and several controlled cessation trials have been published (Addington *et al.*, 1998; Evins *et al.*, 2001; George *et al.*, 2000, 2002; Ziedonis & George, 1997; Evins *et al.*, 2005) using combinations of higher intensity behavioural support and pharmacotherapies (NRT or bupropion) with modest short-term cessation rates. Concurrent alcohol and drug abuse in these patients is high and can complicate cessation efforts, and most studies have attempted cessation in dually diagnosed schizophrenics whose drug use is in recovery and who are psychiatrically stable. Antipsychotic medications which are metabolized via the CYP 1A2 system (e.g. clozapine, olanzapine and chlorpromazine) may be increased within 3–6 weeks of smoking cessation, which necessitates regular monitoring of antipsychotic side effects and plasma levels. There is some evidence that in schizophrenic smokers, prescription of atypical antipsychotic agents (e.g. clozapine) can either reduce smoking in patients not attempting to quit smoking or facilitate smoking cessation in those patients attempting smoking cessation with nicotine patch (George *et al.*, 2000) or bupropion (George *et al.*, 2002), but further studies of this effect are needed in larger samples.

General medical disorders

The presence of an acute medical disorder that comes to medical attention can often be a strong motivator for an individual to consider smoking cessation. As with other smokers, stepped care approaches are appropriate, and if patients fail initial low intensity efforts, more intense behavioural methods and pharmacotherapies should then be considered. There is good evidence that NRTs are useful for smoking cessation in medical patients.

Cardiovascular disease

Smoking is the single most important modifiable risk factor for cardiovascular disease (CVD), and risks of CVD are greatly diminished within 5 years of cessation. The safety of NRTs including nicotine patch has been demonstrated in several clinical trials in cardiac patients.

Pulmonary disease

It is well known that respiratory symptoms are reduced after smoking cessation, and this can be a strong motivator for patients with chronic pulmonary diseases to quit smoking. Many of these pulmonary patients who fail initial quit attempts are highly dependent and often have co-morbid alcoholism, so alcohol use disorders should be screened for in refractory pulmonary smokers, and there is some evidence that NRTs are useful for cessation in these patients.

Cancer

The duration of smoking abstinence is directly related to decreases in risk for developing cancer of various forms, including lung, bowel and breast. In those with cancer, cessation leads to improved quality of life, and thus cancer patients should be encouraged to quit smoking.

Conclusions

It is important to identify smoking in health care settings, particularly populations that are high risk for smoking (e.g. individuals with psychiatric and addictive disorders).

Identifying and urging people to stop smoking and making sure they are aware of the medical consequences of smoking is important. Many smokers are able to quit with minimal therapeutic interventions. Simple advice to give up smoking is one of the most cost effective interventions we can make in medicine, and yet this is not part of routine health care delivery in many settings both in the US and the UK. Initial attempts to assist individuals with smoking cessation should utilize stepped-care approaches, reserving more intensive behavioural therapies and pharmacological interventions for treatment-resistant smokers. More intensive therapies may be needed for smokers who have had multiple failed quit attempts and smokers with co-morbid psychiatric, alcohol or drug, or medical disorders.

There are a number of empirically validated pharmacotherapies for the treatment of nicotine dependence in the USA, including five NRT formulations, varenicline and sustained-release bupropion, as well as a number of non-approved pharmacotherapies which appear promising. Nicotine replacement therapy may be the most cost effective, and it is the treatment that has the largest data base supporting its effectiveness. Bupropion is currently the best non-nicotine treatment, although in a single head-to-head trial, varenicline was superior to bupropion and to placebo. Intensive behavioral support from a trained counsellor is the most effective non-drug treatment for smokers, and it appears equally effective in both an individual and a group setting. The level of evidence for each of the interventions discussed in this chapter are summarized in Table 23.1.

Given that 80% of adult smokers start as teenagers, we should target this age group in order to have a significant impact on smoking cessation. Little real research has taken place with this group.

The issue of passive smoking has received less attention in the UK than in the US in the past, though the recent ban on smoking in pubs and other public places reveals that this issue is taking hold in the UK. Efforts need to continue to be made to make government and business leaders aware of the impact of active as well as passive smoking on morbidity and mortality.

In ever increasing pharmacologic dependent societies, additional research on medications that target neurotransmitter systems involved in nicotine dependence (e.g. selective GABA and DA receptor agonists) may be important for treatment-resistant smokers. If people thought that a simple pill with minimal side effects could help them avoid the discomfort of withdrawal that accompanies smoking cessation, then perhaps greater progress could be made on this important public health issue.

Table 23.1. Effectiveness of treatments for nicotine dependence

Treatment	Form of treatment	Psychiatric disorder/ target audience	Level of evidence for efficacy	Comments
Nicotine replacement therapy	Nicotine gum	Adult smokers	Ia	Gradually and successfully reduces craving and withdrawal (slow absorption)
Nicotine replacement therapy	Transdermal nicotine patch	Adult smokers	Ia	Gradually and successfully reduces craving and withdrawal (slow absorption)
Nicotine replacement therapy	Nasal spray	Adult smokers	Ia	Rapidly reduces craving and withdrawal (rapid absorption)
Nicotine replacement therapy	Nicotine inhaler	Adult smokers	Ia	Rapidly reduces craving and withdrawal (rapid absorption)
Nicotine replacement therapy	Nicotine polacrilex lozenges	Adult smokers	Ib	Gradually and successfully reduces craving and withdrawal (Slow absorption))
Psychopharmacology	Bupropion	Adult smokers	Ia	Significantly better than placebo at short term smoking cessation and at 1-year follow-up. It is dose-dependent in its ability to reduce smoking, weight gain and withdrawal symptoms at the 150 mg and 300 mg (SR) doses.
Psychopharmacology	Varenicline	Adult smokers	Ia	Superior to placebo and bupropion in the short-term (3 months) and at 1-year follow-up. Reduces craving and withdrawal symptoms, but little effect on weight gain. These effects are dose-dependent, with best outcomes at the 2 mg/day divided dosing schedule.
Psychopharmacology	Nortriptyline	Adult smokers	IIa	Listed as a second-line agent but is superior to placebo

Table 23.1. (cont.)

Treatment	Form of treatment	Psychiatric disorder/ target audience	Level of evidence for efficacy	Comments
Psychopharmacology	Clonidine	Adult smokers	IIa	Listed as a second-line agent but is superior to placebo. May be best for people with concomitant anxiety. There are negative reports re effectiveness as well
Psychopharmacology	Mecamylamine	Adult smokers	IIa	Some evidence for efficacy but only in combination with nicotine patch
Psychopharmacology	Naltrexone	Adult smokers	IIa	Some evidence for efficacy but only in combination with nicotine patch
Psychopharmacology	MAOIs	Adult smokers	Ib	Small studies that suggest may be helpful in the short term
Combined treatment	TNP and bupropion	Adult smokers	Ib	Combination not better than bupropion alone and possible side effect of hypertension in the combination. Bupropion alone better than TNP alone.
Psychosocial treatment	Multimodal cognitive behavioral therapy	Adult smokers	Ib	Increases quit rates twofold over control groups. It deserves a Ib because the programmes and populations may differ greatly from study to study
Psychosocial treatment	Self-help and other brief interventions	Adult smokers	IIb	Appear to have a modest but slight increase in quit rates, though little evidence that they work by themselves or with people who are heavy smokers
Psychosocial treatment	Motivational interviewing	Adult smokers	IIb	Appear to have a modest but slight increase in quit rates, real solid methodological studies have yet to be conducted

REFERENCES

Abbot, N. C., Stead, L. F., White, A. R. & Barnes J. (1998). Hypnotherapy for smoking cessation. *Cochrane Database Systematic Reviews.*

Addington, J., el-Guebaly, N., Campbell, W., Hodgins, D. C. & Addington, D. (1998). Smoking cessation treatment for patients with schizophrenia. *American Journal of Psychiatry*, **155**(7), 974–6.

Ahluwalia, J. S., Harris, K. J., Catley, D., Okuyemi, K. S. & Mayo, M. S. (2002). Sustained-release bupropion for smoking cessation in African Americans: a randomized controlled trial. *Journal of the American Medical Association*, **288**(4), 468–74.

Alterman, A. I., Gariti, P. & Mulvaney, F. (2001). Short- and long-term smoking cessation for three levels of intensity of behavioural treatment. *Psychological Addictive Behavior*, **15**(3), 261–4.

American Psychiatric Association (2006). *Practice Guidelines for the Treatment of Patients with Substance Use Disorders*, 2nd edn. Washington, DC: American Psychiatric Association.

Ascher, J. A., Cole, J. O., Colin, J. N. *et al*, (1995). Bupropion: A review of its mechanism of antidepressant activity. *Journal of Clinical Psychiatry*, **56**, 395–401.

Baille, A., Mattick, R. P., Hall, W. & Webster, P. (1994). Meta-analytic review of the efficacy of smoking cessation interventions. *Drug and Alcohol Review*, **13**, 157–70.

Bakkevig, O., Steine, S., von Hafenbradl, K. & Laerum, E. (2000). Smoking cessation. A comparative, randomized study between management in general practice and the behavioural programme SmokEnders. *Scandinavian Journal of Primary Health Care*, **18**(4), 247–51.

Balfour, D. J. K. & Fagerstrom, K. O. (1996). Pharmacology of nicotine and therapeutic use in smoking cessation and neurodegenerative disorders. *Pharmacological Therapy*, **72**, 51–81.

Bartecchi, C. E., MacKenzie, T. D. & Schier, R. W. (1994). The human costs of tobacco use, part II. *New England Journal of Medicine*, **330**, 975–80.

Benowitz, N. (ed.) (1988). Toxicity of nicotine: implications with regard to nicotine replacement therapy. In *Nicotine Replacement: A Critical Evaluation*, ed. P. C. Pomerleau, K. O. Fagerstrom, J. E. Henningfield & J. R. Hughes. Alan R Liss: New York, pp. 187–217.

Berlin, I., Said, S., Spreux-Varoquaux, O. *et al.* (1995). A reversible monoamine oxidase A inhibitor (moclobemide) facilitates smoking cessation and abstinence in heavy, dependent smokers. *Clinical Pharmacological Therapy*, **58**, 444–52.

Blondal, T., Franzon, M. & Westin, A. (1997). A double-blind randomized trial of nicotine nasal spray as an aid in smoking cessation. *European Respiratory Journal*, **10**, 1585–90.

Bolliger, C. T., Zellweger, J. P., Danielsson, T. *et al.* (2000). Smoking reduction with oral nicotine inhalers: double blind, randomised clinical trial of efficacy and safety. *British Medical Journal*, **321**(7257), 329–33.

Borland, R., Segan, C. J., Livingston, P. M. & Owen N. (2001). The effectiveness of callback counseling for smoking cessation: a randomized trial. *Addiction*, **96**(6), 881–9.

Brown, R. A., Goldstein, M. G., Niaura, R., Emmons, K. M. & Abrams, D. B. (1993). Nicotine dependence: assessment and management. In *Psychiatric Care of the Medical Patient*, ed. F. B. Stoudemire. New York: Oxford University Press, 877–901.

Brown, R. A., Kahler, C. W., Niaura, R. *et al.* (2001). Cognitive-behavioral treatment for depression in smoking cessation. *Journal of Consulting and Clinical Psychology*, **69**(3), 471–80.

Brown, R. A., Ramsey, S. E., Strong, D. R. *et al.* (2003). Effects of motivational interviewing on smoking cessation in adolescents with psychiatric disorders. *Tobacco Control*, **12**, 3019 Suppl.

Burke, B. L., Arkowitz, H. & Menchola, M. (2003). The efficacy of motivational interviewing: a meta-analysis of controlled clinical trails. *Journal of Consulting and Clinical Psychology*, **71**, 843–61.

Burling, T. A., Burling, A. S. & Latini, D. A. (2001). A controlled smoking cessation trial for substance-dependent inpatients. *Journal of Consulting and Clinical Psychology*, **69**(2), 295–304.

Butler, C. C., Rollnick, S., Cohen, D., Russel, I., Bachmann, M. & Stott, N. (1999). Motivational consulting versus brief advice for smokers in general practice: a randomised trial. *British Journal of General Practice*, **49**, 611–16.

Carpenter, M. J., Hughes, J. R., Solomon, L. J. & Callas, P. W. (2004). Both smoking reduction with nicotine replacement therapy and motivation advice increase future cessation among smokers unmotivated to quit. *Journal of Consulting and Clinical Psychology*, **72**, 371–81.

Carr A. (2004). *The Easy Way to Stop Smoking.* New York: Sterling.

CDC (2002). Cigarette smoking among adults in the United States. **51**, 300–3.

Cepeda-Benito, A. (1993). Meta-analysis review of the efficacy of nicotine chewing gum in smoking treatment programs. *Journal of Consulting and Clinical Psychology*, **61**, 822–30.

Chengappa, K. N. R., Kambhampati, R. K., Perkins, K. *et al.* (2001). Bupropion sustained release as a smoking cessation treatment in remitted depressed patients maintained on treatment with selective serotonin reuptake inhibitor antidepressants. *Journal of Clinical Psychiatry*, **62**(7), 503–8.

Clarke, P. B. S. (1991). Nicotinic receptor blockade therapy and smoking cessation. *British Journal of Addiction*, **86**, 501–5.

Colby, S. M., Monti, P. M., Barnett, N. P. *et al.* (1998). Brief motivational interviewing in a hospital setting for adolescent smoking: A preliminary study. *Journal of Consulting and Clinical Psychology*, **66**, 574–8.

Cornuz, J., Humair, J. P., Seematter, L. *et al.* (2002). Efficacy of resident training in smoking cessation: a randomized, controlled trial of program based on application of behavioral theory and practice with standardized patients. *Annals of Internal Medicine*, **136**(6), 429–37.

Covey, L. S. & Glassman, A. H. (1991). A meta-analysis of double-blind placebo controlled trials of clonidine for smoking cessation. *British Journal of Addiction*, **86**, 991–8.

Covey, L. S., Glassman, A. H. & Stetner, F. (1999). Naltrexone effects on short-term and long-term smoking cessation. *Journal of Addictive Diseases*, **18**(1), 31–40.

Covey, L. S., Sullivan, M. A., Johnston, A., Glassman, A. H., Robinson, M. D. & Adams, D. P. (2000). Advances in non-nicotine pharmacotherapy for smoking cessation. *Drugs*, **59**(1), 17–31.

Curry, S. (1993). Self-help interventions for smoking cessation. *Journal of Consulting and Clinical Psychology*, **61**, 790–803.

Curry, S. J., McBride, C., Grothaus, L. C., Louie, D., Wagner, E. H. (1995). A randomized trial of self-help materials, personalized feedback, and telephone counseling with nonvolunteer smokers. *Journal of Consulting and Clinical Psychology*, **63**(6), 1005–14.

Dallery, J., Houtsmuller, E. J., Pickworth, W. B. & Stitzer, M. L. (2003). Effects of cigarette nicotine content and smoking pace on subsequent craving and smoking. *Psychopharmacology*, **165**, 172–80.

Department of Health (1998). Smoking kills. *A white paper on tobacco*. London: The Stationery Office.

Dijkstra, A., De Vries, H. & Roijackers, J. (1999). Targeting smokers with low readiness to change with tailored and nontailored self-helo materials. *Preview Medicine*, **28**(2), 203–11.

Doll, R., Peto, R., Wheatley, K., Gray, R. & Sutherland, I. (1994). Mortality in relation to smoking: 40 years' observations on male British doctors. *British Medical Journal*, **309**, 901–11.

Dornelas, E. A., Sampson, R. A., Gray, J. F., Waters, D. & Thompson, P. D. (2000). A randomized controlled trial of smoking cessation counseling after myocardial infarction. *Preview Medicine*, **30**(4), 261–8.

Dunn, C., Deroo, L. & Rivara, F. P. (2001). The use of brief interventions adapted from motivational interviewing across behavioural domains. *Cochrane Database Systematic Review Addiction*, **96**(12), 1725–42.

Edwards, R. (2004). ABC of smoking. The problem of tobacco smoking. *British Medical Journal*, **328**, 217–19.

Ershoff, D. H., Quinn, V. P., Boyd, N. R., Stern, J., Gregory, M. & Wirtschafter, D. (1999). The Kaiser Permanente prenatal smoking cessation trial: When more isn't better, what is enough? *American Journal of Preventive Medicine*, **17**, 161–8.

Etter, J. F. & Perneger, T. B. (2001). Effectiveness of a computer-tailored smoking cessation program. *Archives of Internal Medicine*, **16**(21), 2596–601.

Evins, A. E., Mays, V. K., Rigotti, N. A., Tisdale, T., Cather, C. & Goff, D. C. (2001). A pilot trial of bupropion added to cognitive behavioral therapy for smoking cessation in schizophrenia. *Nicotine and Tobacco Research*, **3**, 397–403.

Evins, A. E., Cather, C., Deckersbach, T. *et al.* (2005). A double-blind placebo-controlled trial of bupropion sustained-release for smoking cessation in schizophrenia. *Journal of Clinical Psychopharmacology*, **25**(3), 218–25.

Fiore, M. C., Novotny, T. E., Pierce, J. P. *et al.* (1990). Methods used to quit smoking in the United States. *Journal of American Medical Association*, **263**, 2760–5.

Fiore, M. C., Jorenby, D. E., Baker, T. B. & Kenford, S. L. (1992). Tobacco dependence and the nicotine patch: clinical guidelines for effective use. *Journal of the American Medical Association,* **268**, 2687–94.

Fiore, M. C., Smith, S. S., Jorenby, D. E. & Baker, T. B. (1994). The effectiveness of the nicotine patch for smoking cessation: a meta-analysis. *Journal of the American Medical Association,* **271**(24), 1940–47.

Fiore, M. C., Bailey, W. C., Cohen, S. J. *et al.* (2000). *Clinical Practice Guideline: Treating Tobacco Use and Dependence.* US Department of Health and Human Services, Rockville, MD: US Public Health Service.

Fiore, M. C., Hatsukami, D. K. & Baker, T. B. (2002). Effective tobacco dependence treatment. *Journal of the American Medical Association,* **288**, 1768–71.

Fisher, E. B. J., Lichtenstein, E., Haire-Joshu, D., Morgan, G. D. & Rehberg, H. R. (1993). Methods, successes, and failures of smoking cessation programs. *Annual Reviews of Medicine,* **44**, 481–513.

Foulds, J. (1996). Strategies for smoking cessation. *British Medical Bulletin,* **52**, 1–17.

Garcia, M. (2000). Evaluation of the amount of therapist contact in a smoking cessation program. *Spanish Journal of Psychology,* **3**(1), 28–36.

Garvey, A. J., Kinnunen, T., Nordstrum, B. L. *et al.* (2000). Effects of nicotine gum dose by level of nicotine dependence. *Nicotine and Tobacco Research,* **2**, 53–63.

George, T. P., Ziedonis, D. M., Feingold, A. *et al.* (2000). Nicotine transdermal patch and atypical antipsychotic medications for smoking cessation in schizophrenia. *American Journal of Psychiatry,* **157**, 1835–42.

George, T. P., Vessicchio, J. C., Termine, A. *et al.* (2002). A placebo-controlled trial of bupropion for smoking cessation in schizophrenia. *Biolological Psychiatry,* **52**, 53–61.

George, T. P., Vessicchio, J. C., Termine, A., Jatlow, P. I., Kosten, T. R. & O'Malley, S. S. (2003). A preliminary placebo-controlled trial of selegiline hydrochloride for smoking cessation. *Biological Psychology,* **53** 136–43.

Giovino, G. A. (2002). Epidemiology of tobacco use in the United States. *Oncogene,* **21**, 7326–40.

Glasgow, R. (1987). Long-term effects of behavioral smoking cessation interventions. *Behavior Therapy,* **18**, 297–324.

Glasgow, R., Whitlock, E. Eakin, E. & Lichtstein, E. (2000). A brief smoking cessation intervention for women in low-income planned parenthood clinics. *American Journal of Public Health,* **90**, 786–9.

Glassman, A. H. (1993a). Cigarette smoking: implications for psychiatric illness. *American Journal of Psychiatry,* **150**, 546–53.

Glassman, A. H., Stetner, F., Walsh, B. T. *et al.* (1988). Heavy smokers, smoking cessation, and clonidine. Results of a double-blind, randomized trial. *Journal of the American Medical Association,* **259**(19), 2863–6.

Glassman, A. H., Covey, L. S., Dalack, G. W. *et al.* (1993b). Smoking cessation, clonidine, and vulnerability to nicotine among dependent smokers. *Clinical Pharmacological Therapy,* **54**, 670–9.

Glover, E. D., Sachs, D. P. L., Stitzer, M. L. *et al.* (1996). Smoking cessation in highly dependent smokers with 4 mg nicotine polacrilex. *American Journal of Health Behavior,* **20**(5), 319–32.

Gonzales, D. H., Nides, M. A., Ferry, L. H. *et al.* (2001). Bupropion SR as an aid to smoking cessation in smokers treated previously with bupropion: a randomized placebo-controlled study. *Clinical Pharmacology and Therapeutics,* **69**(6), 438–44.

Gonzales, D., Rennard, S. I., Nides, M. *et al.* (2006). Varenicline, an $\alpha 4 \beta 2$ nicotinic acetylcholine receptor partial agonist, vs sustained-release bupropion and placebo for smoking cessation: a randomized controlled trial. *Journal of the American Medical Association,* **296**(1), 47–55.

Gourlay, S. G. & Benowitz, N. L. (1995). Is clonidine an effective smoking cessation therapy? *Drugs,* **50**, 197–207.

Gourlay, S. G., Stead, L. F. & Benowitz, N. L. (2001). Clonidine for smoking cessation. *Cochrane Database Systematic Review.* Oxford: Update Software Ltd.

Gritz, E. R., Nielsen, I. R. & Brooks, L. A. (1996). Smoking cessation and gender: the influence of physiological, psychological and beahvioral factors. *Journal of the American Medical Women's Association,* **51**(1–2), 35–42.

Hajek, P., Taylor, T. Z. & Mills, P. (2002). Brief intervention during hospital admission to help patients to give up smoking after myocardial infarction and bypass surgery: randomized controlled trial. *British Medical Journal,* **324**(7329), 87–9.

Hall, S. M., Munoz, R. F., Reus, V. I. *et al.* (1996). Mood management and nicotine gum in smoking treatment: a therapeutic contact and placebo-controlled study. *Journal of Consulting and Clinical Psychology,* **64**(5), 1003–9.

Hall, S. M., Reus, V. I., Munoz, R. F. *et al.* (1998). Nortriptyline and cognitive-behavioral therapy in the treatment of cigarette smoking. *Archives of General Psychiatry,* **55**(8), 683–90.

Hall, S. M., Humfleet, G. L., Reus, V. I., Munoz, R. F., Hartz, D. T. & Maude-Griffin R. (2002). Psychological intervention and anti-depressant treatment in smoking cessation. *Archives of General Psychiatry,* **59**, 930–6.

Hays, J. T., Hurt, R. D., Rigotti, N. A. *et al.* (2001). Sustained-release bupropion for pharmacologic relapse prevention after smoking cessation. *Annals of Internal Medicine,* **135**, 423–33.

Heatherton, T. F., Kozlowski, L. T. Frecker, R. C. & Fagerstrom, K. O. (1991). The Fagerstrom Test for Nicotine Dependence: a revsision of the Fagerstrom Tolerance Questionnaire. *British Journal of Addictions,* **86**, 1119–27.

Henningfield, J. E., Stapleton, J. M., Benowitz, N. L., Grayson, R. F. & London, E. D. (1993). Higher levels of nicotine in arterial than in venous blood after cigarette smoking. *Drug Alcohol Dependency,* **33**, 23–9.

Herrera, N., Franco, R., Herrera, L., Partidas, A., Rolando, R. & Fagerstrom, K. O. (1995). Nicotine gum, 2 and 4 mg, for nicotine dependence. *Chest,* **108**(2), 447–51.

Hjalmarson, A., Franzon, M., Westin, A. & Wiklund, O. (1994). Effect of nicotine nasal spray on smoking cessation. *Archives of Internal Medicine,* **154**, 2567–72.

Hughes, J. R. (1989). Dependence potential and abuse liability of nicotine replacement therapies. *Biomedical Pharmacotherapy*, **43**, 11–17.

Hughes, J. R. (1991). Long-term use of nicotine-replacement therapy. In *New Developments in Nicotine-Delivery Systems*, ed. S. M.. Henningfield, pp. 64–71. New York: Carlton.

Hughes, J. R. (1993). Risk/benefit of nicotine replacement in smoking cessation. *Drug Safety*, **8**, 49–56.

Hughes, J. R. (1994a). Non-nicotine pharmacotherapies for smoking cessation. *Journal of Drug Developments*, **6**, 197–203.

Hughes, J. R. (1994b). An algorithm for smoking cessation. *Archives of Family Medicine*, **3**, 280–5.

Hughes, J. R. (1996a). Treatment of nicotine dependence. In *Pharmacological Aspects of Drug Dependence: Toward an Integrative Neurobehavioral Approach. Handbook of Experimental Psychology Series*, ed. G. S. Schuster & M. J. Kuhar, pp. 599–618. New York: Springer-Verlag.

Hughes, J. R. (1996b). The future of smoking cessation therapy in the United States. *Addiction*, **91**(12), 1797–802.

Hughes, J. R. & Francis, R. J. (1994). Behavioral support programs for smoking cessation. *Modern Medicine*, **62**, 22–6.

Hughes, J. R. & Francis, R. J. (1995). How to help psychiatric patients stop smoking. *Psychiatric Services*, **46**, 435–45.

Hughes, J. R., Stead, L. F. & Lancaster, T. (2003). Antidepressants for smoking cessation. *Cochrane Database Systematic Review.* Oxford: Update Software Ltd.

Hurt, R. D., Sachs, D. P. L., Glover, E. D. *et al.* (1997). A comparison of sustained release bupropion and placebo for smoking cessation. *New England Journal of Medicine* **337**(17), 1195–202.

Irvin, J., Hendricks, P. S. & Brandon, T. H. (2003). The increasing recalcitrance of smokers in clinical trials II: Pharmacotherapy trials. *Nicotine and Tobacco Research*, **5**, 27–35.

Jackson, P., Stapleton, J., Russell, M. & Merriman, R. (1986). Predictors of outcome in a general practitioner intervention against smoking. *Previews of Medicine*, **5**, 244–53.

Jorenby, D. E., Leischow, S. J., Nides, M. A. *et al.* (1999). A controlled trial of sustained-release bupropion, a nicotine patch, or both for smoking cessation. *New England Journal of Medicine*, **340**(9), 685–91.

Jorenby, D. E., Hays, J. T., Rigotti, N. A. *et al.* (2006). Efficacy of varenicline, an α4β2 nicotinic acetylcholine receptor partial agonist, vs placebo or sustained-release bupropion for smoking cessation: a randomized controlled trial. *Journal of the American Medical Association*, **296**(1), 56–63.

Kalman, D., Hayes, K., Colby, S. M., Eaton, C. A., Rohsenow, D. J. & Monti, P. M. (2001). Concurrent versus delayed smoking cessation treatment for persons in early alcohol recovery: a pilot study. *Journal of Substance Abuse Treatment*, **20**, 233–8.

Kalman, D., Morrisette, S. B. & George, T. P. (2005). Co-morbidity of smoking in psychiatric and substance use disorders. *American Journal on Addictions*, **14**, 106–23.

Kornitzer, M., Boutsen, M., Dramaix, M., Thijs, J. & Gustavsson. G. (1995). Combined use of nicotine patch and gum in smoking cessation: a placebo-controlled clinical trial. *Preventive Medicine*, **24**, 41–7.

Krishnan-Sarin, S., Meandjiza, B. & O'Malley, S. S. (2003). Nicotine patch and naltrexone for smoking cessation: a preliminary study. *Nicotine and Tobacco Research*, **5**(6), 851–7.

Lader, D. & Meltzer, H. (2000). Smoking related behaviour and attitudes. Office of National Statistics, UK.

Lancaster, T. & Stead, L. F. (1999a).Individual behavioural counselling for smoking cessation. *Cochrane Database Systematic Review.*

Lancaster, T. & Stead, L. F. (1999b). Self help interventions for smoking cessation. *Cochrane Database Systematic Review.* Oxford: Update Software Ltd.

Lancaster, T. & Stead, L. F. (2002).Mecamylamine (a nicotine antagonist) for smoking cessation. *Cochrane Database Systematic Review.* Oxford: Update Software Ltd.

Lancaster, T., Silagy, C. & Fowler, G. (2000). Training Health Professionals in smoking cessation. *Cochrane Database Systematic Review.* Oxford: Update Software Ltd.

Lasser, K., Boyd, J. W., Woolhander, S., Himmelstein, D. U., McCormick, D. & Bor, D. H. (2000). Smoking and mental illness: a population-based prevalence study. *Journal American Medical Association*, **284**, 2606–10.

Law, M. & Tang, J. L. (1995). An analysis of the effectiveness of interventions intended to help people stop smoking. *Archives of Internal Medicine*, **155**, 1933–41.

Leischow, S. J. (1994). Nicotine vaporiser: review of results. In *Future Directions in Nicotine Replacement Therapy*, pp. 99–103. Chester, UK: Adis.

Lovato, C., Linn, G., Stead, L. F. & Best, A. (2003). Impact of tobacco advertising and promotion on increasing adolescent smoking behaviour. *Cochrane Database Systematic Review.* Oxford: Update Software Ltd.

McChargue, D. E., Gulliver, S. B. & Hitsman, B. (2001). Would smokers with schizophrenia benefit from a more flexible approach to smoking treatment? *Addiction*, **97**, 785–93.

Mermelstein, R. J., Karnatz, T. & Reichmann, S. (1992). Smoking. In *Principles and Practice of Relapse Prevention*, ed. P. H. Wilson, pp. 43–68. New York: Guilford Press.

Miller, W. R. (2004). Motivational interviewing in service to health promotion. *American Journal of Health Promotion*, **18**, A1–A10.

Miller, W. R. & Rollnick, S. (2002). *Motivational Interviewing: Preparing People for Change*, 2nd edn. New York: Guilford Press.

Moher, M., Hey, K. & Lancaster, T. (2003). Workplace interventions for smoking cessation. *Cochrane Database Systematic Review.* Oxford: Update Software Ltd.

Nana, A. & Praditsuwan, R. (1998). Clonidine for smoking cessation. *Journal of Medical Association of Thailand*, **81**(2), 87–93.

Niaura, R., Brown, R. A., Goldstein, M. G., Murphy, J. K. & Abrams, D. B. (1996). Transdermal clonidine for smoking cessation: a double-blind randomized dose-response study. *Experimental and Clinical Psychopharmacology*, **4**(3), 285–91.

Niaura, R., Britt, D. M., Shadel, W. M., Goldstein, M., Abrams, D. & Brown, R. (2001). Symptoms of depression and survival experience among three samples of smokers trying to quit. *Psychological Addictive Behaviour*, **15**(1), 13–17.

NICE (2002). Guidance on the use of nicotine replacement therapy (NRT) & Bupropion for smoking cessation. TA39, ISBN: 1–84257-163-x. National Institute for Clinical Excellence, UK.

Noonan, W. & Moyers, T. (1997). Motivational interviewing: a review. *Journal of Substance Misuse*, **2**, 8–16.

O'Malley, S. S., Cooney, J. L., Krishnan-Sarin, S. *et al.* (2006). A controlled trial of naltrexone augmentation of nicotine replacement therapy for smoking cessation. *Archives of Internal Medicine*, **166**(6), 667–74.

Palmer, K. J. & Faulds, D. (1992). Transdermal nicotine: a review of its pharmacodynamic and pharmacokinetic properties, and therapeutic use as an aid to smoking cessation. *Drugs*, **44**, 498–529.

Parrott, S., Godfrey, C., Raw, M., West, M., West, R. & McNeill, A. (1998). Guidance for commissioners on the cost effectiveness of smoking cessation interventions. *Thorax*, **53** (Suppl. 5, Part 2).

Patten, C. A., Martin, J. E., Myers, M. G., Calfas, K. J. & Williams, C. D. (1998). Effectiveness of cognitive-behavioral therapy for smokers with histories of alcohol dependence and depression. *Journal of Studies of Alcohol*, **59**(3), 327–35.

Perkins, K. A., Grobe, J. E., Stiller, R. L., Fonte, C. & Goettler, J. E. (1992). Nasal spray nicotine replacement suppresses cigarette smoking desire and behavior. *Clinical and Pharmacological Therapy*, **52**, 627–34.

Perkins, K. A., Grobe, J. E., Caggiula, A., Wilson, A. S. & Stiller, R. L. (1997). Acute reinforcing effects of low-dose nicotine nasal spray in humans. *Pharmacology, Biochemistry and Behavior*, **56**(2), 235–41.

Perkins, K. A., Donny, E. & Caggiula, A. R. (1999). Sex-differences in nicotine effects and self-administration: review of human and animal evidence. *Nicotine and Tobacco Research*, **1**, 301–15.

Perkins, K. A., Marcus, M. D., Levine, M. D. *et al.* (2001). Cognitive-behavioral therapy to reduce weight concerns improves smoking cessation outcome in weight-concerned women. *Journal of Consulting and Clinical Psychology*, **69**(4), 604–13.

Platt, S., Tannahill, A., Watson, J. & Fraser, E. (1997). Effectiveness of antismoking telephone helpline: follow up survey. *British Medical Journal*, **314**, 1371–5.

Pomerleau, O. F. & Pomerleau, C. S. (1984). Neuroregulators and the reinforcement of smoking: towards a biobehavioral explanation. *Neuroscience Biobehavior Reviews*, **8**, 503–13.

Prochazka, A. V., Weaver, M. J., Keller, R. T., Fryer, G. E., Licari, P. A. & Lofaso, D. (1998). A randomized trial of nortriptyline for smoking cessation. *Archives of Internal Medicine*, **158**, 2035–9.

Reid, R. D., Pipe, A. & Dafoe, W. A. (1999). Is telephone counseling a useful addition to physician advice and nicotine replacement therapy in helping patients to stop smoking? A randomized controlled trial. *Canadian Medical Associative Journal*, **160**(1), 1577–81.

Resnicow, K., DiIorio, C., Soet, J. E., Borrelli, B., Hecht, J. & Ernst, D. (2002). Movitational interviewing in health promotion: It sounds like something is changing. *Health Psychology*, **21**, 444–51.

Richmond, R. L. (1997). A comparison of measures used to assess effectiveness of the transdermal nicotine patch at 1 year. *Addictive behaviours*, **22**(6), 753–7.

Rigotti, N. A. (2002). Treatment of tobacco use and dependence. *New England Journal of Medicine*, **346**, 506–12.

Rigotti, N. A., Arnsten, J. H., McKool, K. M., Wood-Reid, K. M., Pasternak, R. C. & Singer, D. E. (1997). Efficacy of a smoking cessation program for hospital patients. *Archives in Internal Medicine*, **157**(22), 2653–60.

Roddy, E. (2004). ABC of smoking cessation. Bupropion and other non-nicotine pharmacotherapies. *British Medical Journal*, **328**, 509–11.

Rose, J. E. & Behm, F. M. (1987). Refined cigarette smoke as a method for reducing nicotine intake. *Pharmacological and Biochemical Behaviour*, **28**, 305–10.

Rose, J. E. & Levin, E. D. (1991). Concurrent agonist-antagonist administration for the analysis and treatment of drug dependence. *Pharmacological and Biochemical Behaviour*, **41**, 219–26.

Rose, J. E., Behm, F. M., Westman, E. C., Levin, E. D., Stein, R. M. & Ripka, G. V. (1994). Mecamylamine combined with nicotine skin patch facilitates smoking cessation beyond nicontine patch treatment alone. *Clinical and Pharmacological Therapy*, **56**, 86–99.

Rose, J. E., Behm, F. M. & Westman, E. C. (1998). Nicotine-mecamylamine treatment for smoking cessation: the role of pre-cessation therapy. *Experimental and Clinical Psychopharmacology*, **6**(3), 331–43.

Royal College of Physicians (RCP) (2002). Protecting smokers, saving lives: the case for a tobacco and nicotine regulatory authority. London: RCP.

Russell, M. A. H., Jarvis, M. J., Sutherland, G. & Feyerabend, C. (1987). Nicotine replacement in smoking cessation. *Journal of the American Medical Association*, **257**, 3262–65.

Sachs, D. P. L. (1995). Effectiveness of the 4-mg dose of nicotine polacrilex for the initial treatment of high-dependent smokers. *Archives of Internal Medicine*, **155**(18), 1973–80.

Sachs, D. P. L. (1991). Advances in smoking cessation treatment. *Current Pulmonology*, **12**, 139–98.

Sampablo, L. I., Carreras, J. M., Lores, L., Quesada, M. & Sanchez, A. L. (2002). Smoking cessation and bupropion: anxiety and depression as predictors of therapeutic efficacy. *Archivos de Bronconeumologaia*, **38**(8), 351–5.

Schneider, N. G., Olmstead, R., Mody, F. V. *et al.* (1995). Efficacy of a nicotine nasal spray in smoking cessation: a placebo-controlled, double-blind trial. *Addiction*, **90**, 1671–82.

Schneider, N. G., Olmstead, R., Nilsson, F., Mody, F. V., Franzon, M. & Doan, K. (1996). Efficacy of a nicotine inhaler in smoking cessation: a double-blind, placebo controlled trial. *Addiction*, **91**(9), 1293–306.

Schwartz, J. L. (1992). Methods of smoking cessation. *Medical Clinics of North America*, **76**, 451–76.

Shiffman, S., Dresler, C. M., Hajek, P., Gilburt, S. J. A., Targett, D. A. & Strahs, K. R. (2002). Efficacy of a nicotine lozenge for smoking cessation. *Archives of Internal Medicine*, **162**(11), 1267.

Silagy, C., Mant, D., Fowler, G. & Lodge, M. (1994). Meta-analysis on efficacy of nicotine replacement therapies in smoking cessation. *Lancet*, **343**, 139–42.

Silagy, C., Lancaster, T., Stead, L., Mant, D. & Fowler, G. (2002). Nicotine replacement for smoking cessation. *Cochrane Database Systematic Review*. Oxford: Update Software Ltd.

Slemmer, J. E., Martin, B. R. & Damaj, M. I. (2000). Bupropion is a nicotinic antagonist. *Journal of Pharmacological Experimental Therapy*, **295**, 321–7.

Sowden, A., Arblaster, L. & Stead, L. (2002). Community interventions for preventing smoking in young people. *Cochrane Database Systematic Review*. Oxford: Update Software Ltd.

Stolerman, I. P., Goldfarb, T., Fink, R. & Jarvik, M. E. (1973). Influencing cigarette smoking with nicotine antagonists. *Psychopharmacologia*, **28**, 247–59.

Stotts, A. M., DiClemente, C. C. & Dolen-Mullen, P. (2002). One-to-one – a motivational intervention for resistant pregnant smokers. *Addictive Behaviors*, **27**, 275–92.

Sutherland, G., Russell, M. A. H., Stapleton, J., Feyerabend, C. & Ferno, O. (1992). Nasal nicotine spray: a rapid nicotine delivery system. *Psychopharmacology (Berlin)*, **108**, 512–18.

Sutherland, G., Russell, M. A. H., Stapleton, J. & Feyerabend, C. (1993). Glycerol particle cigarettes: a less harmful option for chronic smokers. *Thorax*, **48**, 385–7.

Sutherland, G., Stapleton, J. A., Russell, M. A. H. & Feyerabend, C. (1995). Naltrexone, smoking behaviour and cigarette withdrawal. *Psychopharmacology (Berlin)*, **120**, 418–25.

Tappin, D. M., Lumsden, M. A., McIntyre, D. *et al.* (2000). A pilot study to establish a randomized trial methodology to test the efficacy of a behavioural intervention. *Health Education Research*, **15**, 491–502.

Tashkin, D. P., Kanner, R., Bailey, W. *et al.* (2001). Smoking cessation in patients with chronic obstructive pulmonary disease: a double-blind, placebo-controlled, randomised trial. *Lancet*, **357**, 1571–5.

Tonnesen, P., Norregaard, J., Mikkelsen, K., Jorgensen, S. & Nilsson, F. (1993). A double-blind trial of a nicotine inhaler for smoking cessation. *Journal of the American Medical Association*, **269**, 1268–71.

Tonstad, S., Tønnesen P., Hajek, P., Williams, K. E., Billing, C. B. & Reeves, K. R. (2006). Effect of maintenance therapy with varenicline on smoking cessation: a randomized controlled trial. *Journal of the American Medical Association*, **296**(1), 64–71.

US Department of Health and Human Services (1988). Treatment of tobacco dependence. In *The Health Consequences of Smoking: Nicotine Addiction*, pp. 459–560. Washington, DC: US Government Printing Office.

Viswesvaran, C. & Schmidt, F. L. (1992). A meta-analytic comparison of the effectiveness of smoking cessation methods. *Journal of Applied Psychology*, **77**, 554–61.

Wallstrom, M., Nilsson, F. & Hirsch, J. M. (2000). A randomized, double-blind, placebo-controlled clinical evaluation of a nicotine sublingual tablet in smoking cessation. *Addiction*, **95**(8), 1161–71.

West, R. & Shiffman, S. (2001). Effects of oral nicotine dosing forms on cigarette withdrawal symptoms and craving: a systematic review. *Psychopharmacologia*, **155**(2), 115–22.

West, R., Hajek, P., Foulds, J., Nilsson, F., May, S. & Meadows, A. (2000). A comparison of the abuse liability and dependence potential of nicotine patch, gum, spray and inhaler. *Psychopharmacologia*, **149**(3), 198–202.

Wetter, D. W., Fiore, M. C., Baker, T. B. & Young, T. B. (1995). Tobacco withdrawal and nicotine replacement influence objective measures of sleep. *Journal of Consulting and Clinical Psychology*, **63**, 658–67.

White, A. R., Rampes, H. & Ernst, E. (2002). Acupuncture for smoking cessation. *Cochrane Database review*. Oxford: Update Software Ltd.

Ziedonis, D. M. & George, T. P. (1997). Schizophrenia and nicotine use: report of a pilot smoking cessation program and review of neurobiological and clinical issues. *Schiophrenia Bulletin*, **23**(2), 247–54.

24

Treatment of co-occurring psychiatric and substance use disorders

Douglas M. Ziedonis, Ed. Day, Erin L. O'Hea, Jonathan Krejci,
Jeffrey A. Berman and David Smelson

Editor's note

The co-morbidity of a concurrent substance use disorder and a non-substance major psychiatric disorder is quite common. Yet there is very little data available to inform the clinician as to what treatment(s) might be best for this particular group of patients with this particular set of substance abuse plus non-substance psychiatric co-morbidity. In general, the limited research available, consensus recommendations and clinical experiences all suggest that integrated treatment, i.e. treatment by the same group of providers that addresses both the substance misuse and the other major mental illness is most effective. However, there are exceptions to this rule and providers must be flexible and offer a combination of services regarding what works best in treating the mental disorder plus what works best in the treatment of the specific substance abuse disorder. While on the surface this appears to be logical and pragmatic, this kind of reasoning does not always work. For example, there is some evidence that lithium is less effective in people with bipolar disorder complicated by substance abuse than it is in bipolar disorder alone. Furthermore, some pharmacological agents used to treat some psychiatric disorders have an increased liability for abuse and dependency, suggesting greater caution in using these interventions when substance abuse is a comorbid issue. The most efficacious treatment approach is probably integrated multi-modal treatment which involves the same group of caregivers providing treatment to both the mental illness and the substance misuse disorder. These integrated treatments draw from and utilize a wide variety of psychosocial interventions that are combined with more specific psychopharmacological strategies that address the specific psychiatric disorder and some of the craving and withdrawal symptoms of the substance misuse. However, much more research needs to be done in this important and common area of practice.

Introduction

Co-occurring mental illness and addiction is common and worsens patient clinical course, treatment compliance, and outcomes (McLellan *et al.*, 1998; SAMSHA, 2003; Westermeyer *et al.*, 2004). Co-occurring disorders are so common that the phenomenon has become the expectation in addiction, mental health, and medical treatment settings. Recent research and clinical experience has improved the system, programme, and clinical interventions that can help these individuals. This chapter will review empirically validated treatment interventions that have been developed to better address co-occurring mental illness and addiction.

Despite being common, the co-occurrence of mental illness and substance use presents a diagnostic and treatment challenge for clinicians and treatment services. The term 'dual diagnosis' is often used to describe this problem, although it lacks precision in describing a very heterogeneous problem. The pattern of co-morbidity may vary between co-morbid mood, anxiety and personality disorders in patients attending substance misuse treatment services, and co-morbid alcohol, cannabis and cocaine misuse in patients accessing general psychiatric services (Abou-Saleh, 2004). Therefore, we prefer the term co-occurring disorder as opposed to dual diagnosis.

The high rate of co-occurring severe mental health and substance use problems has been increasingly recognized in the international research literature over the past 20 years (Maslin, 2003). The National Co-morbidity Study (NCS) and the Epidemiological Catchment Area (ECA) Study both demonstrated that co-occurring mental illness and addiction are very common in the general population, criminal justice system, and treatment system. In the NCS, individuals with alcohol dependence had high rates of clinical depression during their lifetime (24% major depression and 11% dysthymia for men and 49% major depression and 21% dysthymia for women), and individuals with bipolar disorder had high rates of alcohol (61%) and other drug (41%) dependence. High rates of personality disorders have also been reported in patients with substance use disorders, particularly antisocial, narcissistic, and borderline personality disorders (Ross *et al.*, 1988; SAMSHA, 2003; Ziedonis *et al.*, 1994). Personality disorders in substance abuse treatment settings have a poorer response to treatment and a greater risk of suicide (American Psychiatric Association, 1994; SAMSHA, 2003). Finally, tobacco dependence is the most common substance of abuse in the United States and often occurs among individuals being treated for other forms of addiction and mental health problems (Ziedonis & Williams, 2003). Despite methodological problems such as differences in sampling methods, populations and diagnostic systems, these co-morbidity trends appear to be consistent across treatment settings in the USA (Mueser *et al.*, 2000), the UK (Graham *et al.*, 2001; Menezes *et al.*, 1996), Germany (Krausz *et al.*, 1996), and Australia (Fowler *et al.*, 1998).

Individuals with co-occurring mental illness and addiction have more cravings, withdrawal symptoms, cognitive impairment, depressive symptoms, relapses, and poorer responses to traditional treatments compared to individuals with addictive disorders alone (Carol *et al.*, 2001; Smelson *et al.*, 2001, 2002a, 2002b 2003). These individuals often have wide fluctuations in mental status, increased suicide risk, poorer medication compliance, increased hospitalizations and emergency room visits, and increased HIV rates, hepatitis C rates, physical trauma, and other co-existing medical morbidity/mortality. Finally, individuals with dual diagnosis have higher rates of homelessness, greater chances of perpetrating violence and being the victim of traumatic events, and greater incidence of illegal activities compared to individuals with mental illness or addiction alone (SAMHSA, 2003).

Assessment and diagnosis of dual diagnosis

An initial assessment includes a review of parallel time lines of the history of substance use, mood, psychotic and other psychiatric disorders along with any cognitive problems. It should also include an assessment of prior episodes of treatment for co-occurring disorders. The time-line can be used to assess the chronology of symptom development (i.e. whether the signs and symptoms predate or follow the onset of repetitive substance use), whether symptoms were present during extended drug-

free periods (e.g. of 3 months or more), and the impact of each disorder on the presentation, clinical course, and outcome of the other(s). Structured screening instruments and mental status evaluations are also encouraged as they can improve the assessment of psychiatric symptoms in patients with co-occurring disorders. Finally, corroborative information from family members, friends or significant others is invaluable and strongly recommended.

As in the care of any patient with depressive symptoms, suicidal ideation should be assessed regularly and in a systematic manner. The frequency of suicide attempts and completions is substantially higher among patients with substance use disorders than in the general population (Crumley, 1990). The completed suicide rate is approximately 3–4 times that found in the general population (Murphy, 1988), with a lifetime mortality of approximately 15% (Hawton, 1987). Clearly, the presence of a major depressive disorder substantially increases the suicide risk of these patients (Dorpat, 1974).

Substance use disorders are also associated with greater than average risk for other forms of violence, including homicide (Budde, 1989; Langevin *et al.*, 1982). Anxiety, irritability, increased aggression, impaired impulse control, and impaired reality testing may be due either to the direct effects of the substance or to a withdrawal syndrome. Cocaine, hallucinogens, phencyclidine (PCP), stimulants and alcohol (Brecher *et al.*, 1988; Liskow & Goodwin, 1987; Luisada, 1978) are all substances whose use may be associated with aggression. Further, alcohol, opioids, and sedative hypnotics may lead to withdrawal syndromes associated with a greater risk of violence (Liskow & Goodwin, 1987). Finally, patients intoxicated on marijuana or hallucinogens may inadvertently commit violent acts in response to perceptual distortions coupled with high levels of anxiety and paranoia (American Psychiatric Association, 1994).

All patients with substance use disorders should be carefully assessed for the presence of psychiatric symptoms and disorders (Zimmerman *et al.*, 2004). Many symptoms of psychopathology including anxiety, depression, mania, and psychosis are a direct result of substance induced intoxication, withdrawal, or chronic use, and must be addressed during the initial session (Zimmerman *et al.*, 2004). Further, personality traits and disorders often exacerbate the presentation of psychiatric symptoms in individuals with co-morbid substance use disorders. Axis II disorders and traits need to be diagnosed, assessed and formally addressed early in treatment because of their potential impact on the treatment process. In addiction treatment settings, depression, anxiety, and personality disorders are very common. They are more often identified than other disorders, such as PTSD, adult ADHD, learning disabilities, social anxiety disorder, eating disorders, and compulsive behaviours (e.g. gambling), which are also common but often remain undetected. Further, subthreshold mood and anxiety disorders (prominent symptoms of depression or anxiety that do not meet full criteria for DSM diagnoses) can be common; however, due to a lack of research in this area, we are limited to empirically based knowledge as to how to address such issues in treatment. Ongoing monitoring of subthreshold symptoms in treatment, coupled with general mood management and relapse prevention therapy, is a minimum approach.

Motivation to change may vary in an individual depending on the substance of abuse and the form of psychopathology. That is, a patient's motivation for change may be very low for quitting one substance, but not for others. Also, patients may be motivated to quit using substances but not to attend treatment or Twelve Step meetings. It is important to assess such issues separately to avoid the common mistake of dismissing such patients as entirely unmotivated. In general, it is preferable to begin treatment with the problem area for which the patient expresses the greatest level of motivation and self-efficacy (DiClemente *et al.*, 2004).

Treatment models with emphasis on integrated care

Psychiatric treatment services have traditionally been offered separately from services treating substance misuse problems. The two services are often run by different organizations, use separate funding streams, and have differing ideologies and eligibility criteria (Drake & Mueser, 2000). Whereas substance misuse services have required a degree of motivation on the part of the client, psychiatric services are often obliged to treat all patients. Unfortunately the needs of those with severe mental health problems who abuse drugs or alcohol have not always been met by such a system.

Three treatment models have been described for tackling co-morbidity issues and can be classified as follows (Jeffrey *et al.*, 2000):

1. *Serial*: where one treatment, either psychiatric or substance misuse, is followed by the other.
2. *Parallel*: where there is concurrent but separate treatment of both psychiatric and substance misuse disorder.
3. *Integrated*: where the same personnel provide substance misuse and psychiatric treatment concurrently.

The first two models represent the traditional system, and reviews of the literature since the mid-1980s have highlighted a number of problems with such approaches (Drake *et al.*, 1998b). Integrated treatment involves modifications of traditional approaches to both mental health and substance misuse treatment. Over time, a variety of models have evolved and are described below.

There is some evidence from the USA that patients with co-morbid substance misuse problems treated in non-integrated mental health programmes have poor outcomes (Havassy *et al.*, 2000). The Dual Diagnosis Good Practice Guideline issued by the UK Department of Health in 2002 recommended that individuals with both severe mental health and substance misuse problems deserve 'high quality, patient focused and integrated care', and that this should 'be delivered within mental health services' (Department of Health, 2002). It concluded that integrated care by a single team delivers better outcomes than serial or parallel care, but that more UK-based research was required to establish the evidence base. However, the Dual Diagnosis Practice Guideline recommended that well organized parallel care can be used as a stepping stone to integration. Yet although there is a clear movement towards integrated treatment services in the UK (Department of Health, 2002) and Australia (Tesson & Proudfoot, 2003), this is not thus far supported by a strong research evidence base. A Cochrane systematic review of psychosocial treatment programmes for people with both severe mental illness and substance misuse was conducted by Jeffrey *et al.* (2000). It included six randomized trials, four of which were small, and in general the quality of design and reporting was not found to be high. The authors concluded that 'the current momentum for integrated programmes is not based on good evidence'. There was no clear evidence found supporting an advantage of any type of substance misuse programme for those with serious mental illness over the value of standard care.

A broader review by Drake of 36 studies of the effectiveness of integrated treatment for dual diagnosis patients identified 10 studies (six uncontrolled, four controlled) of comprehensive, integrated outpatient treatment programmes that were effective in engaging patients in services, reducing substance use and sustaining remission. Outcomes relating to hospital use, psychiatric symptoms and other domains were less consistent (Drake *et al.*, 1998b). In another study, Drake *et al.* (1998a) performed a large multicentre controlled study comparing the Assertive Community Treatment (ACT) model with standard case management for the delivery of integrated dual disorder treatment. The findings indicated modest advantages for the ACT approach in achieving better outcomes for alcohol use disorders, and good substance abuse treatment outcomes across both programmes, probably due to treatment diffusion. High fidelity to the model was associated with better outcomes. Other studies show a modest benefit for integrated treatment in this patient population (Bond *et al.*, 1991; Hellerstein *et al.*, 1995; Lehman *et al.*, 1993; Mercer-McFadden *et al.*, 1997).

There have been two major randomized trials of integrated treatment packages reported in the UK. Barrowclough *et al.* (2001) conducted a randomized, single-blind controlled comparison of routine care with a programme of routine care integrated with motivational interviewing, cognitive behaviour therapy, and family or a caregiver intervention (Barrowclough *et al.*, 2001; Haddock *et al.*, 2003). Results showed that the intensive treatment package resulted in a significant improvement in the main outcome of patients' general functioning when compared with treatment as usual, and that this improvement persisted up to an 18-month follow-up. There were other benefits to patients, including a significant reduction in positive symptoms, a reduction in symptom exacerbations, and an increase in days abstinent from drugs and alcohol over the 12-month period.

Graham *et al.* adopted a different approach whereby individual assertive outreach teams were treated as whole units for integration (Copello *et al.*, 2001). These teams were provided with training to deliver a cognitive behavioural integrated treatment approach aimed at increasing the awareness of the relationship between psychosis and substance use as well as providing a range of skills to manage these difficulties (Graham *et al.*, 2003c; Graham *et al.*, 2004). Results indicated that the teams increased in their confidence and skills, which were maintained over time. In addition, there were significant improvements in client engagement over the course of the study, and a reduction in alcohol and cannabis consumption (Graham *et al.*, 2006).

In summary, controlled research studies of comprehensive dual diagnosis programmes began to appear in the mid-1990s (Drake *et al.*, 2001), and these studies with experimental or quasi-experimental designs support the effectiveness of integrated dual diagnosis treatments (Brunette *et al.*, 2001; Drake *et al.*, 1997; Ho *et al.*, 1999; Jerrell & Ridgely, 1995). Yet all these research studies published to date have had small sample sizes and have faced a range of methodological problems (Hellerstein *et al.*, 2001). Integrated treatment can be defined in many ways and many different psychiatric and substance use treatment approaches can be tested. The patient group is heterogeneous with varying degrees of psychiatric and substance use severity, and it is not clear that different research samples are comparable. There is a lack of validated outcome measures for both substance abuse and psychotic illness for these patients, and self-report may be particularly unreliable in this group. Most studies have experienced a high drop-out rate, and the small sample sizes and labour-intensive interventions mean limited statistical power and difficulty in blinding raters to treatments. Nonetheless, there is now a substantial body of evidence that suggests that improved outcomes are achieved through integrating a range of treatment strategies and philosophies into a comprehensive treatment package. A number of critical components of integrated treatment have been suggested, including the use of staged interventions, assertive outreach techniques, social support interventions, motivational enhancement approaches and multiple psychotherapeutic modalities (Drake *et al.*, 2001; Mueser & Drake, 2003). Such an approach should also try to be comprehensive, to adopt a long-term perspective, to be aware of cultural issues and to aim primarily at a reduction of negative consequences.

Clinical treatment interventions

The management of co-morbidity is a complex topic with a limited but growing evidence base. It is not realistic to expect a single treatment process to be effective for all types of co-morbidity due of the substantial degree of heterogeneity in both the mental health and substance use problems (Kavanagh *et al.*, 2003a). Furthermore, it is difficult to tease out issues related to the model of service delivery and the actual psychological or pharmacological interventions delivered from the existing evidence base. Several reviewers have concluded that no standardized interventions for co-morbid disorders have been shown in multiple studies to improve outcome (Jeffrey *et al.*, 2000; Teeson & Proudfoot, 2003), but a number of different approaches have been described.

General clinical interventions

Clinicians face many challenges when working with individuals with co-occurring disorders. Research has demonstrated improved outcomes with integrated substance use and mental health treatment interventions (Drake *et al.*, 1998b). Treatment specifically targeting psychiatric co-morbidity is imperative, rather than assuming the psychopathology will spontaneously remit with effective substance abuse treatment. Integrated treatment addresses both mental illness and addiction and often includes both integrated psychosocial approaches and medications (psychiatric and addiction treatment medications). We now consider the general issues regarding medication and psychosocial treatment options, and present specific information for specific co-occurring mental illness subtypes.

Psychopharmacology

There are no official national guidelines for prescribing for patients with co-morbidity in the UK. The National Institute for Health and Clinical Excellence (NICE) produced guidance on the use of newer (atypical) antipsychotic drugs for the treatment of schizophrenia in 2002 (NICE, 2002). This report made no specific recommendations about patients with co-morbidity issues, but did comment that observational studies would provide information on the use of atypical antipsychotics in individuals with schizophrenia and substance abuse disorders.

In 2003 the British Association for Psychopharmacology convened a meeting of experts in the field of addiction and co-morbidity, and a discussion of the important issues identified consensus and areas of uncertainty regarding the quality of the evidence and strength of recommendations. A draft of this discussion and review of the literature was circulated to all participants and other interested parties, and ultimately produced evidence-based guidelines for the pharmacological management of substance misuse, addiction and co-morbidity in 2004 (Lingford-Hughes *et al.*, 2004). The guidelines note a dearth of information and the difficulty in producing guidance. but make the following recommendations.

Medications to treat psychiatric disorders

Regardless of whether an individual is diagnosed solely with a non-substance use related psychiatric disorder or with co-occurring disorders, in most cases the same psychiatric medications are recommended. Although there is limited evidence to guide the choice of medications, clinical issues including liability, safety, and tolerability/side effects must be considered when prescribing traditional psychiatric medications. In treating some psychiatric disorders (e.g., anxiety disorders and ADHD), the most widely used medications may include those with high abuse liability (e.g., benzodiazepines, stimulants) and are therefore a concern with the individual with a substance use disorder. Clinicians are also encouraged to consider overdose risk, seizure risk, sedation, liver toxicity, and the interactions between substances and medications.

Medications to treat substance use disorders

The commonly recommended medications to manage detoxification, protracted abstinence, or agonist maintenance treatment, should be considered for patients with co-occurring mental illness and addiction. There are no available data to suggest different medication treatments for detoxification, protracted abstinence or agonist treatment for this population.

Psychosocial treatments

Integrated psychosocial treatments

Psychosocial treatment continues to be the cornerstone of addiction treatment, and it is equally important in treating co-occurring disorders. Some of the most recent advances in treating co-occurring disorders have been in the development of new psychotherapy approaches. In general, these innovative psychotherapies have been developed for specific subtypes of co-occurring disorders. These approaches integrate and modify the evidence-based core addiction treatments (Motivational Enhancement Therapy, Relapse Prevention/Cognitive Behavioural Therapy, and 12-step Facilitation) with psychotherapy approaches that are evidence-based core therapies for that specific mental illness. Several excellent examples of evidence-based innovative psychotherapy approaches exist to guide clinicians in treating a variety of co-occurring disorders, including PTSD and addiction treatment (Najavits *et al.*, 1998), bipolar disorder and addiction treatment (Weiss *et al.*, 2000), schizophrenia and addiction treatment (Bellack *et al.*, 2001; Carey, 1995; Drake & Mueser, 2000; Roberts *et al.*, 1999; Ziedonis & Stern, 2001) and borderline personality disorder and addiction treatment (Linehan *et al.*, 1999).

Motivational interviewing

Motivational interviewing, when added to standard treatment, appears to increase attendance (Martino *et al.*, 2000; Swanson *et al.*, 1999). There is also evidence that MI cannot only go beyond just enhancing engagement with treatment, but can also produce modest behaviour change in the short term among people with severe mental disorders. Kavanagh *et al.* (2003b) report a brief intervention incorporating motivational interviewing as a primary intervention strategy. A pilot study randomized 25 inpatients in their first to third episode of psychosis to standard care or to a brief intervention called Start Over and Survive or SOS. All participants in the SOS group who received at least one session of motivational interviewing reported less substance use at six months, compared with 58% in routine care. However, nearly 38% of patients allocated to

SOS did not proceed beyond the initial rapport building, and the authors highlight the continuing challenge of initial engagement in sessions with this population. Yet most interventions, even if they have motivational interviewing, are complex packages of care incorporating a variety of elements of treatment.

Cognitive behavioural therapy

The COMPASS Programme in the UK developed an integrated treatment model using C-BIT, a cognitive behavioural manual-based approach (Graham *et al.*, 2003a, 2003b). C-BIT is a structured but flexible integrated psychosocial treatment approach based on the established principles and techniques of cognitive therapy for emotional disorders, substance misuse and psychosis. This integrated treatment approach sought to increase knowledge and awareness amongst mental health treatment staff of the relationship between problem substance use and psychosis. A motivational attitude was adopted, and the C-BIT approach guided clinicians and teams to techniques most suited to a patient's stage of engagement in treatment and motivation to change. A quasi-experimental time-lag design produced evidence that using this approach, staff acquired confidence and skills relevant to working with combined problems, and this in turn yielded beneficial effects for patients in terms of engagement and substance use (Graham, 2004).

Other integrated psychosocial treatments

Studies conducted by Barrowclough *et al.* (2001); Haddock *et al.* (2003) are an example of a synthesis of different treatments to create a comprehensive integrated treatment package. A total of 66 adults with a non-affective psychosis and a substance use disorder who had at least 10 hours contact per week with a caregiver were invited to participate, and 36 (55%) consented. They were then randomly allocated to routine care (case management, medication, monitoring and access to rehabilitation services) or routine care plus integrated intervention. The latter combined three separate treatment approaches: motivational interviewing to increase motivation to change in those who were ambivalent, individual cognitive behaviour therapy modified from approaches used to ameliorate delusions and hallucinations in patients with chronic psychosis, and a family intervention with an emphasis on promoting a family response consistent with the motivational interviewing style. The additional intervention amounted to a median of 22 individual sessions and a median of 11 integrated family sessions over nine months, plus practical advice and assistance from a family support worker. At 12 months, 33% of the integrated treatment group had relapsed, compared with 67% in routine care, but the integrated treatment group did not have consistently better symptom scores at all time points. No significant differences were found between treatment groups in terms of provider or cost outcomes.

Components of integrated treatment

Once the principle of integrated treatment for co-morbid problems is accepted, the next question concerns which elements should form part of a comprehensive treatment package. A wide range of psychosocial treatment approaches have been used to tackle the problem of co-occurring severe mental illness and substance use. Motivational treatments aimed to improve engagement of patients in treatment services have shown considerable promise (Baker *et al.*, 2002; Kavanagh *et al.*, 2003a; Martino *et al.*, 2002). Other than motivational interviewing, it has been difficult to be prescriptive about the specific elements that should be included in a multi-component intervention, although certain elements appear frequently in the literature. These include psychological strategies for managing psychotic symptoms (Barrowclough *et al.*, 2001; Graham *et al.*, 2003b), drug refusal skills training (Bradizza & Stasiewicz, 1997; Shaner *et al.*, 2003), relapse prevention planning (Graham *et al.*, 2003c; Weiss *et al.*, 2003), social network enhancement and family therapy (Barrowclough *et al.*, 2001), and tackling issues surrounding employment and leisure activities (Swanson *et al.*, 1999). Given the complexity of co-occurring disorders, it is likely that combinations of strategies will offer synergistic effects, and that different combinations will prove useful with different patients (Kavanagh *et al.*, 2003a). It may also be useful to try to match symptom severity to treatment intensity (Kavanagh *et al.*, 2003a, 2003b; Timko & Sempel, 2004).

Integrated treatment for specific co-occurring mental illness subtypes

Major depression and dysthymia

Symptoms of depression are common amongst patients in substance abuse treatment. Depression may be a consequence of the effect of substances on the brain, vulnerability to depression alone, and the chaotic and dangerous lifestyle of many substance abusers. Having an addiction is likely to induce sadness, loss of self-esteem and demoralization. Although symptoms of depression that are related to alcohol intoxication or withdrawal often remit in the first few weeks of abstinence (Linnoila, 1989), many patients have a co-occurring mood disorder that requires medication and/or psychosocial treatment of the depression.

Choosing an antidepressant

The literature does not support any particular antidepressant as being more efficacious than another in this population. The choice must be based on tolerability, abuse liability, medication interactions, safety considerations, and favourable responses of family members to a particular medication. For this population, some safety issues include hepatic toxicity, cardiac toxicity, seizure risk, and agitation. Another consideration is that sleep disturbances, primarily insomnia, are common in both depressed patients and individuals with substance abuse disorders (Mackenzie *et al.*, 1999; Stein *et al.*, 2004). These problems may be addressed with non-pharmacological strategies such as stress reduction techniques and good sleep hygiene. However, if an antidepressant is being prescribed for affective symptoms, then it may be advisable to choose a more sedating antidepressant medication that can be taken at bedtime (e.g. mirtazapine or paroxetine) or to add trazodone (a weak antidepressant with strong sedating qualities).

Based on clinical experience and the literature, selective serotonin reuptake inhibitors (SSRIs), as well as other newer antidepressants such as bupropion, mirtazapine, and venlafaxine can be viewed as first line medication treatments for the clinical depression found in this population. These specific antidepressants tend to have better tolerability, less issues related to safety (as discussed above), and less aversive side effects. There is some literature supporting the usefulness of the older tricyclic medications, such as imipramine and desipramine (Kosten *et al.*, 1992; Kranzler *et al.*, 1995; Mason *et al.*, 1996; Nunes & Quitkin, 1997; Roy, 1998); however, few clinicians continue to use these medications due to the side effect risks and risk of toxicity especially in overdose. Of note, depressed patients in methadone maintenance treatment have not done better on an SSRI vs. placebo in treating the depression (Dean *et al.*, 2002; Nunes *et al.*, 1998; Petrakis *et al.*, 1998), and both imipramine and desipramine have been found more effective than placebo in randomized trials in similar samples (Nunes *et al.*, 1998; Ziedonis *et al.*, 1992). Imipramine can reduce cocaine craving and euphoria, but has less effect on cocaine use (Nunes *et al.*, 1995), but it may help the co-morbid depression. A meta-analysis concluded that antidepressant medication exerts a modest beneficial effect for depressive symptoms but concurrent therapy for the substance abuse is necessary (Nunes & Levin, 2004). In summary, the SSRIs are first-line agents and the TCAs are second-line agents in treating opiate agonist maintained depressed patients.

Remission of depressive symptoms should be the goal of medication treatment for individuals with depressive disorders. To date, there are no data that suggest the duration of an antidepressant trial or any other treatment tactics should be different for depression when it occurs in the presence of a substance disorder. Regarding the duration of therapy, patients with co-occurring disorders may need to be seen by the clinician more often than other depressed patients. Continuous and detailed attention to symptom reduction and more frequent incremental medication adjustment must be the cornerstone of medication monitoring. If the patient's pattern of use worsens, sessions may need to be scheduled on a weekly basis. Continuation and maintenance treatment are as important in the co-occurring disorders patient as in all depressed patients, and these should occur for at least six months after depressive symptoms have remitted. However, based on clinical experience, a longer continuation and maintenance phase may be advisable if the patient has a strong family history or if suicidal symptoms have been prominent throughout treatment (Jenike, 1997).

Psychosocial treatment

As with patients without a history of substance abuse, psychosocial interventions are an important component of treatment with this population. Core psychosocial treatments for this population include motivational enhancement therapy (Miller *et al.*, 1995), cognitive therapy (Beck *et al.*, 1993) and interpersonal therapy. Psychosocial treatments target specific aspects of depression, including cognition, behaviour, and affect. Depression might be related to grief, trauma, shame, alienation, loneliness and low self-esteem. In general, targeted therapies are short-term and seek to alleviate the depressive condition per se, rather than to change character.

A few integrated models of substance abuse and depression have been described. Daley *et al.* (2003) developed a recovery-oriented approach that integrates strategies used in addiction counselling, cognitive therapy, interpersonal psychotherapies, motivational interviewing and behavioural skills training. It draws on recovery concepts derived from substance abuse treatment as well as from empirically based mental health and substance abuse treatment approaches.

Bipolar disorder

Substance use disorders co-occur more often with bipolar disorder than with any other mental illness (Regier *et al.*, 1990). Most studies in mental health settings report at least 50% of patients with bipolar disorder have a substance use disorder. Bipolar disorder worsens impulsivity and compliance. Substance abuse worsens the bipolar illness course by increasing the severity and frequency of manic, depressive, and mixed episodes with an earlier age of onset and slower symptom remission (Salloum & Thase, 2000). The few medication studies for this co-occurring disorder subtype found better efficacy and treatment compliance with valproate sodium as a mood stabilizer for bipolar disorder than lithium (Bowden, 2001; Brady *et al.*, 1995; Geller *et al.*, 1998; Nunes *et al.*, 1990; O'Connell *et al.*, 1991; Weiss *et al.*, 1998), though Geller *et al.* (1998) did find that, in adolescents, lithium appeared to help both disorders. Possible reasons why lithium may be less effective in this population are its increased side effects and toxicity and the difficulty of achieving steady blood levels in this population. Carbamazepine's use in this population is supported by a few positive outcomes studies (Brady *et al.*, 2002). Olanzapine, quetiapine and risperidone are now FDA approved to treat bipolar disorder and expert consensus supports their consideration even though there have been only a few pilot studies in this population (Brown *et al.*, 2002).

Based on clinical experience, the first-line pharmacological treatment for severe manic or mixed episodes includes either lithium plus an antipsychotic or valproate plus an antipsychotic. For mixed episodes, valproate may be preferred over lithium. Atypical antipsychotics are preferred over typical antipsychotics because of the relatively benign side effect profile, with most of the evidence supporting the use of olanzapine or risperidone (Sajatovic *et al.*, 2002; Sattar *et al.*, 2003). Short-term adjunctive treatment with a benzodiazepine may also be helpful; however, given the abuse potential of benzodiazepines, the use of this medication should be limited in duration of use. For a depressive episode lithium or lamotrigine are recommended based on clinical experience and antidepressant monotherapy is not recommended. Some clinicians initiate simultaneous treatment with lithium and an antidepressant with the use of bupropion as a first-line antidepressant medication in this situation.

Integrating psychosocial treatments to address both bipolar and substance use disorders is also important. Weiss *et al.* (2000) have developed an effective integrated psychosocial group treatment approach for this population. This approach blends cognitive and behavioural techniques that have been found to be effective in both populations as well as specific ways to enhance motivation to change, coping strategies, and self-efficacy. Interpersonal therapy or cognitive behavioural therapy can be used to target symptoms of bipolar depression.

Anxiety disorders

Anxiety disorders and symptoms commonly co-occur with substance abuse. Different substances during different drug states (intoxication, acute withdrawal, protracted withdrawal) can result in symptoms of anxiety, however. Conversely, substance use may have been an effort to self-medicate anxiety symptoms. Regardless of the pathogenesis, anxiety disorders frequently go undiagnosed in substance abuse treatment settings. Data from the National Comorbidity Study indicate that about one half (41%–65%) of individuals with a substance use disorder, particularly women, may have an anxiety disorder at some time in their lives (Kessler *et al.*, 1996). Careful assessment and integrated treatment, including medications and addiction and mental health psychosocial treatments, are recommended.

Panic disorder

Individuals with co-occurring panic disorder and a substance use disorder tend to respond well to treatment integrating a SSRI and psychosocial therapy (Bakker *et al.*, 2000). Though SSRIs are clearly the first line of pharmacological treatment for these individuals, tricyclic antidepressants may be considered if several SSRIs have been found to be ineffective. Though benzodiazepines are used as a first-line treatment for panic disorder for individuals without substance use disorders, they are not suggested for those with substance use problems as the risks of abuse and dependence are substantial. In some rare cases, benzodiazepines may be considered if the patient has no history of abusing or misusing benzodiazepines, has a strong family history of panic disorder, develops severe depression in the context of ongoing panic symptoms, and is fully informed of the risks of taking benzodiazepines. Prescribing must be judicious and use closely monitored. Each tablet prescribed should be accounted for in a log, and a 'pill count' should be part of every visit.

Similar to generalized anxiety, panic-like symptoms may be experienced by individuals in various stage of substance use (intoxication, withdrawal) or may have been present prior to the substance abuse disorder. Clinicians are encouraged to do a thorough evaluation of patient use of stimulating substances (e.g. cocaine, tobacco) when confronted with a case of panic disorder. Patients may also benefit from psychoeducation regarding the body's autonomic system and its sensitivity to stimulants. Psychosocial treatment for panic disorder includes cognitive behavioural therapy techniques that help the patient develop strategies on how to manage these symptoms, including the knowledge that a panic attack is often not really a medical emergency (O'Hea *et al.*, 2002). Exposure therapy has been found to be efficacious in treating panic disorder in patients without substance use disorders who may have or not have agoraphobia (Barlow, 2002). However, clinicians are advised that exposure therapy will likely be ineffective for those patients continuing to take acute anti-anxiety medications such as alprazolam or diazepam. This is because in order for the exposure therapy to work, the patient must experience the anxiety symptoms, which are often masked by anxiolytics. Finally, more research is needed to assess whether traditional exposure therapy should be a first line treatment with patients with co-occurring substance use and panic disorders.

Post-traumatic stress disorder (PTSD)

PTSD is very common among patients with substance use disorders (12%–34%), particularly among women (30%–59%) (Leskin & Sheikh, 2001). Many women with PTSD and substance use disorders reported childhood physical and/or sexual abuse; men with both disorders more often experienced crime victimization or war trauma (Kessler *et al.*, 1995). Substance abuse is often viewed by the patient as 'self-medication' to cope with the overwhelming emotional pain of PTSD (Chilcoat & Breslau, 1998; Cottler *et al.*, 1992; Grice *et al.*, 1995; Najavits *et al.*, 2003). PTSD symptoms are common triggers for substance use. Unfortunately, people with PTSD and substance abuse are also more likely to experience further trauma than people with substance abuse alone (Dansky *et al.*, 1998). Repeated trauma is common through domestic violence, child abuse, and some substance abuse lifestyles (e.g., prostitution or the drug trade). Helping protect the patient against future trauma may be an important part of work in treatment. Also, becoming abstinent from substances does not resolve PTSD; indeed, some PTSD symptoms worsen with abstinence and are highly likely to trigger a relapse if not successfully treated (Brady, 2001; Kofoed *et al.*, 1993).

Integrated psychosocial treatments for co-occurring PTSD and substance use disorders have been developed (Brady & Clary, 2003; Brady *et al.*, 2001; Najavits *et al.*, 2003; Trifflemann, 1999) and focus on providing education about the disorders and teaching coping skills to gain control over the PTSD symptoms (Jacobson *et al.*, 2001). Helping patients understand the link between their PTSD and substance use also is an important part of treatment. Other skills include activity scheduling, seeking out interpersonal support, identifying and coping with PTSD and substance abuse triggers, and learning to communicate more effectively with others.

Medications for treating PTSD and co-occurring substance use disorders follow the general recommendations for treating PTSD alone from sources such as the APA Practice Guideline for PTSD (Ursano *et al.*, 2004). The SSRIs are considered first-line medication treatment for this disorder with venlafaxine a second-line treatment if the SSRIs prove ineffective or are not well tolerated. Benzodiazepines and other GABA receptor active medications should also be avoided. These include zolpidem and zalepalon. Though benzodiazepines prescribed to help manage PTSD are a particular danger due to their abuse potential, some patients with severe PTSD symptoms may benefit from benzodiazepines if monitored carefully.

Adult attention deficit disorder

Studies have found that about 17 to 50 percent of patients with a substance use disorder have adult attention deficit disorder (ADD). Attention deficit in adults is a controversial area concerning diagnosis and treatment. Although some individuals with this disorder may try to 'self-medicate' with stimulants, most patients with adult ADD who abuse substances do so with tobacco, alcohol, or marijuana. Establishing a diagnosis of ADD can be complicated in a patient with co-occurring addiction as there is considerable symptom overlap with other psychiatric disorders and with effects of substance use and withdrawal (American Psychiatric Association, 1994). Ongoing assessments over a period of prolonged abstinence are important and may uncover other psychiatric disorders including learning disabilities.

Psychiatric medications commonly recommended for ADD are stimulants, which unfortunately have abuse liability. Medications to consider for treating ADD in this population include the recently approved selective norepinephrine reuptake inhibitor atomoxetine or other off-label medications that have been found clinically efficacious in treating ADD such as the antidepressant bupropion. But there are no validated or even standardly recognized treatments for co-morbid ADHD and substance abuse.

Personality disorders

Personality disorders commonly occur in about 50% of individuals with a substance use disorder; however there is some controversy about the accuracy of the rates due to the difficulty of diagnosing personality disorders in individuals with substance use disorders. The most common personality disorders seen with substance use disorders are antisocial, borderline, histrionic, and narcissistic personality disorders (Nace, 1990).

Integrated treatment for this population initially blends behavioural therapy approaches for the personality disorder with traditional substance abuse treatments. During later stages of addiction recovery, patients will often benefit from additional psychotherapy with a therapist experienced in addiction treatment. For some cases medications are used episodically to treat specific psychiatric symptoms. Specific behavioural therapy approaches have been developed to deal with particular personality disorders and associated treatment dilemmas (Ball, 1998; Fisher & Bentley, 1996; Linehan *et al.*, 1999). Linehan's Dialectical Behavioral Therapy (DBT) has been modified to treat co-occurring borderline personality disorder and substance use disorders, and there is some research supporting its effectiveness (Linehan *et al.*, 1999). (See also Chapter 43.)

Schizophrenia

About 40%–60% of individuals with schizophrenia have a current alcohol or other drug disorder and about 60%–85% are tobacco dependent. However, only a minority of patients with schizophrenia who have co-morbid substance abuse enter formal treatment for both disorders (Drake *et al.*, 1998b; George & Krystal, 2000).

Integrated treatment for this population usually occurs in mental health settings and must address both disorders including the positive and negative symptoms of schizophrenia, cognitive limitations, social support, suicidal ideation, and motivation (Maslin, 2003; Mueser *et al.*, 1995). Treatment includes helping the patient with daily living needs such as housing, entitlements, rehabilitation, and community service. Treatment is difficult when the patient is floridly psychotic and such patients often require psychiatric hospitalization in order to achieve the stability necessary to participate in the treatment process. Patients with co-occurring schizophrenia must receive appropriate antipsychotic treatment (Ziedonis & Stern, 2001). Studies and expert consensus support the use of the first-line medications usually prescribed to treat schizophrenia that are cited in the APA Treatment Guidelines for Schizophrenia and the Texas Medication Algorithm Project. In addition, this population should be considered for many of the substance use disorder medications for detoxification, protracted withdrawal, and agonist maintenance treatment.

With respect to the primary antipsychotic medications, studies and expert consensus support the use of approved atypical antipsychotic medications (i.e. aripiprazole, olanzapine, quetiapine, risperidone, or ziprasidone) as a first line intervention, but see Chapter 25 for more information. Compared to traditional antipsychotics, atypical agents are linked with better outcomes, a much lower incidence of extra pyramidal side effects (EPS) and a greater likelihood of improved negative symptoms and cognition. There is some evidence to suggest that the atypical antipsychotics can also reduce substance use symptoms such as craving, protracted withdrawal, and relapse (Littrell *et al.*, 2001).

However, there is insufficient evidence to suggest that one atypical antipsychotic is clearly more effective than another with this population. Expert consensus suggests selecting a medication that is best for the individual, taking into account safety, toxicity and side effects. Individuals with schizophrenia who abuse alcohol and cocaine may have an increased risk for seizures and liver toxicity and may already have QTc prolongation due to the cardiac toxicity of these substances. Some patients who continue to use alcohol or other sedating drugs could have a synergistic reaction with increased somnolence and orthostatic hypotension. Individuals with schizophrenia who abuse substances also appear to be more sensitive to EPS. Tobacco smoking substantially lowers blood levels of clozapine, olanzapine, and numerous traditional antipsychotics (haloperidol, chlorpromazine) by increasing P450 1A2 isoenzyme hepatic metabolism, a moderate effect that may necessitate a medication dosage increase. The metabolism of other atypicals is not significantly affected by changes in smoking status.

Many of the medication studies for individuals with co-occurring schizophrenia and addiction are retrospective, non-randomized, or uncontrolled pilot studies; thus limiting the ability to draw solid conclusions at this time (Siris, 1990). However, several smaller studies have found better outcomes with clozapine (Albanese *et al.*, 1994; Buckley, 1998; Buckley *et al.*, 1994a, 1994b; Drake *et al.*, 2000; Green *et al.*, 2003; Kelly *et al.*, 2003; Lee *et al.*, 1998; Marcus & Snyder, 1995; Tsuang *et al.*, 1999; Zimmet *et al.*, 2000), risperidone (Albanese, 2001; Green *et al.*, 2003; Kosten *et al.*, 2003; Smelson *et al.*, 2002a, 2002b; Tsuang *et al.*, 2002), and olanzapine (Conley *et al.*, 1998; Littrell *et al.*, 2001; Tsuang *et al.*, 2001) than with traditional antipsychotics for patients with co-occurring schizophrenia/psychosis and addiction. However, there is one small randomized controlled trial that compared haloperidol to olanzapine and found that olanzapine was significantly more effective in reducing craving induced in a laboratory and relapse compared to haloperidol (Smelson *et al.*, 2004). While it could be argued that clozapine has an additional advantage in reducing the risk of suicide (Meltzer *et al.*, 2003), given its side effect risks (increased seizure risk, sedation, liver damage), there is still mixed support for clozapine as a first line agent in this population unless used with more motivated patients in well integrated psychosocial treatment programmes. Risperidone, clozapine and olanzapine have all been shown to diminish the pleasure associated with cocaine use in patients with schizophrenia and may be helpful in treating both the symptoms of schizophrenia and the co-morbid substance use disorder. Individuals with schizophrenia and cocaine addiction have a heightened cocaine craving response compared to individuals with cocaine addiction alone (Carol *et al.*, 2001; Smelson *et al.*, 2002a).

As treatment guidelines for schizophrenia spectrum disorders generally recommend novel or atypical antipsychotics as first-line treatment (National Institute for Clinical Excellence, 2002), a large burden of proof is not needed to recommend these agents in patients with co-occurring substance use disorders (Noordsy & Green, 2003). While appropriately sized randomized controlled trials are needed, the current data suggest that management of schizophrenia co-morbid with substance use should include atypical medication such as clozapine (Kavanagh *et al.*, 2003a). However, findings supporting reduced substance use with novel relative to conventional antipsychotics may result from an adverse influence of conventional agents, a beneficial effect of novel agents (or the accompanying treatment programme) or both. There are no studies comparing the new agents with each other, and no data on ziprasidone or aripiprazole.

Another important clinical issue in this population is addressing poor adherence with both pharmacological and psychosocial interventions. The use of long-acting injectable antipsychotic medications can help increase patient adherence with medication regimens. There is now an FDA approved long-acting injectable form of the atypical medication, risperidone. The other two long-acting (depot) injectable antipsychotic medications, haloperidol and fluphenzine, are traditional antipsychotics. Another issue surrounding the use of antipsychotic medications is the use of anticholinergic drugs to minimize certain EPS. The use of anticholinergic medication carries with it the potential for cognitive impairment particularly in an elderly or brain-injured population. Thus the use of these medications (biperiden, benztropine, diphenydramine, procyclidine) should be carefully assessed and discontinued when the need is not evident. Many patients with co-occurring psychotic illnesses are prescribed these medications despite the fact that they have been switched to atypical antipsychotic medications.

Substance abuse treatment medications used during detoxification, protracted abstinence, and maintenance treatment can be safely prescribed in the schizophrenic population, especially naltrexone for alcohol dependence and methadone for opiate dependence (Maxwell & Shinderman, 2000; Petrakis *et al.*, 1998). Given the cognitive difficulties common in schizophrenia, antabuse should be used in select cases where judgement, memory, and impulsivity are adequate.

Integrated psychosocial treatment in the mental health setting begins with clinicians who are optimistic, empathic and hopeful (Drake *et al.*, 1998b). Patients also will require broad-based and comprehensive services. Money management services are often vital since money is a powerful trigger for substance use, and many patients receive social security or social security disability payments in large monthly lump sums. Active outreach and case management in community settings is also important for this population, and because of the low motivational levels of many patients, initial efforts at engagement may focus on small but attainable short-term goals (Carey, 1995; Drake *et al.*, 1998a). New programme models and specific integrated behavioural therapy approaches have been developed for this population, including Assertive Community Treatment Teams and Integrated Stage-Based Motivation-Based Models (Drake *et al.*, 1998b; Hellerstein & Meehan, 1987; Minkoff, 1989; Ziedonis, 1996). Some models emphasize a recovery-orientated perspective while others emphasize a more medical model or behavioural learning model. Most of the integrated therapies, such as Dual Recovery Therapy, blend motivational enhancement therapy, relapse prevention, and social skills training (Roberts *et al.*, 1999; Shaner *et al.*, 2003; Ziedonis & Stern, 2001). Approaches that blend contingency management approaches with skill-based treatment have also demonstrated improved outcomes (Roberts *et al.*, 1999).

Psychosocial and case management treatments can help the difficult transition from acute psychiatry to outpatient care when there is often increased drug craving, relapse and re-hospitalization (Broadnick & Schmitz, 1997). Smelson *et al.* (2004) reported on an integrated psychosocial case management treatment that significantly improved outpatient treatment engagement, reduced re-hospitalization, and increased functional outcome and sobriety compared to those who were discharged as usual to outpatient care during this vulnerable period in recovery.

Summary and conclusions

Psychiatric and substance use disorders commonly co-occur and require the clinician to have additional knowledge and skills in assessing and treating both types of disorders. There are many subtypes of co-occurring mental illness and addiction disorders based on the different types of disorders, the severity of each disorder, and the motivation to address either disorder.

Due to the chronic and often long-standing nature of co-occurring disorders, precise and detailed history taking is critical to accurate diagnoses. The use of collaborative sources of information cannot be overemphasized.

Previously clinicians thought it appropriate to withhold treatment for the psychiatric symptoms until a patient was abstinent for a long period of time. However, now treatment is often initiated much earlier. While each disorder impacts the other, the clinician is often faced with the need to treat withdrawal, intoxication, affective, psychotic and cognitive symptoms without a clear understanding of the exact cause and effect relationships of the presenting symptoms.

More research is needed to study and develop improved treatment approaches for the wide range of co-occurring disorder subtypes in all treatment settings. The use of more than one psychosocial therapy could facilitate better outcomes. For example, the alcoholic with major depression may require motivational enhancement therapy, 12 step facilitation and relapse prevention for the substance abuse or dependence and cognitive behavioural, interpersonal, brief psychodynamic or supportive psychotherapy for the depression. Regular reassessment of the patient will facilitate a more precise diagnosis and better targeted interventions.

The level of evidence for each of the interventions discussed in this chapter is summarized in Table 24.1.

Table 24.1. Effectiveness of treatments for co-occurring psychiatric and substance use disorders

Treatment	Form of treatment	Psychiatric disorder/ Target audience	Level of evidence for efficacy	Comments
Integrated treatment (Psychosocial)	Multimodal treatment that addresses simultaneously substance abuse and psychiatric disorder. An integrated model uses recovery-oriented approaches, motivational interviewing interpersonal psychotherapies and behavioural skills training	Dual diagnosis patients	Ib	There are many different studies using different methodology and since no two studies are exactly alike, Ia is not given here. But the overall impression is that integrated treatment is more effective than serial or parallel treatment across a wide range of psychiatric diagnoses and various substances. The best integrated care is delivered by a single team that approaches 'both' problems
Psychosocial treatment	Motivational interviewing	Dual diagnosis patients	Ib	Attendance in the programme appears to be the main benefit, but also some studies reveal that motivational interviewing can significantly reduce the co-morbid substance misuse
Psychosocial treatment	Dialectical behaviour therapy (DBT)	Co-morbid personality disorder and substance misuse	IIb	Preliminary evidence supports this intervention with at least short-term improvement in use of substances and personality pathology
Pharmacotherapy	Anticonvulsants	Co-morbid bipolar disorder and substance abuse	IIb	Various studies suggest that patients with dual diagnosis tolerate anticonvulsants, particularly valproate, better than lithium
Pharmacotherapy	Antidepressants	Co-morbid depression in substance abuse	Ib–IIa	SSRIs are probably first line and TCAs second line treatment here but some of the evidence is better for the effectiveness of TCAs especially with people on methadone maintenance
Pharmacotherapy	Atypical antipsychotics	Co-morbid schizophrenia and substance abuse	IIb	Atypicals appear more effective than typicals. Some evidence that clozapine, olanzepine and risperidone may be useful to reduce severity of both disorders with the largest evidence base for clozapine

REFERENCES

Abou-Saleh, M. T. (2004). Dual diagnosis: management within a psychosocial context. *Advances in Psychiatric Treatment*, **10**, 352–60.

Albanese, M. J., Khantzian, E. J., Murphy, S. L. *et al.* (1994). Decreased substance use in chronically psychotic patients treated with clozapine. *American Journal of Psychiatry*, **151**(5), 780–1.

Albanese, M. J. (2001). Safety and efficacy of risperidone in substance abusers with psychosis. *American Journal on Addictions*, **10**, 190–1.

American Psychiatric Association (1994). *Diagnostic and Statistical Manual of Mental Disorders, 4th Edn.* Washington, DC: American Psychiatric Association.

Baker, A., Lewin, T., Reichler, H. *et al.* (2002). Motivational interviewing among psychiatric in-patients with substance use disorders. *Acta Psychiatrica Scandinavica*, **106**, 233–40.

Bakker, A., van Balkom, A. J. & van Dyck, R. (2000). Selective serotonin reuptake inhibitors in the treatment of panic disorder and agoraphobia. *International Clinical Psychopharmacology*, **15** (Suppl. 2). S25–30.

Ball, S. A. (1998). Manualized treatment for substance abusers with personality disorders: dual focus schema therapy. *Addictive Behaviors*, **23**(6), 883–91.

Barlow, D. H. (2002). *Anxiety and Its Disorders: The Nature and Treatment of Anxiety and Panic*, 2nd edn. New York: Guilford Press.

Barrowclough, C., Haddock, G., Tarrier, N. *et al.* (2001). Randomized controlled trial of motivational interviewing, cognitive behaviour therapy, and family intervention for patients with comorbid schizophrenia and substance use disorders. *American Journal of Psychiatry*, **158**(10), 1706–13.

Beck, A. T., Wright, F. D., Newman, C. F. & Liese, B. S. (1993). *Cognitive Therapy of Substance Abuse.* New York: Guilford Press.

Bellack, A. S., Buchanan, R. W. & Gold, J. M. (2001). The American Psychiatric Association practice guidelines for schizophrenia: scientific base and relevance for behavior therapy. *Behavior Therapy*, **32**(2), 283–308.

Bond, G. R., McDonel, E. C., Miller, L. D. *et al.* (1991). Assertive community treatment and reference groups: an evaluation of their effectiveness for young adults with serious mental illness and substance abuse problems. *Psychosocial Rehabilitation Journal*, **15**(2), 31–43.

Bowden, C. L. (2001). Clinical correlates of therapeutic response in bipolar disorder. *Journal of Affective Disorders*, **67**(1–3), 257–65.

Bradizza, C. M. & Stasiewicz, P. R. (1997). Integrating substance abuse treatment for the seriously mentally ill into inpatient psychiatric treatment. *Journal of Substance Abuse Treatment*, **14**(2), 103–11.

Brady, K. T. (2001). Comorbid posttraumatic stress disorder and substance use disorders. *Psychiatric Annals*, **31**(5), 313–19.

Brady, K. T. & Clary C. M. (2003). Affective and anxiety comorbidity in post-traumatic stress disorder treatment trials of sertraline. *Comprehensive Psychiatry*, **44**(5), 360–9.

Brady, K. T., Sonne, S. C., Anton, R. *et al.* (1995). Valproate in the treatment of acute bipolar affective episodes complicated by substance abuse: a pilot study. *Journal of Clinical Psychiatry*, **56**(3), 118–21.

Brady, K. T., Dansky, B. S., Back, S. E. *et al.* (2001). Exposure therapy in the treatment of PTSD among cocaine-dependent individuals: preliminary findings. *Journal of Substance Abuse Treatment*, **21**(1), 47–54.

Brady, K. T., Myrick, H., Henderson, S. *et al.* (2002). The use of divalproex in alcohol relapse prevention: a pilot study. *Drug and Alcohol Dependence*, **67**, 323–30.

Brecher, M., Wang, B. W., Wong, H. *et al.* (1988). Phencyclidine and violence: clinical and legal issues. *Journal of Clinical Psychopharmacology*, **8**, 398–401.

Broadnick, P. S. & Schmitz, J. M. (1997). Cocaine craving: an evaluation across treatment phases. *Journal of Substance Abuse*, **10**(1), 9–17.

Brown, E. S., Nejtek, B. A., Perantie, D. C. *et al.* (2002). Quetiapine in bipolar disorder and cocaine dependence. *Bipolar Disorder*, **4**(6), 406–11.

Brunette, M. F., Drake, R. E., Woods, M. *et al.* (2001). A comparison of long-term and short-term residential treatment programs for dual diagnosis patients. *Psychiatric Services*, **52**(4), 526–8.

Buckley, P. F. (1998). Novel antipsychotic medications and the treatment of comorbid substance abuse in schizophrenia. *Journal of Substance Abuse Treatment*, **15**, 113–16.

Buckley, P., Thompson, P., Way, L. *et al.* (1994a). Substance abuse among patients with treatment-resistant schizophrenia: characteristics and implications for clozapine therapy. *American Journal of Psychiatry*, **151**, 385–9.

Buckley, P., Thompson, P. A. & Way, L. (1944b). Meltzer, H. Y., Substance abuse and clozapine treatment. *Journal of Clinical Psychiatry*, **55** (Suppl. B), 114–16.

Budde, R. D. (1989). Cocaine abuse and violent death. *American Journal of Drug and Alcohol Abuse*, **15**, 375–82.

Carey, K. B. (1995). Treatment of substance use disorders and schizophrenia. In *Double Jeopardy: Chronic Mental Illness and Substance Use Disorders*, ed. A. F. Lehman & L. B. Dixon, pp. 85–108. Langhorne, PA: Harwood Academic Publishers/ Gordon and Breach Science Publishers.

Carol, G., Smelson, D. A., Losonczy, M. F. *et al.* (2001) A preliminary investigation of cocaine craving among persons with and without Schizophrenia. *Psychiatric Services*, **52**(8), 1029–31.

Chilcoat, H. D. & Breslau, N. (1988). Posttraumatic stress disorder and drug disorders: testing causal pathways. *Archives of General Psychiatry*, **55**(10), 913–17.

Conley, R. R., Kelly, D. L. & Gale, E. A. (1998). Olanzapine response in treatment-refactory schizophrenic patients with a history of substance abuse. *Schizophrenia Research*, **33**, 95–101.

Copello, A., Graham, H. & Birchwood, M. (2001). Evaluating substance misuse interventions in psychosis: the limitations of the RCT with 'patient' as the unit of analysis. *Journal of Mental Health*, **10**(6), 585–7.

Cottler, L. B., Compton, W. M. 3rd., Mager, D. *et al.* (1992). Posttraumatic stress disorder among substance users from the general population. *American Journal of Psychiatry*, **149**(5), 664–70.

Crumley, F. E. (1990). Substance abuse and adolescent suicidal behavior. *Journal of the American Medical Association*, **163**, 3051–6.

Daley, D. C., Salloum, I. M. & Thase, M. E. (2003). Integrated treatment using a recovery-oriented approach. In *Integrated Treatment for Mood and Substance Disorders*, ed. J. J. Westmeyer, R. D. Weiss & D. M. Ziedonis, pp. 68–89. Baltimore: Johns Hopkins University Press.

Dansky, B. S., Brady, K. T. & Saladin, M. E. (1998). Untreated symptoms of PTSD among cocaine-dependent individuals. Changes over time. *Journal of Substance Abuse Treatment*, **15**(6), 499–504.

Dean, A. J., Bell, J., Mascord, D. J., Gordon, P. *et al.* (2002). A randomised, controlled trial of fluoxetine in methadone maintenance patients with depressive symptoms. *Journal of Affective Disorders*, **72**(1), 85–90.

Department of Health (2002). *Mental Health Policy Implementation Guide: Dual Diagnosis Good Practice Guide*. London: Department of Health.

DiClemente, C. C., Schlundt, D. & Gemmell, L. (2004). Readiness and stages of change in addiction treatment. *American Journal on Addictions*, **13**(2), 103–19.

Dorpat, T. L. (1974). Drug automatism, barbiturate poisoning and suicide behavior. *Archives of General Psychiatry*, **31**, 216–20.

Drake, R. E. & Mueser, K. T. (2000). Psychosocial approaches to dual diagnosis. *Schizophrenia Bulletin*, **26**(1), 105–18.

Drake, R. E., Yovetich, N. A., Bebout, R. R. *et al.* (1997). Integrated treatment for dually diagnosed homeless adults. *Journal of Nervous and Mental Disease*, **185**(5), 298–305.

Drake, R. E., McHugo, G. J., Clark, R. E. *et al.* (1998a). Assertive community treatment for patients with co-occurring severe mental illness and substance use disorder: A clinical trial. *American Journal of Orthopsychiatry*, **68**, 201–15.

Drake, R. E., Mercer-McFadden, C., Mueser, K. T. *et al.* (1998b). Review of integrated mental health and substance abuse treatment for patients with dual disorders. *Schizophrenia Bulletin*, **24**(4), 589–608.

Drake, R. E., Xie, H., McHugo, G. J. *et al.* (2000). The effects of clozapine on alcohol and drug use disorders among patients with schizophrenia. *Schizophrenia Bulletin*, **26**(2), 441–9.

Drake, R. E., Essock, S. M. & Shaner, A. (2001). Implementing dual diagnosis services for clients with severe mental illness. *Psychiatric Services*, **52**(4), 469–76.

Fisher, M. S. & Bentley, K. J. (1996). Two group therapy models for clients with a dual diagnosis of substance abuse and personality disorder. *Psychiatric Services*, **47**(11), 1244–50.

Fowler, I. L., Carr, V. J., Carr, N. T. *et al.* (1998). Patterns of current and lifetime substance use in schizophrenia. *Schizophrenia Bulletin*, **24**, 443–55.

Geller, B., Cooper, T. B., Sun, K. *et al.* (1998). Double-blind and placebo-controlled study of lithium for adolescent bipolar disorders with secondary substance dependency. *Journal of the American Academy of Child and Adolescent Psychiatry*, **37**(2), 171–8.

George, T. P. & Krystal, J. H. (2000). Comorbidity of psychiatric and substance abuse disorders. *Current Opinion in Psychiatry*, **13**, 327–31.

Graham, H. L. (2004). Implementing integrated treatment for co-existing substance use and severe mental health problems in assertive outreach teams: training issues. *Drug and Alcohol Review*, **23**, 463–70.

Graham, H. L., Maslin, J., Copello, A. *et al.* (2001). Drug and alcohol problems amongst individuals with severe mental health problems in an inner city area of the UK. *Journal of Social Psychiatry and Psychiatric Epidemiology*, **36**, 448–55.

Graham, H. L., Copello, A., Birchwood, M. *et al.* (2003a). *Cognitive-Behavioural Integrated Treatment (C-BIT): A Treatment Manual for Substance Misuse in People with Severe Mental Health Problems*. Chichester: John Wiley.

Graham, H. L., Copello, A., Birchwood, M. J. *et al.* (2003b). The combined psychosis and substance use (COMPASS): an integrated shared-care approach. In *Substance Misuse in Psychosis: Approaches to Treatment and Service Delivery*, ed. H. L. Graham, A. Copello, M. J. Birchwood *et al.*, pp. 106–20. Chichester: John Wiley.

Graham, H. L., Copello, A., Birchwood, M. J. *et al.* (2003c). Cognitive-behavioural integrated treatment approach for psychosis and problem substance use. In *Substance Misuse in Psychosis: Approaches to Treatment and Service Delivery*, ed. H. L. Graham, A. Copello, M. J. Birchwood *et al.*, pp. 181–206. Chichester: John Wiley.

Graham, H. L., Copello, A., Birchwood, M. J. *et al.* (2006). A preliminary evaluation of integrated treatment for co-existing substance use and severe mental health problems: impact on teams and service users. *Journal of Mental Health*, **15**(5), 577–91.

Green, A. I., Burgess, E. S., Dawson, R. *et al.* (2003). Alcohol and cannabis use in schizophrenia: effects of clozapine vs. risperidone. *Schizophrenia Research*, **60**, 81–5.

Grice, D. E., Brady, K. T., Dustan, L. R. *et al.* (1995). Sexual and physical assault history and posttraumatic stress disorder in substance-dependent individuals. *American Journal on Addictions*, **4**(4), 297–305.

Haddock, G., Barrowclough, C., Tarrier, N. *et al.* (2003). Cognitive-behavioural therapy and motivational intervention for schizophrenia and substance misuse: 18-month outcomes of a randomised controlled trial. *British Journal of Psychiatry*, **183**(5), 418–26.

Havassy, B. E., Shropshire, M. S. & Quigley, L. A. (2000). Effects of substance dependence on outcomes of patients in a randomized trial of two case management models. *Psychiatric Services*, **51**(5), 639–44.

Hawton, K. (1987). Assessment of suicide risk. *British Journal of Psychiatry*, **150**, 145–53.

Hellerstein, D. J. & Meehan, B. (1987). Outpatient group therapy for schizophrenic substance abusers. *American Journal of Psychiatry*, **144**, 1337–9.

Hellerstein, D. J., Rosenthal, R. N. & Miner, C. R. (1995). A prospective study of integrated outpatient treatment for substance-abusing schizophrenic patients. *American Journal on Addictions*, **4**, 33–42.

Hellerstein, D. J., Rosenthal, R. N. & Miner, C. R. (2001). Integrating services for schizophrenia and substance use. *Psychiatric Quarterly*, **72**(4), 291–306.

Ho, A. P., Tsuang, J. W., Liberman, R. P. *et al.* (1999). Achieving effective treatment of patients with chronic psychotic illness and comorbid substance dependence. *American Journal of Psychiatry*, **156**(11), 1765–70.

Jacobsen, L. K., Southwick, S. M. & Kosten, T. R. (2001). Substance use disorders in patients with posttraumatic stress disorder: a review of the literature. *American Journal of Psychiatry*, **158**, 1184–90.

Jeffrey, D. P., Ley, A., McLaren, S. *et al.* (2000). Psychosocial treatment programmes for people with both severe mental illness and substance misuse (Cochrane Review). In *The Cochrane Library*. Chichester: John Wiley.

Jenike, M. A. (1997). Duration of antidepressant treatment. *Journal of Geriatric Psychiatry and Neurology*, **10**(4), 247.

Jerrell, J. M. & Ridgely, M. S. (1995). Comparative effectiveness of three approaches to serving people with severe mental illness and substance use disorders. *Journal of Nervous and Mental Disease*, **183**(9), 566–76.

Kavanagh, D. J., Mueser, K. T. & Baker, A. (2003a). Management of Comorbidity. In *Comorbid Mental Disorders and Substance Use Disorders: Epidemiology, Prevention and Treatment*, ed. M. Teesson & H. Proudfoot. Canberra, Australia: Commonwealth of Australia.

Kavanagh, D. J., Young, R., White, A. *et al.* (2003b). Start over and survive: a brief intervention for substance misuse in early psychosis. In *Substance Misuse in Psychosis: Approaches to Treatment and Service Delivery*, ed. H. L. Graham, A. Copello, M. D. Birchwood *et al.* Chichester: John Wiley.

Kelly, D., Gale, E. & Conley, R. (2003). Clozapine treatment in patients with prior substance abuse. *Canadian Journal Psychiatry*, **48**(2), 111–14.

Kessler, R. C., Sonnega, A., Bromet, E. *et al.* (1995). Posttraumatic stress disorder in the National Comorbidity Survey. *Archives of General Psychiatry*, **52**(12), 1048–60.

Kessler, R. C., Nelson, C. B., McGonagle, K. A. *et al.* (1996). Comorbidity of DSM-III-R major depressive disorder in the general population: results from the US National Comorbidity Survey. *British Journal of Psychiatry*, **168**(Suppl. 30), 17–30.

Kofoed, L., Friedman, M. J. & Peck, R. (1993). Alcoholism and drug abuse in patients with PTSD. *Psychiatry Quarterly*, **64**(2), 151–71.

Kosten, T. R., Morgan, C. M., Falcione, J. *et al.* (1992). Pharmacotherapy for cocaine-abusing methadone-maintained patients using amantadine or desipramine. *Archives of General Psychiatry*, **49**, 894–8.

Kosten, T. R., Brady, K. T., George, T. P. *et al.* (2003). Risperidone for substance dependent psychotic patients. *CPDD Scientific Meeting Abstracts*.

Kranzler, H. R., Burleson, J. A., Korner, P. *et al.* (1995). Placebo-controlled trial of fluoxetine as an adjunct to relapse prevention in alcoholics. *American Journal of Psychiatry*, **152**(3), 391–7.

Krausz, M., Haasen, C., Mass, R. *et al.* (1996). Harmful use of psychotropic substances by schizophrenics: coincidence, patterns of use and motivation. *European Addiction Research*, **2**, 11–16.

Langevin, R., Paitich, D., Orchard, B. *et al.* (1982) The role of alcohol, drugs, suicide attempts and situational strains in homicide committed by offenders seen for psychiatric assessment: a controlled study. *Acta Psychiatrica Scandinavica*, **66**, 229–42.

Lee, M. L., Dickson, R. A., Campbell, M. *et al.* (1998). Clozapine and substance abuse in patients with schizophrenia. *Canadian Journal of Psychiatry*, **43**, 855–6.

Lehman, A. F., Herron, J. D., Schwartz, R. P. *et al.* (1993). Rehabilitation for adults with severe mental illness and substance use disorders. A clinical trial. *Journal of Nervous and Mental Disease*, **181**(2), 86–90.

Leskin, G. A. & Sheikh, J. I. (2001). Lifetime trauma history and panic disorder: findings from the National Comorbidity Survey. *Journal of Anxiety Disorders*, **16**(6), 599–603.

Linehan, M. M., Schmidt, H. 3rd., Dimeff, L. A. *et al.* (1999). Dialectical behavior therapy for patients with borderline personality disorder and drug-dependence. *American Journal on Addictions*, **8**(4), 279–92.

Lingford-Hughes, A. R., Welch, S. & Nutt, D. J. (2004). Evidence-based guidelines for the pharmacological management of substance misuse, addiction and comorbidity: recommendations from the British Association of Pharmacology. *Journal of Psychopharmacology*, **18**(3), 293–335.

Linnoila, M. I. (1989). Anxiety and alcoholism. *Journal of Clinical Psychiatry*, **50**, 26–9.

Liskow, B. I. & Goodwin, D. (1987). Pharmacological treatment of alcohol intoxication withdrawal and dependence: a critical review. *Journal of Studies on Alcohol*, **48**, 356–70.

Littrell, K. H., Petty, R. G., Hilligoss, N. M. *et al.* (2001). Olanzapine treatment for patients with schizophrenia and substance abuse. *Journal of Substance Abuse Treatment*, **21**, 217–21.

Luisada, P. V. (1978). The phencyclidine psychosis: phenomenology and treatment. *NIDA Research Monograph*, **21**, 241–53.

Mackenzie, A., Funderburk, F. R. & Allen, R. P. (1999). Sleep, anxiety, and depression in abstinent and drinking alcoholics. *Substance Use Misuse*, **34**(3), 347–61.

Marcus, P. & Snyder, R. (1995). Reduction of comorbid substance abuse with clozapine. *American Journal of Psychiatry*, **152**, 959.

Martino, S., Carroll, K. M., O'Malley, S. S. *et al.* (2000). Motivational interviewing with psychiatrically ill substance abusing patients. *American Journal on Addictions*, **9**(1), 88–91.

Martino, S., Carroll, K., Kostas, D. *et al.* (2002). Dual diagnosis motivational interviewing: a modification of motivational interviewing for substance-abusing patients with psychotic disorders. *Journal of Substance Abuse Treatment*, **23**(4), 297–308.

Maslin, J. (2003). Substance misuse in psychosis: contextual issues. In *Substance Misuse in Psychosis: Approaches to Treatment and Service Delivery*, ed. H. L. Graham, A. Copello, M. J. Birchwood *et al.*, pp. 3–23. Chichester, UK: John Wiley.

Mason, B. J., Kocsis, J. H., Ritvo, E. C. *et al.* (1996). A double-blind, placebo-controlled trial of desipramine for primary alcohol dependence stratified on the presence or absence of major depression. *Journal of the American Medical Association*, **275**(10), 761–7.

Maxwell, S. & Shinderman, M. S. (2000). Use of naltrexone in the treatment of alcohol use disorders in patients with concomitant major mental illness. *Journal of Addictive Diseases*, **19**(3), 61–9.

McLellan, A. T. & Hunkeler E. (1998). Patient satisfaction and outcomes in alcohol and drug abuse treatment. *Psychiatric Services*, **49**(5), 573–5.

Meltzer, H. Y., Alphs, L., Green, A. I. *et al.* (2003). Clozapine treatment for suicidality in schizophrenia: International Suicide Prevention Trial (InterSePT). *Archives of General Psychiatry*, **60**(1), 82–91.

Menezes, P. R., Johnson, S., Thornicroft, G. *et al.* (1996). Drug and alcohol problems among individuals with severe mental illnesses in south London. *British Journal of Psychiatry*, **168**, 612–19.

Mercer-McFadden, C., Drake, R. E., Brown, N. B. *et al.* (1997). The community support program demonstrations of services for young adults with severe mental illness and substance use disorders, 1987–1991. *Psychiatric Rehabilitation Journal*, **20**(3), 13–24.

Miller, W. R., Zweben, A., DiClemente, C. C. *et al.* (1995) *Motivational Enhancement Therapy Manual*. Rockville, MD: US Department of Health and Human Services.

Minkoff, K. (1989). An integrated treatment model for dual diagnosis of psychosis and addiction. *Hospital and Community Psychiatry*, **40**(10), 1031–6.

Mueser, K. T. & Drake, R. E. (2003). Integrated dual disorder treatment in New Hampshire (USA). In *Substance Misuse in Psychosis: Approaches to Treatment and Service Delivery*, ed. H. L. Graham, A. Copello, M. J. Birchwood *et al.* Chichester, UK: John Wiley.

Mueser, K. T., Nishith, P., Tracy, J. I. *et al.* (1995). Expectations and motives for substance use in schizophrenia. *Psychiatric Clinics of North America*, **21**(3), 367–78.

Mueser, K. T., Yarnold, P. R., Rosenberg S. D. *et al.* (2000). Substance use disorder in hospitalized severely mentally ill psychiatric patients: prevalence, correlates and subgroups. *Schizophrenia Bulletin*, **26**, 179–92.

Murphy, G. E. (1988). Suicide and substance abuse. *Archives of General Psychiatry*, **45**, 593–4.

Nace, E. P. (1990). Substance abuse and personality disorder. *Journal of Chemical Dependency Treatment*, **3**(2), 183–98.

Najavits, L. M., Weiss, R. D., Shaw, S. R. *et al.* (1998). Seeking safety: outcome of a new cognitive-behavioral psychotherapy for women with posttraumatic stress disorder and substance dependence. *Journal of Traumatic Stress*, **11**(3), 437–56.

Najavits, L. M., Runkel, R., Neuner, C. *et al.* (2003). Rates and symptoms of PTSD among cocaine-dependent patients. *Journal of Studies on Alcohol*, **64**(5), 601–6.

National Institute for Clinical Excellence (2002). *Guidance on the Use of Newer (Atypical) Antipsychotic Drugs for the Treatment of Schizophrenia*. London: National Institute for Clinical Excellence.

Noordsy, D. L. & Green, A. I. (2003). Pharmacotherapy for schizophrenia and co-occurring substance use disorders. *Current Psychiatry Reports*, **5**, 340–6.

Nunes, E. V. & Quitkin, F. M. (1997). Treatment of depression in drug-dependent patients: effects on mood and drug use. In *Treatment of Drug-Dependent Individuals with Comorbid Mental Disorders*, ed. L. S. Onken, J. D. Blaine, S. Genser *et al.*, pp. 61–85. National Institute on Drug Abuse: Rockville, MD.

Nunes, E. V., McGrath, P. J., Quitkin, F. M. *et al.* (1995). Imipramine treatment of cocaine abuse: possible boundaries of efficacy. *Drug and Alcohol Dependence*, **39**(3), 185–95.

Nunes, E. V., Quitkin, F. M., Donovan, S. J. *et al.* (1998). Imipramine treatment of opiate-dependent patients with depressive disorders. *Archives of General Psychiatry*, **55**, 153–160.

Nunes, E. V., McGrath, P. J., Wager, S. *et al.* (1990). Lithium treatment for cocaine abusers with bipolar spectrum disorder. *American Journal of Psychiatry*, **147**(5), 655–7.

Nunes, E. & Levin, F. R. (2004). Treatment of depression in patients with alcohol or other drug dependence: a meta-analysis. *Journal of the American Medical Association*, **291**, 1887–96.

O'Connell, R. A., Mayo, J. A. & Flatlow, L. (1991). Outcome of bipolar disorder on long-term treatment with lithium. *British Journal of Psychiatry*, **159**, 123–9.

O'Hea, E. L., Dutton, G. & Boudreaux, E. D. (2002). Identifying and managing patients with panic disorder in the emergency. *Emergency Psychiatry*, **8**, 21–6.

Petrakis, I., Carroll, K. M., Nich, C. *et al.* (1998). Fluoxetine treatment of depressive disorders in methadone-maintained opioid addicts. *Drug and Alcohol Dependence*, **50**, 221–6.

Regier, D. A., Farmer, M. E., Rae, D. S. *et al.* (1990). Comorbidity of mental disorders with alcohol and other drug abuse. Results from the epidemiologic catchment area (ECA) study. *Journal of the American Medical Association*, **264**, 2511–18.

Roberts, L., Shaner, A. & Eckman, T. A. (1999). *Overcoming Addictions: Skills Training for People With Schizophrenia*. New York: W. W. Norton.

Ross, H. E., Glaser, F. B. & Germanson, T. (1988). The prevalence of psychiatric disorders in patients with alcohol and other drug problems. *Archives of General Psychiatry*, **45**, 1023–31.

Roy, A. (1998). Placebo-controlled study of sertaline in depressed recently abstinent alcoholics. *Biological Psychiatry*, **44**(7), 633–7.

Sajatovic, M., Mullen, J. A. & Sweitzer, D. E. (2002). Efficacy of quetiapine and risperidone against depressive symptoms in outpatients with psychosis. *Journal of Clinical Psychiatry*, **63**(12), 1156–63.

Salloum, I. M. & Thase, M. E. (2000). Impact of substance abuse on the course and treatment of bipolar disorder. *Bipolar Disorders*, **2**, 269–80.

SAMHSA (2003). *SAMHSA report to congress on the prevention and treatment of co-occurring substance abuse disorders and mental disorders*. Washington DC: US Department of Health and Human Services.

Sattar, S. P., Grant, K., Bhatia, S. *et al.* (2003). Potential use of olanzapine in treatment of substance dependence disorders. *Journal of Clinical Psychopharmacology*, **23**(4), 413–15.

Shaner, A., Eckman, T., Roberts, L. J. *et al.* (2003). Feasibility of a skills training approach to reduce substance dependence among individuals with schizophrenia. *Psychiatric Services*, **54**(9), 1287–9.

Siris, S. G. (1990). Pharmacological treatment of substance-abusing schizophrenic patients. *Schizophrenia Bulletin*, **16**, 111–22.

Smelson, D. A., Roy, A., Roy, M. *et al.* (2001). Electroretinogram and cue-elicited craving in withdrawn cocaine-dependent patients: a replication. *American Journal of Drug and Alcohol Abuse*, **27**(2), 391–7.

Smelson, D. A., Losonczy, M., Kaune, M. *et al.* (2002a). Risperidone decreases cue-elicited craving and relapses in withdrawn cocaine-dependent schizophrenics. *Schizophrenia Research*, **53**, 160.

Smelson, D. A., Losonczy, M. F., Davis, C. W. *et al.* (2002b). Risperidone decreases craving and relapses in individuals with schizophrenia and cocaine dependence. *Canadian Journal of Psychiatry*, **47**, 671–5.

Smelson, D. A., Davis, C., Eisenstein, N. *et al.* (2003). Neuropsychological functioning among individuals with schizophrenia and cocaine dependence. *Journal of Substance Abuse Treatment*, **24**, 75–9.

Smelson, D. A., Williams, J., Ziedonis, D. *et al.* (2004). A double-blind placebo-controlled pilot study of risperidone for decreasing cue-elicited craving in recently withdrawn cocaine dependent patients. *Journal of Substance Abuse Treatment* **27**, 45–9.

Stein, M. D., Bishop, S., Lassor, J. A. *et al.* (2004). Sleep disturbances among methadone maintained patients. *Journal of Substance Abuse Treatment*, **26**(3), 175–80.

Swanson, A. J., Pantalon, M. V. & Cohen, K. R. (1999). Motivational interviewing and treatment adherence among psychiatric and dually diagnosed patients. *Journal of Nervous and Mental Disease*, **187**(10), 630–5.

Teesson, M. & Proudfoot, H. (2003). *Comorbid Mental Disorders and Substance Use Disorders: Epidemiology, Prevention and Treatment.* Canberra, Australia: Commonwealth of Australia.

Timko, C. & Sempel, J. M. (2004). Short-term outcomes of matching dual diagnosis patients' symptom severity to treatment intensity. *Journal of Substance Abuse Treatment*, **26**, 209–18.

Triffleman, E., Carroll, K. & Kellogg, S. (1999). Substance dependence posttraumatic stress disorder therapy. An integrated cognitive-behavioral approach. *Journal of Substance Abuse Treatment*, **17**, 3–14.

Tsuang, J. W., Eckman, T. E., Shaner, A. *et al.* (1999). Clozapine for substance-abusing schizophrenic patients. *American Journal of Psychiatry*, **156**(7), 1119–20.

Tsuang, J. W., Eckman, T., Marder, S. *et al.* (2002). Can risperidone reduce cocaine use in substance abusing schizophrenic patients? *Journal of Clinical Psychopharmacology*, **22**, 629–30.

Ursano, R. J., Bell, C., Eth, S. *et al.* (2004). Work Group on ASD and PTSD. Steering Committee on Practice Guidelines. Practice guideline for the treatment of patients with acute stress disorder and posttraumatic stress disorder. *American Journal of Psychiatry*, **161**(11 Suppl), 3–31.

Weiss, R. D., Greenfield, S. F., Najavits, L. M. *et al.* (1998). Medication compliance among patients with bipolar disorder and substance use disorder. *Journal of Clinical Psychiatry*, **59**, 172–4.

Weiss, R. D., Griffin, M. L., Greenfield, S. F. *et al.* (2000). Group therapy for patients with bipolar disorder and substance dependence: results of a pilot study. *Journal of Clinical Psychiatry*, **61**(5), 361–7.

Weiss, R. D., Greenfield, S. F. & O'Leary, G. (2003). Relapse prevention for patients with bipolar and substance use disorders. In *Substance Misuse in Psychosis: Approaches to Treatment and Service Delivery*, ed. H. L. Graham, A. Copello, M. J. Birchwood *et al.* Chichester: John Wiley.

Westermeyer, J., Yargic, I. & Thuras, P. (2004). Michigan assessment-screening test for alcohol and drugs (MAST/AD): evaluation in a clinical sample. *American Journal on Addictions*, **13**(2), 151–62.

Ziedonis, D. M. & Stern, R. (2001). Dual recovery therapy for schizophrenia and substance abuse. *Psychiatric Annals*, **31**(4), 255–64.

Ziedonis, D. & Williams, J. (2003) Management of smoking in people with psychiatric disorders. *Current Opinion in Psychiatry*, **16**(3), 305–15.

Ziedonis, D., Richardson, T., Lee, E. *et al.* (1992). Adjunctive desipramine in the treatment of cocaine abusing schizophrenics. *Psychopharmacology Bulletin*, **28**(3), 309–14.

Ziedonis, D. M., Rayford, B. S., Bryant, K. *et al.* (1994). Psychiatric comorbidity in White and African-American cocaine addicts seeking substance abuse treatment. *Hospital and Community Psychiatry*, **45**, 43–9.

Ziedonis, D. M. & Fisher, W. (1996). Motivation based assessment and treatment of substance abuse in patients with schizophrenia. In *The Hatherleigh Guide to Treating Substance Abuse* (Part II), pp. 269–87. New York, NY: Hatherleigh Press.

Zimmerman, M., Sheeran P., Chelminski, I. *et al.* (2004). Screening for psychiatric disorders in outpatients with DSM-IV substance use disorders. *Journal of Substance Abuse Treatment*, **26**(3), 181–8.

Zimmet, S. V., Strous, R. D., Burgess, E. S. *et al.* (2000). Effects of Clozapine on substance use in patients with schizophrenia and schizoaffective disorder: a retrospective survey. *Journal of Clinical Psychopharmacology*, **20**, 94–8.

Schizophrenia

Section editors

Stephen R. Marder and Peter B. Jones

25

Pharmacological treatments for schizophrenia

Stephen R. Marder and Peter B. Jones

Editor's note

It is interesting that the most researched and possibly most important area of therapeutics in mental illness, the drug treatment of schizophrenia, is covered in less than 4000 words in this chapter. Why is this? Is it that our two authors are so good at précis that they can summarize in 10 words information that would use 100 words in the writing of others, or is it because the information is so diffuse that no conclusions can be drawn? Or is there another reason: that the subject has such a strong evidence base that it is possible to describe it both briefly and fully? Perhaps the last option has it. Lord Moran of Manton, perhaps best known as the personal doctor of Winston Churchill, in his Harveian oration of 1945 put it this way:-

"The physician who knows what is wrong with a patient and has an effective remedy can cut the cackle. He has no need of it". Now we are not suggesting that the other longer chapters are full of cackle, but when there is more doubt, there is more conjecture and this takes up more space. As Adams *et al.* (2006) states, 'the literature on the drug treatment of schizophrenia is actually quite clear and unequivocal; the problem is that in rich countries with powerful drug companies, the constant jockeying for market position tends to confuse by setting up winners and losers on flimsy evidence. Most of the drug treatments for schizophrenia are like racehorses who have identical performances; making conclusions from their positions during the race is of no value to the final outcome'. And I guarantee that virtually all readers will learn something of value to their practice in reading the words below very carefully.

Introduction

The optimal treatment of individuals with schizophrenia will usually focus on managing a diverse group of symptoms and chronic impairments. Treatment plans will be guided by factors including the phase of the person's illness (acute, stable, or stabilization phase), the severity of symptoms, the character of symptoms, the person's functional impairments, and the person's individual treatment goals. In most cases, the plan will include a combination of pharmacological and psychosocial treatments. This chapter describes a number of treatments for schizophrenia that are supported by an evidence-base that in the authors' opinion are sufficient to recommend their implementation for appropriate patients at appropriate stages of their illness. Since most individuals with schizophrenia have symptoms or impairments that do not adequately respond to any single intervention, most will require combinations of pharmacological and psychosocial treatments.

Phases of treatment

The American Psychiatric Association Guidelines for the Treatment of Schizophrenia (Lehman *et al.*, 2004) defines three phases in schizophrenia: acute, stabilization, and stable. Each has its own clinical features and each has its own treatment goals. The acute stage is characterized by psychotic symptoms that may include reality distortions such as hallucinations and delusions as well as disturbed behaviors. Other common features may include mood and anxiety symptoms. The major treatment goal during this phase is the reduction of these disturbing symptoms. Antipsychotic medications represent the most effective intervention at this stage. Psychosocial treatments that are intrusive are likely to be ineffective while patients are acutely psychotic. Following the acute phase, patients will usually enter a stabilization phase in which acute symptoms have been controlled, but patients remain at risk for relapse if treatment is interrupted or if the patient is

Cambridge Textbook of Effective Treatments in Psychiatry, ed. Peter Tyrer and Kenneth R. Silk. Published by Cambridge University Press.
© Cambridge University Press, 2008.

exposed to stress. During this phase, treatment focuses on consolidating therapeutic gains through utilizing similar treatments as those used in the acute stage. This phase may last as long as 6 months following recovery from acute symptoms. During the stabilization phase, patients may benefit from a number of supportive interventions, particularly educational approaches. As in the acute phase, patients may be vulnerable to relapse if intrusive or stressful treatments are implemented. The third stage is the stable or maintenance phase when the illness is in a relative stage of remission. The goals during this phase are to prevent psychotic relapse and to assist patients in improving their level of functioning. This is the phase during which psychosocial treatments and rehabilitation strategies are likely to be most effective.

Antipsychotic medications for acute schizophrenia

Evidence supporting the effectiveness of antipsychotic medications

A large body of evidence supports the effectiveness of antipsychotic medications for treating psychotic symptoms in acute schizophrenia. The introduction of the first antipsychotic medications in the late 1950s and 1960s was greeted with substantial scepticism in the field. This was addressed by the development of standards of research design that have strongly influenced all psychopharmacological research. Among the standards are (1) the demonstration that the agent is more effective than a placebo for the condition; (2) the use of random assignment to the treatments that are being compared; and (3) the reduction of sources of bias by double-blind administration of drugs. Studies carried out in the 1960s by the National Institute of Mental Health and the Department of Veterans Affairs using these methodological advances found that antipsychotics were nearly always more effective than a placebo. Meta-analyses have found that approximately 60% of patients treated with a first-generation antipsychotic (FGA) will demonstrate a substantial remission on an antipsychotic compared to fewer than 20% on a placebo. Studies of second-generation antipsychotics (SGA) (atypical antipsychotics) also find consistent advantages of these agents over placebo.

Antipsychotic drugs are antipsychotic and not antischizophrenic. They are effective for any illness that is characterized by psychotic symptoms. Although relatively few studies have focused on schizoaffective disorder, there is substantial evidence that antipsychotics are effective for this disorder (Levinson et al., 1999; Keck et al., 1999). In

schizophrenia and schizoaffective disorder, they are highly effective for attenuating the psychotic dimension of schizophrenia, which often includes hallucinations and delusions and relatively ineffective for other dimensions. That is, negative symptoms such as blunted affect, emotional withdrawal, and lack of social or vocational interest and cognitive symptoms including impairments in memory, attention, and executive functions tend to improve as psychotic symptoms improve. However, patients often continue to demonstrate negative and cognitive symptoms even after they have achieved a remission of psychotic symptoms. In addition, acute psychosis is often accompanied by symptoms of anxiety and depression. These symptoms commonly improve as psychosis improves. However, when these symptoms persist during antipsychotic treatment, patients may benefit from the addition of an antidepressant or an antianxiety drug.

Typical vs. atypical antipsychotics

When the atypical (second-generation) antipsychotics were first introduced in the early 1990s, there was hope that these agents would be more effective than the first-generation agents against all of the dimensions of schizophrenia. This observation was encouraged by comparisons of clozapine with typical antipsychotics in treatment refractory patients. The comparisons found that clozapine was more effective for a broad range of symptom dimensions including positive, negative, and mood symptoms (Kane et al., 1988). Further support came from early studies of risperidone and olanzapine (for review, see Leucht et al., 1999). However, a meta-analysis by Geddes et al. (2000) concluded that the advantages of the atypical antipsychotic drugs were only apparent when patients received excessive dosages of the comparison drug, which was haloperidol for nearly all of these studies. This suggests that the greater degree of extrapyramidal symptoms (EPS) in the haloperidol-treated group may have given an advantage to the atypical drugs that was not related to intrinsic antipsychotic properties.

Moreover, a careful review of the Leucht meta-analysis (Leucht et al., 1999) indicates that, even when there were statistically significant advantages for the newer drug over haloperidol, the effect sizes were very small. A more recent meta-analysis by Davis and coworkers (Davis et al., 2003) does suggest that there are consistent advantages for clozapine, risperidone and olanzapine (and, perhaps, amisulpride) when compared with haloperidol. These advantages were not present with other atypical antipsychotics. However, these advantages of specific atypical antipsychotics may be related to the time that studies were carried out. That is, drugs that were studied in the early 1990s were likely to include patients who had only received typical antipsychotic drugs and who responded poorly to these agents. On the other hand, patients who participated in studies in the late 1990s may have received both first- and second-generation agents and had entered trials because they did poorly on both.

CATIE and CUtLASS Studies

More recent clinical trials have cast doubt on the proposed advantages of atypical antipsychotics. The first trial was the National Institute of Mental Health CATIE (Clinical Antipsychotic Trial of Intervention Effectiveness) study (Lieberman *et al.*, 2005; McEvoy *et al.*, 2006; Stroup *et al.*, 2006). In the first phase of this study, 1493 patients were randomly assigned to double-blind olanzapine (7.5 to 30 mg per day), perphenazine (8 to 32 mg per day), quetiapine (200 to 800 mg per day), risperidone (1.5 to 6.0 mg per day) or ziprasidone (40 to 160 mg per day) for up to 18 months. The primary outcome was the time that patients remained on their assigned drug. Seventy-four percent of patients discontinued their assigned medication over the entire 18 months. In comparing the different agents, the proportion remaining on their medication was similar, although olanzapine had a statistically significant advantage. Rates of discontinuation were 64% for olanzapine, 75% for perphenazine, 82% for quetiapine, 74% for risperidone, and 79% for ziprasidone. This study is consistent with others in indicating that typical and atypical antipsychotics are similar in their efficacy. Although olanzapine had an advantage for efficacy, more patients were discontinued in the olanzapine condition for adverse effects, particularly metabolic effects. Patients who received perphenazine were more likely to discontinue their medication due to EPS. The study was too brief to evaluate the relative risk of tardive dyskinesia among the agents. In addition, the patients who entered the study were probably not representative of typical patients who receive treatment in clinical settings. On average, patients had been ill for more than 15 years and had received multiple trials with atypical antipsychotics and had still not found a completely satisfactory agent. This could be a partial explanation for the high discontinuation rates. Nevertheless, CATIE also points out a substantial dissatisfaction with antipsychotics.

In a second phase of CATIE (McEvoy *et al.*, 2006), patients who were discontinued for lack of efficacy were randomly assigned to double-blind risperidone, olanzapine, quetiapine, or open label clozapine. In this phase, patients assigned to clozapine had the best outcome with 56% of clozapine patients being discontinued compared to 71% on olanzapine, 86% on risperidone and 93%

on quetiapine. Clozapine treated patients also showed greater symptom improvements than those receiving the other agents. This advantage of clozapine for poor or partial responders is consistent with the findings from a number of other studies (for review, see Marder *et al.*, 2002).

The comparative effectiveness of typical and atypical antipsychotics was also evaluated in the Cost Utility of the Latest Antipsychotic Drugs in Schizophrenia Study #1 (CUtLASS-1). This study from the United Kingdom National Health Service (Jones *et al.*, 2006) randomized 227 patients with schizophrenia to either an SGA or an FGA. Although treatment was open label, raters of the clinical response were blind to the nature of the treating agent. Prior to randomization, the patient's psychiatrist selected the atypical or typical antipsychotic to which each patient would be assigned (i.e. two choices as the randomization actually decided which drug type was given). Among patients who were randomized, 49% of patients in the FGA group received sulpiride and 46% of patients in the SGA group received olanzapine. There was no significant difference in scores on the Quality of Life Scale, the primary outcome instrument. Moreover, there were trends suggesting advantages for the typical antipsychotics. Since sulpiride is not available to psychiatrists in the USA, the findings from CUtLASS-1 are easier to interpret in the UK. Nevertheless, the results do not support any advantage for the newer agents.

Another trial in the UK, CUtLASS-2 (Lewis *et al.*, 2006), randomized 136 patients who had responded poorly to two prior antipsychotics to either clozapine or an SGA selected prior to the randomization. Patients who received clozapine demonstrated greater improvement than those on the comparison drugs.

In summary, if there are advantages of the second-generation antipsychotics over the first, the difference is small and inconsistent. There is evidence that clozapine is more effective for poor responders, and suggestions that risperidone, olanzapine, and amisulpride may have small advantages which, as noted in the section below, need to be balanced with their side effects.

Tolerability and efficacy as interacting factors

Tolerability and efficacy for antipsychotics are closely linked. Most patients with psychotic illnesses will require long-term antipsychotic therapy. As a result, side effects that can be endured by individuals for a relatively brief time can be intolerable for patients who experience chronic discomforts from their medications or for those who have their long-term physical health affected. In addition, patients will often experience a side effect of an antipsychotic before they experience a therapeutic effect. This is because side effects such as drowsiness or restlessness may be experienced during the hours after a medication is started while the antipsychotic effects may be delayed for days or weeks. The side effect may then be interpreted as the effect of the drug.

The effect of extrapyramidal side effects on therapeutic response has been well documented. Akathisia is the most common form of EPS. In its more severe forms it can manifest as an inability to sit still as well as restless pacing. Milder forms can be experienced as anxiety or irritability (Van Putten, 1975). A common dilemma in treating patients with typical antipsychotics was agitation that worsened as patients had their antipsychotic doses increased. The agitation was interpreted by some clinicians as an inadequate antipsychotic dose when it was actually an excessive amount. Other evidence suggests that akinesia, a Parkinsonian variant that is manifest as an inability to initiate movement, can be confused with negative symptoms or even depression.

The introduction of the atypical antipsychotic drugs has substantially decreased EPS as a concern although milder forms of akathisia remain even with these agents. However, other side effects such as sedation or restlessness on these agents can interfere with the effectiveness of the antipsychotic. In addition, antipsychotics can lead to weight gain and other metabolic side effects including type 2 diabetes and hyperlipidemias. These side effects of antipsychotics can interact with an already existing tendency of patients with schizophrenia to be an overweight group with multiple risk factors for heart disease. As a result, the ability of individuals with schizophrenia to adjust in the community is impaired and the effectiveness of the antipsychotic is compromised.

The differences in side effects among the first and second generation antipsychotics were evident in CATIE. In Phase 1 (Lieberman et al., 2005), the agent with an effectiveness advantage, olanzapine, also caused more metabolic side effects including a mean 2 pounds of weight gain per month, as well as elevations in glucose, cholesterol and triglycerides. In a Phase 2 trial for patients who were discontinued for intolerability, patients who gained weight in Phase 1, lost weight when they were changed to ziprasidone or risperidone (Stroup et al., 2006).

Recent treatment guidelines for schizophrenia suggest approaches to managing the metabolic side effects of antipsychotics. These guidelines include the APA Guidelines (Lehman et al., 2004), American Diabetes Association Guidelines (consensus development conference, 2004), and the Mount Sinai Guidelines (Marder et al., 2004). They are similar in that they recommend regular monitoring of weight, glucose, lipids, and blood pressure. Elevations in any of these guidelines should lead to an intervention which can include lifestyle changes or a change in the patient's antipsychotic.

Stable phase pharmacological treatment and maintenance therapy

Goals of long-term treatment

The goals of long-term treatment for schizophrenia have evolved over the past decade. In the past, the focus of long-term treatment was maintaining patients in the community and preventing relapse. Recently, patients and their families have criticized this approach since it fails to focus on the ability of many patients to improve their overall quality of life and community functioning. Instead, these groups are proposing that treatments should be focused on recovery. The recovery approach is associated with the goal of improving life satisfaction, sustaining hope and optimism, and empowering patients to gain greater control of their own treatment (Resnick et al., 2004). In addition, the recovery model recognizes that the relationship between symptoms and functional outcomes such as vocational adjustment are only moderate, and this would suggest that patients can recover even when they sustain symptoms (Anthony et al., 1995).

Promoting recovery in long-term treatment almost always requires a combination of an antipsychotic medication with psychosocial interventions. The following sections provide evidence to support a model in which the most important effect of pharmacotherapy in the stable phase is to support recovery by preventing psychotic relapse. In addition, adverse effects of medication can impair a patient's likelihood of success in psychosocial treatments.

Antipsychotics and relapse prevention

The effectiveness of antipsychotic medications for the prevention of psychotic relapse in schizophrenia has been demonstrated in studies in which stabilized patients on an antipsychotic were randomly assigned to remain on an antipsychotic or were changed to a placebo. Studies with first generation antipsychotics provided compelling evidence that these agents were highly effective. A review of 24 double-blind studies found that in all studies many more patients relapsed when not receiving a drug (Davis, 1975). A meta-analysis that included most of these studies reported that approximately 72% of patients will relapse in a year on a placebo compared to only 23% on a first-generation antipsychotic (Davis *et al.*, 1989). Studies of first-generation drugs also focused on the effectiveness of these agents for patients who had long periods of stability. An important study by Hogarty and coworkers (Hogarty *et al.*, 1976) found that these individuals still had a high likelihood of relapse if antipsychotics were discontinued, again supporting the continuation of antipsychotic medications for most patients who had achieved sustained remissions.

A number of studies have evaluated the effectiveness of atypical antipsychotics in comparison to both placebo and typical antipsychotics. These studies have been reviewed by Leucht and coworkers (Leucht *et al.*, 2003). The six studies that were comparisons to placebos all found advantages for the active drugs. A meta-analysis of the eleven studies that compared an SGA to an FGA found a very modest but statistically significant advantage for the newer agents. This advantage could be attributable to improved adherence to the atypical antipsychotics although these studies were unable to document differences between agents in rates of adherence.

Other studies have focused on the usefulness of continuing medication for patients who have recovered from a first episode of schizophrenia. Although relapse may be somewhat lower for this group, 40–60% of first episode patients will relapse if their medications are discontinued (Lehman *et al.*, 2004). Maintenance antipsychotics were effective in reducing relapse rates. Other studies indicate that atypical antipsychotics may have advantages in first episode patients (Lieberman *et al.*, 2003a, 2003b). Again, it is difficult to determine if the advantage of the atypical antipsychotics is due to an advantage in patient adherence.

Taken together, these studies provide strong support for continuing antipsychotics in patients who have recovered from psychotic episodes. The American Psychiatric Association Treatment Guidelines for Schizophrenia (Lehman *et al.*, 2004) provide reasonable guidance regarding the duration of treatment. Patients with multiple episodes or those with two or more episodes within the past five years should receive indefinite maintenance treatment. For those who do not meet these criteria or for first episode patients, decisions regarding long-term maintenance should be guided by a number of considerations including the long-term risks and side effects of medications and the dangers associated with an individual's psychotic episodes. If a decision is made to attempt the discontinuation of antipsychotics, this should be done through gradual dose reduction combined with close clinical monitoring for prodromal symptoms by the family and the treating clinician.

Treatment resistant schizophrenia

Approximately 60% of patients with schizophrenia will experience complete or nearly complete remission of positive symptoms with antipsychotic medication treatment. The remaining 40% will continue to experience positive symptoms that are resistant to medication. Additionally, patients who experience remission of positive symptoms with treatment may continue to experience negative symptoms, cognitive symptoms or depressive symptoms.

The definition of treatment resistance in schizophrenia has evolved over time. In 1988 Kane *et al.* defined treatment resistance in schizophrenia as including the following criteria: (1) persistent positive psychotic symptoms as defined by a score of greater than or equal to 4 on at least 2 of 4 positive symptom items on the BPRS; (2) moderately severe illness as rated by BPRS score of greater than or equal to 45 and a CGI score of greater than or equal to 4; (3) persistence of illness as evidenced by no stable period of good occupational or social functioning; and (4) illness refractory to medication as evidenced by at least three periods of treatment each of at least 6 weeks' duration with conventional antipsychotics from at least two classes at doses equivalent to 1000 mg chlorpromazine without significant symptom relief and failure to improve by at least 20% in total BPRS score.

The Kane criteria characterized a group of severely ill individuals who had failed to respond to first generation antipsychotics. Approaches to managing treatment resistance have evolved as atypical antipsychotics became widely available. Comparisons between typical and atypical antipsychotics for treatment refractory patients indicate that atypical antipsychotics are more effective for this population (Marder *et al.*, 2002). However, the recent results from CATIE (Lieberman *et al.*, 2005) and CUtLASS-1 (Jones *et al.*, 2006) suggest that there is not an advantage for atypical antipsychotics in groups of patients who are partial responders to their antipsychotics. On the other hand, effect sizes for clozapine tend to be larger than those for other atypical antipsychotics suggesting an advantage for clozapine. As mentioned earlier, the results from Phase 2 of CATIE (McEvoy *et al.*, 2006) and CUtLASS-2 (Lewis *et al.*, 2006) also support an advantage for clozapine. Chakos *et al.* (2001) conducted a review and meta-analysis of studies comparing the efficacy and tolerability of typical and atypical antipsychotics, including clozapine, for treatment-resistant schizophrenia. The studies comparing clozapine to first-generation antipsychotics revealed that treatment with clozapine resulted in more favorable outcomes in terms of both improvement in psychopathology and reduced extrapyramidal side effects. Despite its superior efficacy for treatment resistant schizophrenia, a significant number of treatment refractory patients do not respond to clozapine. The Chakos meta-analysis (Chakos et al., 2001) found that, in most studies, fewer than half of the treatment resistant patients had a response to clozapine. Additionally, many patients who do respond favorably to clozapine continue to have significant symptoms that impairs their functioning in the community.

The recent revision of the Texas Medication Algorithm Project (TMAP) (Miller et al., 2004) provides a reasonable guide for drug selection when patients continue to demonstrate refractory positive symptoms. If patients fail to respond to an adequate trial of a typical antipsychotic he or she should probably receive an adequate trial with an atypical one. A history of two drug trial failures leads to consideration of either a trial of clozapine or a trial of an typical antipsychotic if the patient has not had one. If adherence to oral medication is an issue, a trial of a long-acting depot antipsychotic should be considered.

For patients who are refractory to clozapine in addition to FGAs and other SGAs, there is no clear data to guide treatment. Some clinicians employ high dose antipsychotic treatment for patients who do not respond to typical therapeutic doses. Studies have generally found the use of high dose antipsychotics is not associated with greater improvement than the use of conventional doses (Marder, 1999). Clinicians commonly treat refractory patients with more than one antipsychotic medication. A number of controlled trials have evaluated the effectiveness of adding risperidone to clozapine (Honer et al., 2006; Josiassen et al., 2005; Yagcioglu et al., 2005). Most of the trials failed to find that the combination was effective.

Recently, clinicians also have combined SGAs other than clozapine for the treatment of refractory symptoms. There is little research to support this practice, and studies examining the efficacy of such combinations are needed. Electroconvulsive therapy has been used both as monotherapy and in combination with antipsychotic medications for treatment refractory schizophrenia and there is some data to support its efficacy (Lehman et al., 2004).

Conclusions

It is clear that patients with schizophrenia can benefit greatly by taking antipsychotic medications. This advantage persists through all phases of the illness. There is controversy as to whether SGAs have any real advantage over FGAs, though a number of studies suggest that clozapine may be more effective than the other antipsychotic medications. One major problem with the antipsychotics is the side effects of the medications which probably have a great deal to do with the low compliance rates among these patients. The 'older' side effects of akathisia, akinesia, dyskinesia and tardive dyskinesia, concerns that were prevalent with the FGAs have now been replaced by concerns about weight gain, diabetes, and a full-blown metabolic syndrome with the SGAs. There remains no standard protocol for patients whose symptoms persist at high levels despite rigorous trials of antipsychotic medications.

The level of evidence for each of the interventions discussed in this chapter is summarized in Table 25.1.

Table 25.1. Effectiveness of drug treatment for schizophrenia and related psychoses

Treatment	Form of treatment	Psychiatric disorder	Level of evidence for efficacy	Comments
Typical antipsychotic drugs	Chlorpromazine (also see Appendix) sulpiride	Acute schizophrenia and related acute psychoses (including schizoaffective disorder)	Ia	
Clozapine	Tablets with routine monitoring of blood neutrophil levels	Refractory schizophrenia	Ia	Significantly greater improvement with clozapine than with typical antipsychotic drugs – greater for negative symptoms
Risperidone	Tablets (normal and quick absorption), liquid and depot injection	Acute and maintenance treatment of schizophrenia	Ia	Unequivocal evidence of efficacy with marginal evidence of increased benefit over typical antipsychotic drugs with no conclusive comparative studies yet with injectable form

Table 25.1. (cont.)

Treatment	Form of treatment	Psychiatric disorder	Level of evidence for efficacy	Comments
Olanzapine	Tablets (normal and quick absorption), im injection	Acute and maintenance treatment of schizophrenia	Ia	Unequivocal evidence of efficacy with some evidence of increased benefit over typical antipsychotic drugs offset by greater adverse effects (particularly metabolic ones)
Amisulpride	Tablets	Acute and maintenance treatment of schizophrenia	Ia	Unequivocal evidence of efficacy with marginal evidence of increased benefit over typical antipsychotic drugs
Quetiapine	Tablets	Acute and maintenance treatment of schizophrenia		
All typical and atypical antipsychoticdrugs	Tablets, injections and depot injections	Relapse prevention	Ia	All highly effective and significantly reduces relapse compared with placebo maintenance
Combined antipsychotic drugs (typical plus atypical or in same group)	Both tablets and injections	Treatment refractory schizophrenia	Ia	No clear benefit of polypharmacy
Antipsychotic drugs plus ECT	Any form	Treatment refractory schizophrenia	Ia	Slight benefit of combine therapy

REFERENCES

Adams, C., Tharyan, P., Coutinho, E. S. *et al.* (2006). The schizophrenia drug-treatment paradox: pharmacological treatment based on best possible evidence may be hardest to practise in high-income countries. *British Journal of Psychiatry*, **189**, 391–2.

American Diabetes Association Guidelines (2004). Consensus development conference on antipsychotic drugs and obesity and diabetes. *Diabetes Care*, **27**, 596–601.

Anthony, W. A., Rogers, E. S., Cohen, M. & Davies, R. R. (1995). Relationships between psychiatric symptomatology, work skills, and future vocational performance. *Psychiatric Services*, **46**, 353–8.

Chakos, M., Lieberman, J., Hoffman, E., Bradford, D. & Sheitman, B. (2001). Effectiveness of second-generation antipsychotics in patients with treatment-resistant schizophrenia: a review and meta-analysis of randomized trials. *American Journal of Psychiatry*, **158**, 518–26.

Davis, J. M. (1975). Overview: maintenance therapy in psychiatry: I. Schizophrenia. *American Journal of Psychiatry*, **132**, 1237–45.

Davis, J., Barter, J. & Kane, J. M. (1989). Antipsychotic drugs. In *Comprehensive Textbook of Psychiatry* V, ed. H. I. Kaplan & B. J. Sadock, pp. 1591–1626. Baltimore, Williams and Wilkins.

Davis, J. M., Chen, N. & Glick, I. D. (2003). A meta-analysis of the efficacy of second-generation antipsychotics. *Archives of General Psychiatry*, **60**, 553–64.

Geddes, J., Freemantle, N., Harrison, P. & Bebbington, P. (2000). Atypical antipsychotics in the treatment of schizophrenia: systematic overview and meta-regression analysis. *British Medical Journal*, **321**, 1371–6.

Hogarty, G. E., Ulrich, R. F., Mussare, F. & Aristigueta, N. (1976). Drug discontinuation among long term, successfully maintained schizophrenic outpatients. *Diseases of the Nervous System*, **37**, 494–500.

Honer, W. G., Thornton, A. E., Chen, E. Y. *et al.* (2006). Clozapine alone versus clozapine and risperidone with refractory schizophrenia. *New England Journal of Medicine*, **354**, 472–82.

Josiassen, R. C., Joseph, A., Kohegyi, E. *et al.* (2005). Clozapine augmented with risperidone in the treatment of schizophrenia: a randomized, double-blind, placebo-controlled trial. *American Journal of Psychiatry*, **162**, 130–6.

Jones, P. B., Barnes, T. R., Davies, L. *et al.* (2006). Randomized controlled trial of the effect on Quality of Life of second- vs first-generation antipsychotic drugs in schizophrenia: Cost Utility of the Latest Antipsychotic Drugs in Schizophrenia Study (CUtLASS 1). *Archives of General Psychiatry*, **63**, 1079–87.

Kane, J. M., Honigfeld, G., Singer, J., Meltzer, H. & Group tCCS. (1988). Clozapine for the treatment-resistant schizophrenic: a double-blind comparison versus chlorpromazine/benztropine. *Archives of General Psychiatry*, **45** 789–96.

Keck, P. E. Jr, McElroy, S. L. & Strakowski, S. M. (1999). Schizoaffective disorder: role of atypical antipsychotics. *Schizophrenia Research*, **35** (Suppl. 2), S5–S12.

Lehman, A. F., Lieberman, J. A., Dixon, L. B. *et al.* (2004). Practice guideline for the treatment of patients with schizophrenia, second edition. *American Journal of Psychiatry*, **161**(Suppl. 2), 1–56.

Leucht, S., Pitschel-Walz, G., Abraham, D. & Kissling, W. (1999). Efficacy and extrapyramidal side-effects of the new antipsychotics olanzapine, quetiapine, risperidone, and sertindole compared to conventional antipsychotics and placebo. A meta-analysis of randomized controlled trials. *Schizophrenia Research*, **35**, 51–68.

Leucht, S., Barnes, T. R., Kissling, W., Engel, R. R., Correll, C. & Kane, J. M. (2003). Relapse prevention in schizophrenia with new-generation antipsychotics: a systematic review and exploratory meta-analysis of randomized, controlled trials. *American Journal of Psychiatry*, **160**, 1209–22.

Levinson, D. F., Umapathy, C. & Musthaq, M. (1999). Treatment of schizoaffective disorder and schizophrenia with mood symptoms. *American Journal of Psychiatry*, **156**, 1138–48.

Lewis, S. W., Barnes, T. R., Davies, L. *et al.* (2006). Randomized controlled trial of effect of prescription of clozapine versus other second-generation antipsychotic drugs in resistant schizophrenia. *Schizophrenia Bulletin*, **32**, 715–23.

Lieberman, J. A., Phillips, M., Gu, H. *et al.* (2003a). Atypical and conventional antipsychotic drugs in treatment-naive first-episode schizophrenia: a 52-week randomized trial of clozapine vs chlorpromazine. *Neuropsychopharmacology*, **28**, 995–1003.

Lieberman, J. A., Tollefson, G., Tohen, M. *et al.* (2003b). Comparative efficacy and safety of atypical and conventional antipsychotic drugs in first-episode psychosis: a randomized, double-blind trial of olanzapine versus haloperidol. *American Journal of Psychiatry*, **160**, 1396–404.

Lieberman, J. A., Stroup, T. S., McEvoy, J. P. *et al.* (2005). Effectiveness of antipsychotic drugs in patients with chronic schizophrenia. *New England Journal of Medicine*, **353**, 1209–23.

Marder, S. R. (1999). An approach to treatment resistance in schizophrenia. *British Journal of Psychiatry* (Suppl. 37), 19–22.

Marder, S. R., Essock, S. M., Miller, A. L. *et al.* (2002). The Mount Sinai conference on the pharmacotherapy of schizophrenia. *Schizophrenia Bulletin*, **28**, 5–16.

Marder, S. R., Essock, S. M., Miller, A. L. *et al.* (2004). Physical health monitoring of patients with schizophrenia. *American Journal of Psychiatry*, **161**, 1334–49.

McEvoy, J. P., Lieberman, J. A., Stroup, T. S. *et al.* (2006). Effectiveness of clozapine versus olanzapine, quetiapine, and risperidone in patients with chronic schizophrenia who did not respond to prior atypical antipsychotic treatment. *American Journal of Psychiatry*, **163**, 600–10.

Miller, A. L., Hall, C. S., Buchanan, R. W. *et al.* (2004). The Texas Medication Algorithm Project antipsychotic algorithm for schizophrenia: 2003 update. *Journal of Clinical Psychiatry*, **65**, 500–8.

O'Donnell, C., Donohoe, G., Sharkey, L. *et al.* (2003). Compliance therapy: a randomised controlled trial in schizophrenia. *British Medical Journal*, **327**, 834.

Resnick, S. G., Rosenheck, R. A. & Lehman, A. F. An exploratory analysis of correlates of recovery. *Psychiatric Services*, **55**, 540–7.

Stroup, T. S., Lieberman, J. A., McEvoy, J. P. *et al.* (2006). Effectiveness of olanzapine, quetiapine, risperidone, and ziprasidone in patients with chronic schizophrenia following discontinuation of a previous atypical antipsychotic. *American Journal of Psychiatry*, **163**, 611–22.

Van Putten, T. (1975). The many faces of akathisia. *Comparative Psychiatry*, **16**, 43–7.

Yagcioglu, A. E., Kivircik, A., Turgut, T. I. *et al.* (2005). A double-blind controlled study of adjunctive treatment with risperidone in schizophrenic patients partially responsive to clozapine: efficacy and safety. *Journal of Clinical Psychiatry*, **66**, 63–72.

26

Psychosocial and pharmacological treatments for schizophrenia

Peter B. Jones and Stephen R. Marder

Editor's note

One of the most striking advances in psychiatry in the last 50 years has been the improvement in the outcome of those with schizophrenia. Although it is commonly assumed that the largest part of this has been due to the introduction of effective drug treatments (starting with chlorpromazine), there have been major advances in both society's attitudes to schizophrenia and its psycho-social management that have played a major, if not the most important, part in this shift in outcome and general attitudes. The advances achieved are often difficult to evaluate as many are very complex interventions, but they have been considerable. It is perhaps worth noting that both our distinguished authors are very modest in their descriptions of these, but do not be misled; many are considerable advances that have helped to humanise the problems of those who were in the past regarded as degenerate and irredeemable.

Introduction

Once seen as a separate approach to the treatment of schizophrenia, the interventions under the psycho-social umbrella are now viewed as an essential aspect of modern management. They are partners with pharmacotherapy and form part of a multidisciplinary approach outlined in the previous chapter. Psycho-social interventions are often seen as part of a complex set of interventions, delivered by the range of services outlined in Chapter 8. However, the interventions described in this chapter are, in essence, simple and can be taught to, and delivered by, many individuals in a clinical team, perhaps with supervision from an expert.

Psychosocial interventions (PSI) comprise more than supportive, talking- or psycho-therapies that should accompany any treatment modality. They are often used to target residual positive symptoms, negative symptoms and the debilitating and sometimes puzzling failure of people to return to pre-morbid or predicted levels of functioning despite resolution of symptoms. The role of cognitive impairment in this phenomenon is discussed, below.

Psycho-social interventions involve not only the individual with schizophrenia, but also their family and carers. Indeed, families are often central to the success of a treatment plan, as well as frequently providing the lynch pin of successful community care: accommodation.

There is considerable convergence in terms of the multidisciplinary management of a number of chronic illnesses, not just in the psychological sphere. Education, informed decision making, reducing long-term risks and a focus on increasing function and quality of life, with goals informed by the patient, are central to the modern management of diseases as apparently disparate as diabetes mellitus, asthma, chronic inflammatory conditions and schizophrenia. A sense of optimism and empowerment is common to all, even if the goal is to minimise deterioration or avoid harm. Often the ambitions may be much higher. Concordance, compliance or adherence (all terms are used) with prescribed medication is dismal in many illnesses, with prevalence of full adherence to the prescribed regimen often being below 50% (Sackett, 1978). Those having schizophrenia do not do badly in this context. Some of the most successful talking therapies aim to increase adherence.

A variety of psycho-social interventions is described below, including family interventions, psycho-education, cognitive approaches, social skills training and vocational rehabilitation. First, we review some principles common to them all, and some historical aspects in their development.

Cambridge Textbook of Effective Treatments in Psychiatry, ed. Peter Tyrer and Kenneth R. Silk. Published by Cambridge University Press.

Common principles of psycho-social interventions

Psycho-social interventions should be tailored to individuals' needs, and these are likely to change over time. They should be reviewed periodically. The aims of psycho-social interventions often include increased function, quality of life and recovery, in addition to specific symptom reduction and avoidance of relapse. In many respects PSI, or the people who deliver them, are driven by values. However, there is a firm evidence base to support their success.

Two systematic reviews of psychosocial interventions by Pilling and colleagues (Pilling *et al.*, 2002a, b) contain an excellent summary of trials until the late 1990s. We refer below to systematic reviews undertaken by the Cochrane Collaboration where these are available for the particular intervention described here. Many of these are updated periodically, so include contemporary trials as well as the classic literature. It is worth noting that there is a great deal of evidence available, but it is a very difficult area in which to do good research. Use of a wide variety of outcome measures in different settings and patient groups often makes synthesis of effects difficult or impossible when several trials are compared.

Psychosocial interventions may be targeted not only on the person with schizophrenia; families and carers may be both recipients of specific approaches, and may be allies in management. As such they, themselves, need support, and an attempt should be made to assess and meet their own needs in this context, at least as far as resources will allow.

Finally, many PSI are pragmatic and their principles are easily grasped. However, there is clear evidence that their success may be related to the skill of the therapist, and the sophistication of the service within which they work. In the UK, Europe, Australia and, to a lesser extent, the USA, there has been an increase in training available to mental health professionals, particularly but not exclusively, community psychiatric nurses. Post-graduate courses in PSI for schizophrenia are becoming more common, and nurses may specialise in the treatment of schizophrenia. In general, the services in which they work need to be involved with individuals and their families over the medium to long term, although there are some experiments with brief, focused interventions at particular junctures such as after hospital admission.

Historical points

The fall and rise of the family in the management of schizophrenia is an interesting piece of social and scientific history, and is central to the development of PSI. Families were not always seen in the positive light of modern approaches.

The *hocus pocus* of psychodynamic understanding of schizophrenia that held sway in the mid twentieth century, before antipsychotic drugs or other interventions became widely available, gave rise to a number of analytic theories of aetiology based on a person's relationships with parents, family dynamics and communication (Wynne *et al.*, 1958). Schism and skew in family relationships (Lidz *et al.*, 1965) and the, so-called, double-bind relationship (Bateson *et al.*, 1956) between parent and child were deemed toxic enough to cause schizophrenia as a psychological reaction. Mothers were said to be 'schizophrenogenic' (Fromm-Reichmann, 1954), adding to the obvious trauma and distress brought by a child's mental illness.

These views were grist to the mill for the anti-psychiatrists of the 1960s and 1970s who, themselves, were usually psychiatrists treating people with schizophrenia. These psychiatrists argued that schizophrenia existed only in the minds of observers, not the person deemed ill. The sad irony that their patients didn't respond to the promulgation of these views was lost on their proponents. Kraepelin's original ideas of schizophrenia as a brain illness (Kraepelin, 1919) were forgotten, and the philosophy of empiricism put to one side.

However, careful studies of families where a child had schizophrenia failed to show the differences deemed important by these men (Hirsch & Leff, 1978). At the same time, the closure of the asylums was continuing apace, medication regimens were becoming effective and behavioural views and interventions were overtaking psychodynamic opinions in the USA and much of Europe. It was presumed that people with schizophrenia who were discharged from long-term, institutional care to their family would fare better than those who went to hostels and community-based services. Yet the opposite was true; there were frequently more relapses and readmission in people who had returned to their family, often aging parents. Clinical researchers going into these homes noticed that the emotional tone was often higher in the families of people who had relapsed than in those who had not. In the former, the atmosphere could be cut with a knife, and this tension led to an increase in symptoms, presumably as a stress-related response.

These observations led to the concept of expressed emotion or 'EE', in families and groups, with contributions from domains of hostility, criticism, emotional over-involvement and, having the opposite effect, warmth. Where these elements were high, the risk of relapse of schizophrenia rose, accordingly (Brown, Birley & Wing,

1972). The key step was taken when it was found that EE could be reduced and, with it, the risk of relapse. Moreover, a classic investigation by Vaughn and Leff (1976) showed that there was a positive therapeutic interaction with the use of antipsychotic medication.

Similar, astute clinical observations were important in the development of other approaches. In an asylum context, Brown & Wing (1970) noted that some people with schizophrenia could have a double-edged response to occupation therapy and other activities that were arranged to fill their days. Those with chronic illness and predominant negative symptoms showed a decrease of these features with a carefully tailored programme. However, the dose–response relationship was complex in that if the activity schedule was increased above a certain level, the illness could relapse, with resurgence of both positive and negative features. Not only was this a demonstration that PSI could have an effect on what are considered as more hard-wired aspects of schizophrenia that remain resistant features in terms of pharmacotherapy, it also showed that their use or implementation needs careful planning and monitoring. And like other therapies, they can have side effects.

Family, cognitive and vocational interventions now form part of a suite of multidisciplinary management approaches for schizophrenia. That these approaches are intimately entwined with drug treatments is demonstrated by the fact that two of them, compliance therapy and medications management (see below), have as their goal improved compliance with antipsychotic and other drugs. Some PSI, such as hypnosis (de Izquierdo Santiago et al., 2004) or psychodymamic psychotherapy for schizophrenia (Malmberg & Fenton, 2001), have careful systematic reviews suggesting both no benefit and inadequate evidence, and these are not included here. Similarly, other approaches, such as the token economy (McMonagle & Sultana 2000) are unfashionable, and they also are excluded here, but that does not indicate that well designed trials would not be useful in order clearly to rule them in or rule them out of the management repertoire for this complex disorder.

Specific interventions

Psycho-education

Knowledge and understanding generally lead to better decisions. Improving these two aspects for a patient is amongst the most basic of interventions. Education about illness, its causes and effects may have a positive effect on outcome through a variety of mechanisms. These include improved engagement with services, better

adherence to drug treatments, early detection of signs of relapse, planning strategies to deal with such signs, and ways to deal with or avoid circumstances that may have precipitated illness, either in the first episode or beyond.

In terms of causation of schizophrenia, it is all too common for clinicians to tell people that the causes of the disorder are unknown whereas, on the contrary, much is known. A formulation of aetiology that might encompass vulnerability factors such as a family history or early developmental insults may make the place of possible precipitants, such as drug use, life events or other stressful situations more relevant for a person. A young adult with psychosis who sees their peers smoking cannabis with few apparent ill effects may be more likely to stop or moderate their behaviour if they see reasons why this may have different effects on them. Working out such a formulation with a patient is often a useful process of engagement as well as leading to a better mutual understanding of what has gone on. In the future, we may discuss vulnerability at a more specific level, perhaps at the level of interactions between personal environmental events and a person's genotype.

Information should be shared about symptoms, risks of relapse on and off medication, side effects and their management. People will vary as to how much they want to know at a particular time and, as ever, the information must be tailored to an individual's requirements and wishes. The first episode of schizophrenia or an apparent prodrome are special situations when these issues must be handled with particular care because uncertainty is, necessarily, great in these circumstances.

Education such as this can be done on an individual basis, as well as in a group approach. An example of a special group, the family, is discussed below.

The evidence base for education about schizophrenia is relatively secure, with enough randomised controlled trials (ten by 2002) for a Cochrane review (Pekkala & Merinder, 2002) to conclude that it shows benefits compared with standard care, alone. Psycho-education increased knowledge about schizophrenia and reduced relapse and readmission rates, probably through improved compliance with drug and other treatments, although the results of trials were equivocal on this point. Satisfaction with treatment was improved. It required an educational package to be given to nine people (number needed to treat; NNT) in order to prevent one relapse or readmission. Education for families is considered below.

Family interventions

The time when parents and families were thought to cause schizophrenia has long gone. The tasks of engaging, educating and working with families are now a crucial aspect to the management of schizophrenia because, in general, they are the major support system available outside hospitals. Families are not only an important resource for care, but they can have a major influence on the course and outcome of the disorder. Families need help and support to do this. There is a strong evidence base to underpin a range of interventions targeted on families of someone with schizophrenia, and it is unfortunate that they are often unavailable given this evidence for their effectiveness. This is discussed in more detail below.

Originally, the two main interventions to reduce EE in a family were education about the illness, often reducing criticism of the sufferer through increased understanding, and a reduction in excess face-to-face contact between family members that arises when negative symptoms prevent someone leaving the house. Things are now more sophisticated with greater emphasis on the former in the family component and attention to the latter in other aspects of management.

Whenever possible, family members and others connected to someone with schizophrenia should be involved in the management. There are a number of reasons for this. Families benefit from an intervention that educates them about schizophrenia, its effects on the person with the illness, and on the family, and it provides an avenue of support for them.

Psycho-social family interventions for schizophrenia often have a number of aims. A therapeutic alliance needs to be built with carers so that they will be prepared to take on the work involved in further work. This might include learning to lower the level of EE, the creation of a more positive family atmosphere and attitude, identifying specific problems and learning to solve them rather than feeling non-specifically dissatisfied with events. Through learning about schizophrenia and its effects on their relative, family members may develop and maintain realistic expectations of the performance and ambitions of the person with schizophrenia. On the other hand, they must learn to be able to set limits and to keep appropriate emotional and practical boundaries. This may be difficult when behaviours and family styles have become entrenched over many years of illness, either before or after the initial diagnosis.

In modern services there are generally thought to be three specific components to family interventions for schizophrenia. The first is to engage and build an alliance with the family, the next is to educate and inform them, and the third is to deal with their individual needs as a family.

Engagement with the family is best done early in the first episode, but even then there may have been months or years of abnormal behaviour that may have shattered family relationships. These take time to heal even when parents and siblings gain an understanding of the reasons for the change in their relative. Sometimes drug use and the acquisitive behaviours that support it may have had a very negative effect.

Engagement of the family is, therefore, most likely to be successful when support is provided in the acute phase when they are likely to have many questions and concerns. These issues are likely to vary for the different members of the family, and it is important not to forget siblings and, sometimes, children.

The second component is a relatively structured component that will educate the family about the illness, often referred to as psycho-education, something that is important for the sufferer themselves, and that is considered separately in that context, below. Several studies have demonstrated psycho-educational family interventions to be effective. It is usually begun and maintained by a member of the mental health team, although relatives of other people with schizophrenia may provide additional support and information either individually or through groups for families.

Learning from other families with similar experiences can be useful and provide much needed support to relatives, although it is useful to match families with relatives who have schizophrenia at relatively similar stages of the illness. Tensions can arise if those with relatives who have recovered well meet those whose relative has remained chronically sick, or vice versa. This style of peer support may be relatively informal, arranged through mental health services or, increasingly commonly, through advocacy groups, charities, NGOs or other third sector organisations. However, overall supervision by an expert is best practice.

These two aspects usually need to be supplemented with individual interventions, specifically designed for each family to address their own circumstances. Sometimes this may be formal family therapy from a systems therapist, sometimes ongoing problem solving and support, or reformulation when new problems arise or circumstances change. Either or both may reduce the burden experienced by many families in caring for a relative with schizophrenia, as well as improving the health of that person.

As mentioned above, there is considerable empirical evidence to support this style of family intervention. A Cochrane review (Pharoah et al., 2003) of 14 randomised studies indicated that people's mental state improves with family therapy. However, the improvement was greater with more skilled teams. Drop out rates were low, indicating that family interventions are acceptable to patients and families. No clear effects were defined in the domain of social functioning, but there were positive trends regarding employment and independent living. Families experienced reduced burden of illness, increased knowledge and decreased expressed emotion, as expected from the targets of the interventions.

The review concluded that family interventions lead to a cost saving of about 20% in total costs. The number of families that needed to be treated to prevent one relapse (NNT) was seven. Family therapy has been shown to reduce relapse rates by over 50% compared with medication and case management alone. It has not been shown to have any effect on mortality; the data are simply too sparse to tell. Overall, this is a very difficult area in which to undertake good randomised trials. A number of classic studies typify the field (Berkowitz *et al.*, 1984; Leff *et al.*, 1982, 1984, 1985, 1989; Linszen *et al.*, 1996) though it is important that further trials are undertaken to scrutinise a tendency for effects in more recent trials to approach the null, and for the effect of contemporary social and treatment settings to be investigated.

Cognitive therapy

Cognitive therapy (CT) was originally developed for the treatment of depression. The theoretical framework that underpins this approach to depression cannot be translated directly to the psychotic symptoms and signs of schizophrenia. The depression that is often part of the syndrome may not arise solely from negative automatic thoughts and distorted conclusions and cognitions. People with schizophrenia may be depressed secondary to their very real plight, with hopelessness and suicidal thoughts are actions commonly seen. This aspect of the illness may benefit from conventional CT.

The variant of cognitive therapy known as cognitive-behaviour therapy (CBT) for psychosis has shown positive benefits in schizophrenia, and there are a number of randomised controlled trials, particularly from the UK. This approach maintains many of the traditional elements of CT for depression, but is extended with pragmatic and behavioural elements to encompass the wider schizophrenia syndrome and its sequelae.

The firmest evidence comes from studies of people with chronic positive symptoms refractory to optimum drug therapy, often clozapine. In this group, cognitive therapy techniques focusing on weighing the evidence in favour of delusion or hallucination may result in reduction in symptom scores, and in the grip in which the person is held by the psychotic symptom. However, several recent studies have reported evidence for the efficacy of CBT on depression and negative symptoms, as well as on positive symptoms, and these include studies which have used non-expert case managers as well as those who have used expert therapists.

A Cochrane review of CBT for schizophrenia has reviewed a wide array of trials (Jones *et al.*, 2004). The comparisons are complex, given that there are many potential contrasts: CBT vs. other talking therapies or placebo, improvement in a range of symptom dimensions and service outcomes in the short, medium and long term. Stage of illness is another dimension. In general, the Jones *et al.* review suggested a rather less upbeat message concerning CBT than some of the pioneer trials had suggested.

Thirty papers described 19 randomised controlled trials. CBT plus standard care did not clearly reduce long-term relapse and readmission compared with standard care, but it did decrease the risk of staying in hospital, with four people needing treatment to prevent one delayed discharge. Cognitive-behavioural therapy was associated with improved mental state over the medium term, with a NNT of 4 to prevent one person having no meaningful improvement. However, the difference was not present at 1 year. Conventional, continuous measures of mental state, such as the Beck Depression Inventory and the Brief Psychiatric Rating Scale, showed no consistent effect across the trials. There was little evidence to support an advantage over supportive psychotherapy although, as ever, paucity of evidence does not equate to evidence of no effect. In fact, the effects favoured CBT but not significantly so. Combined with a psychoeducational approach in one RCT, CBT did not significantly reduce readmission rates compared with standard care alone.

Clearly, more research is needed to be sure of the place for CBT as a specific intervention for psychosis. There have been many major, high quality trials (e.g. Drury *et al.*, 1996a, 1996b, 2000; Haddock *et al.*, 1999; Sensky *et al.*, 2000; Lewis *et al.*, 2002; Tarrier *et al.*, 2004), but more are required. A specialised technique, CBT is often unavailable in routine services where clinical psychology is a scarce resource. However, there are moves to educate a broader range of professionals in the technique, as described above. It is certainly an approach that is worthwhile in schizophrenia resistant to drug treatment or where there is anything other than complete recovery, but this must be done in the context of trials if we are to learn the true place of CBT. As clozapine treatment becomes more widespread, the increasingly common situation of schizophrenia resistant to that drug, 'clozapine resistant schizophrenia', should also be an indication for CBT where subjects are motivated enough to try it and, again, where the results can be part of a proper evaluation.

Having said that, there is much psychopathology that the sufferer from schizophrenia has to deal with that is not specifically psychotic. Many have disability from distress, anxiety, depression and problem behaviours that may be part of the syndrome, may be secondary to psychotic phenomena, or may be part of the shared sequelae of chronic ill health. Taken in this light, CBT should not be seen as an antipsychotic intervention but one that is closer to its roots in depression and anxiety and may be useful and effective. This perspective is debated by Birchwood and Trower (2006).

Compliance therapy

The fact that people with schizophrenia may not, for a variety of reasons, continue to take their prescribed anti-psychotic and other drugs leads to a considerable burden of illness and disability. Those established on drugs have a risk of relapse of about 20% over a 2- to 3-year period, rising to 80% if they stop taking them. The NNT in terms of avoiding relapse by maintenance medication is only about two.

Schizophrenia is not particularly associated with lower compliance than many other conditions, but the reasons for non-adherence are likely to be complex given the effects of the illness on insight and on cognitive function, and the side effect profiles of compounds in use. Understanding and improving compliance with effective medication is one of the major challenges for the treatment of schizophrenia.

As discussed above, education is a key aspect to improving compliance, but it is important to make sure people process the information they are given and act upon it. Decisions and plans based on a patient's own conclusions may be easier to maintain than plans they feel have been foisted upon them, or when they feel coerced.

Developed on the basis of motivational interviewing used in substance abuse, compliance therapy uses cognitive therapy techniques to collaborate with and encourage patients to consider their treatment options and to look at evidence for benefits one way or the other in terms of whether or not they take medication, and for how long. The aim is for patients to decide to continue on medication and improve compliance on their own terms and in the light of their own evidence. The same approach can be taken early in the course of illness when someone is deciding for the first time whether to try an antipsychotic or other psychotropic drug.

Compliance therapy is included in a number of Cochrance reviews, as it spans psychoeducation, cognitive approaches, and other techniques. The original RCT by Kemp *et al.* (1996) was followed by an 18-month follow-up and gave encouraging results. Another trial (O'Donnell *et al.*, 2003) showed some supportive results that were statistically inconclusive, perhaps due to small sample size. Recently, using a single-blind four-centre RCT design, Gray *et al.* (2006) compared a compliance therapy (they called it adherence therapy; http://www.adherence therapy.com) with an intervention educating subjects about schizophrenia. They found no difference in quality of life at 1 year, a result that suggested equivalence rather than neither being effective. Perhaps compliance therapy contains much that is educative, and the education package may, in itself, be an effective PSI.

Medications management

Medications management is linked to compliance therapy and the idea of psychoeducation. It aims to inform people with schizophrenia about the effects and side effects of drugs, thus putting them in a better position to be more involved in decisions concerning prescribing. What makes it different from the educative programmes described above is that this task is usually taken on by pharmacists and community nurses who, inevitably, become more involved in the drug management of schizophrenia through this process. Standardised assessment of side effects by using rating scales on a regular basis is usually part of the intervention.

The medications management approach widens the range of professionals involved in this aspect of treatment from solely the physician or psychiatrist. This is seen as helpful in building a treatment alliance and in increasing confidence in this important aspect of treatment. It does have training implications, but medications management is becoming an integral part of specialist courses on PSI.

Cognitive remediation or cognitive rehabilitation

A considerable part of the disability that arises in schizophrenia is now thought to arise secondary to cognitive dysfunction that is much more marked, even in the early stages of the disorder, than was appreciated when contemporary classifications of schizophrenia were made. This contemporary emphasis on a link between cognition and functional outcome is something that had been forgotten. There are clear descriptions in the early literature of the effects of poor attention, concentration problems, distractibility and memory deficits, as well as difficulties with the higher, executive functions of planning, sequencing and decision making. One concern is that these problems may sometimes worsen over the course of the illness, and this is one of the key drivers for emphasis on early intervention.

Cognitive remediation is a set of practical interventions at the interface between clinical neuropsychology, behaviourism, occupational therapy and education. The fusion of approaches is similar to that used in the early stages of dementia. The therapy aims to identify the cognitive impairments and functional sequelae, and thence to help people work around the deficits and to find strategies to improve function in spite of them.

There is an authoritative Cochrane review (Hayes & McGrath, 2000). Three small studies (Medalia et al., 1998; Tompkins et al., 1995; Wykes et al., 1999) met the inclusion criteria. Two compared cognitive rehabilitation with a placebo intervention and the other to occupational therapy. Cognitive rehabilitation was as acceptable as placebo and occupational therapy, with low attrition in both groups, but no effects were demonstrated on measures of mental state, social behaviour or cognitive functioning. An effect in favour of cognitive rehabilitation was shown on self-esteem, something that the authors suggested should be pursued in further trials. A more recent larger trial of 85 patients showed that cognitive remediation produced enduring improvement in working memory and some improvement in cognitive flexibility (Wykes et al., 2007).

This whole area of cognitive remediation is likely to be increasingly studied with either of both psychological and pharmacological interventions.

Social skills training

Reading other people's minds, their reactions, emotions and intentions are probably amongst the most complex cognitive and important processes that we have to do. There is ample evidence that people with schizophrenia can have difficulties with these tasks, even before they develop a psychosis. These difficulties are likely to be due, in part, to the neuro-cognitive impairments described above. It may also be due to, or compounded by, the fact that schizophrenia often begins in late adolescence or early adult life, a period during which humans are learning the finer points of making intimate relationships and developing the skills necessary for independent living and working. Having a severe mental illness is bound to interfere with this learning, particularly if the underlying skills required are already attenuated.

These problems with social skills can be very debilitating and frustrating during recovery. People aspire to having a partner, a job and social life but these barriers prevent success in this most important sphere.

Social skill training targets these impairments. It consists of education about the difficulties, identification of problem areas and simple problem solving techniques.

Behavioural approaches individually and in groups can be helpful with modelling, role play and feedback having been found helpful (See also Chapter 8). Traditional occupational therapy techniques for assessing activities of daily living and teaching those that are deficient are important. These approaches are familiar in psychiatric rehabilitation, but it should be noted that these skills have often never been learnt in the first place where the illness onset was early.

The evidence base is less strong for social skills training than for other psycho-social interventions. Considerable change is often seen, and there is evidence that, as social adjustment improves, social networks can grow and independent living skills develop enough to allow the individual to succeed in living as they would wish. Some effects are non-specific and may be mediated by improvements in medication and symptom management abilities.

However, a systematic review (Pilling et al., 2002) was unable to define an effect when the evidence from existing trials were synthesised. This is likely to have been due, in part, to the difficulty in designing good experiments with such a diffuse set of interventions. This puts the onus on clinicians and researchers to undertake studies to investigate the efficacy and effectiveness of social skills training, and to refine it in the light of the results. This is particularly important now that social skills training has, to a considerable extent, moved from the hospital base to community settings where much less research has been carried out.

In the USA, social skills training is divided into three models: the basic model, the social problem solving model, and the cognitive remediation model. The basic model breaks down social skills into smaller steps that are rehearsed through role playing and then applied to situations in the environment. Social skills training that employs the basic model has been shown to have an effect on improving specific social skills. However, studies have not demonstrated that the skills learned through interventions incorporating the basic model generalise into improved social functioning in the community (Bustillo et al., 2001; Hogarty et al., 1991). Cognitive remediation targets fundamental cognitive impairments such as planning or attention and seeks to improve them prior to the initiation of further skills training. Studies of the efficacy of cognitive remediation have produced mixed results (Bustillo et al., 2001). The evidence is strongest for the efficacy of the social problem-solving model particularly when combined with in vivo skills training (Bustillo et al., 2001; Glynn et al., 2002).

The social problem solving model targets information processing problems that presumably cause social skills impairments. Domains targeted by this model include medication and symptom management, self-care, conversation and recreation. Skills are taught in modules that focus on particular domains. Modules are designed to correct impairments in receptive, processing and sending skills. The social problem solving model has been demonstrated to have an effect on skill enhancement (Marder *et al.*, 1996; Liberman *et al.*, 1998). Marder *et al.* assigned patients to supportive group therapy or problem-solving group therapy for a 2-year period. Subjects attended 90-minute sessions twice weekly for 6 months then weekly. After 2 years, the patients assigned to the problem solving group outperformed the patients in the supportive therapy group in two of six measures of social adjustment. Similarly, Liberman *et al.* followed 80 patients with schizophrenia who were randomly assigned to problem solving model training or occupational therapy over a 6-month period for 3 hours per day 4 days per week. Subjects in the problem-solving group model showed significantly improved independent living skills over a 2-year period. A significantly greater effect was seen in the social skills group in three of ten skills for independent living including management of personal possessions, money management and food preparation. Generalisation of the skills to community functioning was greater in the social skills group than in the occupational therapy group. Patients retained the acquired skills for up to 18 months after the intervention was completed (Liberman 1998). Liberman *et al.* also demonstrated that the problem solving model of skills training could be successfully conducted by paraprofessionals.

Patients obtain greater benefit from skills training with the social problem solving model when it is coupled with in vivo amplified skills training sessions in the community. Glynn *et al.* followed 63 individuals with schizophrenia or schizoaffective disorder who were randomly assigned to 60 weeks of clinic-based skills training alone or clinic-based skills training supplemented with manual-based in vivo amplified skills training sessions in the community. In vivo amplified skills training consisted of 60 specific activities taught simultaneously with skills learned in the clinic. Objectives of this training included the facilitation of completion of clinic assignments in the community, identification of opportunities in the community to employ skills learned in the clinic, and development of a support system through which to maintain the benefits of skills training. In vivo amplified skills training activities included such activities as developing a daily schedule, going to the pharmacy, identifying a nearby emergency facility, attending social gatherings, etc. Both the group receiving clinic-based skills training alone and the group receiving clinic-based skills training plus in vivo amplified skills training demonstrated a modest improvement in social functioning. Transfer of skills to everyday life was enhanced in the group that received augmented skills training (Glynn, 2002).

Vocational rehabilitation

Meaningful and gainful employment is a goal for most adults. Unfortunately, schizophrenia is all too often associated with poor social outcome in terms of this domain. It has also been shown that occupational achievement is often below expectations even before the onset of psychosis, presumably due to subtle developmental impairments and prodromal decline.

This aspect of schizophrenia adds considerably to its economic burden, particularly as it tends to affect people early in their potential working lives. Long-term follow-up studies suggest that only 10%–20% of people return to competitive employment after schizophrenia. This is probably an unduly pessimistic view to give someone in the first episode because many of these studies are biased towards subjects with chronic and more severe illness.

It is an unfortunate irony that much of the economy in the developed world is moving towards information technology and computer-based jobs that require precisely the cognitive skills that are impaired in schizophrenia. A variety of other factors contribute to the incapacity. These include positive psychotic symptoms, negative symptoms, depression and, indirectly, social benefit policies and the societal stigma that still acts as a major barrier to people with schizophrenia entering the labour market.

Placement in sheltered workshops was the original vocational rehabilitation intervention. These were often allied to asylums, more recently moving to local communities. However, these did not lead many people into competitive employment though, as mentioned earlier, the lesson was learned concerning the risks of over-stimulation and precipitation of relapse, particularly in people with residual positive psychotic symptoms.

There are two principal models of vocational rehabilitation. Pre-vocational training involves a period of preparation and training prior to seeking competitive employment. Alternatively, individual placement and support (IPS; also referred to as supported employment) involves some pre-work training, careful tailoring of the working opportunity to the person, and then a period of in-service support. IPS is clearly effective in improving employment outcomes and retaining people in services. However, the improvements in employment outcomes are relatively modest and the effects on symptoms are equivocal.

The Cochrane review of vocational rehabilitation (Crowther *et al.*, 2001) concluded that IPS was a more effective programme than pre-vocational Training. Both, not surprisingly, led to improvements in the prevalence of people at work, in the short term. The NNT for IPS was 4.5 and in this form of vocational rehabilitation, 34% of people were working at 12 months as opposed to 12% in the pre-vocational training conditions.

Individual trials suggest that occupation is likely to have a variety of positive psycho-social consequences. In addition, vocational rehabilitation programmes can reduce re-hospitalisation and may improve insight. Vocational rehabilitation enhances vocational functioning. Modern implementations of IPS rely heavily on relationships with voluntary agencies and NGOs. Often, there are helpful links with educational agencies.

Service configurations

Service configurations are often considered together with PSI. However, there is no great logic to this. Services are quite distinct, being pieces of health technology designed to deliver pharmacological and PSI. They are not interventions themselves, although some aspects of psychological support are inevitably wrapped-up with the service configuration. Moreover, they are very difficult to study.

Tyrer & Milner review the evidence regarding which types of services best deliver complex interventions in Chapter 8. Interested readers are also referred to the relevant Cochrane reviews on subjects such as case management (Marshall & Lockwood, 1998), community mental health teams (Tyrer *et al.*, 1998), day hospitals (Marshall *et al.*, 2001, 2003) and assertive community treatment (Marshall

& Lockwood, 1998). For some, such as early intervention for psychosis, the evidence base is still very limited (Pelosi & Birchwood, 2003), although reviews are complete (Marshall *et al.*, 2005) concerning the possible mediating mechanisms in the form of the link between longer duration of psychosis and poorer outcome. Clinical developments are well advanced, probably because this paradigm unites a number of theoretical approaches and engenders mutual enthusiasm and respect between patients and staff as much as any specific ingredient, although expertise in a specialist patient group must be a factor (http://www.iepa.org.au/).

Conclusions

There is reasonably strong evidence from appropriately designed RCTs that a range of psychosocial interventions have a useful role to play in the management of schizophrenia. They can play a mutually useful adjunct to pharmacotherapy, with the key effective elements of PSI most likely being simple. Most PSI are easily mastered and some, at least, should be available to patients and their families by the majority of mental health services caring for people with schizophrenia.

The level of evidence for each of the interventions discussed in this chapter is summarized in Table 26.1.

Table 26.1. Effectiveness of psychosocial interventions in schizophrenia

Treatment	Form of treatment	Psychiatric disorder	Level of evidence for efficacy	Comments
Psycho-education	Individual	Schizophrenia – all forms	Ia	Reduced relapse and admission compared with standard intervention
Psycho-education	Family	Schizophrenia – all forms	Ia	Reduction of symptoms in patients and reduced burden and expressed emotion in families
Cognitive therapy	Individual	Schizophrenia – all forms	Ia	Modest gains only, with improved mental state over first few months but not after one year
Cognitive therapy	Individual	Schizophrenia – negative symptoms	Ib	Some evidence of greater gain with negative symptoms
Compliance therapy	Individual	Schizophrenia	Ia	Non-specific gains, possibly achieved as much by education as by specific compliance therapy
Medication management	Individual or group	Schizophrenia – acute	III	Insufficient evidence of gain
Cognitive remediation	Individual and group	Schizophrenia – acute to chronic	Ib	Some evidence of improved cognitive function and self-esteem
Social skills training	Group	Schizophrenia – all types	Ib ?	Some inconclusive evidence of specific gains in social functioning
Vocational rehabilitation	Individual or group	Schizophrenia – all types	Ia	Improvement in functioning and possibly insight. Definite evidence of gain (also see Chapter 8)

REFERENCES

Bateson, G., Jackson, D., Haley, J., & Weakland, J. (1956). Towards a theory of schizophrenia: *Behavioural Science*, **1**, 252–264.

Berkowitz, R., Eberlein-Fries, R., Kuipers, L. & Leff, J. (1984). Educating relatives about schizophrenia. *Schizophrenia Bulletin*, **10**, 418–29.

Birchwood, M. & Trower, P. (2006). The future of cognitive–behavioural therapy for psychosis: not a quasi-neuroleptic. *British Journal of Psychiatry*, **188**, 107–8.

Brown, G. W. & Wing, J. (1970). *Institutionalism and Schizophrenia: A Comparative Study of Three Mental Hospitals 1960–1968*. Cambridge: Cambridge University Press.

Brown, G. W., Birley, J. L. & Wing, J. (1972). Influence of family life on the course of schizophrenic disorders: a replication. *British Journal of Psychiatry*, **121**, 241–58.

Bustillo, J., Lauriello, J., Rowland, L. *et al.* (2001). Effects of chronic haloperidol and clozapine treatments on frontal and caudate neurochemistry in schizophrenia. *Psychiatry Research*, **107**(3), 135–49.

Crowther, R., Marshall, M., Bond, G. & Huxley, P. (2001). Vocational rehabilitation for people with severe mental illness. *The Cochrane Database of Systematic Reviews*, Issue 2. Art. No.: CD003080. DOI: 10.1002/14651858.CD003080. Oxford: Update Software Ltd.

de Izquierdo Santiago, A. & Khan, M. (2004). Hypnosis for schizophrenia. *The Cochrane Database of Systematic Reviews*, Issue 3. Art. No.: CD004160.pub2. DOI: 10.1002/14651858.CD004160.pub2.

Drury, V., Birchwood, M., Cochrane, R. & Macmillan, F. (1996a). Cognitive therapy and recovery from acute psychosis: a controlled trial. I. Impact on psychotic symptoms. *British Journal of Psychiatry*, **169**, 593–601.

Drury, V., Birchwood, M., Cochrane, R. & Macmillan, F. (1996b). Cognitive therapy and recovery from acute psychosis: a controlled trial. II. Impact on recovery time. *British Journal of Psychiatry*, **169**, 602–7.

Drury, V., Birchwood, M. & Cochrane, R. (2000). Cognitive therapy and recovery from acute psychosis: a controlled trial. III. Five-year follow-up. *British Journal of Psychiatry*, **117**, 8–14.

Fromm-Reichmann, F., The Academic Lecture Psychotherapy of Schizophrenia group 2. (1954). *American Journal of Psychiatry*.

Glynn, S., Marder, S., Liberman, R. *et al.* (2002). Supplementing clinic-based skills training with manual-based community support sessions: effects on social adjustments of patients with schizophrenia. *American Journal of Psychiatry*, **159**(5), 829–37.

Gray, R., Leese, M., Bindman, J. *et al.* (2006). Adherence therapy for people with schizophrenia. European multicentre randomised controlled trial. *British Journal of Psychiatry*, **189**, 508–14.

Gunderson, J. G., Frank, A. F., Katz, H. M., Vannicelli, M. L., Frosch, J. P. & Knapp, P. H. (1984). [Effects of psychotherapy in schizophrenia. II. Comparative outcome of two forms of treatment]. *Schizophrenia Bulletin*, **10**(4), 564–98.

Haddock, G., Tarrier, N., Morrison, A. P., Hopkins, R., Drake, R. & Lewis, S. (1999). A pilot study evaluating the effectiveness of individual inpatient cognitive-behavioural therapy in early psychosis. *Social Psychiatry and Psychiatric Epidemiology*, **34**, 254–8.

Hayes, R. L. & McGrath, J. J. (2000). Cognitive rehabilitation for people with schizophrenia and related conditions. *The Cochrane Database of Systematic Reviews*, Issue 3. Art. No.: CD000968. DOI: 10.1002/14651858.CD000968. Oxford: Update Software Ltd.

Haynes, R. B., McDonald, H., Garg, A. X. & Montague, P. (2002). Interventions for helping patients to follow prescriptions for medications. *The Cochrane Database of Systematic Reviews*, Issue 2. Art. No.: CD000011. DOI: 10.1002/14651858.CD000011. Oxford: Update Software Ltd.

Hirsch, S. & Leff, J. (1971). Parental abnormalities of verbal communication in the transmission of schizophrenia. *Psychological Medicine*, **1**(2), 118–27.

Hogarty, G., Anderson, C., Reiss, D. *et al.* (1991). Family psycho-education, social skills training and maintenance chemotherapy in the aftercare treatment of schizophrenia. *Archives of General Psychiatry*, **48**(4), 340–7.

Jones, C., Cormac, I., Silveira da Mota Neto, J. I. & Campbell, C. (2004). Cognitive behaviour therapy for schizophrenia. *The Cochrane Database of Systematic Reviews*, Issue 4. Art. No.: CD000524.pub2. DOI: 10.1002/14651858.CD000524.pub2. Oxford: Update Software Ltd.

Kemp, R., Hayward, P., Applewhaite, G., Everitt, B. & David, A. (1996). Compliance therapy in psychotic patients: randomised controlled trial. *British Medical Journal*, **312**, 345–9.

Kraepelin, E. (1919). Dementia praecox and paraphrenia. Translated by R. Mary Barclay from the English Edition of the *Textbook of Psychiatry* vol. iii, Part ii, section on Endogenous Dementias, ed. G. Robertson. Edinburgh: Livingstone.

Leff, J., Kuipers, L., Berkowitz, R., Eberlein-Fries, R. & Sturgeon, D. (1982). A controlled trial of social interventions in the families of schizophrenic patients. *British Journal of Psychiatry*, **141**, 121–34.

Leff, J., Kuipers, L., Berkowitz, R., Eberlein-Fries, R. & Sturgeon, D. (1984). Psychosocial relevance and benefit of neuroleptic maintenance: experience in the United Kingdom. *Journal of Clinical Psychiatry*, **45**, 43–9.

Leff, J., Kuipers, L., Berkowitz, R. & Sturgeon, D. (1985). A controlled trial of social intervention in the families of schizophrenic patients: two-year follow-up. *British Journal of Psychiatry*, **146**, 594–600.

Leff, J., Berkowitz, R., Shavit, N., Strachan, A., Glass, I. & Vaughn, C. (1989). A trial of family therapy versus a relatives' group for schizophrenia. *British Journal of Psychiatry*, **154**, 58–66.

Lewis, S., Tarrier, N., Haddock, G. *et al.* (2002). Randomised controlled trial of cognitive-behavioural therapy in early schizophrenia: acute-phase outcomes. *British Journal of Psychiatry*, **181**(S43), S91–7.

Lidz, T., Flack, S., & Cornelison, A. (1965). *Schizophrenia and the Family*. New York: International Press.

Liberman, R., Wallace, C., Blackwell, G., Kopelowicz, A., Vaccaro, J. & Mintz, J. (1998). Skills training versus psychosocial occupational therapy for persons with persistent schizophrenia. *American Journal of Psychiatry*, **155**(8), 1087–91.

Linszen, D., Dingemans, P., Van der Does, J. W. *et al.* (1996). Treatment, expressed emotion and relapse in recent onset schizophrenic disorders. *Psychological Medicine*, **26**(2), 333–42.

Marder, S., Wirshing, W., Mintz, J. *et al.* (1996). Two-year outcome of social skills training and group psychotherapy for outpatients with schizophrenia. *American Journal of Psychiatry*, **153**(12), 1585–92.

Marshall, M. & Lockwood, A. (1998). Assertive community treatment for people with severe mental disorders. *The Cochrane Database of Systematic Reviews*, Issue 2. Art. No.: CD001089. DOI: 10.1002/14651858.CD001089. Oxford: Update Software Ltd.

Marshall, M., Crowther, R., Almaraz-Serrano, A. M. & Tyrer, P. (2001). Day hospital versus out-patient care for psychiatric disorders. *The Cochrane Database of Systematic Reviews*, Issue 2. Art. No.: CD003240. DOI:10.1002/ 14651858.CD003240. Oxford: Update Software Ltd.

Marshall, M., Crowther, R., Almaraz-Serrano, A. *et al.* (2003). Day hospital versus admission for acute psychiatric disorders. *The Cochrane Database of Systematic Reviews*, Issue 1. Art. No.: CD004026. DOI:10.1002/14651858.CD004026. Oxford: Update Software Ltd.

Marshall, M., Lewis, S., Lockwood, A., Drake, R., Jones, P. & Croudace, T. (2005). Association between duration of untreated psychosis and outcome in cohorts of first-episode patients: a systematic review. *Archives of General Psychiatry*, **62**(9), 975–83.

McMonagle, T. & Sultana, A. (2000). Token economy for schizophrenia. *The Cochrane Database of Systematic Reviews*, Issue 3. Art. No.:CD001473. DOI: 10.1002/14651858.CD001473. Oxford: Update Software Ltd.

Medalia, A., Aluma, M., Tryon, W. & Merriam, A. E. (1998). Effectiveness of attention training in schizophrenia. *Schizophrenia Bulletin*, **24**, 147–52.

O'Donnell, C., Donohoe, G., Sharkey, L. *et al.* (2003) Compliance therapy: a randomised controlled trial in schizophrenia. *British Medical Journal*, **327**, 834.

Pekkala, E. & Merinder, L. (2002) Psychoeducation for schizophrenia. *The Cochrane Database of Systematic Reviews*, Issue 2. Art. No.: CD002831. DOI: 10.1002/14651858.CD002831. Oxford: Update Software Ltd.

Pelosi, A. & Birchwood, M. (2003). Is early intervention for psychosis a waste of valuable resources? *British Journal of Psychiatry*, **182**, 196–8.

Pharoah, F. M., Rathbone, J., Mari, J. J. & Streiner, D. (2003). Family intervention for schizophrenia. *The Cochrane Database of Systematic Reviews*, Issue 3. Art. No.: CD000088. DOI: 10.1002/ 14651858.CD000088. Oxford: Update Software Ltd.

Pilling, S., Bebbington, P., Kuipers, E. *et al.* (2002a). Psychological treatments in schizophrenia II: meta-analyses of randomized controlled trials of social skills training and cognitive remediation. *Psychological Medicine*, **32**, 783–91.

Pilling, S., Bebbington, P., Kuipers, E. *et al.* (2002b). Psychological treatments in schizophrenia: I. Meta-analysis of family intervention and cognitive behaviour therapy. *Psychological Medicine*, **32**, 763–82.

Sackett, D. (1978). Compliance trials and the clinician. *Archives of Internal Medicine*, **138**(1), 23–5.

Sensky, T., Turkington, D., Kingdon, D. *et al.* (2000). A randomized controlled trial of cognitive-behavioural therapy for persistant symptoms in schizophrenia resistant to medication. *Archives of General Psychiatry*, **57**, 165–72.

Tarrier, N., Lewis, S., Haddock, G. *et al.* (2004). Cognitive behavioural therapy in first-episode and early schizophrenia. *British Journal of Psychiatry*, **184**, 231–9.

Tompkins, L. M., Goldman, R. S. & Axelrod, B. N. (1995). Modifability of neuropsychological dysfunction in schizophrenia. *Biological Psychiatry*, **38**, 105–11.

Tyrer, P., Coid, J., Simmonds, S., Joseph, P. & Marriott, S. (1998). Community mental health teams (CMHTs) for people with severe mental illnesses and disordered personality. *The Cochrane Database of Systematic Reviews*, Issue 4. Art. No.: CD000270. DOI:10.1002/14651858.CD000270. Oxford: Update Software Ltd.

Vaughn, C. E. & Leff, J. P. (1976). The influence of family and social factors on the course of psychiatric illness. A comparison of schizophrenic and depressed neurotic patients. *British Journal of Psychiatry*, **129**, 125–37.

Wykes, T., Reeder, C., Corner, J., Williams, C. & Everitt, B. (1999). The effects of neurocognitive remediation on executive processing in patients with schizophrenia. *Schizophrenia Bulletin*, **25**, 292–307.

Wykes, T., Reeder, C., Landau, S. *et al.* (2007). Cognitive remediation therapy in schizophrenia. *British Journal of Psychiatry*, **190**, 421–7.

Wynne, L. C., Ryckoff, I. M., Day, J. & Hirsch, S. (1958). Pseudo-mutuality in the family relations of schizophrenics. *Psychiatry*, **21**(2), 205–20.

Mood disorders

Section editors

William H. Coryell and John Geddes

27

Psychopharmacology of mood disorders

William H. Coryell and John Geddes

Editorial note

As depression has been identified as the fourth leading cause of disease burden, accounting for 12% of total disability worldwide (Üstün *et al.*, 2004), and because drug treatment is one of the most widely used, this chapter is a very important one. There are several messages that need to be disseminated from this chapter. Firstly, antidepressant drugs, despite many improvements over the years, remain drugs with many adverse effects, and selection of a drug is likely to be determined more by its adverse effect profile than by its efficacy rating. Next, depression is often combined with other disorders, and treatment must take into account the nature of these other conditions and the effect of drug treatment upon them. A third message is very important to clinicians; do not increase the dose of an antidepressant too readily. Response, particularly the full response, to an antidepressant is often delayed, and rushing to a high dose will only add to adverse effects at a time when the patient is not well prepared to deal with them. The treatment of bipolar disorder is associated with more controversy than depression alone, especially in the maintenance phase, and here there is a difference between recommendations in the United States and those of other countries, with much greater use of a typical antipsychotics and sodium valproate in the USA and more emphasis on lithium elsewhere, with bigger differences in the maintenance than acute phases of treatment. However, disparity is unlikely to last for long and recommendations are likely to approach consensus in the coming years. The reader will also note that the selection of treatment in the less severe disorders is determined as much by avoidance of undesired effects as by the embracing of desired ones, an important decision with regard to adherence to treatment, particularly in the longer term.

Depressive disorder

The diagnosis of depressive disorder is not as straightforward as it sometimes seems (see Part I of this book). However, in reviewing treatments for this condition, it is assumed that the reader has a working knowledge of current diagnostic practice.

Decision to treat

Despite broad consensus that the causes of depressive syndromes are diverse, there is little agreement as to which patients with depressive episodes derive clear benefit from antidepressants generally or from a specific antidepressant in particular. Nevertheless, three considerations should bear on the decision to prescribe an antidepressant for an as yet untreated patient with a depressive episode.

(1) The clinician should first confirm that the patient does, in fact, meet the criteria for a depressive syndrome. Patients with a level of symptoms that meet diagnostic criteria are more likely to respond to drug therapy and, hence, the hoped for benefits are more likely to outweigh any risks of therapy. Early work by Paykel *et al.* (1988) showed that patients with mild major depression, but not those with minor depression, exhibited a response differential between placebo and tricyclic antidepressant (TCA) similar to that of patients with moderate to severe states. A more recent study found benefits of paroxetine over placebo for dysthymia but not for minor depression (Barrett *et al.*, 2001). A meta-analysis of trials of newer generation antidepressants with the Federal Drug Administration showed that drug/placebo differences grew progressively with increases in baseline symptom severity and that only 10% of patient groups with

a mean Hamilton Rating Scale for Depression score (HRSD) of 24 or less demonstrated superiority of drug over placebo (Khan *et al.*, 2002).

The diagnostic criteria for depressive disorder in DSM-IV and ICD-10 distinguish between depressive symptoms that are severe, persistent and disabling from those causing lesser degrees of symptomatology. In DSM-IV, the criteria for major depressive episode require at least five symptoms present for at least 2 weeks. ICD-10 criteria for depressive episode suggest at least four symptoms for 2 weeks for mild depressive episode and at least 5 symptoms for moderate depressive episode. Diagnostic criteria must be applied correctly. For example, most criteria for a depressive episode, including the DSM-IV criteria for major depression, specify that each of the requisite symptoms have been present during the same period of time and 'most of the day, nearly every day', yet many patients will fail to mention that their symptoms have been quite intermittent or have been present only in certain situations. Patients with this intermittency of symptoms – especially when individual symptoms are of mild severity, may be best considered to have subsyndromal states rather than a clear-cut depressive syndrome.

(2) Episode duration should also be considered in the decision to use an antidepressant. Large, prospective studies of depressed patients and of non-clinical samples have shown a highly reproducible relationship between the pre-existing duration of an episode and the likelihood of a spontaneous remission in the near future, i.e. the longer the duration of episode the less likely is spontaneous recovery (Coryell *et al.*, 1994, 1995; Solomon *et al.*, 2000). In harmony with those findings, placebo-controlled antidepressant trials that examined the relationship between drug effect and episode duration have consistently found that patients with shorter durations of 1 month to 6 months failed to show benefits of drug over placebo, whereas those with larger durations did (Downing & Rickels, 1973; Fairchild *et al.*, 1986; Khan *et al.*, 1991; Brown *et al.*, 1992).

(3) Lastly, patients with major depression are more likely to suffer from many other disorders apart from those of mood. If the physician is entirely focused on the presenting complaint of depressive symptoms, he or she may fail to recognize those cases in which disorders such as substance abuse not only coexist but may have caused the depressive syndrome. In such cases, antidepressants may offer little benefit until the underlying condition is recognized and treated

(Mueller *et al.*, 1994), except when, of course, the second condition is deemed to be a direct consequence of the depressive disorder (e.g. at times with comorbid obsessive-compulsive disorder), and when the treatment may also be effective for the second condition (as in the anxiety disorders – see Chapters 31–36).

Selection of treatment – first line

The critical decision to use antidepressants for treatment is followed by a selection from what has become a wide assortment of options. The clinician strives to match the patient with an antidepressant on the basis of the likely adverse effect profile, potential interactions with drugs the patient is already taking, costs, and the possibility that the patient's demographic or symptom characteristics may predict preferential response to a specific agent.

Adverse effects

The perception of adverse effects varies greatly. The greater likelihood of weight gain associated with the tricyclic antidepressants, monoamine oxidase inhibitors and mirtazapine compared with some related drugs will alarm some patients more than others, but be a potential benefit for those who have lost significant weight as part of their depression. Likewise, patients for whom lack of sexual interest is already a source of chronic difficulty may, because of that, prefer buproprion to a selective serotonin reuptake inhibitor (SSRI). Men who have difficulties with premature ejaculation, on the other hand, may benefit from the orgasmic delay associated with SSRIs (Atmaca *et al.*, 2002). The inhibition of p450 enzymes produced by fluoxetine, fluvoxamine, paroxetine, sertraline and nefazodone may be problematic for patients with medical conditions that require multiple drug treatments, more so if frequent changes in drug type and doses are necessary for controlling the target conditions.

Interactions

Costs

The relative costs of the different antidepressants are likely to be a major factor for those patients responsible for much or all of their medication expense, and in those countries with limited health budgets. In the USA, a month's supply of a second-generation antidepressant may exceed several hundred dollars, while a month of a tricyclic antidepressant such as imipramine may cost under $10.00. The relative tolerability of the SSRIs over the TCAs is well established but the difference may not be as large as is widely assumed, and in poorer countries tricyclic antidepressants are the treatments of choice (Chisholm *et al.*, 2004). The clinician should raise the issue of cost and tolerability, as patients may not volunteer their concerns over out-of-pocket expenses.

Baseline characteristics

The importance of age and sex to antidepressant selection remains uncertain. Although the evidence remains unclear, some consensus has developed that older individuals show a preferential response to TCAs over SSRIs (Parker 2002; Parker *et al.*, 2003); that the reverse is true for younger individuals with SSRIs appearing more effective than TCAs (Kornstein *et al.*, 2000; Joyce *et al.*, 2003); and that this preference of SSRIs over TCAs is particularly true of women (Kornstein *et al.*, 2000; Grigoriadis *et al.*, 2003; Joyce *et al.*, 2003) and of patients with melancholia (Parker, 2002; Joyce *et al.*, 2003; Parker *et al.*, 2003). Some have found superior responses in men given tricyclic antidepressants and women given SSRIs regardless of age (Baca *et al.*, 2004). Because norepinephrine reuptake is the chief pharmacodynamic property that separates TCAs from SSRIs, one would expect age and sex to similarly predict preferential responses to SSRIs versus duloxetine, or to higher doses of venlafaxine. This, however, has yet to be tested.

The SSRIs, but not the tricyclic antidepressants (Soloff *et al.*, 1986), have been found in placebo-controlled studies to be effective for patients with borderline personality disorder (Markovitz, 1995; Salzman *et al.*, 1995; Coccaro and Kavoussi, 1997; Rinne *et al.*, 2002)(see Chapter 43 for further details). Likewise, controlled trials have found that SSRIs (Tollefson *et al.*, 1994), and clomipramine (Thoren *et al.*, 1980), but not other TCAs, benefit obsessive-compulsive disorder. Thus, the SSRIs, rather than most TCAs and, perhaps, other second-generation antidepressants, are preferable when either of these conditions underlies, or represents significant comorbidity to, the depressive disorder. Moreover, because buproprion is one of the few antidepressants shown in a placebo-controlled trial to be ineffective in the treatment of panic disorder (Sheehan *et al.*, 1983), other antidepressants should be used for patients who have experienced panic attacks with depressive episodes.

Attempts to match the side effects typical of particular antidepressants to a patient's more prominent symptoms have intuitive appeal but probably only produce transient benefit. The advantage of sedating over non-sedating antidepressants for insomnia, for instance, has been shown to exist only in the first few weeks of treatment (Rush *et al.*, 2001). Clinicians should therefore take a longer view of side effects as they select an antidepressant to recommend

and should consider the temporary, adjunctive use of an atypical antipsychotic or a benzodiazepine for sleep or sedation.

Dosing and side effect management

Clinicians should tailor the initiation of therapy to the individual patient. Those with a prominent history of anxiety, in particular, may require a very low dose of an SSRI initially and then slow dose progression. Patients in general should be forewarned of the increased anxiety, nausea and sedation they may experience initially and should be reassured that these are typically transient problems (Reimherr *et al.*, 1990). Moderate doses of a benzodiazepine or an atypical antipsychotic may be helpful during the initial weeks of treatment to provide relief of anxiety and insomnia until the antidepressant's benefits become apparent.

Clinicians commonly increase antidepressant doses within the recommended range when patients fail to show substantial improvement within two to four weeks. This view is supported when the patients show subsequent improvement. There are several reasons to believe that such dose increases are very often not causally related to the clinical improvement that follows and a recent meta-analysis has supported this conclusion (Ruhé *et al.*, 2006). Of second-generation antidepressants, only venlafaxine has shown a clear dose–response relationship within the recommended dose range, and this applies only to the lower end of 75–150 mg/day rather than the upper range of 150–325 mg/day (Kelsey, 1996; Rudolph *et al.*, 1998). Second, those few studies that have randomized incompletely responsive patients to either a dose increase or to a continuation of current dose showed that both groups did equally well (Schweizer *et al.*, 1990; Benkert *et al.*, 1997). Third, Quitkin *et al.* (Quitkin *et al.*, 2003) used a placebo-controlled discontinuation strategy to show that improvement delayed as long as 8 weeks is likely to represent a true antidepressant effect. Thus, though the failure of dose-finding studies to show clear differences in efficacy between, for instance, 20 mg/day and 40 mg/day of fluoxetine may obscure the fact that some few individuals do need higher doses to respond, the treating physician will not know this for a given patient unless a trial return to a lower dose is followed by relapse. In our experience such a re-emergence of symptoms typically resolves promptly with a return to the original dose. Such a trial may save a patient the greater expense and side effects associated with unnecessarily higher doses.

Many dose-ranging studies have described higher side effect rates in patients randomized to higher doses.

Because these studies typically grouped side effects that developed early and then resolved, together with side effects that persisted, it is not possible to separate the transient consequences of higher doses from their more enduring consequences. There is some consensus, though, that side effects such as nausea, diarrhoea, delayed orgasm and decreased libido may be insensitive to dose adjustments. The widely recognized, but poorly studied, apathy syndrome associated with SSRIs may, on the other hand, improve with a dose reduction (Hoehn-Saric et al., 1990).

Second-line treatment

The Sequenced Treatment Alternatives to Relieve Depression (STAR*D) trial reported a remission rate following first line monotherapy with citalopram of 28%, a finding that emphasizes that many patients will need second-line therapy (Trivedi et al., 2006) Nonetheless, because true antidepressant drug response can be delayed up to 8 weeks (Quitkin et al., 2003), clinicians should be careful not to abandon a potentially effective drug prematurely, particularly if it is being well tolerated. Efforts to show the predictive relationship between improvement at 2 weeks and recovery at 6 or 8 weeks have generally concluded that the majority of patients who have shown no perceptible improvement in the first 2 weeks will fail to recover by 6 to 8 weeks (Coryell et al., 1982; Katz et al., 1987; Nagayama et al., 1991; Nierenberg et al., 1995). On the other hand, a majority of patients who show at least some early improvement go on to recover (Nierenberg et al., 1995).

The failure of a first-line antidepressant leaves three options: a switch to an alternative, the addition of another antidepressant, or augmentation with agents that are not considered to be antidepressants when used alone. Each approach has certain inherent advantages and disadvantages. A shift to an alternative antidepressant will avoid the added expense and management complexity of an added drug. If the first agent appears to have had some benefit, though, an addition strategy will retain those benefits. Augmentation strategies also introduce new drugs but several of the agents most commonly used for this purpose appear to involve little increase in side effect risk.

Addition

Although open trials have described successes following the addition to SSRI treatment of buproprion (Bodkin et al., 1997; Kennedy et al., 2002), tricyclic antidepressants (Nelson et al., 2004), or buspirone (Joffe & Schuller, 1993), very few randomized trials have been conducted. Fava et al. (2002) assigned patients with partial responses to fluoxetine to an increased dose of fluoxetine, the addition of lithium, or the addition of desipramine. The three groups experienced similar levels of improvement. Two other controlled studies randomly assigned SSRI non-responders to either the continuation of SSRIs at previous doses or to the addition of mianserin (Ferreri et al., 2001; Licht & Quiotzau 2002). In one study the patients given mianserin had significantly better outcomes (Ferreri et al., 2001) and in the other they did not (Licht and Quitzau, 2002). Carpenter et al. (2002) found a significant advantage over placebo with the addition of mirtazepine to antidepressant non-responders.

Thus, only four randomized trials have compared the continuation of SSRI treatment at unchanged doses to the addition of another antidepressant and two found the manoeuvre beneficial.

Level 2 options in STAR*D did not include a placebo-controlled evaluation of the addition of an antidepressant but did compare the addition of buspirone or bupropion to citalopram (Trivedi et al., 2006). In this trial, participants who failed to achieve remission following treatment were randomized to continued citalopram plus buspirone or continued citalopram plus bupropion. Addition of bupropion was associated with a lower withdrawal rate due to adverse effects but there was no difference in efficacy – remission in both groups was 30% (Trivedi et al., 2006).

Substitution

The marketing of each new antidepressant is accompanied by a series of open trials that show the new drug to be useful for patients who have responded inadequately to a standard antidepressant. As of yet there are almost no trials in which patients randomized to the new drug were compared to those maintained on the original one. Ferreri et al. (2001) compared the continuation of fluoxetine to a substitution with mianserin and found only a trend toward better outcomes in the latter group.

One of the level 2 options in STAR*D was to randomize participants who did not remit following open treatment with citalopram to sustained-release bupropion, sertraline or extended-release venlafaxine (Rush et al., 2006). There was no difference in remission rates between the arms of this trial (bupropion 21%, sertraline 18% and venlafaxine 25%) which did not, however, include a continued citalopram arm (Rush et al., 2006) A level 3 option in STAR*D was to randomize participants who had not remitted after level 2 to mirtazepine or nortriptyline: the remission rates were 16% and 20%, respectively, not significantly different (Fava et al., 2006).

Augmentation

In contrast to the literature concerning combination and switching strategies, numerous placebo-controlled, randomized trials have been published on the effects of augmentation with lithium, pindolol and triiodothyronine.

Bauer and Dopfmer (1999) described a meta-analysis of nine placebo-controlled lithium augmentation trials and found good outcomes to be 3.7 times more likely with lithium than with placebo. Clear patterns across the studies favoured doses greater than 600 mg daily and a trial duration of at least 12 days. Nearly all of these reports used lithium to augment TCAs but there are now at least two placebo-controlled trials of lithium augmentation in SSRI therapy for acute treatment (Katona et al., 1995; Baumann et al., 1996), as well as a placebo-controlled discontinuation trial (Bauer et al., 2000). The results of each supported the value of lithium augmentation with the SSRI nonresponders. Not surprisingly, the combination carries an increased risk for diarrhoea (Bauer et al., 1996), but few patients discontinued treatment because of side effects in these trials.

Pindolol is thought to augment SSRI antidepressant effects in so far as it blocks 5HT-1A autoreceptors and thus interrupts the negative feedback produced by increases in intrasynaptic serotonin concentrations. A meta-analysis of nine placebo-controlled studies concluded that the benefits of pindolol augmentation are clear but are limited to a hastening of response rather than to an increase in the likelihood of eventual response (Ballesteros & Callado, 2004). However, the dosing strategy used in nearly all of these studies, 2.5 mg given in three times daily, probably failed to produce consistent occupancy of 5HT-1A receptors as revealed with PET scans, whereas 5 mg three times daily would have resulted in more substantial occupancy (Rabiner et al., 2001). It thus appears that the combination of the daily dose used in earlier studies to a single daily administration may produce a more desirable ratio between pre- and post-receptor 5-HT occupancies (Rabiner et al., 2000). The first study to take this dosing approach has, in fact, shown a robust effect of pindolol given in a single daily dose of 7.5 mg relative to placebo among patients refractory to two or more months of unmodified SSRI treatment (Sokolski et al., 2004).

A meta-analysis of six placebo-controlled trials has concluded that the addition of triiodothyronine also accelerates antidepressant response and that it is much more likely to do so in women than in men (Altshuler et al., 2001). These six studies all used triiodothyronine (T3) to augment tricyclic antidepressants but a more recent review of algorithm-based treatment results shows that this augmentation of second-generation antidepressants is also more likely to succeed in women (Agid & Lerer, 2003).

Only a few controlled trials have tested the value of T3 augmentation in refractory populations. Two used a parallel-group design and one of these found T3 significantly more effective than T4 (Joffe and Singer, 1990). Another found T3 superior to placebo and equal to lithium augmentation (Joffe et al., 1993). The single cross-over study of refractory patients found no difference between T3 and placebo (Gitlin et al., 1987).

There is considerable evidence that patients who have shown a poorer response to either acute or prophylactic antidepressant treatment are more likely to have thyroid indices that tend towards hypothyroidism. Thus, levels of thyroid stimulating hormone (which are raised in secondary hypothyroidism) in the upper half of the normal range (Joffe & Levitt 1992; Cole et al., 2002) or T3 values in the lower half of the normal range (Joffe & Levitt, 1992; Cole et al., 2002; Joffe et al., 2002) were significantly overrepresented in groups of poor responders. This suggests that thyroid indices can be used to select patients most likely to benefit from T3 augmentation. Most of the controlled augmentation trials did not address this possibility but several open trials showed baseline thyroid indices to be predictive of T3 augmentation response (Targum et al., 1984; Agid & Lerer, 2003). Several others found no predictive value (Gitlin et al., 1987; Thase et al., 1989; Fava et al., 1995), but these three studies reported very low overall response rates to T3 augmentation.

A STAR*D level 3 option compared lithium and T3 augmentation and reported a remission rate of 15.9% for lithium and 24.7% with T3 which was not statistically significant, although T3 was better tolerated than lithium (Nierenberg et al., 2006).

Two well-designed trials have shown advantages to the combination of olanzapine and fluoxetine over fluoxetine alone. In the first, the superiority of the combination over the monotherapy was rapid and sustained through the eight-week trial (Shelton et al., 2001). In the second, refractory patients taking the combination experienced significantly more improvement early in the trial but end-point analyses revealed no significant benefits over monotherapy (Shelton et al., 2005).

Maintenance

A meta-analysis of 31 RCTs (4410 patients) investigating continued therapy with antidepressants in patients who had responded to acute phase therapy found that the average relapse rate in the placebo arm was 41% compared to 18% on antidepressants (odds ratio 0.30, 95% confidence interval 0.22 to 0.38, $P < 0.00001$) (Geddes et al., 2003).

There was no material heterogeneity between trials with regard to baseline patient characteristics, specific antidepressant studied or duration of follow-up. Clinically, this result means that, on average, a patient whose acute phase symptoms respond to an antidepressant could expect a halving of their risk of relapse if they continue the drug. The evidence is strongest for up to 2 years continued therapy, although the results are consistent up to 5 years. The decision on whether to use long-term drug therapy will therefore depend on balancing the patient's expected risk of relapse with adverse effect and the patient's preferences. Thus, a patient with a single episode of depression with a low average risk of relapse would tend not to continue therapy beyond 6 months post-treatment response. However, a patient with multiple previous episodes of a single treated episode with other strong risk factors (positive family history, very severe initial severity) may choose continued therapy for at least 2 years. There is currently no robust evidence from head-to-head comparisons between antidepressant agents. The results overall, therefore, do not support the selection of any one specific medication over another on the basis of superior efficacy in relapse prevention.

The average relapse rate on placebo is twice that on active therapy, which represents a very substantial discontinuation effect. This is in contrast to the much smaller drug effects seen in the acute trials of MDD over the past decade (Walsh et al., 2002). This difference may be explained in several ways. Firstly, placebo-controlled trials of acute therapy are difficult to conduct and, for ethical and clinical reasons, tend to recruit mildly ill patients who have high placebo response rates. Baseline depression severity ratings may be inflated by investigators to meet minimum eligibility criteria, and again this can result in high placebo response rates. Lastly, the difference may also reflect the fact that each of these maintenance studies required a median of 4 months of remission on drug before randomization. In eliminating patients with an unstable early response, this criterion is likely to have excluded most partial and placebo responders (Quitkin et al., 1984) and left patients who were, for the most part, well because of drug response rather than because of spontaneous remission. This has practical relevance because the long-term findings of the maintenance studies only directly apply to patients with a true drug response, particularly those who have already maintained this response for a few months. Although studies have not definitively answered the question of how long maintenance should continue, the magnitude of the protective effect observed in the trials remains constant across time and, for many patients, treatment could be indefinite. But any long-term treatment policy should be agreed upon fully with the patient before implementation, preferably as soon as possible after initial response.

Bipolar affective disorder

Acute treatment – mania

Randomized, placebo-controlled trials have shown atypical and conventional antipsychotics (Yatham, 2003), lithium (Goodwin et al., 1969; Stokes et al., 1971), carbamazepine (Ballenger and Post, 1978; Ketter et al., 2004; Weisler et al., 2004, 2005) and valproate (Pope et al., 1991; Bowden et al., 1994; MacRitchie et al., 2000a; Muller-Oerlinghausen et al., 2000) to be effective in the control of acute mania. The risk of recurrence is high in bipolar disorder and the management of acute mania should include the introduction of a long-term mood stabilizer.

Although mood stabilizers such as lithium and valproate are effective antimanic treatments as monotherapy, they are usually prescribed together with antipsychotics to hasten control of manic symptoms. Randomized trials have shown each of the atypical antipsychotics, risperidone, olanzapine, quetiapine, ziprasidone, and aripiprazole to be effective as monotherapy in the acute treatment of mania (Yatham, 2003), and their use seems less likely to be followed by the emergence of depressive symptoms than does the use of typical antipsychotics (Ahlfors et al., 1981; Tohen et al., 2001; 2003; Zarate & Tohen, 2004).

Clinically, it is important to know if some subgroups of patients respond preferentially to one drug or another. There are limited data available, although some subanalyses of trials comparing lithium and valproate suggest that mixed or dysphoric mania may respond preferentially to valproate (Swann et al., 1999) and that a typical or 'classic' mania may more readily improve with lithium (Freeman et al., 1992). Not all trials have found such a differential response (Goldberg et al., 1998), and even if there was a difference between the drugs in the acute phase, it does not follow that there should be a similarly differential efficacy in the maintenance phase. For example, a sub analysis of an RCT comparing valproate, lithium and placebo for maintenance reported an association between dysphoric mania and a better outcome with lithium (Bowden et al., 2000).

Acute treatment – depression

As with the management of acute mania, the treatment of acute bipolar depression also needs to consider medium- and long-term treatment and the selection of an appropriate mood stabilizer for patients not already taking one is clinically important (see Maintenance). Many patients develop depressive episodes despite adhering correctly to treatment with a mood stabilizer. The options are then mood stabilizer dose adjustment, the addition or substitution of another mood stabilizer, an augmentation strategy, or the addition of an antidepressant. The data available to guide clinicians in this choice is unfortunately scant.

One should first consider making no change. As with MDD, depressive episodes that have been, so far, present for only weeks to months are more likely to remit spontaneously than are episodes with longer durations at presentation. Bipolar patients on mood stabilizers are relatively likely to present with such brief depressive episodes because they are likely to have regularly scheduled visits. Watchful reassurance may be particularly advisable early in the course of lithium treatment. In a direct comparison, lithium produced a progressive decline in interepisode morbidity, chiefly depressive symptoms, over a 6-month period, whereas carbamazepine did not (Kleindienst & Greil, 2002).

Blood levels of lithium, valproate and carbamazepine should be brought into their conventional treatment ranges if necessary, but there is little evidence that further adjustment within these boundaries will improve antidepressant effects. Maj et al. (1986), for instance, randomly assigned bipolar patients to four blood level ranges. A range of 0.76–0.90 mmol/l was associated with less manic morbidity, and with more side effects, than was the range of 0.61–0.75 mmol/l, but the two groups experienced identical levels of depressive symptoms. Similarly, a randomized comparison of a 0.4–0.6 mmol/l range to a 0.8–1.0 mmol/l range showed fewer manic recurrences with the higher range but no advantage in the prevention of depressive recurrences (Gelenberg et al., 1989).

The addition of an antidepressant in such cases has the most intuitive appeal but this strategy has been the centre of recent controversy with variations between guideline recommendations in the USA and UK, Europe and Australia (American Psychiatric Association, 2002; Goodwin, 2003a). It has become widely believed that antidepressants not only trigger mania in bipolar patients but also induce and prolong rapid cycling patterns (Wehr & Goodwin 1979; Wehr et al., 1988; Koukopoulos et al., 2003). However, randomized trials comparing antidepressants with placebo do not suggest that the risk is elevated, at least in the short term. A systematic review and meta-analysis of five RCTs found a switch rate of 3.8% for antidepressant and 4.7% for placebo (Gijsman et al., 2003). Moreover, several large naturalistic studies failed to find any association between the use of antidepressants and either switching or the onset of rapid cycling (Frankle et al., 2002; Coryell et al., 2003).

There is also uncertainty if bipolarity is associated with poorer antidepressant response (Kupfer & Spiker 1981; Ghamei et al., 2004, Avery & Winokur 1977; Katz et al., 1987), but a meta-analysis of the randomized studies investigating the effectiveness of antidepressants in bipolar depression suggests that, although the total number of randomized patients is low, antidepressants appear to be similarly effective as they are in unipolar depression, increasing the short-term response rate by 86% (Gijsman et al., 2003). It is also uncertain if antidepressants improve long-term treatment outcomes. Several studies comparing bipolar patients who discontinued antidepressants after depressive symptoms had resolved with bipolar patients who continued taking antidepressants showed significantly fewer relapses in the latter group (Altshuler et al., 2001b; Joffe et al., 2005). However, these studies were not randomized and so the difference in outcome may be due to systematic baseline differences between the patients (for example, more good prognosis patients adhering to long-term therapy), rather than due to the antidepressant. The limited longer-term evidence from controlled studies does not currently suggest a long-term benefit with antidepressant therapy (Ghaemi et al., 2001).

There is some evidence that the atypical antipsychotics quetiapine (Calabrese et al., 2005) and olanzapine (Tohen et al., 2003) are effective antidepressants and may have a role in the treatment of depressive symptoms in bipolar disorder. The acceptability of these drugs may be limited by adverse effects as 19% of patients treated with olanzapine and 10% of patients treated with quetiapine experienced 7 or more kilograms in weight gain during these 8-week trials.

Lamotrigine is increasingly recommended as a first-line treatment for bipolar depression (American Psychiatric Association, 2002; Goodwin, 2003b). Although there is evidence that lamotrigine is effective treatment for preventing depressive relapse (Calabrese et al., 2003; Bowden et al., 2003), the evidence for short-term efficacy is equivocal. Five RCTs have been conducted by GSK comparing lamotrigine with placebo. Although none have found clear-cut evidence of efficacy in the primary analysis (one trial found statistically significant benefit on a key secondary outcome, Calabrese et al., 2005), a meta-analysis of all five trials found a statistically and clinically significant benefit that was consistent across all five trials (Geddes et al., 2006).

Pramipexole, a novel D2/D3 agonist, also shows promise for bipolar depression that arises despite ongoing mood stabilizers. Two such samples, one consisting mostly of bipolar I patients (Goldberg et al., 2004) and the other consisting entirely of bipolar I patients (Zarate et al., 2004) were randomly assigned to 6-week trials of

Table 27.1. Pharmacological treatment of acute and resistant depressive episodes and maintenance treatment

Treatment	Form of treatment	Diagnosis	Level of evidence for efficacy	Comments
Tricyclic antidepressants	Mixed noradrenaline (NA) and 5-HT reuptake inhibitors	Depressive episode	Ia	Choice dependent on adverse effects and risk of overdose
Bupropion		Depressive episode	Ia	
Selective serotonin reuptake inhibitor (SSRI)	Selective 5-HT reuptake inhibition	Depressive episode	Ia	
Selective noradrenaline-serotonin reuptake inhibitors (SNRI)	Selective inhibition of both noradrenaline and 5-HT	Depressive episode	Ia	
Monoamine oxidase inhibitors (MAOI's)	Complete inhibition of mono-amine oxidase (most) and reversible inhibition of mono-amine oxidase (RIMA) (a few)	Resistant depression	II	Not recommended as first line treatments but may be considered when anxiety and panic symptoms are prominent and standard agents have failed
SSRI augmentation with mianserin and mirtazepine		Resistant depression	III	Conflicting trial evidence so firm conclusions impossible
TCA/SSRI augmentation with lithium		Resistant depression	Ia	Effective in lithium dosage of >600 mg daily
SSRI augmentation with pindolol		Resistant depression	Ia	Hastens response rather than changes non-responders into responders
TCA/SSRI augmentation with triiodothyronine		Resistant depression	Ia	Effects stronger in women than men
SSRI-augmention with olanzapine		Resistant depression	Ia	Some evidence of more rapid early response
TCAs, SSRIs, MAOIs and SNRIs		Maintenance treatment of depression after initial recovery	Ia	Difference between drug and placebo greater than for acute treatment (see text)

placebo or pramipexole at flexible doses of 1 to 5 mg/day. Despite small numbers, both studies found significant outcome differences favouring pramipexole. Perhaps because both protocols began with low doses of 0.125 mg/day and then advanced them slowly, dropouts due to adverse events were rare.

Little has been done to test augmentation strategies in bipolar depression. The use of thyroid augmentation is of particular interest because of lithium's effects on the thyroid axis and the likelihood that some of the cognitive difficulties that patients attribute to lithium may be produced by disturbances in this system (Prohaska *et al.*, 1995, 1996).

Maintenance

Of the four mood stabilizers that have been tested in placebo-controlled maintenance trials, lithium has by far

the best support (Goodwin, 2002; Geddes *et al.*, 2004). A recent meta-analysis identified five randomized trials comparing lithium with placebo in bipolar patients (770 participants) and found that lithium was more effective than placebo in preventing all new episodes of mood disturbance (fixed effects relative risk 0.66, 95% CI 0.57 to 0.77; random effects RR 0.65, 95% CI 0.50 to 0.84; $P = 0.001$, chi-square for heterogeneity 10.08, $df = 4$, $P = 0.04$). The statistically significant heterogeneity observed was judged to be quantitative because all the trials found a benefit for lithium over placebo, although this was not always statistically significant. The average risk of relapse in the placebo group was 61% compared to 40% on lithium. This means that one patient would avoid relapse for every five patients who were treated for a year or two with lithium (Laupacis *et al.*, 1988). Lithium was superior to placebo in the prevention of manic episodes (fixed effects RR 0.61; 95% CI 0.39 to 0.95, p = 0.008, chi-square for heterogeneity 3.89, df = 3, $P = 0.27$). The average risk of relapse in the placebo group was 24% compared to 14% on lithium. This means that one patient would avoid relapse for every ten patients who were treated for a year or two with lithium. The effect on depressive relapses appeared smaller and just failed to reach statistical significance (fixed effects RR 0.78, 95% CI 0.60 to 1.01, $P = 0.06$, chi-square for heterogeneity 4.67, df = 3, $P = 0.2$; random effects RR 0.72, 95% confidence interval 0.49 to 1.08). The average risk of relapse in the placebo group was 32% compared to 25% on lithium. This means that that one patient would avoid relapse for 14 patients who were treated for a year or two with lithium.

The single trial done to evaluate valproate failed to differentiate it from placebo on the primary outcome measure though a number of other outcome measures indicated effectiveness (Bowden et al., 2000; MacRitchie et al., 2000b). The only trial that tested carbamazepine for maintenance was insufficiently powered to show a significant advantage of drug over placebo. Trials done to assess lamotrigine for maintenance have targeted bipolar patients with a rapid cycling pattern (Calabrese et al., 2000), patients whose most recent episode was depressive (Calabrese et al., 2003), and patients whose most recent episode was manic (Bowden et al., 2003). All showed significant differences between lamotrigine and placebo in recurrence risk though, for the rapid cycling sample, this was true only for the group with bipolar II disorder (Calabrese et al., 2000). In the other two studies, lamotrigine provided protection against depressive episodes but did not appear to protect against mania (Calabrese et al., 2003).

Evidence that a mood stabilizer is effective as monotherapy in the treatment of bipolar depression is also relevant to its potential value in overall maintenance. Eight of nine placebo-controlled, crossover trials found lithium to be effective as monotherapy for bipolar depression (Zornberg & Pope, 1993). The only placebo-controlled trials to evaluate other mood stabilizers as monotherapy showed efficacy for olanzapine at a mean dose of 10 mg daily (Tohen et al., 2003), quetiapine at 300 or 600 mg/day (Calabrese et al., 2004), and lamotrigine at 50 or 200 mg daily (Calabrese et al., 1999).

To summarize, among mood stabilizers, only lithium has been shown by placebo-controlled studies to be effective in acute mania, in acute bipolar depression and in maintenance treatment of bipolar disorder. Other considerations will, however, also bear on the selection of a mood stabilizer.

The side effects of lithium, divalproex and olanzapine differ qualitatively but direct comparisons of general tolerability have not clearly favoured one over the other. Comparisons of lithium and divalproex have not shown significant differences in rates of discontinuation due to adverse events, whether the agents were being used for acute mania (Bowden et al., 1994) or for maintenance (Bowden et al., 2000). Similarly, a comparison of olanzapine and divalproex in a 47-week study showed no difference in rates of discontinuation due to adverse events (Tohen et al., 2003).

Some patients are particularly wary of weight gain as a potential side effect and these three drugs do appear to differ in this respect. In the maintenance comparisons of lithium and divalproex, only divalproex was significantly more likely than placebo to cause weight gain (Bowden et al., 2000). In turn, olanzapine caused significantly more weight gain than divalproex in two direct comparisons (Zajeka et al., 2002; Tohen et al., 2003).

Of the empirically supported mood stabilizers now in use, lamotrigine appears to produce the fewest side effects. With the use of the currently recommended dose progression, the risk for Stevens–Johnson syndrome, an established adverse muco-cutaneous disorder, appears to be quite small (Wong et al., 1999; Calabrese et al., 2002). In the three monotherapy studies carried out so far, dropouts due to side effects were no more frequent with lamotrigine than they were with placebo and were significantly less likely than with lithium (Calabrese et al., 2000, 2003; Bowden et al., 2003).

It is during the long-term management of bipolar patients that syndromal breakthroughs and persistent side effects lead clinicians to consider the abandonment of one mood stabilizer for another. Because only a few agents have been shown effective for both bipolar depression and for mania, great care should be taken to determine whether poor compliance has preceded breakthroughs and, if so, whether non-compliance occurred in response to ongoing side effects. The lack of sufficient attention to compliance is thought by some to account for the apparent differences in lithium efficacy between research settings and ordinary clinical settings. A number of strategies exists to treat lithium side effects and should be undertaken before the drug is abandoned for an alternative (Coryell, 2002).

Combinations of mood stabilizers are widely used to improve prophylaxis but only a few controlled studies have assessed this approach (Zarate & Quiroz, 2003). The existing literature supports the addition of certain mood stabilizers as well as it does the addition of an antidepressant. The combination of lithium and valproate has been

Table 27.2. Effectiveness of psychopharmacological treatments for mood disorders

Treatment	Duration of treatment	Size of population	Level of evidence for efficacy	Comments
Tricyclic antidepressants	2–5 years	Large	Ia	
Buproprion		Depressive episode	Ia	
Selective serotonin reuptake inhibitor (SSRI)	Selective 5-HT reuptake inhibition	Depressive episode	Ia	
Selective noradrenaline-serotonin reuptake inhibitors (SNRI)	Selective inhibition of both noradrenaline and 5-HT	Depressive episode	Ia	
Monoamine oxidase inhibitors (MAOI's)	Complete inhibition of mono-amine oxidase (most) and reversible inhibition of mono-amine oxidase (RIMA) (a few)	Resistant depression	II	Not recommended as first line treatments but may be considered when anxiety and panic symptoms are prominent and standard agents have failed
SSRI augmentation with mianserin and mirtazepine		Resistant depression	III	Conflicting trial evidence so firm conclusions impossible
TCA/SSRI augmentation with lithium		Resistant depression	Ia	Effective in lithium dosage of >600 mg daily
SSRI augmentation with pindolol		Resistant depression	Ia	Hastens response rather than changes non-responders into responders
TCA/SSRI augmentation with triiodothyronine		Resistant depression	Ia	Effects stronger in women than men. Better tolerated then lithium

evaluated in one randomized trial (Solomon *et al.*, 1997) and a further larger study (the BALANCE trial) is currently in progress (Geddes *et al.*, 2002). There has also been a cross-over study that compared a lithium and carbamazepine combination to 1 year of either drug as monotherapy (Denicoff *et al.*, 1987). The results of both completed trials described lower levels of both depressive and manic morbidity with combination treatment though at the price of higher side effects. As combination therapies are commonly used clinically, further trials are required. One clear example is an assessment of the value of lamotrigine plus lithium, a combination that might optimize control of manic and depressive episodes.

Lithium, valproate and carbamazepine offer advantages in that plasma level monitoring yields an additional check on compliance beyond patient self-report. Spouses can be effective allies in maintenance treatment and it is often only they who are able to report whether an acute manic episode preceded or followed medication noncompliance. Specific instructions in the early recognition of symptoms, and the steps to be taken when they appear, have been shown in a randomized trial to substantially reduce the recurrence of manic, though not depressive, episodes (Perry *et al.*, 1999).

The level of evidence for each of the interventions discussed in this chapter is summarized in Table 27.2.

REFERENCES

Agid, O. & Lerer, B. (2003). Algorithm-based treatment of major depression in an outpatient clinic: clinical correlates of response to a specific serotonin reuptake inhibitor and to triiodothyronine augmentation. *International Journal of Neuropsychopharmacology*, **6**(1), 41–9.

Ahlfors, U. G., Baastrup, P. C. *et al.* (1981). Flupenthixol decanoate in recurrent manic-depressive illness. *Acta Psychiatrica Scandinavica* **64**, 226–37.

Altshuler, L. L., Bauer, M. *et al.* (2001a). Does thyroid supplementation accelerate tricyclic antidepressant response? A review and meta-analysis of the literature. *American Journal of Psychiatry*, **158**(10), 1617–22.

Altshuler, L., Kiriakos, L. *et al.* (2001b). The impact of antidepressant discontinuation versus antidepressant continuation on 1-year risk for relapse of bipolar depression: a retrospective chart review. *Journal of Clinical Psychiatry*, **62**(8), 612–16.

American Psychiatric Association (2002). Practice guideline for the treatment of patients with bipolar disorder (revision). *American Journal of Psychiatry*, **159**, 1–50.

Atmaca, M., Kuloglu, M. *et al.* (2002). The efficacy of citalopram in the treatment of premature ejaculation: a placebo-controlled study. *International Journal of Impotency Research*, **14**(6), 502–5.

Avery, D. & Winokur, G. (1977). The efficacy of electroconvulsive therapy and antidepressants in depression. *Biological Psychiatry*, **12**(4), 507–23.

Baca, E., Garcia-Garcia, M. *et al.* (2004). Gender differences in treatment response to sertraline versus imipramine in patients with nonmelancholic depressive disorders. *Progress in Neuropsychopharmacology and Biolical Psychiatry*, **28**(1), 57–65.

Ballenger, J. C. & Post, R. M. (1978). Therapeutic effects of carbamazepine in affective illness: a preliminary report. *Community Psychopharmacology*, **2**(2), 159–75.

Ballesteros, J. & Callado, L. F. (2004). Effectiveness of pindolol plus serotonin uptake inhibitors in depression: a meta-analysis of early and late outcomes from randomised controlled trials. *Journal of Affective Disorders*, **79**(1–3), 137–47.

Barrett, J. E., Williams, J. W. Jr. *et al.* (2001). Treatment of dysthymia and minor depression in primary care: a randomized trial in patients aged 18 to 59 years. *Journal of Family Practice*, **50**(5), 405–12.

Bauer, M. & Dopfmer, S. (1999). Lithium augmentation in treatment-resistant depression: meta-analysis of placebo-controlled studies. *Journal of Clinical Psychopharmacology*, **19**(5), 427–34.

Bauer, M., Linden, M. *et al.* (1996). Adverse events and tolerability of the combination of fluoxetine/lithium compared with fluoxetine. *Journal of Clinical Psychopharmacology*, **16**(2), 130–4.

Bauer, M., Bschor, T. *et al.* (2000). Double-blind, placebo-controlled trial of the use of lithium to augment antidepressant medication in continuation treatment of unipolar major depression. *American Journal of Psychiatry*, **157**(9), 1429–35.

Baumann, P., Nil, R. *et al.* (1996). A double-blind, placebo-controlled study of citalopram with and without lithium in the treatment of therapy-resistant depressive patients: a clinical, pharmacokinetic, and pharmacogenetic investigation. *Journal of Clinical Psychopharmacology*, **16**(4), 307–14.

Benkert, O., Szepedi, A. *et al.* (1997). Dose escalation versus continued doses of paroxetine and maprotiline: a prospective study in depressed outpatients with an adequate treatment response. *Acta Psychiatrica Scandinavica*, **95**, 288–96.

Biggs, J. T., Chang, S. S. *et al.* (1976). Measurement of tricyclic antidepressant levels in an outpatient clinic. *Journal of Nervous and Mental Diseases*, **162**(1), 46–51.

Bodkin, J. A., Lasser, R. A. *et al.* (1997). Combining serotonin reuptake inhibitors and bupropion in partial responders to antidepressant monotherapy. *Journal of Clinical Psychiatry*, **58**(4), 137–45.

Bowden, C. L., Brugger, A. M. *et al.* (1994). Efficacy of divalproex vs lithium and placebo in the treatment of mania. The Depakote Mania Study Group. *Journal of the American Medical Association*, **271**(12), 918–24.

Bowden, C. L., Calabrese, J. R. *et al.* (2000). A randomized, placebo-controlled 12-month trial of divalproex and lithium in treatment

of outpatients with bipolar I disorder. *Archives of General Psychiatry*, **57**, 481–9.

Bowden, C. L., Calabrese, J. R. *et al.* (2003). A placebo controlled 18-month trial of lamotrigine and maintenance treatment in recently manic or hypomanic patients with bipolar I disorder. *American Journal of Psychiatry*, **60**, 392–400.

Brown, W. A., Johnson, M. F. *et al.* (1992). Clinical features of depressed patients who do and do not improve with placebo. *Psychiatry Research*, **41**(3), 203–14.

Calabrese, J. R., Bowden, C. L. *et al.* (1999). A double-blind placebo-controlled study of lamotrigine monotherapy in outpatients with bipolar I depression. Lamictal 602 Study Group. *Journal of Clinical Psychiatry*, **60**(2), 79–88.

Calabrese, J. R., Suppes, T. *et al.* (2000). A double-blind, placebo-controlled, prophylaxis study of lamotrigine in rapid-cycling bipolar disorder. Lamictal 614 Study Group. *Journal of Clinical Psychiatry*, **61**(11), 841–50.

Calabrese, J. R., Sullivan, J. R. *et al.* (2002). Rash in multicenter trials of lamotrigine in mood disorders: clinical relevance and management. *Journal of Clinical Psychiatry*, **63**(11), 1012–19.

Calabrese, J. R., Bowden, C. L. *et al.* (2003). A placebo-controlled 18-month trial of lamotrigine and lithium maintenance treatment in recently depressed patients with bipolar I disorder. *Journal of Clinical Psychiatry*, **64**(9), 1013–24.

Calabrese, J., Macfadden, W. *et al.* (2005). Double-blind, placebo-controlled study of quetiapine in bipolar depression. *American Journal of Psychiatry*, **162**, 1351–60.

Carpenter, L. L., Yasmin, S. *et al.* (2002). A double-blind, placebo-controlled study of antidepressant augmentation with mirtazapine. *Biological Psychiatry*, **51**(2), 183–8.

Chisholm, D., Sanderson, K., Ayuso-Mateos, J. L. & Saxena, S. (2004). Reducing the global burden of depression: population-level analysis of intervention cost-effectiveness in 14 world regions. *British Journal of Psychiatry*, **184**, 393–403.

Coccaro, E. F. & Kavoussi, R. J. (1997). Fluoxetine and impulsive aggressive behavior in personality-disordered subjects. *Archives of General Psychiatry*, **54**(12), 1081–8.

Cohn, J. B., Collins, G. *et al.* (1989). A comparison of fluoxetine, imipramine and placebo in patients with bipolar depressive disorder. *International Clinical Psychopharmacology*, **4**, 313–22.

Cole, D. P., Thase, M. E. *et al.* (2002). Slower treatment response in bipolar depression predicted by lower pretreatment thyroid function. *American Journal of Psychiatry*, **159**, 116–21.

Coryell, W. (2002). Minimizing the side effects of mood stabilizers. *Primary Psychiatry*, **9**, 47–50.

Coryell, W., Coppen, A. *et al.* (1982). Early improvement as a predictor of response to amitriptyline and nortriptyline: a comparison of 2 patient samples. *Psychological Medicine*, **12**(1), 135–9.

Coryell, W., Akiskal, H. S. *et al.* (1994). The time course of non-chronic major depressive disorder: uniformity across episodes and samples. *Archives of General Psychiatry*, **51**(5), 405–10.

Coryell, W., Endicott, J. *et al.* (1995). Characteristics and significance of untreated major depressive disorder. *American Journal of Psychiatry*, **152**(8), 1124–9.

Coryell, W., Solomon, D. *et al.* (2003). The long-term course of rapid cycling bipolar disorder. *Archives of General Psychiatry.* **60**: 914–20.

Dawson, R., Lavori, P. W. *et al.* (1998). Maintenance strategies for unipolar depression: an observational study of levels of treatment and recurrence. *Journal of Affective Disorders*, **49**(1), 31–44.

Denicoff, K. D., Smith-Jackson, E. E. *et al.* (1987). Comparative prophylactic efficacy of lithium, carbamazepine and the combination in bipolar disorder. *Journal of Clinical Psychiatry*, **58**, 470–8.

Doogan, D. P. & Caillard, V. (1992). Sertraline in the prevention of depression. *British Journal of Psychiatry*, **160**, 217–22.

Downing, R. W. & Rickels, K. (1973). Predictors of response to amitriptyline and placebo in three outpatient treatment settings. *Journal Nervons and Mental Diseases* **156**(2), 109–29.

Fairchild, C. J., Rush, A. J. *et al.* (1986). Which depressions respond to placebo? *Psychiatry Research*, **18**(3), 217–26.

Fava, M., Labbate, L. A. *et al.* (1995). Hypothyroidism and hyperthyroidism in major depression revisited. *Journal of Clinical Psychiatry*, **56**, 186–92.

Fava, M., Alpert, J. *et al.* (2002). Double-blind study of high-dose fluoxetine versus lithium or desipramine augmentation of fluoxetine in partial responders and nonresponders to fluoxetine. *Journal of Clinical. Psychopharmacology*, **22**(4), 379–87.

Fava, M., Rush, A. J., Wisniewski, S. R. *et al.* (2006). A comparison of mirtazapine and nortriptyline following two consecutive failed medication treatments for depressed outpatients: a STAR*D report. *American Journal of Psychiatry*, **163**(7), 1161–72.

Ferreri, M., Lavergne, F. *et al.* (2001). Benefits from mianserin augmentation of fluoxetine in patients with major depression non-responsive to fluoxetine alone. *Acta Psychiatrica Scandinavica*, **103**(1), 66–72.

Frank, E., Kupfer, D. J. *et al.* (1990). Three-year outcomes for maintenance therapies in recurrent depression. *Archives of General Psychiatry*, **47**(12), 1093–9.

Frankle, W. G., Perlis, R. H. *et al.* (2002). Bipolar depression: relationship between episode length and antidepressant treatment. *Psychological Medicine*, **32**(8), 1417–23.

Freeman, T. W., Clothier, J. L. *et al.* (1992). A double-blind comparison of valproate and lithium in the treatment of acute mania. *American Journal of Psychiatry*, **149**(1): 108–11.

Gelenberg, A. J., Kane, J. M. *et al.* (1989). Comparison of standard and low serum levels of lithium for maintenance treatment of bipolar disorder. *New England Journal of Medicine*, **321**(22), 1489–93.

Geddes, J. R., Rendell, J. M. & Goodwin, G. M. (2002). BALANCE: a large simple trial of maintenance treatment for bipolar disorder. *World Psychiatry*, **1**, 48–51.

Geddes, J. R., Carney, S. M., Davies, C. *et al.* (2003). Relapse prevention with antidepressant drug treatment in depressive disorders: a systematic review. *Lancet*, **361**, 653–61.

Geddes, J. R., Burgess, S., Hawton, K., Jamison, K. & Goodwin, G. M. (2004). Long-term lithium therapy for bipolar disorder: systematic review and meta-analysis of randomized controlled trials. *American Journal of Psychiatry*, **161**, 217–22.

Geddes, J. R, Goodwin, G. M. Huffman, R., Paska, W., Evoniuk, G. & Leadbetter, R. (2006). Additional clinical trial data and a retrospective pooled analysis of response rates across alll randomised trials conducted by GSK. *Bipolar Disorders*, **8** (Suppl. 1), 32.

Ghaemi, S. N., Lenox, M. S. & Baldessarini, R. J. (2001). Effectiveness and safety of long-term antidepressant treatment in bipolar disorder. *Journal of Clinical Psychiatry*, **62**, 565–9.

Ghamei, S. N., Rosenquist, K. J. *et al.* (2004). Antidepressant treatment in bipolar versus unipolar depression. *American Journal of Psychiatry*, **161**, 163–5.

Gijsman, H. J., Geddes, J. R., Rendell, J. M., Nolen, W. A. & Goodwin, G. M. (2003). Antidepressants for bipolar depression: a systematic review of randomised controlled trials. *American Journal of Psychiatry*,

Gitlin, M. J., Weiner, H. *et al.* (1987). Failure of T3 to potentiate tricyclic antidepressant response. *Journal of Affective Disorders*, **13**(3), 267–72.

Glassman, A. H., Perel, J. M. *et al.* (1977). Clinical implications of imipramine plasma levels for depressive illness. *Archives of General Psychiatry*, **34**(2), 197–204.

Goldberg, J. F., Garno, J. L. *et al.* (1998). Rapid titration of mood stabilizers predicts remission from mixed or pure mania in bipolar patients. *Journal of Clinical Psychiatry*, **59**(4), 151–8.

Goldberg, J. F., Burdick, K. E. *et al.* (2004). Preliminary randomized, double-blind, placebo-controlled trial of pramipexole added to mood stabilizers for treatment-resistant bipolar depression. *American Journal of Psychiatry*, **161**(3), 564–6.

Goodwin, F. K. (2002). Rationale for long-term treatment of bipolar disorder and evidence for long-term lithium treatment. *Journal of Clinical Psychiatry*, **63**(Suppl.), 5–12.

Goodwin, G. M. (2003). Evidence-based guidelines for treating bipolar disorder: recommendations from the British Association for Psychopharmacology. *Journal of Psychopharmacology* **17**, 149–73.

Goodwin, F. K., Murphy, D. L. *et al.* (1969). Lithium-carbonate treatment in depression and mania. A longitudinal double-blind study. *Archives of General Psychiatry*, **21**(4), 486–96.

Grigoriadis, S., Kennedy, S. H. *et al.* (2003). A comparison of antidepressant response in younger and older women. *Journal of Clinical Psychopharmacology*, **23**(4), 405–7.

Himmelhoch, J. M., Fuchs, C. Z. *et al.* (1982). A double-blind study of tranylcypromine treatment of major anergic depression. *Journal of Nervous and Mental Diseases* **170**(10), 628–34.

Hochstrasser, B., Isaksen, P. M. *et al.* (2001). Prophylactic effect of citalopram in unipolar, recurrent depression: placebo-controlled study of maintenance therapy. *British Journal of Psychiatry*, **178**, 304–10.

Hoehn-Saric, R., Lipsey, J. R. *et al.* (1990). Apathy and indifference in patients on fluvoxamine and fluoxetine. *Journal of Clinical Psychopharmacology*, **10**(5), 343–5.

Joffe, R. T. & Levitt, A. J. (1992). Major depression and subclinical (grade 2) hypothyroidism. *Psychoneuroendocrinology*, **17**(2–3), 215–21.

Joffe, R. T. & Schuller, D. R. (1993). An open study of buspirone augmentation of serotonin reuptake inhibitors in refractory depression. *Journal of Clinical Psychiatry*, **54**(7), 269–71.

Joffe, R. T. & Singer, W. (1990). A comparison of triiodothyronine and thyroxine in the potentiation of tricyclic antidepressants. *Psychiatry Research*, **32**(3), 241–51.

Joffe, R. T., Singer, W. *et al.* (1993). A placebo-controlled comparison of lithium and triiodothyronine augmentation of tricyclic antidepressants in unipolar refractory depression. *Archives of General Psychiatry*, **50**(5), 387–93.

Joffe, R. T., MacQueen, G. M. *et al.* (2002). Induction of mania and cycle acceleration in bipolar disorder: effect of different classes of antidepressant. *Acta Psychiatrica Scandinavica*, **105**(6), 427–30.

Joffe R. T., MacQueen, G. M., Marriot, M. & Young, L. T. (2005). One-year outcome with antidepressant treatment of bipolar depression. *Acta Psychiatrica Scandinavica*, **112**, 105–9.

Joyce, P. R., Mulder, R. T. *et al.* (2003). A differential response to nortriptyline and fluoxetine and melancholic depression: the importance of age and gender. *Acta Psychiatrica Scandinavica*, **108**, 20–3.

Judd, L. L., Akiskal, H. S. *et al.* (1998). Major depressive disorder: a prospective study of residual subthreshold depressive symptoms as predictor of rapid relapse. *Journal of Affective Disorders*, **50**(2–3), 97–108.

Judd, L. L., A. H. S., *et al.* (2002). The long-term natural history of the weekly symptomatic status of bipolar I disorder. *Archives of General Psychiatry*, **59**, 530–7.

Judd, L. L., Schettler, P. J. *et al.* (2003). Long-term symptomatic status of bipolar I versus bipolar II disorders. *International Journal of Neuropsychopharmacology*, **6**, 127–37.

Katona, C. L., Abou-Saleh, M. T. *et al.* (1995). Placebo-controlled trial of lithium augmentation of fluoxetine and lofepramine. *British Journal of Psychiatry* **166**(1): 80–6.

Katz, M. M., Koslow, S. H. *et al.* (1987). The timing, specificity and clinical prediction of tricyclic drug effects in depression. *Psychological Medicine*, **17**(2), 297–309.

Keller, M. B., Kocsis, J. H. *et al.* (1998). Maintenance phase efficacy of sertraline for chronic depression: a randomized controlled trial. *Journal of the American Medical Association*, **280**(19), 1665–72.

Kelsey, J. E. (1996). Dose-response relationship with venlafaxine. *Journal of Clinical Psychopharmacol* **16**(3 Suppl 2): 21S–6S; discussion 26S–8S.

Kennedy, S. H., McCann. S. M. *et al.* (2002). Combining bupropion SR with venlafaxine, paroxetine, or fluoxetine: a preliminary report on pharmacokinetic, therapeutic, and sexual dysfunction effects. *Journal of Clinical Psychiatry*, **63**(3), 181–6.

Ketter, T. A., Kalali, A. H. *et al.* (2004). A 6-month, multicenter, open-label evaluation of beaded, extended-release carbamazepine capsule monotherapy in bipolar disorder patients with manic or mixed episodes. *Journal of Clinical Psychiatry*, **65**(5), 668–73.

Khan, A., Dager, S. R. *et al.* (1991). Chronicity of depressive episode in relation to antidepressant – placebo response. *Neuropsychopharmacology*, **4**, 125–30.

Khan, A., Leventhal, R. M. *et al.* (2002). Severity of depression and response to antidepressants and placebo: analysis of the Food and Drug Administration database. *Journal of Clinical Psychopharmacology*, **22**, 40–5.

Kleindienst, N. & Greil, W. (2002). Inter-episodic morbidity and drop-out under carbamazepine and lithium in the maintenance treatment of bipolar disorder. *Psychological Medicine*, **32**(3), 493–501.

Kocsis, J. H., Friedman, R. A. *et al.* (1996). Maintenance therapy for chronic depression. A controlled clinical trial of desipramine. *Archives of General Psychiatry*, **53**(9), 769–74; discussion 775–6.

Kornstein, S. G., Schatzberg, A. F. *et al.* (2000). Gender differences in treatment response to sertraline versus imipramine in chronic depression. *American Journal of Psychiatry*, **157**(9), 1445–52.

Koukopoulos, A., Sani, G. *et al.* (2003). Duration and stability of the rapid-cycling course: a long-term personal follow-up of 109 patients. *Journal of Affective Disorders* **73**, 75–85.

Kragh-Sorensen, P. & Hansen, E. (1976). Self inhibiting action of nortriptyline antidepressive effect at high plasma levels. *Psychopharmacologia*, **45**, 305–12.

Kupfer, D. J. & Spiker, D. G. (1981). Refractory depression: prediction of non-response by clinical indicators. *Journal of Clinical Psychiatry*, **42**(8), 307–12.

Laupacis, A., Sackett, D. L. & Roberts, R. S. (1988). An assessment of clinically useful measures of the consequences of treatment. *New England Journal of Medicine*, **318**, 1728–33.

Lepine, J. P., Caillard, V. *et al.* (2004). A randomized, placebo-controlled trial of sertraline for prophylactic treatment of highly recurrent major depressive disorder. *American Journal of Psychiatry*, **161**(5), 836–42.

Licht, R. W. & Quitzau, S. (2002). Treatment strategies in patients with major depression not responding to first-line sertraline treatment. *Psychopharmacology*, **161**, 143–51.

MacRitchie, K., Geddes, J. R., Scott, J., Haslam, D. R. & Goodwin, G. M. (2000a). Valproic acid, valproate and divalproex for acute mood episodes in bipolar disorder. Cochrane Library 4[4].

MacRitchie, K., Geddes, J. R., Scott, J., Haslam, D. R. & Goodwin, G. M. (2000b). Valproic acid, valproate and divalproex in the maintenance therapy of bipolar disorder. Cochrane Library 4[4].

Maj, M., Starace, F. *et al.* (1986). Minimum plasma lithium levels required for effective prophylaxis in DSM III bipolar disorder: a prospective study. *Pharmacopsychiatry*, **19**(6), 420–3.

Markovitz, P. (1995). *Pharmacotherapy of Impulsivity, Aggression and Related Disorders*. Chichester, UK: John Wiley.

Montgomery, S. A., Dufour, H. *et al.* (1988). The prophylactic efficacy of fluoxetine in unipolar depression. *British Journal of Psychiatry*, Suppl. (3), 69–76.

Mueller, T. I., Lavori, P. W. *et al.* (1994). Prognostic effect of the variable course of alcoholism on the 10-year course of depression. *American Journal of Psychiatry*, **151**(5), 701–6.

Muller-Oerlinghausen, B., Retzow, A. *et al.* (2000). Valproate as an adjunct to neuroleptic medication for the treatment of acute episodes of mania: a prospective, randomized, double-blind, placebo-controlled, multicenter study. *Journal of Clinical Psychopharmacol*, **20**(2), 195–203.

Nagayama, H., Nagano, K. *et al.* (1991). Prediction of efficacy of antidepressant by 1-week test therapy in depression. *Journal of Affective Disorders*, **23**(4), 213–16.

Nelson, J. C., Mazure, C. M. *et al.* (2004). Combining norepinephrine and serotonin reuptake inhibition mechanisms for treatment of depression: a double-blind, randomized study. *Biological Psychiatry*, **55**(3), 296–300.

Nemeroff, C. B., Evans, D. L. *et al.* (2001). Double-blind, placebo-controlled comparison of imipramine and paroxetine in the treatment of bipolar depression. *American Journal of Psychiatry*, **158**, 906–12.

Nierenberg, A. A., McLean, N. E. *et al.* (1995). Early non-response to fluoxetine as a predictor of poor eight-week outcome. *American Journal of Psychiatry*, **152**, 1500–03.

Nierenberg, A. A., Fava, M., Trivedi, M. H. *et al.* (2006). A comparison of lithinm and T(3) augmentation following two failed medication treatments for depression: a STAR*D report. *American Journal of psychiatry*, **163**(9), 1519–30.

Parker, G. (2002). Differential effectiveness of newer and older antidepressants appears mediated by an age effect on the phenotypic expression of depression. *Acta Psychiatrica Scandinavica*, **106**(3), 168–70.

Parker, G., Parker, K. *et al.* (2003). Gender differences in response to differing antidepressant drug classes: two negative studies. *Psychological Medicine*, **33**(8), 1473–7.

Paykel, E. S., Hollyman, J. A. *et al.* (1988). Predictors of therapeutic benefit from amitriptyline in mild depression: a general practice placebo-controlled trial. *Journal of Affective Disorders*, **14**(1), 83–95.

Perry, A., Tarrier, N. *et al.* (1999). Randomized controlled trial of efficacy of teaching patients with bipolar disorder to identify early symptoms of relapse and obtain treatment. *British Medical Journal*, **318**, 149–53.

Pope, H. G., Jr, McElroy, S. L. *et al.* (1991). Valproate in the treatment of acute mania. A placebo-controlled study. *Archives of General Psychiatry*, **48**(1), 62–8.

Prien, R. F., Kupfer, D. J. *et al.* (1984). Drug therapy in the prevention of recurrences in unipolar and bipolar affective disorders. Report of the NIMH Collaborative Study Group comparing lithium carbonate, imipramine, and a lithium carbonate-imipramine combination. *Archives of General Psychiatry*, **41**(11), 1096–104.

Prohaska, M. L., Stern, R. A. *et al.* (1995). Thyroid hormones and lithium-related neuropsychological deficits: A preliminary test of the lithium-thyroid interactive hypothesis. *Journal of International Neuropsychological Society*, **1**, 134.

Prohaska, M. L., Stern, R. A. *et al.* (1996). The relationship between thyroid status and neuropsychological performance in psychiatric outpatients maintained on lithium. *Neuropsychiatry, Neuropsychology & Behavioral Neurology*, **9**, 30–4.

Quitkin, F. M., Kane, J. *et al.* (1981). Prophylactic lithium carbonate with and without imipramine for bipolar I patients. *Archives of General Psychiatry*, **35**, 902–7.

Quitkin, F. M., Rabkin, J. G. *et al.* (1984). Identification of true drug response to antidepressants. Use of pattern analysis. *Archives of General Psychiatry*, **41**(8), 782–6.

Quitkin, F. M., Petkova, E. *et al.* (2003). When should a trial of fluoxetine for major depression be declared failed? *American Journal of Psychiatry*, **160**, 734–40.

Rabiner, E. A., Gunn, R. N. *et al.* (2000). Beta-blocker binding to human 5-HT(1A) receptors in vivo and in vitro: implications for antidepressant therapy. *Neuropsychopharmacology*, **23**(3), 285–93.

Rabiner, E. A., Bhagwagar, Z. *et al.* (2001). Pindolol augmentation of selective serotonin reuptake inhibitors: PET evidence that the dose used in clinical trials is too low. *American Journal of Psychiatry*, **158**(12), 2080–2.

Reimherr, F. W., Chouinard, G. *et al.* (1990). Antidepressant efficacy of sertraline: a double-blind, placebo- and amitriptyline-controlled, multicenter comparison study in outpatients with major depression. *Journal of Clinical Psychiatry*, **51** (Suppl. B), 18–27.

Rinne, T., deKloet, E. R. *et al.* (2002). Hyperresponsivenesss of hypothalimic pituitary adrenal axis to combined dexamethasone/corticotropin-releasing hormone challenge in female borderline personality disorder subjects with a history of sustained childhood abuse. *Biological Psychiatry*, **52**, 1102–12.

Rudolph, R. L., Fabre, L. F. *et al.* (1998). A randomized, placebo-controlled, dose-response trial of venlafaxine hydrochloride in the treatment of major depression. *Journal of Clinical Psychiatry*, **59**(3), 116–22.

Ruhé, H. G., Huyser, J., Swinkels, J. A. & Schene, A. H. (2006). Dose escalation for insufficient response to standard-dose selective serotonin reuptake inhibitors in major depressive disorder: systematic review. *British Journal of Psychiatry*, **189**, 309–16.

Rush, A. J., Batey, S. R. *et al.* (2001). Does pretreatment anxiety predict response to either bupropion SR or sertraline? *Journal of Affective Disorders*, **64**(1), 81–7.

Rush, A. J., Trivedi, M. H., Wisniewski, S. R. *et al.* (2006). Bupropion-Sr, Sertraline, or venlafaxine-XR after failure of SSRIs for depression. *New England Journal of Medicine*, **354**(12), 1231–42.

Salzman, C., Wolfson, A. N. *et al.* (1995). Effect of fluoxetine on anger in symptomatic volunteers with borderline personality disorder. *Journal of Clinical Psychopharmacology*, **15**(1), 23–9.

Schweizer, E., Rickels, K. *et al.* (1990). What constitutes an adequate antidepressant trial for fluoxetine? *Journal of Clinical Psychiatry*, **51**, 8–11.

Sheehan, D. V., Davidson, J. *et al.* (1983). Lack of efficacy of a new antidepressant (bupropion) in the treatment of panic disorder with phobias. *Journal of Clinical Psychopharmacology*, **3**(1), 28–31.

Shelton, R. C., Williamson, D. J., Corya, S. A. *et al.* (2005). Olanzapine/Fluoxetine combination for treatment-resistant depression: a controlled study of SSRI and nortriptyline resistance. *Journal of Clinical Psychiatry*, **66**, 1289–97.

Sokolski, K. N., Conney, J. C. *et al.* (2004). Once-daily high-dose pindolol for SSRI-refractory depression. *Psychiatry Research*, **125**(2), 81–6.

Soloff, P. H., George, A. *et al.* (1986). Paradoxical effects of amitriptyline on borderline patients. *American Journal of Psychiatry*, **143**(12), 1603–5.

Solomon, D. A., Ryan, C. E. *et al.* (1997). A pilot study of lithium carbonate plus divalproex sodium for the continuation and maintenance treatment of patients with bipolar I disorder. *Journal of Clinical Psychiatry*, **58**(3), 95–9.

Solomon, D. A., Keller, M. B. *et al.* (2000). Multiple recurrences of major depressive disorder. *American Journal of Psychiatry*, **157**(2), 229–33.

Stewart, J. W., Tricamo, E. *et al.* (1997). Prophylactic efficacy of phenelzine and imipramine in chronic atypical depression: likelihood of recurrence on discontinuation after 6 months' remission. *American Journal of Psychiatry*, **154**(1), 31–6.

Stokes, P. E., Shamoian, C. A. *et al.* (1971). Efficacy of lithium as acute treatment of manic-depressive illness. *Lancet*, **1**(7713), 1319–25.

Swann, A. C., Bowden, C. L. *et al.* (1999). Differential effect of number of previous episodes of affective disorder on response to lithium or divalproex in acute mania. *American Journal of Psychiatry*, **156**(8), 1264–6.

Targum, S. D., Greenberg, R. D. *et al.* (1984). Thyroid hormone and the TRH stimulation test in refractory depression. *Journal of Clinical Psychiatry*, **45**(8), 345–6.

Thase, M. E., Kupfer, D. J. *et al.* (1989). Treatment of imipramine-resistant recurrent depression: I. An open clinical trial of adjunctive L-triiodothyronine. *Journal of Clinical Psychiatry*, **50**(10), 385–8.

Thoren, P., Asberg, M. *et al.* (1980). Clomipramine treatment of obsessive-compulsive disorder. I. A controlled clinical trial. *Archives of General Psychiatry*, **37**(11), 1281–5.

Tohen, M., Zhang, F. *et al.* (2001). Olanzapine versus haloperidol in schizoaffective disorder, bipolar type. *Journal of Affective Disorders*, **67**(1–3), 133–40.

Tohen, M., Vieta, E., Calabrese, J. *et al.* (2003a). Efficacy of olanzapine and olanzapine–fluoxetine combination in the treatment of Bipolar I depression. *Archives of General Psychiatry*, **60**, 1079–88.

Tohen, M., Zarate, C. A. Jr *et al.* (2003b). The McLean–Harvard First-Episode Mania Study: prediction of recovery and first recurrence. *American Journal of Psychiatry*, **160**(12), 2099–107.

Tollefson, G. D., Rampey, A. H. Jr. *et al.* (1994). A multicenter investigation of fixed-dose fluoxetine in the treatment of obsessive-compulsive disorder. *Archices of General Psychiatry*, **51**(7), 559–67.

Trivedi, M. H., Rush, A. J., Wisniewski, S. R. *et al.* (2006). Evaluation of outcomes with citalopram for depression using measurement-based care in STARD*D: implications for clinical practice. *American Journal of Psychiatry*, **163**(1), 28–40.

Üstün, T. B., Ayuso-Mateos, J. L., Chatterji, S., Mathers, C. & Murray, C. J. L. (2004). Global burden of depressive disorders in the year 2000. *British Journal of Psychiatry*, **184**, 386–92.

Walsh, B. T., Seidman, S. N. *et al.* (2002). Placebo response in studies of major depression: variable, substantial, and growing. *Journal of the American Medical Association*, **287**(14), 1840–7.

Wehr, T. A. & F. K. Goodwin (1979). Rapid cycling in manic depressives induced by tricyclic antidepressants. *Archives of General Psychiatry*, **36**, 555–9.

Wehr, T. A., Sack, D. Rapid cycling affective disorder: Contributing factors and treatment responses in fifty-one patients. *American Journal of Psychiatry*, **145**, 179–84.

Weisler, R. H., Kalali, A. H. *et al.* (2004). A multicenter, randomized, double-blind, placebo-controlled trial of extended-release carbamazepine capsules as monotherapy for bipolar disorder patients with manic or mixed episodes. *Journal of Clinical Psychiatry*, **65**(4), 478–84.

Weisler, R. H., Keck, P. E., Swann, A. C., Cutler, A. J., Ketter, T. A. & Kalali, A. H. (2005). Extended-release carbamazepine capsules as monotherapy for acute mania in bipolar disorder: a multicenter, randomized, double-blind, placebo-controlled trial. *Journal of Clinical Psychiatry*, **66**, 323–30.

Wong, I. C., Mawer, G. E. *et al.* (1999). Factors influencing the incidence of lamotrigine-related skin rash. *Annales of Pharmacotherapy*, **33**(10), 1037–42.

Yatham, L. N. (2003). Acute and maintenance treatment of bipolar mania: the role of atypical antipsychotics. *Bipolar Disorders*, **5** (Suppl. 2), 7–19.

Zajeka, J. M., Weisler, R. *et al.* (2002). A comparison of the efficacy, safety, and tolerability of divalproex sodium and olanzapine in the treatment of bipolar disorder. *Journal of Clinical Psychiatry*, **63**(12), 1148–55.

Zarate, C. A. J. & Quiroz, J. A. (2003). Combination treatment in bipolar disorder: a review of controlled trials. *Bipolar Disorders*, **5**, 217–25.

Zarate, C. A. J., Payne, J. L. Singh, J. *et al.* (2004). Pramipexole for bipolar II depression: A placebo-controlled proof of concept study. *Biological Psychiatry*, **56**(1), 54–60.

Zarate, C. A. & Tohen, M. (2004). double-blind comparison of the continued use of antipsychotic treatment versus it's discontinuation in remitted manic patients. *American Journal of Psychiatry*, **161**, 169–71.

Zornberg, G. L. & Pope, H. G. Jr (1993). Treatment of depression in bipolar disorder: new directions for research. *Journal of Clinical Psychopharmacology*, **13**(6), 397–408.

28

Efficacy of brain stimulation and neurosurgical procedures for treatment of mood disorders

Kunal K. Patra and Edward Coffey

Editor's note

This chapter should be looked at in conjunction with Chapter 4, where additional justification is given for the rationale behind the newer of these therapies.

In this chapter we review the efficacy of contemporary procedures used in the treatment of mood disorders, including brain stimulation (electroconvulsive therapy (ECT), transcranial magnetic stimulation (TMS), and vagal nerve stimulation (VNS)) and neurosurgical interventions. We focus our review on methodologically sound randomized controlled trials (RCTs), i.e. a prospective comparison of the procedure to either placebo (sham treatment) or an alternative therapy, with random assignment of consecutive patients (rigorously diagnosed) to the treatment groups, and with blinded objective assessment of outcome using sound statistical analyses.

Brain stimulation procedures

Electroconvulsive therapy (ECT)

In ECT, a brief electrical stimulus is applied through the scalp of a patient under general anesthesia, with the goal of inducing a generalized cerebral seizure. Electroconvulsive therapy is a safe medical procedure due in large part to several important medical modifications in the procedure (use of oxygen, anticholinergic premedication where indicated, anesthesia, and muscle relaxation), and recent improvements in technique (e.g., brief pulse stimulus waveform, appropriate stimulus dosage, appropriate stimulus electrode placement, and quantitative seizure monitoring), all of which have lessened cognitive side effects and improved efficacy. Since its inception in 1938, the efficacy of ECT in mood disorders has been documented by an extensive clinical experience and by numerous open and comparative trials (APA, 2001; Abrams, 2002). Published clinical guidelines also recommend the use of ECT in these disorders (APA, 2000, 2002; Rush et al., 1999; Expert Consensus Guideline, 1996, 2001a, b; US Army Report). Several meta-analytic evaluations of the controlled data have also been recently published (see Table 28.1 for a listing of the major RCTs) (Davis et al., 1993; Kho et al., 2003; UK ECT Review Group, 2003; NICE Report, 2003). Together, these data support the following conclusions:

(1) ECT is an effective treatment for an acute depressive episode (e.g., standardized effect size (SES) vs. sham $= -0.91$, 95% CI -1.27 to -0.54) (UK ECT Review Group, 2003).

(2) ECT appears to be more effective than pharmacotherapy (SES -0.80, 95% CI -1.29 to -0.29) (UK ECT Review Group, 2003) for a depressive episode, although there are methodological concerns about these pharmacotherapy studies (Abrams, 2002; Davis et al., 1993; Rifkin, 1988).

(3) The efficacy of ECT for a depressive episode is influenced by stimulus dosage (high-dose suprathreshold dosing more effective than lower dosages) and electrode placement (bilateral more effective than right unilateral), but not by stimulus waveform or concomitant pharmacotherapy (Kho et al., 2003; UK ECT Review Group, 2003; NICE Report, 2003). There is also an interaction between stimulus dosage and electrode placement, with low-dose (relative to seizure threshold) right unilateral ECT being particularly ineffective.

(4) A small literature and extensive clinical experience supports the efficacy of ECT in the treatment of a manic episode (Table 28.1) and of catatonia (APA, 2001; NICE Report, 2003), but much more controlled research is needed. Published treatment guidelines

Cambridge Textbook of Effective Treatments in Psychiatry, ed. Peter Tyrer and Kenneth R. Silk. Published by Cambridge University Press.
© Cambridge University Press, 2008.

Table 28.1. Selected randomized controlled trials of ECT efficacy

Author	Subjects	Method	Findings
Sham ECT studies			
Freeman *et al.*, 1978	40 inpatients; 11 M, 29 F 20–70 years old Dx: depressive illness (HRSD $\geq$ 15; Beck Rating Scale for Depression $\geq$ 15)	Real ECT ($n=20$) Simulated ECT ($n=20$) (the first two ECTs were sham) Partial sine wave (Ectron Duopulse Mk IV); 400 V for 1.5 s. Bilateral ECT, twice weekly Patients received antidepressant medications during trial	(1) After the initial two ECTs, the real ECT group had significantly lower score on the HRSD, the Wakefield, and the VAS scales. (2) The real ECT group received significantly fewer ECTs in the course (mean number 6.0 vs. 7.15 for the simulated ECT group).
Lambourn *et al.*, 1978	32 right-handed inpatients and outpatients; 14 M, 18 F 37–69 years old Dx: depressive psychosis	Real ECT group ($n=16$) Simulated ECT group ($n=16$) Partial sine wave (Ectron Duopulse Mk.4); 10 joules Right temporo-parietal ECT; thrice weekly for a total of 6 ECTs. Patients received benzodiazepines during trial	(1) After 6 ECTs, mean HRSD scores did not differ significantly between the real ECT group and the simulated ECT group. (2) No group differences in non-HRSD scores noted after 6 ECTs.
Johnstone *et al.*, 1980	70 inpatients; 18 M, 52 F 30–69 years old Dx: MRC endogenous depression	Real ECT group ($n=35$) Simulated ECT group ($n=35$) Partial sine wave (Ectron Duopulse Mk), 150 V for 3 s Bifrontal ECT; twice weekly for a total of 8 ECTs Patients received benzodiazepines during trial	(1) Both groups improved on the HRSD score at the end of treatment with significantly greater improvement in the real ECT group (26 points). (2) No group differences in HRSD score at 1-month and 6-month post ECT.
West, 1981	22 inpatients; 13 M, 9 F Dx: primary depressive illness	Real ECT group ($n=11$; 52.0 +/ −3.3 years old) Simulated ECT group ($n=11$; 53.3 +/ − 6.9 years old) Sine wave (Transycon machine); 40 joules Bilateral anterior temporal ECT; twice weekly for a total of 6 ECTs Patients received 50 mg amitryptyline during trial	(1) After 6 ECTs, the real ECT group but not the simulated ECT group had statistically and clinically significant improvement on the physician's VAS, the Beck Depression Inventory, and the nurses' 9-point rating scale. (2) 10/11 patients in the simulated ECT group were later switched to real ECT with significant clinical improvement.
Brandon *et al.*, 1984	95 inpatients; 34 M, 61 F Real ECT group (55.4 years old) Simulated ECT group (53.0 years old) Dx: PSE defined depression with retardation ($n=56$), depression with delusions ($n=26$), and neurotic depression ($n=13$)	Real ECT group ($n=53$) Simulated ECT group ($n=42$) Partial sine wave (Ectron Duopulse Mark IV) on setting 1 Bitemporal ECT; twice weekly for 8 ECTs. Patients received "selected" anxiolytics during trial	(1) The real ECT group had significantly greater improvement on the HRSD scores at 2 weeks and 4 weeks; there were no significant group differences at 12 and 28 weeks. (2) The largest differences between the real ECT and simulated ECT group occurred in the subgroup of depressive patients with delusions.
Gregory *et al.*, 1985	69 inpatients; all right-handed Dx: MRC depressive illness >1 month duration	Bitemporal ECT group ($n=23$) Right tempero-parietal ECT group ($n=23$) Simulated ECT group ($n=23$) Partial sine wave (Ectron Duopulse Mark IV) at waveform 1 Twice weekly ECT Patients received benzodiazepine during trial	(1) After 2, 4, and 6 treatment sessions, both real ECT groups but not the simulated ECT group improved significantly on MADRS and HRSD scores.

Table 28.1. (cont.)

Author	Subjects	Method	Findings
ECT vs. antidepressant drug therapy			
Greenblatt *et al.*, 1964	281 inpatients; 32% M (mean age 46.8), 68% F (mean age 45.4) Dx: severe depression Manic-depressive reactions, depressive type (27%) Schizophrenic reactions, schizoaffective type (20%) Involutional psychotic reactions (18%) Psychoneurotic depressive reactions (18%) Mixed residual type (16%)	ECT group ($n=63$); Thrice weekly for a total of 9 ECTs (no additional details provided) Imipramine group ($n=73$) Phenelzine group ($n=38$) Isocarboxazid group ($n=68$) Placebo group ($n=39$)	(1) A rating of "Marked improvement" on the 3-point clinical ratings was significantly more common in the ECT group (76%) than in imipramine (49%), phenelzine (50%), isocarboxazid (28%), and placebo (46%) groups.
Medical Research Council Trial, 1965	250 inpatients and outpatients; 81 M, 169 F 40–69 years old Dx: depression	ECT group ($n=65$), 4–8 treatments Imipramine group ($n=63$), 200 mg/d (24 wks) Phenelzine group ($n=61$), 60 mg/d (24 wks) Placebo group ($n=61$)	(1) ECT was significantly superior to imipramine in percent improved (84% vs. 72%, respectively) and in percentage of patients showing no or only slight symptoms (71% vs. 52%, respectively) (Rifkin, 1988).
Gangadhar *et al.*, 1982	32 inpatients; 14 M, 18 F Dx: ICD-9 endogenous depression	ECT group + placebo capsule ($n=16$); (46.6 years old); bilateral ECT (no additional details provided); thrice weekly for a total of 6 ECT in first 2 weeks followed by once a week for another 2 weeks and then one maintenance ECT administered during the sixth, eighth, and twelfth week. Imipramine group + simulated ECT ($n=16$); (42.19 years old)	(1) ECT group had a significantly lower HRSD score at 2 weeks (but not at any other time points) and a greater median percentage improvement in HRSD scores at three weeks (but not at any other time).
Dinan *et al.*, 1989	30; 10 M, 20 F 29–77 years old Dx: DSM-III Major depression, HRSD endogenicity >5, resistant to tricyclic antidepressants	ECT group ($n=15$); Bilateral ECT; Twice weekly for a total of 6 ECTs (no additional details provided) TCA + Lithium group ($n=15$); 600–800 mg/d	(1) After 3 weeks of treatment, both groups improved, with no group differences on the HRSD scores.
Folkerts *et al.*, 1997	39 right-handed inpatients with 2 failed trials of antidepressant medications; 18 M, 21 F Dx: ICD-10 Major Depressive episode, single (HRSD* 22) ($n=15$) Major Depressive episode, recurrent ($n=19$) Bipolar disorder ($n=5$)	ECT group ($n=21$) Paroxetine group ($n=18$), average 44 mg/d Brief-pulse (Thymatron-DGx); right unilateral ECT; suprathreshold stimulus dosage (2.5-fold seizure threshold); thrice weekly for a total of 6–9 ECTs. Patients received tranquilizer, sedative, and sedative neuroleptic medications during trial.	(1) At 4 weeks the ECT group had significantly greater reduction on the HRSD score (59% vs. 29%), and a significantly higher proportion of responders (71.4% vs. 27.8%).

Table 28.1. (cont.)

Author	Subjects	Method	Findings
Sham ECT studies for mania			
Small *et al.*, 1988	34 inpatients; 21 M, 13 F Dx: RDC Bipolar Disorder I, in manic or mixed phases (SDMS-D&M 7, GAS 60)	Lithium carbonate group ($n = 17$); (plasma levels 0.6–1.5 mmol/l) Brief pulse, bitemporal ECT; thrice weekly (mean ECTs 9.3) ($n = 17$), followed by continuation therapy with lithium carbonate. Patients received neuroleptic medications during trial.	(1) Both groups improved during the first 8 weeks of treatment, but such improvement was greater in the ECT group at weeks 6, 7, and 8, as measured by CGI severity of illness scale, the GAS, and several mania rating scales. (2) There were no group differences in ratings after 8 weeks, and the groups were comparable in terms of relapse, recurrence, and re-hospitalization during the 2 years follow-up period.
Mukherjee *et al.*, 1994	Inpatients (27) from two combined studies Dx: RDC Bipolar Disorder, manic with a Modified Mania Scale score * 30.	Randomly assigned to ECT (right unilateral, left unilateral, or bitemporal) ($n = 22$) or lithium-haloperidol drug therapy ($n = 5$) Brief pulse (MECTA SRI) waveform; stimulus dosing at 150% initial seizure threshold; 3–5 times/week Patients received no additional psychotropic medications during trial.	(1) Complete clinical remission was achieved in 13 (59%) of the ECT group compared with none (0%) in the lithium–haloperidol drug group.
Sikdar *et al.*, 1994	30 inpatients and outpatients Dx: DSM-III-R Bipolar Disorder, manic with Mania Rating Scale score 14	Real ECT + Chlorpromazine 600 mg/d ($n = 15$) Simulated ECT + Chlorpromazine 600 mg/d ($n = 15$) Sine waveform at 110 V for 0.6 s. Bifronto-temporal ECT thrice weekly for a total of 8 ECTs Patients received no concomitant drug therapy other than chlorpromazine	(1) 12 (80%) patients in the real ECT group achieved complete recovery compared with 1 (7%) in the simulated ECT group. (2) Real ECT group had significantly greater and faster improvement on the MRS scores compared with simulated ECT group.

recommend such use for ECT (APA, 2002; Rush *et al.*, 1999; Expert Consensus Guideline Series, 1996).

(5) There are no published RCTs on the use of ECT for continuation or maintenance therapy after successful ECT for either acute depression or mania, although such use is supported by extensive clinical experience and open trials, and is recommended in published treatment guidelines (APA, 2000, 2001, 2002; Expert Consensus Guideline, 1996, 2001a, b).

(6) There are no published RCTs on the use of ECT for dysthymic or cyclothymic disorder.

Transcranial magnetic stimulation (TMS)

In transcranial magnetic stimulation (TMS), a handheld electrical coil is used to generate a pulsed magnetic field, which passes unimpeded through the scalp and skull of an awake individual, and which in turn induces electric fields in the brain that depolarize neurons (George *et al.*, 2003). A basic neuroscience research instrument, TMS, is used for non-invasively stimulating the brain (George *et al.*, 2003), but repetitive TMS (rTMS) may also have potential clinical applications in neuropsychiatry (George *et al.*, 1999, 2003; Gershon *et al.*, 2003; Daskalakis *et al.*, 2002). At the time of this writing, rTMS is considered an investigational procedure in the USA, although it was recently approved in Canada for treatment of depression, and it is being used with increasing frequency as an anti depressant treatment in Europe, Australia, and Israel.

In January 2007, the US Food and Drug Administration recommended against approval of TMS for treatment of depression. Panel members found the device safe but questioned its efficacy based upon the results of a clinical trial program sponsored by a TMS manufacturer. In that still-to-be-published multi-site study, 325 medication-free outpatients with treatment-resistant depression were randomized to a 6-week, sham-controlled, double-blind study. At both the 4 and 6 week assessments, patients in both groups showed significant improvement in depression severity scores (Montgomery Asberg Depression Rating Scale), but there was no significant difference between groups (www.fda.gov/obrms/dockets/ac/07/briefing/2007-4273b1_00-index.htm).

A number of studies have examined the efficacy of rTMS in major depression (Garcia-Toro et al., 2001; Berman et al., 2000; George et al., 1997, 2000). Six meta-analyses have analyzed the relevant RCTs (Holtzheimer et al., 2001; Kozel & George, 2002; Burt et al., 2002; McNamara et al., 2001; Martin et al., 2003; 2004) of TMS in major depression. Together these data support the following conclusions:

(1) Current trials are of low quality, and provide insufficient evidence to support the use of rTMS in the treatment of depression (Martin et al., 2003, 2004).

(2) Although the effect sizes in favor of rTMS are generally statistically significant, the magnitude of the therapeutic effects is of questionable clinical significance (Burt et al., 2002).

(3) For patients with psychotic symptomatology, a small literature suggests that ECT is superior to rTMS, although there are methodological concerns about these studies (Gershon et al., 2003; Martin et al., 2004). There are only limited data on the use of rTMS for continuation or maintenance therapy for depression (George et al., 2003; Nahas et al., 2000).

(4) There are no published RCTs on the use of rTMS for dysthymic or cyclothymic disorder.

(5) One recent trial showed rTMS to be significantly better than sham treatment in those with resistant depression when given three times weekly for 4–6 weeks (Anderson et al., 2007).

Vagal nerve stimulation (VNS)

In VNS, a pulse generator implanted subcutaneously in the left anterior chest wall is used to stimulate the left vagus nerve at the cervical level (Kosel & Schlaepfer, 2003).

Vagal nerve stimulation has been available in Europe since 1994 and in the USA since 1997, as an add-on treatment for partial-onset seizures which have been refractory to medications. It has been approved for management of treatment resistant depression (TRD) and bipolar disorder in Europe and Canada since 2001.

Early studies by Elger et al. noted improvement on the Montgomery-Asberg Depression Rating Scale (MADRS) at 3 and 6 months poststimulation. (Elgar et al., 2000) Similarly, studies conducted by Harden et al. in epileptic patients treated with VNS noted improvement on the Beck Depression Rating (BDS) and Hamilton Depression Rating Scale (HDRS) at 3-month follow up. (Harden et al., 2000) These studies conducted in epileptic populations revealed mood improvement regardless of anti-seizure efficacy.

Vagal nerve stimulation was approved by the FDA in 2005 in the USA for adjunctive long-term treatment of chronic or recurrent treatment-refractory major depression in adults 18 years or older. This approval was based in part upon the results of a 10-week open-label pilot study of 60 patients with major depression, of which 18 (30.5%) responded to the treatment (defined as a 50% or greater reduction in baseline HDRS-28 total score) and 9 (15.3%) achieved remission (defined as a score of 10 or less on the HDRS-28 total score). (Rush et al., 2000; Sackeim et al., 2001) At one year follow-up, 26 (44.1%) of the test subjects developed response on the HDRS-28 and the percent of remitters increased to 16 (27.1%). A 2-year outcome LOCF analysis revealed a 42.4% response rate and a 22% remission rate implying sustained but not increased benefit. Given the study design, it was unclear if the observed improvement was simply a placebo effect or related to spontaneous remission or concomitant medications. (Marangell et al., 2002; Nahas et al., 2005)

A subsequent larger ($n = 235$), sham-controlled, double-masked, 10-week registration trial of patients with treatment-resistant major or bipolar depression with mean baseline HDRS-24 score of 29.3 found no significant between-group differences in HDRS-24 response rates (defined as per above) of 15.2% and 10% for the active and sham control groups, respectively, Clinical Global Impression-Improvement (CGI), or the MADRS. Despite significant improvement in the 30-item Inventory of Depressive Symptomatology-Self Report (IDS-SR-30), this study failed to demonstrate efficacy for VNS in treatment-resistant depression. (Rush et al., 2005a) This sample was then followed in an open fashion for an additional 9 months, during which time the patients in the sham group were crossed over to a 9-month course of active VNS treatment while the active VNS treatment group continued an additional 9 months of treatment. In addition to the VNS treatment, all patients continued to receive "treatment as usual" (ongoing antidepressant regimens and doses could be changed; ECT, rTMS, or changes in psychotherapy were allowed). At 12 months follow-up, results revealed a doubling of the response rate (27.2%) and the remission rate (15.8%) using LOCF analysis. (Rush *et al.*, 2005b) Despite increased antidepressant effect with VNS over 12 months, this study suffered from lack of active treatment comparator and that subject population was allowed 'treatment as usual'.

In a naturalistic comparison study, George *et al.* compared open label extension phase patients after 12 months of VNS with a 'treatment as usual' (TAU) group whereby both groups received any combination of anti-depressant therapies but the TAU group did not receive VNS. Using the IDS-SR-30 as primary outcome measure, the VNS + TAU group not only had a greater decline (mean decline −9.9 vs. −3.7) in their IDS-SR-30 scores but also had a greater response (19.6% vs. 12.1%) and remission rate (15% vs. 3.6%) compared to the TAU group. The VNS + TAU group also achieved improvement in the secondary outcome HDRS-24 measure. However, certain factors may have confounded the findings such as difference in use of psychotropic medications, number of lifetime major depressive episodes, and likelihood of receiving ECT during the current episode. (George *et al.*, 2005)

Together these data support the following conclusions.

(1) In the USA, approval of VNS for depression has been shrouded in controversy. (US Senate Committee on Finance, 2006) Despite an FDA scientific advisory panel's support for premarket approval in 2004, the FDA initially rejected that recommendation though in early 2005 it reversed itself stating that the device would be considered approvable and gave premarket approval in July 2005 for treatment-resistant depression (TRD).

(2) VNS is the first implantable device used to treat depression and the first approved therapy for TRD.

(3) It failed to differentiate from sham in the 3-month, randomized control trial for TRD based on its primary outcome measure. In absence of a double-blind randomized placebo-controlled comparator administered in parallel, the true efficacy of this treatment modality in major depression remains uncertain at best.

(4) The antidepressant benefit from VNS seems to be gradual and accrue over weeks or months. It may therefore be more useful as a long-term maintenance for chronic depression rather than for acute stabilization of an episode.

(5) Its advantages include high adherence rate and absence of drug interactions while potential disadvantages include delay in seeing appreciable antidepressant effect, absence of guidelines in terms of where VNS fits in treatment algorithms for TRD, and that many third-party payers do not currently reimburse VNS treatment for depression.

Neurosurgical procedures

Ablative procedures

Surgery remains a last resort for severely incapacitated patients who have failed to respond to all other established treatments. Patients with intractable OCD and major affective disorder (i.e., major depression or bipolar disorder) are considered for these procedures (Cosgrove, 2000). A history of personality disorder, substance abuse, or other axis II symptomatology is a relative contraindication to surgery. Presently, surgical approaches consist of one of four distinct procedures performed bilaterally using stereotactic techniques: cingulotomy, subcaudate tractotomy, limbic leucotomy, and anterior capsulotomy (Cosgrove, 2000). Although results are generally promising (especially when considering the severity of the psychopathology), none of the published studies meet the criteria described above for a contemporary RCT (Binder & Iskandar, 2000; Ovsiew & Frim, 1997).

Deep brain stimulation (DBS)

Deep brain stimulation consists of stereotactic implantation of a small stimulus electrode into specific brain targets with magnetic resonance (MRI) imaging guidance. Deep brain stimulation is established as a therapy for intractable movement disorders (Pollak *et al.*, 2002; Greenberg & Rezai, 2003), and it is an investigational treatment in intractable obsessive-compulsive disorder (Nuttin *et al.*, 1999; Mallet *et al.*, 2002). There are no controlled studies of DBS for treatment of mood disorders. Uncontrolled studies of a small number of patients with severe depression have reported sustained antidepressant effects from deep brain stimulation in the subgenual cingulate (area 25) (Mayberg *et al.*, 2005).

The level of evidence for each of the interventions discussed in this chapter is summarized in Table 28.2.

Table 28.2. Effectiveness of brain stimulation procedures in mood disorders

Treatment	Form of treatment	Psychiatric disorder	Level of evidence for efficacy	Comments
Bilateral ECT	Suprathreshold dosage	Severe depressive episodes	Ia	Unequivocal efficacy with only one negative study
Unilateral ECT	Suprathreshold dosage	Severe depression in elderly	Ia	Less effective than bilateral treatment but less memory disturbance
Bilateral ECT	Suprathreshold dosage	Mania	III	No clear trial evidence despite many reported clinical successes
Bilateral ECT	Not known	Maintenance treatment of depression	IV	No evidence of efficacy despite repeated use
rTMS	Up to three times weekly	Severe depression	Ib	Trials small and difficult to evaluate, but growing evidence of some efficacy
Vagal nerve stimulation	Pulse generator treatment	Treatment resistant depression	III	Open studies only, but results promising

REFERENCES

Abrams, R. (2002). *Electroconvulsive Therapy*, 4th edn. New York: Oxford University Press.

American Psychiatric Association (APA) (2000). Practice Guideline for the Treatment of Patients with Major Depressive Disorder (Revision). *American Journal of Psychiatry*, **157** (April Suppl.) [G]

American Psychiatric Association (APA). (2001). *The Practice of Electroconvulsive Therapy: Recommendations for Treatment, Training, and Privileging*, 2nd edn. Washington DC: American Psychiatric Association.

American Psychiatric Association (APA). (2002). Practice Guideline for the Treatment of Patients with Bipolar Disorder (Revision). *American Journal of Psychiatry*, **159** (April Suppl. 4).

Anderson, I. M., Delvai, N. A., Ashim, B. S. *et al.* (2007). Adjunctive fast repetitive transcranial magnetic stimulation (rTMS) in the treatment of depression. *British Journal of Psychiatry*, **190**, 533–4.

Berman, R. M., Narasimhan, M., Sanacora, G. *et al.* (2000). A randomize clinical trial of repetitive transcranial magnetic stimulation in the treatment of major depression. *Biological Psychiatry*, **47**(4), 332–37.

Binder, D. K. & Iskandar, B. J. (2000). Modern neurosurgery for psychiatric disorders. *Neurosurgery*, **47**(1), 9–23.

Brandon, S., Cowley, P., McDonald, C. *et al.* (1984). Electroconvulsive therapy: results in depressive illness from the Leicestershire trial. *British Medical Journal*, **288**, 22–5.

Burt, T., Lisanby, S. H. & Sackeim, H. A. (2002). Neuropsychiatric applications of transcranial magnetic stimulation. *International Journal of Neuropsychopharmacology*, **5**, 73–103.

Cosgrove, G. R. (2000). Surgery for psychiatric disorders. *CNS Spectrums*, **5**(10), 43–52.

Daskalakis, Z. J., Christensen, B. K., Fitzgerald, P. B. & Chen, R. (2002). Transcranial magnetic stimulation: a new investigational and treatment tool in psychiatry. *Journal of Neuropsychiatry and Clinical Neuroscience*, **14**, 406–15.

Davis, J. M., Wang, Z. & Janicak, P. G. (1993). A quantitative analysis of clinical drug trials for the treatment of affective disorders. *Psychopharmacology Bulletin*, **29**, 175–81.

Dinan, T. G. & Barry, S. (1989). A comparison of electroconvulsive therapy with a combined lithium and tricyclic combination among depressed nonresponders. *Acta Psychiatria Scandinavica*, **80**, 97–100.

Elger, G., Hoppe, C., Falkai, P. *et al.* (2000). Vagus nerve stimulation is associated with mood improvements in epilepsy patients. *Epilepsy Research*, **42**(2–3), 203–10.

Expert Consensus Guideline (2001a). Treatment of depression in women. *Postgraduate Medicine*.

Expert Consensus Guideline Series (2001b). Pharmacotherapy of depressive disorders in older patients. *Postgraduate Medicine*.

Folkerts, H. W., Michael, N., Tolle, R. *et al.* (1997). Electroconvulsive therapy vs. paroxetine in treatment-resistant depression – a randomized study. *Acta Psychiatrica Scandinavica*, **96**, 334–42.

Freeman, C. P. L., Basson, J. V. & Crighton, A. (1978). Double-blind controlled trial of electroconvulsive therapy (E.C.T.) and simulated E.C.T. in depressive illness. *The Lancet*, **1**, 738–40.

Gangadhar, B. N., Kpaur, R. L. & Kalyanasundaram, S. (1982). Comparison of electroconvulsive therapy with imipramine in endogenous depression: a double blind study. *British Journal of Psychology*, **141**, 367–71.

Garcia-Toro, M., Mayol, A., Arnillas, H. *et al.* (2001). Modest adjunctive benefit with transcranial magnetic stimulation in medication resistant depression. *Journal of Affective Disorders*, **64**(2–3), 271–5.

George, M. S., Wassermann, E. M., Williams, W. E. *et al.* (1997). Mood improvements following daily left prefrontal repetitive transcranial magnetic stimulation in patients with depression:

a placebo-controlled crossover trial. *American Journal of Psychiatry*, **154**, 1752–6.

George, M. S., Lisanby, S. H. & Sackeim, H. A. (1999). Transcranial Magnetic Stimulation: applications in neuropsychiatry. *Archives of Genernal Psychiatry*, **56**, 300–11.

George, M. S., Nahas, Z., Molloy, M. *et al.* (2000). A controlled trial of daily prefrontal cortex TMS for treating depression. *Biological Psychiatry*, **48**(10), 962–70.

George, M. S., Nahas, Z., Bohning, D. *et al.* (2002). Vagus nerve stimulation therapy: a research update. *Neurology*, **59** (Suppl. 4), S56–S61.

George, M. S., Nahas, Z., Kozel, F. A. *et al.* (2003). Mechanisms and the current state of transcranial magnetic stimulation. *CNS Spectrums*, **8**(7), 496–514.

George, M. S., Rush, A. J., Marangell, L. B. *et al.* (2005). A one year comparison of vagus nerve stimulation with treatment as usual for treatment-resistant depression. *Biological Psychiatry*, **58**(5), 364–73.

Gershon, A. A., Dannon, P. N. & Grunhaus, L. (2003). Transcranial Magnetic Stimulation in the treatment of depression. *American Journal of Psychiatry*, **160**(5), 835–45.

Greenberg, B. D. & Rezai, A. R. (2003). Mechanisms and the current state of deep brain stimulation in neuropsychiatry. *CNS Spectrums*, **8**(7), 522–6.

Greenblatt, M., Grosser, G. H. & Wechsler, H. (1964). Differential response of hospitalized depressed patients to somatic therapy. *American Journal of Psychology*, **120**, 935–43.

Gregory, S., Shawcross, C. R. & Gill, D. (1985). The Nottingham ECT Study. A double-blind comparison of bilateral, unilateral and simulated ECT in depressive illness. *British Journal of Psychiatry*, **146**, 520–4.

Harden, C. L., Pulver, M. C., Ravdin, L. D. *et al.* (2000). A pilot study of mood in epilepsy patients treated with vagus nerve stimulation. *Epilepsy Behavior*, **1**(2), 93–9.

Holtzheimer, P. E., Russo, J. & Avery, D. (2001). A meta-analysis of repetitive transcranial magnetic stimulation in the treatment of depression. *Psychopharmacology Bulletin*, **35**, 149–69.

Johnstone, E. C., Deakin, J. F. W., Lawler, P. *et al.* (1980). The Northwick Park electroconvulsive therapy trial. *The Lancet*, **2**, 1317–20.

Kho, K. H., Vreeswijk, M. F., Simpson, S. & Zwinderman, A. H. (2003). A meta-analysis of electroconvulsive therapy efficacy in depression. *Journal of ECT*, **19**(3), 139–47.

Kozel, F. A. & George, M. S. (2002). Meta-analysis of left prefrontal repetitive transcranial magnetic stimulation to treat depression. *Journal of Psychiatric Practice*, **8**, 270–5.

Kosel, M. & Schlaepfer, T. E. (2003). Beyond the treatment of epilepsy: new applications of vagus nerve stimulation in psychiatry. *CNS Spectrums*, **8**(7), 515–21.

Lambourn, I. & Gill, D. (1978). A controlled comparison of simulated and real ECT. *British Journal of Psychiatry*, **133**, 514–19.

McNamara, B., Ray, J. L., Arthurs, O. J. *et al.* (2001). Transcranial magnetic stimulation for depression and other psychiatric disorders. *Psychological Medicine*, **31**, 1141–6.

Mallet, L., Mesnage, V. *et al.* (2002). Compulsions, Parkinson's disease, and stimulation. *Lancet*, **360**, 1302–4.

Marangell, L. B., Rush, A. J., George, M. S. *et al.* (2005). Vagus nerve stimulation (VNS) for major depressive episodes: one year outcomes. *Biological Psychiatry*, **51**(4), 280–7.

Martin, J. L. R., Barbanoj, M. J., Schlaepfer, T. E. *et al.* (2003). Repetitive transcranial magnetic stimulation for the treatment of depression: systematic review and meta-analysis. *British Journal of Psychiatry*, **182**, 480–91.

Martin, J. L. R., Barbanoj, M. J., Schlaepfer, T. E. *et al.* (2004). Transcranial magnetic stimulation for treating depression [Review]. *The Cochrane Database of Systematic Reviews*, **1**. Oxford: Update Software Ltd.

Mayberg, H. S., Lozano, A. M., Voon, V. *et al.* (2005). Deep brain stimulation for treatment-resistant depression. *Neuron*, **45**, 651–60.

Medical Research Council (1965). Clinical trial of the treatment of depressive illness. *British Medical Journal*, **5439**, 881–6.

Mukherjee, S., Sackeim, H. A. & Schnur, D. B. (1994). Electroconvulsive therapy of acute manic episodes: a review of 50 years' experience. *American Journal of Psychiatry*, **151**, 169–76.

Nahas, Z., Oliver, N. C., Johnson, M. *et al.* (2000). Feasibility and efficacy of left prefrontal rTMS as a maintenance antidepressant [abstract]. *Biological Psychiatry*, **57**.

Nahas, Z., Marangell, L. B., Husain, M. M. *et al.* (2005). Two year outcome of vagus nerve stimulation (VNS) for treatment of major depressive episodes. *Journal of Clinical Psychiatry*, **66**(9), 1097–104.

National Institute for Clinical Excellence (NICE) Report (April 2003). www.nice.org.uk/pdf/Final_assessment_report ECT.pdf.

Nuttin, B., Cosyns, P. *et al.* (1999). Electrical stimulation in anterior limbs of internal capsules in patients with obsessive-compulsive disorder. *Lancet*, **354**, 1526.

Ovsiew, F. & Frim, D. M. (1997). Neurosurgery for psychiatric disorders. *Journal of Neurology, Neurosurgery and Psychiatry*, **63**, 701–5.

Pollak, P., Fraix, V., Krack, P. *et al.* (2002). Treatment results: Parkinson's disease. *Movement Disorders*, **17**(Suppl. 3), S75–S83.

Rifkin, A. (1988). ECT versus tricylic antidepressants in depression: a review of the evidence. *Journal of Clinical Psychiatry*, **49**, 3–7.

Rush, A. J., Rago, W. V., Crismon, M. L. *et al.* (1999). Medication treatment for the severely and persistently mentally ill: the Texas medication algorithm project. *Journal of Clinical Psychiatry*, **60**(5), 284–91.

Rush, A. J., George, M. S., Sackeim, H. A. *et al.* (2000). Vagus nerve stimulation (VNS) for treatment-resistant depression: a multicenter study. *Biological Psychiatry*, **47**, 276–86.

Rush, A. J., Linden, M. & Zobel, A. (2002). Vagus stimulation. Eine Neue Behaldlungsoption fur chronifizierte depressive Erkrankungen. *Fortschrift Neurologie Psychiatrie*, **70**, 297–302.

Rush, A. J., Marangell, L. B., Sackeim, H. A. *et al.* (2005a) Vagus nerve stimulation for treatment-resistant depression: a randomized, controlled acute-phase trial. *Biological Psychiatry*, **58**(5), 347–54.

Rush, A. J., Sackeim, H. A., Marangell, L. B. *et al.* (2005b). Effects of 12 months of vagus nerve stimulation in treatment-resistant depression: a naturalistic study. *Biological Psychiatry*, **58**, 355–63.

Sackeim, H. A., Rush, A. J., George, M. S. *et al.* (2001). Vagus nerve stimulation (VNS) for treatment-resistant depression: efficacy, side effects, and predictors of outcome. *Neuropsychopharmacology*, **25**(5), 713–28.

Sikdar, S., Kulhara, P., Avasthi, A. & Singh, H. (1994). Combined chlorpromazine and electroconvulsive therapy in mania. *British Journal of Psychology*, **164**, 806–10.

Small, J. G., Klapper, M. H., Kellams, J. J. *et al.* (1988). Electroconvulsive treatment compared with lithium in the management of manic states. *Archives in General Psychology*, **45**, 727–32.

The Expert Consensus Guideline Series (1996). Treatment of bipolar disorder. *Journal of Clinical Psychiatry*, **57**(12A), 11–88.

UK ECT Review Group (2003). Efficacy and safety of electroconvulsive therapy in depressive disorders: a systematic review and meta-analysis. *The Lancet*, **361**, 799–808.

US Army MEDCOM Report. http://www.cs.amedd.army.mil/qmo/depress/depress.htm.

US Senate Committee on Finance (2006). Review of the FDA's approval process for the vagus nerve stimulation therapy system for treatment resistant depression. February 2006. Available at: http://finance.senate.gov/press/Gpress/02report.pdf.

West, E. D. (1981). Electric convulsion therapy in depression: a double-blind controlled trial. *British Medical Journal*, **282**, 355–7.

29

Psychotherapy for depression: current empirical status and future directions

Scott Temple and John Geddes

Editor's note

The treatment of the most common of mental disorders by the means most patients prefer, psychotherapy, is likely to be one of the most frequently referenced chapters in this book. Here we see a common message writ clear; psychological treatments are in the same league as drug treatments for depression and tend to be better in the long term in maintaining a stable mood. Not all psychological therapies are similar in efficacy, but both cognitive therapy and interpersonal therapy can be championed as contenders for preferred treatment for all forms of mild to moderate depression. While drug treatment may have the edge in more severe depression, when combined with psychological treatments they do even better. The only negative issues are the paucity of skilled therapists and the delay in reaching improvement, the latter being generally greater with psychological therapy. But we are still at the relative dawn of good evidence in this subject and in particular the specific place of the different psychological treatments has yet to be determined.

Introduction

There is perhaps more high-quality evidence for the efficacy of psychotherapy in the treatment of depression than in any other mental disorder. A large number of randomized controlled trials (RCTs) have demonstrated that psychological treatments work, and research is beginning to shed light on possible active mechanisms of treatment. Therapies evaluated in this chapter will follow the grading criteria established initially by a task force of the American Psychological Association (1995) but the evidence table at the end of the chapter maintains the same criteria as Appendix II.

(1) Efficacious treatments, which are those treatments that have been found to be effective in more than one RCT, including at least one at a site other than where the therapy was developed.

(2) Probably efficacious treatments, which are promising treatments, found to be effective in at least one high-quality RCT, but in need of replication by further RCTs.

(3) Efficacious and specific treatments for depression, is a designation reserved for therapies which have not only established efficacy, but have shown effects that are superior to other active treatments for depression.

Two psychotherapies qualify as efficacious treatments for depression, using the APA guidelines above, Interpersonal Psychotherapy (IPT) and Beck's cognitive therapy (CT).

Cognitive therapy

The best validated and most widely known psychological treatment for depression remains that developed by Aaron T. Beck and associates (Beck *et al.*, 1979). Known simply as cognitive therapy or cognitive behaviour therapy, Beck's model posits that changes in thinking mediate changes in behaviour. Specifically, Beck's model posits that depression arises in the context of depressive cognitive biases, the modification of which relieves depressive symptoms. The model incorporates behavioural techniques through the use of what are called 'behavioural experiments', which are intended to help the patient assess and modify thinking processes which are believed to be distorted by depression. There is small-scale, but consistent, randomized evidence that cognitive therapy is superior to wait-list control in mild–moderate DSM major depression (NICE, 2003). There is more substantial randomized evidence that cognitive therapy is equally as effective as antidepressant drug therapy for mild–moderate

Cambridge Textbook of Effective Treatments in Psychiatry, ed. Peter Tyrer and Kenneth R. Silk. Published by Cambridge University Press. © Cambridge University Press, 2008.

DSM major depression (NICE, 2003). Combination therapy with cognitive therapy plus antidepressant drugs is superior to monotherapy for people with severe depression and chronic depression (NICE, 2003).

In addition, Beck's early model posits that core beliefs and schemas, possibly dormant during periods of remission, become activated in depression and remain predisposing risk factors for relapse. While the evidence regarding the role of core beliefs and schemas is mixed, in terms of their relationship to depressive relapse (Clark & Steer, 1996; Clark et al., 1999), Cognitive therapy for depression also targets such beliefs during the treatment of acute depressive episodes. Whether through moderation of schemas or through training patients to manage early onset of depressive symptoms, cognitive therapy is thought to provide a moderate prophylactic effect on recurrence of MDD (Evans et al., 1992; Jarrett et al., 1999).

Interpersonal psychotherapy (IPT)

IPT was derived from the more interpersonally orientated psychodynamic therapies, such as Harry Stack Sullivan (Sullivan, 1953). Intended as a short-term treatment for depression, IPT targets key areas of interpersonal functioning as a means of understanding the factors which maintain, though not necessarily cause, unipolar MDD. IPT believes that depression is an etiologically complex mix of psychological and interpersonal factors, but focuses primarily on the interpersonal factors believed implicated in the origins and maintenance of depression (Klerman et al., 1984). Key areas for intervention include role transitions, interpersonal disputes, unresolved grief, and interpersonal deficits, including isolation and/or withdrawal from others. IPT was subject to one early RCT (DiMascio et al., 1979; Weissman et al., 1979); the results supported the efficacy of IPT, imipramine, and IPT + imripramine over a control condition. But it was the treatment of depression collaborative research program (TDCRP) (Elkin et al., 1989; Elkin, 1994) which elevated the status of IPT to one of parity with CBT. The prophylactic effects of IPT have been tested in several studies. Acute treatment with IPT did not provide prophylactic benefits in terms of relapse prevention (Weissman et al., 1981), or in the TDCRP study (Elkin, 1994), the latter showing no prophylactic effects of any acute treatment (medication, IPT, CBT) versus pill placebo at 18 months. However, IPT has demonstrated efficacy in reducing relapse of MDD when used as a maintenance therapy, usually including monthly sessions (Frank et al., 1990). In addition, IPT is a probably efficacious treatment for postpartum depression (Stuart, 1999; O'Hara et al., 2000). In summary, there is limited but consistent evidence that IPT is more effective than pill placebo and usual primary medical care (NICE, 2003). There is some evidence that combination therapy with IPT plus antidepressant drug therapy is superior to IPT monotherapy in reducing relapse rates over three years (NICE, 2003).

Treatment of depression collaborative research program (TDCRP)

The TDCRP was a large multi-centre study, conceived in the late 1970s and carried out at three sites, each at separate universities. Project coordinators and therapist trainers from three additional universities in the USA and Canada were also involved. The TDCRP remains a study whose results were equivocal in important respects, and whose design and findings have generated substantial controversy ever since (Elkin, 1994; Jacobson & Hollon, 1996). Among its goals, the TDCRP was intended to provide a test of the relative efficacies of two psychotherapies, CT and IPT, versus tricyclic antidepressant medication versus placebo. The TDCRP eventually enrolled 250 patients, who were assigned to one of four treatment arms (CT, IPT, imipramine + clinical management (IMI-CM), pill placebo + clinical management (PLA-CD)), for a treatment duration of 16 weeks.

Among the key findings from the TDCRP study are the following.

(1) For mild to moderate MDD, 'there is no evidence of any differences between the two psychotherapies in their ability to reduce depressive and general symptomatology or to improve functioning' (Elkin, 1994, p. 119).

(2) On the Hamilton Rating Scale for Depression (HRSD) and the Beck Depression Inventory (BDI), medication (IMI-CM) 'clearly had more rapid effects (than either psychotherapy), with consistently significant differences ... by the 12th week of treatment. (ibid, p. 122)'

(3) By the conclusion of treatment, at 16 weeks, there was a 'general lack of significant differences in mean scores between either of the psychotherapies and PLA-CM' (ibid, p. 130), which the author attributes not to the weakness of either CT or IPT, but to the surprising improvements noted in the PLA-CM condition. This improvement may have reflected the fact that mild to moderate depression is responsive to supportive clinical management provided by skilled clinicians, even when they are dispensing placebo medication.

(4) Despite the fact that IPT and CT are based on significantly different theories and intervention strategies, remarkable little in the way of specific treatment

effects were achieved in the TDCRP. Perhaps counter-intuitively, patients low on social dysfunction had lower depression severity scores at treatment completion when receiving IPT; CT patients with lower scores on cognitive dysfunction, using the Dysfunctional Attitude Scale, achieved lower depression severity scores at the completion of treatment. Sotsky *et al.* (1991) posited that 'patients with good social function may be better able to take advantage of interpersonal strategies to recover from depression, while patients without severe dysfunctional attitudes may better utilize cognitive techniques to restore mood and behaviour (p. 1006).'

(5) An analysis of recovery from depression, as measured by cut-off scores on the HRSD, revealed that the percentage of recovered patients was significantly higher in the three presumably active treatment conditions (IMI-CM, CT, IPT) than in the PLA-CM condition.

(6) For more severe MDD, as measured by the HSRD and the BDI, significant differences emerged between IMI-CM and psychotherapy, particularly CT, which lagged behind both IMI-CM and IPT as a treatment for severe depression. IPT performed better with more severe MDD than did CT. CT's relatively poorer performance for severe MDD reflected treatment × site effects, in that one center in which CBT was conducted performed significantly better than the other, for those patients with GAS scores of 50 or less. A reverse pattern was found for IPT. In contrast, IMI-CM performed comparably across centers in which it was tested. The variability of CT's performance with severe MDD was also found in a study by Hollon *et al.* (1992), which found comparable site × treatment effects. In addition, very small severe MDD subgroup sample sizes and the well-known hazards of post-hoc subgroup analyses limit the interpretability of these findings.

(7) Prophylactic effects of all treatment conditions, among treatment completers, was limited. Craighead *et al.* (2002) conclude that 'none of the acute treatment differences was maintained over the follow-up, and none of the treatments was superior even to PLA-CM (p. 253)' at 18 months.

Prophylactic effects of treatments

With respect to the prophylactic effects of IPT, Frank *et al.* (1990) found that ongoing maintenance therapy, providing IPT once a month, reduced relapse at 36 months.

In contrast to the lack of prophylactic effects for CT demonstrated in the TDCRP study, such effects for CT have been demonstrated in a variety of studies (Kovacs *et al.*, 1981;

Simons *et al.*, 1986; Evans *et al.*, 1992), with relapse being reduced by nearly half in comparison to patients receiving antidepressant medication (Hollon, 2001).

Although considering that there may be differences in treatments for more severe MDD, Elkins (1994) notes that 'it is important to remember that IPT did not do significantly better than CT on any measures, so one cannot conclude that IPT is more effective than CT (p. 132).' She concludes as follows:

We should also point out that although IMI-CM is not significantly superior to the psychotherapies, even for the more severe patients, its results for these patients are more consistent across sites, while the psychotherapies are quite variable, probably depending more on the particular patient, therapist, and therapist-patient interaction (p. 132).

TDCRP conclusions regarding treatment of severe depression

Despite Elkin's caveats about the two psychotherapies studied in the TDCRP, including their relative efficacies with moderate to severe MDD, the TDCRP's results had a swift and in some ways unfortunate impact on the establishment of 'depression guidelines' (Depression Guideline Panel, 1993; American Psychiatric Association, 1993). For example, the American Psychiatric Association's *Practice Guidelines for the Treatment of Depression in Adults* (2000) recommends antidepressant medications, and not cognitive therapy, as a first-line treatment for moderate to severe MDD. However, the uniformity and quality of the CT provided in the TDCRP has been questioned (Jacobson & Hollon, 1996), as has the role of an allegiance effect in treatment outcome (Jacobson, 1999). Craighead *et al.*, 2002) suggest that the guidelines from the APA or the AHCPR were premature. As Jacobson & Hollon (1996b) wryly note, 'Now that the verdict is in, the jury can hear the evidence.' On the other hand, if quality of CT varies to this extent within a clinical trial, it is likely to do so within routine clinical practice. This highlights one of the key difficulties of making CT widely available for the treatment of depression.

Studies of cognitive therapy following the TDCRP

Two much awaited multi-centre studies of cognitive therapy have been recently completed, designed to test CT's efficacy compared to antidepressant medication for patients with moderate to severe MDD. Hollon and DeRubeis, at Vanderbilt University and the University of Pennsylvania, respectively, assessed CT in comparison to paroxetine, in both the acute phase and for their prophylactic effects at 2-year follow-up (DeRubeis *et al.*, 2005).

Overall findings from the acute phase study showed that paroxetine was statistically superior to pill placebo at 16 weeks and that CT approached – but did not reach – statistical superiority (DeRubeis *et al.*, 2005). Treatment-by-site differences also emerged in the study, just as occurred in the TDCRP. Post-hoc analysis suggested differing experience levels at the two sites which led DeRubeis and Hollon to propose that CT is an effective treatment for moderate to severe depression when provided by highly experienced cognitive therapists.

A 2-year follow-up study of treatment completers revealed that a limited continuation phase of CT (three sessions spread over 12 months) had significant prophylactic effects at 24 months (Hollon *et al.*, 2005). In particular, CT provided at least as much protection as continuation medication therapy at 2 years for treatment completers. Thus, it appears that reasonable evidence is accruing to suggest that CT, as well as IPT, confers protective benefits, in terms of relapse, for patients with MDD. In summary, the findings suggest the possibility of an alternative strategy to long-term drug treatment as recommended in the American Psychiatric Association guidelines (2000), although, of course, this recommendation is based on trials of antidepressant drugs including several thousand randomized patients (Geddes *et al.*, 2003).

One additional new adaptation of cognitive therapy is under development as a method for addressing relapse prevention. Mindfulness-based cognitive therapy (MBCT) combines cognitive therapy and mindfulness meditation as a means of reducing relapse in patients in remission from MDD. MBCT was designed as an 8-session group intervention for patients currently in remission from MDD. It combines psychoeducation, cognitive therapy, and meditation practice into a group administered treatment that is intended to disrupt the process of depressive rumination thought to be implicated in the onset and maintenance of depression relapse.

A preliminary multi-centre randomized controlled trial was conducted, involving 145 recovered MDD patients (Teasdale *et al.*, 2000). The results showed that MBCT significantly reduced depression relapse over the course of an 8-week trial, followed by 52 weeks of follow-up, for patients with three or more prior episodes of depression. However, MBCT did not reduce relapse rates for patients with two prior episodes of MDD.

A second study was conducted to determine whether MBCT's poorer effects on patients with two prior episodes would be replicated. Consistent with the first clinical trial, the second (Ma & Teasdale, 2004) found that relapse rates at one year follow-up were reduced from 78% to 36% in patients with three or more prior episodes. For patients with four or more prior episodes of MDD, the results were especially striking; only 38% of MBCT patients relapsed, compared to 100% of patients in the treatment-as-usual condition. However, in patients with only two prior MDD episodes, relapse rates were again not reduced.

Ma and Teasdale speculate about qualitative differences between the depression groups which may account for the differential response to MBCT. In particular, they contend that depressive rumination, which is a target of intervention in MBCT, is most evident in the three or more prior episode group. Patients with two prior episodes were more likely to have life events as triggers for depression, less childhood adversity, and a later onset than the group with three or more prior episodes.

Further studies are clearly needed to determine why patients with three or more prior MDD episodes respond better to MBCT than do those with two prior episodes. However, at this point, with two randomized controlled trials completed, MBCT has established that it is an efficacious treatment for depression relapse for those with three or more prior episodes of MDD.

The recent Christchurch Psychotherapy of Depression Study (CPDS) conducted in New Zealand compared CBT with IPT in depressed outpatients and found no statistically significant differences between the therapies on the primary outcome of percentage improvement in symptoms, although the results suggested a consistent benefit to CBT that was almost significant overall and a clearer benefit in more severely depressed patients (Luty *et al.*, 2007). The CDPS also reported that comorbid personality disorder adversely affected treatment outcomes with IPT compared to CBT (Joyce *et al.*, 2007). The finding that more severely depressed patients respond better to CBT than IPT contrast with the TDCRP but emphasizes the difficulty of interpreting subgroup effects. The magnitude of the difference in the proportion of responders (14%) suggests that, although one of the largest comparative trials to date, it may still have been somewhat underpowered to detect a clinically important difference. In general the evidence for CBT is more substantial and more convincing than that for IPT.

Given the evidence that CT is efficacious when provided by an expert therapist and possibly preferred by many patients compared to drug therapy, one of the main challenges is to make CT widely available to all who may benefit from it. In many countries, the availability of suitably trained therapists is inadequate to meet potential need. For this reason, current clinical practice guidelines often recommend a stepped approach to care with brief CT-based therapies based on self-help or provided by computer, for most patients (e.g. NICE, 2003). In the stepped-care model, therapist-administered CT would then be reserved for more severely affected patients (in combination with antidepressant drugs), and patients who strongly preferred a psychological treatment and who had failed to respond to first-line therapy.

Probably efficacious treatments

Probable efficacious treatments include various forms of behaviour therapy. More recently, psychodynamically oriented psychotherapies for depression have been subjected to RCTs.

Behaviour therapy has a long history as a treatment for depression, including reported success in clinical trials. Lewinsohn, in particular, developed an early model which focused on helping depressed patients re-engage in pleasant activities, as a means of increasing rates of positive reinforcement in daily life (Lewinsohn, 1974). He later developed a group-administered protocol, consisting of 20 sessions (Lewinsohn *et al.*, 1984; Lewinsohn & Gotlib, 1995). Although there have been numerous relatively small clinical trials supporting the efficacy of Lewinsohn *et al.*'s approach, until recently, behaviour therapies have been generally eschewed in favour of Beck's CT and IPT in the larger randomized trials. This relative exclusion of behavioural approaches has been described by Craighead *et al.* (2002) as 'due primarily to the sociology of science and to no small extent the exclusion of behaviour therapy from the well-publicized NIMH clinical trial (p. 248).'

The eclipsing of behavioural treatments for depression is being rectified by two sets of studies, each involving a new and highly innovative approach to depression, developed initially by the late Neil S. Jacobson and associates, at the University of Washington (Martell *et al.*, 2001; Jacobson *et al.*, 2001). Called *Behavioural Activation (BA)*, it was originally intended to be used as the solely behavioural component of CBT in a dismantling study of the components of Beck's cognitive therapy. Jacobson postulated that depression was best conceptualized from the perspective of a negative reinforcement paradigm, in which the patient's withdrawal and avoidance was seen as a means of escaping painful feared consequences of engagement in life. He offered the cogent observation that 'people are not depressed because they have depressing thoughts; they're depressed because they have depressing lives (Dimidjian, 2003).' One feature that makes BA uniquely behavioural is its emphasis on the function of depressive ideation, rather than on its content. This difference is highly significant in terms of intervention strategies. Beck's model, for example, views cognition as a significant mediator of change in therapy, though Beck has always recognized that behavioural change can precede a change in cognition (Beck *et al.*, 2004). Still, Beck's model relies heavily on exploring and modifying the content of depressive thinking.

By contrast, Jacobson *et al.* focus more on direct re-engagement of the patient not just in pleasant activities but in activities that are both meaningful and necessary in the patient's daily life. They do so without exploring the content of the patient's depressive appraisals. Thus, patients in BA are helped to recognize that periods of depressive rumination actually work at cross-purposes with their stated goals of living their lives more fully and meaningfully.

Since CT employs behavioural activation early in treatment, especially for more severe depression, Jacobson *et al.* set out to explore whether the behavioural or cognitive components of CBT were the 'active' ingredient in treatment outcome. A large multi-centre randomized trial was conducted, involving 150 outpatients, assigned to either a course of complete cognitive therapy (behavioural activation + automatic thought modification + schema therapy), to behavioural activation + automatic thought modification, or to behavioural activation, alone. Jacobson *et al.* (1996) found that the more purely behavioural approach, BA, performed as well at the termination of acute treatment (20 sessions) and at 6-month follow-up as did a full course of cognitive therapy. They concluded that there was 'no evidence that CT is any more effective than either of its components (p. 302),' raising questions 'as to the theory of change put forth in the CT book by Beck and his associates (p. 303).' A 2-year follow-up study showed that BA was equally effective at preventing relapse as CT (Gortner *et al.*, 1998).

Jacobson *et al.* went on to develop BA as a 'stand-alone' treatment model for depression, with its own theory of depression, treatment, and change (Martell *et al.*, 2001). The results of a second multi-centre trial of BA, this time especially targeting more severely depressed outpatients, has been completed, and the results are consistent with the earlier RCT (Martell *et al.*, 2003; Dimidjian *et al.*, 2006). This randomized controlled trial compared antidepressant medication with behavioural activation and cognitive therapy. Two hundred and forty-one patients were randomized to the treatment groups. For the more severely depressed patients, BA was equivalent to medication. Both were statistically significantly superior to cognitive therapy. The results of this trial add to the complexity of determining which psychological treatments are efficacious for severer depression. In addition, these findings add a further challenge, if not to cognitive therapy's overall efficacy as a treatment for depression, then to its claim that cognitive mediation is the active mechanism of change. Finally, with the results of this study published, it appears that BA should be considered an efficacious, rather than probably efficacious treatment for depression.

Cognitive behavioural analysis system of psychotherapy (CBASP) for chronic depression

McCullough (2000) developed a model of psychotherapy which is intended to address chronic, rather than episodic, depression. CBASP is a blend of behavioural, cognitive, and interpersonal therapies, and it is included as a form of behaviour therapy for two reasons: (1) it shares BA's emphasis on the function, rather than the content, of thought, and (2) social problem-solving is employed, which shares premises in common with BA.

CBASP is intended to help patients become more aware of the consequences of their depressive cognitions and coping behaviours. Rather than encouraging the patient to consider the accuracy or validity of their depressive appraisals and coping behaviours, the therapist asks the patient to delineate what they wanted from a specific situation, and whether their thoughts and behaviours in that situation got them their intended outcome, or an undesirable outcome. A social problem-solving approach is encouraged, to assist patients in obtaining desired goals, rather than the unintended outcomes, in key situations. In addition, CBASP encourages a specific focus on the therapeutic relationship as a means of altering depressogenic interpersonal patterns in the patient's life.

A large 12-center study was conducted, which involved random assignment of 681 adults to 12-weeks of treatment with CBASP, nefazadone, or combined CBASP and nefazodone. Inclusionary criteria included MDD with poor remission for 2 years' duration, or MDD superimposed on pre-existing dysthymia. The results indicated that CBASP performed as well as nefazodone in the acute phase of treatment. The combination of CBASP and nefazodone, however, was superior to either treatment alone, with a response rate of 85% being achieved for treatment completers (Keller et al., 2000).

This study remains the only RCT of CBASP, making it a 'probably efficacious' treatment for chronic depression. A new randomized trial is currently underway, involving more than 900 patients. It will be completed in 2006, and its results will be eagerly awaited.

Finally, a form of psychodynamic therapy, psychodynamic-interpersonal therapy (PI), was found to be equivalent to CT as a treatment of depression in one multi-center RCT (Shapiro et al., 1994). The sole outcome measure on which an advantage for CT was found was the Beck Depression Inventory. Another psychodynamic treatment, supportive-expressive psychotherapy, is currently being tested in an RCT at the University of Pennsylvania, although no data are available at this time.

Conclusions

Two psychotherapies have established efficacy as treatments for depression. The psychotherapies are Beck's cognitive therapy (CT) and Interpersonal Psychotherapy (IPT). Both treatments demonstrate efficacy in the acute phase of treatment. Both CT and IPT show promise as maintenance therapies in reducing relapse of recurrent MDD. In addition, mindfulness-based cognitive therapy (Segal et al., 2002) has emerged as a probably efficacious relapse mitigation treatment for patients with three or more prior episodes of MDD.

Among the therapies with probable efficacy as treatments for acute MDD are several behaviour therapies. Currently, both behavioural activation (BA) and the cognitive-behavioural analytic system of psychotherapy (CBASP) are being subjected to replication in large multicenter RCTs. In addition, a single psychoanalytically orientated therapy, psychodynamic-interpersonal psychotherapy (PI), is also close to established efficacy.

Among the more interesting issues emerging in the depression literature is the question of whether there are 'efficacious and specific treatments' for depression. It appears that at present, despite the relative success of a variety of different treatments, no treatment has displayed clear and specific effects. Initially, it was posited that cognitive therapy (CT) had displayed such efficacy relative to other treatments. However, DeRubeis & Crits-Christoph (1998) cite studies of CT in comparison to interpersonal psychotherapy (Elkin, 1994), behavioural activation (Jacobson et al., 1996) and a psychodynamic interpersonal psychotherapy (Shapiro et al., 1994), in which CT fares no better than any of these other treatment models. They conclude that 'the inference that CT is especially effective relative to other psychological treatments that are targeted for depression is premature (DeRubeis & Hollon, 1998, p. 39).'

This lack of specific treatment effects for *any* psychotherapeutic treatment of depression remains a puzzling, yet important, issue. A novel method of assessing the role of therapy processes in treatment outcome sheds light on possible reasons for this rough equivalence of numerous therapies in the treatment of MDD. Ablon & Jones (1999, 2002) describe a Q-sort methodology, in which experts in CT and IPT were asked to sort items into 'ideal' prototypes of their respective therapies. Then, using tapes from the TDCRP study, independent raters rated CT and IPT sessions, separately, using the Q-sort. Then, comparisons were made to establish the degree to which IPT and CT actually conformed to the 'ideal' prototype. In fact, Ablon and Jones (2002) found that, despite stated differences between IPT and CT, 'the nature of the interaction between therapist and patient might be quite similar (p. 781).' While differences were found between the two therapies, considerable overlap between the therapies exists when independent raters code the two therapies. Ablon & Jones (2002) conclude that 'in both treatments, the therapies assumes an authoritative role and coaches patients to think or conduct themselves differently and encourages them to test out these new ways of thinking and behaviour in everyday life (ibid).' A comparison of psychodynamic and cognitive therapies revealed other areas of overlap, including a developmental focus, which

Jones & Pulos (1992) speculate may be the common therapeutic element in the two treatments.

Wampold (2001) suggests that the rough equivalence of various treatments is due to their conformity to a common factors model. Both Wampold and Ablon & Jones would suggest that a common factors model, or 'meta-model', as outlined by Frank and Frank in their seminal work *Persuasion and Healing* (1991), may explain the equivalence of various empirically supported therapies for depression. Further efforts to dismantle various components of successful treatment may eventually shed light on such issues as a common factors model, which may explain what makes for an efficacious short-term treatment. At this point, while we do know that several psychotherapies are efficacious treatments of depression, we have yet to discern why and how they help. Depression research has advanced to the point that further RCTs may yet shed light on these complex issues.

The level of evidence for each of the interventions discussed in the chapter is summarized in Table 29.1

Table 29.1. Effectiveness of treatments for psychotherapies in depression

Treatment	Form of treatment	Psychiatric disorder	Level of evidence for efficacy	Comments
Cognitive therapy	Individual	Mild to moderate depression	Ia	Cognitive therapy superior to placebo and equivalent to antidepressant therapy
Cognitive therapy	Individual	Severe depression	?	Good evidence lacking
Cognitive therapy in combination with antidepressant drugs	Individual	Severe and resistant depression	Ia	Consistent evidence of superiority for cognitive therapy
Cognitive therapy	Individual	Long term maintenance of improvement	Ia	Effect of cognitive therapy persists for longer and prevents relapse to a greater extent than antidepressant drugs once treatment is completed
Interpersonal psychotherapy	Individual	Acute treatment for mild/moderate depression	Ia	Superior to placebo and equivalent to antidepressant drugs
Interpersonal psychotherapy	Individual	Severe depression	Ia	Not as effective as antidepressant drugs
Interpersonal psychotherapy and antidepressants	Individual	Prevention of relapse	Ib	Slight evidence in favour of drug/IPT combination in reducing relapse compared with IPT alone and for IPT alone given in maintenance form to be superior to antidepressants
Mindful based cognitive therapy	Individual	Prevention of relapse in depression	Ib	Only effective for those with three or more prior episodes
Behaviour therapy and activation	Group	Moderate depression	Ib	Effects may be similar to cognitive therapy
Cognitive behavioural analysis system of psychotherapy	Individual	Chronic depression	Ib	Possible equivalent to antidepressant therapy
Psychodynamic interpersonal therapy	Individual	Moderate depression	Ib	Uncertain evidence of efficacy in one trial

REFERENCES

Ablon, J. S. & Jones, E. E. (1999). Psychotherapy process in the NIMH Treatment of Depression Collaborative Research Program. *Journal of Consulting and Clinical Psychology*, **67**(1), 64–75.

Ablon, J. S. & Jones, E. E. (2002). Validity of controlled clinical trials of psychotherapy: findings from the NIMH Treatment of Depression Collaborative Research Program. *American Journal of Psychiatry*, **159** (5), 775–83.

American Psychiatric Association (1993). Practice guidelines for major depressive disorder in adults. *American Journal of Psychiatry*, **150** (Suppl.), 1–26.

American Psychiatric Association (2000). Practice guidelines for patients with major depressive disorder (revision). *American Journal of Psychiatry*, **157** (Suppl.), 1–45.

Beck, A. T., Rush, A. J., Shaw, B. F. & Emery, G. (1979). *Cognitive Therapy of Depression: A Treatment Manual*. New York: Guilford Press.

Beck, A. T., Freeman, A. & Davis, D. D. (2004) *Cognitive Therapy of Personality Disorders*, 2nd edn. New York: Guilford.

Chambless, D. L. & Hollon, S. D. (1998). Defining empirically supported therapies. *Journal of Consulting and Clinical Psychology*, **66**(1), 7–18.

Clark, D. A. & Steer, R. A. (1996). Empirical status of the cognitive model of anxiety and depression. In *Frontiers of Cognitive therapy*, ed. P. M. Salkovskis. New York: Guilford Press.

Clark, D. A., Beck, A. T. & Alford, B. (1999). *Scientific Foundations of Cognitive Theory and Therapy of Depression*. New York: John Wiley.

Craighead, W. E., Hart, A. B., Craighead, L. W. & Ilardi, S. S. (2002). Psychosocial treatments of major depressive disorder. In *A Guide to Treatments that Work*, 2nd edn. ed. P. E. Nathan & J. M. Gorman. New York: Oxford University Press.

Depression Guideline Panel (1993). *Clinical Practice Guideline Number 5: Depression in Primary Care, 2: Treatment of Major Depression*. Rockville, MD: United States Department of Health and Human Services, Agency for Health Care Policy and Research (AHCPR Publication #93-0551).

DeRubeis, R. J. & Crits-Cristoph, P. (1998). Empirically supported individual and group psychological treatments for adult mental disorders. *Journal of Consulting and Clinical Psychology*, **66**(1), 37–52.

DeRubeis, R. J., Amsterdam, J. D., O'Reardon, J. P. & Young, P. R. (2004). Cognitive therapy versus medications: acute treatment of severe depression. In *Cognitive Therapy versus Medications: Treatment and prevention of severe depression*, Chair S. D. Hollon. Symposium conducted at the annual meeting of the American Psychological Association, Honolulu.

DeRubeis, R., Hollon, S. D., Amsterdam, J. D. *et al.* (2005). Cognitive therapy vs medications in the treatment of moderate to severe depression. *Archives of General Psychiatry*, **62**(4), 409–16.

DiMascio, A., Weissman, M. M., Prusoff, B. A., Neu, C., Zwilling, M. & Klerman, G. L. (1979). Differential symptom reduction by drugs and psychotherapy in acute depression. *Archives of General Psychiatry*, **36**, 1450–6.

Dimidjian, S. (2003). Clinical applications of behavioral discussion. Panel Discussion, 37th Annual Convention, Association for Advancement of Behavior Therapy, Reno, Nevada.

Dimidjian, S., Hollon, SD, Dobson, K. S. *et al.* (2006). Randomized trial of behavioral activation, cognitive therapy, and antidepressant medication in the acute treatment of adults with major depression. *Journal of Consulting and Clinical Psychology*, **74**, 658–70.

Elkin, I. (1994). The NIMH treatment of depression collaborative research program: where we began and where we are. In *Handbook of Psychotherapy and Behavior Change*, 4th edn, pp. 114–38, ed. A. E. Bergin & S. L. Garfield. New York: John Wiley.

Elkin, I., Shea, M. T., Watkins, J. T. *et al.* (1989). National Institute of Mental Health treatment of depression collaborative research program: general effectiveness of treatments. *Archives of General Psychiatry*, **46**, 971–82.

Evans, M. D., Hollon, S. D., DeRubeis, R. J. *et al.* (1992). Differential relapse following cognitive therapy and pharmacotherapy for depression. *Archives of General Psychiatry*, **49**, 802–8.

Frank, E., Kupfer, D. J., Perel, T. M. *et al.* (1990). Three-year outcomes for maintenance therapies in recurrent depression. *Archives of General Psychiatry*, **47**, 1093–9.

Frank, J. D. & Frank, J. B. (1991). *Persuasion and Healing: A Comparative Study of Psychotherapy*. Baltimore: Johns Hopkins Press.

Geddes, J. R., Carney, S. M., Davies, C. *et al.* (2003). Relapse prevention with antidepressant drug treatment in depressive disorders: a systematic review. *Lancet*, **361** (9358), 653–61.

Gortner, E. T., Gollan, J. K., Dobson, K. S. & Jacobson, N. S. (1998). Cognitive-behavioral treatment for depression: relapse prevention. *Journal of Consulting and Clinical Psychology*, **66**, 377–84.

Hollon, S. D., DeRubeis, R. J., Evans, M. D. *et al.* (1992). Cognitive therapy and pharmacotherapy for depression: singly and in combination. *Archives of General Psychiatry*, **49**, 774–81.

Hollon, S. D., DeRubeis, R., Shelton, C. *et al.* (2005). Prevention of relapse following cognitive therapy vs medications in moderate to severe depression. *Archives of General Psychiatry*, **62**(4), 417–22.

Jacobson, N. S. (1999). The role of the allegiance effect in psychotherapy research: controlling and accounting for it. *Clinical Psychology: Science and Practice*, **6**(1), 116–19.

Jacobson, N. S. & Hollon, S. D. (1996a). Prospects for future comparisons between drugs and psychotherapy: lessons from the CBT-versus-pharmacotherapy exchange. *Journal of Consulting and Clinical Psychology*, **64**, 104–8.

Jacobson, N. S. & Hollon, S. D. (1996b). Cognitive-behavior therapy versus pharmacotherapy: Now that the jury's returned its verdict, it's time to present the rest of the evidence. *Journal of Consulting and Clinical Psychology*, **64**, 74–80.

Jacobson, N. S., Dobson, K. S., Truax, P. A. *et al.* (1996). A component analysis of cognitive-behavioral treatment for depression. *Journal of Consulting and Clinical Psychology*, **64**, 295–304.

Jacobson, N. S., Martell, C. R. & Dimidjian, S. (2001). Behavioral activation treatment for depression: returning to contextual roots. *Clinical Psychology: Science and Practice*, **8**(3), 255–68.

Jarrett, R. B., Schaffer, M., McIntire, D. Witt-Browden, A., Kraft, D., & Risser, R. C. (1999). Treatment of atypical depression with cognitive therapy or phemelzein: a double-blind placebo-controlled trial. *Archives of General Psychiatry*, **56**, 431–7.

Jones, E. E. & Pulos, S. M. (1993). Comparing the process in psychodynamic and cognitive-behavioral therapies. *Journal of Consulting and Clinical Psychology*, **61**(2), 306–16.

Joyce, P. R., McKenzie, J. M., Carter, J. D. *et al.* (2007). Temperament, character and personality disorders as predictors of response to interpersonal psychotherapy and cognitive behaviour therapy for depression. *British Journal of Psychiatry*, **190**, 503–8.

Keller, M. B., McCullough, J. P., Klein, D. N. *et al.* (2000). A comparison of nefazodone, the cognitive behavioral-analysis system of psychotherapy, and their combination for the treatment of chronic depression. *New England Journal of Medicine*, **342**, 1462–70.

Klerman, G. L., Weissman, M. M., Rousaville, B. J. & Chevron, E. S. (1984). *Interpersonal Psychotherapy of Depression*. New York: Basic Books.

Lewinsohn, P. M. (1974). A behavioral approach to depression. In *The Psychology of Depression: Contemporary Theory and Research*, ed. R. J. Friedman & M. M. Katz, pp. 176–8. Washington, DC: Winston-Wiley.

Lewinsohn, P. M. & Gotlib, I. H. (1995). Behavioral theory and treatment of depression. In *Handbook of Depression*, ed. E. E. Becker & W. R. Leber. New York: Guilford Press.

Lewinsohn, P. M., Antonuccio, D. O., Breckenridge, J. S. & Teri, L. (1984). *The Coping With Depression Course*. Eugene, Oregon: Castalia.

Luty, S. E., Carter, J. D., McKenzie, J. M. *et al.* (2007). Christchurch Psychotherapy of Depression Study: a randomised controlled trial of interpersonal psychotherapy and cognitive behaviour therapy. *British Journal of Psychiatry* **190**, 496–502.

Ma, H. & Teasdale, J. D. (2004). Mindfulness-based cognitive therapy for depression: replication and exploration of differential relapse prevention effects. *Journal of Consulting and Clinical Psychology*, **72**(1), 31–40.

Martell, C. R., Addis, M. E. & Jacobson, N. S. (2001). *Depression in Context: Strategies for Guided Action*. New York: W.W. Norton.

Martell, C. R., Dimidjian, S., Mulick, P. S., Roberts, L. J., & Wagner, A. (2003). Clinical applications of behavioral discussion. Panel Discussion, 37th Annual Convention, Association for Advancement of Behavior Therapy, Reno, Nevada.

McCullough, J. P. (2000). *Treatment for Chronic Depression: Cognitive Behavioral Analysis System of Psychotherapy*. New York: Guilford Press.

Murphy, G. E., Simons, A. D., Wetzel, R. D. & Lustman, P. J. (1984). Cognitive therapy and pharmacotherapy: singly and together in the treatment of depression. *Archives of General Psychiatry*, **41**, 33–41.

National Institute of Clinical Excellence (2003). Management of depression in primary and secondary care http://www.nice.nhs.uk/page.aspx?o=236667.

O'Hara, M. W., Stuart, S., Gorman, L. L. & Wenzel, A. (2000). Efficacy of interpersonal psychotherapy for postpartum depression. *Archives of General Psychiatry*, **57**, 1039–45.

Rush, A. J., Beck, A. T., Kovacs, M. & Hollon, S. D. (1977). Comparative efficacy of cognitive therapy in the treatment of depressed outpatients. *Cognitive Therapy and Research*, **1**, 17–36.

Segal, Z. S., Williams, J. M. G. & Teasdale, J. D. (2002). *Mindfulness-Based Cognitive therapy for Depression: A New Approach to Preventing Relapse*. New York: Guilford Press.

Shapiro, D. A., Barkham, M., Rees, A., Hardy, G., Reynolds, S. & Startup, M. (1994). Effects of treatment duration and severity of depression on the effectiveness of cognitive-behavioral and psychodynamic-interpersonal psychotherapy. *Journal of Consulting and Clinical Psychology*, **62**, 522–34.

Simons, A. D., Murphy, G. E., Levine, J. L. & Wetzel, R. D. (1986). Cognitive therapy and pharmacotherapy for depression. *Archives of General Psychiatry*, **43**, 43–8.

Sotsky, S. M., Glass, D. R., Shea, M. T. *et al.* (1991). Patient predictors of response to psychotherapy and pharmacotherapy: findings in the NIMH treatment of depression collaborative research program. *American Journal of Psychiatry*, **148**, 997–1008.

Stuart, S. P. (1999). Interpersonal psychotherapy for postpartum depression. In *Postpartum Mood Disorders*, ed. L. J. Miller. Washington: American Psychiatric Press, Inc.

Sullivan, H. S. (1953). *The Interpersonal Theory of Psychiatry*. New York: W.W. Norton & Company.

Task Force on Promotion and Dissemination of Psychological Procedures (1995). Training in and dissemination of empirically-validated psychological treatments: Report and recommendations. *Clinical Psychologist*, **48**, 3–23.

Teasdale, J. D., Segal, Z. V., Williams, J. M. G., Ridgeway, V. A., Sousby, J. M. & Lau, M. A. (2000). Prevention of relapse/recurrence in major depressin by mindfulness-based cognitive therapy. *Journal of Consulting and Clinical Psychology*, **68**(4), 615–23.

Wampold, B. E. (2001). *The Great Psychotherapy Debate: Models, Methods, and Findings*. Mahwah, New Jersey: Lawrence Erlbaum Publishers.

Weissman, M. M., Prusoff, B. A., DiMascio, A., Neu., C., Goklaney, M. & Klerman, G. L. (1979). The efficacy of drugs and psychotherapy in the treatment of acute depressive episodes. *American Journal of Psychiatry*, **136**, 555–8.

Weissman, M. M., Klerman, G.L, Prusoff, B. A., Sholomskas, D. & Padian, N. (1981). Depressed outpatients: results 1-year after treatment with drugs and/or interpersonal psychotherapy. *Archives of General Psychiatry*, **38**, 51–5.

30

Alternative therapies for mood disorders

William H. Coryell

Editors' note

As depression is so common, it is hardly surprising that there are a large number of alternative treatments in psychiatry for this condition. We now have good evidence for the efficacy of light therapy, where naturally it is chosen primarily for the treatment of seasonal affective disorder. It is of particular interest that efficacy is almost at its greatest when the light of an early dawn is being simulated. Sleep deprivation is only effective in the very short term but it undoubtedly does have benefit over a 48–72 hour period and may be combined with other treatments for this condition. There is an increasing literature on the benefits of omega-3 supplements in the treatment of depression and, for those who want to have the specific compounds, an alternative name for eicosapentaenoic acid might have to be found to avoid confusion. Whilst the benefits of essential fatty acids appear to be ascending, the opposite applies to St John's Wort, which, despite a very large number of trials, does not yet have unequivocal evidence of benefit.

Introduction

The high prevalence of affective disorders, together with the frequent inadequacy of conventional treatments, has produced a long-standing interest in alternative approaches. The following summarizes the evidence for those approaches that are supported by at least two prospectively randomized and controlled, parallel-design studies.

Light therapy

The observation that many persons regularly experience depressive symptoms during winter months, and that the prevalence of this pattern increases with latitude, led to the use of light exposure as a treatment for seasonal affective disorder (Rosenthal et al., 1984). Many controlled studies have followed (Terman et al., 1989), and the results support conclusions that the symptomatic improvement following bright light exposure far exceeds that following dim light exposure, with greater benefits for morning than for evening exposures. Atypical depressive symptoms such as hypersomnia, evening worsening and carbohydrate craving predict response to light therapy, while melancholic symptoms such as psychomotor retardation, morning worsening and terminal insomnia predict non-response (Terman et al., 1996). The amount of improvement with morning light appears to correlate with the degree to which melatonin onset is advanced by the exposure, and it is thought to be optimal when timed to begin 2 1/2 hours after the sleep midpoint (Terman et al., 2001). There is an interesting finding from research in northern Norway where in mid-winter there is no light during the day and where a much lower proportion of the population (around 1 in 5) have problems relating to sleep or mood during the winter months (Hansen et al., 1998). This suggest that, when daylight is absent, different mechanisms are operating.

Earlier studies applied 2500 lux of light for 2 hours in the morning, but most recent trials have used 10 000 lux for 30 minutes. No direct comparisons of these two approaches have appeared as yet, but compliance is likely to be greater with the shorter time commitment. Still better compliance may be expected with dawn simulation, a gradual increase in ambient light to 250 lux over a 1 1/2 hour period beginning at 4:30 a.m. (Avery et al., 2001). Relatively few controlled studies have tested this dosing, though, and direct comparisons to conventional bright light exposure have had inconsistent results that, in balance, have favoured bright light exposure (Avery et al., 1992, 2001).

Cambridge Textbook of Effective Treatments in Psychiatry, ed. Peter Tyrer and Kenneth R. Silk. Published by Cambridge University Press.
© Cambridge University Press, 2008.

Though light treatment was first applied to seasonal affective disorder, it may be no less effective for patients with a non-seasonal temporal pattern (Kripke, 1998). Moreover, a substantial proportion of individuals with seasonal affective disorder prove, on follow-up, to have assumed a non-seasonal course (Schwartz et al., 1996). Of six randomized studies that have compared bright light to dim light as monotherapy for non-seasonal depression, three showed a significant advantage for bright light (Kripke et al., 1992; Yamda et al., 1995; Beauchemin & Hays, 1997; Lam et al., 1999). One of the two negative studies had low statistical power (Mackert et al., 1991). The other found no difference between bright and dim light exposures but noted much more improvement in bipolar than in unipolar patients regardless of the light intensity (Deltito et al., 1991). This may have reflected a hypersensitivity to melatonin suppression by dim light present in bipolar, but not unipolar disorders (Nathan et al., 1999). A differential sensitivity was also revealed in a naturalistic study of inpatients in which those with bipolar depression assigned to rooms facing east (i.e. towards the dawn light in the northern hemisphere) had significantly shorter stays in the hospital than those given rooms facing west, while no such difference emerged for patients with unipolar depression (Benedetti et al., 2001).

Controlled studies have also shown bright light exposure to be a useful adjunct to antidepressant treatment (Beauchemin & Hays, 1997; Benedetti et al., 2003). The adjunctive use of bright light treatment with partial sleep deprivation may be particularly important (Neumeister et al., 1996).

Sleep deprivation

Numerous studies have shown that the deprivation of sleep for a 36-hour period (total sleep deprivation or TSD), or for the second half of the night (partial sleep deprivation or PSD), produces an immediate improvement in depressive symptoms in a substantial proportion of patients. Symptoms return at their previous severity after a night of sleep when sleep deprivation is used as monotherapy. The combined use of sleep deprivation with antidepressant drugs, however, appears to offer clear and practical advantages over either treatment alone.

Two prospectively randomized studies (Colombo et al., 2000; Baxter et al., 1986) and two naturalistic studies (Grube & Hartwich, 1990; Benedetti et al., 1999) have described bipolar I patients given sleep deprivation with or without lithium. One used partial sleep deprivation on two consecutive nights (Baxter et al., 1986), two used three

TSDs over a 1-week period (Colombo et al., 2000; Benedetti et al., 1999) and one used a single TSD (Grube & Hartwich, 1990). Despite these treatment differences, all described significantly lower depression scores after the final recovery night. The only study to provide follow-up data found that those who had received sleep deprivation while taking lithium had significantly lower depressive symptom scores 3 months later than did those who had received sleep deprivation without lithium, even though the latter group had begun taking lithium following the TSD course (Benedetti et al., 1999). Only one report compared patients randomized to lithium with sleep deprivation to those given lithium alone. Outcome measured 5 days later significantly favoured the combined therapy (Baxter et al., 1986).

An equivalent literature pertains to the use of sleep deprivation in conjunction with antidepressants. Two trials compared clomipramine initiated with one (Loosen et al., 1976) or two (Elsenga & Van den Hoofdakker, 1982) TSDs to clomipramine alone. Another compared fluoxetine begun with a week of three TSD nights to fluoxetine used alone (Benedetti et al., 1997). All found that those given TSD had experienced significantly more improvement after one week of drug treatment. Only two studies provided a longer observation period, and both found that group differences disappeared after 2 or 3 weeks (Loosen et al., 1976).

There is thus substantial evidence that sleep deprivation can at least hasten antidepressant responses to lithium and to other antidepressants. This potential has particular applicability to inpatient settings. Evidence that the benefits of sleep deprivation combined with lithium may be sustained well beyond the first week in bipolar patients, together with findings that bipolar I patients are more likely than bipolar II or unipolar patients to have sustained improvement with TSD monotherapy (Barbini et al., 1998), suggest that bipolar I patients who develop depression despite lithium prophylaxis may derive particular benefit from a trial sleep deprivation.

Omega-3 supplementation

A diverse body of evidence indicates that deficits in certain of the essential fatty acids (EFAs) both raise the risk of affective disorder and worsen its course. Epidemiological studies have shown inverse correlations between national levels of fish consumption and the prevalence of depressive symptoms (Hibbeln, 1998; Tanskanen et al., 2001), postpartum depression (Hibbeln, 2002) and bipolar spectrum disorders (Noaghiul & Hibbeln, 2003). In case-controlled

Table 30.1. Placebo-controlled studies of omega-3 in affective disorders

MDD	Patient group	N omega-3/placebo	Daily dose	Study length (wks)	Results
Peet et al., 2002[a]	TR[b]	15/15	1 g EPA	12	50% ↓ in HDRS[c] in 53% vs. 29%
Nemets et al., 2002	TR	10/10	2 g EPA	4	– ↓ in HDRS sig. greater for omega-3 group – (final means = 11.6 vs. 20.0)
Merengell et al., 2003	non-TR	18/17	2 g DHA	6	no diff. In change from baseline
Su et al., 2003	TR	12/10	9.6 g omega-3	8	– ↓ in HDRS sig. greater for omega-3 group – (final means = 8.9 vs. 15.7)
Bipolar AD					
Stoll et al., 1999	some TR	15/15	9.6 g omega-3	16	– omega-3 group had longer time before symptoms forced exit from protocol
Frangou et al., 2006	unselected	49/26 (omega-EPA 1 g (Elsenga & Van den Hoofdakker, 1982), 2 g (Benedetti et al., 1997)	1–2 g	12	significantly greater reduction in depression with omega-3 group
Borderline PD					
Zanarini & Frankenburg, 2003	drug-free	20/10	1 g EPA	8	– ↓ in MADRS[d] sig. greater for EPA group

[a] also included doses of 2 and 4 g daily; differences favoring 0–3 over placebo approached significance for 4 g but were absent for 2 g.
[b] TR = treatment resistant.
[c] HDRS = Hamilton Depression Rating Scale.
[d] MADRS = Montgomery–Asberg Depression Rating Scale.

comparisons, depressed patients had significantly lower tissue concentrations of various components of the omega-3 pathway than did well controls (Edwards et al., 1998; Peet et al., 1998; Maes et al., 1996, 1999; Mamalakis et al., 2002; Frasure-Smith et al., 2004).

These findings led to placebo-controlled trials designed to determine whether omega-3 supplementation might augment antidepressants or mood stabilizers (Table 30.1). In six of seven such studies, patients assigned to omega-3 supplementation had significantly superior outcomes to those given placebo. Most commercially available omega-3 supplements consist principally of eicosapentaenoic acid (EPA) and docosahexaenoic acid (DHA) and the above studies used either the combination of EPA and DHA or one of the two alone. The fact that the only negative study of major depression was also the only one to use DHA alone suggests that EPA may be the effective component of various omega-3 preparations, possibly because EPA is incorporated into tissues much more rapidly than is DHA (Brown et al., 1991). Some of these trials used high doses of 9 g and others used doses of only 1 to 2 g per day.

A comparison across studies (Table 30.1) suggests no benefit of high doses over low doses though direct comparisons have not been undertaken.

Exercise therapy

Carefully controlled trials have repeatedly shown benefits of supervised exercise programs for depressive symptoms. Most have used educational lectures or occupational therapy sessions of equivalent duration and frequency as control conditions and most have targeted older individuals. The earliest well-controlled study described a sample of inpatients with major depressive disorder and a mean age of 40. Those randomized to 9 weeks of aerobic exercise experienced significantly larger decreases in depressive symptoms than did those given equivalent number of occupational therapy sessions (Martinsen et al., 1985). Among those who received exercise the degree of improvement in depressive symptoms correlated significantly with improvements in maximum oxygen uptake.

Another three studies compared an exercise program to a series of health-related lectures given to samples of older individuals (Singh *et al.*, 2001; Penninx *et al.*, 2002; Mather *et al.*, 2002). In all studies individuals in the exercise groups experienced significantly larger decreases in depression scores. Though one study also compared aerobic to resistance exercise and found the former to be superior, the other two used weight-lifting or weight-bearing exercises and also noted significant benefits over equivalent numbers of educational sessions. Notably, one of these limited participation to patients with depressive disorders that had persisted despite six weeks of antidepressant treatment (Mather *et al.*, 2002).

Another trial randomized outpatients with MDD to a 16-week aerobic exercise program, to treatment with sertraline, or to a combination of the two (Blumenthal *et al.*, 1999). Decreases in depressive symptom scores were similarly large in the three groups. On follow-up 6 months later, though, the two groups assigned to exercise had significantly lower recurrence rates than the group that had been assigned to sertraline alone (Babyak *et al.*, 2000). The difference was particularly large for those patients who had continued with regular exercise in the interval.

A recent controlled trial tested the biophilia hypothesis, that good health is maintained only by a positive relationship with the natural environment, by comparing the treatment of depression by swimming with dolphins with a control group having time-equivalent water-based therapy only. The results showed significantly greater benefit in the dolphin-assisted therapy group (Antonioli & Reveley, 2005). Exercise levels were roughly similar in both groups.

Estrogen replacement in perimenopausal depression

A meta-analysis of the extensive literature on hormone replacement treatment and mood symptoms concluded that estrogen replacement benefits mood symptoms in mixed samples of perimenopausal and postmenopausal women (Zweifel & O'Brien, 1997). Results varied considerably across studies and drug–placebo differences were not significant for the 12 samples consisting entirely of postmenopausal women. There are now at least three placebo-controlled, parallel-design studies of estrogen replacement for women with depressive symptoms in the perimenopausal period and all showed robust differences between those given replacement treatment and those given placebo (Montgomery *et al.*, 1987; Schmidt

et al., 2000; Soares *et al.*, 2001). The results leave quite unclear the ideal hormonal dose or delivery, or the duration of an adequate trial. In one study, improvement after 6 weeks was no greater than improvement after three weeks (Schmidt *et al.*, 2000). In another, differences between estrogen replacement and placebo increased throughout the 12-week trial (Soares *et al.*, 2001). The benefits of estrogen replacement persisted after a 4-week washout in one report (Soares *et al.*, 2001) but neither of the other two studies tested for the persistence of benefit.

Androgens

The previously mentioned meta-analysis of hormone replacement therapy in mixed samples also found that androgen replacement, with or without estrogen, was associated with substantially more improvement in mood symptoms than hormone replacement therapy with estrogen alone (Zweifel & O'Brien, 1997). This has implications for the management of postmenopausal women who experience persistent depressive symptoms despite estrogen-only HRT.

Numerous reports have demonstrated an association between depressive disorders in males and low testosterone concentrations (Margolese, 2000) and the relationship appears to be particularly robust for free testosterone concentrations (Barrett-Connor *et al.*, 1999). This has led to trials of testosterone replacement as a treatment of depression in men.

In perhaps the earliest placebo-controlled study depressed men who received the synthetic androgen, mesterolone, for 6 weeks had outcomes similar to those who received placebo. The participants had a mean age of 43 and baseline testosterone concentrations were not assessed. Another more recent trial required a baseline testosterone concentration of 350 ng/ml or less and used weekly intramuscular injections of 200 mg testosterone for active treatment (Seidman *et al.*, 2001), but again, improvement with androgen treatment resembled that for treatment with placebo. In contrast to these two trials was one that used placebo or 10 g of testosterone gel applied daily for 8 weeks in a sample of men who had failed to improve with an SSRI trial and who had testosterone concentrations less than 300 ng/dl. Response was significantly more likely with testosterone treatment. The difference in depression scores between testosterone and placebo increased throughout the 8-week trial and responses were limited to those whose testosterone concentrations increased by more than 200 ng/dl.

Another administered 400 mg testosterone or placebo in bi-weekly intramuscular injections to HIV positive men with low baseline testosterone concentrations and clinical evidence of 'hypogonadal mood symptoms' (Rabkin et al., 2000). Among the 26 with an Axis-I mood disorder at baseline, those who received testosterone were four times (58% vs. 14%) more likely to be much, or very much, improved than were those given placebo. Yet another trial randomized HIV positive men who had had clinical signs of hypogonadism and who had responded to a 12-week open trial of the same testosterone regime to either continue with testosterone or to receive placebo injections instead, for an additional 6-week trial (Rabkin et al., 2000). Nine in ten of those switched to placebo lost their responses compared to only two of ten of those maintained on testosterone.

In summary, three placebo-controlled trials found that testosterone supplementation benefited depressed men; two did not. Of the two negative studies, one did not confine inclusion to hypogonadal men and both described high placebo response rates. In contrast, two of the positive acute treatment studies yielded placebo-response rates of zero (Pope et al., 2003) and 14% (Rabkin et al., 2000). The discontinuation study (Rabkin et al., 1999) probably eliminated placebo responders by requiring a sustained and stable response to active treatment in the initial, open phase of the trial (Quitkin et al., 1984).

Hypericum extract (Saint John's wort)

A meta-analysis of fourteen placebo-controlled studies concluded that hypericum extract, or St John's wort, is significantly superior to placebo with a responder-rate ratio of 2.67 (CI = 1.78 – 4.01) (Linde et al., 1996). Nearly all of the samples were composed of fewer than 100 subjects, most of whom were thought to have 'neurotic depression'. Three more recent, multicenter studies described larger samples of 200–300 subjects, all of whom had MDD (Lecrubier et al., 2002; Group HDTS, 2002; Shelton et al., 2001) and results were much less supportive. Of the two that simply compared hypericum to placebo, one found no significant difference in the primary outcome measure (Shelton et al., 2001). The other did find differences, but the hypericum and placebo groups had ITT changes in HRS scores that differed by less than 2 points (−9.9 and −8.1, respectively) (Lecrubier et al., 2002). The third study included a group assigned to sertraline and found that neither hypericum nor sertraline

resulted in better outcomes than placebo on the primary measure.

The literature thus does not yet permit a firm conclusion on the efficacy of hypericum in depressive disorders. The earlier, more positive, studies have been faulted because of small sample sizes, non-standardized outcome measures, and diagnostically mixed patient samples. Such shortcomings would tend toward false-negative results rather than the falsely positively ones, however. A bias against the publication of negative studies, the 'file drawer effect', may have been in play but there is little reason to believe that this effect has not played an equal or greater role in shaping the literature on SSRIs and other conventional antidepressants. Moreover, the failure of the Hypericum Depression Trial Study Group to show differences in outcome between placebo and either hypericum or sertraline suggests that the larger, more recent trials may have been affected by the substantial and steady increase in placebo response rates noted in antidepressant trials over the past 20 years (Walsh et al., 2002). Indeed, 32% of FDA registered trials done from 1985 through 1997 failed to find significant outcome differences between established antidepressants and placebo (Khan et al., 2002).

Whether or not a clinician recommends St John's Wort to his patients, he or she should at least inquire whether they are taking it, or plan to do so. Because of its effects on cytokine p450 enzymes and on serotonin reuptake hypericum it can lower blood levels of certain medications and can result in a serotonin syndrome when combined with others (Izzo, 2004).

Conclusions

There are many different alternative treatments for depression and, on the surface, all or almost all look to have some merit. Light therapy, exercise therapy and even sleep deprivation (at least in the short-term), all seem to have some effectiveness, and compounds such as St John's Wort (in mild depression) and omega-3 essential fatty acids also seem to be able to improve some depressions. What we do not know is how these treatments stand up to rigorous methodologically sound studies and how they can augment existing treatment. More work needs to be done, but many of the alternative treatments are not as alternative as they may first seem.

The level of evidence for each of the interventions discussed in this chapter is summarized in Table 30.2.

Table 30.2. Effectiveness of alternative treatments (excluding dietary supplements) for mood disorders

Treatment	Form of treatment	Psychiatric disorder	Level of evidence for efficacy	Comments
Light therapy alone	2500 lux for 2 h to 10 000 lux for 30 min	Depression (mainly seasonal affective disorder)	Ib	Undoubtedly effective as an antidepressant treatment
Light therapy with antidepressant drugs	As above with antidepressants in conventional dosage	Depression (mainly seasonal affective disorder)	Ib	Undoubtedly effective and may be of greater superiority to antidepressants in this group
Sleep deprivation	Total sleep deprivation for 36 hours or partial sleep deprivation for 5 hours	Depression	IIa	Antidepressant effect short-lived
Sleep deprivation with mood stabilizers (lithium)	As above	Bipolar I	Ib	Effective but more information needed on persistence of benefit
Omega 3 free fatty acids	Compounds containing docoshexaenoic acid (DCA) and eicosapentaenoic acid (EPA)	Depression	Ia	Clearly effective in depression and may be effective in bipolar depression. EPA may be the more effective preparations
Sleep deprivation with antidepressant drugs	As above with conventional doses of drugs	Depression	Ib	Effects short-lived and after 3 weeks no difference between groups
Exercise therapy	Variable periods of mainly aerobic exercise (3–12 weeks) often with maintenance exercise	Depression	Ib	Undoubted efficacy with equivalent benefit to antidepressant drugs (boosted by dolphin assistance)
Estrogen replacement	3–12 weeks	Perimenopausal and postmenopausal women with depression	Ia	Limited evidence of efficacy with any benefits mainly in perimenopausal group (with possible gains from added androgens)
Testosterone and related compounds (e.g. mesterolone)	6–10 weeks	Depression	IIa	Very mixed results with no clear benefit
St John's Wort (Hypericum extract)	4–12 weeks	Depression	Ia	Early evidence of benefit thrown into doubt by recent larger studies (see also Chapter 7)

REFERENCES

Antonioli, C. & Reveley, M. A. (2005). Randomised controlled trial of animal facilitated therapy with dolphins in the treatment of depression. *British Medical Journal*, **331**, 1231.

Avery, D., Bolte, M. A. & Millet, M. (1992). Bright dawn simulation compared with bright morning light in the treatment of winter depression. *Acta Psychiatrica Scandinavica*, **85**(6), 430–4.

Avery, D. H., Eder, D. N., Bolte, M. A. *et al.* (2001). Dawn simulation and bright light in the treatment of SAD: a controlled study. *Biological Psychiatry*, **50**(3), 205–16.

Babyak, M., Blumenthal, J. A., Herman, S. *et al.* (2000). Exercise treatment for major depression: maintenance of therapeutic benefit at 10 months. *Psychosomatic Medicine*, **62**(5), 633–8.

Barbini, B., Colombo, C., Benedetti, F., Campori, E., Bellodi, L. & Smeraldi, E. (1998). The unipolar–bipolar dichotomy and the response to sleep deprivation. *Psychiatry Research*, **79**(1), 43–50.

Barrett-Connor, E., Von Muhlen, D. G. & Kritz-Silverstein, D. (1999). Bioavailable testosterone and depressed mood in older men: the Rancho Bernardo Study. *Journal of Clinical Endocrinology and Metabolism*, **84**(2), 573–7.

Baxter, L. R., Jr, Liston, E. H., Schwartz, J. M. *et al.* (1986). Prolongation of the antidepressant response to partial sleep deprivation by lithium. *Psychiatry Research*, **19**(1), 17–23.

Beauchemin, K. M. & Hays, P. (1997). Phototherapy is a useful adjunct in the treatment of depressed in-patients. *Acta Psychiatrica Scandinavica*, **95**(5), 424–7.

Benedetti, F., Barbini, B., Lucca, A., Campori, E., Colombo, C. & Smeraldi, E. (1997). Sleep deprivation hastens the antidepressant action of fluoxetine. *European Archives of Psychiatry and Clinical Neuroscience*, **247**(2), 100–3.

Benedetti, F., Colombo, C., Barbini, B., Campori, E. & Smeraldi, E. (1999). Ongoing lithium treatment prevents relapse after total sleep deprivation. *Journal of Clinical Psychopharmacology*, **19**(3), 240–5.

Benedetti, F., Colombo, C., Barbini, B., Campori, E. & Smeraldi, E. (2001). Morning sunlight reduces length of hospitalization in bipolar depression. *Journal of Affective Disorders*, **62**(3), 221–3.

Benedetti, F., Colombo, C., Pontiggia, A., Bernasconi, A., Florita, M. & Smeraldi, E. (2003). Morning light treatment hastens the antidepressant effect of citalopram: a placebo-controlled trial. *Journal of Clinical Psychiatry*, **64**(6), 648–53.

Blumenthal, J. A., Babyak, M. A., Moore, K. A. *et al.* (1999). Effects of exercise training on older patients with major depression. *Archives of Internal Medicine*, **159**(19), 2349–56.

Brown, A. J., Pang, E. & Roberts, D. C. R. (1991). Persistent changes in the fatty acid composition of erythrocyte membranes after moderate intake of *n*-3 polyunsaturated fatty acids: study design implications. *American Journal of Clinical Nutrition*, **54**, 668–73.

Colombo, C., Lucca, A., Benedetti, F., Barbini, B., Campori, E. & Smeraldi, E. (2000). Total sleep deprivation combined with lithium and light therapy in the treatment of bipolar depression: replication of main effects and interaction. *Psychiatry Research*, **95**(1), 43–53.

Deltito, J. A., Moline, M., Pollak, C., Martin, L. Y. & Maremmani, I. (1991). Effects of phototherapy on non-seasonal unipolar and bipolar depressive spectrum disorders. *Journal of Affective Disorders*, **23**(4), 231–7.

Edwards, R., Peete, M., Shay, J. & Horrobin, D. F. (1998). Omega-3 polyunsaturated fatty acid levels in the diet and in red blood cell membranes of depressed patients. *Journal of Affective Disorders*, **48**, 149–55.

Elsenga, S. & van den Hoofdakker, R. H. (1982). Clinical effects of sleep deprivation and clomipramine in endogenous depression. *Journal of Psychiatry Research*, **17**(4), 361–74.

Frangou, S., Lewis, M. & McCrone, P. (2006). Efficacy of ethyl-eicosapentaenoic acid in bipolar depression: randomised, double-blind, placebo-controlled study. *British Journal of Psychiatry*, **188**, 46–50.

Frasure-Smith, N., Lesperance, F. & Julien, P. (2004). Major depression is associated with lower omega-3 fatty acid levels in patients with recent acute coronary syndromes. *Biological Psychiatry*, **55**(9), 891–6.

Group HDTS (2002). Effect of *Hypericum perforatum* (St John's wort) in major depressive disorder: a randomized controlled trial. *Journal of the American Medical Association*, **287**(14), 1807–14.

Grube, M. & Hartwich, P. (1990). Maintenance of antidepressant effect of sleep deprivation with the help of lithium. *European Archives in Psychiatry and Clinical Neuroscience*, **240**(1), 60–1.

Izzo, A. A. (2004). Drug interactions with St. John's wort (*Hypericum perforatum*): a review of the clinical evidence. *International Journal of Clinical Pharmacology Therapy*, **42**, 139–48.

Hansen, V., Lund, E. & Smith-Sivertsen, T. (1998). Self-reported mental distress under the shifting daylight in the high north. *Psychological Medicine*, **28**, 447–52.

Hibbeln, J. R. (1998). Fish consumption and major depression. *Lancet*, **351**(9110), 1213.

Hibbeln, J. R. (2002). Seafood consumption, the DHA content of mother's milk and prevalence rates of post-partum depression. A cross-national, ecological analysis. *Journal of Affective Disorders*, **69**, 15–29.

Khan, A., Leventhal, R. M., Khan, S. R. & Brown, W. A. (2002). Severity of depression and response to antidepressants and placebo: Analysis of the Food and Drug Administration database. *Journal of Clinical Psychopharmacology*, **22**, 40–5.

Kripke, D. F. (1998). Light treatment for nonseasonal depression: speed, efficacy, and combined treatment. *Journal of Affective Disorders*, **49**(2), 109–17.

Kripke, D. F., Mullaney, D. J., Klauber, M. R., Risch, S. C. & Gillin, J. C. (1992). Controlled trial of bright light for nonseasonal major depressive disorders. *Biological Psychiatry*, **31**(2), 119–34.

Lam, R. W., Carter, D., Misri, S., Kuan, A. J., Yatham, L. N. & Zis, A. P. (1999). A controlled study of light therapy in women with late luteal phase dysphoric disorder. *Psychiatry Research*, **86**(3), 185–92.

Lecrubier, Y., Clerc, G., Didi, R. & Kieser, M. (2002). Efficacy of St. John's wort extract WS 5570 in major depression: a double-blind, placebo-controlled trial. *American Journal of Psychiatry*, **159**(8), 1361–6.

Linde, K., Ramirez, G., Mulrow, C. D., Pauls, A., Weidenhammer, W. & Melchart, D. (1996). St John's wort for depression – an overview and meta-analysis of randomised clinical trials. *British Medical Journal*, **313**(7052), 253–8.

Loosen, P. T., Merkel, U. & Amelung, U. (1976). [Combined sleep deprivation/chlorimipramine therapy of endogenous depression (author's transl)]. *Arzneimittelforschung*, **26**(6), 1177–8.

Mackert, A., Volz, H. P., Stieglitz, R. D. & Muller-Oerlinghausen, B. (1991). Phototherapy in nonseasonal depression. *Biological Psychiatry*, **30**(3), 257–68.

Maes, M., Smith, R., Christophe, A., Cosyns, P., Desnyder, R. & Meltzer, H. Y. (1996). Fatty acid composition in major depression: decreased omega-3 fractions in cholesteryl esters and increased C-20: 4 omega-six/C-20:5 omega-3 ratio in cholesteryl esters and phospholipids. *Journal of Affective Disorders*, **38**, 35–46.

Maes, M., Christophe, A., Delanghe, J., Altemura, C., Neels, H. & Meltzer, H. Y. (1999). Lowered omega-3 polyunsaturated fatty acids in serum phospholipids and cholesteryl esters of depressed patients. *Psychiatry Research*, **85**, 275–91.

Mamalakis, G., Tornaritis, M. & Kafatos, A. (2002). Depression and adipose essential polyunsaturated fatty acids. *Prostaglandins, Leukotrienes and Essential Fatty Acids*, **67**(5), 311–18.

Margolese, H. C. (2000). The male menopause and mood: testosterone decline and depression in the aging male – is there a link? *Journal of Geriatric Psychiatry and Neurology*, **13**(2), 93–101.

Martinsen, E. W., Medhus, A. & Sandvik, L. (1985). Effects of aerobic exercise on depression: a controlled study. *British Medical Journal (Clinical Research Education)*, **291**(6488), 109.

Mather, A. S., Rodriguez, C., Guthrie, M. F., McHarg, A. M., Reid, I. C. & McMurdo, M. E. (2002). Effects of exercise on depressive symptoms in older adults with poorly responsive depressive disorder: randomised controlled trial. *British Journal of Psychiatry*, **180**, 411–15.

Montgomery, J. C., Appleby, L., Brincat, M. *et al.* (1987). Effect of oestrogen and testosterone implants on psychological disorders in the climacteric. *Lancet*, **1**(8528), 297–9.

Nathan, P. J., Burrows, G. D. & Norman, T. R. (1999). Melatonin sensitivity to dim white light in affective disorders. *Neuropsychopharmacology*, **21**(3), 408–13.

Neumeister, A., Goessler, R., Lucht, M., Kapitany, T., Bamas, C. & Kasper, S. (1996). Bright light therapy stabilizes the antidepressant effect of partial sleep deprivation. *Biological Psychiatry*, **39**(1), 16–21.

Noaghiul, S. & Hibbeln, J. R. (2003). Cross-national comparisons of seafood consumption and rates of bipolar disorders. *American Journal of Psychiatry*, **160**(12), 2222–7.

Peet, M., Murphy, B., Shay, J. & Horrobin, D. (1998). Depletion of omega-3 fatty acid levels in red blood cell membranes of depressive patients. *Biological Psychiatry*, **43**, 315–19.

Penninx, B. W., Rejeski, W. J., Pandya, J. *et al.* (2002). Exercise and depressive symptoms: a comparison of aerobic and resistance exercise effects on emotional and physical function in older persons with high and low depressive symptomatology. *Journal of Gerontology: B. Psychological Science and Social Science*, **57**(2), P124–32.

Pope, H. G., Cohane, G. H., Kanayama, G., Siegel, A. J. & Hudson, J. I. (2003). Testosterone gel supplementation for men with refractory depression: A randomized, placebo-control trial. *American Journal of Psychiatry*, **160**, 105–11.

Quitkin, F. M., Rabkin, J. G., Ross, D. & Stewart, J. W. (1984). Identification of true drug response to antidepressants. *Use of pattern analysis. Archives of General Psychiatry*, **41**(8), 782–6.

Rabkin, J. G., Wagner, G. J. & Rabkin, R. (1999). Testosterone therapy for human immunodeficiency virus-positive men with and without hypogonadism. *Journal of Clinical Psychopharmacology*, **19**(1), 19–27.

Rabkin, J. G., Wagner, G. J. & Rabkin, R. (2000). A double-blind, placebo-controlled trial of testosterone therapy for HIV-positive men with hypogonadal symptoms. *Archives of General Psychiatry*, **57**(2), 141–7; discussion 155–6.

Rosenthal, N. E., Sack, D. A., Gillin, J. C. *et al.* (1984). Seasonal affective disorder. A description of the syndrome and preliminary findings with light therapy. *Archives of General Psychiatry*, **41**(1), 72–80.

Schwartz, P. J., Brown, C., Wehr, T. A. & Rosenthal, N. E. (1996). Winter seasonal affective disorder: a follow-up study of the first 59 patients of the National Institute of Mental Health Seasonal Studies Program. *American Journal of Psychiatry*, **153**(8), 1028–36.

Schmidt, P. J., Nieman, L., Danaceau, M. A. *et al.* (2000). Estrogen replacement in perimenopause-related depression: a preliminary report. *American Journal of Obstetrics & Gynecology*, **183**(2), 414–20.

Seidman, S. N., Spatz, E., Rizzo, C. & Roose, S. P. (2001). Testosterone replacement therapy for hypogonadal men with major depressive disorder: a randomized, placebo-controlled clinical trial. *Journal of Clinical Psychiatry*, **62**(6), 406–12.

Shelton, R. C., Keller, M. B., Gelenberg, A. *et al.* (2001). Effectiveness of St John's wort in major depression: a randomized controlled trial. *Journal of the American Medical Association*, **285**(15), 1978–86.

Singh, N. A., Clements, K. M. & Singh, M. A. (2001). The efficacy of exercise as a long-term antidepressant in elderly subjects: a randomized, controlled trial. *Journal of Gerontology: A. Biological Science and Medical Science*, **56**(8), M497–504.

Soares, C. N., Almeida, O. P., Joffe, H. & Cohen, L. S. (2001). Efficacy of estradiol for the treatment of depressive disorders in perimenopausal women: a double-blind, randomized, placebo-controlled trial. *Archives of General Psychiatry*, **58**(6), 529–34.

Tanskanen, A., Hibbeln, J. R., Tuomilehto, J. *et al.* (2001). Fish consumption and depressive symptoms in the general population in Finland. *Psychiatric Services*, **52**(4), 529–31.

Terman, M., Terman, J. S., Quitkin, F. M., McGrath, P. J., Stewart, J. W. & Rafferty, B. (1989). Light therapy for seasonal affective disorder. A review of efficacy. *Neuropsychopharmacology*, **2**(1), 1–22.

Terman, M., Amira, L., Terman, J. S. & Ross, D. C. (1996). Predictors of response and nonresponse to light treatment for winter depression. *American Journal of Psychiatry*, **153**(11), 1423–9.

Terman, J. S., Terman, M., Lo, E. S. & Cooper, T. B. (2001). Circadian time of morning light administration and therapeutic response in winter depression. *Archives of General Psychiatry*, **58**(1), 69–75.

Walsh, B. T., Seidman, S. N., Sysko, R. & Gould, M. (2002). Placebo response in studies of major depression: variable, substantial, and growing. *Journal of the American Medical Association*, **287**(14), 1840–7.

Yamda, N., Martin-Ivrson, M. T., Daimon, K., Tsujimoto, T. & Takashashi, S. (1995). Clinical and chronobiological affects of light therapy on non-seasonal affective disorders. *Biological Psychiatry*, **37**, 866–73.

Zweifel, J. E. & O'Brien, W. H. (1997). A meta-analysis of the effect of hormone replacement therapy upon depressed mood. *Psychoneuroendocrinology*, **22**(3), 189–212.

Anxiety and neurotic disorders

Section editors

Peter Tyrer and Randall D. Marshall

31

Treatment of generalised anxiety and somatoform disorders

Peter Tyrer and David Baldwin

Editor's note

This subject, as indicated in the first section of this book, is a somewhat controversial one as generalised anxiety disorder has only recently achieved a level of diagnostic acceptability in the medical profession. The doubts have been expressed particularly in primary care where most of these disorders are treated. What is undoubtedly true is that generalised anxiety however, it is formulated in diagnostic terms, is extremely common and the syndrome is probably the most common seen in clinical practice. It is closely accompanied by somatoform disorders in terms of frequency so these two disorders cover most of mental illness. Common diseases usually offer hundreds of remedies and these two disorders do not disappoint this expectation. The account below indicates a good degree of consensus over general strategies of management, but the detail is all important and it is likely that a set of combined treatments at different times will be needed for these common and persistent conditions.

Generalised anxiety disorder is a persistent, common and pervasive condition of unfocused worry and anxiety, twice as common in women than men, that is not restricted to a particular setting or event, although changes in circumstances may aggravate the symptoms. Like all anxiety disorders (see Part I) it has both psychological (restlessness, irritability, sleep disturbance, feelings of threat and nervous tension) and somatic or bodily feelings (palpitations, difficulty in breathing, dizziness, nausea, dry mouth and sweating), the latter being recognised as part of the anxiety syndrome in generalised anxiety disorder but independent in the case of the somatoform disorders. Both these conditions overlap considerably with other common mental disorders (you will notice from Part I that the diagnosis has a low clinical utility score), and it is possible to regard the conditions as more like diatheses

for mood and related disorders than completely separate conditions. The course of most generalised anxiety and somatoform disorders is a relapsing one, and intervening successfully to effect a complete resolution of symptoms is uncommon, but in the short and medium term, effective treatments include psychological therapies, primarily cognitive-behavioural therapy (CBT); self-help approaches based on CBT principles; and drug treatments, principally selective serotonin reuptake inhibitors (SSRIs).

Assessment

All forms of anxiety are relatively easy to identify in clinical practice but it is a much more difficult task to disentangle primary from secondary symptoms, which in the case of somatoform disorders are inverted, so that patients invariably claim that their anxiety is a consequence, not a cause of their physical symptoms. This represents a major hurdle in treatment as the attributions of the patients are, at least at first, completely different from those of the therapists (Tyrer, 1973).

In addition to this general policy of clinical management there is some scope for screening patients for primary anxiety or somatoform disorders. Although in general psychiatric practice the clinician can normally be relied upon to make adequate assessments, in other settings, particularly general or specialised medical clinics where the main focus of treatment and assessment is on physical symptoms, such screening measures may be helpful. One of the most widely used scales is the Hospital Anxiety and Depression Scale, which includes anxiety and depression sub-scales (7 items each), is both sensitive and specific in identifying pathological anxiety (Zigmond & Snaith, 1983), and uses symptoms that are not scored positively by those who have physical symptoms related to other medical conditions.

Cambridge Textbook of Effective Treatments in Psychiatry, ed. Peter Tyrer and Kenneth R. Silk. Published by Cambridge University Press.
© Cambridge University Press, 2008.

Table 31.1. Diagnosis of generalisation anxiety disorder

Feature	ICD-10	DSM-IV-TR™
Duration of symptoms	At least 6 months	At least 6 months
Main symptom	Prominent tension, worry and feelings of apprehension about everyday events and problems	Excessive anxiety and worry (apprehensive expectation) about a number of events or activities
Additional major feature		The person finds it difficult to control the worry
Specific symptoms (minimum requirement)	At least four, including one from autonomic arousal list	At least three
	Autonomic arousal: palpitations, sweating, trembling, dry mouth	No equivalent
	Chest and abdomen: difficulty in breathing, feeling of choking, chest pain, nausea	No equivalent
	Mental state symptoms: feeling dizzy, feelings of unreality (depersonalisation and derealisation), fear of losing control, fear of dying	Difficulty in concentration or mind going blank
	General symptoms: hot flushes or cold chills, numbness or tingling, muscle tension or aches and pains, restlessness and inability to relax, feeling keyed up (mentally tense), sensation of lump in throat (difficulty in swallowing)	Restlessness or feeling keyed up or on edge, being easily fatigued, irritability, muscle tension
	No equivalent	Sleep disturbance (difficulty falling or staying asleep, or restless unsatisfying sleep)
Exclusion criteria related to overlapping symptoms	Does not meet the criteria for panic disorder, phobic anxiety disorders, obsessive-compulsive disorder, or hypochondriacal disorder	Focus of worry not confined to features of an associated (Axis I) disorder, such as panic disorder, social phobia, obsessive-compulsive disorder, separation anxiety disorder, anorexia nervosa, somatisation disorder or post-traumatic stress disorder
Other exclusion criteria	Symptoms not due to a physical disorder such as hyperthyroidism, an organic mental disorder, or substance-related disorder (e.g. benzodiazepine withdrawal)	Disturbance not due to direct physiological effects of a substance or medication, or to a general medical condition (e.g. hyperthyroidism), or exclusively during a mood disorder, psychotic or pervasive developmental disorder
Social functioning	Not included	Clinically significant distress or impairment in social, occupational or other important areas of functioning

It is therefore particularly useful in identifying pathological anxiety and depression in medical patients and is now recommended as a valuable screen for this purpose (Bambauer *et al.*, 2005). A score of 8 of more on either of the sub-scales indicates likely pathological anxiety or depression (or both) (Bjelland *et al.*, 2002). The best-known instrument for assessing severity in research practice is the Hamilton Rating Scale for Anxiety (Hamilton, 1959) but this may include too many physical symptoms, is cumbersome to use, and alternatives are becoming more widely employed; some of these are more specific to generalised anxiety disorder (Meyer *et al.*, 1990; Newman *et al.*, 2002).

Somatoform disorders constitute one of the most unsatisfactory groups of disorders in psychiatry with regard to both diagnosis and treatment but the scheme outlined in Table 31.1, whilst not universally accepted, is a useful pragmatic guide. There are no simple screening measures for conversion disorder or dissociative states, as this is one area where clinical acumen is particularly important. Somatisation is an area where current attempts to screen are very difficult. Scales such as the Illness Behaviour Questionnaire (IBQ) (Pilowsky, 1969) can discriminate between individuals who somatise and those who do not, but this appears to be highly correlated with general neuroticism (Zonderman *et al.*, 1985). More and more these conditions are recognised to be anxiety-related and the diagnosis of hypochondriasis is now often replaced by the less pejorative term 'health anxiety'. Whilst anxiety is not a universal requirement – the delusions of bodily absence in Cotard's syndrome being an example where depression over-rides all other symptoms dramatically – in most of those with non-psychotic disorders who suffer from hypochondriasis, anxiety is a prominent symptom. The Health Anxiety Inventory (HAI) (Salkovskis *et al.*, 2002) is a useful self-rated questionnaire that when scored at 18 or above is likely to indicate a hypochondriacal syndrome of either transient or persistent nature with a duration of at least 6 months. Medically unexplained physical symptoms are the most amorphous of all the somatoform disorders, but may have one of the best prospects of rapid successful treatment. An assessment instrument, the Schedule for Evaluating Persistent Symptoms (SEPS) (Seivewright & Tyrer, 2005), is currently being evaluated and it is probably too early for this to be recommended. Scales of this nature can only be a guide to assessment and they should not be regarded as diagnostic instruments.

Theoretical models of treatment of anxiety and somatoform disorders

As with most treatments in psychiatry, pharmacological and psychological treatments vie with each other for supremacy in anxiety disorders and both have sound backing from theory and evidence. Most sedative drugs (i.e. those that are prescribed for anxiety and have an immediate or rapid onset of action) are facilitators of gamma-amino butyric acid (GABA), which is the most powerful inhibitory neurotransmitter within the nervous system. So it is to be expected that GABA-facilitating drugs such as alcohol, barbiturates, chloral derivatives, cyclo-pyrrolones (e.g. zopiclone), and benzodiazepines should all be effective in reducing anxiety. Unfortunately, the negative consequences of prolonged or excessive GABA enhancement include depression of brain stem centres that can lead to cardiac and respiratory failure after overdose, and the phenomenon of tolerance which is a common problem with some of these drugs, itself leading to dependence and withdrawal problems (see Chapter 18).

Benzodiazepines and cyclopyrrolones represent an advance over earlier drugs and this is illustrated by the existence of the GABA-benzodiazepine receptor complex. In 1977 it was found that benzodiazepines interacted with a specific binding site, which suggested a natural substance (endogenous ligand) linked to benzodiazepines must be present in the brain. The $GABA_A$ receptor complex allows drugs to act more selectively if they can bind preferentially with the benzodiazepine binding site, and both benzodiazepines and cyclopyrrolones are able to do this.

The azaspirodecanediones, of which the best known is buspirone, act quite differently as partial agonists of $5\text{-}HT_{1A}$ receptors, but as yet these drugs have yet to achieve widespread use. They are not associated with euphoriant effects and have little propensity to tolerance or dependence, so they can be withdrawn without major adverse effects (Rickels *et al.*, 1988; Murphy *et al.*, 1989).

Psychological treatments for anxiety have developed from psychodynamic, cognitive and learning theory. Anxiety was recognised by Freud as one of the most important problems to be overcome in psychoanalysis and was postulated to be at the core of psychiatric pathology (Freud, 1926). Cognitive theory has emphasised the distortions in thinking that tend to reinforce pathological anxiety (Beck, 1976) and this approach has generally been of more value than simple behavioural ones in generalised anxiety disorder, as there is no specific connection with symptoms and setting unlike phobic disorders. The underlying mechanisms of somatoform disorders remain uncertain but there are theoretical justifications for both drug and psychological treatments in these conditions (Lipowski, 1988).

General principles of treatment

Most anxiety and somatoform disorders are seen and managed in primary care. This is therefore the best setting to treat people who suffer from these often long-term disorders. Epidemiological studies suggest a large proportion of the 7% of the general population with anxiety disorders remain untreated (Regier *et al.*, 1990). There is general agreement that this represents a failure of services, but provided that people are given adequate assessment (clearly not the case at present), there is no reason why people should necessarily start or persist with treatments which are not ideal. The growth of self-help and internet treatments probably means that many may obtain help without going to more traditional health services. Despite most treatment being delivered in primary care, there has long been concern that the necessary time and services for all treatments are not readily available in such settings (Deans & Skinner, 1992). Psychological therapies are generally considered to be preferable to drug treatments (and may be preferred as treatments in the case of depressive disorders (Paykel & Priest, 1992)), but frequently they cannot be given because of limited resources. For the immediate future it is likely that, in most Western countries, drug treatment will be the most commonly given treatment, but in the UK there is currently a major thrust towards developing cognitive-behavioural therapy across the health service for all (Layard, 2006).

Drug treatment of generalised anxiety disorder (GAD)

Acute treatment

This has the longest history of good evaluation and there have been many systematic reviews of randomised placebo-controlled trials in generalised anxiety disorder since 1980. Many important treatment studies were carried out before 1980 into 'anxiety neurosis' and similar disorders but cannot be included in such reviews as they do not satisfy the right diagnostic criteria. The efficacy of these drugs is summarised in Table 31.2. It will immediately be clear from other chapters in this section that the recommendations are similar to those for other disorders. Despite initial claims (sometimes called 'pharmacological dissection') that panic disorder was a specific indication for antidepressant therapy and that generalised anxiety disorder was not responsive (Klein, 1964, 1967), there is now clear evidence that antidepressants are effective treatments in both GAD and in the closely related panic disorder. This was first demonstrated by Kahn et al. (1986) with imipramine, and similar benefit has been shown with other tricyclic antidepressants (Casacalenda & Boulenger, 1998) (although, as most of these were introduced long before the diagnosis of generalised anxiety disorder, they are now seldom included within randomised controlled trials).

Tricyclic antidepressants

As noted in Chapter 27 potential adverse effects of tricyclic antidepressants, such as sedation, may represent an advantage in the treatment of anxiety. However, tricyclic antidepressants in general are not regarded as first-line treatments for generalised anxiety. Although this is good general advice, it may not always be so for particular patients, and in a patient who is agitated, underweight and has gastrointestinal symptoms associated with anxiety, a tricyclic antidepressant may be the best treatment, at least initially. One of the major concerns over tricyclic antidepressants is that of their toxicity in overdose (Nutt, 2005), but this is somewhat less of a risk in anxiety disorders and the two agents, lofepramine and clomipramine, are unlikely to have fatal consequences if taken in overdose alone. However, the most sedative antidepressants (trimipramine and amitriptyline), and dosulepin (dothiepin) are toxic in overdose and need to be avoided in patients at risk of self-harm.

Selective serotonin reuptake inhibitors (SSRIs)

This class of drugs, commonly abbreviated to its acronym (SSRI), includes citalopram and its enantiomer escitalopram, paroxetine, sertraline, fluoxetine, and fluvoxamine, although only escitalopram and paroxetine are licensed for the treatment of generalised anxiety disorder (see individual drugs in Appendix). Treatment effects, as with tricyclic antidepressants, are delayed but as the therapeutic doses of the drugs are easier to achieve with SSRIs more patients prescribed these drugs, particularly in primary care where most anxiety is treated, are likely to complete a therapeutic course (Lawrenson et al., 2000). The SSRIs have a range of potentially troublesome adverse effects, including initial increased nervousness, insomnia, and nausea (NICE, 2004) and sexual dysfunction (Baldwin, 2004). There is a small but important risk of increasing suicidal behaviour, particularly in younger people (Whittington et al., 2004; Dubicka et al., 2006). When stopped abruptly, most SSRIs can produce a discontinuation syndrome characterised by mood disturbance, dizziness, insomnia and flu-like symptoms (Schatzberg et al., 2006).

Other effective treatments include the serotonin–noradrenaline reuptake inhibitors (SNRIs) venlafaxine and duloxetine, some benzodiazepines (alprazolam, diazepam), the tricyclic imipramine, the 5-HT$_{1A}$ partial agonist buspirone, the antipsychotic trifluoperazine, the antihistamine hydroxyzine, and the anticonvulsant pregabalin (Ballenger et al., 2001; Baldwin et al., 2004, 2005, 2006). Most treatments are of similar efficacy: differences have been shown in occasional treatment studies, but these could be explained in terms of dosage and, when meta-analyses of many studies are compared, these differences diminish.

Benzodiazepines and cyclopyrrolones

Benzodiazepines can be effective within 15–60 minutes of administration, whereas buspirone takes up to 72 hours to act and is often preceded by mild dysphoria (Tyrer & Owen, 1984; Chessick et al., 2006). Antidepressants typically take up to 4 weeks to demonstrate efficacy but significant improvement may be noted after 2 weeks and it has been claimed the conventional wisdom is wrong (Mitchell, 2006). However, benzodiazepines are associated with risk of dependence after long-term usage (Tyrer et al., 1983; Rickels et al., 1988) and, although there may sometimes be withdrawal problems ('discontinuation symptoms') with antidepressants (Haddad, 1997), they are less likely to lead to persistent consumption than benzodiazepines. Because of this, the general guidance is to give benzodiazepines only for short-term treatment up to 4 weeks (Priest & Montgomery, 1988; Ballenger et al., 2001; NICE, 2004; Baldwin et al., 2005). Although this statement is frequently repeated, it is often ignored by many who prescribe in general practice. It is also worth adding that, as both generalised anxiety disorder and somatoform disorders are chronic conditions, it is highly unlikely that less than 4 weeks treatment would be of value. In practice, because both patients and practitioners find benzodiazepines to be of some value, they continue to be prescribed, either regularly or intermittently, over long periods and this applies even when the risks of dependence are known and explained. Short-term regular prescriptions of benzodiazepines are often of limited benefit and if followed by immediate withdrawal this benefit disappears (Tyrer *et al.*, 1988) and so intermittent irregular but long-term use becomes the norm, even when patients are fully aware of the risk of dependence (Holton & Tyrer, 1990).

Compounds such as zolpidem, zopiclone and zaleplon have many similarities to benzodiazepines, but are all prescribed for insomnia rather than anxiety. They too carry a risk of tolerance in continued use, and discontinuation symptoms have been reported.

Antidepressants

Differences between antidepressants, whilst demonstrated to small degrees in individual studies (Baldwin *et al.*, 2006; Bielski *et al.*, 2005), are probably not sufficiently strong to lead to firm conclusions regarding the superiority of one class or individual drug over another. Most consensus guidelines and reviews suggest that tricyclic, SSRI and SNRI classes have similar overall efficacy (Ballenger *et al.*, 2001; Baldwin *et al.*, 2005; NICE, 2004). The choice of treatment is usually determined more by the spectrum of adverse effects than by anxiolytic supremacy. Thus, if insomnia and restlessness are major symptoms it may sometimes be more appropriate to choose a sedative tricyclic drug such as amitriptyline or trimipramine rather than an SSRI or SNRI, as an increase in anxiety and restlessness is not uncommon in the early stages of treatment with these classes. Because the spectrum of adverse effects with SSRIs (nausea, dizziness, anorexia) is generally considered to be less troubling than those of tricyclic antidepressants (dry mouth, sedation, postural hypotension, difficulty in micturition) it is now generally recommended that an SSRI (e.g. escitalopram or paroxetine) is chosen as first-line treatment (NICE, 2005; Baldwin & Polkinghorn, 2005; Baldwin *et al.*, 2005). Escitalopram is certainly efficacious in acute treatment (Goodman *et al.*, 2000) and in the prevention of relapse (Allgulander *et al.*, 2006) and, despite a degree of cynicism regarding its introduction, it seems superior to citalopram in major depression and panic disorder (Stahl *et al.*, 2003), and possibly to paroxetine

generalised anxiety disorder (Baldwin *et al.*, 2006), although these studies require independent replication.

Venlafaxine

The serotonin–noradrenaline reuptake inhibitor (SNRI), venlafaxine, is licensed for generalised anxiety disorder and is undoubtedly effective in short-term studies (Allgulander *et al.*, 2001; Kapczinski *et al.*, 2003; Baldwin *et al.*, 2005). Interestingly, it also appears to be effective at all doses from 37.5 mg to 150 mg daily (Allgulander *et al.*, 2001). It is also effective in older people (Katz *et al.*, 2002). A large systematic review of randomised controlled trials of venlafaxine and comparator antidepressants in major depression indicated there was a higher rate of remission compared with SSRIs (45% vs. 35%)(Thase *et al.*, 2001) and has led to a general notion that venlafaxine is more effective than other antidepressants.

However, previous concerns regarding potential cardiotoxic effects (Drent *et al.*, 2003), discontinuation symptoms after abrupt withdrawal, and potential danger in overdose, led the Committee of Safety of Medicines in the UK (CSM) to recommend that venlafaxine treatment should only be initiated by specialist mental health practitioners, with a requirement for pre-treatment ECG and blood pressure measurement, and avoidance in patients with cardiac disease (CSM, 6th December, 2004, www.mhra.gov.uk). These recommendations were subsequently revised, largely on the basis that venlafaxine tends to be used in patients with more serious or 'resistant' conditions, although the CSM still argues that the risks of venlaxine overdose are greater than those with SSRIs (with 8.5 fatalities per million prescriptions following overdose with venlafaxine, compared with 1.0 per million for the SSRIs [combined] (www.mhra.gov.uk/).

Long-term treatment

Because generalised anxiety disorder is a chronic condition, long-term treatment should be anticipated at the outset and planned accordingly. Most of the evidence of efficacy is derived from acute treatment studies and recommendations beyond 12 weeks are based on rather limited data. The SSRIs escitalopram and paroxetine have both been found efficacious in placebo-controlled relapse-prevention studies (Stocchi *et al.*, 2003; Allgulander *et al.*, 2006). Continued double-blind treatment with venlafaxine offers advantages over continued treatment with placebo, in both the proportion of patients that achieve symptomatic remission, and who avoid relapse (Montgomery *et al.*, 2002a). What is clear is that relapse is frequent after drugs are withdrawn, even after the period normally covered by discontinuation syndromes has passed (Montgomery *et al.*, 2002b). What is also of interest is that, when randomised trials include both treatment and withdrawal components, the effectiveness of placebo increases markedly (Tyrer *et al.*, 1988; Montgomery *et al.*, 2002b). The concern over dependence on benzodiazepines leads to recommendations that these drugs are generally avoided in the long-term (Ballenger *et al.*, 2001; NICE, 2004; Baldwin *et al.*, 2005) but the alternative of continuous antidepressant therapy is currently supported by rather limited evidence.

Buspirone, as a non-addictive anxiolytic drug, has been recommended to be of particular value in the long-term treatment of those who are at risk of problems with other drugs, such as patients with alcohol dependence, but again only limited evidence supports this use (Fawcett *et al.*, 2000). A recent Cochrane review (Chessick *et al.*, 2006) has confirmed its efficacy over placebo, but it appears to be particularly ineffective and disliked by those who have been treated with benzodiazepines previously, and conspicuously unhelpful in those who have benzodiazepine dependence (Ashton *et al.*, 1990).

Second-line drug treatments

Other drugs may also have a place in the treatment of generalised anxiety disorder. Beta-blockers, such as propranolol, account for up to 10% of prescriptions for anxiety symptoms in primary care (Seivewright *et al.*, 1991). Although previous studies carried out before generalised anxiety disorder was delineated suggested some value in patients with marked somatic anxiety symptoms mediated through beta-adrenergic receptors (Granville-Grossman & Turner, 1966; Kellner *et al.*, 1974; Tyrer & Lader, 1974; Tyrer, 1992) beta blockers are of unproven efficacy (Meibach *et al.*, 2001). Propranolol combined with a benzodiazepine may be more effective than a benzodiazepine alone in generalised anxiety disorder (Hallstrom *et al.*, 1981) and this may also assist the subsequent withdrawal of the benzodiazepine (Tyrer *et al.*, 1981).

Monoamine oxidase inhibitors (MAOIs) such as phenelzine may also have a place in the treatment of intractable generalised anxiety disorder but they should never be first-line treatments. They can be highly effective in severe anxiety but potential adverse effects with tyramine-containing foods (cheese, principally) and sympathomimetic drugs has restricted their use and they have not been formally tested in generalised anxiety disorder. However, their clear efficacy in what was termed 'endogenous anxiety' (Sheehan *et al.*, 1980) (which shares some of the properties of Lopez Ibor's 'vital anxiety' (1950)) suggests a role for these drugs in secondary care settings when other treatments have failed. The safer reversible MAOI, moclobemide has proven efficacy in social phobia (Versiani *et al.*, 1992) but does not have the same level of efficacy as the irreversible MAOI phenelzine (Baldwin *et al.*, 2005).

Psychological symptoms of anxiety may respond better to antidepressant drugs than to benzodiazepines, but there have been few comparator-controlled studies, and most reveal no significant differences in efficacy between active compounds (Mitte *et al.*, 2005). Benzodiazepines have only limited efficacy against depressive symptoms, and given the comorbidity of GAD with depression and potential hazards associated with prolonged use of benzodiazepines, antidepressant treatment is preferable to prescription of benzodiazepine anxiolytics in 'cothymia' and other mixed conditions (Ballenger *et al.*, 2001; Baldwin *et al.*, 2005; Mitte *et al.*, 2005). There has been some reaction against the general advice that benzodiazepines should only be prescribed for up to 4 weeks in regular dosage and then tapered off as this can be less efficacious than taking a placebo (Tyrer *et al.*, 1988); it being argued that some patients who respond well to benzodiazepines have chronic disorders for whom continued treatment is desirable and justifiable (Taylor, 1989; Romach *et al.*, 1995), but this remains a minority view.

Although low-doses of antipsychotic drugs have often been used in primary care settings to treat anxiety symptoms, formal evidence of efficacy is limited to a single placebo-controlled study of the conventional agent trifluoperazine: although superior to placebo from the first week, it was poorly tolerated (Mendels *et al.*, 1986). Similarly, the sedative effects of antihistamines have sometimes been used to quell troublesome anxiety symptoms, this strategy being supported by the proven efficacy of hydroxyzine, at least in short-term treatment (Darcis *et al.*, 1995; Llorca *et al.*, 2002).

Despite the plethora of guidelines there is still much confusion over the best way of treating generalised anxiety disorder with drug treatment. What appears to have happened in practice is that patients formerly treated with benzodiazepines alone are now being treated with benzodiazepines and antidepressants, usually SSRIs (Salzman *et al.*, 2001) with the intention, not always achieved, of stopping the benzodiazepine treatment in advance of the antidepressant.

Although it is very important to know about the management of patients who have not responded to first-line treatment, the evidence here is very limited. There is no clear evidence for response improving by raising the dose (Ruhé *et al.*, 2006), although there is some equivocal support for this provided treatment has been given for at least four weeks in regular dosage. Switching between treatments with proven efficacy may also be helpful (Baldwin *et al.*, 2005). Two recent small placebo-controlled augmentation studies suggest the antipsychotic drugs olanzapine and risperidone may enhance the response to fluoxetine (Pollack *et al.*, 2006) and other SSRIs or anxiolytics (Brawman-Mintzer *et al.*, 2005).

Withdrawal of drugs in generalised anxiety disorder

There is now a reasonable body of evidence, including one meta-analysis of 29 studies (Oude Voshaar *et al.*, 2006) suggesting that sedative anxiolytic drugs can be withdrawn more successfully if two strategies are employed. The first is a minimal one of giving simple advice in the form of a letter or meeting to a large group of people that is well suited to primary care (Cormack *et al.*, 1994). The second is gradual tapering of medication, with no evidence indicting the preferred duration of taper. Further discussion of this subject is developed in Chapter 16 but it is worth mentioning here than many with generalised anxiety disorder who take long-term medication do not have any problems in withdrawing from their drugs, and many that do have similar ('pseudowithdrawal') problems that occur even if the drug is not being withdrawn (Tyrer *et al.*, 1983).

Withdrawal of antidepressants has much less evidence behind it. No clear guidelines can be given but an expert group have recently concluded that a combination of clinical monitoring to determine the progress of withdrawal, education about the likely drug withdrawal effects and gradual tapering of drugs, is the best strategy (Schatzberg *et al.*, 2006).

Psychological treatment

Acute treatment of generalised anxiety disorder

Some psychological therapies have proven efficacy in the treatment of generalised anxiety disorder. Older treatments, such as hypnosis, have rarely been tested in formal trials but have some evidence of efficacy (Ashton *et al.*, 1997) that deserves further exploration. The most common psychological treatments used for generalized anxiety disorder are cognitive-behavioural therapy, various forms of dynamic psychotherapy and more behaviourally-based treatments such as anxiety-management training. A review of 14 studies of psychological treatment in generalised anxiety disorder revealed generally modest improvement in symptoms, with 50% relief of somatic symptoms and a similar proportion attaining normal function after treatment (Durham & Allan, 1993). However, this compares well with drug treatment and the most effective of the psychological treatments, cognitive-behaviour therapy, in a review of 35 studies, was shown to have a similar effect size (0.7) to that of drug treatment (0.6) (Gould *et al.*, 1997). Comparison of cognitive-behaviour therapy, analytic psychotherapy and anxiety management training showed that cognitive-behaviour therapy was both superior at the end of treatment and at 6 month follow-up and could be delivered effectively in 8–10 sessions (Durham *et al.*, 1994).

Unfortunately, many psychological treatment studies have deficiencies in study design that reduce the confidence that can be placed in the findings. The use of a 'waiting list' group for comparison with an active treatment group, rather than a proper psychological placebo treatment, is a flaw that undermines the results of some studies (Butler *et al.*, 1991; Barlow *et al.*, 1992). There have been few comparisons of pharmacological and psychological treatment approaches, and the studies which have made this comparison have used benzodiazepines for short periods rather than antidepressants with proven efficacy in GAD.

Long-term treatment of generalised anxiety disorder

Psychological treatments may be better at maintaining their efficacy than drug treatments, but there have been few long-term comparisons between treatment approaches. Relapse is less frequent after stopping cognitive-behaviour therapy (although booster treatment sessions may be necessary) and initial improvement may be maintained for up to 2 years, particularly if the therapists giving the original treatment were more competent (reference needed). However, in the long term (8–14 years) only around a third of patients make a good recovery and a similar proportion, particularly those with more severe symptoms referred from primary care, do not show any substantial improvement (Durham *et al.*, 2003).

Pharmacological treatments in somatoform disorders

There have been few formal evaluations of the efficacy of pharmacological treatments in patients with somatoform disorder, with a dearth of randomised double-blind placebo-controlled treatment studies. In an early cross-over study, there was no evidence of efficacy for the anti-depressant mianserin in a small group ($n = 11$) of patients with somatoform pain and accompanying depression, although it was efficacious in a smaller group ($n = 8$) of pain-free depressed patients (Onghena et al., 1993). The selective serotonin reuptake inhibitor fluvoxamine has been found efficacious in the treatment of a larger group ($n = 42$) of men with prostatodynia (a male somatoform disorder characterised by urogenital pain and urinary symptoms) (Turkington et al., 2002), and the SNRI venlafaxine was recently found efficacious in reducing pain and somatic physical symptoms in depressed and anxious patients with multisomatoform disorder (Kroenke et al., 2006), this finding echoing that of a previous systematic review and meta-analysis, in which anti-depressants were found efficacious in relieving pain in patients with psychogenic pain or somatoform pain disorder (Fishbain et al., 1998). Other pharmacological treatments with evidence of efficacy in randomised placebo-controlled studies include a preparation of the medicinal herb, St John's wort (Muller et al., 2004; Volz et al., 2002) and opipramol (Volz et al., 2000).

Psychological treatments of somatoform disorders

In contrast to drug treatments, psychological therapies have a much better evidence base than drug treatments in patients with somatoform disorders. In a systematic review of 31 controlled trials (29 randomised and 2 non-randomised) (Kroenke & Swindle, 2000) consistent benefits of cognitive-behaviour therapy were identified. The evidence suggested greater effectiveness with physical symptoms, of which chronic fatigue was the best example, with 71% showing greater improvement with the psychological treatment. Improvement in function (47% superiority) and psychological distress (38% superiority) was less marked. There was evidence of maintenance of improvement up to 12 months, and interventions as brief as 5 sessions were also effective.

Several further published reports support these general conclusions, including group therapy for chronic fatigue (Bazelmans et al., 2005), with extension of the treatment to adolescent sufferers with good results (Stulemeijer et al., 2005), support for cost-effectiveness (Severens et al., 2004), good sustained response in those with health anxiety in primary care and genitourinary medical clinics (Barsky & Ahern, 2004; Seivewright et al., 2007), and in the treatment of chronic pain (Morley et al., 1999), where there is now a significant evidence base for this intervention developing.

Combined drug and psychological treatments

Although it may seem reasonable to combine psychological and drug treatments in generalised anxiety disorder the evidence for added benefit with combination treatment is slim. This may be because of patient choice; those who wish for one type of treatment are often averse to the other and avoid it where possible. However, there is some slight evidence of greater benefit. In one study buspirone improved the symptoms of both generalised anxiety and panic disorder when combined with cognitive-behaviour therapy (Cottraux et al., 1995), but this was not shown in another study with buspirone in generalised anxiety disorder (Lader & Bond, 1998). A primary care study found that combination of diazepam with CBT was more efficacious than either treatment given alone (although there was no significant difference between diazepam and placebo) (Power et al., 1990), but another study suggested that combination treatment was less efficacious than psychological treatment alone (Durham & Turvey, 1987). There is some evidence that combined therapy is more effective in patients who also have a personality disorder (Kool et al., 2003) but this needs to be replicated in specific anxiety disorders.

Guidelines based on full reviews of the literature all, somewhat disappointingly, suggest that there is insufficient evidence to recommend combined treatment initially, although this can be considered when initial (single) treatment fails (NICE, 2004; Baldwin et al., 2005; Mitte et al., 2005). However, it could be argued that in clinical practice it is not difficult to predict who will fail with an individual treatment so an experienced practitioner should not be unduly inhibited from giving combined treatment without going through the experience of failure first.

Self-help

The sometimes disappointing effects of pharmacological and psychological treatments and consumer preferences for more convenient or 'natural' remedies have encouraged the development of many self-help therapies across the range of anxiety disorders. However, there have been few randomised controlled trials of the efficacy and acceptability of self-help approaches in diagnostically homogenous groups that have used reliable outcome measures and robust statistical analysis.

A systematic review of six randomised controlled trials indicates that self-help is efficacious in primary care patients with mixed anxiety disorders, greater efficacy being seen with more detailed instruction in use of self-help manuals (Van Boeijen *et al.*, 2005). Much better results were found in those patients without any evidence of personality disturbance, and in this group self-help may be superior to both drug therapy and cognitive-behaviour therapy (Tyrer *et al.*, 1993). Systematic review of complementary therapies found some evidence for the efficacy in GAD of relaxation training, exercise, and use of kava (now withdrawn because of hepatotoxicity) (Jorm *et al.*, 2004). In primary care patients who present with a range of emotional problems that clearly included generalised anxiety disorder (anxiety, depression, and 'stress'), counselling was more effective in the short term (but not in the long term) than standard general practitioner care, with or without antidepressant treatment (Bower *et al.*, 2001.

More recently, cognitive-behaviour therapy has been adapted to be delivered in computerised format, which essentially constitutes a self-help approach. Early results with this treatment have been encouraging and show that the treatment may be particularly adapted to primary care (Marks *et al.*, 2003). In 2002, the UK National Institute for Health and Clinical Excellence previously concluded that there was insufficient evidence to recommend the general introduction of computerised cognitive-behaviour therapy for anxiety symptoms or disorders (NICE, 2002). However, this treatment shows considerable promise and a recent large controlled trial in both anxious and depressed patients showed that computer-aided therapy was significantly more effective than usual treatment (Proudfoot *et al.*, 2004), and markedly more cost-effective. The mean service costs of providing the treatment was £40 but the saving in terms of lost employment regained was £407 (McCrone *et al.*, 2004). As use of computers and the internet continues to grow it is likely that this will become a widespread and useful application of an effective treatment that is feasible in primary care. As the demand for psychological treatments is never likely to be met satisfactorily from face-to-face treatment with therapists this could be a valuable alternative.

Prevention of generalised anxiety disorder

Apart from studies of tertiary prevention in those with an already established disorder (principally maintenance pharmacological or psychological treatment to avoid relapse), there is little evidence that generalised anxiety disorder can be prevented effectively. The link between personality trait status and generalised anxiety disorder is developed early in life and Akiskal and colleagues (Akiskal, 1998;

Akiskal *et al.*, 2005) have suggested the condition is best regarded as an anxious temperament. The links between generalised anxiety disorder and the personality dimension of 'neuroticism' are very strong and influenced heavily by genetic factors. Hettema *et al.* (2004) found correlations of 0.80 between the two conditions and concluded that 'the genetic factors underlying neuroticism are nearly indistinguishable from those that influence liability to generalised anxiety disorder' (p. 1585).

In this context it is also important to acknowledge the importance of anxiety as a fundamental drive that has evolutionary value. Its removal should not just be regarded as relief of a distressing and unwanted symptom. Many patients with generalised anxiety disorder are able to function well, often better than those with other disorders (Casey *et al.*, 1985), and it is only when symptoms interfere with normal social function that it may be appropriate to intervene. With the growth of self-help through the internet and group psychoeducational community interventions for anxiety and depression (Brown *et al.*, 2004), it is likely that people could receive earlier help at a time when it may be more valuable. As generalised anxiety disorder is not a condition that tends to improve with age – data suggest that anxiousness as both a personality and clinical problem becomes more prominent with increasing age (Larkin *et al.*, 1992; Seivewright *et al.*, 2002; Flint, 2005) – any intervention with preventive value would be highly valued.

When and when not to treat

Generalised anxiety disorder is a broad diagnosis and it would be highly unwise to respond to its detection simply by an automatic treatment intervention. Many patients who fulfil diagnostic criteria are likely to respond to minimal intervention (e.g. assessment and recognition of the problem); in others, symptoms will resolve spontaneously, particularly in primary care (Mann *et al.*, 1981; Seivewright *et al.*, 1998). It is unwise to rush into treatment approaches that carry some risk. This has been shown in the use of some SSRIs in the treatment of depression in children and adolescents, where the evidence base of efficacy has been found wanting (Whittington *et al.*, 2004). In deciding when and how to treat it is wise to be open in discussing the varying treatment options and to share decision-making between therapist and patient, as recommended in recent guidelines (NICE, 2004; Baldwin *et al.*, 2005). This should also include a frank discussion of the placebo effect, as this can be high and at a level that is greater than some drug/placebo differences (Piercy *et al.*, 1996).

Conclusions

Anxiety in both its somatic and psychological manifestations is so common in life as to be considered 'normal'. However, although many are able to tolerate and adapt to the high levels of background anxiety that are common in generalised anxiety disorder and somatoform disorders, the conditions lead to much morbidity. In deciding on effective treatments, although we acknowledge that there is a good evidence base for many of our interventions, they are usually only partial in their effects and how we treat the non-responders is a more difficult question. Because so many of the treatments we describe have similar effects the choice of intervention demands attention to the clinical features of the patient (for example, the presence of comorbid depression and a history of a good response to a previous treatment), patient preferences and the local availability of particular services. With both drug and psychological treatments, patients should be told that they will not respond immediately, that symptoms can sometimes briefly worsen during treatment, and that long-term treatment may be needed to maintain an initial response. For psychological treatment, resources are more limited, but cognitive-behaviour therapy, the most effective form of psychological treatment, is likely to be adapted further for computerised use without the need for live interaction, and offers much hope for optimism, particularly for chronic somatisation problems that are almost the most persistently difficult to treat in primary care.

Because of the relative rarity of both generalised anxiety disorder and specific somatoform disorders to exist as 'pure' conditions without comorbidity, and their well-established tendency to persist over time, it is wise to select treatments that have the potential to be given long term and to choose one with a wide spectrum of activity that might also be effective in treating depression, other anxiety disorders, and somatoform disorders. For this reason, current guidelines (NICE, 2004, Baldwin et al., 2005), that recommend use of either CBT or an SSRI as first choice treatments, with a general bias towards CBT if readily available, are understandable and probably wise in our present state of knowledge. Despite the wide prevalence of this disorder in clinical practice, the importance of regular monitoring when treatment is first started is now becoming of much greater importance in management, as even in these chronic conditions the introduction of a new treatment can lead to a temporary disequilibrium. There is room for a final word. Like the story of the tortoise and the hare, psychological treatments for these disorders are increasingly being shown to win when the race is a marathon, whereas drugs always win over the sprints. Both clinician and patient have to be clear when the starting gun is fired that they have planned the same distance.

The level of evidence for each of the interventions discussed in this chapter is summarised in Table 31.2.

Table 31.2. Effectiveness of treatments for generalised anxiety disorder (GAD) and somatoform disorder (SD)

Treatment and (diagnosis)	Form of treatment	Duration of treatment	Level of evidence for efficacy	Comments
Benzodiazepines (eg diazepam, alprazolam, clonazepam) (GAD)	tablets, liquid or im.iv injection	Acute and long term	Ia	Clinically effective in short term and also in long term, but dangers of dependence in long term tend to preclude usage (but see Chapter 21 on sedative-hypnotic dependence
Tricyclic antidepressants (best evidence with clomipramine)(GAD)	Oral (im preparations available but no evidence of value)	Medium and long term	Ib	Effective but preferred less than others because of adverse effects and toxicity
Selective serotonin reuptake inhibitors (GAD)(and SD – fluvoxamine only)	tablets	Medium, long term and relapse prevention	Ia	Demonstrably effective in both acute and long-term treatment
Serotonin-noradrenaline reuptake inhibitor (SNRI) (e.g. venlafaxine)(GAD and SD)	tablets	Medium and long term	Ia	Concern over potential cardiotoxicity has blunted strong evidence of efficacy
Azaspirodecanediones (e.g. buspirone)(GAD)	tablets (10–60 mg)	Medium to long-term	Ib	Effective but not well liked by patients, lack dependence risk

Table 31.2. (cont.)

Treatment and (diagnosis)	Form of treatment	Duration of treatment	Level of evidence for efficacy	Comments
Antihistamine (e.g. hydroxyzine)(GAD)	tablets	Medium to long term	Ib	Definite evidence of efficacy but comparative studies lacking
Low dose antipsychotic drugs (e.g. trifluoperazine) (GAD)	Tablets or im injections (not indicted for this disorder)	Medium term	Ib	Certainly effective and not addictive, but dangers of movement disorders in prolonged dosage
Anticonvulsants (pregabalin)(GAD)	tablets	Medium term and relapse prevention	Ib	Certainly efficacious but have some advantages early in treatment.
St John's wort (Hypericum)(SD)	Extract in tablet form	Acute treatment	Ib	Some value but see Part II, Chapter 7
Cognitive-behaviour therapy (GAD and SD)	Individual treatment	Acute and medium term treatment	Ia	Highly efficacious for GAD, health anxiety, chronic fatigue and pain symptoms
Self-help and bibliotherapy (GAD)	Personal choice	Acute and long term	Ia	Effective with particular value in those with no personality disturbance
Relaxation training (and hypnosis)(GAD)	Group or individual	Acute	IIa	Some evidence of benefit but not as strong as for other therapies
Counselling (GAD)	Individual	Acute	Ib	Only works in short term, effect probably lost later
Internet and computerised cognitive-behaviour therapy	Individual	Acute	IIa	Increasing evidence of efficacy but more information needed

(This paper is an expansion of a paper first published in the *Lancet* (Tyrer & Baldwin, 2006) and is published with the agreement of the Editor and publishers of that journal.)

REFERENCES

Akiskal, H. S. (1998). Towards a definition of GAD as an anxious temperament type. *Acta Psychiatrica Scandinavica*, **Suppl. 393**, 66–73.

Akiskal, H. S., Mendlowicz, M. V., Jean-Louis, G. *et al.* (2005). TEMPS-A: validation of a short version of a self-rated instrument designed to measure variations in temperament. *Journal of Affective Disorders*, **85**, 45–52.

Allgulander, C., Hackett, D. & Salinas, E. (2001). Venlafaxine extended release (ER) in the treatment of generalised anxiety disorder. Twenty-four-week placebo-controlled dose-ranging study. *British Journal of Psychiatry*, **179**, 15–22.

Allgulander, C., Florea, I. & Huusom, A. K. T. (2006). Prevention of relapse in generalized anxiety disorder by escitalopram treatment. *International Journal of Neuropsychopharmacology*, **9**, 495–505.

Ashton, C. H., Rawlins, M. D. & Tyrer, S. P. (1990). A double-blind placebo-controlled study of buspirone in diazepam withdrawal in chronic benzodiazepine users. *British Journal of Psychiatry*, **157**, 232–8.

Ashton, C., Whitworth, G. C., Seldomrdge, J. A. *et al.* (1997). Self-hypnosis reduces anxiety following coronary artery bypass surgery – a prospective, randomized trial. *Journal of Cardiovascular Surgery*, **38**, 69–75.

Baldwin, D. S. (2004). Sexual dysfunction associated with antidepressant drugs. *Expert Opinion on Drug Safety*, **3**, 457–70.

Baldwin, D. S. & Polkinghorn, C. (2005). Evidence-based pharmacotherapy of generalized anxiety disorder. *International Journal of Neuropsychopharmacology*, **8**, 293–302.

Baldwin, D. S., Anderson, I. M., Nutt, D. J. *et al.* (2005). Evidence-based guidelines for the pharmacological treatment of anxiety disorders: recommendations from the British Association for Psychopharmacology. *Journal of Psychopharmacology*, **19**, 567–96.

Baldwin, D. S., Huusom, A. K. & Maehlum, E. (2006). Escitalopram and paroxetine in the treatment of generalised anxiety disorder: randomised, placebo-controlled, double-blind study. *British Journal of Psychiatry*, **189**, 264–72.

Ballenger, J. C., Davidson, J. R. T., Lecrubier, Y. *et al.* (2001). Consensus statement on generalized anxiety disorder from the international consensus group on depression and anxiety. *Journal of Clinical Psychiatry*, **62** (suppl. 11), 53–8.

Bambauer, K. Z., Locke, S. E., Aupont, O., Mullan, M. G. & McLaughlin, T. J. (2005). Using the Hospital Anxiety and Depression Scale to screen for depression in cardiac patients. *General Hospital Psychiatry*, **27**, 275–84.

Barlow, D. H., Rapee, R. M. & Brown, T. A. (1992). Behavioral treatment of generalized anxiety disorder. *Behavior Therapy*, **23**, 551–70.

Barsky, A. J. & Ahern, D. K. (2004). Cognitive behavior therapy for hypochondriasis: a randomized controlled trial. *Journal of the American Medical Association*, **291**, 1464–70.

Bazelmans, E., Prins, J. B., Lulofs, R., van der Meer, J. W. M., Bleijenberg, G. & the Netherlands Fatigue Research Group Nijmegen (2005). Cognitive behaviour group therapy for chronic fatigue syndrome: a non-randomised waiting list controlled study. *Psychotherapy and Psychosomatics*, **74**, 218–24.

Beck, A. T. (1976). *Cognitive Therapy and the Emotional Disorders*. New York: International Universities Press.

Bielski, R. J., Bose, A. & Chang, C. C. (2005). A double-blind comparison of escitalopram and paroxetine in the long-term treatment of generalized anxiety disorder. *Annals of Clinical Psychiatry*, **17**, 65–9.

Bjelland, I., Dahl, A. A., Haug, T. T. & Neckelmann, D. (2002). The validity of the Hospital Anxiety and Depression Scale. An updated literature review. *Journal of Psychosomatic Research*, **52**, 69–77.

Bower, P., Richards, D. & Lovell, K. (2001). The clinical and cost-effectiveness of self-help treatments for anxiety and depressive disorders in primary care: a systematic review. *British Journal of General Practice*, **51**, 838–45.

Brawman-Mintzer, O., Knapp, R. G. & Nietert, P. J. (2005). Adjunctive risperidone in generalized anxiety disorder: a double-blind, placebo-controlled study. *Journal of Clinical Psychiatry*, **66**, 1321–5.

Brown, J. S. L., Elliott, S. A., Boardman, J., Ferns, J. & Morrison, J. (2004). Meeting the unmet need for depression services with psycho-educational self-confidence workshops: preliminary report. *British Journal of Psychiatry*, **185**, 511–15.

Butler, G., Fennell, M., Robson, P. & Gelder, M. (1991). Comparison of behavior therapy and cognitive behavior therapy in the treatment of generalized anxiety disorder. *Journal of Consulting and Clinical Psychology*, **59**, 167–75.

Casacalenda, N. & Boulenger, J. P. (1998). Pharmacologic treatments effective in both generalized anxiety disorder and major depressive disorder: clinical and theoretical implications. *Canadian Journal of Psychiatry*, **43**, 722–30.

Casey, P. R., Tyrer, P. J. & Platt, S. (1985). The relationship between social functioning and psychiatric symptomatology in primary care. *Social Psychiatry*, **20**, 5–9.

Chessick, C. A., Allen, H. A., Thase, M. E. *et al.* (2006). *Cochrane Database of Systematic Reviews*, **3**, CD006115 2006. Oxford: Update Software.

Cormack, M. A., Sweeney, K. G., Hughes-Jones, H. & Foot, G. A. (1994). Evaluation of an easy, cost-effective strategy for cutting benzodiazepine use in general practice. *British Journal of General Practice*, **44**, 5–8.

Cottraux, J., Note, I. D., Cungi, C. *et al.* (1995). A controlled study of cognitive behaviour therapy with buspirone or placebo in panic disorder with agoraphobia. *British Journal of Psychiatry*, **167**, 635–41.

Darcis, T., Ferreri, M., Natens, J., Burtin, B., Deram, P. and the French GP Study Group for Hydroxyzine (1995). A multicenter double-blind placebo-controlled study investigating the efficacy of hydroxyzine in patients with generalized anxiety disorder. *Human Psychopharmacology*, **10**, 181–7.

Deans, H. G. & Skinner, P. (1992). Doctors views on anxiety management in general practice. *Journal of the Royal Society of Medicine*, **85**, 83–6.

Drent, M., Singh, S., Gorgels, A. P. M. *et al.* (2003). Drug-induced pneumonitis and heart failure simultaneously associated with venlafaxine. *American Journal of Respiratory and Critical Care Medicine*, **167**, 958–61.

Dubicka, B., Hadley, S. & Roberts, C. (2006). Suicidal behaviour in depressed youths treated with new-generation antidepressants: meta-analysis. *British Journal of Psychiatry*, **189**, 393–8.

Durham, R. C. & Allan, T. (1993). Psychological treatment of generalized anxiety disorder: a review of the clinical significance in outcome studies since 1980. *British Journal of Psychiatry*, **163**, 19–26.

Durham, R. C. & Turvey, A. A. (1987). Cognitive therapy versus behaviour therapy in the treatment of chronic generalised anxiety. *Behavior Research and Therapy*, **25**, 229–34.

Durham, R. C., Murphy, T., Allan, T., Richard, K., Treliving, L. R. & Fenton, G. W. (1994). Cognitive therapy, analytic psychotherapy and anxiety management training for generalized anxiety disorder. *British Journal of Psychiatry*, **165**, 315–23.

Durham, R. C., Chambers, J. A., MacDonald, R. R., Power, K. G. & Major, K. (2003). Does cognitive-behavioural therapy influence the long-term outcome of generalized anxiety disorder? An 8–14 year follow-up of two clinical trials. *Psychological Medicine*, **33**, 499–509.

Fawcett, J., Kravitz, G., McGuire, M. *et al.* (2000). Pharmacological treatments for alcoholism: revisiting lithium and considering buspirone. *Alcohol Clinical and Experimental Research*, **24**, 666–74.

Fishbain, D. A., Cutler, R. B., Rosomoff, H. L. & Rosomhoff, R. S. (1998). Do antidepressants have an analgesic effect in psychogenic pain and somatoform pain disorder? A meta-analysis. *Psychosomatic Medicine*, **60**, 503–9.

Flint, A. J. (2005). Generalized anxiety disorder in elderly patients: epidemiology, diagnosis and treatment options. *Drugs and Aging*, **22**, 101–14.

Freud, S. (1924). On the grounds for detaching a particular syndrome from neurasthenia under the description 'anxiety neurosis'. English translation in *Complete Psychological Works*, ed. J. T. Strachey, Vol. 3, pp. 85–117. London: Hogarth Press.

Freud, S. (1926). Inhibitions, symptoms and anxiety. In *Complete Psychological Works*, ed. J. T. Strachey, Vol. 20, pp. 75–174. London: Hogarth Press.

Goodman, W. K., Bose, A. & Wang, Q. (2000). Treatment of generalized anxiety disorder with escitalopram: pooled results from double-blind, placebo-controlled trials. *Journal of Affective Disorders*, **87**, 161–7.

Gould, R. A., Otto, M. W., Pollack, M. H. & Yap, L. (1997). Cognitive behavioural and pharmacological treatment of generalised anxiety disorder: a preliminary meta-analysis. *Behavior Therapy*, **28**, 285–305.

Granville-Grossman, K. L. & Turner, P. (1966). The effect of propranolol on anxiety. *Lancet*, **i**, 788–90.

Haddad, P. (1997). Newer antidepressants and the discontinuation syndrome. *Journal of Clinical Psychiatry*, **58** (Suppl 7), 17–21.

Hallstrom, C., Treasaden, I., Edwards, J. G. & Lader, M.(1981). Diazepam, propranolol and their combination in the management of chronic anxiety. *British Journal of Psychiatry*, **139**, 417–21.

Hamilton, M. (1959). The assessment of anxiety states by rating. *British Journal of Medical Psychology*, **32**, 50–5.

Hettema, J. M., Prescott, C. A. & Kendler, K. S. (2004). Genetic and environmental sources of covariation between generalized anxiety disorder and neuroticism. *American Journal of Psychiatry*, **161**, 1581–7.

Holton, A. & Tyrer, P. (1990). Five year outcome of patients withdrawn from long term treatment with diazepam. *Biritish Medical Journal*, **300**, 1241–2.

Jorm, A. F., Christensen, H., Griffiths, K. M., Parslow, R. A., Rodgers, B. & Blewitt, K. A. (2004). Effectiveness of complementary and self-help treatments for anxiety disorders. *Medical Journal of Australia*, **181**(Suppl), S29–46.

Kahn, R. J., McNair, D. M., Lipman, R. S. *et al.* (1986). Imipramine and chlordiazepoxide in depressive and anxiety disorders: II. Efficacy in anxious out-patients. *Archives of General Psychiatry*, **43**, 79–85.

Kapczinski, F., Schmitt, R. & Lima, M. S. (2003). The use of antidepressants for generalized anxiety disorder. *Cochrane Database of Systematic Reviews*, **2**, CD003592. Oxford: Update Software Ltd.

Katz, I. R., Reynolds, C. F. 3rd, Alexopoulos, G. S. & Hackett, D. (2002). Venlafaxine ER as a treatment for generalized anxiety disorder in older adults: pooled analysis of five randomized placebo-controlled clinical trials. *Journal of the American Geriatric Society*, **50**, 18–25.

Kellner, R., Collins, A. C., Shulman, R. S. & Pathak, D. (1974). The short-term antianxiety effects of propranolol HCl (1974). *Journal of Clinical Pharmacology*, **14**, 301–4.

Klein, D. F. (1967). Importance of psychiatric diagnosis in prediction of clinical drug effects. *Archives of General Psychiatry*, **16**, 118–25.

Kool, S., Dekker, J., Duijsens, I. J., de Jonghe, F. & Puite, B. (2003). Efficacy of combined therapy and pharmacotherapy for depressed patients with or without personality disorders. *Harvard Review of Psychiatry*, **11**, 133–41.

Kroenke, K. & Swindle, J. (2000). Cognitive-behavioral therapy for somatization and symptom syndromes: a critical review of controlled clinical trials. *Psychotherapy and Psychosomatics*, **69**, 205–15.

Kroenke, K., Messina, N. 3rd, Benattia, I., Graepel, J. & Musgnung, J. (2006). Venlafaxine extended release in the short-term treatment of depressed and anxious primary care patients with multisomatoform disorder. *Journal of Clinical Psychiatry*, **67**, 72–80.

Lader, M. H. & Bond, A. J. (1998). Interaction of pharmacological and psychological treatments of anxiety. *British Journal of Psychiatry*, **Suppl**. **34**, 42–48.

Larkin, B. A., Copeland, J. R. M., Dewey, M. E. *et al.* (1992). The natural history of neurotic disorder in an elderly urban population: findings from the Liverpool study of continuing health in the community. *British Journal of Psychiatry*, **160**, 681–6.

Lawrenson, R. A., Tyrer, F., Newson, R. B. & Farmer, R. D. (2000). The treatment of depression in UK general practice: selective serotonin reuptake inhibitors and tricyclic antidepressants compared. *Journal of Affective Disorders*, **59**, 149–57.

Layard, R. (2006). The case for psychological treatment centres. *British Medical Journal*, **332**, 1030–2.

Lipowski, Z. J. (1988). Somatization: the concept and its clinical application. *American Journal of Psychiatry*, **145**(11), 1358–68.

Llorca, P. M., Sapdine, C., Sol, O. *et al.* (2002). Efficacy and safety of hydroxyzine in the treatment of generalized anxiety disorder: a three-month double-blind study. *Journal of Clinical Psychiatry*, **63**, 1020–7.

Mann, A. H., Jenkins, R. & Belsey, E. (1981). The twelve-month outcome of patients with neurotic illness in general practice. *Psychological Medicine*, **11**, 535–50.

Marks, I. M., Mataix-Cols, D., Kenwright, M., Cameron, R., Hirsch, S. & Gega, L. (2003). Pragmatic evaluation of computer-aided self-help for anxiety and depression. *British Journal of Psychiatry*, **183**, 57–65.

McCrone, P., Knapp, M., Proudfoot, J. *et al.* (2004). Cost-effectiveness of computerized cognitive behaviour therapy for anxiety and depression in primary care: randomized controlled trial. *British Journal of Psychiatry*, **185**, 55–62.

Meibach, R. C., Dunner, D. M., Wilson, L. G., Ishiki, D. & Dager, S. R. (2001). Comparative efficacy of propranolol, chlordiazepoxide, and placebo in the treatment of anxiety: a double-blind trial. *Journal of Clinical Psychiatry*, **62**, 523–39.

Mendels, J., Krajewski, T. F., Huffer, V. *et al.* (1986). Effective short-term treatment of generalised anxiety with trifluoperazine. *Journal of Clinical Psychiatry*, **47**, 170–4.

Meyer, T. J., Miller, M. L., Metzger, R. L. & Borkovec, T. D. (1990). Development and validation of the Penn State Worry Questionnaire. *Behavior Research and Therapy*, **28**, 487–95.

Mitchell, A. J. (2006). Two-week delay in onset of action of antidepressants: new evidence. *British Journal of Psychiatry*, **188**, 105–6.

Mitte, K., Noack, P., Steil, R. & Hautzinger, M. (2005). A meta-analytic review of the efficacy of drug treatment in generalized anxiety disorder. *Journal of Clinical Psychopharmacology*, **25**, 141–50.

Montgomery, S. A., Sheehan, D. V., Meoni, P., Haudiquet, V. & Hackett, D. (2002a). Characterization of the longitudinal course of improvement during long term treatment with venlafaxine XR. *Journal of Psychiatric Research*, **36**, 209–17.

Montgomery, S. A., Mahe, V., Haudiquet, V. & Hackett, D. (2002b). Effectiveness of venlafaxine, extended release formulation, in short-term and long-term treatment of generalized anxiety disorder: results of a survival analysis. *Journal of Clinical Psychopharmacology*, **21**, 561–7.

Morley, S., Eccleston, C. & Williams, A. (1999). Systematic review and meta-analysis of randomized controlled trials of cognitive behaviour therapy and behaviour therapy for chronic pain in adults, excluding headache. *Pain*, **80**, 1–13.

Muller, T., Mannel, M., Murck, H. & Rahlfs, V. W. (2004). Treatment of somatoform disorders with St. John's wort: a randomized, double-blind and placebo-controlled trial (2004). *Psychosomatic Medicine*, **66**, 538–47.

Murphy, S. M., Owen, R. & Tyrer, P. (1989). Comparative assessment of efficacy and withdrawal symptoms after 6 and 12 weeks' treatment with diazepam or buspirone. *British Journal of Psychiatry*, **154**, 529–34.

National Institute for Clinical Excellence (NICE) (2002). *Guidance on the use of computerised cognitive behavioural therapy for anxiety and depression.* Health Technology Appraisal Guidance 51. London: NICE.

National Institute for Clinical Excellence (NICE) (2004). *The management of panic disorder and generalised anxiety disorder in primary and secondary care.* London: National Collaborating Centre for Mental Health.

Newman, M. G., Zuellig, A. R., Kachin, K. E. *et al.* (2002). Preliminary reliability and validity of the Generalized Anxiety Disorder Questionnaire IV: a revised self-report diagnostic measure of generalized anxiety disorder. *Behavior Therapy*, **28**, 215–33.

Nutt, D. J. (2005). Death by tricyclic: the real antidepressant scandal? *Journal of Psychopharmacology*, **19**, 123–4.

Onghena, P., De Cuyper, H., Van Houdenhove, B. & Verstraeten, D. (1993). Mianserin and chronic pain: a double-blind placebo-controlled process and outcome study. *Acta Psychiatrica Scandinavica*, **88**, 198–204.

Oude Voshaar, R. C., Couvée, J. E., Van Balkom, A. J. L. M., Mulder, P. G. H. & Zitman, F. G. (2006). Strategies for discontinuing long-term benzodiazepine use: meta-analysis. *British Journal of Psychiatry*, **189**, 213–20.

Paykel, E. S. & Priest, R. G. (1992). Recognition and management of depression in general practice: consensus statement. *British Medical Journal*, **305**, 1198–202.

Piercy, M. A., Sramek, J. J., Kurtz, N. M. & Cutler, N. R. (1996). Placebo response in anxiety disorders. *Annals of Pharmacotherapy*, **30**, 1013–19.

Pilowsky, I. (1969). Abnormal illness behaviour. *British Journal of Medical Psychology*, **42**, 347–51.

Pollack, M. H., Simon, N. M., Zalta, A. K. *et al.* (2006). Olanzapine augmentation of fluoxetine for refractory generalized anxiety disorder: a placebo-controlled study. *Biological Psychiatry*, **59**, 211–15.

Power, K. G., Simpson, R. J., Swanson, V. & Wallace, L. A. (1990). Controlled comparison of pharmacological and psychological treatment of generalized anxiety disorder in primary care. *British Journal of General Practice*, **40**, 289–94.

Priest, R. G. & Montgomery, S. A. (1988). Benzodiazepines and dependence: a College statement. *Psychiatric Bulletin*, **12**, 107–8.

Proudfoot, J., Ryden, C., Everitt, B. *et al.* (2004). Clinical effectiveness of computerized cognitive behaviour therapy for anxiety and depression in primary care. *British Journal of Psychiatry*, **185**, 46–54.

Regier, D. A., Narrow, W. E. & Rae, D. S. (1990). The epidemiology of anxiety disorders: the Epidemiologic Catchment Area (ECA) experience. *Journal of Psychiatric Research*, **24** (Suppl. 2), 3–14.

Rickels, K., Schweizer, E., Csanalosi, I., Case, W. G. & Chung, H. (1988). Long-term treatment of anxiety and risk of withdrawal: prospective study of clorazepate and buspirone. *Archives of General Psychiatry*, **45**, 444–50.

Romach, M., Busto, U., Somer, G., Kaplan, H. l. & Sellers, E. (1995). Clinical aspects of chronic use of alprazolam and lorazepam. *American Journal of Psychiatry*, **152**, 1161–7.

Ruhé, H. G., Huyser, J., Swinkels, J. A. & Schene, A. H. (2006). Dose escalation for insufficient response to standard-dose selective serotonin reuptake inhibitors in major depressive disorder: systematic review. *British Journal of Psychiatry*, **189**, 309–16.

Salkovskis, P. M., Rimes, K. A., Warwick, H. M. C. & Clark, D. M. (2002). The Health Anxiety Inventory: development and validation of scales for the measurement of health anxiety and hpochondriasis. *Psychological Medicine*, **32**, 843–53.

Salzman, C., Goldenberg, I., Bruce, S. E. & Keller, M. B. (2001). Pharmacologic treatment of anxiety disorders in 1989 versus 1996: Results from the Harvard/Brown anxiety disorders research program. *Journal of Clinical Psychiatry*, **62**, 149–52.

Schatzberg, A. F., Blier, P., Delgado, P. L., Fava, M., Haddad, P. M. & Shelton, R. C. (2006). Antidepressant discontinuation syndrome: consensus panel recommendations for clinical management and additional research. *Journal of Clinical Psychiatry*, **67** (Suppl. 4), 27–30.

Seivewright, H. & Tyrer, P. (2005). *Schedule for Evaluating Persistent Symptoms (SEPS).* London: Imperial College, Department of Psychological Medicine.

Seivewright, H., Tyrer, P., Casey, P. & Seivewright, N. (1991). A three-year follow-up of psychiatric morbidity in urban and rural primary care. *Psychological Medicine*, **21**, 495–503.

Seivewright, H., Tyrer, P. & Johnson, T. (1998). Prediction of outcome in neurotic disorder: a five year prospective study. *Psychological Medicine*, **28**, 1149–57.

Seivewright, H., Tyrer, P. & Johnson, T. (2002). Change in personality status in neurotic disorders. *Lancet*, **359**, 2253–4.

Seivewright, H., Green, J., Salkovskis, P., Barrett, B., Nur, U. & Tyrer, P. (2007). Randomised controlled trial of cognitive behaviour therapy in the treatment of health anxiety in a genito-urinary medicine clinic. (in press)

Severens, J. L., Prins, J. B., van der Wilt, G. J., van der Meer, J. W. M. & Bleijenberg, G. (2004). Cost-effectiveness of cognitive behaviour therapy for patients with chronic fatigue syndrome. *QJM: An International Journal of Medicine*, **97**, 153–61.

Sheehan, D. V., Ballenger, J. & Jacobsen, G. (1980). Treatment of endogenous anxiety with phobic, hysterical, and hypochondriacal symptoms. *Archives of General Psychiatry*, **37**, 51–9.

Stahl, S. M., Gergel, I. & Li, D. (2003). Escitalopram in the treatment of panic disorder: a randomized, double-blind, placebo-controlled trial. *Journal of Clinical Psychiatry*, **64**, 1322–7.

Stocchi, F. G., Nordera, G., Jokinen, R. H. *et al.* (2003). Efficacy and tolerability of paroxetine for the long-term treatment of generalized anxiety disorder. *Journal of Clinical Psychiatry*, **64**, 250–8.

Stulemeijer, M., de Jong, L. W. A. M., Fiselier, T. J. W., Hoogveld, S. W. B. & Bleijenberg, G. (2005). Cognitive behaviour therapy for adolescents with chronic fatigue syndrome: randomised controlled trial. *British Medical Journal*, **330**, 14–17.

Taylor, F. K. (1989). The damnation of benzodiazepines. *British Journal of Psychiatry*, **154**, 353–60.

Thase, M. E., Entsuah, A. R. & Rudolph, R. L. (2001). Remission rates during treatment with venlafaxine or selective serotonin reuptake inhibitors. *British Journal of Psychiatry*, **178**, 234–41.

Turkington, D., Grant, J. B., Ferrier, I. N., Rao, N. S., Linsley, K. R. & Young, A. H. (2002). A randomized controlled trial of fluvoxamine in prostatodynia, a male somatoform pain disorder. *Journal of Clinical Psychiatry*, **63**, 778–81.

Tyrer, P. (1973). Relevance of bodily feelings in emotion. *Lancet*, **i**, 915–16.

Tyrer, P. (1992). Anxiolytics not acting at the benzodiazepine receptor: beta-blockers. *Progress in Neuropsychopharmacology and Biological Psychiatry*, **16**, 17–26.

Tyrer, P. & Baldwin, D. (2006). Generalized anxiety disorder. *Lancet*, **368**, 2156–66.

Tyrer, P. & Lader, M. H. (1974). Response to propranolol and diazepam in somatic and psychic anxiety. *British Medical Journal*, **2**, 14–16.

Tyrer, P. & Owen, R. (1984). Anxiety in primary care: is short-term drug treatment appropriate? *Journal of Psychiatric Research*, **18**, 73–8.

Tyrer, P., Rutherford, D. & Huggett, T. (1981). Benzodiazepine withdrawal symptoms and propranolol. *Lancet*, **i**, 520–2.

Tyrer, P., Owen, R. & Dawling, S. (1983). Gradual withdrawal of diazepam after long-term therapy. *Lancet*, **i**, 1402–6.

Tyrer, P., Seivewright, N., Murphy, S. *et al.* (1988). The Nottingham study of neurotic disorder: comparison of drug and psychological treatments. *Lancet*, **ii**, 235–40.

Tyrer, P., Seivewright, N., Ferguson, B., Murphy, S. & Johnson, A. L. (1993). The Nottingham study of neurotic disorder: impact of personality status on response to drug treatment, cognitive therapy and self-help over two years. *British Journal of Psychiatry*, **162**, 219–26.

van Boeijen, C. A., van Balkom, A. J., van Oppen, P., Blankenstein, N., Cherpanath, A. & van Dyck, R. (2005). Efficacy of self-help manuals for anxiety disorders in primary care: a review. *Family Practice*, **22**, 192–6.

Versiani, M., Nardi, A. E., Mundim, F. D., Alves, A. B., Liebowitz, M. R. & Amrein, R. (1992). Pharmacotherapy of social phobia. A controlled study with moclobemide and phenelzine. *British Journal of Psychiatry*, **161**, 353–60.

Volz, H. P., Murck, H., Kasper, S. & Moller, H. J. (2002). St John's wort extract (LI 160) in somatoform disorders: results of a placebo-controlled trial. *Psychopharmacology*, **164**, 294–300.

Volz, H. P., Moller, H. J., Reimann, I. & Stoll, K. D. (2000). Opipramol for the treatment of somatoform disorders. Results from a placebo-controlled trial. *European Neuropsychopharmacology*, **10**, 211–17.

Whittington, C. J., Kendall, T., Fonagy, P., Cottrell, D., Cotgrove, A. & Boddington, E. (2004). Selective serotonin reuptake inhibitors in childhood depression: systematic review of published versus unpublished data. *Lancet*, **363**, 1341–5.

Zigmond, A. S. & Snaith, R. P. (1983). The Hospital Anxiety and Depression Scale. *Acta Psychiatrica Scandinavica*, **57**, 361–70.

Zonderman, A. B., Heft, M. W. & Costa, P. T. (1985). Does the Illness Behavior Questionnaire measure abnormal illness behaviour? *Health Psychology*, **4**, 425–36.

32

Panic disorder

Stacy Shaw Welch, Michelle Craske, Murray B. Stein,
Phil Harrison-Read and Peter Roy-Byrne

Editor's note

Panic disorder is a relatively new diagnosis that did not
exist formally before 1980, when it was first introduced
into DSM-III. Its introduction divided the primary anxiety
disorders into panic and generalized anxiety disorder. The
assets of the diagnosis are also its handicaps. The experience of a panic attack is so profound that it cannot but be
remembered starkly and clearly, and so the definition of a
panic attack is remarkably easy. However, most psychiatrists never see someone having a severe panic attack, and
so the reporting of symptoms is for the most part retrospective and possibly distorted by the experience. This has
led to difficulty in defining panic disorder, and the official
classifications of DSM and ICD differ to some extent in
that ICD-10 maintains that the panic attacks in panic disorder 'are not consistently associated with a specific
symptom or object' (as when they are symptoms
forming part of a phobic disorder), whereas in DSM IV,
the exclusion clause that 'they are not better accounted
for by another mental disorder' is much more open to interpretation. Panic attacks are said to be 'uncued' (i.e. they
come 'out of the blue'), but increasingly, as this chapter
illustrates, they are often associated with a variety of cues.
It is a condition which is not so much treated, but prevented, as the successful treatments prevent the disorder
(i.e. stop) the panic attacks rather than treat them.

Introduction

Panic disorder (PD) is a prevalent and disabling mental
disorder that affects up to 5% of the population at some
point in their lives, and around 3% in any given year
(Kessler *et al.*, 2005a, 2005b). Its costs are serious from
both an individual and public health perspective, and

include reduced quality of life, increased health care utilization, reduced workplace productivity and absenteeism
(Greenberg *et al.*, 1999; Barlow, 2002). Several very efficacious and well-validated classes of treatment (cognitive-
behavioral and pharmacological treatments) exist. Still,
the etiology and precise mechanisms involved in PD are
not clear, despite growing identification of genetic and early
experiential risk factors. Along with the need for greater
understanding of the causes and mechanisms of PD, adapting and disseminating evidence-based treatments effectively are major new challenges for the field.

Clinical features

Panic attacks are characterized by sudden, paroxysmal
bursts of severe anxiety, accompanied by a range of physical (cardiorespiratory, autonomic, gastrointestinal, and/
or otoneurologic) as well as cognitive (fears of losing control, dying, or going crazy) symptoms. The diagnosis of
panic disorder requires the presence of recurrent panic
attacks accompanied by either (1) worry about the possibility of future attacks or (2) development of phobic avoidance or other change in behavior due to the attacks.
Phobic avoidance typically includes staying away from
location or situations the individual fears will elicit a
panic attack. Alternatively, the individual might avoid
situations where escaping or obtaining help would be
difficult (i.e. driving on a bridge, crowded places, etc.).
Other changes in behavior due to the attacks, such as visits
to the hospital or physician due to concern about heart
attacks or other physical ailments may be observed
(APA, 1994).

Panic attacks in panic disorder often have a dramatic
initial presentation, as well as an unexpected quality,
with onset sometimes unaccompanied by an obvious trigger. However, recent evidence suggest that a substantial

Cambridge Textbook of Effective Treatments in Psychiatry, ed. Peter Tyrer and Kenneth R. Silk. Published by Cambridge University Press.
© Cambridge University Press, 2008.

proportion of panic attacks in PD patients are not unexpected or unanticipated but have clear cut, identifiable cues (Kessler *et al.*, 2006), much like panic attacks occurring as part of other disorders such as phobias and PTSD. Panic attacks as isolated phenomena are quite common, and are thought to occur occasionally over the last year in about 3%–5% of the general population (Norton *et al.*, 1992) and include a similar physical and cognitive symptom constellation. In clinical settings, panic disorder is almost always accompanied by comorbid conditions. A greater prevalence of PD in patients with other axis I psychiatric disorders, particularly major depression (Kessler *et al.*, 1998), bipolar illness, (Goodwin & Hoven, 2002) other anxiety disorders (Goisman *et al.*, 1995) and possibly alcohol abuse (Zimmermann *et al.*, 2003) has been consistently reported.

A growing body of evidence underlines the importance of panic disorder in children and adolescents where it tends to have a chronic course and is frequently comorbid with other anxiety, mood and disruptive disorders (Biederman *et al.*, 1997). Studies suggest that childhood panic (Biederman *et al.*, 2005), as well as its possible precursor, "behavioural inhibition" (Rosenbaum *et al.*, 2000) (which is also a risk factor for social anxiety disorder), are more common in offspring of parents with panic disorder. Separation anxiety is distinct from childhood panic, and does not reliably develop into adult panic, though it is also more common in offspring of parents with panic disorder (Aschenbrand *et al.*, 2003).

Agoraphobia

Agoraphobia co-exists with panic disorder in approximately 50% of cases. Agoraphobia involves fear and avoidance of places where panic may occur, particularly situations where escape or help would be difficult to obtain (even staying at home alone). Functional impairment is high and might include travel restrictions, need for accompaniment by others, or becoming partially or completely house-bound. Although agoraphobia tends to increase with duration of PD, many patients continue to experience panic attacks for many years without increasing agoraphobic avoidance.

A current area of controversy involves the conceptualization and classification of agoraphobia *without* panic attacks. Interestingly, this is extremely uncommon in clinical settings, but is commonly found in community samples (Wittchen *et al.*, 1998). In about 30% of cases, agoraphobia appears before the onset of panic, and this suggests that it may not always be a complication or consequence of PD (Bienvenu *et al.*, in press).

Chronicity and course

Panic disorder tends to be chronic, and only about a third of patients remit within a few years without relapse. A slightly higher percentage, about 35%, experience a waxing and waning course which includes times of significant improvement (Roy-Byrne & Cowley, 1995; Katschnig & Amering, 1998). It does appear, however, that the course of panic disorder is less chronic than in the case of generalized and social anxiety disorders, both of which take longer to initially remit and also take a shorter time to recur. This is particularly true for PD without agoraphobia (Bruce *et al.*, 2005). These poor outcomes could be modified if the low rates of receiving evidence-based treatment in the community could be improved (Wang *et al.*, 2000).

Etiology and explanatory models

As with most psychiatric disorders, a 'diathesis stress' model is commonly used to explain the genesis and maintenance of PD. Diathesis stress models emphasize disorder as produced by the interaction of a vulnerable hereditary predisposition that interacts and is triggered by environment/life events. The greater the underlying vulnerability, the less stress is needed to trigger the behavior/disorder.

Heritability
As with many other disorders, panic disorder is thought to be a genetically complex disorder with multiple genes determining vulnerability through pathways that are not yet understood (Kendler, 2005). Interestingly, while many earlier neurobiological theories of anxiety have focused on the two most well-known and studied neurotransmitters, noradrenaline and serotonin, there has been only minimal evidence that genes involved in the synthesis, degradation, or transport of these neurotransmitters, or the receptors that mediate their effects, are linked to, or associated with, panic disorder (Roy-Byrne *et al.*, 2006).

Risk factors
There is a large literature examining risk factors for PD. Research suggests that stressful life events likely contribute to both the onset and maintenance of PD (Watanabe *et al.*, 2005; Roy-Byrne *et al.*, 1986). Childhood trauma/maltreatment has been identified as a specific risk factor (Stein *et al.*, 1996). Recent studies have implicated cigarette smoking and nicotine dependence in adolescence as a risk factor for later PD onset, although the causal nature of this association has been questioned (Isensee *et al.*, 2003). Temperament, which of course can be conceptualized as

both a risk factor and a predisposing factor, also appears important. An anxious temperament characterized by "neuroticism", (Roth, 1984) and "anxiety sensitivity", may be especially important as a risk factor through increasing the salience of bodily sensations that are central to the onset of panic disorder (McNally, 2002; Reiss, 1980).

Development and maintenance of panic disorder

Psychological processes

Central to the development of panic disorder is acute "fear of fear," referring to the fear of the physical sensations of panic that develops in vulnerable individuals after initial attacks. This is generally attributed to two factors, interoceptive conditioning and catastrophic misappraisals of bodily sensations, both of which have cognitive and neurobiological underpinnings. Interoceptive conditioning refers to conditioned fear responses to internal cues such as elevated heart rate or shortness of breath. Once these internal cues are paired with the terror of panic, even early or subtle cues of a stereotypic physical anxiety response elicit, in turn, more acute bursts of anxiety or panic (Bouton *et al.*, 2001). Such slight changes in bodily functions are not necessarily consciously recognized (Block *et al.*, 1987; Craske *et al.*, 2002), but may explain the unexpected quality of panic in PD. This conditioned fear and panic then adds to the terror of panic (Bouton *et al.*, 2001; Barlow, 1988). Such changes in bodily function might result from "subclinical" cardiorespiratory or vestibular dysfunction. However, the testability of the interoceptive conditioning model has been questioned.

The second factor is catastrophic misappraisals of bodily sensations (e.g., imminent death or loss of control) (Clark, 1986) which can operate subconsciously (as might occur in nocturnal panic attacks or in panic attacks in which specific catastrophic thoughts are not recalled), but mostly are consciously accessible even when panic attacks are perceived as happening from "out of the blue." While the theoretical validity of this factor has been questioned, it is argued that catastrophic misappraisals may become conditioned stimuli that trigger panic (Bouton *et al.*, 2001). There is some direct evidence for this phenomenon (Clark *et al.*, 1988) as well as evidence for a cognitive style that is more attentive to physical threat (Hope *et al.*, 1990) and to increased fear of procedures eliciting sensations similar to panic (Jacob *et al.*, 1992). These factors may explain observations of the "fear of fear" response that dates back to 1967 when Pitt observed that hyperosmolar sodium lactate provoked panic attacks

in patients with PD but not controls (Pitts *et al.*, 1967). The same effects have been shown using anxiogenic pharmacologic agents with distinct action mechanisms (e.g., caffeine, isoproterenol, yohimbine, carbon dioxide, CCK). In some cases these studies have produced panic in PD patients but not in non-panicking patients with other anxiety or mood disorder (Krystal *et al.*, 1996).

Neurobiological processes

Current models of panic disorder emphasize the amygdala and related structures (pre-frontal, orbito-frontal and temporal cortices, hippocampus) as part of a dysfunctional anxiety evaluation and response system. (Gorman *et al.*, 2000). Reports of abnormalities in these structures are numerous though not specific to panic disorder (i.e. they are also seen in PTSD and social anxiety) (Kent & Rauch, 2003). These include reduced volumes in the amygdala and temporal lobe (Massana *et al.*, 2003; Uchida *et al.*, 2003), lowered amounts of creatine and phosphocreatine metabolites in the medial temporal lobe (Massana *et al.*, 2002), and reduced metabolic activity in amygdala and hippocampus, as well as in thalamus and brainstem areas (Sakai *et al.*, 2005). Reduced orbitofrontal blood flow predicts panic response to the respiratory stimulant doxapram (Kent *et al.*, 2005), which is consistent with the modulating effect of this area on the amygdala hyperactivity that presumably results from this anxiogenic stimulus.

Finally, a number of studies show abnormalities in GABA, benzodiazepine and serotonin pathways that subserve the two major anti-panic medication classes, SSRIs and benzodiazepines. For the former system, studies have shown reductions in benzodiazepine receptor density in peri-hippocampal and amygdala areas, reductions in cortical GABA at baseline (Goddard *et al.*, 2001), and reduced cortical GABA decreases in response to benzodiazepine challenge (Goddard *et al.*, 2004). For the latter, a recent neuroimaging study showed reductions in $5HT_{1a}$ receptors (Neumeister *et al.*, 2004) consistent with animal knock-out models of this same receptor resulting in pathological anxiety and changes in GABA (Sibille *et al.*, 2000), thereby establishing a link with these two neurochemical systems so relevant to panic.

Psychosocial treatment

Cognitive-behavioural therapy (CBT)

By far the most extensively validated psychotherapeutic treatment for PD is cognitive-behavioral therapy (CBT) in its various forms. The treatment has been subjected to multiple randomized controlled trials and is recommended as a first-line treatment for panic disorder internationally (National Institute for Health and Clinical Excellence (NICE), 2004, American Psychiatric Association guidelines (APA, 1998). Other psychotherapeutic treatments frequently used in clinical practice (insight-oriented therapies, supportive therapies, relaxation training without exposure, hypnosis, eye movement desensitization and reprocessing therapy (EMDR), and stress management) have not found good empirical support and will therefore not be described in detail here.

Two large meta-analyses of CBT for PD found large effect sizes for the treatment of 1.55 and 0.90 (Western & Morrison, 2001; Mitte, 2005). Large percentages of patients are panic-free after a course of CBT (Craske, 1999); one recent long-term follow up found gains maintained after 6–8 years (Kenardy & Dob, 2005). The percentages of patients free of excessive anxiety are also high but somewhat lower than for panic attacks. Gains appear to be maintained or improved after the active treatment phase, and the improvements significantly improve quality of life (Telch *et al.*, 1995). Cognitive-behavioural therapy is also effective when comorbid conditions are present and may, in fact, improve the outcome of the comorbid conditions themselves (Tsao *et al.*, 2002).

CBT is based on both the interoceptive conditioning and cognitive theories reviewed above, and several manuals/treatment protocols exist (Craske, 1999). Treatment is typically conducted individually in 11–16 hour-long sessions, although it has also been adapted for group formats. Elements of CBT for PD emphasize the following components: psychoeducation, cognitive restructuring, interoceptive exposure and in vivo exposure.

Psychoeducation and breathing retraining

In early CBT sessions, patients are taught about panic and anxiety, including their cognitive, behavioral, and physiological attributes. These sessions tend to be quite didactic and accompanied by bibliotherapy. The "fear of fear" model is presented, and the harmless nature of acute panic is emphasized. Breathing retraining is also typically presented early on in treatment. The breathing techniques are taught in order to decrease symptoms of hyperventilation that occur in some PD patients, reduce vulnerability to the phenomenon, and assist patients in developing a self-control technique that can help them cope with anxiety (as opposed to eliminate it). Some data have found this to be useful regardless of whether patients actually hyperventilate or not (Garssen *et al.*, 1992), but others have questioned the necessity of breathing retraining (de Beurs

et al., 1995). Several studies also indicate the effectiveness of applied relaxation techniques as part of an exposure-based CBT package (Arntz & van den Hout, 1996).

Cognitive restructuring

In cognitive restructuring for panic disorder, patients are taught methods of identifying automatic patterns of anxious thinking (for instance, assuming that any elevation of heart rate is dangerous). They also learn two major ways of categorizing and challenging anxiety-based errors in thinking: probability overestimation, or risk inflation (for instance, the likelihood of fainting during a panic attack when one has never fainted before), and catastrophic interpretations (for example, the assumption that fainting during a panic attack would be unmanageable or disastrous). These can be more familiarly referred to as "jumping to conclusions" and "blowing things out of proportion".

Interoceptive exposure and in vivo exposure

Interoceptive exposure refers to the set of techniques used by a CBT therapist to weaken "fear of fear" conditioning, specifically through decreasing the association of specific physiological cues with panic attacks. These physiological cues (elevated heart rate, hyperventilation, dizziness) are elicited in the office. The patient might run in place, breathe through a straw, or spin around the room, for instance, and repeat the experience until anxiety decreases. In vivo exposure targets agoraphobic avoidance. Here, the therapist plans with the patient areas where they will gradually practice eliciting and tolerating their anxiety. For instance, a patient might practise shopping at a previously avoided mall, and then shopping at the mall when it is very crowded. Practice outside the office is always prescribed for both types of exposure, and the emphasis is on the patient learning to experience and tolerate the anxiety.

Pharmacotherapy

Selective serotonin reuptake inhibitors (SSRIs)

The SSRIs are the current medication of choice for PD. Six different agents, fluoxetine, fluvoxamine, sertraline, paroxetine, citalopram and escitalopram, have been shown effective in randomized clinical trials (Roy-Byrne & Cowley, 2002). Meta-analyses/reviews have indicated medium to large effect sizes compared to placebo for several SSRIs (Otto *et al.*, 2001; Boyer, 1995; Mitte, 2005; Bakker *et al.*, 2002), and there is no evidence of differential efficacy within this class of medications. All SSRIs tend to cause an initial dose-related increase in anxiety, so starting doses should be low and built up slowly. Differences do appear in side effect profiles, drug interactions, and half-life. Perhaps the most relevant distinctions, however, are in costs which are driven by availability of the generic forms. The majority of SSRI trials have confirmed efficacy up to 1 year through the use of placebo-controlled discontinuation designs after a period of successful acute treatment (Pollack *et al.*, 2003). Placebo controlled trials also support efficacy for an extended-release form of venlafaxine, an SNRI (Bradwejn *et al.*, 2005). Other second-generation antidepressants have either no evidence for efficacy (duloxetine, mirtazepine, nefazodone) or data suggesting lack of efficacy (trazodone (Charney *et al.*, 1986), buproprion (Sheehan *et al.*, 1983)). The older class of tricyclic antidepressants is less commonly used because of increased side effects (Bakker *et al.*, 2002). However, they are both less expensive and comparably effective. In fact, in cases of SSRI-nonresponse, they may yield beneficial effects. Multiple studies have demonstrated efficacy for imipramine, desipramine, clomipramine, nortriptyline and amitriptyline (Roy-Byrne & Cowley, 2002), and MAO inhibitors were effective in six pre-DSM III studies in panic-like populations ("phobic anxiety") (Roy-Byrne & Cowley, 2002). These older agents, particularly the MAOIs, can be useful in treatment-refractory patients.

Benzodiazepines

The second class of medications for PD are the benzodiazepines. They have a number of advantages: they are very effective, work rapidly, may be even better tolerated than the SSRI class of agents (though systematic comparisons are lacking), and are widely available generically (Bruce *et al.*, 2003). Limitations of benzodiazepines include a more narrow range of efficacy across disorders (PD, GAD and SAD, but no demonstrated efficacy in OCD, PTSD or major depression), the risk of physiological dependence and withdrawal (although apparently without the development of tolerance to the anti-panic effect), and the risk of abuse. This profile has made benzodiazepine use in PD controversial. While the recent NICE guidelines suggest that long term use is contraindicated (NICE, 2004), others suggest that fears about abuse are exaggerated and may limit use of these medications to the disadvantage of patients who would otherwise benefit (APA, 1998). Because many anxious patients do not fully respond to SSRIs, the co-prescription of benzodiazepines is extremely common (Bruce *et al.*, 2003). Co-administration of a benzodiazepine can also be used to more quickly reduce panic during the window of weeks it can take for an SSRI to take effect (Goddard *et al.*, 2001).

Numerous studies show clearly that discontinuation of medication results in relapse in a significant proportion of patients, with placebo-controlled discontinuation studies showing rates between 25% and 50% within 6 months, depending on study design (Roy-Byrne & Cowley, 2002). In addition, SSRIs, SNRIs, TCAs, and benzodiazepines are associated with a time limited withdrawal syndrome (considerably worse for the benzodiazepines (Rickels *et al.*, 1993)), which itself may serve as an interoceptive stimulus that promotes or contributes to panic disorder relapse.

Other issues

Data is limited for other medications for PD. Buspirone (Sheehan *et al.*, 1993) and beta-blockers (Noyes *et al.*, 1984) have not demonstrated efficacy in controlled studies. Other medications with theoretically relevant mechanisms of action (e.g., corticotropin-releasing factor receptor-1 antagonists and glutamate antagonists) are still in development. A major need for the future is research that specifically targets PD that is non-responsive to standard care, as has been done for major depression in the recently published US-based STAR-D trial (Trivedi *et al.*, 2006). While it is common practice to switch agents either within or between antidepressant classes, this has not been evaluated in placebo-controlled trials. Augmenting SSRIs with benzodiazepines, other antidepressants, or even atypical neuroleptics in partial responders has also not been evaluated systematically. In the absence of such data, a course of CBT appears to be the best option for non-responders to pharmacotherapy. A recent study found that nearly two-thirds of non-responders who received a course of CBT met remission criteria. Significant benefits were sustained for up to 1 year and were associated with reductions in medication use (Heldt *et al.*, 2006). In the case of CBT non-response, one controlled study indicated a better response to paroxetine than placebo (Kampman *et al.*, 2002), and another showed paroxetine superior to placebo in augmenting the impact of brief CBT (Stein *et al.*, 2000).

Comparative and combination treatments

A recent review of the literature found clear evidence for CBT-based exposure in extending the treatment effects of medication. However, only modest support appears for adding pharmacotherapy to comprehensive CBT (Smits *et al.*, 2006). It appears that some medications may initially augment the effects of CBT but later detract from them. For instance, a study of the benzodiazepine alprazolam alone or in combination with exposure in patients with PD and agoraphobia revealed that alprazolam marginally improved the effects of exposure in the short term but that, following taper and discontinuation, patients who had received alprazolam with their exposure had worse outcome than patients receiving exposure with a placebo (Marks *et al.*, 1993). Another major multicenter study compared imipramine, CBT, or placebo to combinations of CBT (with imipramine and with placebo) (Barlow *et al.*, 2000). At 6 months, the combination of imipramine and CBT was marginally superior to either treatment alone at 6 months (consistent with prior reports of the superiority of combined treatment in more complicated panic) (Telch & Lucas, 1994). Following discontinuation, however, patients receiving the CBT plus imipramine combination were somewhat worse. One hypothesis is that attributions and state- (or context)-dependent learning that occurs when treatments are combined might attenuate the new learning that would otherwise cause sustained benefit in CBT (Smits *et al.*, 2006).

Once active treatment is discontinued, CBT effects are generally more durable than those of medication, as reflected in recent NICE guidelines (NICE, 2004). Meta-analyses show that cognitive-behavioral treatments yield larger mean effect sizes (averaging over all dependent variables) (ES = 0.88–0.90) than either antidepressants (ES = 0.40–0.55) or benzodiazapines (ES = 0.40). However, patient samples might not be comparable across these studies (Mitte, 2005; Craske, 1999). It is not yet clear from the current evidence base, then, whether most patients with PD should begin with medication, CBT, or combination treatment. It does seem clear, however, that adding CBT at some point in the treatment of PD is likely to optimize long-term positive impact.

Treatment delivery challenges

Unfortunately, typical treatment delivery does not often include CBT. The approach is widely under utilized in the United States, especially when compared to medications (Young *et al.*, 2001). While there seems to be increased interest in the application of CBT for anxiety and depression in the UK (Bower & Gilbody, 2005), CBT is under utilized there as well (Bebbington *et al.*, 2000). Low rates of use are likely due to the public's unfamiliarity with its nature and efficacy relative to medication, limited access to specialty mental health treatment, and limited training/ proficiency with CBT on the part of many mental health professionals who currently treat PD patients.

Furthermore, most patients with PD receive care in the primary care setting (Roy-Byrne *et al.*, 1999), where it is associated with significant disability and work

impairment even when accounting for the impact of comorbid physical and depressive illness (Pignone *et al.*, 2002). Typically patients perceive PD to be a physical ailment, and as such go to their physician or to the emergency room when symptoms arise (Roy-Byrne *et al.*, 1999). The difficulty with diagnosis in this setting provides a strong argument for more population-based screening efforts in primary care (Roy-Byrne *et al.*, 2000), similar to current recommendations for major depression (Pignone *et al.*, 2002). Perhaps more compelling is the fact that only 19%–40% of primary care patients receive minimally acceptable levels of evidence-based treatment (Young *et al.*, 2001; Stein *et al.*, 2004). Many difficulties have contributed to the state of affairs. In addition to detection/ diagnosis difficulties, there is widespread uncertainty about where to seek help. The primary care system is still insufficiently organized to treat chronic disease, and, at least in the USA, problems with insurance coverage and concerns about cost of care compound the problem (Craske *et al.*, 2005).

To overcome these barriers, there is increasing interest in adapting treatments to primary care. Emerging evidence indicates that models emphasizing a primary role for the primary care physician but with added support from a mental health provider to deliver medications (effect sizes 0.42–0.69) (Roy-Byrne *et al.*, 2001), managed care in general (Rollman *et al.*, 2003), and/or to provide CBT specifically adapted for that setting are effective (effect sizes 0.23–0.51) (Roy-Byrne *et al.*, 2005), and cost-effective (Katon *et al.*, 2006). Other promising approaches that may supplement care provided by PCPs, or that may serve as stand-alone approaches for some patients, include the use of self-help treatments for which computer (web-based) delivery approaches are being increasingly proposed (Proudfoot *et al.*, 2004).

Several reports of computer or internet-assisted treatments for PD have emerged in the past few years (Barlow *et al.*, 2005) including several comparisons to traditional CBT. One randomized trial compared 10 weekly sessions of CBT to 10 modules of a web-based self-help program which included email interactions with a therapist (Carlbring *et al.*, 2005). Results indicated that the treatments were comparable in efficacy, although there were slight advantages to the live CBT. Marks and colleagues (Marks *et al.*, 2004) compared patients with phobia or panic disorder who were randomized to exposure therapy guided by a clinician or mainly by a computer system with a computer-guided relaxation condition (included as a placebo). In this study, the two exposure treatments showed comparable improvement and satisfaction post-treatment and at follow-up one month later, while the relaxation treatment was associated with low efficacy and satisfaction. However, it had lower dropout rates than the clinician-assisted or computer-assisted exposure treatments (6, 24, and 43%, respectively). The authors estimate that the computer condition cut clinician time per patient by 73%. A multi-site, randomized trial by Kenardy and colleagues (Kenardy *et al.*, 2003) compared standard (12 sessions) and brief (6 sessions) therapist delivered CBT, a computer augmented CBT protocol (6 sessions) and a wait-list control condition. Unlike a previous report, (Clark *et al.*, 1999) the outcome for the 12-session CBT was significantly better than the 6-session CBT. While the outcomes for the computer-augmented treatment were in between the 12 and 6 session therapist-delivered conditions, it did not differ statistically from either. At a 6-month follow up, none of the active treatments were statistically distinct. While more research is clearly needed, these trials are a very promising beginning and point to the possibilities of adding computer or internet-assisted treatment into primary care.

Prevention

Unfortunately, only a handful of studies to date have evaluated prevention. One ER-based study found benefits for a brief exposure instruction as compared to a reassurance condition. All recipients randomized to the exposure group showed benefits on measures of panic/anxiety 6 months later (no improvements were found in the reassurance group) (Swinson *et al.*, 1992). Another study examined undergraduates who reported having at least one panic attack in the past year and moderate anxiety sensitivity. The students were randomized to either a wait-list or a CBT workshop (Gardenswarz & 2001). At 6-month follow-up, 1.8% of the intervention group had developed panic disorder compared to 13.6% in the wait-list group. Another study targeted undergraduates who were high on a measure of anxiety sensitivity, a risk factor for PD; they were randomly assigned to a 6-week internet-based intervention or a wait-list control. Positive outcomes for the intervention group included anxiety-related cognitions and depression, but only a trend towards decreases in anxiety sensitivity, and treatment gains continued at a 6-month follow up (Kenardy & Rosa, 2006).

Hopefully, large-scale prevention efforts will increase in the future. Research in this area should prioritize improvement of detection and identification of at-risk populations. Other prevention efforts for children at risk for anxiety disorders more generally have been promising, and suggest that earlier interventions may be key (Barrett & Farrell, 2005).

Conclusions

Panic disorder has many different treatment approaches. SSRIs and/or CBT, most often presented in a package combined with psychoeducation, cognitive restructuring and exposure, are considered first line approaches with large effect sizes. These treatments can lead to the prevention of the attacks rather than to the treatment of the attacks if and when they occur. This can then minimize the 'fear-of-fear', which may be the main route to the significant impairment associated with this disorder.

The level of evidence for each of the interventions discussed in this chapter is summarized in Table 32.1.

Table 32.1. Effectiveness of treatments for panic disorder

Treatment	Form of treatment	Psychiatric disorder	Level of evidence for efficacy	Comments
Psychotherapy	Cognitive-behavioural therapy (CBT) 10–16 sessions, but with some studies demonstrating efficacy with fewer sessions	Panic disorder with and without agoraphobia	Ia	Undoubtedly as effective as medications. May be slightly more effective long-term if medication is discontinued. First-line treatment
Psychopharmacology	Selective serotonin reuptake inhibitors (SSRIs) Standard doses but start with lower doses to avoid initial increase in anxiety	Panic disorder with and without agoraphobia	Ia	Undoubtedly effective. First-line treatment

Table 32.1. (cont.)

Treatment	Form of treatment	Psychiatric disorder	Level of evidence for efficacy	Comments
Psychopharmacology	Tricyclic antidepressants (TCAs) Standard antidepressant doses but starting with lower doses	Panic disorder with and without agoraphobia	Ia	Undoubtedly effective. Increased and more uncomfortable side effects compared to SSRIs
Psychopharmacology	Benzodiazepines 2–4 mg alprazolam equivalents	Panic disorder with and without agoraphobia	Ia	Undoubtedly effective. Some risk of physiologic dependence/withdrawal/abuse. Greater chance of abuse in those with substance abuse history. Cognitive impairment can occur
Psychotherapy plus Psychopharmacology	Combined CBT and SSRIs	Panic disorder with and without agoraphobia	Ia	Undoubtedly effective but more information needed on persistence of benefit compared to CBT alone
Computer assisted or delivered CBT	Computer-assisted delivery of CBT; recommended dose is not yet established	Panic disorder with and without agoraphobia	Ib	Probably efficacious. Efficacy compared to therapist-delivered CBT needs further study

REFERENCES

American Psychiatric Association (APA) (1994). *DSM-IV Diagnostic and Statistical Manual of Mental Disorders*, 4th edn. Washington, DC: American Psychiatric Association.

American Psychiatric Association (APA) (1998). Practice guideline for the treatment of patients with panic disorder. Work Group on Panic Disorder. American Psychiatric Association. *American Journal of Psychiatry*, **155**(5 Suppl), 1–34.

Arntz, A. & van den Hout, M. (1996). Psychological treatments of panic disorder without agoraphobia: cognitive therapy versus applied relaxation. *Behaviour Research Therapy*, **34**(2), 113–21.

Aschenbrand, S. G., Kendall, P. C., Webb, A., Safford, S. M. & Flannery-Schroeder, E. (2003). Is childhood separation anxiety disorder a predictor of adult panic disorder and agoraphobia? A seven-year longitudinal study. *Journal of the American Academy of Child and Adolescent Psychiatry*, **42**(12), 1478–85.

Bakker, A., van Balkom, A. J. & Spinhoven, P. (2002). SSRIs vs. TCAs in the treatment of panic disorder: a meta-analysis. *Acta Psychiatrica Scandinavica*, **106**(3), 163–7.

Barlow, D. H. (1988). *Anxiety and its Disorders: The Nature and Treatment of Anxiety and Panic*. New York, NY: Guilford Press.

Barlow, D. H. (2002). *Anxiety and its Disorders: The Nature and Treatment of Anxiety and Panic*. New York, NY: Guilford Press.

Barlow, D. H., Gorman, J. M., Shear, M. K. & Woods, S. W. (2000). Cognitive-behavioral therapy, imipramine, or their combination for panic disorder: a randomized controlled trial. *Journal of the American Medical Association*, **283**(19), 2529–36.

Barlow, J. H., Ellard, D. R., Hainsworth, J. M., Jones, F. R. & Fisher, A. (2005). A review of self-management interventions for panic disorders, phobias and obsessive-compulsive disorders. *Acta Psychiatrica Scandinavica*, **111**(4), 272–85.

Barrett, P. M. L., Lock, S. & Farrell, J. (2005). Developmental differences in universal preventive intervention for child anxiety. *Clinical Child Psychology and Psychiatry*, **10**(4), 539–55.

Bebbington, P. E., Brugha, T. S., Meltzer, H. *et al.* (2000). Neurotic disorders and the receipt of psychiatric treatment. *Psychological Medicine*, **30**(6), 1369–76.

Biederman, J., Faraone, S. V., Marrs, A. *et al.* (1997). Panic disorder and agoraphobia in consecutively referred children and adolescents. *Journal of the American Academy of Child and Adolescent Psychiatry*, **36**(2), 214–23.

Biederman, J., Petty, C., Faraone, S. V. *et al.* (2005). Parental predictors of pediatric panic disorder/agoraphobia: a controlled study in high-risk offspring. *Depression and Anxiety*, **22**(3), 114–20.

Bienvenu, O. J., Onyike, C. U., Stein, M. B. *et al.* (2006). Agoraphobia in general population adults: incidence and longitudinal relationships with panic, with clinical reappraisal. *British Journal of Psychiatry*, **188**, 432–8.

Block, R. I., Ghoneim, M. M., Fowles, D. C., Kumar, V. & Pathak, D. (1987). Effects of a subanesthetic concentration of nitrous oxide on establishment, elicitation, and semantic and phonemic generalization of classically conditioned skin conductance responses. *Pharmacological and Biochemical Behaviour*, **28**(1), 7–14.

Bouton, M. E., Mineka, S. & Barlow, D. H. (2001). A modern learning theory perspective on the etiology of panic disorder. *Psychological Review*, **108**(1), 4–32.

Bower, P. & Gilbody, S. (2005). Stepped care in psychological therapies: access, effectiveness and efficiency. Narrative literature review. *British Journal of Psychiatry*, **186**, 11–17.

Boyer, W. (1995). Serotonin uptake inhibitors are superior to imipramine and alprazolam in alleviating panic attacks: a meta-analysis. *International Clinical Psychopharmacology*, **10**(1), 45–9.

Bradwejn, J., Ahokas, A., Stein, D. J., Salinas, E., Emilien, G. & Whitaker, T. (2005). Venlafaxine extended-release capsules in panic disorder: flexible-dose, double-blind, placebo-controlled study. *British Journal of Psychiatry*, **187**, 352–9.

Bruce, S. E., Vasile, R. G., Goisman, R. M. *et al.* (2003). Are benzodiazepines still the medication of choice for patients with panic disorder with or without agoraphobia? *American Journal of Psychiatry*, **160**(8), 1432–8.

Bruce, S. E., Yonkers, K. A., Otto, M. W. *et al.* (2005). Influence of psychiatric comorbidity on recovery and recurrence in generalized anxiety disorder, social phobia, and panic disorder: a 12-year prospective study. *American Journal of Psychiatry*, **162**(6), 1179–87.

Carlbring, P., Nilsson-Ihrfelt, E., Waara, J. *et al.* (2005). Treatment of panic disorder: live therapy vs. self-help via the Internet. *Behavior Research Therapy*, **43**(10), 1321–33.

Charney, D. S., Woods, S. W., Goodman, W. K. *et al.* (1986). Drug treatment of panic disorder: the comparative efficacy of imipramine, alprazolam, and trazodone. *Journal of Clinical Psychiatry*, **47**(12), 580–6.

Clark, D. M. (1986). A cognitive approach to panic. *Behaviour Research Therapy*, **24**(4), 461–70.

Clark, D. M., Salkovskis, P. M., Gelder, M. *et al.* (1988). Test of a cognitive theory of panic. In *Panic and Phobias II: Treatments and Variables Affecting Course and Outcome*, ed. I. Hand & H. V. Wittchen, pp. 71–90. Berlin: Springer-Verlag.

Clark, D. M., Salkovskis, P. M., Hackmann, A., Wells, A., Ludgate, J. & Gelder, M. (1999). Brief cognitive therapy for panic disorder: a randomised controlled trial. *Journal of Consulting and Clinical Psychology*, **67**, 583–9.

Craske, M. G. (1999). *Anxiety Disorders: Psychological Approaches to Theory and Treatment*. Boulder, CO: Westview Press.

Craske, M. G., Lang, A. J., Rowe, M. *et al.* (2002). Presleep attributions about arousal during sleep: nocturnal panic. *Journal of Abnormal Psychology*, **111**(1), 53–62.

Craske, M. G., Edlund, M. J., Sullivan, G. *et al.* (2005). Perceived unmet need for mental health treatment and barriers to care among patients with panic disorder. *Psychiatric Services*, **56**(8), 988–94.

de Beurs, E., Lange, A., van Dyck, R. & Koele, P. (1995). Respiratory training prior to exposure in vivo in the treatment of panic disorder with agoraphobia: efficacy and predictors of outcome. *Australian and N Z Journal of Psychiatry*, **29**(1), 104–13.

Gardenswarz, C. & Craske, M. (2001). Prevention of panic. *Behavior Therapy*, **32**, 725–38.

Garssen, C. & Van Dyck, R. (1992). Breathing retraining: a rational placebo? *Clinical Psychology Review*, **12**(2), 141–53.

Goddard, A. W., Brouette, T., Almai, A., Jetty, P., Woods, S. W. & Charney, D. (2001). Early coadministration of clonazepam with sertraline for panic disorder. *Archives of General Psychiatry*, **58**(7), 681–6.

Goddard, A. W., Mason, G. F., Almai, A. *et al.* (2001). Reductions in occipital cortex GABA levels in panic disorder detected with 1h-magnetic resonance spectroscopy. *Archives in General Psychiatry*, **58**(6), 556–61.

Goddard, A. W., Mason, G. F., Appel, M. *et al.* (2004). Impaired GABA neuronal response to acute benzodiazepine administration in panic disorder. *American Journal of Psychiatry*, **161**(12), 2186–93.

Goisman, R. M., Goldenberg, I., Vasile, R. G. & Keller, M. B. (1995). Comorbidity of anxiety disorders in a multicenter anxiety study. *Comparative Psychiatry*, **36**(4), 303–11.

Goodwin, R. D. & Hoven, C. W. (2002). Bipolar-panic comorbidity in the general population: prevalence and associated morbidity. *Journal of Affective Disorders*, **70**(1), 27–33.

Gorman, J. M., Kent, J. M., Sullivan, G. M. & Coplan, J. D. (2000). Neuroanatomical hypothesis of panic disorder, revised. *American Journal of Psychiatry*, **157**(4), 493–505.

Gould, R. A., Otto, M. & Pollack, M. (1995). A meta-analysis of treatment outcome for panic disorder. *Clinical Psychology Review*, **15**, 819–44.

Greenberg, P. E., Sisitsky, T., Kessler, R. C. *et al.* (1999). The economic burden of anxiety disorders in the 1990s. *Journal of Clinical Psychiatry*, **60**(7), 427–35.

Heldt, E. M., Gisele G., Kipper, L., Blaya, C., Isolan, L. & Otto, M. W. (2006). One-year follow-up of pharmacotherapy-resistant patients with panic disorder treated with cognitive-behavior therapy: Outcome and predictors of remission. *Behaviour Research and Therapy*, **44**(5), 657–65.

Hope, D. A., Rapee, R. M., Heimberg, R. G. & Dombeck, M. J. (1990). Representations of the self in social phobia: vulnerability to social threat. *Cognitive Therapy and Research*, **14**(2), 177–89.

Isensee, B., Wittchen, H. U., Stein, M. B., Hofler, M. & Lieb, R. (2003). Smoking increases the risk of panic: findings from a prospective community study. *Archives in General Psychiatry*, **60**(7), 692–700.

Jacob, R. G., Furman, J. M., Clark, D. B. & Durrant, J. D. (1992). Vestibular symptoms, panic, and phobia: overlap and possible relationships. *Annals of Clinical Psychiatry*, **4**(3), 163–74.

Kampman, M., Keijsers, G. P. J., Hoogduin, C. A. L. & Hendriks, G.-J. (2002). A randomized, double-blind, placebo-controlled study of the effects of adjunctive paroxetine in panic disorder patients unsuccessfully treated with cognitive-behavioral therapy alone. *Journal of Clinical Psychiatry*, **63**(9), 772–7.

Katon, W., Russo, J., Sherbourne, C. *et al.* (2006). Incremental cost-effectiveness of a collaborative care intervention for panic disorder. *Psychological Medicine*, **36**(3), 353–63.

Katschnig, H. & Amering, M. (1998). The long-term course of panic disorder and its predictors. *Journal of Clinical Psychopharmacology*, **18**(6 Suppl. 2), 6S–11S.

Kenardy, J. A., Dow, M. G., Johnston, D. W., Newman, M. G., Thomson, A. & Taylor, C. B. (2003). A comparison of delivery methods of cognitive-behavioral therapy for panic disorder: an international multicenter trial. *Journal of Consulting and Clinical Psychology*, **71**(6), 1068–75.

Kenardy, J. R. S. & Dob, R. (2005) Cognitive behaviour therapy for panic disorder: long-term follow-up. *Cognitive Behaviour Therapy*, **34**(2), 75–8.

Kenardy, J. M. K. & Rosa, V. (2006). Internet-delivered indicated prevention for anxiety disorders: six-month follow-up. *Clinical Psychologist*, **10**(1), 39–42.

Kendler, K. S. (2005). "A gene for" the nature of gene action in psychiatric disorders. *American Journal of Psychiatry*, **162**(7), 1243–52.

Kent, J. M. & Rauch, S. L. (2003). Neurocircuitry of anxiety disorders. *Current Psychiatry Reports*, **5**(4), 266–73.

Kent, J. M., Coplan, J. D., Mawlawi, O. *et al.* (2005). Prediction of panic response to a respiratory stimulant by reduced orbitofrontal cerebral blood flow in panic disorder. *American Journal of Psychiatry*, **162**(7), 1379–81.

Kessler, R., Stang, P., Wittchen, H., Ustun, B., Roy-Byrne, P. & Walters, E. (1998). Lifetime panic-depression comorbidity in the national comorbidity survey. *Archives of General Psychiatry*, **55**, 801–8.

Kessler, R. C., Berglund, P., Demler, O., Jin, R., Merikangas, K. R. and Walters, E. E. (2005a). Lifetime prevalence and age-of-onset distributions of DSM-IV disorders in the National Comorbidity Survey Replication. *Archives in General Psychiatry*, **62**(6), 593–602.

Kessler, R. C., Chiu, W. T., Demler, O., Merikangas, K. R. & Walters, E. E. (2005b). Prevalence, severity, and comorbidity of 12-month DSM-IV disorders in the National Comorbidity Survey Replication. *Archives in General Psychiatry*, **62**(6), 617–27.

Kessler, R. C., Chiu, W. T., Jin, R., Ruscio, A. M., Shear, K. & Walters, E. E. (2006). The Epidemiology of Panic Attacks, Panic Disorder, and Agoraphobia in the National Comorbidity Survey Replication. *Archives of General Psychiatry*, **63**, 415–24.

Krystal, J. H., Deutsch, D. N. & Charney, D. S. (1996). The biological basis of panic disorder. *Journal of Clinical Psychiatry*, **57** (Suppl. 10), 23–31; discussion 32–3.

McNally, R. J. (2002). Anxiety sensitivity and panic disorder. *Biological Psychiatry*, **52**(10), 938–46.

Marks, I. M., Swinson, R. P., Basoglu, M. *et al.* (1993). Alprazolam and exposure alone and combined in panic disorder with agoraphobia. A controlled study in London and Toronto. *British Journal of Psychiatry*, **162**, 776–87.

Marks, I. M., Kenwright, M., McDonough, M., Whittaker, M. & Mataix-Cols, D. (2004). Saving clinicians' time by delegating routine aspects of therapy to a computer: a randomized controlled trial in phobia/panic disorder. *Psychological Medicine*, **34**(1), 9–17.

Massana, G., Gasto, C., Junque, C. *et al.* (2002). Reduced levels of creatine in the right medial temporal lobe region of panic disorder patients detected with (1)H magnetic resonance spectroscopy. *Neuroimage*, **16**(3 Pt 1), 836–42.

Massana, G., Serra-Grabulosa, J. M., Salgado-Pineda, P. *et al.* (2003). Amygdala atrophy in panic disorder patients detected by volumetric magnetic resonance imaging. *Neuroimage*, **19**(1), 80–90.

Mitte, K. (2005). A meta-analysis of the efficacy of psycho- and pharmacotherapy in panic disorder with and without agoraphobia. *Journal of Affective Disorders*, **88**(1), 27–45.

Neumeister, A., Bain, E., Nugent, A. C. *et al.* (2004). Reduced serotonin type 1A receptor binding in panic disorder. *Journal of Neuroscience*, **24**(3), 589–91.

NICE (2004). Anxiety: management of anxiety (panic disorder, with or without agoraphobia, and generalised anxiety disorder) in adults in primary, secondary and community care. London: National Collaborating Centre for Primary Care. (www.nice.org.uk/CG022fullguideline)

Norton, C. R., Cox, B. J. & Malan, J. (1992). Nonclinical panickers: a critical review. *Clinical Psychology Review*, **12**, 121–39.

Noyes, R., Jr, Anderson, D. J., Clancy, J. *et al.* (1984). Diazepam and propranolol in panic disorder and agoraphobia. *Archives in General Psychiatry*, **41**(3), 287–92.

Otto, M. W., Tuby, K. S., Gould, R. A., McLean, R. Y. & Pollack, M. H. (2001). An effect-size analysis of the relative efficacy and tolerability of serotonin selective reuptake inhibitors for panic disorder. *American Journal of Psychiatry*, **158**(12), 1989–92.

Pignone, M. P., Gaynes, B. N., Rushton, J. L. *et al.* (2002). Screening for depression in adults: a summary of the evidence for the U.S. Preventive Services Task Force. *Annales of Internal Medicine*, **136**(10), 765–76.

Pitts, F. N., Jr. & McClure, J. N., Jr (1967). Lactate metabolism in anxiety neurosis. *New England Journal of Medicine*, **277**(25), 1329–36.

Pollack, M. H., Allgulander, C., Bandelow, B. *et al.* (2003). WCA recommendations for the long-term treatment of panic disorder. *CNS Spectrums*, **8**(8 (Suppl. 1), 17–30.

Proudfoot, J., Ryden, C., Everitt, B. *et al.* (2004). Clinical efficacy of computerised cognitive-behavioural therapy for anxiety and depression in primary care: randomised controlled trial. *British Journal of Psychiatry*, **185**, 46–54.

Reiss, S. (1980). Pavlovian conditioning and human fear: an expectancy model. *Behavior Therapy*, **11**(3), 380–96.

Rickels, K., Schweizer, E., Weiss, S. & Zavodnick, S. (1993). Maintenance drug treatment for panic disorder. II. Short- and long-term outcome after drug taper. *Archives of General Psychiatry*, **50**(1), 61–8.

Rollman, B. L., Belnap, B. H., Reynolds, C. F., Schulberg, H. C. & Shear, M. K. (2003). A contemporary protocol to assist primary care physicians in the treatment of panic and generalized anxiety disorders. *General Hospital Psychiatry*, **25**, 74–82.

Rosenbaum, J. F., Biederman, J., Hirshfeld-Becker, D. R. *et al.* (2000). A controlled study of behavioral inhibition in children of parents with panic disorder and depression. *American Journal of Psychiatry*, **157**(12), 2002–10.

Roth, M. (1984). Agoraphobia, panic disorder and generalized anxiety disorder: some implications of recent advances. *Psychiatric Developments*, **2**(1), 31–52.

Roy-Byrne, P. P. & Cowley, D. S. (1995). Course and outcome in panic disorder: A review of recent follow-up studies. *Anxiety*, **1**, 151–60.

Roy-Byrne, P. P., & Cowley, D. (2002). Pharamcologic treatments for panic disorder, generalized anxiety disorder, specific phobia and social anxiety disorders. In *A Guide to Treatments that*

Work, ed. P. E. Nathan and J. Gorman, pp. 337–65. New York: Oxford University Press.

Roy-Byrne, P. P., Geraci, M. & Uhde, T. W. (1986). Life events and the onset of panic disorder. *American Journal of Psychiatry*, **143**(11), 1424–7.

Roy-Byrne, P. P., Stein, M. B., Russo, J. *et al.* (1999). Panic disorder in the primary care setting: comorbidity, disability, service utilization, and treatment. *Journal of Clinical Psychiatry*, **60**(7), 492–9.

Roy-Byrne, P. P., Katon, W., Cowley, D. S. *et al.* (2000). Panic disorder in primary care: Biopsychosocial differences between recognized and unrecognized patients. *General Hospital Psychiatry*, **22**, 405–11.

Roy-Byrne, P. P., Katon, W. J., Cowley, D. S. & Russo, J. (2001). A randomized trial of collaborative care for patients with panic disorder in primary care. *Archives of General Psychiatry*, **58**, 869–76.

Roy-Byrne, P. P., Craske, M. G., Stein, M. B. *et al.* (2005). A randomized effectiveness trial of cognitive-behavioral therapy and medication for primary care panic disorder. *Archives of General Psychiatry*, **62**(3), 290–8.

Roy-Byrne, P. P., Craske, M. G. & Stein, M. B. (2006). Panic disorder. *Lancet*, **368**, 1023–32.

Sakai, Y., Kumano, H., Nishikawa, M. *et al.* (2005). Cerebral glucose metabolism associated with a fear network in panic disorder. *Neuroreport*, **16**(9), 927–31.

Sheehan, D. V., Davidson, J., Manschreck, T. & Van Wyck Fleet, J. (1983). Lack of efficacy of a new antidepressant (bupropion) in the treatment of panic disorder with phobias. *Journal of Clinical Psychopharmacology*, **3**(1), 28–31.

Sheehan, D. V., Raj, A. B., Harnett-Sheehan, K., Soto, S. & Knapp, E. (1993). The relative efficacy of high-dose buspirone and alprazolam in the treatment of panic disorder: a double-blind placebo-controlled study. *Acta Psychiatrica Scandinavica*, **88**(1), 1–11.

Sibille, E., Pavlides, C., Benke, D. & Toth, M. (2000). Genetic inactivation of the Serotonin(1A) receptor in mice results in downregulation of major GABA(A) receptor alpha subunits, reduction of GABA(A) receptor binding, and benzodiazepine-resistant anxiety. *Journal of Neuroscience*, **20**(8), 2758–65.

Smits, J. A. J. O. C., Conall, M. & Otto, M. W. (2006). Combining cognitive-behavioral therapy and pharmacotherapy for the treatment of panic disorder. *Journal of Cognitive Psychotherapy*, **20**(1), 75–84.

Stein, M. B., Walker, J. R., Anderson, G. *et al.* (1996). Childhood physical and sexual abuse in patients with anxiety disorders and in a community sample. *American Journal of Psychiatry*, **153**(2), 275–7.

Stein, M. B., Norton, G. R., Walker, J. R., Chartier, M. J. & Graham, R. (2000). Do SSRIs enhance the efficacy of very brief cognitive behavioral therapy for panic disorder? A pilot study. *Psychiatry Research*, **94**, 191–200.

Stein, M. B., Sherbourne, C. D., Craske, M. G. *et al.* (2004). Quality of care for primary care patients with anxiety disorders. *American Journal of Psychiatry*, **161**(12), 2230–7.

Swinson, R. P., Soulios, C., Cox, B. J. & Kuch, K. (1992). Brief treatment of emergency room patients with panic attacks. *American Journal of Psychiatry*, **149**(7), 944–6.

Telch, M. & Lucas, R. (1994). Combined pharmacological and psychological treatment of panic disorder: current status and future directions. In *Treatment of Panic/Disorder: A Consensus Development Conference*. American Psychiatric Press.

Telch, M. J., Schmidt, N. B., Jaimez, T. L., Jacquin, K. M. & Harrington, P. J. (1995). Impact of cognitive-behavioral treatment on quality of life in panic disorder patients. *Journal of Consulting Clinical Psychology*, **63**(5), 823–30.

Trivedi, M., Fava, M., Wisniewski, S. R. *et al.* (2006). Augmentation after the Failure of SSRIs for Depression. *New England Journal of Medicine*, **354**(12), 1243–52.

Tsao, J. C. I., Mystkowski, J., Zucker, B. & Craske, M. G. (2002). Effects of cognitive-behavioral therapy for panic disorder on comorbid conditions: replication and extension. *Behavior Therapy*, **33**, 493–509.

Uchida, R. R., Del-Ben, C. M., Santos, A. C. *et al.* (2003). Decreased left temporal lobe volume of panic patients measured by magnetic resonance imaging. *Brazilian Journal of Medical and Biological Research*, **36**(7), 925–9.

Wang, P. S., Berglund, P. & Kessler, R. C. (2000). Recent care of common mental disorders in the United States: prevalence and conformance with evidence-based recommendations. *Journal of General Internal Medicine*, **15**(5), 284–92.

Watanabe, A., Nakao, K., Tokuyama, M. & Takeda, M. (2005). Prediction of first episode of panic attack among white-collar workers. *Psychiatry and Clinical Neuroscience*, **59**(2), 119–26.

Westen, D. & Morrison, K. (2001). A multidimensional meta-analysis of treatments for depression, panic, and generalized anxiety disorder: an empirical examination of the status of empirically supported therapies. *Journal of Consulting Clinical Psychology*, **69**(6), 875–99.

Wittchen, H. U., Reed, V. & Kessler, R. C. (1998). The relationship of agoraphobia and panic in a community sample of adolescents and young adults. *Archives of General Psychiatry*, **55**(11), 1017–24.

Young, A. S., Klap, R., Sherbourne, C. D. & Wells, K. B. (2001). The quality of care for depressive and anxiety disorders in the United States. *Archives of General Psychiatry*, **58**(1), 55–61.

Zimmermann, P., Wittchen, H. U., Hofler, M., Pfister, H., Kessler, R. C. & Lieb, R. (2003). Primary anxiety disorders and the development of subsequent alcohol use disorders: a 4-year community study of adolescents and young adults. *Psychological Medicine*, **33**(7), 1211–22.

33

Specific phobias and agoraphobia

Sonya B. Norman and Ariel J. Lang

Editor's note

It is pleasant to note that in this short chapter the most common psychiatric disorder, specific phobia, can be effectively treated, often with as little as one session of exposure therapy, so effectively giving the lie to the common belief that, once affected with mental illness, recovery is rare. Because the evidence for this simple behavioural intervention is so strong, other treatments almost become redundant, with only blood phobias being treated successfully in a novel way, although at present the evidence base is a little limited. Agoraphobia without panic is an interesting condition that is somewhat similar to avoidant personality disorder; the absence of panic allows coping strategies to be developed that allow adjustment to the phobic symptoms and preclude the need to seek help, although as the authors note, this is often at the expense of significant impairment in relationships. It is also worth noting that these conditions have no evidence base for drug treatment and thereby occupy an almost unique position in this book, and the absence of competing claims from other forms of management make the recommendations in the evidence table below absolutely unequivocal.

Introduction

Specific phobia (formerly known as simple phobia) and agoraphobia are prevalent and disabling psychiatric disorders. Individuals with specific phobia have a persistent, excessive, and unreasonable fear of a particular object or situation. The feared stimulus is often something that commonly evokes some fear or disgust, for example, small, enclosed places, open wounds or tarantulas. In the individual with specific phobia, however, the fear response is excessive, the feared stimulus is avoided or

endured with great distress, and the fear causes significant interference in functioning. Although specific phobia is among the most prevalent of any psychiatric disorders (Kessler et al., 2005; Regier et al., 1998; Iancu et al., 2006), it is also one of the least studied (Norton et al., 1995). The treatments available, however, are some of the most effective. Patients can be treated successfully in as little as one session. In this chapter, we review treatments for specific phobias that have received support through meta-analysis and randomized, controlled trials (RCTs).

Agoraphobia is most commonly associated with panic disorder. It has traditionally been held that agoraphobia develops as a response to spontaneous panic, but new evidence suggests that agoraphobia not only occurs with some regularity without a history of panic (Andrews & Slade, 2006) but also predicts the development of panic disorder (Bienvenu et al., 2006). Based on this, it has been argued that agoraphobia should be viewed as a stand-alone diagnostic entity (Bienvenu et al., 2006). Agoraphobia is associated with significant impairment and disability (Sareen et al., 2006). It is also a source of increased medical costs because agoraphobic patients have higher than average rates of medical utilization (Swinson et al., 1992), which may be offset, however, by successful treatment (Roberge et al., 2005). The chapter by Welch et al. presents a review of treatment of panic disorder with agoraphobia (PDA). This chapter focuses on treatment issues specific to agoraphobia and on agoraphobia without a history of panic disorder (AWP).

Prevalence and public health impact

Specific phobia (SP)

The 12-month prevalence rate of specific phobia among adults in the US has been estimated at 8.7% and 9.9%

(Kessler *et al.*, 2005; Regier *et al.*, 1998). Similar prevalence rates were found among Swedish children (Lichtenstein & Annas, 2000). Among European adults, reported rates are lower, 3.5% for the past 12 months and 8% for lifetime (Alonso *et al.*, 2004). However, in both the USA and Europe, rates of specific phobia tend to be higher than those of other psychiatric disorders (Kessler *et al.*, 2005; Regier *et al.*, 1998; Iancu *et al.*, 2006). Specific phobia is frequently comorbid with social anxiety disorder (Iancu *et al.*, 2006), substance use disorders (Sareen *et al.*, 2006), and depression (Bittner *et al.*, 2004). Having a specific phobia in childhood may be a risk factor for developing an eating disorder (Kaye *et al.*, 2004). The disorder is associated with a high number of work loss days (Alonso *et al.*, 2004) and, among medical patients, a high level of disability (Sareen *et al.*, 2006). However, the data suggest that specific phobias are less impairing than other anxiety disorders (Mataix-Cols *et al.*, 2006) and associated with smaller (although still significant) reductions in life satisfaction (Meyer *et al.*, 2004). The mean duration of specific phobia is 24.5 years, longer than that of most psychiatric disorders. (Meyer *et al.*, 2004).

Agoraphobia

The prevalence of and demographic risk factors for PDA have been discussed by Welch and colleagues in this volume. Many studies do not produce estimates of AWP, so the prevalence of this condition is less well established. The 12-month rate of AWP ranged from 0.1%–3.1% in a review of European epidemiological studies (Goodwin *et al.*, 2005) and was recently estimated at 0.5% and 0.8% in two US samples. (Kessler *et al.*, 2005; Hand, 2000; Wittchen *et al.*, 1998). Because agoraphobia has been so closely linked to panic, some structured interviews instruct the interviewer to skip out when panic is not endorsed. This may have led to underestimates of the true prevalence of AWP. Estimates are higher when interviews are specifically designed to assess AWP. For example, Wittchen and colleagues (Wittchen *et al.*, 1998) found a 12-month prevalence of 2.8% endorsing only one prototypical triggering situation and 1.4% endorsing two or more triggering situations.

Agoraphobia itself is impairing and disabling, but it also increases the risk of other mental health problems. Agoraphobia increases the risk of developing major depression (Bittner *et al.*, 2004). As compared to individuals with no anxiety disorder, patients with agoraphobia without a history of panic disorder (AWP) have four times the odds of having had lifetime suicidal ideation and five times the odds of having made a suicide attempt in their lifetime (Sareen *et al.*, 2005).

Clinical features

Specific phobias

Individuals with specific phobia have a persistent, excessive and unreasonable fear of a specific object or situation. Anticipation of exposure to the feared stimulus and actual exposure both cause immediate onset of anxiety, which may include panic attacks. To meet DSM-IV criteria for a diagnosis of specific phobia, an individual must recognize that the fear is excessive, must go to great lengths to avoid the stimulus or endure it with great distress, and must exhibit significant interference in functioning due to the fear (APA, 1994). Similar requirements are made for the diagnosis of specific (or isolated) phobia in ICD-10, with marked fear or avoidance of the object or situation, marked anxiety when placed in the situation of the phobic stimulus that is confined to that situation, and considerable distress that is recognized by the subject as unreasonable. An individual may also spend a great deal of time and energy preparing in case the feared stimulus is encountered, even when the likelihood of encountering the stimulus is extremely low. The main types of specific phobias are animal (e.g., dogs, spiders), natural environmental (e.g. heights, lightening), situational (e.g. fear of enclosed places), blood-injury (e.g. shots, wounds, blood), and an 'other' category. Blood-injury phobias differ from the other types in that individuals may have a fainting response when exposed to their feared stimulus.

Agoraphobia

Agoraphobia is characterized by fear of being in situations that would be difficult to escape or in which help might not be available in the event of panic or panic-like symptoms. Such situations are avoided or found to be very distressing if endured (APA, 1994). There is evidence for gender differences in agoraphobia, with women reporting more severe avoidance as well as more catastrophic thinking and more fear-provoking bodily sensations (Turgeon *et al.*, 1998). Cultural differences in the expression of PDA have been described as well. For example, African Americans have been shown to differ from Caucasian Americans in terms of the manifestation of anxiety symptoms, rates of co-occurring disorders (e.g. PTSD), naturalistic coping strategies and culturally based explanations of symptoms (Bittner *et al.*, 2004). Hinton and colleagues have shown that symptoms of panic among Cambodian refugees often focus on different symptoms and have different culturally based explanations for their symptoms than are typical among individuals of European descent

(Hinton *et al.*, 2006a, 2006b, 2006c), which may lead to different patterns of avoidance.

Another special population to be considered in relation to agoraphobia is older adults. Whereas agoraphobia in younger adults is nearly always associated with panic (Horwath *et al.*, 1993), agoraphobia in the elderly is less often associated with spontaneous panic (McCabe *et al.*, 2006). Agoraphobia among older adults is more common in individuals with chronic health problems, (McCabe *et al.*, 2006) leading to the hypothesis that agoraphobia develops in relation to fears about medical problems or changes in functioning. An individual may become fearful about his or her ability to remain safe outside of their home (e.g. fearing falls), leading to avoidant behaviour (Flint, 1999).

Agoraphobia is also associated with increased difficulties within close relationships (Marcaurelle *et al.*, 2003). One strategy that individuals with agoraphobia may use to cope with their fears is delegating feared tasks to others (Marcaurelle *et al.*, 2003). For example, an agoraphobic patient may ask friends or family to drive her to appointments or to accompany her to the store. This level of dependence may contribute to discord in close relationships. Alternatively, marital distress may contribute to the development or maintenance of agoraphobia (Daiuto *et al.*, 1998). Chronic stress associated with difficulty in intimate relationships may be a risk factor for the disorder (Franklin & Andrews, 1989; Scocco *et al.*, 2006), and marital adjustment and difficulties in problem solving predict the severity of PDA (Hinton *et al.*, 2006; Marcaurelle *et al.*, 2005).

Treatment

Psychosocial treatment: specific phobias

Specific phobias are considered to be the most treatable of the anxiety disorders, sometimes responding in as little as one session of treatment (Antony & Barlow, 2001). Few studies have looked across cultures, but at least one study indicates that treatments tend to be equivalent between European-Americans and Hispanics/Latinos (Pina *et al.*, 2003). Exposure therapy has shown the most effectiveness in treating phobias (Table 33.1).

Exposure-based treatments

A meta-analysis of 35 RCTs of specific phobia concluded that exposure-based therapies outperformed all other types of psychotherapy (Horowitz *et al.*, 2005). The theory

behind exposure therapy is that catastrophic beliefs regarding the feared stimuli maintain escape and avoidance behaviours. These behaviours prevent the patient from obtaining new information to correct the false belief. Exposure to the feared stimuli sets up a series of tests for the patient to get new information regarding the feared stimuli.

Therapy can be delivered in one massed exposure session lasting several hours or over five or more sessions of gradual exposure. Several RCTs have shown that massed or gradual exposure have similar outcomes, (Ost *et al.*, 1997, 2001), although there are theoretical reasons to prefer spacing exposure trials (Lang *et al.*, 1999) and there is some evidence to support this approach (Rowe & Craske, 1998). Massed exposure generally follows the following format (Ost *et al.*, 1997, Ost, 1989): the patient and therapist create a hierarchy of feared and/or disgust inducing situations related to the feared stimuli (Smits *et al.*, 2002). The treatment then consists of prolonged, therapist-directed exposure to the two or three most anxiety arousing situations on the patient's hierarchy. There must be a significant drop (many clinicians aim for 50% reduction) in subjective level of anxiety before moving on the next situation on the hierarchy.

Gradual treatment generally consists of several 1-hour sessions of therapist-directed exposure to at least four or five anxiety-arousing situations from the patient's hierarchy. Between sessions, the patient repeats the same exposure as was completed in session for homework. Again, it is generally recommended that the patient's anxiety drop about 50% before moving up the hierarchy (Ost *et al.*, 1997).

Many phobic patients have safety seeking behaviours that may be used as crutches to 'get through' exposure to a feared stimulus. For example, a person with a fear of heights may only go up an elevator with a cell phone or if accompanied by a spouse. Treatment outcomes are improved when patients are counselled not to use safety behaviours (Kamphuis & Telch, 2000; Sloan & Telch, 2002; Telch *et al.*, 2004). In fact, even the perception that safety behaviours are available has been shown to be detrimental to treatment outcomes (Powers *et al.*, 2004). This may be because patients misattribute their failure to be harmed during exposure to the safety behaviour rather than using the exposure to disconfirm their original faulty threat (Telch *et al.*, 2004; Öst *et al.*, 1991).

It is important to match the focus of the exposure assignments to the patient's core threat (Kamphuis & Telch, 2000). For example, subtypes of driving phobia have been found where some patients are primarily focused on danger expectancies (e.g. car accidents) while others are focused on anxiety expectancies and unpleasant driving situations (Taylor *et al.*, 2000). Using guided threat appraisal by identifying a participant's core threat relative to a situation, instructing the participant to focus all of their available attention during exposure on the core threat, and testing the accuracy of the threat perception during exposure, has been shown to have better outcomes than therapy without a focus on the core threat (Kamphuis & Telch, 2000).

Exposure therapy for specific phobia is generally delivered in individual psychotherapy. One study (Ost, 1996) found a single session group treatment to be effective in treating spider phobias. This study did not compare group treatments to individual treatments, however, so relative performance cannot be assessed. Individual therapy is believed to perform better than therapy with a self-help manual (Hellstrom & Ost, 1995). Computer guided self-exposure therapy worked as well as therapist-guided therapy in one RCT (Marks *et al.*, 2004), but this study did not have a follow-up assessment.

Varying the context of exposure therapy, such as going to different places and varying the stimuli used during exposure, such as bringing in different types of snakes, is helpful (Rowe & Craske, 1998; Gros & Antony, 2006; Rowe & Craske, 1998).

Exposure treatment for specific phobias in children and adolescents

An RCT by Ost and colleagues (Ost *et al.*, 2001) showed exposure therapy to be effective in treating specific phobia in children. Sixty children, ages 7–17, were randomized to one 3-hour session of exposure therapy alone, exposure therapy with a parent present, or a waitlist control. The therapy was adapted to the developmental level of the children. For example, more play-based activities were included for the younger children. The two active conditions outperformed the control condition on self-report, behavioural, and physiological measures at 1-month and 1-year follow-up. Exposure therapy was well-accepted by the children as well (Svensson *et al.*, 2002). Most children reported the therapy was a positive experience.

Exposure plus other psychosocial treatments

Other psychosocial treatments of specific phobias generally include exposure therapy plus an additional element (Gros & Antony, 2006). For example, K. B. Wolitzky and M. J. Telch (unpublished data) compared exposure alone to exposure plus 'opposite action' in an RCT and found the latter group to have better outcomes on self-report and behavioural measures. Opposite action meant doing the opposite of what a patient would normally do during exposure, such as folding hands behind back while looking over a ledge rather than clasping the ledge.

Cognitive therapy helps patients to identify and challenge distorted beliefs that may contribute to anxiety and impede exposure. Two review papers (Gros & Antony, 2006; Craske & Rowe, 1997) and a meta-analysis, (Horowitz *et al.*, 2005), however, have concluded that exposure therapy alone performs as well without the addition of cognitive therapy.

Virtual reality exposure therapy (VRET)

Integrating virtual reality into exposure has received a great deal of attention in recent years. Virtual reality exposure therapy (VRET) involves exposing patients to their feared stimuli using an integration of computer graphics, body tracking devises, visual displays, and other sensory input that immerses a patient into a virtual environment that changes in a natural way with head and body motion (Gros & Antony, 2006; Pull, 2006). Most VRET studies have examined flying, acrophobia, driving, claustrophobia, and fear of spiders (Pull, 2006). Studies comparing exposure therapy with and without VR show comparable results for both conditions in acrophobia and spider phobia (Pull, 2006; Krijn *et al.*, 2004; Garcia-Palacios *et al.*, 2002). Thus, it is up to clinicians to decide if it is worth the extra expense to acquire VR technology. Virtual reality can be a viable alternative, however, if the feared stimulus for in vivo exposure is not available. Critiques of VRET question if the computer graphics are real enough to trigger anxiety levels comparable to the actual feared stimuli (Walshe *et al.*, 2005). RCTs across more specific phobias are necessary to answer this question.

Psychotherapeutic treatment of blood-injection-injury phobias

Unlike other specific phobias, exposure therapy is not the treatment of choice for blood phobias (Ost *et al.*, 1991). Applied tension or tension only therapies outperformed in vivo exposure therapy in one RCT (Ost *et al.*, 1991). Tension is a technique to prevent the fainting response common to blood phobias by raising blood pressure at the first sign of a drop in blood pressure in response to a blood or injury stimulus. Specifically, a patient is instructed to tense the muscles of the arms, chest, and legs until there is a feeling of warmth rising to the face (usually 15–20 seconds). The patient is then instructed to release the tension to return to the starting level of tension, pause, and then repeat the procedure five times (Ost & Sterner, 1987). Applied tension is when the tension technique is used during an in vivo exposure exercise (Ost & Sterner, 1987).

Five session of applied tension, a single session of applied tension, and a single session of tension only have equivalent efficacy in treating blood-related phobias (Hellstrom *et al.*, 1996). When delivered in five 1-hour sessions, the first session is used to teach the technique. Sessions 2–3 are used to practise the technique while viewing slides of blood phobia-related stimuli. In Session 4 the patient observes people donating blood, and in Session 5, the patient observes thoracic surgery. When the treatment is delivered in a single session, the patient is taught the technique then practises it while viewing fear-provoking slides for up to 2 hours. In single session tension only, the patient practises the technique until he or she can successfully increase their systolic blood pressure by at least 15 mm Hg, for up to 2 hours. The patient is then encouraged to practise the technique when exposed to blood stimuli in the future. In an RCT with 30 patients randomized to one of the three tension treatments, all techniques showed clinically significant improvement post-treatment and at 1-year follow-up ranging from 60 to 70% (Hellstrom *et al.*, 1996).

Psychosocial treatment: agoraphobia

Treatment of PDA has been reviewed by Welch and colleagues in this text, so this chapter will focus on aspects of treatment that are specific to agoraphobia. Little has been done to determine how to best manage AWP, perhaps because patients with AWP are less likely to seek care than agoraphobic patients with panic (Andrews & Slade, 2006; Wittchen *et al.*, 1998).

Although there is no evidence that either individual or group psychotherapy leads to better outcomes, it has been argued that good cohesiveness within a treatment group can be a powerful motivator to continue with difficult exposure tasks (Hand, 2000). It also may be useful to continue treatment until avoidant behaviour is completely resolved. One study of long-term outcomes after exposure for PDA showed that continued remission was more likely if there was no residual agoraphobic avoidance after treatment (Fava *et al.*, 1995). Craske and colleagues (Craske *et al.*, 2003) dismantled CBT for PDA to examine whether or not agoraphobic avoidance needs to be targeted directly. They compared panic control treatment with and without in vivo exposure to avoided situations. They found no significant differences between these conditions in terms of agoraphobic avoidance or overall distress and impairment, suggesting that it is not necessary to target

avoidance directly in treatment. This result should be replicated before clinical practice is altered. The analyses were not completed on an intent-to-treat basis. Although the rate of attrition did not significantly differ between conditions, the rate was higher in the group that did not receive exposure (21% vs. 12%), and missing data on specific measures further limited the analysable data set for some measures.

As has been described, agoraphobia is associated with increased relational difficulties, which may serve as a risk factor for the development or maintenance of avoidant behaviour. Multiple studies also have documented increased marital difficulty after treatment for agoraphobic symptoms (Marcaurelle *et al.*, 2003). A spouse who felt positively reinforced for the care-giving role may react negatively to no longer being 'needed.' As a result, a couple's ability to adapt to changes in their relationship may be important in both treatment outcome and quality of the marital relationship (Marcaurelle *et al.*, 2003). Specific adaptations to treatment have been suggested to address relational issues, including training the partner to assist with exposure and focusing directly on the couple's problems (Daiuto *et al.*, 1998). Simply engaging a spouse in treatment without attention to marital communication or other problematic aspects of the relationship does not appear to be helpful (Marcaurelle *et al.*, 2003; Daiuto *et al.*, 1998). The addition of problem solving and communications skills to exposure-based treatment, on the other hand, may be useful, particularly in terms of long-term maintenance of changes (Daiuto *et al.*, 1998). Some authors have reported better outcomes with the added components, although others have found no positive effect (Marcaurelle *et al.*, 2003). It may be that the effectiveness of adding problem solving and communication skills depends on the couple's ability to resolve conflict prior to treatment. There is insufficient evidence to conclude whether or not behavioural treatment for the couple, rather than as an adjunct to exposure, would effectively reduce agoraphobic symptoms (Daiuto *et al.*, 1998). Future studies will be necessary to determine the optimal way to adapt treatment based on pre-treatment marital functioning.

Alternative means of delivering treatment may also be important to consider for agoraphobia. Cognitive-behaviour therapy, which is the best-supported treatment for PDA, may not be accessible to patients because they live in an area where this type of treatment is not available or because their mobility is significantly impacted by their disorder. For such individuals, self-directed treatment may be the best option. Self-directed therapy likely would not be sufficient to fully address severe symptoms, but it may be effective for those with mild to moderate symptoms (London & Barlow, 2004) or provide enough relief for a previously housebound patient to be able to receive care outside the home. Several studies have shown that self-directed treatment using the Mastery of Your Anxiety and Panic manual can be as effective as if the intervention is delivered in person (Landon & Barlow, 2004). Delivering CBT by telephone may also be a reasonable option. A trial of telephone-based CBT for PDA in rural patients showed that this type of treatment delivery was an effective way of reducing symptoms for those who would not otherwise be able to engage in CBT (Swinson et al., 1995). Administration of treatment materials by computer (Kenwright et al., 2001) and over the Internet (Kenwright & Marks, 2004) also has been shown to be feasible and to effectively reduce symptoms. Although computers may increase accessibility and affordability of treatment, this modality may not be as satisfying to patients (Jacobs et al., 2001) and may lead to higher drop-out rates (Landon & Barlow, 2004).

A patient's culture may also be an important consideration in treatment of agoraphobia. One study showed that African-Americans did not respond as well to exposure-based treatment as did a Caucasian comparison group (Chambless & Williams, 1995). It has been argued that treatment should be adapted for other cultural groups (Takriti & Ahmad, 2000) and for women (Mohlman, 2000). Cultural differences in symptoms or coping strategies may influence the way in which an intervention is received by a patient and speak to the need for therapists to be aware of such issues. Linguistic and cultural compatibility is also important in increasing rates of mental health utilization among minority groups (Vega et al., 2001).

Pharmacotherapy: specific phobias

There have been very few studies that look at pharmacotherapy treatments for specific phobias (Antony & Barlow, 2001; Gros & Antony, 2006; Stein & Matsunaga, 2006). One double-blind pilot study randomized eleven patients to paroxetine up to 20/mg day or a placebo condition. One out of six patients responded to placebo compared to three out of five patients to paroxetine. These results should be interpreted with caution, however, because all outcome measures used a self-report format and because of the preliminary nature of this study.

Pharmacotherapy: agoraphobia

In their earlier chapter, Welsh and colleagues reviewed pharmacological management of panic disorder with agoraphobia. There are no separate specific pharmacologic recommendations for AWP.

Comparative and combination treatments

Combination treatments have also received little attention in the study of SP and AWP. A study with benzodiazepines in combination with exposure therapy compared to exposure therapy alone show no added benefits of adding pharmacoptherapy (Zoellner et al., 1996). Another similar study found that the benzodiazepine plus exposure condition had higher rates of relapse than exposure alone (Thom et al., 2000).

A double-blind RCT of 28 patients randomized to VRET plus D-cycloserine (DCS), a partial agonist at the N-methyl-D-aspratate receptor, versus VRET alone, found that subjects in the pharmacotherapy condition had significantly greater symptom reduction and significantly more improvement and physiological and behavioural measures than participants in VRET only post-treatment and at 3-month follow-up (Ressler et al., 2004). Participants completed two sessions of VRET and took DCS or placebo prior to both sessions. This preliminary data is promising, but should be followed up with a larger RCT. To date, the research in total provides little support for using pharmacotherapy as a stand-alone treatment or in conjunction with psychotherapy in the treatment of specific phobia (Gros & Antony, 2006).

Treatment delivery challenges

The biggest obstacle to delivering treatment is that individuals rarely present for treatment if specific phobia or agoraphobia alone are their primary diagnoses (Gros & Antony, 2006; Brown et al., 2001). Instead, people tend to work around their phobias, avoiding for example crowded places or locations where they may encounter spiders.

In addition, there is a scarcity of healthcare professionals trained in delivering exposure therapy for SP or agoraphobia. Such training is perceived to be time consuming and costly (Gega et al., 2006). One promising recent development is the availability of computer training in exposure therapy. Gega et al. (2006) randomized 92 nursing students to computer instruction or teacher-led instruction in exposure therapy for SP and panic. Both conditions showed similar improvements in knowledge and skills and similar satisfaction ratings. Future research is necessary to see if treatment outcomes are similar by clinicians trained in both methods.

Future directions

There are several psychotherapeutic and pharmaco-logical add-ons to exposure therapy that appear promising and deserve further study. These include opposite action, guided threat appraisal, VRET, and DCS pharmacotherapy.

Longer follow-ups may reveal more information about the effectiveness of treatments for specific phobias and shed light on how we can further improve outcomes. Most of the studies reviewed in this chapter have follow-ups up to one year post-treatment. Lipsitz and colleagues (Lipsitz et al., 1999) followed up with 28 patients who had participated in a treatment study of specific phobia 10–16 years later. Of those that had originally been categorized as responders, 62% had significant avoidance or endurance with dread of their feared stimuli. Forty-five per cent had clinically significant symptoms. This study challenges the notion that specific phobia treatments lead to long-lasting symptom remission and highlights the need for more research on therapies and characteristics associated with long-term outcomes.

There is already evidence that VRET is effective in the treatment of specific phobias. Other developing technologies show promise as well and should be studied for their utility in treatment. One possibility is augmented reality therapy where virtual elements are introduced into the real world where, for example, a scurrying cockroach is virtually superimposed into the actual therapy room. This technology may have several benefits over what is currently available: it is less expensive than VR because most of it is set in the real world, also because it

is set in the real world, it may facilitate a feeling of reality and presence, thus helping resolve the issue of whether VR is realistic enough to invoke fear and disgust. A single case study of cockroach phobia showed promising results (Botella et al., 2005). This technology deserves and will surely receive further attention in the treatment of specific phobia.

Finally, most treatment outcomes research to date has been conducted with very few phobias (Gros & Antony, 2006), and AWP in particular has received little attention (Andrews & Slade, 2006; Wittchen et al., 1998). More research is needed with other phobias.

Summary and guidelines

Specific phobias and agoraphobia are highly prevalent in the community. Empirically supported psychosocial treatments are efficacious and quick. Based on available evidence, exposure therapy should be considered the first-line treatment for specific phobia. More research is needed to understand how pharmacotherapy can be used in tandem with exposure or as a stand-alone treatment for phobias. Developing technologies may change the face of some of the available treatments in coming years. Our greatest challenge, however, will be to disseminate our already available and effective treatments so that they are readily available to patients who would benefit from them.

The level of evidence for each of the interventions discussed in this chapter is summarized in Table 33.1.

Tabel 33.1. Effectiveness of treatments for specific phobia and agoraphobia

Treatment	Form of treatment	Psychiatric disorder	Level of evidence for Efficacy	Comment
In vivo exposure therapy	Individual treatment	Specific phobias except blood phobias	Ia	Can be delivered in single session or over multiple sessions
Applied Tension	Individual treatment	Blood phobias	Ib	Can be delivered in single session or over five sessions
Exposure therapy with virtual reality	Individual with VR technology	Specific phobias	Ib	
Cognitive-behaviour therapy (CBT) including exposure	Individual treatment	Agoraphobia	Ia	
CBT including exposure	Self-directed	Agoraphobia	Ia	
CBT including exposure	Internet	Agoraphobia	Ib	

REFERENCES

Alonso, J., Angermeyer, M. C., Bernert, S. *et al.* (2004). Prevalence of mental disorders in Europe: results from the European Study of the Epidemiology of Mental Disorders (ESEMeD) project. *Acta Psychiatrica Scandinavia,* **Suppl. 420**, 21–7.

Alonso, J., Angermeyer, M. C., Bernert, S. *et al.* (2004). Disability and quality of life impact of mental disorders in Europe: results from the European Study of the Epidemiology of Mental Disorders (ESEMeD) project. *Acta Psychiatrica Scandinavia,* **Suppl. 420**, 38–46.

American Psychiatric Association. (APA) (1994). *Diagnostic and Statistical Manual of Mental Disorders,* 4th edn. Washington, DC: APA.

Andrews, G. & Slade, T. (2006). Agoraphobia without a history of panic disorder may be part of the panic disorder syndrome. *Journal of Nervous and Mental Disease,* **190**, 624–30.

Antony, M. & Barlow, D. (2001). Specific phobias. *Anxiety and its Disorders: The Nature and Treatment of Anxiety and Panic,* ed. D. Barlow, pp. 380–417. New York: Guilford Publications.

Bienvenu, O., Onyike, C. & Stein, M. (2006). Agoraphobia in adults: incidence and longitudinal relationship with panic. *British Journal of Psychiatry,* **188**, 432–8.

Bittner, A., Goodwin, R., Wittchen, H., Beesdo, K., Hofler, M. & Lieb, R. (2004). What characteristics of primary anxiety disorders predict subsequent major depressive disorder? *Journal of Clinical Psychiatry,* **65**, 618–26.

Botella, C. M., Juan, M. C., Banos, R. M., Alcaniz, M., Guillen, V., & Rey, B. (2005). Mixing realities? An application of augmented reality for the treatment of cockroach phobia. *Cyberpsychological Behavior,* **8**(2), 162–71.

Brown, T. A., Campbell, L. A., Lehman, C. L., Grisham, J. R. & Mancill, R. B. (2001). Current and lifetime comorbidity of the DSM-IV anxiety and mood disorders in a large clinical sample. *Journal of Abnormal Psychology,* **110**(4), 585–99.

Chambless, D. & Williams, K. (1995). A preliminary study of African Americans with agoraphobia: symptom severity and outcome of treatment with in vivo exposure. *Behavior Therapy,* **26**, 501–15.

Craske, M. & Rowe, M. (1997). A comparison of behavioral and cognitive treatments for phobias. In *Phobias: A Handbook of Theory, Research, and Treatment,* ed. G. Davey, pp. 247–80. Chichester, UK: John Wiley.

Craske, M., DeCola, J., Sachs, A. & Pontillo, D. (2003). Panic control treatment for agoraphobia. *Journal of Anxiety Disorders,* **17**, 321–33.

Daiuto, A., Baucom, D., Epstein, N. & Dutton, S. (1998). The application of behavioral couples therapy to the assessment and treatment of agoraphobia: Implications of empirical research. *Clinical Psychology Review,* **18**, 663–87.

Fava, G., Zielezny, M., Savron, G. & Grandi, S. (1995). Long-term effects of behavioural treatment for panic disorder with agoraphobia. *British Journal of Psychiatry,* **166**, 87–92.

Flint, A. J. (1999). Anxiety disorders in late life. *Canadian Family Physician,* **45**, 2672–9.

Franklin, J. and Andrews, G. (1989). Stress and the onset of agoraphobia. *Australian Psychologist,* **24**, 203–19.

Garcia-Palacios, A., Hoffman, H., Carlin, A., Furness, T. A., III & Botella, C. (2002). Virtual reality in the treatment of spider phobia: a controlled study. *Behaviour Research and Therapy,* **40**(9), 983–93.

Gega, L., Norman, I. J. & Marks, I. M. (2006). Computer-aided vs. tutor-delivered teaching of exposure therapy for phobia/panic: randomized controlled trial with pre-registration nursing students. *International Journal of Nursing Studies,* **44**(3), 397–405.

Goodwin, R., Faravelli, C., Rosi, S. *et al.* (2005). The epidemiology of panic disorder and agoraphobia in Europe. *European Neuropsychopharmacology,* **15**, 435–43.

Gros, D. F. & Antony, M. M. (2006). The assessment and treatment of specific phobias: a review. *Current Psychiatry Reports,* **8**(4), 298–303.

Hand, I. (2000). Group exposure in vivo for agoraphobics (1974): a multifaceted pilot study and its impact on subsequent agoraphobia research. *Behavioural and Cognitive Psychotherapy,* **28**(335), 351.

Hellstrom, K. & Ost, L. G. (1995). One-session therapist directed exposure vs two forms of manual directed self-exposure in the treatment of spider phobia. *Behaviour Research and Therapy,* **33**(8), 959–65.

Hellstrom, K., Fellenius, J. & Ost, L. G. (1996). One versus five sessions of applied tension in the treatment of blood phobia. *Behaviour Research and Therapy,* **34**(2), 101–12.

Hinton, D., Chhean, D., Fama, J., Pollack, M. & McNally, R. J.. (2006). Gastrointestinal-focused panic attacks among Cambodian refugees: associated psychopathology, flashbacks, and catastrophic cognitions. *Journal of Anxiety Disorders,* E pub ahead of print.

Hinton, D., Chhean, D., Pich, V., Um, K., Fama, J. & Pollack, M. (2006). Neck-focused panic attacks among Cambodian refugees: a logistic and linear regression analysis. *Journal of Anxiety Disorders,* **20**, 119–38.

Hinton, D., Hinton, L., Tran, M., Nguyen, L., Hsia, C. & Pollack, M. (2006). Orthostatically induced panic attacks among Vietnamese refugees: associated psychopathology, flashbacks, and catastrophic cognitions. *Journal of Anxiety Disorders,* **23**, 113–15.

Horwath, E., Lish, J., Johnson, J., Hornig, C. & Weissman, M. (1993). Agoraphobia without panic: clinical reappraisal of an epidemiologic finding. *American Journal of Psychiatry,* **150**, 1496–501.

Horowitz, J., Wolitzky, K. & Powers, M. (2005). *Psychosocial Treatments for Specific Phobias: A Meta-analysis.* Washington, DC.

Iancu, I., Levin, J., Hermesh, H. *et al.* (2006). Social phobia symptoms: prevalence, sociodemographic correlates, and overlap with specific phobia symptoms. *Comparative Psychiatry,* **47**(5), 399–405.

Jacobs, M., Christensen, A., Snibbe, J., Dolezal-Wood, S., Huber, A. & Polterok, A. (2001). A comparison of computer-based versus traditional individual psychotherapy. *Professional Psychology: Research and Practice,* **32**, 92–6.

Kamphuis, J. H. & Telch, M. J. (2000). Effects of distraction and guided threat reappraisal no fear reduction during exposure based treatments for specific fears. *Behaviour Research and Therapy*, **38**, 1163–81.

Kaye, W. H., Bulik, C. M., Thornton L., Barbarich, N., Masters K. (2004). Comorbidity of anxiety disorders with anorexia and bulimia nervosa. *American Journal of Psychiatry*, **161**(12), 2215–21.

Kenwright, M., Liness, S. & Marks, I. (2001). Reducing demands on clinicians by offering computer-aided self-help for phobia/panic: feasibility study. *British Journal of Psychiatry*, **179**, 456–9.

Kenwright, M. & Marks I. Computer-aided self-help for phobia/panic via internet at home: a pilot study. *British Journal of Psychiatry*, 2004; **184**, 448–9.

Kessler, R., Chiu, W., Demler, O. & Walters, E. (2005). Prevalence, severity, and comorbidity of 12-month DSM-IV disorders in the National Comorbidity Survey Replication. *Archives of General Psychiatry*, **62**, 617–627.

Krijn, M., Emmelkamp, P. M., Biemond, R., de Wilde de, L. C., Schuemie, M. J. & van der Mast, C. A. (2004). Treatment of acrophobia in virtual reality: the role of immersion and presence. *Behaviour Research and Therapy*, **42**(2), 229–39.

Landon, T. & Barlow, D. H. (2004). Cognitive-behavioral treatment for panic disorder: Current status. *Journal of Psychiatric Practice*, **10**, 211–26.

Lang, A. J., Craske, M. G. & Bjork, R. A. (1999). Implications of a new theory of disuse for the treatment of emotional disorders. *Clinical Psychology: Science and Practice*, **6**, 80–94.

Lichtenstein, P. & Annas, P. (2000). Heritability and prevalence of specific fears and phobias in childhood. *Journal of Child Clinical Psychiatry*, **41**(7), 927–37.

Lipsitz, J. D., Mannuzza, S., Klein, D. F., Ross, D. C. & Fyer, A. J. (1999). Specific phobia 10–16 years after treatment. *Depression and Anxiety*, **10**(3), 105–11.

McCabe, L., Cairney, J., Veldhuizen, S., Herrmann, N. & Streiner, D. (2006). Prevalence and correlates of agoraphobia in older adults. *American Journal of Geriatric Psychiatry*, **14**, 515–22.

Marcaurelle, R., Belanger, C. & Marchand, A. (2003). Marital relationship and the treatment of panic disorder with agoraphobia: a critical review. *Clinical Psychology Review*, **23**, 247–76.

Marcaurelle, R., Belanger, C., Marchand, A., Katerelos, T. & Mainguy, N. (2005). Marital predictors of symptom severity in panic disorder with agoraphobia. *Journal of Anxiety Disorders*, **19**, 211–32.

Marks, I. M., Kenwright, M., McDonough, M., Whittaker, M. & Mataix-Cols, D. (2004). Saving clinicians' time by delegating routine aspects of therapy to a computer: a randomized controlled trial in phobia/panic disorder. *Psychological Medicine*, **34**(1), 9–17.

Mataix-Cols, D., Cowley, A. J., Hankins, M. *et al.* (2006). Reliability and validity of the work and social adjustment scale in phobic disorders. *Comparative Psychiatry*, **46**(3), 223–8.

Meyer, C., Rumpf, H. J., Hapke, U. & John, U. (2004). Impact of psychiatric disorders in the general population: satisfaction with life and the influence of comorbidity and disorder duration. *Social Psychiatry and Psychiatric Epidemiology*, **39**(6), 435–41.

Mohlman, J. (2000). Taking our housebound sisters to the mall: What can a feminist perspective add to CBT for panic and agoraphobia? *Behavior Therapist*, **23**, 30–41.

Norton, G., Cox, B., Asmundson, G. J. G. & Maser, J. (1995). The growth of research on anxiety disorders during the 1980s. *Journal of Anxiety Disorders*, **9**, 75–85.

Ost, L. G. (1989). One-session treatment for specific phobias. *Behaviour Research and Therapy*, **27**(1), 1–7.

Ost, L. G. (1996). One-session group treatment of spider phobia. *Behaviour Research and Therapy*, **34**(9), 707–15.

Ost, L. G. & Sterner, U. (1987). Applied tension. A specific behavioral method for treatment of blood phobia. *Behaviour Research and Therapy*, **25**(1), 25–9.

Ost, L. G., Fellenius, J. & Sterner, U. (1991). Applied tension, exposure in vivo, and tension-only in the treatment of blood phobia. *Behaviour Research and Therapy*, **29**(6), 561–74.

Öst, L., Salkovskis, P. & Hellström, K. (1991). One-session therapist-directed exposure vs. self-exposure in the treatment of spider phobia. *Behavior Therapy*, **22**, 407–22.

Ost, L. G., Brandberg, M. & Alm, T. (1997). One versus five sessions of exposure in the treatment of flying phobia. *Behaviour Research and Therapy*, **35**(11), 987–96.

Ost, L. G., Alm, T., Brandberg, M. & Breitholtz, E. (2001). One vs five sessions of exposure and five sessions of cognitive therapy in the treatment of claustrophobia. *Behaviour Research and Therapy*, **39**(2), 167–83.

Ost, L. G., Svensson, L., Hellstrom, K. & Lindwall, R. (2001). One-session treatment of specific phobias in youths: a randomized clinical trial. *Journal of Consulting Clinical Psychology*, **69**(5), 814–24.

Pina, A. A., Silverman, W. K., Fuentes, R. M., Kurtines, W. M. & Weems, C. F. (2003). Exposure-based cognitive-behavioral treatment for phobic and anxiety disorders: treatment effects and maintenance for Hispanic/Latino relative to European-American youths. *Journal of the American Academy for Child and Adolescent Psychiatry*, **42**(10), 1179–87.

Powers, M. B., Smits, J. A. J. & Telch, M. J. (2004). Disentangling the effects of safety-behavior utilization and safety-behavior availability during exposure-based treatment: a placebo-controlled trial. *Journal of Consulting and Clinical Psychology*, **72**(3), 448–54.

Pull, C. B. (2006). Current status of virtual reality therapy in anxiety disorders. *Current Opinion in Psychiatry*, **18**, 7–14.

Regier, D. A., Kaelber, C. T., Rae, D. S. *et al.* (1998). Limitations of diagnostic criteria and assessment instruments for mental disorders: implications for research and policy. *Archives in General Psychiatry*, **55**, 109–15.

Ressler, K. J., Rothbaum, B. O., Tannenbaum, L. *et al.* (2004). Cognitive enhancers as adjuncts to psychotherapy: use of D-cycloserine in phobic individuals to facilitate extinction of fear. *Archives in General Psychiatry*, **61**(11), 1136–44.

Roberge, P., Marchand, A., Reinharz, D. *et al.* (2005). Healthcare utilization following cognitive-behavioral treatment for panic disorder with agoraphobia. *Cognitive and Behavioral Therapy*, **34**, 79–88.

Rowe, M. K. & Craske, M. G. (1998). Effects of an expanding-spaced vs massed *exposure* schedule on fear reduction and return of fear. *Behaviour Research and Therapy*, **36**(7–8), 701–17.

Rowe, M. K. & Craske, M. G. (1998). Effects of varied-stimulus exposure training on fear reduction and return of fear. *Behaviour Research and Therapy*, **36**(7–8), 719–34.

Sareen, J., Cox, B., Afifi, T. *et al.* (2005). Anxiety disorders and risk for suicidal ideation and suicide attempts. *Archives of General Psychiatry*, **62**, 1249–57.

Sareen, J., Jacobi, F., Cox, B., Belik, S., Clara, I. & Stein, M. (2006). Disability and poor quality of life associated with comorbid anxiety disorders and physical conditions. *Archives of Internal Medicine*, **166**(19), 2109–16.

Sareen, J., Jacobi, F., Cox, B., Belik, S., Clara, I. & Stein, M. (2006). Disability and poor quality of life associated with comorbid anxiety disorders and physical conditions. *Archives of Internal Medicine*, **166**, 2109–16.

Scocco, P., Barbieri, I. & Frank, E. (2006). Interpersonal problem areas and onset of panic disorder. *Psychopathology*, **40**, 8–13.

Sloan, T. & Telch, M. J. (2002). The effects of safety-seeking behavior and guided threat reappraisal on fear reduction during exposure: an experimental investigation. *Behaviour Research and Therapy*, **40**, 235–51.

Smits, J. A. J., Telch, M. J. & Randall, P. K. (2002). An examination of the decline in fear and disgust during exposure-based treatment. *Behaviour Research and Therapy*, **40**, 1243–53.

Stein, D. J. & Matsunaga, H. (2006). Specific phobia: a disorder of fear conditioning and extinction. *CNS Spectrum*, **11**(4), 248–51.

Svensson, L., Larsson, A. & Ost, L. G. (2002). How children experience brief-exposure treatment of specific phobias. *Journal of Clinical and Child and Adolescent Psychology*, **31**(1), 80–9.

Swinson, R., Cox, B. & Woszczyna, C. (1992). Use of medical services and treatment for panic disorder with agoraphobia and for social phobia. *Canadian Medical Association Journal*, **147**, 878–83.

Swinson, R., Fergus, K., Cox B. & Wickwire, K. (1995). Efficacy of telephone-administered behavioral therapy for panic disorder with agoraphobia. *Behaviour Reseach and Therapy*, **33**, 465–9.

Takriti, A. & Ahmad, T. (2000). Anxiety disorders and treatment in Arab-Muslim culture. In *Al-Junun: Mental Illness in the Islamic World*, ed. I. Al-Issa, p. 235–50. Madison, WI: International Universities Press, Inc.

Taylor, J. E., Deane, F. P. & Podd, J. V. (2000). Determining the focus of driving fears. *Journal of Anxiety Disorders*, **14**(5), 453–70.

Telch, M. J., Valentiner, D. P., Ilai, D., Young, P. R., Powers, M. B. & Smits, J. A. J. (2004). Fear activation and distraction during the emotional processing of claustrophobic fear. *Journal of Behavior Therapy and Experimental Psychology*, **35**, 219–32.

Thom, A., Sartory, G. & Johren, P. (2000). Comparison between one-session psychological treatment and benzodiazepine in dental phobia. *Journal of Consulting Clinical Psychology*, **68**(3), 378–87.

Turgeon, L., Marchand, A. & Dupuis, G. (1998). Clinical features in panic disorder with agoraphobia: a comparison of men and women. *Journal of Anxiety Disorders*, **12**, 539–53.

Vega, W., Vega, W. & Aguilar-Gaxioa, S. (2001). Help seeking for mental health problems among Mexican Americans. *Journal of Immigrant Health*, **3**, 133–40.

Walshe, D., Lewis, E., O'Sullivan, K. & Kim, S. I. (2005). Virtually driving: are the driving environments "real enough" for exposure therapy with accident victims? An explorative study. *Cyberpsychological Behavior*, **8**(6), 532–7.

Wittchen, H., Reed, V. & Kessler, R. C. (1998). The relationship of agoraphobia and panic in a community sample of adolescents and young adults. *Archives of General Psychiatry*, **55**, 1017–24.

Zoellner, L., Craske, M., Hussain, A., Lewis, M. & Echeveri, A. (1996). Contextual effects of alprazolam during exposure therapy. Paper presented at the 30th Anual Convention of the Association for Advancement of Behavior Therapy. New York, Nov. 21–24, 1996.

34

Social phobia

Laura Campbell-Sills and Murray B. Stein

Editor's note

The evidence base for treatments of social phobia is one of the most rapidly expanding ones in psychiatry. The recent interest in the subject arose primarily from epidemiological studies that showed large numbers of untreated people severely handicapped by shyness who were not seeking help. Despite strong evidence of effective treatments with both psychological (CBT) and psychopharmacological interventions, only about half of the people with this disorder seek treatment and usually only after 15–20 years of being symptomatic. Pharmacological and non-pharmacological interventions are equally effective, but pharmacological interventions appear to act more quickly while CBT is longer lasting. Nonetheless, response rates remain in the 50%–70% range, and more studies and research are needed to find ways to help those who do not respond to our current treatments.

Introduction

Social phobia (also known as social anxiety disorder) is a common and often disabling mental disorder. Individuals with social phobia strongly fear social or performance situations in which they might be exposed to unfamiliar people or be scrutinized by others (American Psychiatric Association, 2000). When confronted with feared situations, individuals with social phobia experience symptoms of anxiety that may reach the level of a panic attack. The discomfort provoked by social encounters or performance situations leads many people with the disorder to avoid interactions with others. Avoidance can produce a marked effect on psychosocial functioning, causing disruptions in occupational, academic, interpersonal, and other daily activities.

Social phobia can present in many different ways and at varying levels of severity. Some individuals fear and avoid just one or two social situations, which are typically performance situations like public speaking or more challenging interpersonal situations like asserting oneself. In diagnosing these cases of social phobia, a usual question is whether the fear causes enough distress and/or impairment to merit a clinical diagnosis. In contrast, individuals who fear a broad range of social situations are characterized as having 'generalized' social phobia (GSP). Though not always the case, GSP tends to be more disabling than the non-generalized variant. GSP is highly overlapping with another DSM-IV-TR diagnostic entity, avoidant personality disorder (AvPD). AvPD is conceptualized as a pervasive pattern of social inhibition, feelings of inadequacy, and preoccupation with negative evaluation that begins by age 18 and is present in a variety of contexts (American Psychiatric Association, 2000). DSM-IV-TR acknowledges that GSP and AvPD may be alternative conceptualizations of the same condition, and it has been suggested that AvPD simply represents a more severe version of GSP (Chavira & Stein, 2002).

The most recent large-scale epidemiological survey estimated the 12-month prevalence of social phobia at 6.8% and the lifetime prevalence at 12.1% (Kessler et al., 2005a, b). The disorder typically begins by adolescence (median age of onset = 13; Kessler et al., 2005a) and follows a chronic course (Bruce et al., 2005). Although social phobia is relatively common across demographic groups, lifetime risk is higher for women than for men (Kessler et al., 1994), and higher for non-Hispanic Whites than for Hispanics and non-Hispanic Blacks (Breslau et al., 2006).

Social phobia has high rates of comorbidity with other mental disorders (Kessler et al., 2005b; Magee et al., 1996). In many cases, social phobia is temporally primary and

Cambridge Textbook of Effective Treatments in Psychiatry, ed. Peter Tyrer and Kenneth R. Silk. Published by Cambridge University Press.
© Cambridge University Press, 2008.

may increase risk for developing other problems such as mood disorders (Kessler *et al.*, 1999). Individuals suffering from social phobia often experience impairment in major life roles and report high levels of life dissatisfaction (Stein & Kean, 2000). Despite the degree of suffering and impairment associated with social phobia, only about half of individuals with the disorder ever seek treatment and in most cases treatment is sought after 15–20 years of experiencing symptoms (Wang *et al.*, 2005).

These statistics suggest that social phobia negatively impacts individuals and the community, and that effective treatment of this disorder should be considered a public health priority. In this chapter, we present an overview of effective pharmacological and psychological treatments for social phobia (See Table 34.1). In the majority of cases, the treatments we review are supported by randomized controlled trials (RCTs), with minimal consideration of uncontrolled studies. We also consider the evidence pertaining to maintenance treatment, comparative efficacy of treatments, combining pharmacological and psychological treatments, and predictors of treatment outcome. Given that treatment of social phobia in children and adolescents is addressed elsewhere (Chapter 57), we restrict our focus to treatment of adults with social phobia.

Pharmacological treatments

Twenty years ago a review of the evidence base for the treatment of social phobia would have been limited to the simple statement that monoamine oxidase inhibitors (MAOIs) were possibly efficacious (Solyom *et al.*, 1986). We now know from a number of RCTs that several pharmacological treatments are efficacious in the treatment of social phobia.

Selective serotonin reuptake inhibitors (SSRIS)

The literature supports the use of SSRIs as first-line treatments for social phobia. Randomized controlled trials support the efficacy and tolerability of citalopram (Furmark *et al.*, 2005), escitalopram (Kasper *et al.*, 2005; Lader *et al.*, 2004), fluoxetine (Davidson *et al.*, 2004; but cf. Kobak *et al.*, 2002), fluvoxamine (Stein *et al.*, 1999; van Vliet *et al.*, 1994), paroxetine (Allgulander, 1999; Baldwin *et al.*, 1999; Stein *et al.*, 1998; Stein *et al.*, 1999), controlled release paroxetine (Lepola *et al.*, 2004), and sertraline (Katzelnick *et al.*, 1995; Liebowitz *et al.*, 2003; Van Ameringen *et al.*, 2001). Meta-analyses also offer strong

support for the efficacy of SSRIs (Blanco *et al.*, 2003; Fedoroff & Taylor, 2001; Gould *et al.*, 1997).

Dosages of SSRIs for treatment of social phobia are generally in the same range as those used to treat major depression. It is important to continue SSRI treatment long enough to achieve maximum therapeutic response and to prevent relapse. With respect to length of treatment, one study showed that many patients who were nonresponders after 8 weeks of paroxetine treatment were classified as responders at week 12 (Stein *et al.*, 2002). Therefore, 3 months or longer may be necessary for an adequate trial of an SSRI. Moreover, several studies support continuation of SSRI treatment for 3 months or longer after remission of social phobia. Responders to escitalopram, paroxetine, and sertraline have been shown to have significantly higher rates of relapse when switched to placebo for 3 to 6 months following acute treatment than when continued on the active medication (Montgomery *et al.*, 2005; Stein *et al.*, 1996; Stein *et al.*, 2002; Walker *et al.*, 2000). Finally, a study in which responders were maintained on fluvoxamine CR or switched to placebo for 3 months after acute treatment showed that the active medication group achieved additional reduction in social anxiety symptoms whereas the placebo group did not (Stein *et al.*, 2003).

Monoamine oxidase inhibitors (MAOIS)

Phenelzine has demonstrated efficacy for treatment of social phobia in several RCTs (Gelernter *et al.*, 1991; Heimberg *et al.*, 1998; Liebowitz *et al.*, 1992; Versiani *et al.*, 1992). However, the risk of hypertensive crisis and the requirement of a low-tyramine diet decrease the clinical utility of phenelzine and other irreversible MAOIs (e.g. tranylcypromine). These constraints on their use, as well as their less than favourable side-effect profile (i.e. frequent postural hypotension and weight gain) have relegated their use in recent years to situations of treatment-resistance (where, it should be noted, there is no strong evidence that they are especially useful, but expert practitioners still believe they may be). Reversible selective MAOIs such as brofaromine and moclobemide are considered safer and also have demonstrated some benefit for reducing symptoms of social phobia. Brofaromine has demonstrated efficacy in three RCTs (Fahlen *et al.*, 1995; Lott *et al.*, 1997; van Vliet *et al.*, 1992). Results with moclobemide have been mixed: three RCTs found moclobemide to be superior to placebo (International Multicenter Clinical Trial Group on Moclobemide in Social Phobia, 1997; Stein *et al.*, 2002; Versiani *et al.*, 1992); however, another large RCT (Noyes *et al.*, 1997) and a smaller RCT did not support its efficacy (Schneier *et al.*, 1998).

Other antidepressants

Venlafaxine ER is an extended release, dual serotonin-norepinephrine reuptake inhibitor. It has been demonstrated to be safe, well tolerated, and superior to placebo for social phobia in several RCTs (Leibowitz *et al.*, 2005; Rickels *et al.*, 2004; Stein *et al.*, 2005). The therapeutic benefit of Venlafaxine ER is comparable to that of paroxetine (Allgulander *et al.*, 2004; Leibowitz *et al.*, 2005). Venlafaxine ER at a low dose (75 mg) has comparable efficacy to a flexible higher dose (150–225 mg), suggesting that norepinephrine reuptake blockade may not contribute substantially to alleviation of social phobia symptoms (Stein *et al.*, 2005).

Mirtazapine, a noradrenergic and serotonergic antidepressant, was effective in reducing symptoms of social phobia in women in one moderately sized, placebo-controlled RCT (Muehlbacher *et al.*, 2005). Other antidepressants, including tricyclics such as imipramine and clomipramine, have not demonstrated substantial benefit in reducing symptoms of social phobia (e.g. Versiani *et al.*, 1988; Zitrin *et al.*, 1983).

Benzodiazepines

Benzodiazepine monotherapy
Clonazepam has demonstrated efficacy in two placebo-controlled investigations (Davidson *et al.*, 1993; Otto *et al.*, 2000). Alprazolam and other benzodiazepines do not have strong empirical support for treatment of social phobia. For instance, alprazolam produced a response rate of 38% compared to a 69% response rate associated with phenelzine in one study (Gelernter *et al.*, 1991). Although there are limited empirical data (e.g. compared to the much larger evidence base for antidepressants), the overall clinical consensus appears to be that these agents can be useful in some cases of social phobia; therefore, they may be considered as alternatives to SSRIs and MAOIs on a case-by-case basis.

Adjunctive benzodiazepine treatment
Patients taking antidepressants for social phobia are sometimes prescribed adjunctive benzodiazepines to boost or accelerate treatment response. Although the research literature is limited, existing studies do not suggest a clear benefit for the antidepressant-benzodiazepine combination. One small pilot study did not show more rapid resolution of social anxiety symptoms in individuals treated with clonazepam plus paroxetine, compared to those treated with paroxetine alone (Seedat & Stein, 2004). The two treatments also yielded statistically similar results on major outcome measures, although there was a trend toward greater global improvement in the clonazepam plus paroxetine group (79% classified as responders in the clonazepam plus paroxetine group compared to 43% in the placebo plus paroxetine group). The difference in response rates may have been statistically significant with a larger sample size, suggesting that further evaluation of the benefits of combining SSRIs and benzodiazepines is warranted.

Other agents

In a multicentre RCT, the anticonvulsant gabapentin was superior to placebo in treating social phobia (Pande *et al.*, 1999). The novel anxiolytic pregabalin, currently approved in some markets for the treatment of neuropathic pain, has demonstrated efficacy in one RCT for social phobia (Pande *et al.*, 2004). The anticonvulsants topiramate (Van Ameringen *et al.*, 2004) and valproic acid (Kinrys *et al.*, 2003) appeared to benefit some patients with social phobia in open-label trials, but data from RCTs are lacking. Although the anticonvulsant levetiracetam showed some promise in an open-label pilot study of 20 patients with generalized social phobia (Simon *et al.*, 2004), results of an as-yet unpublished multicenter RCT did not show levetiracetam to be superior to placebo (Data on file, UCB Pharma, unpublished data, 2006).

One very small RCT showed that the atypical antipsychotic olanzapine was superior to placebo in reducing symptoms of social phobia (Barnett *et al.*, 2002). As part of an open-label trial of low doses (0.25–3.0 mg/d) of the atypical antipsychotic risperidone to augment treatment of patients with refractory anxiety disorders, several patients with social phobia were found to benefit (Simon *et al.*, 2006). Much more work needs to be done to determine whether risperidone or other atypical antipsychotics will have a role to play – either as monotherapy or as adjunctive therapy – for social phobia.

Although commonly believed to ameliorate the symptoms of performance anxiety, beta-blockers such as atenolol do not appear efficacious for treatment of GSP (Liebowitz *et al.*, 1992; Turner *et al.*, 1994). Moreover, pindolol failed to augment treatment response in patients with GSP when added to paroxetine in a double-blind, placebo-controlled crossover study (Stein *et al.*, 2001).

Psychological treatments

The psychological treatment with the largest evidence base for its efficacy in treating social phobia is cognitive-behavioural therapy (CBT). This most commonly includes a combination of patient education, modification of anxious thinking, and exposure to feared social situations. Some CBT packages also include other elements such as social skills training (SST), in which specific skills for navigating social situations are taught to patients. Evidence suggests that some components of CBT, such as exposure, are effective when conducted as stand-alone treatments rather than as one element of a CBT package.

Cognitive-behavioural therapy

According to most CBT models, two major factors maintain social phobia: (1) anxious thoughts that are predominantly focused on negative social evaluation, and (2) avoidance of feared social situations. Cognitive-behavioural therapy directly targets anxious thinking and situational avoidance using a combination of patient education, cognitive restructuring, and in vivo exposure. The educational component of treatment focuses on explaining the cognitive-behavioural model of social anxiety and providing a rationale for treatment. Patients learn about the nature and purpose of anxiety, the relationship between thoughts, feelings, and behaviours, and the use of cognitive restructuring and exposure to interrupt the anxiety cycle. During the cognitive component of treatment, patients are taught to recognize anxious thoughts, identify mistakes in thinking that contribute to anxiety, and generate alternative, evidence-based interpretations of social situations. Finally, patients develop a list of feared social situations and confront each situation repeatedly during the exposure phase of treatment.

Many RCTs support the efficacy of CBT for social phobia (Clark et al., 2003; Clark et al., 2006; Cottraux et al., 2000; Davidson et al., 2004; Gelernter et al., 1991; Heimberg et al., 1990; Heimberg et al., 1998; Hofmann, 2004; Otto et al., 2000). Cognitive-behavioural therapy has demonstrated superiority to pill placebo and credible therapeutic placebo conditions such as education-based treatments and supportive therapy (Cottraux et al., 2000; Heimberg et al., 1998). Meta-analyses further show that CBT is consistently superior to placebo and associated with moderate to large effect sizes (see Butler et al., 2006 and Rodebaugh et al., 2004 for reviews of meta-analytic findings). Importantly, the effects of CBT for social phobia are durable, lasting one year or more after treatment withdrawal (Clark et al., 2003; Clark et al., 2006; Heimberg et al., 1993; Scholing & Emmelkamp, 1996).

Most controlled trials demonstrating the efficacy of CBT for social phobia have delivered the treatment in a group format. Assumed benefits of the group modality for socially phobic patients have included the normalization of social concerns, social support, and opportunities for naturalistic exposure to social situations inherent in the group format. However, meta-analyses suggest that individual and group CBT produce at least equivalent effects (Rodebaugh et al., 2004), and in one head-to-head study individual treatment produced stronger effects than group treatment (Stangier et al., 2003). This study tested a form of CBT based on a specific cognitive model of social phobia (Clark & Wells, 1995); therefore, it is not yet clear if the superiority of individual treatment would extend to other CBT packages.

Recently, efforts have been made to test versions of CBT that require less direct therapist contact. One RCT showed that internet-delivered CBT with minimal therapist contact was superior to a waiting list control in reducing symptoms of social phobia, and that treatment gains were maintained one year later (Andersson et al., 2006). The empirical validation of self-administered versions CBT may eventually increase the accessibility of this effective form of treatment for individuals with limited financial or insurance resources, or for those who live in geographic regions that have few CBT specialists.

Exposure therapy

Exposure therapy primarily targets avoidance of social situations. Exposure is hypothesized to facilitate habituation, or the natural abatement of the fear response that occurs with increased experience with a situation. Although cognitions are not directly targeted in exposure therapy, this treatment may impact patients' beliefs about social situations by allowing them to gather new evidence and learn that their worst fears do not typically come true in social situations. In exposure therapy, patients develop a hierarchy of feared situations that are later confronted during the course of treatment. Most exposure treatment is conducted in a gradual fashion, with patients confronting situations of increasing difficulty. For instance, a patient might begin by conversing with a familiar person for a few minutes and work up to speaking in front of a group.

Exposure treatment is effective in reducing symptoms of social phobia, and treatment gains can be sustained for six months or longer (Hofmann, 2004; Hope et al., 1995; Mersch, 1995; Scholing & Emmelkamp, 1993; Turner et al., 1994). Exposure has generally compared favourably to CBT in the acute term. Several studies have shown that group exposure treatment produces equivalent effects to group CBT at post-treatment (Hofmann, 2004; Hope et al., 1995; Mersch, 1995). However, one recent study showed that individual CBT was superior to individual exposure therapy plus relaxation training at post-treatment and at 12-month follow-up (Clark et al., 2006). Moreover, in another study patients who received CBT continued to improve in the 6 months following treatment withdrawal, whereas patients who received exposure therapy did not (Hofmann, 2004). These more recent findings suggest some advantage for more comprehensive CBT packages that directly target anxious thinking over exposure therapy alone.

Social skills training (SST)

The theoretical assumption that underlies SST is that individuals with social phobia have deficits in social skills that contribute to their anxiety in social situations. Social skills training therefore focuses on teaching and practising social skills. Empirical research has produced equivocal findings regarding the presence of social skills deficits in individuals with social phobia (Baker & Edelmann, 2002; Rapee & Lim, 1992; Stopa & Clark, 1993). Therefore, it is probably necessary to assess the social skills of patients on a case-by-case basis in order to determine if SST is necessary. One study did show that addition of SST to standard CBT augmented treatment response in individuals with GSP and AvPD (Herbert et al., 2005). This result suggests that the combination of CBT and SST may be particularly relevant for patients whose highly avoidant tendencies may have prevented them from developing adequate social skills.

Comparative efficacy of pharmacological and psychological interventions

Overall, empirically supported psychological treatments compare favourably to first-line pharmacotherapies for treating social phobia in head-to-head comparisons. A recent multi-site RCT compared group CBT that included SST to fluoxetine, CBT plus fluoxetine, placebo, and CBT plus placebo (Davidson et al., 2004). At the end of acute treatment (14 weeks), CBT and fluoxetine were superior to placebo and produced equivalent effects on major treatment outcome measures, including percentage of patients classified as responders. Approximately 50% of patients responded to each active treatment compared to 32% response to placebo (see further discussion of the combined CBT and fluoxetine treatment in 'Combining Pharmacological and Psychological Interventions' below).

Another study compared an individual CBT programme to fluoxetine plus weekly self-exposure assignments, and placebo plus weekly self-exposure assignments (Clark et al., 2003). Cognitive-behavioural therapy was superior to fluoxetine plus self-exposure and placebo plus self-exposure at post-treatment, whereas fluoxetine plus self-exposure and placebo plus self-exposure were equivalent. In this study, patients receiving CBT or fluoxetine plus self-exposure were followed for 12 months after acute treatment withdrawal, and CBT also was superior to fluoxetine plus self-exposure at the 12-month follow-up.

Cognitive-behavioural therapy also has compared relatively favourably to the MAOI phenelzine (Heimberg et al., 1998; Gelernter et al., 1991). A multicentre RCT compared CBT to phenelzine, placebo, and an educational support group that was rated as equally credible to CBT (Heimberg et al., 1998). After 12 weeks of treatment, CBT and phenelzine both produced response rates that were higher than those of the placebo and educational support groups; however, CBT and phenelzine did not differ from one another (75% of CBT completers and 77% of phenelzine completers achieved responder status). More individuals achieved responder status by mid-treatment in the phenelzine group than in the CBT group, suggesting that phenelzine produced its beneficial effects more quickly than CBT. In addition, the quality of response in the phenelzine-treated group appeared superior as indicated by clinician ratings and self-report measures of social phobia symptoms. However, more patients who responded to phenelzine relapsed after treatment was withdrawn compared with those who responded to CBT (50% vs. 17% relapse; Leibowitz et al., 1999).

Finally, a direct comparison of CBT and clonazepam showed that the two treatments produced comparable rates of remission in the intent-to-treat sample (Otto et al., 2000). There was some suggestion of better quality of response in the clonazepam responders; however, this effect may have been a byproduct of differential attrition. This study also was limited by lack of a placebo control group.

Two comparative studies suggest an advantage for psychological treatment over medication after treatment is withdrawn (Haug et al., 2003; Leibowitz et al., 1999). In one case, individuals receiving exposure continued to improve during the follow up period whereas those treated with sertraline reached a plateau or deteriorated during follow up (Haug et al., 2003). The other study showed greater rates of relapse in phenelzine responders compared to CBT responders during the follow-up period (Leibowitz et al., 1999).

Meta-analytic studies have differed in their conclusions regarding the relative efficacy of pharmacological and psychological treatments. Gould et al. (1997) found equivalent effect sizes for pharmacological treatments and CBT (0.62 and 0.74, respectively). In contrast, Fedoroff and Taylor (2001) found SSRIs and benzodiazepines to be more effective than CBT overall.

When meta-analytic and direct comparison studies are considered in conjunction, pharmacological and psychological treatments seem roughly equivalent in their effects. However, pharmacotherapy may produce a quicker and better quality of response in some cases while psychological treatment may produce more durable effects.

Combining pharmacological and psychological interventions

Very few studies have been designed to adequately evaluate the benefits of combining pharmacological and psychological treatments. However, one study that was mentioned above included a CBT plus fluoxetine condition (Davidson *et al.*, 2004). Although this combined treatment was superior to placebo, it performed no better than CBT alone, fluoxetine alone, or CBT plus placebo (Davidson *et al.*, 2004). Therefore, to date, no benefit has been observed in regard to combining the two first-line treatments of SSRIs and CBT.

In contrast, one recent study suggests that the effects of exposure therapy can be augmented by addition of D-cycloserine (DCS; Hofmann *et al.*, 2006). Extinction learning, which is the proposed mechanism of exposure therapy, is blocked by antagonists at the glutamatergic NMDA receptor. In contrast, DCS (a partial agonist at the NMDA receptor) has been shown to facilitate extinction of conditioned fear in animals (Ledgerwood *et al.*, 2003; Walker *et al.*, 2002). A recent RCT with 27 socially phobic patients compared exposure therapy plus DCS to exposure therapy plus placebo (Hofmann *et al.*, 2006). Patients who received DCS 1 hour before exposure therapy sessions demonstrated greater reductions in social anxiety symptoms than those given placebo one hour before exposure therapy sessions at both post-treatment and 1-month follow up. Studies with larger sample sizes are needed to confirm the benefit of combining DCS with exposure therapy; however, these initial results suggest that facilitation of extinction learning via DCS administration may augment the efficacy of traditional exposure-based treatments.

Predictors of treatment outcome

Little has been established regarding characteristics in individuals with social phobia that predict response to different psychotropic medications. One study that investigated more than 800 patients who participated in RCTs of paroxetine found no significant effect of a variety of demographic, physiologic, and clinical variables on treatment outcome; only duration of treatment with paroxetine was a significant predictor of treatment response (Stein *et al.*, 2002). Another study showed that only early age of onset of social phobia predicted less robust response to sertraline (Van Ameringen *et al.*, 2004).

Several studies have shown that pre-treatment depression negatively impacts CBT outcome (Chambless *et al.*, 1997; Ledley *et al.*, 2005; Scholing & Emmelkamp, 1999). One of these studies showed that pre-treatment depression had a similarly negative outcome on all treatment conditions including fluoxetine and a fluoxetine plus CBT combination, suggesting that the impact of depression on treatment outcome is not specific to CBT (Ledley *et al.*, 2005). Therefore, evaluating the effects of depressive symptoms on treatment is important with both pharmacotherapy and psychotherapy. Other comorbid Axis I disorders have not been consistently shown to impact CBT outcome (Rodebaugh *et al.*, 2004). Moreover, social phobia subtype does not seem to predict degree of response to CBT, and results regarding the predictive value of AvPD have been equivocal (Brown *et al.*, 1995; Feske *et al.*, 1996; Hope *et al.*, 1995, Turner *et al.*, 1996).

There is also a dearth of well-designed studies focused on treating patients who fail to respond to first-line treatments such as SSRIs or CBT. Some studies that have established the efficacy of first-line treatments for social phobia show response rates of only 50%, and even the best response rates are in the range of 75%. These statistics underscore the need for research on interventions for treatment-resistant social phobia, as well as further research on novel methods for treating this disorder.

Conclusions

Tremendous advances in the treatment of social phobia have been made in the past two decades. Psychopharmacological treatments such as SSRIs and SNRIs have accrued a substantial evidence base for their efficacy, and they have become mainstays of treatment for social phobia in the community. Similarly, CBT has been proven efficacious and more enduring in its efficacy than medications. But CBT is more difficult to administer and access given our current systems of healthcare delivery. Though primarily studied as a group treatment, preliminary evidence suggests that particular applications of individual CBT may prove more efficacious; this remains to be further studied.

Only approximately 50% of patients derive significant benefit from the first treatment for social phobia they receive, and virtually nothing is known about treatment sequences that should be applied to increase overall response rates. Preliminary studies of combining CBT and SSRIs have failed to show additional benefits of the combination, but such studies have not been conducted in subjects who fail monotherapy (i.e. either CBT or SSRI alone). In this regard, the field is in need of studies of 'stepped care' approaches that would provide information about optimal sequences of the application of treatments with the combined goals of increasing overall efficacy, providing benefits to patients who are refractory to standard treatments, and enhancing the durability of responses for this chronic anxiety disorder. Finally, remarkable advances in the translational neuroscience of extinction learning offer possibilities for developing new treatment modalities that may yield substantially better outcomes than existing treatments.

The level of evidence for each of the interventions discussed in this chapter is summarized in Table 34.1.

Table 34.1. Effectiveness of treatments for social phobia

Treatment	Form of treatment	Psychiatric disorder/target audience	Level of evidence for efficacy	Comments
Psychopharmacology	SSRIs	Social phobia	Ia	Effectiveness shown across all the SSRIs. Effective in antidepressant dosages. May take up to 12 weeks for full effectiveness
Psychopharmacology	MAOIs	Social phobia	Ia	Irreversible have more consistent results than reversible but both are effective. Dietary restrictions and drug-drug interactions, especially with irreversible, limit usage
Psychopharmacology	SNRIs	Social phobia	Ia	Venlafaxine ER comparable to SSRIs in efficacy. May work as well in low doses as in higher doses
Psychopharmacology	Other serotonergic compounds (mirtazepine)	Social phobia	Ib	Small evidence base, but effective in some cases
Psychopharmacology	TCAs	Social phobia	IIb	No evidence of substantial benefit. Side effects more troublesome than with SSRIs
Psychopharmacology	Benzodiazepines	Social phobia	IIa	Little evidence for effectiveness except with clonazepam. Not as effective as SSRIs
Psychosocial	CBT	Social phobia	Ia	Combines patient education, modification of anxious beliefs, and exposure to feared social situations. Effectiveness has been shown in many studies. Treatment gains maintained at least one year after treatment has ended. Equally efficacious in group or individual formats
Psychosocial	Exposure therapy	Social phobia	Ia	Often included as one component of CBT but can be equally effective as a stand-alone treatment
Psychosocial	Social skills training	Social phobia	IIb	Some versions of CBT include a social skills training component. Not usually presented in isolation. Indicated when patient presents with social skills deficits in addition to social anxiety
Psychopharmacological and psychosocial	SSRI plus CBT	Social phobia	IIb	The few available studies do not show this combination to be superior to SSRIs or CBT alone. More research is needed

REFERENCES

Allgulander, C. (1999). Paroxetine in social anxiety disorder: a randomized placebo-controlled study. *Acta Psychiatrica Scandinavica*, **100**, 193–8.

Allgulander, C., Mangano, R., Zhang, J. *et al.* & SAD 388 study group (2004). Efficacy of venlafaxine ER in patients with social anxiety disorder: a double-blind, placebo-controlled, parallel-group comparison with paroxetine. *Human Psychopharmacology*, **19**, 387–96.

American Psychiatric Association (2000). *Diagnostic and Statistical Manual of Mental Disorders, 4th edn. – Text Revision (DSM-IV-TR)*. Washington, DC: APA.

Andersson, G., Carlbring, P., Holmstrom, A. *et al.* (2006). Internet-based self-help with therapist feedback and in vivo group exposure for social phobia: a randomized controlled trial. *Journal of Consulting and Clinical Psychology*, **74**, 677–86.

Baker, S. R. & Edelmann, R. J. (2002). Is social phobia related to lack of social skills? Duration of skill-related behaviours and ratings of behavioural adequacy. *British Journal of Clinical Psychology*, **41**, 243–57.

Baldwin, D., Bobes, J., Stein, D. J., Scharwachter, I. & Faure, M. (1999). Paroxetine in social phobia/social anxiety disorder: randomised, double-blind, placebo-controlled study. *British Journal of Psychiatry*, **175**, 120–6.

Barnett, S. D., Kramer, M. L., Casat, C. D., Connor, K. M. & Davidson, J. R. (2002). Efficacy of olanzapine in social anxiety disorder: a pilot study. *Journal of Psychopharmacology*, **16**, 365–8.

Blanco, C., Schneier, F. R., Schmidt, A. *et al.* (2003). Pharmacological treatment of social anxiety disorder: a meta-analysis. *Depression and Anxiety*, **18**, 29–40.

Breslau, J., Aguilar-Gaxiola, S., Kendler, K. S., Su, M., Williams, D. & Kessler, R. C. (2006). Specifying race-ethnic differences in risk for psychiatric disorder in a USA national sample. *Psychological Medicine*, **36**, 57–68.

Brown, E. J., Heimberg, R. G. & Juster, H. R. (1995). Social phobia subtype and avoidant personality disorder: effect on severity of social phobia, impairment, and outcome of cognitive-behavioral treatment. *Behavior Therapy*, **26**, 467–86.

Bruce, S. E., Yonkers, K. A., Otto, M. W. *et al.* (2005). Influence of psychiatric comorbidity on recovery and recurrence in generalized anxiety disorder, social phobia, and panic disorder: a 12-year prospective study. *American Journal of Psychiatry*, **162**, 1179–87.

Butler, A. C., Chapman, J. E., Forman, E. M. & Beck, A. T. (2006). The empirical status of cognitive-behavioral therapy: a review of meta-analyses. *Clinical Psychology Review*, **26**, 17–31.

Chambless, D. L., Tran, G. Q. & Glass, C. R. (1997). Predictors of response to cognitive-behavioral group therapy for social phobia. *Journal of Anxiety Disorders*, **11**, 221–40.

Chavira, D. A. & Stein, M. B. (2002). Phenomenology of social phobia. In *The American Psychiatric Publishing Textbook of Anxiety Disorders*, ed. D. J. Stein & E. Hollander, pp. 289–300. Washington, DC: American Psychiatric Publishing, Inc.

Clark, D. M. & Wells, A. (1995). A cognitive model of social phobia. In *Social Phobia: Diagnosis, Assessment, and Treatment*, ed.

R. Heimberg, M. Liebowitz, D. A. Hope & F. R. Schneier, pp. 69–93. New York: Guilford Press.

Clark, D. M., Ehlers, A., McManus, F. *et al.* (2003). Cognitive therapy versus fluoxetine in generalized social phobia: a randomized placebo-controlled trial. *Journal of Consulting and Clinical Psychology*, **71**, 1058–67.

Clark, D. M., Ehlers, A. Hackman, A. *et al.* (2006). Cognitive therapy versus exposure and applied relaxation in social phobia: a randomized controlled trial. *Journal of Consulting and Clinical Psychology*, **74**, 568–78.

Cottraux, J., Note, I., Albuisson, E. *et al.* (2000). Cognitive behavior therapy versus supportive therapy in social phobia: a randomized controlled trial. *Psychotherapy and Psychosomatics*, **69**, 137–46.

Davidson, J. R., Potts, N., Richichi, E. *et al.* (1993). Treatment of social phobia with clonazepam and placebo. *Journal of Clinical Psychopharmacology*, **13**, 423–8.

Davidson, J. R. T., Foa, E. B., Huppert, J. D. *et al.* (2004). Fluoxetine, comprehensive cognitive behavioral therapy, and placebo in generalized social phobia. *Archives of General Psychiatry*, **61**, 1005–13.

Fahlen, T., Nilsson, H. L., Borg, K., Humble, M. & Pauli, U. (1995). Social phobia: The clinical efficacy and tolerability of the monoamine-oxidase-A and serotonin uptake inhibitor brofaromine. A double-blind placebo-controlled study. *Acta Psychiatrica Scandinavica*, **92**, 351–8.

Fedoroff, I. C. & Taylor, S. T. (2001). Psychological and pharmacological treatments of social phobia: a meta-analysis. *Journal of Clinical Psychopharmacology*, **21**, 311–24.

Feske, U., Perry, K. J., Chambless, D. L., Renneberg, B. & Golstein, A. (1996). Avoidant personality disorder as a predictor for treatment outcome among generalized social phobics. *Journal of Personality Disorders*, **10**, 174–84.

Furmark, T., Appel, L., Michelgard, A. *et al.* (2005). Cerebral blood flow changes after treatment of social phobia with the neurokinin-1 antagonist GR205171, citalopram, or placebo. *Biological Psychiatry*, **15**, 132–42.

Gelernter, C. S., Uhde, T. W., Cimbolic, P. *et al.* (1991). Cognitive-behavioral and pharmacological treatments of social phobia: a controlled study. *Archives of General Psychiatry*, **48**, 938–45.

Gould, R. A., Buckminster, S., Pollack, M. H., Otto, M. & Yap, L. (1997). Cognitive-behavioral and pharmacological treatment for social phobia: a meta-analysis. *Clinical Psychology: Science and Practice*, **4**, 291–306.

Haug, T. T., Blomhoff, S., Hellstrom, K. *et al.* (2003). Exposure therapy and sertraline in social phobia: 1-year follow-up of a randomized controlled trial. *British Journal of Psychiatry*, **182**, 312–18.

Heimberg, R. G., Dodge, C. S., Hope, D. A., Kennedy, C. R., Zollo, L. & Becker, R. E. (1990). Cognitive-behavioral group treatment of social phobia: comparison to a credible placebo control. *Cognitive Therapy and Research*, **14**, 1–23.

Heimberg, R. G., Salzman, D. G., Holt, C. S. & Blendell, K. A. (1993). Cognitive-behavioral group treatment for social phobia: effectiveness at five-year follow-up. *Cognitive Therapy and Research*, **17**, 325–39.

Heimberg, R. G., Liebowitz, M. R., Hope, D. A. *et al.* (1998). Cognitive behavioral group therapy vs phenelzine for social phobia. *Archives of General Psychiatry*, **55**, 1133–41.

Herbert, J. D., Gaudiano, B. A. Rheingold, A. A., Myers, V. H., Dalrymple, K. & Nolan, E. M. (2005). Social skills training augments the effectiveness of cognitive behavioral group therapy for social anxiety disorder. *Behavior Therapy*, **36**, 125–38.

Hofmann, S. G. (2004). Cognitive mediation of treatment change in social phobia. *Journal of Consulting and Clinical Psychology*, **72**, 392–9.

Hofmann, S. G., Meuret, A. E., Smits, J. A. J. *et al.* (2006). Augmentation of exposure therapy with D-cycloserine for social anxiety disorder. *Archives of General Psychiatry*, **63**, 298–304.

Hope, D. A., Heimberg, R. G. & Bruch, M. A. (1995a). Dismantling cognitive-behavioral group therapy for social phobia. *Behaviour Research and Therapy*, **33**, 637–50.

Hope, D. A., Herbert, J. D. & White, C. (1995b). Diagnostic subtype, avoidant personality disorder, and efficacy of cognitive-behavioral group therapy for social phobia. *Cognitive Therapy and Research*, **19**, 399–417.

International Multicenter Clinical Trial Group on Moclobemide in Social Phobia (1997). Moclobemide in social phobia: a double-blind, placebo-controlled study. *European Archives of Psychiatry and Clinical Neuroscience*, **247**, 71–80.

Kasper, S., Stein, D. J., Loft, H. & Nil, R. (2005). Escitalopram in the treatment of social anxiety disorder: randomized, placebo-controlled, flexible-dosage study. *British Journal of Psychiatry*, **186**, 222–6.

Katzelnick, D. J., Kobak, K. A., Greist, J. H., Jefferson, J. W., Mantle, J. M. & Serlin, R. C. (1995). Sertraline for social phobia: a double-blind, placebo-controlled crossover study. *American Journal of Psychiatry*, **152**, 1368–71.

Kessler, R. C., McGonagle, K. A., Zhao, S. *et al.* (1994). Lifetime and 12-month prevalence of DSM-III-R psychiatric disorders in the United States: results from the National Comorbidity Survey. *Archives of General Psychiatry*, **51**, 8–19.

Kessler, R. C., Stang, P., Wittchen, H. U., Stein, M. B. & Walters, E. E. (1999). Lifetime comorbidities between social phobia and mood disorders in the National Comorbidity Survey. *Psychological Medicine*, **29**, 555–67.

Kessler, R. C., Berglund, P., Demler, O., Jin, R., Merikangas, K. R. & Walters, E. E. (2005a). Lifetime prevalence and age-of-onset distributions of *DSM-IV* disorders in the National Comorbidity Survey Replication. *Archives of General Psychiatry*, **62**, 593–602.

Kessler, R. C., Chiu, W. T., Demler, O. & Walters, E. E. (2005b). Prevalence, severity, and comorbidity of 12-month *DSM-IV* disorders in the National Comorbidity Survey Replication. *Archives of General Psychiatry*, **62**, 617–27.

Kinrys, G., Pollack, M. H., Simon, N. M., Worthington, J. J., Nardi, A. E. & Versiani, M. (2003). Valproic acid for the treatment of social anxiety disorder. *International Clinical Psychopharmacology*, **18**, 169–72.

Kobak, K. A., Greist, J. H., Jefferson, J. W. & Katzelnick, D. J. (2002). Fluoxetine in social phobia: a double-blind, placebo-controlled pilot study. *Journal of Clinical Psychopharmacology*, **22**, 257–62.

Lader, M., Stender, K., Burger, V. & Nil, R. (2004). Efficacy and tolerability of escitalopram in 12- and 24-week treatment of social anxiety disorder: randomised, double-blind, placebo-controlled, fixed-dose study. *Depression and Anxiety*, **19**, 241–8.

Ledgerwood, L., Richardson, R. & Cranney, J. (2003). D-cycloserine facilitates extinction of conditioned fear as assessed by freezing in rats. *Behavioral Neuroscience*, **117**, 341–9.

Ledley, D. R., Huppert, J. D., Foa, E. B., Davidson, J. R. T., Keefe, F. J. & Potts, N. L. S. (2005). Impact of depressive symptoms on the treatment of generalized social anxiety disorder. *Depression and Anxiety*, **22**, 161–7.

Lepola, U., Bergtholdt, B., St. Lambert, J., Davy, K. L. & Ruggiero, L. (2004). Controlled-release paroxetine in the treatment of patients with social anxiety disorder. *Journal of Clinical Psychiatry*, **65**, 222–9.

Liebowitz, M. R., Schneier, F., Campeas, R. *et al.* (1992). Phenelzine vs atenolol in social phobia: a placebo-controlled comparison. *Archives of General Psychiatry*, **49**, 290–300.

Liebowitz, M. R., Heimberg, R. G., Schneier, F. R. *et al.* (1999). Cognitive-behavioral group therapy versus phenelzine in social phobia: long-term outcome. *Depression and Anxiety*, **10**, 89–98.

Liebowitz, M. R., DeMartinis, N. A., Weihs, K. *et al.* (2003). Efficacy of sertraline in severe generalized social anxiety disorder: results of a double-blind, placebo-controlled study. *Journal of Clinical Psychiatry*, **64**, 785–92.

Liebowitz, M. R., Gelenberg, A. J. & Munjack, D. (2005a). Venlafaxine extended release vs placebo and paroxetine in social anxiety disorder. *Archives of General Psychiatry*, **62**, 190–8.

Liebowitz, M. R., Mangano, R. M., Bradwejn, J., Asnis, G. & SAD study group (2005b). A randomized controlled trial of venlafaxine extended release in generalized social anxiety disorder. *Journal of Clinical Psychiatry*, **66**, 238–47.

Lott, M., Greist, J. H., Jefferson, J. W. *et al.* (1997). Brofaromine for social phobia: a multicenter, placebo-controlled, double-blind study. *Journal of Clinical Psychopharmacology*, **17**, 255–60.

Magee, W. J., Eaton, W. W., Wittchen, H. U., McGonagle, K. A. & Kessler, R. C. (1996). Agoraphobia, simple phobia, and social phobia in the National Comorbidity Survey. *Archives of General Psychiatry*, **53**, 159–68.

Mersch, P. P. A. (1995). The treatment of social phobia: the differential effectiveness of exposure *in vivo* and an integration of exposure *in vivo*, rational emotive therapy and social skills training. *Behaviour Research and Therapy*, **33**, 259–69.

Muehlbacher, M., Nickel, M. K., Nickel, C. *et al.* (2005). Mirtazapine treatment of social phobia in women: a randomized, double-blind, placebo-controlled study. *Journal of Clinical Psychopharmacology*, **25**, 580–3.

Montgomery, S. A., Nil, R., Durr-Pal, N., Loft, H. & Boulenger, J. P. (2005). A 24-week randomized, double-blind, placebo-controlled study of escitalopram for the prevention of generalized social anxiety disorder. *Journal of Clinical Psychiatry*, **66**, 1270–8.

Noyes, R., Moroz, G., Davidson, J. R. *et al.* (1997). Moclobemide in social phobia: a controlled dose-response trial. *Journal of Clinical Psychopharmacology*, **17**, 247–54.

Otto, M. W., Pollack, M. H., Gould, R. A., Worthington, J. J., McArdle, E. T. & Rosenbaum, J. F. (2000). A comparison of the efficacy of clonazepam and cognitive-behavioral group therapy for the treatment of social phobia. *Journal of Anxiety Disorders*, **14**, 345–58.

Pande, A. C., Davidson, J. R., Jefferson, J. W. *et al.* (1999). Treatment of social phobia with gabapentin: a placebo-controlled study. *Journal of Clinical Psychopharmacology*, **19**, 341–8.

Pande, A. C., Feltner, D. E., Jefferson, J. W. *et al.* (2004). Efficacy of the novel anxiolytic pregabalin in social anxiety disorder: a placebo-controlled, multicenter study. *Journal of Clinical Psychopharmacology*, **24**, 141–9.

Rapee, R. M. & Lim, L. (1992). Discrepancy between self- and observer ratings of performance in social phobics. *Journal of Abnormal Psychology*, **101**, 728–31.

Rickels, K., Mangano, R. & Khan, A. (2004). A double-blind, placebo-controlled study of a flexible dose of venlafaxine ER in adult outpatients with generalized social anxiety disorder. *Journal of Clinical Psychopharmacology*, **24**, 488–96.

Rodebaugh, T. L., Holaway, R. M. & Heimberg, R. G. (2004). The treatment of social anxiety disorder. *Clinical Psychology Review*, **24**, 883–908.

Schneier, F. R., Goetz, D., Campeas, R., Fallon, B., Marshall, R. & Liebowitz, M. R. (1998). Placebo-controlled trial of moclobemide in social phobia. *British Journal of Psychiatry*, **172**, 70–7.

Scholing, A. & Emmelkamp, P. M. G. (1993). Exposure with and without cognitive therapy for generalized social phobia: effects of individual and group treatment. *Behaviour Research and Therapy*, **31**, 667–81.

Scholing, A. & Emmelkamp, P. M. G. (1996). Treatment of generalized social phobia: results at long-term follow-up. *Behaviour Research and Therapy*, **34**, 447–52.

Scholing, A. & Emmelkamp, P. M. G. (1999). Prediction of treatment outcome in social phobia: a cross-validation. *Behaviour Research and Therapy*, **37**, 659–70.

Seedat, S. & Stein, M. B. (2004). Double-blind, placebo-controlled assessment of combined clonazepam with paroxetine compared with paroxetine monotherapy for generalized social anxiety disorder. *Journal of Clinical Psychiatry*, **65**, 244–8.

Simon, N. M., Hoge, E. A., Fischmann, D. *et al.* (2006). An open-label trial of risperidone augmentation for refractory anxiety disorders. *Journal of Clinical Psychiatry*, **67**, 381–5.

Simon, N. M., Worthington, J. J., Doyle, A. C. *et al.* (2004). An open-label study of levetiracetam for the treatment of social anxiety disorder. *Journal of Clinical Psychiatry*, **65**, 1219–22.

Solyom, L., Ledwidge, B. & Solyom, C. (1986). Delineating social phobia. *British Journal of Psychiatry*, **149**, 464–70.

Stangier, U., Heidenreich, T., Peitz, M., Lauterbach, W. & Clark, D. M. (2003). Cognitive therapy for social phobia: individual versus group treatment. *Behaviour Research and Therapy*, **41**, 991–1007.

Stein, D. J., Berk, M., Els, C. *et al.* (1999). A double-blind placebo-controlled trial of paroxetine in the management of social phobia (social anxiety disorder) in South Africa. *South African Medical Journal*, **89**, 402–6.

Stein, D. J., Cameron, A., Amrein, R., Montgomery, S. A. & Moclobemide Social Phobia Clinical Study Group (2002a). Moclobemide is effective and well tolerated in the long-term pharmacotherapy of social anxiety disorder with or without comorbid anxiety disorder. *International Clinical Psychopharmacology*, **17**, 161–70.

Stein, D. J., Stein, M. B., Pitts, C. D., Kumar, R. & Hunter, B. (2002b). Predictors of response to pharmacotherapy in social anxiety disorder: an analysis of 3 placebo-controlled paroxetine trials. *Journal of Clinical Psychiatry*, **63**, 152–5.

Stein, D. J., Versiani, M., Hair, T., & Kumar, R. (2002c). Efficacy of paroxetine for relapse prevention in social anxiety disorder: a 24-week study. *Archives of General Psychiatry*, **59**, 1111–18.

Stein, M. B. & Kean, Y. M. (2000). Disability and quality of life in social phobia: epidemiologic findings. *American Journal of Psychiatry*, **157**, 1606–13.

Stein, M. B., Chartier, M. J., Hazen, A. L. *et al.* (1996). Paroxetine in the treatment of generalized social phobia: open-label treatment and double-blind, placebo-controlled discontinuation. *Journal of Clinical Psychopharmacology*, **16**, 218–22.

Stein, M. B., Liebowitz, M. R., Lydiard, R. B., Pitts, C. D., Bushnell, W. & Gergel, I. (1998). Paroxetine treatment of generalized social phobia (social anxiety disorder): a randomized controlled trial. *Journal of the American Medical Association*, **280**, 708–13.

Stein, M. B., Fyer, A. J., Davidson, J. R., Pollack, M. H. & Wiita, B. (1999). Fluvoxamine treatment of social phobia (social anxiety disorder): a double-blind, placebo-controlled study. *American Journal of Psychiatry*, **156**, 756–60.

Stein, M. B., Sareen, J., Hami, S. & Chao, J. (2001). Pindolol potentiation of paroxetine for generalized social phobia: a double-blind, placebo-controlled, crossover study. *American Journal of Psychiatry*, **158**, 1725–27.

Stein, D. J., Westenberg, H. G., Yang, H., Li, D. & Barbato, L. M. (2003). Fluvoxamine CR in the long-term treatment of social anxiety disorder: the 12- to 24-week extension phase of a multicentre, randomized, placebo-controlled trial. *International Journal of Neuropsychopharmacology*, **6**, 317–23.

Stein, M. B., Pollack, M. H., Bystritsky, A., Kelsey, J. E. & Mangano, R. M. (2005). Efficacy of low and higher dose extended-release venlafaxine in generalized social anxiety disorder: a 6-month randomized controlled trial. *Psychchopharmacology (Berlin)*, **177**, 280–8.

Stopa, L. & Clark, D. M. (1993). Cognitive processes in social phobia. *Behaviour Research and Therapy*, **31**, 255–67.

Turner, S. M., Beidel, D. C. & Jacob, R. G. (1994). Social phobia: a comparison of behavior therapy and atenolol. *Journal of Consulting and Clinical Psychology*, **62**, 350–8.

Turner, S. M., Beidel, D. C., Wolff, P. L., Spaulding, S. & Jacob, R. G. (1996). Clinical features affecting treatment outcome in social phobia. *Behaviour Research and Therapy*, **10**, 795–804.

Van Ameringen, M. A., Lane, R. M., Walker, J. R. *et al.* (2001). Sertraline treatment of generalized social phobia: a 20-week, double-blind, placebo-controlled study. *American Journal of Psychiatry*, **158**, 275–81.

Van Ameringen, M., Mancini, C., Pipe, B., Oakman, J. & Bennett, M. (2004a). An open trial of topiramate in the treatment of generalized social phobia. *Journal of Clinical Psychiatry*, **65**, 1674–8.

Van Ameringen, M., Oakman, J., Mancini, C., Pipe, B. & Chung, H. (2004b). Predictors of response in generalized social phobia: effect of age of onset. *Journal of Clinical Psychopharmacology*, **24**, 42–8.

van Vliet, I. M., den Boer, J. A. & Westenberg, H. G. (1992). Psychopharmacological treatment of social phobia: Clinical and biochemical effects of brofaromine, a selective MAO-A inhibitor. *European Neuropsychopharmacology*, **2**, 21–9.

van Vliet, I. M., den Boer, J. A. & Westenberg, H. G. (1994). Psychopharmacological treatment of social phobia: a double-blind placebo controlled study with fluvoxamine. *Psychopharmacology (Berlin)*, **115**, 128–34.

Versiani, M., Mundim, F. D., Nardi, A. E. & Liebowitz, M. R. (1988). Tranylcypromine in social phobia. *Journal of Clinical Psychopharmacology*, **8**, 279–83.

Versiani, M., Nardi, A. E., Mundim, F. D., Alves, A. B., Liebowitz, M. R. & Amrein, R. (1992). Pharmacotherapy of social phobia: a controlled study with moclobemide and phenelzine. *British Journal of Psychiatry*, **161**, 353–60.

Walker, D. L., Ressler, K. J., Lu, K. T. & Davis, M. (2002). Facilitation of conditioned fear extinction by systemic administration or intra-amygdalar infusions of D-cycloserine as assessed with fear-potentiated startle in rats. *Journal of Neuroscience*, **22**, 2243–351.

Walker, J. R., Van Ameringen, M. A., Swinson, R. et al. (2000). Prevention of relapse in generalized social phobia: results of a 24-week study in responders to 20 weeks of sertraline treatment. *Journal of Clinical Psychopharmacology*, **20**, 636–44.

Wang, P. S., Lane, M., Olfson, M., Pincus, H. A., Wells, K. B. & Kessler, R. C. (2005). Twelve-month use of mental health services in the United States: results from the National Comorbidity Survey Replication. *Archives of General Psychiatry*, **62**, 629–40.

Zitrin, C. M., Klein, D. F., Woerner, M. G. & Ross, D. C. (1983). Treatment of phobias I. Comparison of imipramine hydrochloride and placebo. *Archives of General Psychiatry*, **40**, 125–38.

35

Obsessive-compulsive disorder

Helen Blair Simpson and Phil Harrison-Read

Editor's note

You will note from Part I that obsessive-compulsive disorder, formerly called obsessional neurosis before the word neurosis was eliminated from usage, has the highest clinical utility score of the disorders within the neurotic spectrum. It is therefore not surprising that we have much clearer guidelines and evidence for treatment than for others within the spectrum. The arguments in favour of both drug and psychological treatments are strong and are often complementary across the range of clinical indications in OCD. There are some disparities between the UK and USA but most are matters of emphasis rather than fundamental disagreements. We need more evidence from studies on combinations of drug and psychological interventions as this is a very common position in clinical practice.

Introduction

Obsessive-compulsive disorder (OCD) is a relatively common, usually chronic and sometimes very disabling condition, which by convention excludes clinically similar syndromes caused by psychoactive drugs or by a general medical condition. It is characterized by obsessions, compulsions or a combination of both. Obsessions are recurrent and persistent ideas, images or impulses that cause pronounced anxiety and which are usually recognized by the person affected as being self-produced, and yet irrational. Compulsions are intentional repetitive behaviours or mental acts (rituals) performed in response to obsessions or in response to self-imposed rules which are aimed at reducing distress or at preventing unacceptable or anxiety-provoking outcomes. Compulsive rituals are usually recognized as unreasonable, pointless or time-wasting and are also usually resisted by the individual

affected. Some patients have poor insight into the irrationality of their symptoms and can appear delusional about their OCD beliefs (Kozak & Foa, 1994; Tolin et al., 2001).

Although all patients with OCD have obsessions and/or compulsions, the specific content of obsessions and compulsions can vary greatly between patients. For example, obsessions can include fears of harming others or being harmed, fears of contamination, intrusive sexual or religious thoughts, the excessive need for symmetry or exactness, and/or the excessive need to keep or collect possessions. Compulsions can include repetitive checking, washing, repeating, ordering and arranging and/or hoarding of objects. Many patients have multiple obsessions and multiple compulsions (Mataix-Cols et al., 2005).

Diagnostic criteria for obsessive compulsive disorder are similar in ICD-10 and DSM-IV.

Recognition of the disorder can be problematic as people affected by OCD may conceal their symptoms usually because of embarrassment but sometimes out of fear of being stigmatized or judged insane or dangerous. Diagnosis may therefore be delayed by many years. Co-existent symptoms or syndromes, especially depression and anxiety, are common and may be the presenting complaints in a significant minority (over one-third). Patients presenting with other common psychiatric disorders, particularly those with atypical features, which are not responding well to treatment, should therefore be asked about problems with obsessions and compulsions.

Intrusive thoughts and repetitive behaviours are also common in a number of other psychiatric disorders, and features of many other mental disorders may be confused with OCD (e.g. anankastic personality disorder, Asperger's syndrome, depressive disorder, anxiety disorders, hypochondriasis, paraphilias). Approximately 15% of people suffering from schizophrenia qualify for a diagnosis of OCD, and this is associated with a poor outcome of both conditions.

Cambridge Textbook of Effective Treatments in Psychiatry, ed. Peter Tyrer and Kenneth R. Silk. Published by Cambridge University Press.
© Cambridge University Press, 2008.

The etiology of OCD is unknown, but behavioural, cognitive, neurobiological and genetic factors have all been implicated. Obsessive-compulsive disorder-like syndromes occur in various brain syndromes such as Sydenham's chorea, temporal lobe epilepsy and encephalitis lethargica. Patients suffering from tic disorders such as Tourette's syndrome can show features of OCD, and tics are not uncommon in established OCD. Dopamine, noradrenaline, various neuropeptides and especially serotonin are neurotransmitters implicated in the pathophysiology of OCD, as is a malfunctioning brain circuit involving the orbito-frontal cortex, the basal ganglia and the thalamus (Saxena et al., 2001).

In a subgroup of children, the onset of OCD is linked to Group-A beta-hemolytic streptococcal (GAS) infection. The working hypothesis is that the GAS infection in a susceptible host incites the production of antibodies to GAS that cross-react with the cellular components of the basal ganglia, leading to obsessions, compulsions, tics, and other neuropsychiatric symptoms (Snider & Swedo, 2004). A recent study found that 42% of a group of children with OCD had antibasal ganglia antibodies (as seen in Sydenham's chorea) compared with 2%–10% of a control group (Dale et al., 2005). This has not yet led to changes in treatment strategy in clinical practice, but researchers are examining immunomodulatory treatments.

Obsessions and compulsions as isolated symptoms occur, respectively, in at least 80% and 50% of the general population (Muris et al., 1997; Salkovskis & Harrison, 1984). For DSM-IV OCD, the 12-month prevalence in adults ranges from 0.6% to 1.0% (Crino et al., 2005; Kessler et al., 2005). In the recently completed US National Comorbidity Survey Replication, the lifetime prevalence of OCD in adults was estimated to be 1.6%; in this large sample, the median age of onset was 19, with at least 25% of people developing the disorder by the age of 14 (Kessler et al., 2005). Obsessive-compulsive disorder tends to develop earlier in males than females.

In the early stages of the disorder, relapses and remissions often occur (Skoog & Skoog, 1999). After several years, a chronic waxing and waning course is more common with most patients suffering from moderate or severe symptoms (Kessler et al., 2005). Approximately 10% get worse over time, and these are typically males with an insidious onset in childhood.

Drug and psychological (behavioural and cognitive) treatments are the mainstays of management of OCD. Even when OCD is recognized and diagnosed appropriately, patients may be reluctant to start treatment, and in particular to continue with it over the prolonged periods which are often required. Drug treatment may seem more appealing as an initial strategy because, although typically slow to reach full effectiveness, it does not require patients' active participation and is less likely to exacerbate distress due to patients having to confront their obsessional fears or disrupt their compulsive behaviour. Furthermore, while some obsessional fears (e.g. those concerning rarely occurring events) and obsessional doubt and slowness may be relatively difficult to tackle with psychological approaches, they represent ready targets for drug treatment. However, long-term treatment with medication may cause understandable concern about drug dependency and delayed adverse drug reactions, and unlike psychological treatment, the benefits of drug treatment probably do not persist beyond its administration.

All drugs recommended as first-line treatments for OCD are potent inhibitors of the neuronal reuptake of serotonin, an indoleamine neurotransmitter widely distributed in the brain. Serotonin reuptake inhibitors (SRIs) include clomipramine, a tricyclic antidepressant that also has potent effects on other neurotransmitter systems and the selective serotonin reuptake inhibitors, drugs with a more or less selective action on serotonin neuronal reuptake (i.e. citalopram, escitalopram, fluoxetine, fluvoxamine, paroxetine and sertraline). All SSRIs, except for citalopram and escitalopram, are currently licensed in the UK and approved by the Food and Drug Administration in the USA for the treatment of OCD.

The best established psychological intervention for OCD is behaviour therapy including exposure to ritual-provoking stimuli and response prevention, often called ERP in the literature. In ERP, patients are taught to confront situations and objects they fear (i.e. exposure) and to refrain from performing compulsions (i.e. ritual prevention). Exposures may include live confrontations with feared situations (e.g. touching objects in public bathrooms) and imaginal confrontations of feared consequences (e.g. imagining becoming ill from 'contamination'). Exposures that provoke moderate anxiety/discomfort are confronted first, followed by exposures of increasing difficulty. Patients are expected to face their fears for a prolonged period without ritualizing, and this allows the initial anxiety or discomfort to dissipate on its own ('habituation'). The goal is to weaken the connections between feared stimuli and distress and between ritualizing and relief from distress. In the process, mistaken OCD beliefs (e.g. that compulsive rituals prevent harm, that anxiety/discomfort will persist forever, that feared consequences will occur) are corrected. An important aspect of behaviour therapy is 'homework' in which the patient continues ERP outside the formal therapy sessions. ERP has been delivered in different formats. Some programmes involve in-patient or intensive treatment (e.g. 2-hour sessions five days a week for a month). Other treatment programmes involve little or no direct contact with a therapist, and the patient may instead rely on a treatment manual or interactive computer program to guide their therapy. It is thought that the most effective variant of ERP includes not just habituation but discussion of distorted beliefs and feared consequences (Huppert & Franklin, 2006).

Notwithstanding the many other variables that are likely to be of relevance, it appears that the effectiveness of psychological treatment depends partly on the amount of time spent in direct contact with a therapist. Thus interventions involving less than 10 therapist hours per patient are categorized as low intensity treatment whereas 30 or more therapist hours constitute high intensity treatment in the NICE guidelines (see below).

Several standardized rating scales for features of OCD have been developed for research studies. This includes the widely used Yale–Brown Obsessive Compulsive Scale (Y-BOCS, (Goodman *et al.*, 1989)), which is observer-rated and well validated. The Y-BOCS considers obsessions and compulsions separately in five dimensions: time taken up, interference with normal functioning, distress, resistance, and patient's ability to control. Thus as well as measuring OCD symptoms, the Y-BOCS assesses emotional well-being and social functioning. The maximum score on the Y-BOCS is 40; a score of 16 or above is generally considered clinically significant OCD warranting treatment.

Different criteria for treatment response and remission have been used in clinical trials for OCD (Simpson *et al.*, 2006). Often, response is defined as 25% decrease from baseline in the Y-BOCS score. However an improvement of 35% or more in the baseline Y-BOCS score is probably necessary for patients to feel substantially improved. Different criteria for remission have also been proposed e.g. a total Y-BOCS score of 16 or less (Pallanti *et al.*, 2002) or of 12 or less (Simpson *et al.*, 2006). Lower Y-BOCS scores appear to be positively associated with better quality of life and functioning (Huppert *et al.*, in review).

Official UK treatment guidelines

Comprehensive clinical practice guidelines for the recognition and management of OCD in primary and secondary care in the UK were issued by the National Institute of Health and Clinical Excellence (NICE) in November 2005,

with a revised publication in January 2006 (NICE, 2006). At the time of writing, there are no other official UK treatment guidelines for OCD apart from those published electronically as 'PRODIGY Guidance' by the National Electronic Library for Health (NeLH) under the auspices of the Department of Health. However, these guidelines were withdrawn in the latter part of 2004, presumably pending release of the NICE guidelines. PRODIGY guidelines dealt only with patients aged 16 or over and were explicity aimed at primary healthcare professionals with advice on when OCD patients should be referred to secondary care services.

The only other UK national treatment guidelines for OCD are those implicit in the review of evidence about treatment effectiveness published as 'Clinical Evidence' jointly by the National Library for Health, and the BMJ Publishing Group (Soomro, 2004). Clinical Evidence summarises 'the current state of knowledge and uncertainty' about the treatment of OCD in adults based on published systematic reviews, randomized controlled trials (RCTs) and other referenced sources. Although there are no explicit treatment guidelines in Clinical Evidence, evidence regarding treatment outcomes is grouped under headings such as 'beneficial treatments', 'treatments likely to be effective' and 'treatments of unknown effectiveness'. Clinical Evidence does not make a distinction between treatments in primary and secondary care settings.

NICE guidelines

The NICE guidelines concerning OCD deal with 'core interventions' for the treatment of both OCD and body dysmorphic disorder in children and adults. (NICE, 2006). The NICE guidelines eschew specifying first-line and second-line treatments, and instead adopt a graded or 'stepped care' approach. In this, the least intrusive and intensive interventions are used first except for the most severely affected individuals, with progression to more intensive treatments if there is insufficient or unsatisfactory treatment response. Initial low intensity treatment strategies for adults with OCD are likely to be delivered in primary care and are specified in ascending order as:

- Low intensity (up to 10 therapist hours per patient) cognitive-behaviour therapy (CBT) is recommended for adults with mild functional impairment due to OCD. In the NICE guidelines CBT for OCD is defined as always involving a component of exposure and response or ritual prevention (ERP), and for low intensity treatment, may include structured self-help materials, treatment over the telephone, or group CBT.

- For adults who reject, do not engage with, or fail to respond to low intensity CBT, or for patients with moderate functional impairment, the guidelines recommend either (a) a course of an SSRI drug (all are considered to be equally effective) or (b) moderately intensive CBT (including ERP) as defined as involving between 10 and 30 therapist hours per patient. Special monitoring is advised for young adults treated with SSRI drugs in view of concerns regarding increased risk of deliberate self -harm and suicide. If response to an SSRI is inadequate after 4 to 6 weeks of treatment, dose increases should be considered up to the recommended maximum for each drug, with treatment lasting for at least 12 weeks at the optimal dose.

- For adults suffering from OCD with severe functional impairment, or for whom SSRI medication or moderately intensive psychological treatment as monotherapy have been ineffective, combined SSRI medication and CBT (including ERP) should be offered.

- If treatment response is still unsatisfactory, consider treating in a specialist care multidisciplinary setting and combining CBT (including ERP) and drug therapy using a different SSRI from that used previously, or use clomipramine. Clomipramine (an SRI) should be used next if the patient has previously responded well to it and/or requested it, but clomipramine is likely to be less well tolerated than SSRIs.

In the event of an inadequate response to the above in terms of a clinically significant improvement in both OCD symptoms and overall functioning, further treatment strategies involving mangement by multidisciplinary teams in secondary (specialist) settings care will be necessary.

- Further specialist treatment options for adults with OCD include intensive CBT (including ERP) (more than 30 therapist hours per patient), and adding an atypical antipsychotic drug to an SSRI or clomipramine.

The NICE guidelines make some recommendations about the duration of treatment with medication. If effective, medication should be continued for at least 12 months 'to prevent relapse and allow for further improvements'. The decision to prolong treatment beyond 1 year is a clinical judgement based on patient choice and preference, the severity and duration of previous OCD episodes, the presence of residual symptoms and concurrent psychosocial difficulties.

Summary and comment on the UK guidelines for OCD
Older UK guidelines for OCD such as the PRODIGY and Clinical Evidence Guidelines failed to provide clear, and unambiguous advice regarding the setting, type and order in which different treatments should be tried. In the case of medication, they did not help in the choice between SSRIs and SRI (clomipramine) or whether to combine psychological and pharmacological approaches. By contrast, the 'stepped-care' approach used in the very comprehensive NICE guidelines makes for clear and coherent sequential recommendations to guide treatment. The NICE guidelines also cover the not uncommon situation in which OCD patients show a poor response to treatment, both initially and at later stages. However, the expectation by NICE that many patients (maybe the majority) will be managed in primary care settings is probably unrealistic, given the current scarcity of appropriately trained staff and resources to deliver psychological treatments for OCD in primary care.

All of the guidelines considered are somewhat vague regarding the optimal duration of treatment, especially regarding medication, reflecting inadequacies in the available evidence. This is an important point considering the likelihood that a substantial minority of OCD patients will still show significant symptomatology and dysfunction following a period of treatment, and have a relatively low prospect of achieving a complete and lasting remission of illness, even if the treatment is continued indefinitely.

Official US treatment guidelines

Comprehensive clinical practice guidelines for the recognition and management of OCD in the USA have been prepared by the American Psychiatric Association (APA) and published in 2007 in the *American Journal of Psychiatry*. These guidelines address how to treat OCD patients aged 18 and older and are aimed at psychiatrists in clinical practice. APA guidelines are developed by an expert work group and are based upon a systematic review of the scientific literature; the guidelines then undergo wide review by experts and allied organizations.

Previous US treatment guidelines included the Expert Consensus Guideline Series. Treatment guidelines for OCD were published in 1997 and provided a detailed algorithym of first and second-line treatments for OCD (March *et al.*, 1997). These guidelines were based on a synthesis of the opinions of a large group of experts. Since 1997, several of the strategies advocated in these guidelines have been subjected to additional study. Several key research findings are highlighted below and are reflected in the new APA guidelines.

Efficacy of selective serotonin reuptake inhibitors (SSRIs)
Since 1997, controlled trials continue to demonstrate the efficacy of SRIs and clomipramine for OCD, including

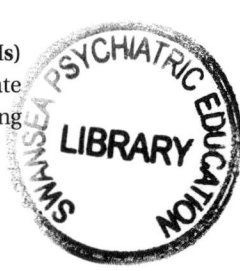

a multi-site RCT of citalopram in OCD (Montgomery et al., 2001). However, the limitations of the SRIs have also been highlighted in the literature. For example, although up to 65% of OCD patients respond to an SRI trial, the mean reduction in OCD symptoms (measured by the Y-BOCS) has ranged from 20% to 40% across studies (Pigott & Seay, 1999). Thus, many SRI responders continue to have clinically significant OCD symptoms that can affect their functioning and quality of life (Simpson et al., 2006).

For OCD patients with a partial or no response to SSRIs, two strategies were advocated in the Expert Consensus Guideline Series for OCD: switching to another SRI or augmenting the SSRI with either psychotherapy or another medication. The data in support of switching to another SRI is limited. Case series indicate that SRI non-responders are unlikely to respond to another SRI (Fineberg & Gale 2005). In the only controlled switching trial, 19% of paroxetine non-responders responded when switched to venlafaxine (Denys et al., 2004b). In contrast, the data that has accumulated since 1997 for SRI augmentation is compelling. As reviewed below, the addition of antipsychotic medications (e.g. risperidone, olanzapine, quetiapine) has been shown in several randomized controlled trials to benefit up to 50% of OCD patients with minimal response to an SRI (Bloch et al., 2006). Moreover, data from open trials (Simpson et al., 1999; Tolin et al., 2004), one controlled trial (Tenneij et al., 2005) and a multi-site trial that has just been completed (trial described in Simpson & Liebowitz 2005) indicate that ERP can also successfully augment SRI response in many OCD patients.

Efficacy of clomipramine (CMI)

The Expert Consensus Guideline Series for OCD suggest that after failing 2–3 trials of selective serotonin uptake inhibitors (SSRIs), an OCD patient should be switched to the non-selective serotonin reuptake inhibitor drug CMI, based on the notion that CMI may be more efficacious than SSRIs because of its broader mode of action. Indeed, meta-analyses (Abramowitz, 1997; Ackerman & Greenland, 2002; Eddy et al., 2004) have found that CMI is more efficacious than SSRIs. However, head-to-head comparisons have not found a significant difference between CMI and SSRIs (Freeman et al., 1994; Koran et al., 1996; Lopez-Ibor et al., 1996; Mundo et al., 2000). Thus, it remains unclear whether CMI is more effective than the SSRIs for OCD or not. Because of the greater potential for adverse side effects from CMI, SSRIs continue to be the medication treatment to try first.

On the other hand, clinicians in the USA are sometimes using venlafaxine in place of clomipramine, assuming it has similar efficacy (due to its inhibition of both norepinephrine and serotonin uptake like clomipramine) and

fewer side effects (because it lacks anticholinergic, antihitaminergic, and α_1-adrenergic blocking effects). In the only randomized placebo-controlled trial in OCD (Yaryura-Tobias & Neziroglu, 1996), venlafaxine was not significantly different from placebo, but this study had important limitations (e.g. small sample size, short trial duration, low dose). In active comparison trials that did not include a placebo arm, venlafaxine and venlafaxine XR, respectively, have also been shown to have equivalent efficacy to CMI (Albert et al., 2002) and to paroxetine (Denys et al., 2003). In several open trials, venlafaxine has also been found effective for OCD (Hollander et al., 2003b; Rauch et al., 1996; Sevincok & Uygur, 2002). Although used, venlafaxine is not currently approved by the US Food and Drug Administration for the treatment of OCD.

Efficacy of psychosocial treatments

Since 1997, findings from controlled trials continue to demonstrate the efficacy of cognitive-behavioural therapy consisting primarily of ERP in the treatment of OCD. For example, ERP has been shown to be superior to pill placebo and SRI pharmacotherapy in OCD patients without comorbid depression (Foa et al., 2005) as well as to be superior to anxiety management therapy (Lindsay et al., 1997), self-guided relaxation therapy (Greist et al., 2002), and wait-list control (Cordioli et al., 2003; McLean et al., 2001; van Balkom et al., 1998). ERP that focuses primarily on habituation (i.e. without formal discussion of dysfunctional cognitions) has been shown to have similar efficacy to cognitive therapy that includes behavioural experiments (van Balkom et al., 1998; Whittal et al., 2005). Current studies are addressing whether the addition of formal cognitive procedures to ERP improves outcome (e.g. Vogel et al., 2004).

It has been argued that the attempt to distinguish behavioural and cognitive therapy is somewhat artificial, given that some ERP variants include informal cognitive procedures, and cognitive therapy (CT) typically includes behavioural experiments that can resemble exposures. Both ERP and CT can change cognitions (Whittal et al., 2005). Some experts have concluded that the question of cognitive vs. behavioural therapy is not clinically useful; they advocate that OCD therapists use an integrated cognitive-behavioural approach that includes exposure, ritual prevention, and discussion of distorted beliefs (Huppert & Franklin 2006).

Summary and comment on the US guidelines for OCD

Treatment guidelines for OCD have been developed by the American Psychiatric Association to assist US psychiatrists in clinical decision-making and to improve patient care; these guidelines reflect the latest scientific information. However, the challenge in the USA is how to encourage the use of these guidelines in routine clinical practice. Of note, OCD treatment guidelines have been available since 1997, yet many OCD patients still do not receive appropriate care (Blanco *et al.*, 2006; Eisen *et al.*, 1999; Koran *et al.*, 2000). The reasons for this remain unclear, but are likely to include patient, clinician, and system barriers. OCD treatment in the USA continues to be an area with substantial opportunity for quality improvement.

Evidence for treatment effectiveness in OCD

With OCD patients, unlike other anxiety disorders or depression, the rate of response to control treatments is typically small (5%–20% compared to 30%–50% in studies in depression), reflecting the relatively refractory and enduring nature of OCD. Nonetheless, current treatments for OCD assessed in groups of patients typically produce clinically important and statistically significant improvements relative to controls, as assessed by increased response or remission rates (typically 30%–50%) (dichotomous outcomes) or by greater mean reductions in symptoms (continuous outcomes). However, the proportions of patients not responding to treatments may be considerable (a quarter or more), and even many treatment responders fail to achieve remission (i.e. no more than minimal symptoms at the end of treatment (Simpson *et al.*, 2006)).

Psychological treatments

Most of the evidence available for the effectiveness of psychological treatments in OCD applies to behavioural and cognitive approaches or combinations of the two in the form of cognitive behaviour therapy (CBT).

Behaviour therapy including ERP

Behaviour therapy for OCD mainly comprises exposure to situations or stimuli, which evoke obsessive-compulsive symptoms (i.e. exposure) combined with response (ritual) prevention; this treatment has often been referred to as ERP in the literature. Some ERP variants examined in controlled trials focus only on habituation (e.g. McLean *et al.*, 2001; Whittal *et al.*, 2005); others also include informal cognitive interventions to target dysfunctional beliefs and/or to prevent relapse (e.g. Foa *et al.*, 2005).

In comparison with relaxation therapy or general anxiety management, individual behaviour therapy, generally lasting about 12 weeks, has been convincingly shown to be effective in OCD (Fals-Stewart *et al.*, 1993; Greist *et al.*, 2002; Lindsay *et al.*, 1997). Individual behaviour therapy has also been shown to be superior to wait-list control (van Balkom *et al.*, 1998; Whittal *et al.*, 2005) and to pill placebo (Foa *et al.*, 2005). Group behaviour therapy which obviously has advantages in making efficient use of scarce resources also has been shown to be more effective than progressive muscle relaxation (Fals-Stewart *et al.*, 1993), group CT (McLean *et al.*, 2001), and wait-list control (Cordioli *et al.*, 2003). Even behaviour therapy guided by a computer has been found to help patients if they adhere to the procedures (Greist *et al.*, 2002).

Several controlled studies have compared the efficacy of ERP, SRI medication, and/or their combination in OCD (Franklin *et al.*, 2005). In OCD patients without comorbid depression, one study found that ERP optimally delivered was superior to SRI monotherapy (Foa *et al.*, 2005). However, in OCD patients with comorbid depression, another study found that combination treatment was superior to ERP alone (Hohagen *et al.*, 1998).

In contrast to drug treatment, the benefits of behaviour therapy are likely to persist beyond the period of actual treatment (Marks *et al.*, 1975; Foa & Goldstein, 1978). In the study by Marks *et al.* (1975) 20 OCD patients who had successfully received ERP in a randomized-controlled trial were followed up over 2 years, with nearly 80% sustaining their improvement. However, few randomized controlled studies have systematically evaluated the long-term durability of ERP, controlling for interim treatment. In one study that examined the post-treatment effects of ERP after sustained treatment discontinuation using evaluators blind to original treatment assignment (Simpson *et al.*, 2004), 88% of patients who responded to ERP (with or without concomitant medication) maintained their gains up to 12 weeks after treatment discontinuation. Clinical experience suggests that patients can maintain their gains from ERP if they continue to confront feared situations in their daily life and to avoid ritualizing.

Although ERP can be a highly effective treatment for OCD, its effects may be reduced by certain patient factors. These include: poor adherence with the exposure procedures (Abramowitz *et al.*, 2002), the presence of certain comorbid conditions (e.g. severe depression or comorbid anxiety disorders, (Abromowitz *et al.*, 2000; Gershuny *et al.*, 2002; Steketee *et al.*, 2001), and poor insight about the irrationality of the obsessive fears (Foa *et al.*, 1999). As with drug treatment, up to half of OCD patients may show an unsatisfactory or incomplete response to behaviour therapy, with some not responding at all (Stanley & Turner 1995; Simpson *et al.*, 2006). Another problem with ERP is the lack of sufficient numbers of skilled providers. As a result, some have proposed a stepped-care approach to the treatment of OCD, in which self-help ERP approaches are disseminated and used first as a way to help more patients and to save resources (Mataix-Cols & Marks, 2006).

Cognitive therapy (CT)

Cognitive therapy for OCD mainly comprises identifying, challenging and modifying faulty beliefs. Most CT variants include behavioural experiments, which can resemble exposure techniques. In several head-to-head comparisons, CT that included behavioural experiments had similar efficacy to ERP that focused on habituation only (e.g. Cottraux *et al.*, 2001; van Balkom *et al.*, 1998; Whittal *et al.*, 2005), although one found ERP superior (McLean *et al.*, 2001). On the other hand, it is thought that the most effective variant of ERP includes not just habituation but discussion of distorted beliefs and feared consequences (Huppert and Franklin 2006). Whether the systematic integration of CT and ERP leads to better outcome than optimally delivered ERP alone is currently under study (Vogel *et al.*, 2004). Cognitive therapy has also been used as an adjunct to standard ERP for certain types of OCD patients, like those without overt rituals (Freeston *et al.*, 1997). There are little data to support the use of cognitive therapy in OCD in the absence of exposure or behavioural experiments.

A systematic review of all psychological treatment interventions for OCD that include an ERP or cognitive therapy component with respect to the number of therapist hours per patient was carried out by the group responsible for producing the NICE guidelines (NICE, 2006). The systematic review included 29 studies and considered three levels of intensity of intervention; low intensity (less than 10 therapist hours per patient, 8 studies); medium intensity interventions (between 10 and 29 therapist hours per patient, 13 studies); and high intensity studies (30 or more therapist hours per patient, 8 studies). The effect size (standard mean difference) for each sub-group was −0.93, −1.44, and −1.65 for low, medium and high intensity groups respectively, with the number of therapist hours per patient significantly ($P < 0.05$) predicting treatment outcome after allowing for some but not all potentially confounding variables.

Pharmacological treatments

Clomipramine

Early anecdotal reports of tricyclic antidepressants being effective in OCD soon focused on one drug in particular, clomipramine. Clomipramine is a potent non-selective serotonin reuptake inhibitor (SRI). The effectiveness of this drug in OCD was first reported in 1967, and has since been confirmed in numerous randomized placebo-controlled trials. By contrast, tricyclic antidepressant drugs lacking a potent effect on serotonin reuptake are not effective treatments in OCD (Thoren *et al.*, 1980; Leonard *et al.*, 1989), although venlafaxine (a potent reuptake inhibitor of both serotonin and catecholamines) may be as effective as clomipramine in OCD (Albert *et al.*, 2002).

The early studies of clomipramine in OCD were mostly carried out in relatively small groups of patients with stable, severe, previously untreated illness who typically showed a low placebo response (less than 5% vs. the 30%–50% typical of studies in depression), and a marked specific treatment response to clomipramine, reflected by a 50% or more reduction in rating scores. In these early studies, many OCD patients had marked depressive symptoms, and it was argued by some that the benefits of clomipramine on OCD symptoms were dependent on the drug's antidepressant effect. However, depressive symptoms in OCD tend to respond relatively early on during treatment, whereas obsessional symptoms continue to improve over weeks, months and even years of treatment. In order to exclude an interfering effect of depressive symptoms on the anti-obsessional action of clomipramine, later studies excluded patients suffering from comorbid depression and yet still demonstrated a large specific treatment effect relative to placebo. Nonetheless, the established effectiveness of clomipramine as an anti-obsessional drug in depressed patients with OCD has led to it being regarded as particularly beneficial in these cases.

Two large multicentre placebo-controlled studies of clomipramine using variable dosages of up to 300 mg a day in non-depressed adults have demonstrated a gradual improvement in obsessions and compulsions starting in the first week of treatment and continuing throughout the 10 to 12 weeks of each trial. Reductions of 40–50% from baseline in obsessive compulsive ratings were typically found compared to improvements of less than 10% in the placebo-treated groups (Katz *et al.*, 1990; Clomipramine Collaborative Study Group, 1991). The high doses of clomipramine that were used in these studies were surprisingly well tolerated. In the study by Katz *et al.*, 1990, over half of the 142 patients who received clomipramine (placebo group $n = 140$) were no longer experiencing significant social dysfunction as a result of their obsessional symptoms by the end of the trial. Benefits of clomipramine over placebo continued to accrue in those patients who were entered into a 1-year double-blinded extension study. In the Clomipramine Collaborative Study (1991) involving 520 subjects in 21 sites in the USA, there was a 40% reduction in OCD scores due to drug treatment. Fifty-eight percent of the clomipramine group ($n = 60$) rated themselves as much or very much improved by the end of the 10-week trial, compared to 3% of placebo-treated patients ($n = 260$).

A meta-analysis of six placebo-controlled RCTs of clomipramine in OCD was published in treatment guidelines for anxiety disorders produced by the New Zealand National Health Committee (1998). This meta-analysis included the Katz *et al.*, 1990 and Clomipramine Collaborative Study Group 1991 study mentioned above and involved various measures of response rate (percentage improvement) in a total sample of 1057 patients receiving doses of between 50 and 300 mg per day of clomipramine over 5 to 12 weeks. The pooled NNT was 2 (95% CI = 2–3), which represents a potent treatment effect.

Selective serotonin reuptake inhibitors

Following the introduction of selective serotonin reuptake inhibitors (SSRIs) in the mid-1980s, approximately 10 placebo-controlled studies have been conducted involving over 2500 OCD patients. Placebo-controlled RCTs of currently licensed SSRIs in OCD, using various measures of response rate have yielded NNT values of between 2 and 11. Controlled direct comparisons of various SSRIs in OCD have failed to detect statistically significant differences between them (Bergeron *et al.*, 2002; Mundo *et al.*, 1997). However, these studies have been insufficiently powered to rule out clinically important differences in the effectiveness of different SSRIs in OCD.

Most of the studies of the effectiveness of SSRIs carried out in the 1990s obtained a somewhat smaller reduction in baseline OCD scores compared to the earlier clomipramine studies (about 30% vs. 40%–50%). Furthermore, the placebo response in these later studies was higher (20% vs. less than 10% in earlier studies). This suggests that the later OCD trials using SSRIs studied milder, often previously treated cases of OCD, which showed smaller specific drug responses. This is an important consideration when judging the comparative efficacy of SSRIs versus clomipramine (Greist & Jefferson 1998). Recent 'head-to-head' comparisons of clomipramine and SSRIs have failed to confirm the results of earlier meta-analyses showing superior efficacy of clomipramine over SSRIs. In one RCT involving 167 patients, the SSRI sertraline appeared, if anything, superior to clonipramine (Bisserbe *et al.*, 1997). The safest conclusion is that until further evidence becomes available, clomipramine and all SSRIs should be regarded as having comparable efficacy in OCD, with both obsessions and compulsions responding equally well to drug treatment.

A number of studies have demonstrated that SSRIs are associated with less adverse effects and are better tolerated compared to clomipramine (Bisserbe *et al.*, 1997; Mundo *et al.*, 2000; Mundo *et al.*, 2001). However, the differences may not be clinically important and for example do not necessarily result in fewer patients withdrawing from treatment with SSRIs compared to clomipramine (Kobak *et al.*, 1998).

Clinical tips in using SRIs

In most RCTs of anti-obsessional SSRI drug treatment, variable dose schedules have been used in an attempt to optimize the clinical outcome. This applies to all the RCTs involving clomipramine. There are a limited number of RCTs of SSRIs in which fixed doses of the various drugs have been used in order to clarify dose-response relationships. In the case of citalopram, fluoxetine and paroxetine, there is some evidence that higher doses (60 mg per day) may be more effective than the usual starting dose (20 mg per day), and somewhat paradoxically, higher doses may be associated with fewer withdrawals from treatment owing to adverse effects. (e.g. see Montgomery *et al.*, 1993, 2001; Tollefson *et al.*, 1994). Despite the limited evidence on this subject, it is often recommended that when an individual patient fails to responsed adequately to a starting dose of clomipramine or SSRI, the dose should be gradually increased to the maximum recommended dose in order to improve efficacy.

In the limited number of studies that have examined continuation treatment with SRIs, the results suggest that some subjects who have responded to initial treatment lasting approximately 12 weeks, will show further improvement in symptoms for treatment periods of between 6 and 12 months (e.g. Montgomery *et al.*, 1993; Tollefson *et al.*, 1994; Greist *et al.*, 1995). However, the differences from placebo in these continuation studies are not striking.

When the issue of optimal treatment duration is investigated by estimating relapse rates in OCD patients who remain on SRI medication, several RCTs indicate that maintenance treatment with SSRIs for periods of up to 1 year has a protective effect against relapses compared to placebo. In some studies, the effect appears to be relatively weak (Koran *et al.*, 2002), and may only occur at higher doses (e.g. 60 mg per day of fluoxetine) (Romano *et al.*, 2001).

Favourable treatment responsiveness to SRIs has been associated with later age of onset of OCD and lack of previous drug treatment, whereas poor response to SRIs tends to occur in patients with comorbid tic disorder or schizotypal personality disorder (see Soomro, 2004). Patients whose predominant or only symptom is hoarding (the accumulation or acquisition of items beyond reasonable need or items of little objective value) may be less likely to benefit from SRIs than patients with other symptom patterns (Abramowitz *et al.*, 2003; Black *et al.*, 1998; Mataix-Cols *et al.*, 2002).

Given the impression that up to a half of OCD patients are only partially or non-responsive to SRI treatment, even after treatment periods exceeding 1 year, it is hardly surprising that alternative or augmenting drug treatment regimes have been tried and tested. In addition to tricyclic antidepressants other than clomipramine, monoaminoxidase inhibitors, lithium, antipsychotic drugs, benzodiazepines and electro-convulsive therapy have all proved ineffective as monotherapy for OCD (Fineberg, 1999).

In contrast, the addition of haloperidol (McDougle *et al.*, 1994), risperidone (Erzegovesi *et al.*, 2005; Hollander *et al.*, 2003a; McDougle *et al.*, 2000), olanzapine (Bystritsky *et al.*, 2004), or quetiapine (Denys *et al.*, 2004a) has been shown in randomized placebo-controlled trials to augment SRI response in OCD. In these trials, the addition of antipsychotics caused a further reduction in Y-BOCS scores in up to 50% of OCD patients; significant differences between the antipsychotic and placebo were observed within 4–6 weeks. Although a few controlled trials did not find significant differences between antipsychotic and placebo augmentation (olanzapine (Shapira *et al.*, 2004); quetiapine (Carey *et al.*, 2005)), design limitations likely contributed to the negative findings.

The long-term efficacy of antipsychotic augmentation has not been systematically studied. A retrospective chart review found that 15 of 18 patients (83%) who responded to antipsychotic augmentation relapsed within two months after the antipsychotic was discontinued (Maina *et al.*, 2003). Other unanswered questions include: what is the optimal dose for each agent, why do only some patients benefit, and do the agents differ in their effects? One study (McDougle *et al.*, 1994) found that haloperidol only benefited OCD patients with comorbid tic disorders. Although effective for many OCD patients, antipsychotic augmentation comes with the known risks of exposure to antipsychotic medications (Marder *et al.*, 2004).

Neurosurgery and repetitive transcranial magnetic stimulation

In the 5%–10% of patients with very severe treatment refractory OCD, neurosurgery may be considered. The most frequently used neurosurgical procedures are cingulotomy, capsulotomy, leucotomy and subcaudate tractotomy. Evaluation of outcome is difficult because the patients referred for neurosurgery are already at the extreme end of symptom severity and disability. Not surprisingly there have been no prospective controlled trials

carried out in this field, and the long term results are particularly uncertain. Given the risk of short term postoperative complications, epilepsy and personality change, it is obvious that neurosurgery should only be considered for the most difficult cases in which other treatments have been exhaustively evaluated and have failed (Jenike, 1998).

Transcranial magnetic stimulation is an established technique to non-invasively stimulate the cerebral cortex (Barker *et al.*, 1985). No anaesthetic is required, and the procedure appears safe, with a low risk of inducing seizures over 2 to 3 weeks of daily treatments. Preliminary evidence suggests that repetitive transcranial magnetic stimulation may have benefit in OCD (Greenberg *et al.*, 1997; Mantovani *et al.*, 2005), but further studies are needed (Martin *et al.*, 2003).

Combined psychological and pharmacological treatment in OCD

Both ERP and SRI monotherapy have been shown in randomized controlled trials to be efficacious for adults with OCD. However, only a handful of trials directly address whether the combination of SRIs and ERP is superior to either treatment alone. Despite methodological limitations in these studies (Franklin *et al.*, 2005), the available data suggest that combination treatment (SRI + ERP) can be superior to monotherapy in some OCD patients, but that combination treatment is not necessary for all OCD patients. For example, some studies found that combination therapy was superior to ERP alone in OCD patients with comorbid depression.(Cottraux *et al.*, 1990; Hohagen *et al.*, 1998). On the other hand, other studies found that ERP alone was as efficacious as combination treatment in OCD patients with minimal depression (Foa *et al.*, 2005; van Balkom *et al.*, 1998).

Most studies have examined the efficacy of combination treatment when psychotherapy and SRI medication are started at the same time. However, given that medication can take 6–10 weeks to take effect, this design might not be the best to demonstrate the superiority of combination treatment. Several open and controlled trials (Simpson *et al.*, 1999; Tenneij *et al.*, 2005; Tolin *et al.*, 2004) indicate that OCD patients who have received an adequate SRI trial but who have clinically significant residual symptoms can benefit significantly from the sequential addition of ERP.

Some data suggest that combination treatment may reduce SRI relapse. Following treatment responders after treatment discontinuation, Simpson *et al.* (2004) found that responders to intensive ERP or to combination treatment (CMI + ERP) had a lower relapse rate and longer time to relapse 12 weeks after treatment discontinuation

Table 35.1. Effectiveness of treatments for obsessive-compulsive disorder

Treatment	Form of treatment	Psychiatric Disorder/ Target audience	Level of evidence for efficacy	Comments
Psychopharmacology	SSRIs	OCD	Ia	Effectiveness shown across all the SSRIs. May need higher doses than for depression. About 65% of patients have symptoms reduced between 40% and 50%
Psychopharmacology	Clomipramine	OCD	Ia	Effective as well. Many RCTs to support it. Unclear whether it is more or less effective than the SSRIs. Has more side effects than the SSRIs
Psychopharmacology	Typical and atypical antipsychotics	OCD	Ia	Are effective as augmentation in helping up to 50% of patients further diminish OCD symptoms
Psychosocial	CBT	OCD	Ia	Numerous studies support its effectiveness. Two versions of CBT have been examined in OCD: one focused on behavioural techniques (ERP) and one focused on cognitive techniques (CT)
	ERP			Effective as monotherapy. Unclear whether more effective when formally combined with CT but difficult to test because ERP contains some cognitive components
	CT		Ib	Some evidence for efficacy when CT contains behavioral experiments. Little evidence supporting CT in the absence of behavioral experiments
Psychopharmacology and Psychosocial Treatments (Combination)	ERP and SRIs		Ia	Combination treatment is highly effective. Available data suggest that there are specific clinical situations where it is preferable to SRIs or ERP alone
Somatic	Psychosugery Transcranial Magnetic Stimulation	OCD	IIb	May be somewhat effective in the most difficult cases. Subject pool remains small and definitive studies have yet to be conducted

than did responders to CMI alone. In a clinical case report, others (Baer *et al.*, 1994) found that CBT helped some OCD patients taper and discontinue their SSRI.

In sum, combination treatment may be warranted in certain clinical situations: to treat OCD patients with comorbid conditions (like depression) that are responsive to SSRIs and that can interfere with CBT (Cottraux *et al.*, 1990; Hohagen *et al.*, 1998), to augment partial response to monotherapy, (Simpson *et al.*, 1999; Tolin *et al.*, 2004), and to minimize SSRI relapse. (Baer *et al.*, 1994; Simpson *et al.*, 2004). Finally, some patients may be unwilling to embark upon long term SSRI treatment for OCD because of concerns about drug-related side effects and drug dependency. A significant minority (25%) of OCD patients may be

reluctant to start behavioural therapy because of the initial high level of anxiety that ERP engenders. Starting treatment with SRIs and then introducing behaviour therapy later when OCD symptoms have improved may be an appropriate strategy in these patients, with the option of phasing out medication if behaviour therapy is successful.

Conclusions

Obsessive-compulsive disorder can be a very debilitating disorder. Yet there are very effective treatments, both in the psychopharmacological as well as the psychosocial spheres. Nonetheless, not all patients respond, and those that do respond, do not always respond completely. Augmentation and combination strategies require more study. Nonetheless, guidelines in the UK as well as in the USA are quite similar in their approach to this disorder.

The level of evidence for each of the interventions discussed in this chapter is summarized in Table 35.1.

REFERENCES

Abramowitz, J. S. (1997). Effectiveness of psychological and pharmacological treatments for obsessive-compulsive disorder: a quantitative review. *Journal of Consulting and Clinical Psychology*, **65**, 44–52.

Abramowitz, J. S., Franklin, M. E., Street, G. P., Kozak, M. J. & Foa, E. B. (2000). Effects of comorbid depression on response to treatment for obsessive-compulsive disorder. *Behavior Therapy*, **31**, 517–28.

Abramowitz, J. S., Franklin, M. E., Zoellner, L. A. & DiBernardo, C. L. (2002). Treatment compliance and outcome in obsessive-compulsive disorder. *Behavior Modification*, **26**, 447–63.

Abramowitz, J. S., Franklin, M. E., Schwartz, S. A. & Furr, J. M. (2003). Symptom presentation and outcome of cognitive-behavioral therapy for obsessive-compulsive disorder. *Journal of Consulting and Clinical Psychology*, **71**, 1049–57.

Ackerman, D. L. & Greenland, S. (2002). Multivariate meta-analysis of controlled drug studies for obsessive-compulsive disorder. *Journal of Clinical Psychopharmacology*, **22**, 309–17.

Albert, U., Aguglia, E., Maina, G. & Bogetto, F. (2002). Venlafaxine versus clomipramine in the treatment of obsessive-compulsive disorder: a preliminary single-blind, 12-week, controlled study. *Journal of Clinical Psychiatry*, **63**, 1004–9.

American Psychiatric Association (APA) (2007). Practice guideline for the treatment of patients with obsessive-compulsive disorder. *American Journal of Psychiatry*, **164** (suppl.), 1–56.

Baer, L., Ricciardi, J., Keuthen, N. *et al.* (1994). Discontinuing obsessive-compulsive disorder medication with behavior therapy. *American Journal of Psychiatry*, **151**, 1842.

Barker, A. T., Jalinous, R. & Freeston, H. (1985). Non-invasive stimulation of the human motor cortex, *Lancet*, **I**, 1106–7.

Bergeron, R., Ravindran, A. V., Chaput, Y. *et al.* (2002). Sertraline and fluoxetine treatment of obsessive-compulsive disorder: results of a double-blind, 6 month treatment study. *Journal of Clinical Psychopharmacology*, **22**, 148–54.

Bisserbe, J. C., Lane, R. M. & Flament, M. F. (1997). A double blind comparison of sertraline and clomipramine in outpatients with obsessive compulsive disorder. *European Psychiatry*, **12**, 82–93.

Black, D. W., Monahan, P., Gable, J., Blum, N., Clancy, G. & Baker, P. (1998). Hoarding and treatment response in 38 non-depressed subjects with obsessive-compulsive disorder. *Journal of Clinical Psychiatry*, **59**, 420–5.

Blanco, C., Olfson, M., Stein, D., Simpson, H. B., Gameroff, M. J. & Narrow, W. E. (2006). Treatment of obsessive-compulsive disorder by U.S. Psychiatrists. *Journal of Clinical Psychiatry*, **67**, 946–51.

Bloch, M. H., Landeros-Weisenberger, A., Kelmendi, B., Coric, V., Bracken, M. B. & Leckman, J. F. (2006). A systematic review: antipsychotic augmentation with treatment refractory obsessive-compulsive disorder. *Molecular Psychiatry*, **11**, 622–32.

Bystritsky, A., Ackerman, D. L., Rosen, R. M. *et al.* (2004). Augmentation of serotonin reuptake inhibitors in refractory obsessive-compulsive disorder using adjunctive olanzapine: a placebo-controlled trial. *Journal of Clinical Psychiatry*, **65**, 565–8.

Carey, P. D., Vythilingum, B., Seedat, S., Muller, J. E., van Ameringen, M. & Stein, D. J. (2005). Quetiapine augmentation of SRIs in treatment refractory obsessive-compulsive disorder: a double-blind, randomised, placebo-controlled study [ISRCTN83050762]. *BMC Psychiatry*, **5**, 5.

Chouinard, G., Goodman, W., Greist, J. *et al.* (1990). Results of a double-blind placebo controlled trial of a new serotonin uptake inhibitor, sertraline in the treatment of obsessive-compulsive disorder. *Psychophamacology Bulletin*, **26**, (3).

Clomipramine Colloborative Study Group (De Veaugh-Geiss, J., Katz, R., Landau, P. *et al.*) (1991). Clomipramine in the treatment of patients with obsessive disorder. *Archives of General Psychiatry*, **48**, 730–8.

Cordioli, A. V., Heldt, E., Bochi, D. B. *et al.* (2003). Cognitive-behavioral group therapy in obsessive-compulsive disorder: a randomized clinical trial. *Psychotherapy and Psychosomatics*, **72**, 211–16.

Cottraux, J., Mollard, E., Bouvard, M. *et al.* (1990). A controlled study of fluvoxamine and exposure in obsessive-compulsive disorder. *International Clinical Psychopharmacology*, **5**, 17–30.

Cottraux, J., Note, I., Yao, S. N. *et al.* (2001). A randomized controlled trial of cognitive therapy versus intensive behavior therapy in obsessive compulsive disorder. *Psychotherapy and Psychosomatics*, **70**, 288–97.

Crino, R., Slade, T. & Andrews, G. (2005). The changing prevalence and severity of obsessive-compulsive disorder criteria from DSM-III to DSM-IV. *American Journal of Psychiatry*, **162**, 876–82.

Dale, R. C., Heyman, I., Giovannoni, G. & Church, A. W. J. (2005). Incidence of anti-brain antibodies in children with obsessive-compulsive disorder. *British Journal of Psychiatry*, **187**, 314–19.

Denys, D., van der Wee, N., van Megen, H. J. & Westenberg, H. G. (2003). A double blind comparison of venlafaxine and paroxetine in obsessive-compulsive disorder. *Journal of Clinical Psychopharmacology*, **23**, 568–75.

Denys, D., De Geus, F., Van Megen, H. J. & Westenberg, H. G. (2004a). A double-blind, randomized, placebo-controlled trial of quetiapine addition in patients with obsessive-compulsive disorder refractory to serotonin reuptake inhibitors. *Journal of Clinical Psychiatry*, **65**, 1040–8.

Denys, D., van Megen, H. J., van der Wee, N. & Westenberg, H. G. (2004b). A double-blind switch study of paroxetine and venlafaxine in obsessive-compulsive disorder. *Journal of Clinical Psychiatry*, **65**, 37–43.

Eddy, K. T., Dutra, L., Bradley, R. & Westen, D. (2004). A multidimensional meta-analysis of psychotherapy and pharmacotherapy for obsessive-compulsive disorder. *Clinical Psychology Review*, **24**, 1011–30.

Eisen, J. L., Goodman, W. K., Keller, M. B. *et al.* (1999). Patterns of remission and relapse in obsessive-compulsive disorder: a 2-year prospective study. *Journal of Clinical Psychiatry*, **60**, 346–51.

Erzegovesi, S., Guglielmo, E., Siliprandi, F. & Bellodi, L. (2005). Low-dose risperidone augmentation of fluvoxamine treatment in obsessive-compulsive disorder: a double-blind, placebo-controlled study. *European Neuropsychopharmacology*, **15**, 69–74.

Fals-Stewart, W., Marks, A. P. & Schafer, J. (1993). A comparison of behavioral group therapy and individual behavior therapy in treating obsessive-compulsive disorder. *Journal of Nervous and Mental Diseases*, **181**, 189–93.

Fineberg, N. (1999). Evidence-based pharmacotherapy for obsessive compulsive disorder. *Advances in Psychiatric Treatment*, **5**, 357–65.

Fineberg, N. A. & Gale, T. M. (2005). Evidence-based pharmacotherapy of obsessive-compulsive disorder. *International Journal of Neuropsychopharmacology*, **8**, 107–29.

Foa, E. B. & Goldstein, A. (1978). Continuous exposure and complete response prevention in obsessive compulsive neurosis. *Behaviour Therapy*, **9**, 821–9.

Foa, E. B., Abramowitz, J., Franklin, M. E. & Kozak, M. J. (1999). Feared consequences, fixity of beliefs, and treatment outcome in patients with obsessive-compulsive disorder. *Behavior Therapy*, **30**, 717–24.

Foa, E. B., Liebowitz, M. R., Kozak, M. J. *et al.* (2005). Randomized, placebo-controlled trial of exposure and ritual prevention, clomipramine, and their combination in the treatment of obsessive-compulsive disorder. *American Journal of Psychiatry*, **162**, 151–61.

Franklin, M. E., Simpson, H. B. & Blair, H. (2005). Combining pharmacotherapy and exposure plus ritual prevention for obsessive compulsive disorder: research findings and clinical applications. *Journal of Cognitive Psychotherapy*, **19**, 317–30.

Freeman, C. P., Trimble, M. R., Deakin, J. F., Stokes, T. M. & Ashford, J. J. (1994). Fluvoxamine versus clomipramine in the treatment of obsessive compulsive disorder: a multicenter, randomized, double-blind, parallel group comparison. *Journal of Clinical Psychiatry*, **55**, 301–5.

Freeston, M. H., Ladouceur, R., Gagnon, F. *et al.* (1997). Cognitive-behavioral treatment of obsessive thoughts: a controlled study. *Journal of Consulting and Clinical Psychology*, **65**, 405–13.

Gershuny, B. S., Baer, L., Jenike, M. A., Minichiello, W. E. & Wilhelm, S. (2002). Comorbid posttraumatic stress disorder: impact on treatment outcome for obsessive-compulsive disorder. *American Journal of Psychiatry*, **159**, 852–4.

Goodman, W. K., Price, L. H., Rasmussen, S. A. *et al.* (1989). The Yale-Brown obsessive scale. I development, use and reliability. *Archives of General Psychiatry*, **46**, 1006–11.

Greenberg, B. D., George, M. S., Martin, J. D. *et al.* (1997). Effect of prefrontal repetitive transcranial magnetic stimulation in obsessive-compulsive disorder: a preliminary study. *American Journal of Psychiatry*, **154**, 867–9.

Greist, J. H. & Jefferson, J. W. (1998). Pharmacotherapy for obsessive compulsive disorder. *British Journal of Psychiatry*, **173** (Suppl. 35), 64–70.

Greist, J. H, Chouinard, G., DuBuff, E. *et al.* (1995). Double-blind comparison of three doses of sertraline and placebo in the treatment of outpatients with obsessive compulsive disorder. *Archives of General Psychiatry*, **52** (4), 289–95.

Greist, J. H., Marks, I. M., Baer, L. *et al.* (2002). Behaviour therapy for obsessive-compulsive disorder guided by a computer or by a clinician compared with relaxation as a control. *Journal of Clinical Psychiatry*, **63**, 138–45.

Hohagen, F., Winkelmann, G., Rasche-Raeuchle, H. *et al.* (1998). Combination of behaviour therapy with fluvoxamine in comparison with behaviour therapy and placebo: results of a multicentre study. *British Journal of Psychiatry*, **173** (Suppl. 35), 71–8.

Hollander, E., Baldini Rossi, N., Sood, E. & Pallanti, S. (2003a). Risperidone augmentation in treatment-resistant obsessive-compulsive disorder: a double-blind, placebo-controlled study. *International Journal of Neuropsychopharmacology*, **6**, 397–401.

Hollander, E., Friedberg, J., Wasserman, S., Allen, A., Birnbaum, M. & Koran, L. M. (2003b). Venlafaxine in treatment-resistant obsessive-compulsive disorder. *Journal of Clinical Psychiatry*, **64**, 546–50.

Huppert, J. D. & Franklin, M. E. (2006). Cognitive behavioral therapy for obsessive-compulsive disorder: an update. *Current Psychiatry Reports*, **7**, 268–73.

Jenike, M. A. (1998). Neurosurgical treatment of obsessive treatment of obsessive compulsive disorder. *British Journal of Psychiatry*, **173** (Suppl 35), 79–90.

Katz, R. J., De Veaugh-Geiss, J. & Landau, P. (1990). Clomipramine in obsessive compulsive disorder. *Biological Psychiatry*, **28**, 401–14.

Kessler, R. C., Berglund, P., Demler, O., Jin, R., Merikangas, K. R. & Walters, E. E. (2005). Lifetime prevalence and age-of-onset distributions of DSM-IV disorders in the National Comorbidity Survey Replication. *Archives of General Psychiatry*, **62**, 593–602.

Kobak, K. A., Greist, J. H., Jefferson, J. W., Katzelnick, D. J. & Henk, H. J. (1998). Behavioural versus pharmacological treatments of obsessive-compulsive disorder: a meta-analysis. *Psychopharmacology* (*Berlin*), **136**, 205–16.

Koran, L. M., McElroy, S. L., Davidson, J. R. & Rasmussen, S. A. (1996). Fluvoxamine versus clomipramine for obsessive-compulsive disorder: a double-blind comparison. *Journal of Clinical Psychopharmacology*, **16**, 121–9.

Koran, L. M., Leventhal, J. L., Fireman, B. & Jacobson, A. (2000). Pharmacotherapy of obsessive-compulsive disorder in a health maintenance organization. *American Journal of Health System Pharmacy*, **57**, 1972–8.

Koran, L. M., Hackett, E., Rubin, A. *et al.* (2002). Efficacy of sertraline in the long-term treatment of obsessive-compulsive disorder. *American Journal of Psychiatry*, **159**, 88–95.

Kozak, M. J. & Foa, E. B. (1994). Obsessions, overvalued ideas, and delusions in obsessive-compulsive disorder. *Behaviour Research and Therapy*, **32**, 343–53.

Leonard, H., Swedo, S. & Rapoport, J. L. (1989). Treatment of childhood obsessive compulsive disorder with clomipramine and desmethylimipramine. A double blind crossover comparison. *Psychopharmacology Bulletin*, **24**, 93–5.

Lindsay, M., Crino, R. & Andrews, G. (1997). Controlled trial of exposure and response prevention in obsessive-compulsive disorder. *British Journal of Psychiatry*, **171**, 135–9.

Lopez-Ibor, J. J., Jr, Saiz, J., Cottraux, J. *et al.* (1996). Double-blind comparison of fluoxetine versus clomipramine in the treatment of obsessive compulsive disorder. *European Neuropsychopharmacology*, **6**, 111–18.

Maina, G., Albert, U., Ziero, S. & Bogetto, F. (2003). Antipsychotic augmentation for treatment resistant obsessive-compulsive disorder: what if antipsychotic is discontinued? *International Clinical Psychopharmacology*, **18**, 23–8.

Mantovani, A., Lisanby, S. H., Fulvio, P., Ulivelli, M., Castrogiovanni, P. & Rossi, S. (2005). Repetitive transcranial magnetic stimulation (rTMS) in the treatment of obsessive-compulsive disorder (OCD) and Tourette's syndrome (TS). *International Journal of Neuropsychopharmacology*, **9**, 95–100.

March, J. S., Frances, A., Kahn, D. A. & Carpenter, D. (1997). The Expert Consensus Guideline Series: treatment of obsessive-compulsive disorder. *Journal of Clinical Psychiatry*, **58**.

Marder, S. R., Essock, S. M., Miller, A. L. *et al.* (2004). Physical health monitoring of patients with schizophrenia. *American Journal of Psychiatry*, **161**, 1334–49.

Marks, I. M., Hodgson, R. & Rachman, S. (1975). Treatment of chronic obsessive compulsive neurosis by in-vivo exposure. A two-year follow up and issues in treatment. *British Journal of Psychiatry*, **127**, 349–64.

Martin, J. L., Barbanoj, M. J. & Perez, V. (2003). Transcranial magnetic stimulation for the treatment of obsessive-compulsive disorder. In *The Cochrane Library*, **3**, CD003387.

Mataix-Cols, D. & Marks, I. M. (2006). Self-help with minimal therapist contact for obsessive-compulsive disorder: a review. *European Psychiatry*, **21**, 75–80.

Mataix-Cols, D., Marks, I. M., Greist, J., Kobak, K. A. & Baer, L. (2002). Obsessive-compulsive symptom dimensions as predictors of compliance with and response to behavior therapy: results from a controlled trial. *Psychotherapy and Psychosomatics*, **71**, 255–62.

Mataix-Cols, D., Rosario-Campos, M. C. & Leckman, J. F. (2005). A multidimensional model of obsessive-compulsive disorder. *American Journal of Psychiatry*, **162**, 228–38.

McDougle, C. J., Goodman, W. K., Leckman, J. F., Lee, N. C., Heninger, G. R. & Price, L. H. (1994). Haloperidol addition in fluvoxamine-refractory obsessive-compulsive disorder. A double-blind, placebo-controlled study in patients with and without tics. *Archives of General Psychiatry*, **51**, 302–8.

McDougle, C. J., Epperson, C. N., Pelton, G. H. *et al.* (2000). A double-blind, placebo-controlled study of risperidone addition in serotonin reuptake inhibitor-refractory obsessive-compulsive disorder. *Archives of General Psychiatry*, **57**, 794–801.

McLean, P. D., Whittal, M. L., Thordarson, D. S. *et al.* (2001). Cognitive versus behavioural therapy in the group treatment of obsessive-compulsive disorder. *Journal of Consulting and Clinical Psychology*, **69**, 205–14.

Montgomery, S. A., McIntyre, A. & Osterheider, M. and the Lilly European OCD Study Group. (1993). A double-blind, placebo-controlled study of fluoxetine in patients with DSM-III-R obsessive compulsive disorder. *European Neuropsychopharmacology*, **3**, 143–52.

Montgomery, S. A., Kasper, S., Stein, D. J., Bang Hedegaard, K. & Lemming, O. M. (2001). Citalopram 20 mg, 40 mg and 60 mg are all effective and well tolerated compared with placebo in obsessive-compulsive disorder. *International Clinical Psychopharmacology*, **16**, 75–86.

Mundo, E., Bianchi, L. & Bellodi, L. (1997). Efficacy of fluvoxamine, paroxetine, and citalopram in the treatment of obsessive-compulsive disorder: a single blind study. *Journal of Clinical Psycyhopharmacology*, **17**, 267–71.

Mundo, E., Maina, G. & Uslenghi, C. (2000). Multicentre, double-blind, comparison of fluvoxamine and clomipramine in the treatment of obsessive-compulsive disorder. *International Clinical Psychopharmacology*, **15**, 69–76.

Mundo, E., Rouillon, F., Figuera, L. *et al.* (2001). Fluvoxamine in obsessive-compulsive disorder. Similar efficacy but superior tolerability in comparison with clomipramine. *Human Psychopharmacology*, **16**, 461–8.

Muris, P., Merckelbach, H. & Clavan, M. (1997). Abnormal and normal compulsions. *Behaviour Research and Therapy*, **35**, 249–52.

NICE (2006). Obsessive-compulsive disorder: core interventions in the treatment of obsessive-compulsive disorder and body dysmorphic disorder. National clinical practice giudeline number 31. National Institute of Health and Clinical Excellence. London, pp. 1–350. (http://guidance.nice.org.UK/CG31/guidance/pdf/English) (accessed 12-6-2007).

New Zealand National Health Committee. Guidelines for assessing and treating anxiety disorders. National Health Committee Guidelines Group (1998). www.nzgg.org.nz/guidelines/0038/anxiety (accessed 15-1-2005, no longer available).

Pallanti, S., Hollander, E., Bienstock, C. *et al.* (2002). Treatment non-response in OCD: methodological issues and operational definitions. *International Journal of Neuropsychophamacology*, **5**, 181–91.

Pigott, T. A. & Seay, S. M. (1999). A review of the efficacy of selective serotonin reuptake inhibitors in obsessive-compulsive disorder. *Journal of Clinical Psychiatry*, **60**, 101–6.

Rauch, S. L., O'Sullivan, R. L. & Jenike, M. A. (1996). Open treatment of obsessive-compulsive disorder with venlafaxine: a series of ten cases. *Journal of Clinical Psychopharmacology*, **16**, 81–4.

Romano, S., Goodman, W., Tamura, R. *et al.* (2001). Long-term treatment of obsessive-compulsive disorder after an acute response: a comparison of fluvoxamine versus placebo. *Journal of Clinical Psychopharmalogy*, **21**, 46–52.

Salkovskis, P. M. & Harrison, J. (1984). Abnormal and normal obsessions – a replication. *Behaviour Research and Therapy*, **22**, 549–52.

Saxena, S., Bota, R. G. & Brody, A. L. (2001). Brain–behavior relationships in obsessive-compulsive disorder. *Seminary Clinical Neuropsychiatry*, **6**, 82–101.

Sevincok, L. & Uygur, B. (2002). Venlafaxine open-label treatment of patients with obsessive-compulsive disorder. *Australian and New Zealand Journal of Psychiatry*, **36**, 817.

Shapira, N. A., Ward, H. E., Mandoki, M. *et al.* (2004). A double-blind, placebo-controlled trial of olanzapine addition in fluoxetine-refractory obsessive-compulsive disorder. *Biological Psychiatry*, **55**, 553–5.

Simpson, H. B., Liebowitz, M. R. (2005). Best practice in treatment obsessive-compulsive disorder: what the evidence says. In *Pathological Anxiety: Emotional Processing in Etiology and Treatment*, ed. B. Rothbaum. New York: Guilford Publications, Inc.

Simpson, H. B., Gorfinkle, K. S. & Liebowitz, M. R. (1999). Cognitive-behavioral therapy as an adjunct to serotonin reuptake inhibitors in obsessive-compulsive disorder: an open trial. *Journal of Clinical Psychiatry*, **60**, 584–90.

Simpson, H. B., Liebowitz, M. R., Foa, E. B. *et al.* (2004). Post-treatment effects of exposure therapy versus clomipramine in OCD. *Depression and Anxiety*, **19**, 225–33.

Simpson, H. B., Huppert, J. D., Petkova, E., Foa, E. & Liebowitz, M. (2006). Response versus remission in obsessive-compulsive disorder. *Journal of Clinical Psychiatry*, **67**, 269–76.

Skoog, G. & Skoog, I. (1999). A 40-year follow-up of patients with obsessive-compulsive disorder. *Archives in General Psychiatry*, **56**, 121–7.

Snider, L. A. & Swedo, S. E. (2004). PANDAS: current status and directions for research. *Molecular Psychiatry*, **9**, 900–7.

Soomro, G. M. (2004). Obsessive compulsive disorder. *Clinical Evidence*, **12**, 1458–73 (also available on www.clinicalevidence.com).

Stanley, M. A. & Turner, S. M. (1995). Current status of pharmacological and behavioural treatment of obsessive-compulsive disorder. *Behaviour Therapy*, **26**, 163–86.

Steketee, G., Chambless, D. L. & Tran, G. Q. (2001). Effects of axis I and II comorbidity on behavior therapy outcome for obsessive-compulsive disorder and agoraphobia. *Comprensive Psychiatry*, **42**, 76–86.

Tenneij, N. H., van Megen, H. J., Denys, D. A. & Westenberg, H. G. (2005). Behavior therapy augments response of patients with obsessive-compulsive disorder responding to drug treatment. *Journal of Clinical Psychiatry*, **66**, 1169–75.

Thoren, P., Asberg, M., Cronholm, E., Jornestedt, L. & Traskman, L. (1980). Clomipramine treatment of obsessive-compulsive disorder. I. A clinical controlled trial. *Archives of General Psychiatry*, **37**, 1281–5.

Tolin, D. F., Abramowitz, J. S., Kozak, M. J. & Foa, E. B. (2001). Fixity of belief, perceptual aberration, and magical ideation in obsessive-compulsive disorder. *Journal of Anxiety Disorders*, **15**, 501–10.

Tolin, D. F., Maltby, N., Diefenbach, G. J., Hannan, S. E. & Worhunsky, P. (2004). Cognitive-behavioral therapy for medication nonresponders with obsessive-compulsive disorder: a wait-list-controlled open trial. *Journal of Clinical Psychiatry*, **65**, 922–31.

Tollefson, G. D., Rampey, A. H., Potvin, J. H. *et al.* (1994). A multicenter investigation of fixed-dose fluoxetine in the treatment of obsessive-compulsive disorder. *Archives of General Psychiatry*, **51**, 559–67.

van Balkom, A. J., de Haan, E., van Oppen, P., Spinhoven, P., Hoogduin, K. A. & van Dyck, R. (1998). Cognitive and behavioral therapies alone versus in combination with fluvoxamine in the treatment of obsessive compulsive disorder. *Journal of Nervous and Mental Disorders*, **186**, 492–9.

Vogel, P. A., Stiles, T. C. & Gotestam, K. G. (2004). Adding cognitive therapy elements to exposure therapy for obsessive compulsive disorder: a controlled study. *Behavioural and Cognitive Psychotherapy*, **32**, 275–90.

Whittal, M. L., Thordarson, D. S. & McLean, P. D. (2005). Treatment of obsessive-compulsive disorder: cognitive behavior therapy vs. exposure and response prevention. *Behaviour and Research Therapy*, **43**, 1559–76.

Yaryura-Tobias, J. A. & Neziroglu, F. A. (1996). Venlafaxine in obsessive-compulsive disorder. *Archives of General Psychiatry*, **52**, 53–60.

36

Post-traumatic stress disorders and adjustment disorders

Randall D. Marshall, Steven B. Rudin and Peter Tyrer

Editor's note

Stress reactions run from Acute Stress Reactions and Adjustment Disorders to Post-traumatic Stress Disorder (PTSD). The first two, in many instances, may be thought of as time limited in their impact and respond to many different types of psychosocial interventions. The primary purpose of intervening in these disorders is to facilitate more effecting coping with the stressor, reduce functional impairment, and return the individual to his previous level of active functioning in the community. PTSD has been shown to respond to both trauma-focused cognitive-behavioral psychotherapies and to pharmacological agents, particularly the SSRIs, though other pharmacologic interventions may impact some of the disturbed affect, anxiety, and lability, and to psychosocial interventions. As with many other disorders, there is a treatment resistant group that remain significantly impaired despite treatment, and long-term management of symptoms becomes the primary goal.

Introduction: differences in classification of stress disorders

The adjustment disorders, acute stress disorder, and post-traumatic stress disorder (DSM-IV) all share the common feature of occurring as a response to an adverse environmental event or cluster of events. The distinction appears clear cut; post-traumatic stress disorders follow extreme stressors that are operationally defined, whereas adjustment disorders may follow any kind of stressor of a less serious degree.

Adjustment disorders are defined as "clinically significant emotional or behavioral symptoms in response to an identifiable psychosocial stressor or stressors" (DSM-IV), and must develop within 3 months of the stressor (DSM-IV).

Clinical significance is determined by the presence of marked distress "in excess of what would be expected" or by significant impairment. If another Axis I disorder is present, the diagnosis is not given. Subtypes are specified based on the primary presenting symptom constellation (anxiety, mixed anxiety and depressed mood, disturbance of conduct, mixed disturbance of emotions and conduct, or unspecified).

Post-traumatic stress disorder (PTSD) not only follows more severe stress but is a debilitating psychiatric condition that is relatively common, and occurs in approximately twice as many women as men. Symptoms include persistent fear, anxiety, and increased vigilance, unwanted recollections of the event, avoidance of many activities that evoke memories or emotions related to the trauma, social isolation, emotional numbing, and problems with concentration, sleep, and irritability. Untreated PTSD is associated also with disruption of interpersonal relationships, inability to work, high rates of health problems, and suicide (Marshall *et al.*, 2001a; Riggs *et al.*, 1998; Davidson *et al.*, 1991; Blanchard *et al.*, 1998).

Some of the most significant differences between the American (DSM-IV) and International (ICD-10) diagnostic systems can be found in the conceptual models for organizing diagnoses judged to be the direct consequence of environmental stressors or trauma. In general, the DSM-IV model emphasizes the importance of *phenomenology* – the type of reactions, symptoms and problems that are manifest in the patient – whereas the ICD-10 emphasizes the fact of an observed *relationship* between an environmental event and the onset of a patient's reactions, symptoms and problems. This is a major problem in the state of our science, in that it is extremely difficult to reconcile clinical and descriptive research from the two literatures. In application, however, the research literature has inclined heavily toward use of the DSM-IV diagnoses.

For example, in the ICD-10, the category "Reactions to severe stress, and adjustment disorders" groups the diagnoses with the common feature of being clearly precipitated by severe stressors, across the full range of symptoms, problems, and severity . These are acute stress reaction, post-traumatic stress disorder, and the adjustment disorders, with a residual category of "unspecified." The DSM-IV has separate sections for adjustment disorder, groups PTSD with the anxiety disorders, and formally distinguishes between stressors and traumas, trauma being a special category of stressor. Only a traumatic event, by definition, can produce PTSD, but traumatic events can also increase risk for other disorders and reactions that are precipitated by stressors (e.g., major depressive disorder).

The definition of PTSD in the American DSM has changed substantially through the DSM-III, -IIIR, and IV editions (Marshall *et al.*, 1999). In contrast, the ICD-10 definition of PTSD still resembles the DSM-III definition in that it does not require a minimum duration of symptoms, whereas DSM-IV requires symptom duration of 1 month to make the diagnosis. Acute stress reaction (ICD-10), by contrast, requires immediate onset of symptoms (within 1 hour), and relatively rapid diminution of symptoms after the stressor is relieved (within 8 hours). If the stressor is ongoing, diminution of symptoms must begin after not more than 48 hours. Thus, this syndrome essentially describes an immediate, transient *reaction* to a traumatic experience which may differ from normative reactions only in degree. In DSM-IV, an acute reaction to a traumatic event would be captured by the diagnoses of either adjustment disorder, or acute stress disorder. For the latter to be diagnosed, however, the patient must also present with significant dissociative symptoms. The strength of the diagnosis is that it does identify persons with acute symptoms who are at increased risk for chronic PTSD. The primary shortcoming of the diagnosis is that it fails to identify approximately one third of persons who will develop chronic PTSD because they do not present with prominent dissociative symptoms (Marshall *et al.*, 1999; Bryant, 2003). In ICD-10, acute stress reaction can be diagnosed following "an exceptional mental or physical stressor," and provides three levels of severity with different criteria sets for each and a complex method for assigning the diagnosis. Thus, it captures a broad range of peri-traumatic responses with varying degrees of dissociation, anxiety, affective instability, and confusion.

The primary strength of the ICD-10 approach is that it provides a coherent system for capturing a wide range of reactions to life events that may become the focus of clinical attention, and has greater diagnostic coverage for a broader range of post-traumatic responses associated with impairment and distress. This is accomplished through inclusion of both non-specific acute responses to trauma (in the diagnoses of acute stress reaction and adjustment disorder), and the specific, well-validated constellation of symptoms included in PTSD. It differs from the DSM approach in that there is probably substantial overlap with normal emotional reactions, since the milder form of acute stress reaction describes an emotional upheaval that resolves relatively rapidly after trauma.

This chapter, as a summary and discussion of the literature describing syndromes that have a direct relationship to stressors, uses the ICD-10 conceptual model but draws primarily from research using DSM-IV diagnoses since this nosology dominates the research literature. It is striking, however, that the substantial body of research to date in the adjustment disorders originates in Europe. This may be in part because adjustment disorders have been identified as a major economic burden in European economies, primarily because of its high prevalence and its association with sick leave and disability claims (van der Klink, 2003), but it is also possible that many adjustment disorders could be regarded as post-traumatic stress disorders in a different context, and vice versa. Although adjustment disorders do seem to be as prevalent in the USA as in Europe (Strain *et al.*, 1998) this area remains neglected as a research focus in the USA.

It is also fair to add that virtually all concerned with the classification of stress and adjustment disorders are to some extent dissatisfied with the current ICD and DSM systems and a major effort is being made to tighten up the diagnoses in DSM-V (Spitzer *et al.*, 2007).

Adjustment disorder

A major criticism of evidence-based treatment has been the charge that research patients are so carefully selected that the research literature is not representative of real-world clinical treatment. To address this issue, Stirman *et al.* (2003) studied a random selection of outpatients ($n = 500$) from a large behavioral healthcare company managing the care of approximately 20 000 patients per year. The authors found that, if a diagnosis had been studied in the literature, 80% of patients would have been eligible for study, demonstrating that the above criticism is not a valid reason to ignore the recommendations of evidence-based treatment. On the other hand, the majority of outpatients (58%) had primary diagnoses that had not yet been studied in randomized controlled trials of psychotherapy: adjustment disorder was the most common diagnosis in this group, found in nearly one third (29%) of outpatients. This remarkable finding, which also appears consistent with the published European literature, highlights possibly *the most glaring deficiency in the interventions research literature. That is, at present, the research literature does not offer sufficient evidence-based guidance for the treatment of one of the most common diagnoses in outpatient mental health services and almost certainly the most common in primary care.*

Naturalistic observations and treatment outcomes in community settings

A consortium of seven university teaching hospitals in the USA conducted a large ($n = 1039$) multi-site study of the utilization of the adjustment disorder diagnosis in the consultation-liaison setting (Strain *et al.*, 1998). Among these consecutive referrals for consultation-liaison psychiatry services, adjustment disorder was diagnosed in 12.0% of cases. It was the sole diagnosis in 7.8% of cases, and a comorbid diagnosis in 4.2%. Comorbidity occurred most frequently with personality disorder and organic mental disorder. Findings were consistent with the construct of a maladaptive reaction to a significant stressor, in that the diagnosis was associated with problems with anxiety, coping, and depression; but also associated with higher functioning and less psychiatric illness than other Axis I disorders. Despite the above, these patients required as much treatment time (mean of 3 visits requiring 2.4 hours) and received similar rates of recommendation for psychological intervention as other disorders. The stressor was typically serious medical illness.

A large study of psychiatric outpatients across the spectrum of depressive disorders ($n = 812$) examined health status, functioning, and quality of life using the 36-item Short-Form Health Status Survey (SF-36) before entering treatment and again after 6 months (Jones *et al.*, 1999). Adjustment disorder patients showed the highest level of overall functioning, and major depressive disorder patients the lowest, with adjustment disorder patients showing physical health scores equivalent to the US population but considerable impairment in emotional health scores. Similar evidence of better functioning in adjustment disorders has been found in a UK study (Casey *et al.*, 1985). At 6 month follow-up in the US study, all patient groups showed equivalent improvement from individualized treatment in the clinic, and thus demonstrated that community-based treatment was associated with clinically significant improvement in adjustment disorder symptoms.

Trials of clinical interventions

The first published randomized controlled trial in persons with Adjustment Disorder that appeared in the literature was conducted in the Netherlands among persons on first sick leave because of an Adjustment Disorder (van der Klink *et al.*, 2003). This remarkable study was conducted within the Dutch Postal and Telecom Services Company (Royal KPN) that employs more than 100 000 persons, with cluster randomization by occupational physician within this network. Subjects were eligible if on sick leave for 2 weeks because of an adjustment disorder; if this was the first such occurrence; and if there were no medical or more severe psychiatric explanations for the absenteeism. A checklist for the DSM-IV diagnosis of Adjustment Disorder was used and included the requirement that a recent (<3 months) psychosocial stressor be present, as well as 8/17 distress symptoms. Patients were randomized to receive either treatment-as-usual from occupational physicians ($n = 83$) or a new 5–6 session 90-minute intervention based on Stress Inoculation Training, a validated and highly effective cognitive therapy ($n = 109$), for a total of $n = 192$ subjects. This therapy was a three-stage intervention that first provided psychoeducation about "loss of control"; assistance in identifying stressors and the development of problem-solving strategies; and, finally, encouragement to put these problem-solving strategies into practice as well as instruction to increase activities. The authors state that "the patients' own responsibility and active role in the recovery process was emphasized." Thus, it appears that cognitive-behavioral strategies were employed to shift the patient's locus of control toward greater mastery by helping the patient structure his or her thinking and behavior in this direction.

Outcome was assessed using measures of work functioning (e.g. days until returning to work) and psychological symptoms (depressive, anxiety, and general psychopathology). The intervention group showed superior outcome as measured by duration of sick leave and days to return to work. Mean time to return to work was 36 days vs. 53 days, and mean time to full return to work was 69 vs. 91 days, an approximately 30% superiority. Despite this clearly superior outcome from both functional and societal perspectives, there was no difference in symptom improvement between groups; both groups showed clinically significant improvement at both the 3-month and 12-month evaluations.

These results are notable for several reasons. First, this is the first randomized clinical trial in a disorder that has been dramatically neglected despite being probably the single most common mental health diagnosis in the community, and a significant source of economic loss and functional disability in the post-industrial world. Second, the study's design is illustrative of new research priorities that emphasize real-world relevance, use of community providers where possible, and more rigorous comparison groups than "no treatment" wait-lists, which has unfortunately dominated the psychotherapy outcome literature. In fact, the authors note that treatment-as-usual by occupational physicians in this company was already considerably better than the national average, making this a particularly rigorous comparison. Third, the uncoupling of psychological symptoms from functional impairment in study results is unusual for clinical trials in psychiatry. This might be seen as further validation of the adjustment Disorder diagnosis as a "problem in living" rather than a putative disease process. It might be considered an illness, but not a disease. An illness is an involuntary condition with clear implications for functioning and well-being, that is resistant to self-instruction and persists despite clear negative implications for the individual (Marshall & Klein, 2002; Klein, 1978).

If something has gone wrong within the organism (as in *disease*), it permits the individual to claim the sick role, which distinguishes illness from simple deviance from the norm and ordinary human unhappiness. The fact that disease states are involuntary leads to exemptions from normal obligations that the sick role provides. When disease is hypothesized without objective, obvious pathology, the suspicion of exploitative malingering arises. This has been a problem throughout the history of psychiatry, and in particular, the history of disorder resulting from stressors and trauma (Herman, 1997). As mental health professionals, we address stigma both through our work with patients – by providing education about the fact and consequences of mental disorder – and our interactions in society at large.

Awareness of the dimensional nature of mental illness has been much more widespread in recent years and the boundary between adjustment disorders and mood disorders has come under scrutiny. In the Nottingham Study of Neurotic Disorder, a long-term cohort study begun as a randomized trial in 1983, patients with anxiety and depressive disorders seen in general practice psychiatric clinics diagnosed according to DSM criteria using a structured interview (SCID) were treated with drug and psychological treatments for 6 weeks and then had their treatment slowly withdrawn by 10 weeks. The symptoms of one in four of those allocated to placebo were dramatically reduced over the initial 10 weeks (Tyrer *et al.*, 1988) and, more significantly, these symptoms remained largely absent 5 years later, when improvement with all treatments at 10 weeks was a strong predictor of 5-year outcome (Seivewright *et al.*, 1998). Thus the initial improvement with placebo, and by

extrapolation with the other treatments too, was quite untypical of a placebo reaction which classically is magnified initially and then wears off. It is therefore possible to postulate that a proportion (up to one in four) of patients with common anxiety and depressive disorders really have an adjustment disorder that will improve (or completely resolve) either spontaneously or with minimal intervention. These conditions might be described as short-term adjustment disorders masquerading as depressive and anxiety disorders and be treated unnecessarily (Tyrer *et al.*, 2005). This remains a speculative hypothesis as it was developed by *post hoc* analysis and prospective studies are needed to establish whether this is a viable explanation of the generally 30% good outcome that one sees in common mental disorders almost irrespective of treatment. It is also far too early to comment on, or attempt to formulate, treatment guidelines for these conditions.

Treatment guidelines recommendations for adjustment disorder

There is little in the way of formal guidelines for the treatment of adjustment disorders but the British Association for Psychopharmacology consensus statement recommends that antidepressants are avoided and "education, support and simple problem solving" (Anderson *et al.*, 2000) are recommended. Based on the single large clinical trial above, stress translation training is currently the treatment of choice.

Acute stress disorder

Psychosocial treatment

A few single-site psychosocial trials have addressed the two primary questions in the field of secondary prevention: (1) Can treatment accelerate recovery after a traumatic experience? (2) Can treatment reduce risk for developing chronic disorder?

In the first pilot study of these important questions, Foa *et al.* (1995) treated women with full PTSD for less than 30 days ($n = 20$) by providing a brief (4 session) CBT intervention developed out of established PTSD treatments (Foa *et al.*, 1995). Outcome was compared in non-randomized design to a parallel assessment-only group. Two months after the assault, the CBT group was significantly more improved, but this difference had disappeared by about 6 months post-assault.

The first randomized trial was conducted by Bryant *et al.* (1998), who randomized patients with acute stress disorder to five sessions of either brief trauma-focused CBT or supportive counseling. At the end of treatment and at 6 month follow-up, PTSD rates were significantly lower in the CBT group than in the counseling group. In contrast to the first study of Foa *et al.* patients showed both accelerated recovery and reduced rates of chronic PTSD. In a subsequent study ($n = 45$) comparing two versions of CBT (exposure therapy plus cognitive therapy or exposure therapy alone) to supportive counseling, rates of PTSD 6 months later were approximately 20% in both CBT groups, compared to 67% in the control condition (Bryant *et al.*, 1999).

Though considerably more research is needed, these preliminary studies provide evidence that the same treatment models shown effective for PTSD can also be effective for persons experiencing the acute severe responses to traumatic events that are captured by the diagnosis of acute stress disorder.

Pharmacological treatment

Pitman & Delahanty (2005) have synthesized a growing body of animal conditioning research by hypothesizing specific relationships between stressful events and the evoked hormonal and neurobiological activation that produces robust memory traces of adverse events. Such memories are particularly difficult to extinguish, are easily reactivated, and presumably drive fear-related behaviors and pathological states. Their model postulates that stress hormones released during the event lead to over-consolidation of the memory, theoretically increasing the chance of survival if the organism encounters similar stimuli in the future. By analogy, humans experiencing traumatic events may be left with "supermemories" of the event. The affective links between fear centers such as the amygdala and key aspects of the trauma memory then generate intrusive memories of the event spontaneously and in the presence of reminders. This leads to further consolidation of the memory such that in some persons the result is a positive feedback loop that reinforces the fear-memory connection, ("overconsolidation"), in contrast to the pattern seen in the majority of persons who recover gradually and spontaneously after a traumatic event.

Pitman has reasoned that blocking this initial adrenergic loop immediately after trauma might theoretically interfere with overconsolidation and therefore reduce risk of PTSD. Pitman *et al.* conducted a small RCT (Pitman *et al.*, 2002) in which propranolol was administered at 40 mg QID, begun within 6 hours of the traumatic event, for 10 days after the trauma. There were no group differences in PTSD symptoms at 3 months follow-up. The authors did find physiologic differences between groups

using script-driven imagery, however, in that the placebo group had higher physiologic responses to trauma-related cues. This suggests that there may have been a prevention effect on physiologic arousal, but this had no impact on patient symptoms. A second small non-randomized study found that propranolol prescribed as 40 mg TID for 7 days, followed by an 8–12 week taper, reduced rates of PTSD in the propranolol group (1/11) compared to the non-treated group (3/8) (Vaiva *et al.*, 2003). Further work is needed in this potentially promising area.

Treatment guidelines recommendations for acute stress disorder

At present, no pharmacological treatment is available that can be given in the acute post-traumatic setting to accelerate recovery from the traumatic experience or reduce-risk of chronic disorder. Replicated research demonstrates that brief trauma-focused cognitive-behavioral models as developed by Bryant and Foa can accelerate recovery in symptomatic individuals, and possibly reduce long-term risk in persons meeting criteria for acute stress disorder (that is, with both prominent PTSD symptoms and dissociative symptoms).

Post-traumatic stress disorder

Pharmacotherapy

This section will provide the clinician with an overview and guidance in the use of medication for persons suffering from post-traumatic stress disorder. First, the evidence to support the use of psychotropic medications will be presented. Next a review of the scientific literature will be described, including the evidence for each class of medication that has been studied. Finally, clinical issues such as comorbidity, adherence, symptom cluster response, and continuation, maintenance, and termination recommendations will be presented.

Evidence from investigators in basic science, neuro-imaging, neuroimmunology, and other areas supports the existence of neurobiological alterations in PTSD. Alterations have been observed in the autonomic nervous system, the hypothalamic-pituitary-adrenal axis, endogenous opioid regulation and function, the catecholaminergic and serotonergic systems, and various aspects of the immune system (Marshall & Garakani, 2002). This may be the underlying basis for the changes in brain structures that have been observed in some PTSD patients (Vermetten & Bremner, 2002). So far, these observations have been mostly isolated findings, many unreplicated, and not completely understood. However, most experts agree that the memory and fear dysregulation in PTSD patients has an underlying neurobiological basis.

In addition to the neurobiological findings in PTSD, there are numerous studies confirming that medication can be effective in PTSD. This literature is comprised of case reports, open trials, retrospective studies, and double-blind placebo-controlled trials. Almost every class of medication has been tried in the treatment of PTSD, both as monotherapy and adjunctively. In particular, several multi-site studies demonstrate that the SSRIs are effective with supportive clinical management.

Although the early research literature was based primarily on war veteran populations, this is not the case for the most technologically advanced studies of the last decade that have primarily been conducted with SSRIs. Studies with monoamine oxidase inhibitors and tricyclic antidepressants are older, less rigorous, single-site studies, with war veterans. Because of differences in subject population, it was recognized that studies with US war veterans may not be generalizable to the general population (Marshall & Klein, 1995).

There are no direct comparisons to date between pharmacotherapy and psychosocial treatment. For some patients (e.g. those with severe symptoms, limited coping skills, or severe avoidance), pharmacotherapy may be the treatment of choice. There is no evidence that medication interferes with psychosocial treatment (with the possible exception of high-dose benzodiazepines). Many experts believe that the combination of medication with behavioral therapy may yield superior results than either modality alone with some patients, based on extensive clinical experience in this population, and this hypothesis is currently being tested in ongoing research.

Serotonin reuptake inhibitors (SSRIs) and serotonin–noradrenaline reuptake inhibitors (SNRIs)

The SSRIs are considered first-line agents for the treatment of PTSD. Studies with SSRIs have benefited from the use of state of the art standardized clinical assessments (Clinician Administered PTSD Scale (CAPS), Davidson Trauma Scale), superior design (double-blind and crossover), and broadening of subject population to non-combat related PTSD. The SSRIs have been shown to target the entire syndrome of PTSD. In addition, SSRIs are safe, well tolerated, and very familiar to psychiatrists as well as other physicians. One caveat is that most of the published studies have been industry funded.

Several large, controlled trials have shown efficacy for sertraline (Brady *et al.*, 2000; Davidson, Rothbaum *et al.*,

2001) and paroxetine (Marshall *et al.*, 2001; Tucker *et al.*, 2001). Currently, sertraline and paroxetine are approved by the United States Food and Drug Administration FDA for the treatment of PTSD. There are two randomized placebo controlled studies for fluoxetine, one positive (Martenyi *et al.*, 2002) and one negative (Hertzberg *et al.*, 2000). Most studies with SSRIs have used the same dosing strategies as those typically used for the treatment of major depressive disorder and panic disorder. In addition, some studies reported improvement as early as week 2.

Brady *et al.* (2000) reported that treatment with sertraline in subjects with mixed traumas and multiple comorbidities resulted in a responder rate of 53% at study end point compared with 32% for placebo. Response was defined as a greater than 30% reduction of symptoms as measures by the CAPS or a CGI-I of very much improved or much improved. Improvement was evident as early as week 2. Using similar endpoint measures, Davidson *et al.* (2001) reported somewhat more robust findings of 60% response rate for sertraline vs. 38% response rate for placebo. Both studies used flexible dosing for sertraline (50–200 mg/day). Davidson *et al.* (2004) reviewed these two 12 week trials and estimated rates of remission ranging from 23.1%–26.3% for sertraline and 13.9%–14.9% for placebo.

Marshall *et al.* (2001) reported that treatment with paroxetine resulted in response rates of 62% ($n = 113$, 20-mg/day group) and 54% ($n = 99$, 40-mg/day group), compared to approximately 37% ($n = 67$) for those in the placebo group. Interestingly, outcomes did not vary according to patients' gender, trauma type, time since onset of trauma, or the severity of PTSD or depressive symptoms at baseline. Tucker *et al.* (2001) reported similar findings in a 12-week randomized placebo controlled trial of subjects with chronic PTSD with mixed traumas. Despite high rates of associated symptoms and comorbid disorders, pharmacological trials typically do not measure outcome in these domains. Moreover, the vast majority of research has been conducted in Caucasians. Recent research, however, shows both higher rates of trauma and PTSD among urban minorities in the USA, and increased vulnerability to developing PTSD among Hispanics compared to Caucasians or African-Americans (Galea *et al.*, 2002). To address these deficiencies in the literature, Marshall *et al.* (2006) conducted a single-site trial of paroxetine for chronic PTSD. Consistent with previous research, paroxetine was superior to placebo in alleviating PTSD symptoms. In addition, paroxetine was superior for dissociative symptoms and interpersonal problems over the 10-week period. Adverse effects of SSRIs include gastrointestinal discomfort (nausea, bloating, vomiting), restlessness/internal agitation, insomnia, somnolence, weight gain, weight loss, apathy, sweating, and sexual dysfunction. Recently, there have been reports of increased suicide risk associated with SSRIs in children, and warnings about this rare but possible serious adverse effect have been issued in both the USA and the UK.

Patients with PTSD can be very sensitive to side effects, possibly secondary to fear, hypervigilance, and somatic worries. Thus, lower starting doses and cautious titration is advised. In addition, patients should be warned that precipitous discontinuation of an SSRI may be associated with uncomfortable discontinuation symptoms such as nausea, malaise, dysphoria, and flu-like symptoms.

Serotonin–noradrenergic reuptake inhibitors (venlafaxine, mirtazepine)

Venlafaxine was effective for chronic PTSD symptoms in a large multi-site 12-week RCT comparing venlafaxine, sertraline, and placebo in $n = 538$ patients (Davidson et al., 2006a). Venlafaxine treatment led to remission of PTSD in 30.2% of patients, compared to 24.3% for sertraline and 19.6% for placebo. A second important international study continued treatment for 24 weeks in $n = 329$ patients with chronic PTSD and found venlafaxine superior to placebo on primary outcome measures (Davidson et al., 2006b). Remission rates were notable at 50.9% for venlafaxine, and 37.5% for placebo.

Adverse effects of venlafaxine include nausea, insomnia, sedation, and dizziness. Venlafaxine has also been noted to increase systolic blood pressure in some patients.

Mirtazepine showed promise in a small RCT (n = 26) of drug vs placebo in a patient population with relatively severe PTSD, in which it was superior to placebo on global ratings of improvement and on general anxiety measures, but failed to reach significance on PTSD measures (Davidson et al., 2003). A larger RCT of mirtazapine vs sertraline, an established medication for PTSD, found the two medications showed equivalent efficacy (Chung et al., 2004).

Tricyclic antidepressants (TCAs)

At present, there is insufficient evidence to recommend TCAs as fist-line agents for PTSD. Two randomized controlled trials have demonstrated moderate efficacy for amitriptyline (Davidson et al., 1990) and imipramine (Kosten et al., 1991) in treating PTSD. One randomized controlled study showed that desipramine was not effective, but in retrospect was too small to detect the expected differences (Reist et al., 1989). Open studies, retrospective studies, and case reports have yielded mixed results.

The literature regarding the use of TCAs in PTSD is limited by several factors. Firstly, many studies were conducted prior to the development of rating scales that specifically measure improvement in PTSD, such as the CAPS and the DTS. Secondly, all three randomized trials were conducted with adult male war veterans, a population that may not be representative of the entire population with PTSD. Thirdly, the randomized trials were relatively short in duration (i.e. 4–8 weeks), which may be too brief to note significant improvement. Finally, the trials used three different agents with different pharmacodynamic properties, which limits the ability to extrapolate these findings to the whole class of TCAs.

Expert consensus is that TCAs are a reasonable alternative as adjunctive or monotherapy in patients that have not responded to other more validated treatments. Clinicians should be aware that TCAs are lethal in overdose and contraindicated in patients with certain types of cardiac disease (e.g. electrical conduction defects). In addition, TCAs are associated with bothersome side effects such as dry mouth, constipation, blurred vision, tachycardia, sedation, weight gain, dizziness, and orthostatic hypotension. Dosing of TCAs for PTSD follows the same guidelines as for major depressive disorder (e.g. imipramine 150–300 mg/day).

Monoamine oxidase inhibitors (MAOIs)

Non-selective, irreversible MAOIs

Phenelzine, an irreversible monoamine oxidase inhibitor, was the first medication to be considered as a possible treatment for PTSD (Hogben & Cornfield, 1981). However, MAOIs are currently reserved for patients that have not responded to other treatments. This is due partly to their potential to cause fatal reactions if not used properly. Specifically, this class of medications can have life-threatening food–drug and drug–drug interactions. MAOIs are also not considered first-line treatment for PTSD because of the paucity of literature demonstrating their efficacy.

One randomized trial (Kosten et al., 1991) showed superiority of phenelzine over both imipramine and placebo, in contrast to a previous trial with negative results (Shestatsky et al., 1987). Similar to the case with TCAs, studies with MAOIs were conducted prior to the development of specific rating scales that measure the full PTSD syndrome (e.g. the Impact of Events Scale). In addition, the three randomized controlled studies have been criticized for their short duration of treatment, small sample size, inclusion of less globally symptomatic subjects, and exclusive focus on US war veterans (Marshall & Klein, 1995).

Patients who take MAOIs must adhere to special diets free of tyramine (an amino acid found in ripe cheeses, fortified wine, and other foods). In addition, they must avoid certain medications (e.g. Meperidine (Demerol), pseudoephedrine, SSRI antidepressants, and others). Ingestion of even small amounts of these substances can result in hypertensive crisis or the serotonin syndrome. Both can be fatal. Adverse effects of MAOIs include hypotension, headache, insomnia, weight gain, sexual dysfunction, peripheral edema, somnolence, agitation, and dry mouth.

Selective, reversible MAOIs
One randomized placebo-controlled study demonstrated that brofaromine, a selective, reversible MAOI, was moderately effective for the treatment of PTSD (Baker *et al.*, 1995). Two other open trials with brofaromine (Katz *et al.*, 1995) and moclobemide (Neal *et al.*, 1997) showed positive findings. These agents, which are not available in the United States, are promising but warrant further investigation. A benefit of these medications are that they most likely do not require such strict precautions as the non-selective, irreversible subtype. Adverse effects include mild headache, transient gastrointestinal upset, and loss of appetite.

Other antidepressants
A growing number of other medications exist that have antidepressant and anti-anxiety properties, but whose mechanism of action is different than the SSRIs, TCAs, and MAOIs. Nefazodone has promising open trials, and the rest only case reports (reviewed briefly below). Bupropion does not appear useful for PTSD based on open trials. At present, there have been no published placebo-controlled double-blind studies using these medications for the treatment of PTSD. However, a few open label trials and case reports suggest that these medications might be efficacious.

For now, it is reasonable to consider these medications as alternative medication treatments that could be given on a rational basis if a patient has failed to respond to the other validated medications. Given their better tolerability profiles as well as safety in overdose, many clinicians consider these classes of medication prior to a trial of TCA or MAOIs.

Multiple open label studies have shown promise for nefazadone as a treatment of PTSD (Davis *et al.*, 2000; Garfield *et al.*, 2001; Zisook *et al.*, 2000). Pooled results of six open-label trials of nefazodone for treatment of PTSD showed a 31.3% reduction of symptoms overall, with similar reductions in each symptom cluster (Hidalgo *et al.*, 1999). Nefazadone has the advantage of rarely causing sexual dysfunction. However, nefazadone was recently pulled from the European market due to the risk of

irreversible liver damage. The United States Food and Drug Administration issued a similar warning. Other adverse effects of nefazodone include sedation, nausea, constipation, dizziness, headache and blurred vision.

Bupropion is an antidepressant that is not likely to cause sexual side effects or weight gain. Indications for bupropion include major depression, smoking cessation, and attention deficit disorder. One open label study (Canive *et al.*, 1998) found that bupropion was minimally helpful for hyperarousal but did improve comorbid depression. However, adverse effects of increased anxiety, agitation, and insomnia may limit its utility in PTSD. Other adverse effects include headache and the potential to cause seizures at high doses in some vulnerable populations (i.e. patients with bulimia and alcohol abuse).

Trazodone was found to be helpful in one open label study with veterans (Hertzberg *et al.*, 1996). Trazodone's tendency to cause sedation, even at low doses, makes it a popular choice for insomnia. However, as monotherapy, the doses that are most likely needed for therapeutic effect in PTSD (i.e. 400–600 mg/day) may be too sedating for most patients. Adverse effects of trazodone include dizziness and priapism (1/1000–1/10 000) in men.

Buspirone is indicated for the treatment of generalized anxiety disorder. Two case reports found it useful for PTSD (Fichtner & Crayton, 1994; LaPorta & Ware, 1992; Wells *et al.*, 1991). Cyproheptidine is an antihistamine and partial serotonin antagonist; it is mainly used for allergic reactions. Three case reports (Brophy, 1991; Harsch, 1986; Gupta *et al.*, 1998a) and one retrospective study (Gupta *et al.*, 1998b) found that cyproheptadine was beneficial in reducing PTSD-associated nightmares.

Benzodiazepines
At present, benzodiazepines are not indicated for the treatment of PTSD, at least as monotherapy for the core symptoms (i.e. reliving, avoidance, hyperarousal). Some studies using benzodiazepines have shown mild non-specific improvement (Dunner *et al.*, 1986; Lowenstein *et al.*, 1998; Mellman *et al.*, 1998). One randomized trial with alprazolam showed no therapeutic advantage, but was too small to detect group differences based on what is known now about placebo response in PTSD (Braun *et al.*, 1990). More importantly, benzodiazepines if given in the acute aftermath of a traumatic event (for example, by a physician in the Emergency Room) may actually worsen the condition. Gelpin *et al.* (1996) found in a case-control design that high-dose benzodiazepines given within days after a traumatic event and continued for several months appeared to increase the risk of developing PTSD. A well known case report (Risse *et al.*, 1990)

observed that eight patients with chronic PTSD developed prominent rage reactions while withdrawing from alprazolam. Clearly, these studies have multiple flaws, and it remains difficult to extrapolate from this literature. In general, however, most experts do not recommend benzodiazepines as a treatment for PTSD. It can sometimes be useful to produce quick improvement from comorbid conditions such as severe generalized anxiety or comorbid panic disorder.

Clinicians should be aware of several clinical issues that make the use of benzodiazepines problematic in the PTSD population. For one, there are high rates of comorbid substance abuse in PTSD patients, and the most common comorbid addiction involves prescription medications (Kessler et al., 1995). Secondly, adverse effects of sedation, ataxia, and memory disturbance may be quite distressing to patients with PTSD, especially for patients who are hypervigilant and fearful of any agent that alters their sense of alertness. Thirdly, there is a risk of paradoxical disinhibition in some patients, which may put them at risk for dangerous reactions. Lastly, benzodiazepines are known to interfere with new learning (anterograde memory). Learning and reappraisal of trauma-related fears and schema are believed to be integral to recovery in PTSD.

Mood stabilizers

Mood stabilizers are a class of medications that includes lithium as well as the anticonvulsants valproate, carbamazepine, gabapentin, lamotrigine, topiramate, and others. Only one small randomized placebo controlled study has been published. In a 12-week study using lamotrigine (50–500 mg/day), five of ten subjects were rated as much or very much improved according to the Duke Global Rating for PTSD Scale, compared to one of four on placebo (Hertzberg et al., 1999). Improvements were noted specifically in intrusive and avoidance/numbing symptoms. Most of the evidence behind the use of mood stabilizers in PTSD includes open label studies and case reports involving treatment refractory combat veterans with problems in impulse control and affective regulation (Yehuda et al., 2002). The open studies on valproate are contradictory; the most recent open trial ($n = 10$) of civilians with PTSD showed no benefit (Otte et al., 2004). Open studies using lithium, carbamazepine, gabapentin, and topiramate (as add-on or monotherapy) have observed some therapeutic benefit for non-core PTSD symptoms (Kitchner & Greenstein, 1985). The Expert Consensus Guidelines suggest adding a mood stabilizer if the patient has had only a partial response after 8 weeks of treatment with an SSRI (Foa et al., 1999). However, agents in the class may be helpful for irritability, impulsivity, anger, and affective lability, which are symptoms that are often associated with PTSD. The adverse effects for these medications vary considerably depending on the particular agent. In addition, if used improperly these medications can have serious or even fatal consequences.

Antipsychotics

Antipsychotic medications, also called neuroleptics, are a class that falls into two categories: older generation and newer generation. Older generation antipsychotics include haloperidol, chlorpromazine, fluphenazine, perphenazine, and others. Newer generation antipsychotics (also called atypical or second generation antipsychotics) include clozapine, risperidone, olanzapine, quetiapine, ziprasidone, and aripiprazole. Newer agents have the advantage of being less likely to cause neurological problems (i.e. dystonia or tardive dyskinesia), cognitive dulling, or reproductive hormonal abnormalities. Some of the newer antipsychotics have applications for mood disorders (including bipolar mania and depression), and are being studied for some anxiety disorders. Quetiapine is approved for treatment of bipolar disorder in the USA. Weight gain, glucose regulation, and lipid abnormalities have been associated with the use of some newer generation antipsychotics.

There have been no formal studies using older generation antipsychotics in PTSD. Expert opinion strongly discourages using the older generation antipsychotics. There is no evidence they are effective in PTSD; they may exacerbate numbing and dysphoria; they perpetuate the impression of an incorrect diagnosis; and they have serious long-term adverse effects . Despite this recommendation, older generation antipsychotics are not used uncommonly for PTSD, at least in veteran populations (Sernyak et al., 2001). This trend is hopefully changing as a result of the widespread use of newer generation antipsychotics.

One 8-week randomized placebo controlled trial reported that risperidone (0.5–8 mg/day) was associated with a significantly greater reduction in intrusive and hyperarousal symptoms in subjects with chronic PTSD related to childhood abuse, when compared to placebo (Reich et al., 2004). Several case reports and two open label trials have studied second-generation antipsychotics as add-on treatment. The case reports have noted improvement for symptoms such as insomnia, hyperarousal, nightmares, intrusive thoughts, anger and aggression (Burton & Marshall., 1999; Krashin & Oats, 1999; Leyba & Wampler, 1998; Monelly & Ciraulo, 1999). Two open label trials have been conducted using olanzapine as monotherapy; one was promising (Petty et al., 2001) and one showed no benefit (Butterfield *et al.*, 2001). At present, the role of newer generation antipsychotics in the treatment of PTSD is still not entirely clear.

Autonomic nervous system modulators

The development of PTSD most likely involves a dysregulation of the acute stress response, which is associated with increased locus ceruleus activity, sympathetic arousal and cortisol and opioid release (Marshall & Garakani, 2002). This, combined with the finding of short-term clinically significant heart rate elevations and increased catecholamine metabolites in urine and serum of PTSD patients, leads to the idea that autonomic nervous system modulators could be helpful for PTSD (Shalev, 1998; Marshall *et al.*, 2002; Bryant *et al.*, 2000; Kosten *et al.*, 1987; Yehuda, *et al.*, 1992).

There is some evidence that the non-selective beta adrenergic receptor blocker (i.e. beta blocker) propranolol (120–160 mg/day) may be helpful for explosiveness, nightmares, intrusive recollection, hyperalertness, startle, and psychosocial functioning (Kolb *et al.*, 1984; Famularo *et al.*, 1998). Similarly, the alpha-2 noradrenergic receptor blockers clonidine (0.1–0.6 mg/day) and guanfacine may also be helpful for aggression, impulsivity, emotional outbursts, mood lability, hyperarousal, insomnia, nightmares, and generalized anxiety (Harmon & Riggs, 1996; Horrigan, 1996). Beta blockers should be used with caution with patients with asthma and cardiac failure. Adverse effects of both beta blockers and alpha-2 noradrenergic receptor blockers include hypotension, dizziness, fatigue, depressed mood, and sexual dysfunction.

Opiate antagonists

There is some evidence that naloxone, naltrexone, and nalmefene may be somewhat helpful (Pitman, 1990; Glover, 1993; Bills & Kreisler, 1993; Ibarra *et al.*, 1994). At present, however, the benefit of these medications in PTSD is still theoretical. It is rarely used in practice, however, because the amount of endogenous opoids released under stress are micromolar in relation to the amounts needed to induce dependence. Furthermore, the sudden incapacitation of naturally occurring regulatory functions can have additional effects (such as a sudden increase in somatic pain and discomfort) that causes more distress than is necessary in comparison to more effective treatments.

Clinical issues in pharmacotherapy

Comorbidity

The majority of patients with PTSD suffer from comorbid psychiatric disorders. For example, in a study conducted by Breslau *et al.* (1991), 83% of subjects in an urban population also met criteria for one or more additional DSM diagnoses. This is consistent with findings in the National Comorbidity Survey (Kessler *et al.*, 1995). The most common psychiatric disorders co-occurring in PTSD patients include major depressive disorder, panic disorder, generalized anxiety disorder, somatization disorder, substance abuse, and personality disorders (Brady *et al.*, 1995; Breslau *et al.*, 1991; Kessler *et al.*, 1995). Although largely underrecognized, the prevalence of traumatic experiences in the lives of patients with psychotic disorders and bipolar disorder is significant enough to warrant screening for PTSD in this population as well, although there is an insufficient evidence base that could guide treatment of comorbid PTSD and psychotic disorder at present (Mueser *et al.*, 2002). Although SSRI medications are considered first line for the treatment of PTSD, choice of pharmacologic agent also depends on the presence of a comorbid psychiatric disorder. For bipolar patients, a mood stabilizer at effective doses must be prescribed prior to an SSRI, to guard against iatrogenic complications. For comorbid panic disorder and PTSD, education about the actual dangers of panic attacks, and some exposures to panic (proving to the client that she will not lose her mind or have a cardiac event, and that the feelings always pass) may be necessary in addition to SSRI treatment to inspire the agoraphobic client to venture beyond the feared thresholds of his "safe" space. It is essential in treating both panic disorder and PTSD that the client enter the feared situations, and then *remain* there, until the anxiety subsides.

Adherence

It is not clear whether treatment drop out is more common in PTSD when compared to other psychiatric disorders. However, some patients with PTSD may be difficult to engage. This may be due to a variety of factors, including mistrust, avoidance, fear, and shame. For example, many patients who have been victimized may be mistrustful of others, especially those in authority positions with power over others. They may have had prior negative experiences with healthcare providers, whom they perceived as uncaring or not supportive. In other cases, mental and behavioral avoidance may be so severe that the treatment itself serves as a powerful reminder of the trauma. In this case, the person fears not the clinical care itself, but the traumatic memory that the care evokes. This may be especially prominent if the traumatic experience involved a visit to the hospital. Fear is also a prominent feature of PTSD. Patients with PTSD are often very sensitive to somatic cues. Many view hypervigilance as a way to cope with the perception of perpetual threat. Some patients may equate relaxation via medication with being put dangerously off-guard. In addition, any side effect that alters the senses (i.e. dizziness, blurred vision, sedation) can be overwhelming. Shame can be a strong barrier to treatment for people suffering from PTSD. In addition, some patients may interpret the suggestion of pharmacotherapy as evidence of personal failure or as the clinician's wish to suppress their feelings.

Placebo response
Placebo response has been consistently high in large PTSD trials, at approximately 1/3. Placebo treatment might be considered a form of supportive psychotherapy in these clinical trials, in that the patient receives a careful, thorough evaluation; is offered support and encouragement at regular visits; and is assessed repeatedly, calling attention to symptoms or problems that are the source of suffering. In particular, calling attention to avoidance might encourage the patient to attempt to reverse these behaviors and thus reduce their symptoms according to contemporary theory.

Refractory symptoms
There is good evidence that SSRI medications treat all symptom clusters in PTSD (i.e. reexperiencing, avoidance, and hyperarousal), although the majority of patients will show improvement but not complete recovery. In most cases, an adequate trial of SSRI medication should be attempted prior to augmenting with another medication to address associated symptoms. This is dependent on the individual patient. Some patients may benefit from adjunctive medication for insomnia, aggression, impulsivity, mood lability, nightmares, and generalized anxiety. However, at present, there is no standardized approach to refractory symptoms in the treatment guidelines literature.

Continuation, maintenance and termination
At present, there are only a few studies in the literature regarding when to consider tapering medication in a patient who has achieved a therapeutic response. In a double-blind placebo-controlled study of 92 patients with chronic, severe PTSD, Davidson *et al.* (2001) showed that those subjects maintained on sertraline for 6 months were 6.5 times less likely to experience relapse or clinical deterioration compared to those switched to placebo in double-blind fashion after 6 months of open treatment (Davidson, 2004). Clinical deterioration among the placebo group occurred most frequently within the first two months after the switch to placebo and was equivalent across all three symptom clusters.

The Expert Consensus Guidelines (Foa *et al.*, 1999) suggest considering tapering medication at the following time periods: 6–12 months for acute PTSD, 12–24 months for chronic PTSD with excellent response, and at least 24 months for chronic PTSD with residual symptoms. Factors to consider include presence of effective concomitant psychosocial treatment, duration of illness, time and course of recovery, and any substantial change in psychosocial factors. Current life stressors, suicide risk (past or present), history of violence, and comorbid conditions may be additional indications to continue treatment beyond the suggested guidelines (Foa *et al.*, 1999).

Summary
Pharmacotherapy is rational and effective in the treatment of PTSD. Numerous studies have confirmed that SSRI medications are safe, well tolerated, and effective for all symptom clusters in PTSD. At present, SSRI are considered first line agents for the treatment of PTSD. The evidence for tricyclic antidepressants and MAO inhibitors is limited by multiple factors, but these classes are reasonable alternatives for patients who have not responded to SSRIs. Other antidepressants (venlafaxine, mirtazepine, trazodone, and nefazadone) may be useful as an alternative monotherapy or as adjunctive treatment for partial responders. Mood stabilizers and second generation antipsychotics may be helpful for patients with impulsivity, affective dysregulation, anger, or sleep problems. Autonomic nervous system modulators may have a role in attenuating symptoms related to physiologic hyperarousal (aggression, impulsivity, emotional outbursts, mood lability, hyperarousal, insomnia, nightmares, and generalized anxiety). Benzodiazepines are generally not helpful in PTSD and may be harmful, especially in vulnerable populations and patients with a history of substance abuse. The evidence for opiate antagonists is largely theoretical.

Medication may be helpful alone or in combination with psychosocial treatment. Pharmacological treatment should be considered more strongly in patients with severe and/or chronic symptoms, patients who continue to have symptoms despite psychosocial treatments, and patients with comorbid psychiatric disorders that are responsive to medication. Identification of comorbid psychiatric disorders is essential in PTSD. In addition awareness of factors that influence adherence such as trust, avoidance, fear, and shame may optimize outcome. Important questions regarding approaches to refractory symptoms, length of treatment, and relapse rate after discontinuation of medication remain.

Psychosocial treatments

Introduction

At present, trauma-focused treatments derived from cognitive-behavioral treatments are considered the first-line treatment for PTSD. There are no randomized comparisons of a medication vs. psychosocial treatment in PTSD at present.

Therapies derived from the principles of exposure therapy have consistently been shown effective for PTSD. Prolonged exposure therapy (PE) and Cognitive Processing Therapy are perhaps the best-studied of these, and may result in high-end-state functioning in as many as 50% of patients (Cahill *et al.*, 2006; Foa *et al.*, 1991, 1999; Marks *et al.*, 1998; Tarrier *et al.*, 1990). There is also evidence that it produces continued gains after termination (Foa *et al.*, 1999a, b; Marks *et al.*, 1998).

Trauma-focused psychodynamic therapy

Brom *et al.* (1989) in a pioneering comparative psychotherapy study randomized patients to one of four groups: desensitization therapy (similar to Prolonged Exposure), hypnotherapy, brief dynamic therapy (based on the model of Horowitz), or wait-list control ($n = 112$) in individuals with DSM-III PTSD of no more than 5 years' duration. Patients met DSM-III criteria for PTSD, with the restriction that no more than 5 years had elapsed since the incurring event. For most subjects, the traumatic event was loss of an immediate family member (74%). The psychodynamic treatment used was based on manualized treatment guidelines developed by Horowitz that integrate principles from psychodynamic, information-processing and cognitive theory (Horowitz, 1986). In application, the therapy involves an active, supportive-interpretive therapy that aims to work through trauma-related themes as they arise using the usual techniques of supportive dynamic therapy (i.e. clarification and interpretation of defenses, motives, and responses to fears). The explicit goal is to restore function to pre-event levels, and to maintain a focus on the traumatic event wherever possible.

In the overall analysis, all treatments appeared equally effective, and superior to wait-list control, on multiple measures of post-traumatic symptoms, general psychopathology, and personality functioning. No differences emerged in direct comparisons of the different treatments. The authors note that clinically significant improvement was observed in 60% of treated patients, vs. 26% of the untreated group. On the Impact of Event Scale (Horowitz *et al.*, 1979), desensitization therapy reduced symptoms by 41.4% (47.4 to 28), compared to reductions of 33.7% (50.8 to 33.7) for hypnotherapy and 29.4% for dynamic therapy

(46.3 to 32.7). That is, desensitization therapy produced the largest acute reduction in PTSD symptoms, although differences were not statistically significant.

This early study possesses a number of limitations, including absence of structured diagnostic interviews, lack of direct monitoring of the treatments provided, absence of ratings to ensure adherence to treatment protocols and difference between treatments, and the study of a population of individuals mostly suffering from loss as the criterion A trauma. Comorbid psychiatric diagnoses were also not reported. This limits generalizability of the study, since comorbidity in PTSD is common and significant comorbidity may limit outcome. Furthermore, the exclusion of individuals with more than 5 years' duration of symptoms limits generalizability to more chronic PTSD.

Exposure therapies

All exposure- and cognitive-based therapies are based on the principle that the client must focus on the memory of the trauma in order to facilitate both cognitive and emotional processing. This is usually accomplished through a combination of telling and retelling the story of the trauma in progressively greater detail, so that the client is eventually no longer overwhelmed by the memories; writing down the traumatic memories and going over them alone and with the therapist (CPT); or calling images of the trauma to mind, and then substituting alternative thoughts or images that can neutralize fear, most commonly in the form of eye movement desensitization and reprocessing (EMDR), a controversial treatment that has both strong advocates and sceptics. Before this phase of the treatment is reached, however, all therapists spend time forming an alliance with the patient; educating him about the nature of PTSD and linking his or her personal experiences with aspects of the disorder; and educating him or her about the treatment itself. The goal of these early meetings is to offer the patient hope by demonstrating the therapists' interest in her and the therapist's competence. Finally, it is important to persuade the patient that the treatment makes sense and can be helpful to avoid the patient feeling she is being "forced to do something against her will." This is a common cognition (or transference reaction) in trauma survivors who have in reality often been abused, coerced, or otherwise used like an object by some more powerful other.

Early controlled studies of exposure therapy in PTSD were conducted with male Vietnam veterans. Exposure therapy was found to be modestly effective compared to standard treatment alone (weekly group/individual therapy (Cooper & Clum 1989); compared to no treatment

(Keane *et al.*, 1989), and compared to traditional psychotherapy (Boudewyns *et al.*, 1991).

Foa has conducted two clinical trials in female assault victims with PTSD. In the first, Foa *et al.* (1991) randomly assigned rape victims with chronic PTSD to nine sessions of prolonged exposure (PE), stress inoculation training (SIT), supportive counseling (SC), or wait-list (WL) control (5 weeks). The supportive counseling treatment emphasized problem-solving in the here-and-now and discouraged detailed discussion of the traumatic experience. Only a completer analysis was reported ($n = 45$). Immediately post-treatment, SIT was superior on a measure of PTSD severity to the WL and SC groups. When clinically significant improvement was defined as 2 standard deviations below total sample baseline scores, 71% of the SIT patients and 40% of the PE patients were significantly improved compared to 18% of supportive counseling and 20% of the wait-list group (chi square = 10.18, 3df, $P < 0.05$). At follow-up however, there were no significant differences between the active treatment groups (67% SIT, 56% PE, and 33% SC). It is of interest that in the supportive counseling and wait-list groups, arousal symptoms improved, but not intrusion and avoidance symptoms, suggesting that confronting the trauma in therapy is important to reduce intrusion and avoidance specifically.

Foa *et al.* (1999) conducted a second randomized study comparing the efficacy of nine twice-weekly sessions of the same treatments (PE, SIT), their combination (PE/SIT), and a wait-list comparison group (WL) in 96 female assault victims with PTSD. The authors had hypothesized that combination treatment might be more effective than either treatment alone. However, at completion of the trial there were no differences between active treatments, and all were superior to wait-list. In the intent-to-treat sample, high end-state functioning (defined as scores on the PSS-I < 20, STAI-S < 40, and BDI < 10) was achieved by 52% in PE, 31% in SIT, 27% in the PE/SIT, and 0% in the WL groups. These differences achieved trend significance between PE and SIT, and PE and PE/SIT on chi square analyses ($P = 0.12$, and $P = 0.05$, respectively). At 1 year follow-up ($n = 46$), there were no statistically significant differences between active treatments on high end-state functioning (52% PE, 42% SIT, 36% in PE/SIT).

In a similar study in the UK, Marks *et al.* (1998) compared exposure therapy (E), cognitive restructuring (C), exposure therapy combined with cognitive restructuring (EC), and relaxation training(R) in adults with PTSD of at least 6 months duration, due to mixed trauma. Unfortunately, intent-to-treat analyses were not reported; data on those completing at least 6 weeks of treatment were analyzed ($n = 76$). Immediately post-treatment, the E,C, and E + C groups all appeared superior to relaxation training (RT). When high end-state function was defined stringently as a 50% drop in PTSD symptoms, BDI < 7, and STAI < 35, response rates were 53% for E, 32% for C, 32% for E/C, and 15% for R (chi square not significant). This study used CAPS scores, making comparisons to other studies easier. The PE group scores were reduced from approximately 62 to 32, a 48% reduction. Symptom reductions in the other cells were 48% (C), 51% (E + C), and 25% (R).

Tarrier and colleagues (1999) conducted a randomized trial of imaginal exposure (IE) vs. cognitive therapy (CT) after a 4-week evaluation and monitoring period (randomized $n = 72$). Both treatments resulted in significant improvement compared to baseline with no differences between treatments. Pre- post-CAPS score changes were 71 to 48 for Imaginal Exposure (32% reduction), vs. 77 to 50 for Cognitive Therapy (35% reduction). Percentage of patients rated as having none or slight symptoms post-treatment were the following: 41% for IE, vs. 33% for CT (a non-significant difference). The authors concluded there were no significant differences in the efficacy of PE vs. CT. This study includes two interesting observations about clinical process and range of treatment response. First, patients' average attendance was actually biweekly due to patients missing sessions. The authors interpreted this anecdotally as due to the stressful nature of sessions. Second, they found that significantly more patients in the IE cell ($n = 9$) worsened on CAPS score compared to the CT cell ($n = 3$) (chi square = 5.42, 1df, $P = 0.02$). These patients found therapy as significantly less credible ($P = 0.009$) and missed more therapy sessions ($P = 0.012$) compared to those who improved in treatment. Initial severity of those who showed worsening was not reported.

EMDR (formerly known as Eye Movement Desensitization and Reprocessing)

Although EMDR has received an extraordinary amount of attention in the press and has been successfully disseminated to thousands of practicing clinicians, insufficient research has been conducted on this treatment. Devilly & Spence (1999) compared Eye Movement Desensitization and Reprocessing (EMDR, 8 sessions) to exposure-based therapy (Trauma Treatment Protocol, TTP, nine sessions) for individuals with non-combat related PTSD ($n = 32$). This relatively small study has a number of significant limitations, including the absence of randomized assignment and structured diagnostic interviews, non-standardization of concurrent treatment (43% were also taking medication), small sample size, and analysis of only a completer sample.

The exposure-based treatment, called the Trauma Treatment Protocol (TTP), also included elements of cognitive restructuring during and immediately after exposure. Both treatments produced significant improvement relative to baseline, and there were no significant differences between treatments on multiple analyses. Symptom reduction measured by the PSS-SR (Foa *et al.*, 1993) was 60% for TTP and 29.8% for EMDR. At 3-month follow-up, treatment gains in the TTP were stable, whereas the EMDR group showed a non-significant increase in symptoms. Following the method of Foa *et al.* (1991) to identify subjects with minimal symptoms at completion, the authors found that TTP was significantly superior to EMDR on four PTSD measures both immediately post-treatment, and at 3-month follow-up.

Rothbaum *et al.* (2005) conducted a rigorous randomized clinical trial comparing the relative efficacy of Prolonged Exposure (PE), Eye Movement Desensitization and Reprocessing (EMDR), and a no-treatment wait-list control (WAIT) in the treatment of PTSD in adult female rape victims ($n = 74$). Improvement in PTSD as assessed by blind independent assessors. Improvement in PTSD symptoms, depression, dissociation, and state anxiety was significantly greater in both the PE and EMDR group than the WAIT group ($n = 20$ completers per group). PE and EMDR did not differ significantly at the end of treatment, or at the 6-month follow-up assessment.

A recent meta-analysis of the effects of EMDR (Davidson & Parker, 2001) concludes that it offers no specific advantages over other psychotherapies.

Cognitive-processing therapy

This study randomized $n = 171$ female rape victims with PTSD and major depression to treatment with Cognitive Processing Therapy, Prolonged Exposure Therapy, and a minimal attention condition (Resick *et al.*, 2002). Both 12-week active treatments were highly efficacious and superior to the control condition, with minimal differences between the two effective treatments. These differences persisted through 3-and 9-month follow-up. The CPT begins with education about PTSD and about the treatment model. The patient then writes a statement about the meaning of the traumatic event, which is read and discussed with the therapist. The next sessions pursue these memories in greater detail. The therapist then examines the derived meanings of the trauma using the cognitive dysfunction model, particularly regarding self-blame and guilt, but also safety, trust, and intimacy, and power, with the goal of working toward internalizing the process and achieving more balanced, less grim self-statements. Pre- Post-scores on the CAPS (intent-to-treat analysis)

were 74.7 – 39.08 for CPT (46.7% improvement), and 76.6 – 44.9 (41.4% improvement) for PE, with essentially no change in the minimal attention control. These are both large effect sizes. When secondary measures were analyzed, CPT showed small effect size superiority for PTSD, depression, and guilt symptoms relative to PE.

Skills training in affective and interpersonal regulation followed by exposure: a phase-based treatment for PTSD related to childhood abuse

Cloitre *et al.* (2002) randomized $n = 58$ women with PTSD related to childhood abuse to either a two-phase cognitive-behavioral treatment or a minimal attention wait-list. The active treatment group (STAIR) improved significantly in affect dysregulation, interpersonal skills deficits, and PTSD symptoms, with persistent gains at 3-and 9-month follow-up. The two phases included eight sessions of skills training in affect and interpersonal regulation, followed by eight sessions of modified prolonged exposure. The skills training phase focuses on particular skills deficits identified in this population from the literature: (1) labeling and identifying feelings; (2) emotion management (especially anger/anxiety); (3) distress tolerance; (4) acceptance of feelings and enhanced experience of positive emotions; (5) identification of trauma-based schemas and how they are enacted in daily life; (6) identifying conflicts between personal goals and trauma-generated feelings; (7) role plays related to power, control, and flexibility. Phase II was a modified exposure technique that eliminated homework-based in vivo exposure, and included cognitive processing after exposures to reinforce skills and concepts from Phase I. Only completer analyses were shown, making it difficult to compare to other studies, but the STAIR group did show improvement from CAPS 69 – 31, a 55% improvement. Notably, there was additional significant improvement at 3-and 9-month follow-up.

Limitations of exposure-based therapy

A number of investigators have noted anecdotally that PE is limited in its applicability to a subset of patients due to symptom exacerbation, high drop-out rates, or inability to engage in the treatment due to high levels of depression, anger, or dissociation (Chemtob *et al.*, 1997; Riggs *et al.*, 1998; Jaycox *et al.*, 1998). Case reports have described adverse reactions to exposure therapy. Pitman *et al.* (1991) reported serious adverse consequences of guilt, shame, and feelings of failure (rather than amelioration of such feelings); relapse of substance abuse; and worsening of panic disorder. A high rate of non-compliance with exposure exercises in cognitive therapy of PTSD was recently reported in a small series of outpatients

(Scott & Stradling, 1997), and was associated with greater severity of both PTSD and depressive symptoms.

The only study to examine this question empirically found that a minority (10–30%) of individuals receiving PE in a clinical trial experienced transient increases in anxiety and depression, but this was unrelated to drop-out or treatment outcome (Foa *et al.*, 2002). This finding is reassuring in that it suggests that a transient increase in anxiety and depression, which is predicted by exposure theory, does not mitigate the success of PE if patients persist in treatment.

Discussion

Common techniques across trauma-focused psychotherapies

Taken together, this literature demonstrates that a wide spectrum of problems and disorders are the direct result of adverse experiences that are extremely common in adulthood. It also fortunately offers a number of clinical guidelines to helping patients reduce symptoms and overcome functional impairment.

Formulate a diagnosis

The importance of diagnosis cannot be overemphasized. All research to date that makes use of modern scientific methods is keyed to a specific type of problem that all the patients have in common. For example, after a traumatic event, a patient might be experiencing a wide range of possible problems, including a normative reaction; an adjustment disorder; PTSD; major depression; or generalized anxiety disorder. Treatment planning must be organized around the disorder being treated, and then tailored to the individual case.

Focus on the problem

All empirically validated treatments for stress and trauma-related disorders create a very supportive treatment framework that helps the patient articulate the problem, and then provides an optimistic model for overcoming it. These treatments openly enlist the patient as a collaborative partner in this process ("collaborative empiricism") and encourage the patient to develop and pursue effortful activities both within and outside treatment sessions that will help him overcome the disorder. Much of the actual training of therapists in conducting these treatments involves learning ways to educate patients about their problems and about how treatment can work, and then to motivate them to make use of the therapeutic model. This is a critical aspect of the treatment process, since most persons seeking treatment are demoralized and feel helpless in the face of their situation. In addition, therapists learning these treatments also need a great deal of support and supervision if it is available, since it is a particularly emotional experience to hear these very personal examples of man's inhumanity to man. New therapists typically fear that they will overwhelm the patient by encouraging him to focus on the trauma (this is typically the patient's fear that the therapist is absorbing through the transference in most cases). Once a therapist has seen a treatment work effectively a few times, these kinds of fears tend to recede, and in place of these, the therapist feels optimistic about being able to help relieve suffering using these techniques.

Maintain the treatment focus

Therapists often experience a tension between maintaining the focus on the presenting problem, and allowing the patient to talk about day-to-day concerns or crises or even other serious problems in living. In treating PTSD, patients typically have multiple problems with relationships, with psychosocial circumstances, and with symptoms. Even if the therapist has successfully communicated her understanding of the nature of the patient's disorder, and won the patient over to the treatment approach being recommended, she will inevitably find her attention drawn to other problems, particularly if she has shown herself to be helpful and insightful. However, the therapist should be mindful of the possibility that allowing his focus to become diffuse may simply allow the patient to overwhelm the therapy with a flood of problems, leaving no time for finding solutions. In effect, the patient communicates to the therapist his experience of being overwhelmed with adversity and suffering, as well as his helpless inability to find solutions and relief.

In the case of PTSD, by definition the patient experiences negative affect whenever reminded of the traumatic experience. The same may be true of adjustment disorder, in that patients may feel overwhelmed, hopeless, or frustrated whenever discussing the stressor. The therapist must be confident enough in her knowledge of treatment efficacy, and her own ability to help the patient, to support the patient through this initial reaction.

Therapeutic themes that become a focus of exploration and reframing

All empirically validated therapies encourage the patient to focus consciously on the traumatic experience in detail. Exposure-based, cognitive, and psychodynamic approaches emphasize the importance of verbalizing the traumatic experience, and EMDR primarily uses mental imagery. Therapists using any of these techniques will identify themes that are common to trauma survivors with PTSD: feelings and cognitions related to helplessness, guilt, rage, defectiveness, lack of safety, and personal failure. The approach to these themes varies across therapies, but in all cases the therapist will facilitate and often explicitly provide reframing interpretations that relieve the patient of excessive negative affect. In cognitive therapy, a well-articulated model for addressing these thoughts as cognitive distortions is particularly useful to the trainee. In Prolonged Exposure therapy, supportive psychoeducation is used to identify common themes of incompetence and defectiveness, i.e. pointing out to the patient that feeling defective is a symptom that afflicts many trauma survivors, not because he is actually defective. In EMDR, a more positive image or interpretation is encouraged (relying on the mechanism of reciprocal inhibition).

Conclusions

Mechanisms of therapeutic efficacy in PTSD: psychosocial vs. pharmacologic treatments

The application of clinical trials methodology to psychosocial treatments has greatly enhanced knowledge of both the efficacy and limitations of psychosocial approaches. For PTSD, several forms of psychotherapy have been developed and found to be effective compared to no treatment. Fewer studies have found superiority compared to an active control group, and no study has compared any psychotherapy to any medication treatment.

The few studies that have compared different psychotherapies for individuals with chronic PTSD have found minimal differences. That is to say, most treatments with a clear rationale and theoretical foundation (cognitive, behavioral, psychodynamic) for a survivor of trauma have been shown to be helpful. Small variations in the superiority of one psychosocial treatment over another have been found, and only replication will demonstrate whether such findings are valid. It is widely held that an important ingredient of trauma-focused psychotherapy is the facilitation of "emotional processing" of the traumatic experience (Foa & Kozak, 1986), although this process is poorly understood and subject to wide-ranging speculation from multiple theoretical perspectives. Models of the mechanism of action of psychosocial treatment must also encompass the fact that supporting counseling, as well as placebo plus clinical management, have moderate efficacy. Supportive clinical contact can facilitate working through of overgeneralized and frightening cognitions about the trustworthiness of others, the sense of the self as defective, and perception of the environment as dangerous (Foa & Kosak, 1986). Regardless, it is likely that

psychosocial treatment primarily exerts its effect through mechanisms of *learning*, including basic processes of desensitization and memory modification, and as re-appraisal of complex cognitive schema linked to the traumatic experience. In essence, what is learned during successful PTSD treatment is that the memory itself is not dangerous, and that the trauma need not continue to be feared or held in mind in order to protect the individual from it happening again.

Limitations of Psychosocial Treatment for PTSD

The lack of availability of mental health providers in the community who are well-trained in these specialized techniques is a major problem in both the US and the UK. Just as with medication treatments, all psychosocial treatments to date leave a significant proportion of patients with residual symptoms after brief treatment. There are many possible explanations for this (including the fact that PTSD is often a highly chronic disorder of many years duration, and probably requires more than brief treatment, and a more comprehensive approach to treatment in many persons). There is also concern in the field about whether exposure-based therapies are appropriate for all patients; and some patients are simply too avoidant or symptomatic to tolerate a therapy that emphasizes talking about the traumatic experience (Marshall & Cloitre, 2000). Medication treatment is an alternative for such patients, but public health would also benefit if alternative approaches can be found. It is also possible that conscious processing of the trauma is ultimately the most beneficial component for many patients and should be the conceptual core of treatment modifications. For example, treatment planning might involve increasing the therapeutic time devoted to forming an alliance and psychoeducation prior to narrative reconstruction of the trauma; more time might be devoted to cognitive processing of the trauma; or other components might be added such as skills-building interventions (Cloitre et al., 2002) and exploration of interpersonal trauma-related schema.

Although the mechanism of action for effective medications in PTSD is also unknown, we would argue that its mechanism of action is likely to differ from, and thus be more complementary to, that of a psychosocial treatment, although the final common pathways may overlap considerably. Symptom improvement with medications is likely secondary to stabilization of CNS networks regulating mood, fear, anxiety, and sleep. If the SSRIs exert their effects through altering serotonin transmission (rather than other neurotransmitter systems in a cascade effect), the critical pathways involved may be serotonergic pathway projections to brain centers implicated in PTSD such as the amygdala, hippocampus, and locus ceruleus (Charney *et al.*, 1998). Dampening of overactivity and/or restoration of homeostasis in these neural circuits presumably result in decreased hyperarousal, diminished sensitivity to potentially aversive stimuli, and perhaps reduced activation of memory traces linked to conditioned aversive stimuli.

Treatment Guidelines recommendations

In the first expert consensus report on the treatment of PTSD, the first-line treatment recommendation for adults with chronic PTSD was either psychotherapy alone or the combination of medication and psychotherapy (Foa *et al.*, Expert Consensus Guidelines, 1999). This recommendation is striking in light of the fact that there were no studies to date examining either combined psychosocial and pharmacological treatment in PTSD, or comparing a

psychosocial treatment to medication treatment. Experts recommended combination treatment if psychiatric comorbidity was present, including major depressive disorder and other anxiety disorders. Medications recommended were SSRIs, nefazodone, or venlafaxine. Of note, medication without supportive psychotherapy was not a recommendation, although this may change after results of multi-center trials are more widely known. Promotion of the SSRIs as an approved treatment for PTSD may also increase the frequency of SSRI prescription as a primary treatment among non-psychiatrist physicians. Whether this can represent adequate treatment in the community is unknown, as the study of real-world application of evidence-based trauma treatments is still in its infancy.

The level of evidence for each of the interventions discussed in this chapter is summarized in Table 36.1.

Table 36.1. Effectiveness of treatments for post-traumatic stress disorders and adjustment disorders

Treatment	Form of treatment	Psychiatric disorder	Level of evidence for efficacy	Comments
Community Treatment	Non-specified	Adjustment Disorder	IIb	At 6 months, all patient groups showed improvement. Is this an effect of community treatment or "natural course" of the disorder
Stress Inoculation Training	CBT involving psychoeducation, problem-solving strategies and implementation of those strategies	Adjustment Disorder	IIb	30% superiority in mean time to return to work, but both groups showed significant clinical improvement in psychological symptoms at 3 and 12 month evaluations
Psychosocial Treatment	5 sessions CBT	Acute Stress Disorder	Ib	Reduced rates of PTSD at 6 months (20% v 67 %)
Pharmacotherapy	SSRIs Sertraline 50–200 mg Paroxetine 20–40 mg	PTSD	Ia	Response rates 1.5x-2.0x placebo
Pharmacotherapy	TCAs Amitriptyline and imipramine 150–300 mg	PTSD	IIa	Methodological problems in studies and side effects and lethality limits usage
Pharmacotherapy	Irreversible MAOIs	PTSD	IIb	Study results are contradictory and limited by side effects and dietary restrictions of the medications
Pharmacotherapy	Reversible MAOIs	PTSD	Ib	Growing evidence that they may be useful. Only available in USA
Pharmacotherapy	Other antidepressants (nefazadone, venlafaxine, mirtazepine, trazodone, bupropion)	PTSD	III	Case study reports but no controlled trials
Pharmacotherapy	Benzodiazepines	PTSD	III	Little evidence. May assist with ancillary anxiety symptoms

Table 36.1. (cont.)

Treatment	Form of treatment	Psychiatric disorder	Level of evidence for efficacy	Comments
Pharmacotherapy	Mood stabilisers	PTSD	III	May help with impulsivity, irritability, affect lability, anger. One RCT with lamotrigine
Pharmacotherapy	Antipsychotics	PTSD	IV	May help with impulsivity, irritability, affect lability, anger. Atypicals favoured over neuroleptics
Pharmacotherapy	Autonomic nervous system modulators	PTSD	IIb	Some evidence that beta blockers and alpha-2 noradrenergic agents may attenuate some physiologic hyperarousal
Psychosocial	Exposure therapies, desensitization therapy, stress inoculation training	PTSD	Ia	Clearly superior to wait-list or relaxation but not necessarily better than other active treatments
Psychosocial	Cognitive therapies including cognitive restructuring and cognitive processing therapy	PTSD	Ia	Equivalent to exposure therapies
Psychosocial	Eye movement desensitization and reprocessing (EMDR)	PTSD	Ia	Most studies claiming large specific effects are flawed. No clear evidence of special value

REFERENCES

Anderson, I. M., Nutt, D. J. & Deakin, J. F. (2000). Evidence-based guidelines for treating depressive disorders with antidepressants: a revision of the 1993 British Association for Psychopharmacology guidelines. British Association for Psychopharmacology. *Journal of Psychopharmacology*, **14**, 3–20.

Baker, D. G., Diamond, B. I., Gillette, G. *et al.* (1995). A double-blind randomized placebo-controlled multi-center study of brofaromine in the treatment of post-traumatic stress disorder. *Psychopharmacology*, **122**, 386–9.

Bills, L. J. & Kreisler, K. (1993). Treatment of flashbacks with naltrexone. *American Journal of Psychiatry*, **150**, 1430.

Blanchard, E. B., Buckley, T. C., Hickling, E. J. & Taylor A. E. (1998). Posttraumatic Stress disorder and comorbid major depression: is the correlation an illusion? *Journal of Anxiety Disorder*, **12**, 21–37.

Brady, K. T., Sonne, S. C. & Roberts, J. M. (1995). Sertraline treatment of comorbid posttraumatic stress disorder and alcohol dependence. *Journal of Clinical Psychiatry*, **56**(11), 502–5.

Brady, K., Pearlstein, T., Asnis, G. M. *et al.* (2000). Efficacy and safety of sertraline treatment of posttraumatic stress disorder: a randomized controlled trial. *Journal of the American Medical Association*, **283**, 1837–44.

Braun, P., Greenberg, D., Dasberg, H. & Lerer, B. (1990). Core symptoms of posttraumatic stress disorder unimproved by alprazolam treatment. *Journal of Clinical Psychiatry*, **51**, 236–8.

Breslau, N., Davis, G. C., Andreski, P. & Peterson, E. (1991). Traumatic events and posttraumatic stress disorder in an urban population of young adults. *Archives of General Psychiatry*, **48**(3), 216–22.

Brophy, M. H. (1991). Cyproheptadine for combat nightmares in post-traumatic stress disorder and dream anxiety disorder. *Military Medicine*, **156**, 100–1.

Bryant, R. A., Harvey, A. G., Dang, S. T., Sackville, T. & Basten, C. (1998). Treatment of acute stress disorder: a comparison of cognitive-behavioral therapy and supportive counseling. *Journal of Consulting and Clinical Psychology*, **66**, 862–6.

Bryant, R. A. (2003). Early predictors of post-traumatic stress disorder. *Biological Psychiatry*, **53**, 789–95

Bryant, R. A., Sackville, T., Dang, S. T., Moulds, M. & Guthrie, R. (1999). Treating acute stress disorder: an evaluation of cognitive behavior therapy and supportive counseling techniques. *American Journal of Psychiatry*, **11**, 1780–6.

Bryant, R. A., Harvey, A. G., Guthrie, R. M. & Moulds, M. L. (2000). A prospective study of psychophysiological arousal, acute stress disorder, and posttraumatic stress disorder. *Journal of Abnormal Psychology*, **109**, 341–4.

Boudewyns, P. A., Albrecht, J. W., Talbert, F. S. & Hyer, L. A. (1991). Comorbidity and treatment outcome of inpatients with chronic combat-related PTSD. *Hospital and Community Psychiatry*, **42**(8), 847–849.

Burton, J. K. & Marshall, R. D. (1999). Categorizing fear: the role of trauma in clinical formulation. *American Journal of Psychiatry*, **156**(5), 761–6.

Butterfield, M. I., Becker, M. E., Connor, K. M., Sutherland, S., Churchill, L. E. & Davidson, J. R. (2001). Olanzapine in the treatment of post-traumatic stress disorder: a pilot study. *International Clinical Psychopharmacology*, **16**(4), 197–203.

Cahill, S. P., Foa, E. B., Hembree, E. A., Marshall, R. D. & Nacash, N. (2006). Dissemination of exposure therapy in the treatment of PTSD. *Journal of Traumatic Stress*, **19**(5), 1–14.

Casey, P. R., Tyrer, P. & Platt, S. (1985). The relationship between social functioning and psychiatric symptomatology in primary care. *Social Psychiatry*, **20**, 5–9.

Chemtob, C. M., Novaco, R. W., Hamada, R. S. & Gross, D. M. (1997). Cognitive-behavioral treatment for severe anger in post-traujatic stress disorder. *Journal of Consulting and Clinical Psychology*, **65**, 184–9.

Chung, M. Y., Min, K. H., Jun, Y. J., Kim, S. S., Kim, W. C. & Jun, E. M. (2004). Efficacy and tolerability of mirtazapine and sertraline in Korean veterans with posttraumatic stress disorder: a randomized open label trial. *Human Psychopharmacology*, **19**(7), 489–94.

Cloitre, M., Cohen, L. R., Koenen, K. C. & Han, H. (2002). Skills training in affective and interpersonal regulation followed by exposure: a phase-based treatment for PTSD related to childhood abuse. *Journal of Consult Clinical Psychology*, **70**, 1067–74.

Connor, K. M., Davidson, J. R., Weisler, R. H. & Ahearn, E. (1999). A pilot study of mirtazapine in post-traumatic stress disorder. *International Clinical Psychopharmacology*, **14**(1), 29–31.

Cooper, N. A. & Clum, G. A. (1989). Imaginal flooding as a supplementary treatment for PTSD in combat veterans: a controlled study. *Behavior Therapy*, **20**, 381–91.

Davidson, J. R. (2004). Remission in post-traumatic stress disorder (PTSD): effects of sertraline as assessed by the Davidson Trauma Scale, Clinical Global Impressions and the Clinician Administered PTSD scale. *International Clinical Psychopharmacology*, **19**(2), 85–7.

Davidson, P. R. & Parker, K. C. (2001). Eye movement desensitization and reprocessing (EMDR): a meta-analysis. *Journal of Consulting and Clinical Psychology*, **69**, 305–16.

Davidson, J., Kudler, H., Smith, R. *et al.* (1990). Treatment of posttraumatic stress disorder with amitriptyline and placebo. *Archives of General Psychiatry*, **47**, 259–66.

Davidson, J. R. T., Hughes, D., Blazer, D. & George, L. K. (1991a). Posttraumatic stress disorder in the community: an epidemiological study. *Psychological Medicine*, **2**, 1–19.

Davidson, J., Pearlstein, T., Londborg, P. *et al.* (2001b). Efficacy of sertraline in preventing relapse of posttraumatic stress disorder: results of a 28-week double-blind, placebo-controlled study. *American Journal of Psychiatry*, **158**, 12, 1974–81.

Davidson, J. R., Rothbaum, B. O., van der Kolk, B., Sikes, C. R. & Farfel, G. M. (2001d). Multi-center double-blind comparison of sertraline and placebo in the treatment of posttraumatic stress disorder. *Archives of General Psychiatry*, **58**, 485–92.

Davidson, J. R., Weisler, R. H., Butterfield, M. I. *et al.* (2003). Mirtazapine vs. placebo in posttraumatic stress disorder: a pilot trial. *Biological Psychiatry*, **53** (2), 188–91.

Davidson, J., Rothbaum, B. O., Tucker, P., Asnis, G., Benattia, I. & Musgnung, J. J. (2006a). Venlafaxine extended release in posttraumatic stress disorder: a sertraline- and placebo-controlled study. *Journal of Clinical Psychopharmacology*, **26**(3), 259–67.

Davidson, J., Baldwin, D., Stein, D. J. *et al.* (2006b). Treatment of posttraumatic stress disorder with venlafaxine extended release: a 6-month randomized controlled trial. *Archives of General Psychiatry*, **63**(10), 1158–65.

Davis, L. L., Nugent, A. L., Murray, J., Kramer, G. L. & Petty, F. (2000). Nefazodone treatment for chronic posttraumatic stress disorder: an open trial. *Journal of Clinical Psychopharmacology*, **20**(2), 159–64.

Devilly, G. J. & Spence, S. H. (1999). The relative efficacy and treatment distress of EMDR and a cognitive-behavior trauma treatment protocol in the amelioration of posttraumatic stress disorder. *Journal of Anxiety Disorders*, **13**(1–2), 131–57.

Dunner, D. L., Ishiki, D., Avery, D. H., Wilson, L. G. & Hyde, T. S. (1986). Effects of alprazolam and diazepam on anxiety and panic attacks in panic disorder: a controlled study. *Journal of Clinical Psychiatry*, **47**, 458–460.

Famularo, R., Kinscherff, R. & Fenton, T. (1998). Propranolol treatment for childhood post-traumatic stress disorder, acute type: a pilot study. *American Journal of Diseases of Children*, **142**, 1244–7.

Foa, E. B., Rothbaum, R. O., Riggs, D. S. & Murdock, T. B. (1991). Treatment of posttraumatic stress disorder in rape victims: a comparison between cognitive-behavioral procedures and counseling. *Journal of Consulting and Clinical Psychology*, **59**, 715–23.

Foa, E. B., Hearst-Ikeda, D. & Perry, K. J. (1995). Evaluation of a brief cognitive-behavioral program for the prevention of chronic PTSD in recent assault victims. *Journal of Consulting and Clinical Psychology*, **63**, 948–55.

Foa, E. B., Dancu, C. V., Hembree, E. A., Jaycox, L. H., Meadows, E. A. & Street, G. P. (1999a). A comparison of exposure therapy, stress inoculation training, and their combination for reducing posttraumatic stress disorder in female assault victims. *Journal of Consulting and Clinical Psychology*, **67**, 194–200.

Foa, E. B., Davidson, J. R. T. & Frances, A. (1999b). The expert consensus guideline series: treatment of posttraumatic stress disorder. *Journal of Clinical Psychiatry*, **60** (Suppl.) 16, 1–76.

Galea, S., Ahern, J., Resnick, H. *et al.* (2002). Psychological sequelae of the September 11 terrorist attacks in New York City. *New England Journal of Medicine*, **346**, 982–7.

Garfield, D. A., Fichtner, C. G., Leveroni, C. & Mahableshwarkar, A. (2001). Open trial of nefazodone for combat veterans with post-traumatic stress disorder. *Journal of Traumatic Stress*, **14**(3), 453–60.

Gelpin, E., Bonne, O., Peri, T., Brandes, D. & Shalev, A. Y. (1996). Treatment of recent trauma survivors with benzodiazepines: a prospective study. *Journal of Clinical Psychiatry*, **57**(9), 390–4.

Glover, H. (1993). A preliminary trial of nalmefene for the treatment of emotional numbing in combat veterans with post-traumatic stress disorder. *Israel Journal of Psychiatry and Related Sciences*, **30**(4), 255–63

Gupta, S., Austin, R., Cali, L. A. & Bhatara, V. (1998a). Nightmares treated with cyproheptadine. *Journal of the American Academy of Child and Adolescent Psychiatry*, **37**(6), 570–2.

Gupta, S., Popli, A., Bathhurst, E., Hennig, L., Droney, T. & Keller, P. (1998b). Efficacy of cyproheptadine for nightmares associated with posttraumatic stress disorder. *Comprehensive Psychiatry*, **39**(3), 160–4.

Harmon, R. J. & Riggs, P. D. (1996). Clonidine for posttraumatic stress disorder in preschool children. *Journal of the American Academy of Child and Adolescent Psychiatry*, **35**, 1247–9.

Harsch, H. H. (1986). Cyproheptadine for recurrent nightmares. *American Journal of Psychiatry*, **143**, 1491–2.

Herman, J. (1997). "A forgotten history." in *Trauma and Recovery: The Aftermath pf Violence – from Domestic Abuse to Political Terror*, pp. 7–32. New York: BasicBooks.

Hertzberg, M. A., Feldman, M. E., Beckham, J. C. & Davidson, J. R. (1996). Trial of trazadone for posttraumatic stress disorder using a multiple baseline group design. *Journal of Clinical Psychopharmacology*, **16**(4), 294–8.

Hertzberg, M. A., Butterfield, M. I., Feldman, M. E. *et al.* (1999). A preliminary study of lamotrigine for the treatment of posttraumatic stress disorder. *Biological Psychiatry*, **45**, 1226–9.

Hertzberg, M. A., Feldman, M. E., Beckham, J. C., Kudler, H. S. & Davidson, J. R. (2000). Lack of efficacy for fluoxetine in PTSD: a placebo controlled trial in combat veterans. *Annals of Clinical Psychiatry*, **12**(2), 101–5.

Hidalgo, R., Hertzberg, M. A., Mellman, T. *et al.* (1999). Nefazodone in post-traumatic stress disorder: results from six open-label trials. *International Journal of Clinical Psychopharmacology*, **14**(2), 61–8.

Hogben, G. L. & Cornfield, R. B. (1981). Treatment of neurotic war neurosis with phenelzine. *Archives of General Psychiatry*, **38**, 440–5.

Horrigan, J. P. (1996). Guanfacine for PTSD nightmares. *Journal of the American Academy of Child and Adolescent Psychiatry*, **35**, 975–6.

Jaycox, L. H., Foa, E. B. & Morral, A. R. (1998). Influence of emotional engagement and habituation on exposure therapy for PTSD. *Journal Consulting Clinical and Psychology*, **66**, 185–192.

Jones, R., Yates, W., Williams, S., Zhou, M., & Hardman, L. (1999). Outcome for adjustment disorder with depressed mood: comparison with other mood disorders. *Journal of Affective Disorders*, **55**, 55–61.

Ibarra, P., Bruehl, S. P., McCubbin, J. A. *et al.* (1994). An unusual reaction to opioid blockade with naltrexone in a case of post-traumatic stress disorder. *Journal of Traumatic Stress*, **7**(2), 303–9.

Katz, R. J., Lott, M. H., Arbus, P. *et al.* (1995). Pharmacotherapy of post-traumatic stress disorder with a novel psychotropic. *Anxiety*, **1**, 169–74.

Keane, T. M., Fairbank, J. A., Caddell, J. M. & Zimmering, R. T. (1989). Implosive (flooding) therapy reduces symptoms of PTSD in Vietnam combat veterans. *Behavior Therapy*, **20**, 245–60.

Kessler, R. C., Sonnega, A., Bromet, E., Hughes, M. & Nelson, C. B. (1995). Posttraumatic stress disorder in the National Comorbidity Survey. *Archives of General Psychiatry*, **52**, 1048–60.

Kitchner, L. & Greenstein, R. (1985). Low dose lithium carbonate in the treatment of post traumatic stress disorder: brief communication. *Military Medicine*, **150**, 378–81.

Klein, D. F. (1978). A proposed definition of mental illness. In *Critical Issues in Psychiatric Diagnosis*, ed. R. L. Spitzer, & D. F. Klein, New York: Raven Press.

Kolb, L. C., Burris, B. C. & Griffiths, S. (1984). Propranolol and clonidine in the treatment of the chronic post-traumatic stress disorders of war. In *Post-traumatic Stress Disorder: Psychological and Biological Sequelae*, ed. B. A. Van der Kolk, pp. 98–105. Washington, DC: American Psychiatric Press.

Kosten, T. R., Frank, J. B., Dan, E., McDougle, C. J. & Giller, E. L. (1991). Pharmacotherapy for posttraumatic stress disorder using phenelzine or imipramine. *Journal of Nervous and Mental Disease*, **179**, 366–70.

Kosten, T. R., Mason, J. W., Giller, E. L., Ostroff, R. B. & Harkness, L. (1987). Sustained urinary norepinephrine and epinephrine elevation in posttraumatic stress disorder. *Psychoneuroendocrinology*, **12**, 13–20.

Krashin, D. & Oates, E. W. (1999). Risperidone as an adjunct therapy for post-traumatic stress disorder. *Military Medicine*, **164**(8), 605–6.

Leyba, C. M. & Wampler, T. P. (1998). Risperidone in PTSD. *Psychiatric Service*, **49**(2), 245–6.

Lowenstein, R. J., Hornstein, N. & Farber, B. (1988). Open trial of clonazepam in post-traumatic stress symptoms in multiple personality disorder. *Dissociation*, **1**, 3–12.

Marks, I., Lovell, K., Noshirvani, H., Livanou, M. & Thrasher, S. (1998). Treatment of posttraumatic stress disorder by exposure and/or cognitive restructuring. *Archives of General Psychiatry*, **55**, 317–25.

Marshall, R. D. & Klein, D. F. (1995). Pharmacotherapy in the treatment of Posttraumatic Stress Disorder. *Psychiatric Annals*, **25**, 588–97.

Marshall, R. D. & Garakani, A. (2002). Psychobiology of the acute stress response and its relationship to the psychobiology of post-traumatic stress disorder. *Psychiatric Clinics of North America*, **25**, 385–95.

Marshall, R. D., & Klein, D. F. (2002). Conceptual antecedents of the Anxiety Disorders. In *Anxiety*, ed. D. J. Nutt & J. C. Ballenger. Oxford: Blackwell Science Limited.

Marshall, R. D., Spitzer, R. & Liebowitz, M. R. (1999). A Review and critique of the new DSM-IV diagnosis of acute stress disorder. *American Journal of Psychiatry*, **156**, 1677–85.

Marshall, R. D., Olfson, M., Hellman, F., Blanco, C., Guardino, M., Struening, E. (2001a). Comorbidity, impairment and suicidality in subthreshold PTSD. *American Journal of Psychiatry*, **158**: 1467–73

Marshall, R. D., Beebe, K. L., Oldham M, and Zaninelli R (2001b). Efficacy and safety of paroxetine treatment for chronic PTSD: a fixed-dose, placebo-controlled study. *American Journal of Psychiatry*, **158**(12), 1982–88.

Marshall, R. D., Blanco, C., Printz, D., Liebowitz, M. R., Klein, D. F. & Coplan, J. (2002). Noradrenergic and HPA axis functioning in PTSD vs. Panic Disorder. *Psychiatry Research*, **110**(3), 219–30.

Marshall, R. D., Lewis-Fernandez, R., Blanco, C. *et al.* (2006). A controlled trial of Paroxetine for chronic PTSD, dissociation and interpersonal problems in urban, mostly minority adults. *Depression and Anxiety*, **0**, 1–8.

Mellman, T. A., Byers, P. M. & Augenstein, J. S. (1998). Pilot evaluation of hypnotic medication during acute traumatic stress response. *Journal of Traumatic Stress*, **11**, 563–9.

Martenyi, F. Brown, E. B.. Zhang, H., Prakash, A. & Koke, S. C. (2002). Fluoxetine versus placebo in posttraumatic stress disorder. *Journal of Clinical Psychiatry*, **63**(3), 199–206.

Monnelly, E. P. & Ciraulo, D. A. (1999). Risperidone effects on irritable aggression in posttraumatic stress disorder. *Journal of Clinical Psychopharmacology*, **19**(4), 377–8.

Mueser, K. T., Rosenberg, S. D., Goodman, L. A. & Trumbetta, S. L. (2002). Trauma, PTSD, and the course of severe mental illnesss: an interactive model. *Schizophrenia Research*, **53**, 123–43.

Neal, L. A., Shapland, W. & Fox C (1997). An open trial of moclobemide in the treatment of post-traumatic stress disorder. *International Clinical Psychopharmacology*, **12**, 231–237.

Otte, C., Wiedemann, K., Yassouridis, A. & Kellner, M. (2004). Valproate monotherapy in the treatment of civilian patients with non-combat-related posttraumatic stress disorder: an open-label study. *Journal of Clinical Psychopharmacology*, **24**(1), 106–8.

Pitman, R. K. & Delahanty, D. L. (2005). Conceptually driven pharmacologic approaches to acute trauma. *CNS Spectrums*, **10**, 99–106.

Pitman, R. K., van der Kolk, B. A., Orr, S. P. & Greenberg, M. S. (1990). Naloxone-reversible analgesic response to combat-related stimuli in posttraumatic stress disorder. *Archives of General Psychiatry*, **47**, 541–4.

Pitman, R. K., Altman, B., Greenwald, E. *et al.* (1991). Psychiatric complications during flooding therapy for posttraumatic stress disorder. *Journal of Clinical Psychiatry*, **52**, 17–20.

Pitman, R. K., Sanders, K. M., Zusman, R. M. *et al.* (2002). Pilot study of secondary prevention of posttraumatic stress disorder with propanolol. *Biological Psychiatry*, **51**, 189–92.

Petty, F., Brannan, S., Casada, J. *et al.* (2001). Olanzapine treatment for post-traumatic stress disorder: an open-label study. *International Clinical Psychopharmacology*, **16**, 331–7.

Reich, D. B. Winternitz, S. Hennen, J. Watts, T. & Stanculescu, C. (2004). A preliminary study of risperidone in the treatment of posttraumatic stress disorder related to childhood abuse in women. *Journal of Clinical Psychiatry*, **65**(12),1601–6.

Reist, C., Kauffman, C. D., Haier, R. J. *et al.* (1989). A controlled trial of desipramine in 18 men with posttraumatic stress disorder. *American Journal of Psychiatry*, **146**, 513–16.

Resick, P. A., Nishith, P., Weaver, T. L., Astin, M. C. & Feuer, C. A. (2002). A comparison of cognitive-processing therapy with prolonged exposure and a waiting condition for the treatment of chronic posttraumatic stress disorder in female rape victims. *Journal of Consulting Clinical Psychology*, **70**, 867–79.

Riggs, D. S., Byrne, C. A., Weathers, F. W. & Litz, B. T. (1998). The quality of the intimate relationships of male Vietnam veterans: problems associated with posttraumatic stress disorder. *Journal of Traumatic Stress*, **11**, 87–101.

Risse, S. C., Whitters, A., Burke, J., Chen, S., Scurfield, R. M. & Raskind, M. A. (1990). Severe withdrawal symptoms after discontinuation of alprazolam in eight patients with combat-induced posttraumatic stress disorder. *Journal of Clinical Psychiatry*, **51**(5), 206–9.

Rothbaum, B. O., Astin, M. C. & Marsteller, F. (2005). Prolonged exposure therapy versus Eye Movement Desensitization and Reprocessing (EMDR) for PTSD rape victims. *Journal of Traumatic Stress*, **18**, 607–16.

Scott, M. J. & Stradling, S. G. (1997). Client compliance with exposure treatments for Posttraumatic Stress Disorder. *Journal of Traumatic Stress*, **10**, 523–6.

Seivewright, H., Tyrer, P. & Johnson, T. (1998). Prediction of outcome in neurotic disorder: a five year prospective study. *Psychological Medicine*, **28**, 1149–57.

Sernyak, M. J., Kosten, T. R., Fontana, A. & Rosenheck, R. (2001). Neuroleptic use in the treatment of post-traumatic stress disorder. *Psychiatric Quarterly*, **72**(3), 192–213.

Shalev, A. Y., Sahar, T., Freedman, S. *et al.* (1998). A prospective study of the heart rate response following trauma and the subsequent development of posttraumatic stress disorder. *Archives of General Psychiatry*, **55**, 553–9.

Shestazky, M., Greenberg, D. & Lerer, B. (1987). A controlled trial of phenelzine in posttraumatic stress disorder. *Psychiatric Research*, **24**, 149–55.

Smajkic, A., Weine, S., Djuric-Bijedic, Z., Boskailo, E., Lewis, J. & Pavkovic, I. (2001). Sertraline, paroxetine, and venlafaxine in refugee posttraumatic stress disorder with depression symptoms. *Journal of Traumatic Stress*, **14**(3), 445–52.

Spitzer, R. L., First, M. B. & Wakefield, J. C. (2007). Saving PTSD from itself in DSM-V. *Journal of Anxiety Disorders*, **21**, 233–41.

Stirman, S. W., DeRubeis, R. J., Crits-Christoph, P. & Brody, P. E. (2003). Are samples in randomized controlled trials of psychotherapy representative of community outpatients? A new methodology and initial findings. *Journal of Consulting and Clinical Psychology*, **71**, 963–72.

Strain, J. J., Smith, G. C., Hammer, J. S. *et al.* (1998). Adjustment disorder: a multi-site study of its utilization and interventions in the consultation-liaison psychiatry setting. *General Hospital Psychiatry*, **20**: 139–49.

Tarrier, N., Pilgrim, H., Sommerfield, C. *et al.* (1999). A randomized trial of cognitive therapy and imaginal exposure in the treatment of chronic posttraumatic stress disorder. *Journal of Consulting and Clinical Psychology*, **67**, 13–18.

Tucker, P., Zaninelli, R., Yehuda, R., Ruggiero, L., Dillingham, K. & Pitts, C. D. (2001). Paroxetine in the treatment of chronic posttraumatic stress disorder: results of a placebo-controlled, flexible-dosage trial. *Journal of Clinical Psychiatry*, **62**(11), 86–868.

Tyrer, P., Seivewright, N., Murphy, S. *et al.* (1988). The Nottingham study of neurotic disorder: comparison of drug and psychological treatments. *Lancet*, **ii**, 235–40.

Tyrer, P., Seivewright, H. & Johnson, T. (2005). Long-term outcome of anxiety and depressive disorders: the Nottingham Study of Neurotic Disorder. *Directions in Psychiatry*, **25**, 269–80.

Vaiva, G., Ducrocq, F., Jezequel, K. *et al.* (2003). Immediate treatment with propranolol decreases posttraumatic stress disorder two months after trauma. *Biological Psychiatry*, **54**, 947–9.

Van der Klink, J. J. L., Blonk, R. W. B., Schene, A. H. & Dijk, F. J. H. (2003). Reducing long term sickness absence by an activating intervention in adjustment disorders: a cluster randomized controlled design. *Occupational and Environmental Medicine*, **60**, 429–37.

Vermetten, E. & Bremner, J. D. (2002). Circuit and systems in stress II. Applications to neurobiology and treatment in posttraumatic stress disorder. *Depression and Anxiety*, **16**, 14–38.

Yehuda, R., Marshall, R. M., Penkower, A. & Wong, C. M. (2002). Pharmacological treatments for posttraumatic stress disorder. In *A Guide to Treatments that Work, 2nd edn*, ed. P. E. Nathan & J. M. Gorman, pp. 411–45. New York: Oxford University Press.

Yehuda, R., Southwick, S. M. & Giller, E. L. (1992). Urinary catecholamine excretion and severity of PTSD symptoms in Vietnam combat veterans. *Journal of Nervous and Mental Disease*, **180**, 321–5.

Zisook, S., Chentsova-Dutton, Y. E., Smith-Vaniz, A. *et al.* (2000). Nefazodone in patients with treatment-refractory posttraumatic stress disorder. *Journal of Clinical Psychiatry*, **61**(3), 203–8.

Eating disorders

Section editors

Ulrike Schmidt and Katherine Halmi

37

Psychopharmacology of eating disorders

Andrew Bennett, Rishi Caleyachetty and Janet Treasure

Editor's note

Most people do not think much about drug treatment when eating disorders are mentioned. However, it has a long history, and 30–40 years ago drug treatments, particularly tricyclic antidepressants and typical antipsychotic drugs such as chlorpromazine, were regarded by many as essential treatments for anorexia nervosa (Dally & Sargant, 1966; Mills, 1976). A brief look at the evidence table tells us where we are today with these and other treatments, and shows the great turn-around of the last 20 years. The authors illustrate the difficulties in constructing an evidence base common to specialties in which numbers of patients are relatively few, but the results of this review are impressive, particularly in regard to bulimia nervosa, where there is now a solid range of effective treatments.

Introduction

The aim of this chapter is to synthesize the evidence from systematic reviews and various national clinical guidelines on the use of medication in the management of people with eating disorders and to set it in the context of clinical practice. A variety of National Guidelines for eating disorders have been published including those from the USA (American Psychiatric Association, 2000), UK (National Collaborating Centre for Mental Health, 2004), Australia and New Zealand (Beumont et al., 2004) and Finland (Ebeling et al., 2003). Most of these make some reference to the use of medication. Some of these guidelines (such as those from the UK and Australia) are built upon a systematic synthesis of all the evidence in the literature. In addition there are systematic reviews within the Cochrane library on the use of medication for bulimia nervosa (Hay & Bacaltchuk, 2003) and there is also a protocol for a systematic review on

anorexia nervosa. As part of the *British Medical Journal*'s Clinical Evidence series a systematic synthesis of the literature is updated on an annual basis for anorexia nervosa (Treasure & Schmidt, 2002) and bulimia nervosa (Hay & Bacaltchuk, 2001). Thus there is no shortage of high quality reviews. However, the evidence is often not translated into clinical practice for a variety of reasons.

The use of medication in the management of anorexia nervosa

The gap between evidence based approaches and clinical practice is most marked in the case of anorexia nervosa. First of all there are insufficient data. Furthermore, those data that are available may not apply to all cases of anorexia nervosa. Anorexia nervosa comes in many clinical forms ranging from presentations in childhood to older adults, and from a severe, high risk, medical state through to mildly compromised well being. The balance of risk and benefits of medication varies between these clinical forms. Most of the trials of medication for anorexia nervosa have been conducted with adults and it is often unwise to extrapolate to their use in children or adolescents. The QT interval of the electrocardiogram is prolonged by starvation and electrolyte imbalance (Cooke et al., 1994) and thus there is the potential for adverse interactions with drugs which have an independent effect on cardiac rhythmicity.

There are also two forms of anorexia nervosa, the restricting subtype and the binge/purge subtype and it is difficult to provide clear guidelines of treatment for these separately. A key differentiating factor is the behaviour related to food: binge/purge subtypes exhibit the characteristic of disinhibited eating and robust hunger, whereas a weaker constrained appetite is associated with restricting anorexia nervosa. Evidence is accumulating that suggests the subtypes differ

Cambridge Textbook of Effective Treatments in Psychiatry, ed. Peter Tyrer and Kenneth R. Silk. Published by Cambridge University Press.
© Cambridge University Press, 2008.

in their biological aetiology (Collier & Treasure, 2004). Indeed there is also evidence that binge/purge and restricting subtypes of anorexia nervosa respond differently to medication (Halmi *et al.*, 1986). Unfortunately in many treatment studies either there is no information on the clinical subtypes of the sample or the power of the study is inadequate to reliably estimate the effect size for each subtype. Thus drug treatment may need to be tailored to the phenotype, phase of illness and age of the patient.

Evidence based efficacy

The Cochrane systematic review of the literature for the use of medication in the treatment of anorexia nervosa is not completed. Both the UK (National Collaborating Centre for Mental Health, 2004) and the Australian and New Zealand guidelines (Beumont *et al.*, 2004) however do include a systematic review of the literature.

The conclusions from the UK NICE guidelines(National Collaborating Centre for Mental Health, 2004) were as follows:

Effect of treatment on weight gain

- There is evidence suggesting that it is unlikely there is a clinically significant benefit of antidepressant drugs versus placebo in promoting weight gain by the end of multi-modal inpatient treatment (Halmi *et al.*, 1986a; Attia *et al.*, 1998; Biederman *et al.*, 1985; Lacey & Crisp, 1980).
- There is insufficient evidence to determine whether antipsychotics or antihistamines have any impact on weight compared with placebo during multi-modal inpatient treatment (Vandereycken, 1984; Vandereycken & Pierloot, 1982) There is insufficient evidence to determine whether there is any difference between antipsychotics and antidepressants with regard to weight gain (Ruggiero *et al.*, 2001).

Effect of treatment on relapse/clinical deterioration

- There is limited evidence suggesting that there is a clinically significant difference between an SSRI (fluoxetine) and placebo with fewer patients with restricting anorexia nervosa deteriorating clinically (which for the majority of patients was defined as a worsening or no improvement in symptoms) following inpatient weight restoration if given fluoxetine for one year (Kaye *et al.*, 2001).

Clinical practice

Many people with anorexia nervosa do not adhere to medication as they are fearful of many aspects of such treatment, including the loss of control inherent in drug treatment, the additional calories in the coating of drugs,

and the threat of weight gain itself. Thus time needs to be given to strategies to improve adherence to medication. In the following we have divided the clinical section according to phase and severity of the illness.

Patients with high medical risk

In their most acute state, patients with anorexia nervosa are frequently admitted to a form of intensive care where they may exhibit anxious or depressed mood and agitated or compulsive behaviours. Thus medication may be considered for these other symptoms rather than for weight gain. It is prudent, however, to forego the use of psychotropic drugs in the severely underweight patient until disturbances in electrolytes and liver function tests, among others, have resolved. At this stage of treatment, issues of rehydration and refeeding predominate. Even when medically stable, underweight patients are more prone to experience side effects and even toxicity. Therefore, medications with a low therapeutic index (TI) (the TI is the ratio between the toxic and therapeutic doses) should be used with caution and the dosage may need to be adjusted according to weight.

Nevertheless, through perceived necessity, low doses of neuroleptics are frequently used to treat obsessional and anxious symptoms in this setting. In the severely emaciated patient with anorexia nervosa, resistance to eating is the norm and anxiolytics are sometimes prescribed before meals to reduce these anticipatory fears. There is no anxiolytic that has been shown to be particularly helpful in the resistant patient. Chlorpromazine, however, is sometimes useful for the motivated patient who suffers from a high degree of nausea around meals, especially the purging anorexic.

Chlorpromazine possesses anti-emetic as well as anxiolytic properties, but it is important to monitor for hypotension and for changes in the electrocardiogram. There is widespread use in the USA of the newer atypical antipsychotics such as olanzapine and risperidone, but as yet there are no controlled trials to support their use. There are case reports and open-label trials to support the use of both olanzapine (Powers & Santana, 2002) and risperidone (Newman-Toker, 2000), but we still do not know whether atypical antipsychotics add anything to nutritional and behavioural interventions.

Cyproheptadine is an antihistamine with anti-serotonergic and anti-cholinergic properties and is an appetite stimulant. In one of three controlled trials, it was shown to be of some mild benefit to hospitalized patients in promoting weight gain and relieving depression particularly those with restricting subtype of anorexia nervosa (Halmi *et al.*, 1986). This subtype specific response may apply to other appetite stimulating drugs and further research which addresses the possibility of a differential clinical response between the two anorexia nervosa subtypes is warranted. The use of this drug is not advocated in the UK(National Collaborating Centre for Mental Health 2004) and Australian guidelines (Beumont *et al.*, 2004).

It is possible that some of the negative effects of drug trials in patients with anorexia nervosa in the intensive care setting are due to the much greater effects of intensive care nursing obscuring any smaller drug contribution.

Patients with moderate medical risk

In the medically stable, ambulatory patient, less caution is needed. However, there are only a few research studies that can inform management in these settings. Most of these are open studies which fail to meet the quality standards needed to be accepted for an evidence based approach (Ruggiero *et al.*, 2003).

Patients with anorexia nervosa commonly exhibit depressive symptoms and obsessive attitudes about shape and weight and also frank obsessive compulsive comorbidity which in theory could respond to medications such as SSRIs and TCAs. Some argue that SSRIs should be started only after the patient has undergone nutritional rehabilitation and attained oestrogen levels within the normal range. In the acute state nutritional deficiencies, e.g. tryptophan or the secondary consequences of malnutrition such as oestrogen deficiency may render medication ineffective. However, in an interesting study which addressed this hypothesis in part it was found that nutritional supplements (tryptophan, vitamin, minerals and essential fatty acids) did not enhance the effectiveness of fluoxetine in underweight patients with anorexia nervosa (Barbarich *et al.*, 2004). In addition, little is known about how people with anorexia nervosa absorb and metabolize antidepressants or any medications, raising the possibility that there may be inadequate penetration to the brain. Thus more research into the use of medication in ambulatory care is needed.

Relapse prevention

There are two roles for psychopharmacological treatment after the anorexic patient has restored weight. The first is to treat those psychiatric symptoms associated with anorexia nervosa that persist after weight restoration. In the USA guidelines it is recommended that because symptoms associated with anorexia nervosa, such as depression, or OCD may remit with weight restoration, the practitioner should if possible defer decisions concerning the use of medications until the person with anorexia nervosa has reached an appropriate weight. Clomipramine is sometimes used for weight-restored patients with comorbid obsessive compulsive disorder as second-line treatment if SSRIs have failed. Because of its anticholinergic properties, constipation is a frequent side effect.

The second role for psychopharmacology is the use of antidepressants for weight maintenance in anorexia nervosa. The limited evidence so far on the effect of fluoxetine to reduce the risk of relapse is promising and worthy of further study.

The newest atypical antipsychotics, such as aripiprazole and ziprasidone, are also used in the USA, although there is even less evidence to support their use. They may have some use in the weight maintenance phase of treatment when weight gain is no longer the goal of treatment but the patient remains focused on body image distortions and fear of additional weight gain. Because weight gain does not appear to be a common side effect of these medications, they are frequently used for patients who reject any medication that may cause weight gain even when this is precisely the goal of treatment.

Contraindications

Although not widely used, buproprion is sometimes prescribed to depressed patients with anorexia nervosa who have not responded to SSRIs. As discussed below, buproprion is contraindicated in the treatment of bulimia nervosa because of the high risk of generalized seizures. The manufacturer of buproprion has extended its contraindication to anorexia nervosa, regardless of subtype. The American Psychiatric Association also recommends extending this contraindication to patients with the purging subtype of anorexia nervosa.

It is prudent to avoid TCAs in the underweight patients because of their potential to prolong the QT-interval on the electrocardiogram. In addition, TCAs increase the risk of hypotension and of arrhythmia, particularly in purging patients who may be dehydrated. Cisapride which has been used to improve gastric motility is not recommended because of the risk of cardiac toxicity.

The use of medication in the management of bulimia nervosa

Within the Cochrane library there is a systematic review and a meta-analysis of the studies which address the use of medication for bulimia nervosa and binge eating disorders comparing antidepressants with placebo (Bacaltchuk & Hay, 2003). This was updated and reanalysed as part of the process of constructing the NICE guidelines (National Collaborating Centre for Mental Health, 2004). In the latter process some studies were excluded as they did not reach the quality standards set by the committee. In this section we also report on how such evidence can be applied in clinical practice.

In contrast to anorexia nervosa it is more satisfactory to use an evidence based approach in the management of bulimia nervosa. The clinical presentation is less diverse and the context of treatment is more uniform, i.e. typically these patients are treated in outpatient settings. Also the higher incidence, prevalence and better prognosis means that fewer resources are required to undertake treatment studies. Thus, there is a greater amount of high quality evidence. Nevertheless, there are limitations in the evidence. Most placebo-controlled trials of medication have only examined the response over a period of 8 weeks or less, which may not be sufficient time to assess efficacy. Little is known about how people with eating disorders absorb and metabolize drugs. A poor response may occur because medication is lost due to purging. There are subtypes of bulimia nervosa, e.g. purging and non-purging but there is less evidence than in anorexia nervosa that these may represent aetiologically distinct variants.

The majority of the numerous medication trials were undertaken in adults and the results may not generalize to children or adolescents. It remains to be seen how the recent warnings about SSRIs and suicidality in adolescents will affect prescribing practices.

Evidence based efficacy

We outline the conclusions from the NICE guidelines as this is the most recent systematic review and meta-analysis we have found.

Effect of treatment on remission from binge eating/purging

- There is limited evidence suggesting that there is a clinically significant difference between antidepressants and placebo, in terms of antidepressants being superior in terms of remission from binge eating/purging (defined as cessation of binge eating/purging) by the end of treatment (McCann & Agras 1990; Mitchell et al., 1990; Pope et al., 1983; Walsh et al., 1991), four studies compared SSRIs with placebo (Goldstein et al., 1995; Kanerva et al., 1994; Mitchell et al., 2001), two compared MAOIs with placebo (Walsh et al., 1987; Carruba et al., 2001), and three compared other

antidepressants with placebo (Horne et al., 1988; Pope et al., 1989a; Pope et al., 1989b).
- There is limited evidence suggesting that there is a clinically significant difference between the MAOIs and placebo, with MAOIs being superior in terms of remission from binge eating (defined as cessation of binge eating) by the end of treatment (Walsh et al., 1987).
- There is insufficient evidence to determine whether SSRIs or tricyclics are preferable in improving remission rates by the end of treatment.

Effect of treatment on frequency of binge eating and purging

- There is strong evidence suggesting that there is a clinically significant difference between antidepressants and placebo with antidepressants being superior in terms of clinical improvement (defined as at least a 50% reduction in the frequency of binge eating) by the end of treatment (Arnold et al., 2002; Hudson et al., 1998; Laederach-Hofmann et al., 1999; McElroy et al., 2000).
- There is strong evidence from three trials that SSRIs when compared to placebo produce clinical improvement in binge eating and purging by the end of treatment (Arnold et al., 2002; Hudson et al., 1998b; McElroy et al., 2000).
- There is strong evidence suggesting that there is a clinically significant difference between tricyclics and placebo with tricyclics being superior in terms of clinical improvement (defined as at least a 50% reduction in the frequency of binge eating) by the end of treatment (Laederach-Hofmann et al., 1999).
- Both SSRIs and TCA were found to be acceptable and tolerated.
- There was insufficient evidence to conclude whether supplementing psychotherapy with medication improved the outcome compared to either treatment alone.

Guideline recommendation

The conclusion from the NICE guidelines was that medication appeared to be less effective at the end of treatment than psychotherapy (National Collaborating Centre for Mental Health, 2004). Also, in contrast to the availability of data on long-term results of psychotherapy, there was no information about the long-term effects following pharmacological treatment. Therefore, it was suggested that antidepressants might be used as an alternative or additional first step in the management of bulimia nervosa.

Clinical practice

Fluoxetine is the only drug which the US Food and Drug Administration have approved for the treatment of bulimia nervosa at a dose of 60 mg/day. It is possible that any SSRI or any other antidepressant may be helpful in reducing episodes of binge eating and purging. There are, however, no studies directly comparing two classes of antidepressants, e.g. SSRIs vs. TCAs.

Some clinicians start fluoxetine for bulimia nervosa at 60 mg/day and titrate downwards if not tolerated. Because of this data involving fluoxetine, other SSRIs are frequently dosed in the high normal range. In contrast, the APA recommends dosing tricyclic antidepressants for treating bulimia nervosa as one would when treating depression.

The recommended course of a successful treatment with an antidepressant is six months to one year. It is unclear if antidepressant treatment produces a lasting remission if it is discontinued after 6 months. However, relapse while continuing an effective medication is common. If a patient relapses during antidepressant treatment, clinicians should assess whether the patient is taking the medication shortly before purging. If there is no problem in achieving effective blood levels, then switching to another medication is indicated.

There is also evidence to support switching to a different antidepressant if the first medication does not help reduce the frequency of binge eating and purging. This evidence came from a trial in which non-responders to desipramine were switched to fluoxetine (Mitchell *et al.*, 1989). In practice, if the initial SSRI fails, the next medication will often be another SSRI or venlafaxine because of their generally favourable side-effect profiles. In the USA, some clinicians recommend against paroxetine for bulimia nervosa because of its relative propensity for causing weight gain.

The side effect profile of tricyclic antidepressants (TCA) is particularly problematic for people with bulimia nervosa. The main problem is that TCAs in general are likely to produce some degree of weight gain (see Chapter 27), and, not surprisingly, bulimic patients do not tolerate this well. In addition, TCAs may exacerbate orthostatic hypotension and constipation caused by restrictive eating and fluid balance abnormalities caused by purging. Reduced salivation may exacerbate the dental erosion caused by purging. TCAs may also increase the risk of arrhythmias caused by hypokalaemia from excessive purging. Finally it is important to assess the suicide risk and level of impulsive self harm in patients being prescribed TCAs as these drugs (apart from the possible exceptions of lofepramine and clomipramine) are toxic in overdose. These limitations mean that, other SSRIs or venlafaxine are commonly tried before a TCA.

There are no studies concerning augmentation strategies when a bulimic patient has shown a partial response to an antidepressant. Since all antidepressants appear efficacious in reducing bulimic symptoms, TCA augmentation is one option. There is no evidence regarding the addition of mirtazapine, a common augmenting strategy in treating depression. It should be noted that agranulocytosis is a rare but potentially lethal side effect of mirtazapine, and that bulimics may exhibit some degree of compromised immune systems. There is also no data about combining medications of different classes, e.g. an SSRI and topiramate. It is important to note that people with bulimia nervosa commonly have comorbidity with major affective disorder and substance abuse. Often, these are used as exclusion criteria for formal research studies of treatment. Therefore, a pragmatic clinical approach is needed that takes account of evidence derived from several quarters.

Atypical neuroleptics are commonly added to SSRIs in patients with comorbid personality disorder or traits, usually for self-injurious behaviour such as cutting or suicidality. Although they may have some effect in reducing 'non-bulimic' self-injurious behaviour (see Chapter 42), they have not been shown to have any effect in reducing the frequency of binge eating or purging.

It can be difficult to choose a mood-stabilizer for a patient with bulimia nervosa, which may be necessary in the treatment of comorbid bipolar disorder. Bulimics are prone to lithium toxicity because of rapid shifts in fluid volume. Both lithium carbonate and valproic acid can produce weight gain, which people with bulimia nervosa tolerate poorly. Recent mood stabilizers, such as lamotrigine and oxcarbazepine, may be less likely to produce undesirable weight gain, although this has not been systematically examined.

Clinical common sense would suggest that those who have failed or partially responded to psychological treatment might benefit if medication is added. In practice, those patients who present as very depressed would most commonly receive an SSRI, provided that nausea and vomiting are not major adverse effects; clinicians may wait and see if milder forms of depression respond to CBT alone.

New approaches

Two randomized controlled studies have shown that topiramate, an anticonvulsant, reduced binge eating and purging in patients with bulimia nervosa when compared with placebo (Hedges *et al.*, 2003; Hoopes *et al.*, 2003). Its side-effect profile, however, may limit its use. Paraesthesias and cognitive difficulties are the most common side effects, and because of this a slow titration is recommended, e.g.

25–50 mg per week. Caution is advised, especially when using topiramate with those bulimics who are below normal weight, even if they do not meet criteria for anorexia nervosa as weight loss is a common side effect. The mechanism of weight loss due to topiramate is unknown.

Rarely used approaches

The use of the opiate antagonist naltrexone is not common. One small study, however, did show some efficacy when used in higher doses of 200–300 mg/day, which is higher than doses used to prevent alcohol relapse and opiate addiction (Marrazzi et al., 1995). The risk of nausea, however, may preclude use at such doses for most patients. There are some case reports of using naltrexone to augment SSRIs. It is more likely to be used when a history of self-injurious behaviour, such as cutting, is present. Liver function tests must be monitored because of the risk of hepatotoxicity at high doses.

Irreversible MAOIs are rarely used because of the dietary restrictions necessary to avoid tyramine reactions, although weight gain can be very marked with these drugs.

Contraindications

Because of the risk of generalized seizures, buproprion is contraindicated in patients with bulimia nervosa. This contraindication extends to its use for any reason, including smoking cessation. This contraindication also applies to non-purging bulimics as well as to anyone with a past history of bulimia nervosa.

The use of medication in the management of binge eating disorder (atypical eating disorder)

Introduction

The history of binge eating disorder is less extensive than that of the other conditions as it has not been accorded the status of a separate condition in diagnostic manuals. However, it has been considered as a separate topic in the UK National Guidelines and a systematic review and meta analysis of the literature was undertaken. In this section in addition to reporting on the systematic literature reviews and studies completed since these have appeared we also report on the information in guidelines and clinical practice.

Evidence based efficacy

The following statements are taken from the NICE guidelines (National Collaborating Centre for Mental Health 2004):

Effect of treatment on remission

- There is limited evidence suggesting that there is a clinically significant difference between antidepressants (SSRIs) and placebo with antidepressants being superior in terms of remission (defined as cessation of binge eating) by the end of treatment (Arnold et al., 2002; Hudson et al., 1998; McElroy et al., 2000).
- There is limited evidence suggesting that there is a clinically significant difference between topiramate and placebo with topiramate being superior in terms of remission (defined as cessation of binge eating) by the end of treatment (McElroy et al., 2003; McElroy et al., 2004).

Effect of treatment on symptoms

There is limited evidence suggesting that there is a clinically significant difference between antidepressants and placebo with antidepressants being superior on mean frequency of binge eating by the end of treatment (Arnold et al., 2002; Hudson et al., 1998; Laederach-Hofmann et al., 1999; McElroy et al., 2000).

Effect of treatment on weight

- There is insufficient evidence to determine whether antidepressants have any impact on weight when compared with placebo at the end of treatment (McElroy et al., 2000).

New approaches

Sibutramine, a specific reuptake noradrenaline and serotonin inhibitor (SNRI) has been used in the treatment of obese patients with binge eating disorder and was found to reduce both weight and binge frequency. Dry mouth and constipation were side effects (Appolinario et al., 2003). NICE guidelines suggest it is only given to those who have seriously tried to lose weight by other methods and who are being carefully monitored. It is only licensed for use for 1 year, and rebound weight gain may follow its cessation.

Clinical approaches

Much of what was written for the clinical management of bulimia nervosa can probably be transferred into binge eating disorder in that there are uncertainties about the long-term effects, and the strategies to be made with resistant or relapsing cases. Issues such as the sequencing or supplementation of therapeutic approaches are unknown.

Conclusions

In the main, psychotherapeutic approaches have been both more effective and acceptable in the management of eating disorders than drug treatments. However, it is possible that tailoring medication to the type, severity and duration of the illness may improve both outcome and clinical utility. Thus research with new drugs such as sibutramine and others specifically marketed for these disorders, each with a more comprehensive risk benefit profile, and more trials in which both the type and severity of the disorder is characterized more carefully, may widen their use in this patient population.

The level of evidence for each of the interventions discussed in this chapter is summarized in Table 37.1.

Table 37.1. Effectiveness of drug treatments for eating disorders

Treatment	Form of treatment	Psychiatric disorder	Level of evidence for efficacy	Comments
Tricyclic antidepressants (TCAs)	(e.g. amitriptyline, clomipramine) Conventional treatment (up to 6 weeks acute treatment and then maintenance dosage)	Anorexia nervosa	IIIa	No incremental value when combined with full multi-modal treatment. Care to be taken with very emaciated patients with electrolyte disturbance or suicidal risk
Selective serotonin reuptake inhibitors (SSRIs)	(e.g. fluoxetine)	Anorexia nervosa (particularly in restricting sub-group)	Ib	Randomized trial evidence that fluoxetine aids maintenance of weight after successful initial (non-pharmacological) treatment
Typical antipsychotic drugs	(e.g. chlorpromazine) May be useful as anti-nausea drug	Anorexia nervosa	IV	No firm evidence of efficacy
Atypical antipsychotic drugs	(e.g. aripiprazole, ziprasidone)	Anorexia nervosa	IV	Possible use to maintain weight gain
Anti-anxiety drugs	(e.g. diazepam)	Anorexia nervosa	IV	Use as required at times of great distress but not regularly
Monoamine oxidase inhibitors	Up to 8 weeks initially	Bulimia nervosa	Ib	Evidence favouring MAOIs in remission from binge eating
Tricyclic antidepressants	(e.g. clomipamine) in conventional dosage up to 1yr	Bulimia nervosa	Ia	Significantly superior to placebo in reducing binge eating
Selective serotonin reuptake inhibitors (SSRIs)	(e.g. fluoxetine in higher than conventional dosage) 40–60 mg daily for up to 8 weeks and subsequent maintenance treatment up to 1 yr	Bulimia nervosa	Ia	Significantly superior to placebo in reducing binge eating and maintaining remission. Paroxetine avoided because of weight gain
Selective noradrenaline and serotonin reuptake inhibitors (SNRIs)	Sibutramine	Bulimia nervosa	Ib	Significant reduction in weight and binge frequency
Anticonvulsants	Topiramate (in gradual increasing dosage)	Bulimia nervosa	Ib	Significant reduction of binging and purging but effects compromised by adverse effects
Opiate antagonists	Natrexone	Bulimia nervosa	Ib	

REFERENCES

American Psychiatric Association (2000). Practice guideline for the treatment of patients with eating disorders (revision). American Psychiatric Association Work Group on Eating Disorders, *American Journal of Psychiatry*, **157**(1) Suppl, 1–39.

Appolinario, J. C., Bacaltchuk, J., Sichieri, R. (2003). A randomized, double-blind, placebo-controlled study of sibutramine in the treatment of binge-eating disorder. *Archives of General Psychiatry*, **60**(11), 1109–16.

Arnold, L. M., McElroy, S. L., Hudson, J. I., Welge, J. A., Bennett, A. J. & Keck, P. E. (2002). A placebo-controlled, randomized trial of fluoxetine in the treatment of binge-eating disorder. *Journal of Clinical Psychiatry*, **63**(11), pp. 1028–33.

Attia, E., Haiman, C., Walsh, B. T. & Flater, S. R. (1998). Does fluoxetine augment the inpatient treatment of anorexia nervosa? *American Journal of Psychiatry*, **155**(4), 548–51.

Bacaltchuk, J. & Hay, P. (2003). Antidepressants versus placebo for people with bulimia nervosa. *Cochrane Database Systematic Review*, **4**, CD003391. Oxford: Update Software Ltd.

Barbarich, N. C., McConaha, C. W., Halmi, K. A. *et al.* (2004). Use of nutritional supplements to increase the efficacy of fluoxetine in the treatment of anorexia nervosa. *International Journal of Eating Disorders*, **35**(1), 10–15.

Beumont, P., Hay, P., Beumont, D. (2004). Australian and New Zealand clinical practice guidelines for the treatment of anorexia nervosa. *Australia and New Zealand Journal of Psychiatry*, **38**(9), 659–70.

Biederman, J., Herzog, D. B., Rivinus, T. M. *et al.* (1985). Amitriptyline in the treatment of anorexia nervosa: a double-blind, placebo-controlled study. *Journal of Clinical Psychopharmacology*, **5**(1), 10–16.

Carruba, M. O., Cuzzolaro, M., Riva, L. *et al.* (2001). Efficacy and tolerability of moclobemide in bulimia nervosa: a placebo-controlled trial. *International Clinical Psychopharmacology*, **16**(1), 27–32.

Collier, D. A. & Treasure, J. L. (2004). The aetiology of eating disorders. *British Journal of Psychiatry*, **185**, 363–5.

Cooke, R. A., Chambers, J. B., Singh, R. *et al.* (1994). QT interval in anorexia nervosa. *British Heart Journal*, **72**(1), 69–73.

Dally, P. & Sargant, W. (1966). Treatment and outcome of anorexia nervosa. *British Medical Journal*, **2**, 793–5.

Ebeling, H., Tapanainen, P., Joutsenoja, A. *et al.* (2003). A practice guideline for treatment of eating disorders in children and adolescents. *Annals of Medicine*, **35**(7), 488–501.

Fluoxetine Bulimia Nervosa Collaborative Study Group (1992). Fluoxetine in the treatment of bulimia nervosa. A multicenter, placebo-controlled, double-blind trial. *Archives of General Psychiatry*, **49**(2), 139–47.

Goldstein, D. J., Wilson, M. G., Thompson, V. L., Potvin, J. H. & Rampey, A. H., Jr (1995). Long-term fluoxetine treatment of bulimia nervosa. Fluoxetine Bulimia Nervosa Research Group. *British Journal of Psychiatry*, **166**(5), 660–6.

Halmi, K. A., Eckert, E., LaDu, T. J. & Cohen, J. (1986). Anorexia nervosa. Treatment efficacy of cyproheptadine and amitriptyline. *Archives of General Psychiatry*, **43**(2), 177–81.

Hay, P. J. & Bacaltchuk, J. (2001). Extracts from "Clinical evidence": bulimia nervosa. *British Medical Journal*, **323**(7303), 33–7.

Hay, P. J. & Bacaltchuk, J. (2003). Psychotherapy for bulimia nervosa and binging (Cochrane Review). *Cochrane Database Systematic Review*, **1**, CD000562. Oxford: Update Software Ltd.

Hedges, D. W., Reimherr, F. W., Hoopes, S. P. *et al.* (2003). Treatment of bulimia nervosa with topiramate in a randomized, double-blind, placebo-controlled trial, part 2: improvement in psychiatric measures. *Journal of Clinical Psychiatry*, **64**(12), 1449–54.

Hoopes, S. P., Reimherr, F. W., Hedges, D. W. *et al.* (2003). Treatment of bulimia nervosa with topiramate in a randomized, double-blind, placebo-controlled trial, part 1: improvement in binge and purge measures. *Journal of Clinical Psychiatry*, **64**(11), 1335–41.

Horne, R. L., Ferguson, J. M., Pope, H. G., Jr *et al.* (1988). Treatment of bulimia with bupropion: a multicenter controlled trial. *Journal of Clinical Psychiatry*, **49**(7), 262–6.

Hudson, J. I., McElroy, S. L., Raymond, N. C. *et al.* (1998). Fluvoxamine in the treatment of binge-eating disorder: a multicenter placebo-controlled, double-blind trial. *American Journal of Psychiatry*, **155**(12), 1756–62.

Kanerva, R., Rissanen, A. & Sarna, S. (1994). Fluoexetine in the treatment of anxiety, depressive symptoms and eating-related symptoms in bulimia nervosa. *Journal of Psychiatry*, **11**(3), 239–57.

Kaye, W. H., Nagata, T., Weltzin, T. E. (2001). Double-blind placebo-controlled administration of fluoxetine in restricting- and restricting-purging-type anorexia nervosa. *Biological Psychiatry*, **49**(7), 644–52.

Lacey, J. H. & Crisp, A. H. (1980). Hunger, food intake and weight: the impact of clomipramine on a refeeding anorexia nervosa population. *Postgraduate Medical Journal*, **56** (Suppl. 1), 79–85.

Laederach-Hofmann, K., Graf, C., Horber, F. *et al.* (1999). Imipramine and diet counseling with psychological support in the treatment of obese binge eaters: a randomized, placebo-controlled double-blind study. *International Journal of Eating Disorders*, **26**(3), 231–44.

Marrazzi, M. A., Bacon, J. P., Kinzie, J. & Luby, E. D. (1995). Naltrexone use in the treatment of anorexia nervosa and bulimia nervosa. *International Clinical Psychopharmacology*, **10**(3), 163–72.

McCann, U. D. & Agras, W. S. (1990). Successful treatment of nonpurging bulimia nervosa with desipramine: a double-blind, placebo-controlled study [see comments]. *American Journal of Psychiatry*, **147**(11), 1509–13.

McElroy, S. L., Arnold, L. M., Shapira, N. A. *et al.* (2003). Topiramate in the treatment of binge eating disorder associated with obesity: a randomized, placebo-controlled trial. *American Journal of Psychiatry*, **160**(2), 255–61.

McElroy, S. L., Casuto, L. S., Nelson, E. B. *et al.* (2000). Placebo-controlled trial of sertraline in the treatment of binge eating disorder. *American Journal of Psychiatry*, **157**(6), 1004–6.

McElroy, S. L., Shapira, N. A., Arnold, L. M. (2004). Topiramate in the long-term treatment of binge-eating disorder associated with obesity. *Journal of Clinical Psychiatry*, **65**(11), 1463–9.

Mills, I. H. (1976). Amitriptyline therapy in anorexia-nervosa. *Lancet*, **2**, 687.

Mitchell, J. E., Pyle, R. L., Eckert, E. D., Hatsukami, D., Pomeroy, C. & Zimmerman, R. (1989). Response to alternative antidepressants in imipramine nonresponders with bulimia nervosa. *Journal of Clinical Psychopharmacology*, **9**(4), 291–3.

Mitchell, J. E., Pyle, R. L., Eckert, E. D., Hatsukami, D., Pomeroy, C. & Zimmerman, R. (1990). A comparison study of antidepressants and structured intensive group psychotherapy in the treatment of bulimia nervosa. *Archives of General Psychiatry*, **47**(2), 149–57.

Mitchell, J. E., Fletcher, L., Hanson, K. *et al.* (2001). The relative efficacy of fluoxetine and manual-based self-help in the treatment of outpatients with bulimia nervosa. *Journal of Clinical Psychopharmacology*, **21**(3), 298–304.

National Collaborating Centre for Mental Health. (2004). *National Clinical Practice Guideline: Eating Disorders: Core interventions in the treatment and management of anorexia nervosa, bulimia nervosa, and related eating disorders.* National Institute for Clinical Excellence. Electronic Citation.

Newman-Toker, J. (2000). Risperidone in anorexia nervosa [letter]. *Journal of the American Academy for Child and Adolescent Psychiatry*, **39**(8), 941–2.

Pope, H. G., Jr, Hudson, J. I., Jonas, J. M. & Yurgelun-Todd, D. (1983). Bulimia treated with imipramine: a placebo-controlled, double-blind study. *American Journal of Psychiatry*, **140**(5), 554–8.

Pope, H. G., Jr Keck, P. E., Jr, McElroy, S. L. & Hudson, J. I. (1989). A placebo-controlled study of trazodone in bulimia nervosa. *Journal of Clinical Psychopharmacology*, **9**(4), 254–9.

Powers, P. S. & Santana, C. A. (2002). Eating disorders: a guide for the primary care physician. *Primary Care*, **29**(1), 81–98, vii.

Ruggiero, G. M., Laini, V., Mauri, M. C. (2001). A single blind comparison of amisulpride, fluoxetine and clomipramine in the treatment of restricting anorectics. *Progress in Neuropsychopharmacological and Biological Psychiatry*, **25**(5), 1049–59.

Ruggiero, G. M., Mauri, M. C., Omboni, A. C. (2003). Nutritional management of anorexic patients with and without fluoxetine: 1-year follow-up. *Progress in Neuropsychopharmacological and Biological Psychiatry*, **27**(3), 425–30.

Treasure, J. & Schmidt, U. (2002). Anorexia nervosa. *Clinical Evidence*, **7**, 824–33.

Vandereycken, W. (1984). Neuroleptics in the short-term treatment of anorexia nervosa. A double-blind placebo-controlled study with sulpiride. *British Journal of Psychiatry*, **144**, 288–92.

Vandereycken, W. & Pierloot, R. (1982). Pimozide combined with behavior therapy in the short-term treatment of anorexia nervosa. A double-blind placebo-controlled cross-over study. *Acta Psychiatrica Scandinavica*, **66**(6), 445–50.

Walsh, B. T., Gladis, M., Roose, S. P., Stewart, J. W. & Glassman, A. H. (1987). A controlled trial of phenelzine in bulimia. *Psychopharmacology Bulletin*, **23**(1), 49–51.

Walsh, B. T., Hadigan, C. M., Devlin, M. J., Gladis, M. & Roose, S. P. (1991). Long-term outcome of antidepressant treatment for bulimia nervosa. *American Journal of Psychiatry*, **148**(9), 1206–12.

38

Other somatic physical treatments and complex interventions for eating disorders

Philippa Hugo and Scott Crow

Editor's note

There are many practices that are common in the management of eating disorders that do not have a satisfactory evidence base yet are still accepted as reasonable practice. Although it should not be assumed that what is reasonable is necessarily appropriate or true, it is important to acknowledge these areas of the subject, and this chapter is open and frank about the issues concerned. The chapter also points to other areas in which evaluative research is needed.

Introduction

Potential somatic treatments for eating disorders include medications, feeding, light and heat treatments, exercise, electroconvulsive therapy and psychosurgery. Apart from feeding and psychopharmacology, these have been studied rarely for the treatment of eating disorders. The evidence base for these types of treatments for other disorders is discussed in Part II of this book. The literature regarding these interventions is mostly confined to case reports and case series, and many of these at this point are relatively old. With few exceptions, reports involve short-term rather than long-term outcomes. Apart from feeding, these approaches appear to be rarely used, infrequently advocated and have limited empirical support. Medication treatments are covered elsewhere in this volume. The existing literature for other somatic treatments is summarized below.

Intensive feeding

Refeeding is a necessary component of the treatment of anorexia nervosa. The methods, setting and rate of refeeding are much debated and there is little evidence to aid clinical practice. Guidelines are available in a number of countries and there is general agreement that oral refeeding in the context of a psychotherapeutic programme is preferred (National Collaborating Centre for Mental Health, 2004; Position of the American Dietetic Association, 1994). The overwhelming majority of patients will be refed orally with skilled support. For details on preferred methods and recommended rates of weight gain, please see the chapter on complex treatments of eating disorders.

More intensive methods of feeding need to be considered if the patient is non-compliant with the above and if warranted by the patient's physical health. Most clinicians concur that, in this instance, refeeding should take place in a setting which has the expertise to manage it safely. Close medical monitoring, vitamin and mineral supplementation, particularly phosphate, is recommended to prevent 'refeeding syndrome' (Solomon & Kirby, 1990, Birmingham et al., 1996). The complex legal and ethical issues should always be considered, and carers or parents involved in the decision if possible (Goldner et al., 1997; Bentovim, 2000).

Nasogastric (NG) tube feeding is the preferred route, should more invasive refeeding be considered. Nasogastric feeding has few medical complications, is easily halted and thus can support a return to normal eating as soon as possible. Other routes of feeding that have been described are via gastrostomy or jejunostomy (Pesenti et al., 1999; Neiderman et al., 2000) and total parenteral nutrition (TPN) (Mehler & Weiner, 1993). The latter has been shown to produce significantly more rapid weight gain in 11 subjects when compared to a matched group receiving behaviourally orientated inpatient therapy (Pertschuk et al., 1981). However, complications are common and TPN is rarely recommended for this reason.

There are very few studies examining the efficacy and acceptability of nasogastric feeding. Case series document the biochemical and anthropometric changes (Bufano *et al.*, 1990, Birmingham *et al.*, 1996), and describe nocturnal supplementary feeding in a domiciliary setting (Greaves *et al.*, 1991). Although it is a commonly held view that nasogastric feeding can be experienced as abusive with negative long-term outcomes, Serfaty & McCluskey (1998) found that it was not detrimental to the therapeutic relationship. Neiderman *et al.*'s (2001) study of patients' and parents' experiences of NG feeding showed diverse views, with reactions being more positive than anticipated. Even those with wholly negative views accept that, given the severity of the medical condition, there had been no feasible alternative.

More extensive studies have recently been published. Two retrospective studies compare nasogastric in addition to oral feeding to oral feeding alone within an inpatient treatment setting. Robb *et al.* (2002) compared nocturnal supplementary nasogastric feeding to enhance oral feeding in 52 patients with 48 oral feeding controls. Zuercher *et al.* (2003) reported the comparison between 155 patients receiving nasogastric feeding voluntarily in addition to oral feeds with 226 patients having oral feeds only. Both studies reported significantly greater increases in weight in the nasogastric feeding group. There were no differences in length of hospital stay (Robb *et al.*, 2002), EDI 2 scores and patient satisfaction (Zuercher *et al.*, 2003). It should be noted that these patients were volunteering, were not randomly assigned and long-term outcomes are not available. These studies therefore provide limited evidence that supplementary nasogastric feeding produces clinically significant weight increases in the short term. The impact of nasogastric feeding on long-term outcome, on other parameters (e.g. quality of life) and on involuntary patients remains uncertain.

Exercise

A number of reports describe use of exercise as an adjunct to treatment of patients with eating disorders. The exercise programmes described vary considerably from the educational to relying on the patient to adhere to a prescribed exercise programme, to more supervised activities. The majority of reports are descriptive.

Two studies report the use of exercise in the treatment of binge-eating disorder. Levine *et al.* (1996) compared 44 patients in an active treatment group, which included an exercise component, to 33 in a delayed treatment control group. At the end of treatment there were significantly greater increases in exercise frequency and overall calorie expenditure in the active treatment group. Binge abstinent subjects showed significant increases in exercise frequency compared to those who were not abstinent post-treatment.

Pendleton *et al.* (2002) evaluated the effects of adding exercise to CBT for binge-eating disorder. There was a significant decrease in binge-eating frequency and an increase in abstinence rates in the exercise group, post-treatment and at follow up at 16 months. In contrast to the previous study, exercise was also associated with weight loss and an improvement in mood.

Patients with bulimia nervosa tend to adopt a chaotic approach to exercise, oscillating between excessive exercise and no exercise at all. Beumont *et al.* (1994) commented that the introduction of regular exercise including aerobic, non-aerobic and social sport may benefit these patients in increasing confidence, maintaining a healthy weight and through it effect decreasing anxiety and depression. Sundgot-Borgen *et al.* (2002) evaluated the effectiveness of exercise as compared to CBT and nutritional advice in a randomized controlled trial of 69 patients with bulimia nervosa. Patients were followed up for 6 and 18 months after the end of treatment. Physical exercise appeared more effective than CBT in reducing the drive for thinness scale on the EDI, and frequency of binge eating, purging and laxative abuse. Abstinence rates were not reported.

In anorexia nervosa, the treatment of excessive exercise has been reported but little is written on the use of exercise within treatment. Most treatment programmes restrict exercise or use exercise as a reinforcement for weight gain. Physical therapies like dance movement therapy, yoga, Tai Chi, and horse riding are used in some European countries (Vandereycken *et al.*, 1987). There are a few reports describing structured exercise programmes as an adjunct to treatment of anorexia nervosa (Beumont *et al.*, 1994; Carraro *et al.*, 1998; Thien *et al.*, 2000; Szabo & Green, 2002). Two of these studies attempted to evaluate the effectiveness of prescribed exercise. In their pilot study, Thien *et al.* examined the impact of a graded exercise programme on quality of life in 8 patients with anorexia nervosa as compared to eight anorexic controls. The exercise was prescribed but not supervised. Zabo & Green (2002) assessed the impact of resistance training on mood and EDI scores. Both studies included a small number of subjects and show non-significant improvements in psychological parameters. Exercise programmes do not appear to impact on weight gain (Touyz *et al.*, 1993; Thien *et al.*, 2000; Szabo & Green 2002) and may enhance staff and patient satisfaction.

In conclusion, there is limited evidence to support the notion that exercise improves outcome in the treatment of patients with eating disorders. The inclusion of an exercise programme as an adjunct to treatment may have some benefits on patient satisfaction and adherence to treatment.

Heat treatment

William Gull, the discoverer of anorexia nervosa, was the first to note the therapeutic effect of heat treatment. Four reports consider the use of heat treatment in anorexia nervosa. The first reported three patients with anorexia nervosa in which hyperactivity decreased followed by progressive recovery following three different methods of heat treatment (Gutierrez & Vazquez, 2001). The same authors consider the use of sauna baths as an adjunct to the treatment of anorexia nervosa (Gutierrez et al., 2002). Subsequently these researchers investigated whether warming (by wearing a heating vest) increases the rate of weight gain in patients with anorexia nervosa (Birmingham et al., 2004). Ten women were randomized to a treatment group and 11 to a control arm. There was no difference in change of BMI. Finally, a small randomized, controlled trial compared the combination of heat and a computerized eating monitor to waiting list control. Higher remission rates were seen in the heat plus computer monitoring group (Bergh et al., 2002). To date, therefore, the evidence does not support the use of heat treatment in anorexia nervosa.

Light therapy

Four case reports describe the treatment of patients with eating disorders with bright light therapy, two patients with bulimia nervosa (Lam, 1989; Schwitzer et al., 1994), one with night eating syndrome (Friedman et al., 2002) and an adolescent with restrictive atypical eating disorder (Ash et al., 1997). All of these patients had concurrent depression, and treatment improved both mood and eating symptoms.

Four studies investigate this further. All of these have limitations in that the treatment periods are brief, and eating symptomatology is largely measured using self report diaries. Three controlled studies examine the effect of bright light treatment on binge eating, purging and mood (Lam et al., 1996; Blouin et al., 1996; Braun et al., 1999). In a cross-over design study of 17 women, Lam et al. (1996) found a significant improvement in binge eating, purging and depressive symptoms, but only one patient was abstinent from binge eating at the end of 2 weeks of treatment. Contrasting results were found in a randomized control study of 18 patients treated for a 1 week period (Blouin et al., 1996). They showed a significant

effect on mood but not on binge eating or purging. In both of these studies a large number of subjects suffered a concurrent depressive illness, with 47% in one study (Lam et al., 1996) and 72% in the other (Blouin et al., 1996). A subsequent trial of 34 patients, only 23.5% of whom were depressed, demonstrated an effect on binge frequency but not on mood or purging (Braun et al., 1999).

In an open study of 22 women with bulimia nervosa and seasonal affective disorder, treated with 4 weeks of light therapy, mood and binge purge frequency significantly improved (Lam et al., 2001). Only two patients were abstinent of bulimic symptoms at the end of the treatment period.

All these results may reflect a primary effect on depressive symptoms with any improvement in bulimic symptoms as a secondary occurrence. The authors also note that those patients with seasonal symptoms make the greatest improvement. From the available evidence, therefore, light therapy cannot be recommended as a standard treatment for patients with bulimia nervosa.

Electroconvulsive therapy

A handful of case reports describe the use of electroconvulsive therapy (ECT) for the treatment of anorexia nervosa. Most of this literature is old, with only two reports being published in the last 20 years. LaBoucherie, in 1954 reported a series of 19 patients with anorexia nervosa receiving ECT. A second report of 15 cases was added in 1959 by Wall. He asserted that 'electric shock therapy usually hastens the improvement' and further reported that 10 of the 15 subjects did 'fairly well' over an unspecified follow-up period. Subsequently, a variety of case reports of good response to ECT in anorexia nervosa followed (Bernstein, 1964; Bernstein, 1972; Grounds, 1982; Ferguson, 1993; Hill et al., 2001; Morgan et al., 1983). Notably, a number of these cases appear to have been somewhat atypical; for example, subjects with onset of illness in their seventies (Hill et al., 2001) or nineties (Bernstein, 1972). Furthermore, it appears that in many cases these individuals had, in addition to anorexia nervosa, substantial depressive symptoms, raising some question as to whether positive effects observed with ECT related to direct effects on the pathophysiology of anorexia nervosa or were merely related to improvements in comorbid psychopathology.

No published reports of the use of ECT for the treatment of bulimia nervosa are available, except for one case report of a patient with both depression and bulimia nervosa who developed myoclonic jerks following the treatment (Dibble & Tandon, 1992). Based on this very limited literature, it is impossible to recommend ECT as a treatment for eating disorders at present.

Psychosurgery

The literature on psychosurgery for anorexia nervosa is similar to that observed for ECT in that it consists entirely of case reports or small case series. Several papers have examined the use of leukotomy (Drury, 1950; Glazebrook *et al.*, 1956; Sifneos, 1952; Sargant, 1951; Kay, 1953; Hemphill, 1944; Zamboni *et al.*, 1993; Kelly & Mitchell-Heggs, 1973; Carmody & Vibbler, 1952). All of these case reports or small series have reported improved illness status after surgery. Additionally, a particularly useful report is that of Crisp & Kalucy (1973) who reported on the outcome of four cases of leukotomy. In the short run, those patients displayed some improvement. One, however, died of suicide after partial weight restoration; the other three became relatively weight restored. Follow-up data were published in 2000 on those same cases (Morgan & Crisp, 2000). At longer-term follow-up, disordered eating cognitions persisted, although weight loss had ceased. These authors concluded that, in certain instances, leukotomy may be 'a justifiable recommendation of last resort'. Much as with ECT, the existing literature does not support recommendations for the use of psychosurgery in the treatment of anorexia nervosa.

Conclusions

Although feeding is clearly a critical component of eating disorder treatment, it has received surprisingly little research attention. The few studies into exercise, light and heat treatments have limitations and offer no conclusive evidence for effectiveness. A number of case reports and small case series are found which have examined the use of ECT and/or psychosurgery in the treatment of eating disorders. The great majority of these mostly old reports share weaknesses: sample sizes are very small, the reports are uncontrolled, and data for eating disorder symptoms apart from weight restoration are not available. Based on this existing literature, no recommendations can be made for the use of these somatic physical treatments for the treatment of eating disorders at this time.

The level of evidence for each of the interventions discussed in this chapter is summarized in Table 38.1.

Table 38.1. Effectiveness of other somatic treatments for eating disorders

Treatment	Form of Treatment	Psychiatric disorder	Level of evidence	Comments
Refeeding	Nasogastric tube feeding	Anorexia nervosa	III	Supplementary NG feeding produces significant weight increases in the short term. The impact of NG feeding on long term outcome is unknown
Refeeding	Total parenteral nutrition	Anorexia nervosa	III	Complications are common
Exercise	Graded prescribed physical exercise	Anorexia nervosa	III	Inconclusive
Exercise	Graded prescribed physical exercise	Bulimia nervosa	Ib	One small RCT found a physical exercise regime to be more effective than CBT in reducing bulimic symptoms Abstinence rates were not reported
Exercise	Graded prescribed physical exercise	Binge eating disorder	Ib	Adding exercise to treatment of BED enhances outcome and contributes to reductions in binge eating and BMI
Heat treatment	e.g. Sauna, heating vests or heated environment	Anorexia nervosa	Ib	Evidence inconclusive
Light therapy		Bulimia nervosa	Ib	Some effects on mood or eating disorder symptoms. Evidence inconclusive
Electroconvulsive therapy		Anorexia nervosa	IV	Case reports only

REFERENCES

American Dietetic Association (1994). Nutrition intervention in the treatment of anorexia nervosa, bulimia nervosa and binge eating. *Journal of the American Dietetic Association*, **94** (8), 902–7.

Ash, J. B., Piazza, E. & Anderson, J. L. (1997). Light therapy in the clinical management of an eating-disordered adolescent with winter exacerbation. *International Journal of Eating Disorders*, **23**(1), 93–7.

Bentovim, M. (2000). Ethical and legal issues. In *Anorexia Nervosa and Related Eating Disorders in Childhood and Adolescence*, ed. B. Lask & R. Bryant–Waugh, 2nd edn, pp. 349–60, London: Psychology Press.

Bergh, C., Brodin U., Lindberg, G. & Södersten, P. (2002). Randomized controlled trial of a treatment for anorexia and bulimia nervosa. *Proceedings of the National Academy of Sciences*, **99**(14), 9486–91.

Bernstein, I. C. (1964). Anorexia nervosa treated successfully with electroshock therapy and subsequently followed by pregnancy. *American Journal of Psychiatry*, **120**, 1021–5.

Bernstein, I. C. (1972). Anorexia nervosa: 94-year-old woman treated with electroshock. *Minnesota Medicine*, **55**, 552–3.

Beumont, P. J., Beumont, C. C., Touyz, S. W. & Williams, H. (1997). nutritional counselling and supervised exercise. In *Handbook of Treatment for Eating Disorders*, ed. D. M. Garner & P. E. Garfinker, 2nd edn, pp. 178–87. New York: Guilford Press.

Beumont, P. J., Arthur, B., Russel, J. D. & Touyz, S. W. & Stephen W. (1994). Excessive physical activity in dieting disorder patients: Proposals for a supervised exercise program. *International Journal of Eating Disorders*, **15**(1), 21–36.

Birmingham, C. L., Alothman, A. F. & Goldner, E. M. (1996). Anorexia nervosa: refeeding and hypophosphatamia. *International Journal of Eating Disorders*, **20**(2), 211–13.

Birmingham, C. L., Guitierrez, E., Jonat, L. & Beumont, P. (2004). Randomized controlled trial of warming in anorexia nervosa. *International Journal of Eating Disorders*, **35**(2), 234–8.

Blouin, A. G., Blouin, J. H. *et al.* (1996). Light therapy in bulimia nervosa: a double-blind, placebo-controlled study. *Psychiatry Research*, **60**(1), 1–9.

Braun, D. L., Sunday, S. R., Fornari, V. M. & Halmi, K. A. (1999). Bright light therapy decreases winter binge frequency in women with bulimia nervosa: a double-blind, placebo-controlled study. *Comprehensive Psychiatry*, **40**(6), 442–8.

Bufano, G., Bellini, C. Cervellin, G. & Coscelli, C. (1990). Enteral nutrition in anorexia nervosa. *Journal of Parenteral and Enteral Nutrition*, **14**(4), 404–7.

Carmody, J. T. B. & Vibbler, F. L. (1952). Anorexia nervosa treated by prefrontal lobotomy. *Annals of Internal Medicine*, **36**, 647–52.

Carraro, A., Cognolato, S. & Fiorellini Bernadis, A. L. (1998). Evaluation of a program of adapted physical activity for ED patients. *Eating Weight Disorders*, **3**, 110–14.

Crisp, A. H. & Kalucy, R. S. (1973). The effect of leucotomy in intractable adolescent weight phobia (primary anorexia nervosa). *Postgraduate Medical Journal*, **49**, 883–93.

Dibble, L. & Tandon, R. (1992). Post-ECT myoclonic jerks in a depressed patient with bulimia. *Convulsive Therapy*, **8**(4), 285–9.

Drury, M. O. (1950). An emergency leucotomy. *British Medical Journal*, **2**, 609.

Ferguson, J. M. (1993). The use of electroconvulsive therapy in patients with intractable anorexia nervosa. *International Journal of Eating Disorders*, **13**(2), 195–201.

Friedman, S., Even, C., Dardennes, R. & Guelfi, J. D. (2002). Light therapy, obesity and night-eating syndrome. *American Journal of Psychiatry*, **159**(5), 875–6.

Glazebrook, A. J., Matas, J. & Prosen, H. (1956). Compulsive neurosis with cachexia. *Canadian Medical Association Journal*, **75**, 40–2.

Goldner E. M., Birmingham, C. L. & Smye, V. (1997). Addressing treatment refusal in anorexia nervosa: clinical, ethical and legal considerations. In *Handbook of Treatment for Eating Disorders*, ed. D. M. Garner & P. E. Garfinkel, 2nd edn. New York: Guilford Press.

Greaves, E., Blades, M., Christie, R. A. S., Machen, J., Ryecart, C. N., Baird-Smith, S. (1991). Short communication. Anorexia nervosa: nocturnal supplementary nasogastric feeding in the community. *Journal of Human Nutrition and Dietetics*, **4**, 165–70.

Grounds, A. (1982). Transient psychoses in anorexia nervosa: a report of 7 cases. *Psychological Medicine*, **12**, 107–13.

Gutierrez, E. Vazquez, R. (2001). Heat in the treatment of patients with anorexia nervosa. *Eating and Weight Disorders*, **6**, 49–52.

Gutierrez, E., Vazquez, R. & Beumont, P. (2002). Do people with anorexia nervosa use sauna baths? A reconsideration of heat treatment in anorexia nervosa. *Eating behaviors*, **3**, 133–42.

Hemphill, R. E. (1944). Return of virility after prefrontal lencotomy. *Lancet*, **2**, 345–6.

Hemphill, R. E. & Dubl, M. D. (1944). Return of virility after prefrontal leucotomy. *Lancet*, **2**, 345–6.

Hill, R., Haslett, C. & Kumar, S. (2001). Anorexia nervosa in an elderly woman. *Australian and New Zealand Journal of Psychiatry*, **35**, 246–8.

Kay, D. W. K. (1953). Anorexia nervosa: a study in prognosis. *Proceedings of the Royal Society of Medicine*, **46**, 669–74.

Kelly, D. & Mitchell-Heggs, N. (1973). Stereotactic limbic leucotomy. A follow-up study of thirty patients. *Postgraduate Medical Journal*, **49**, 852–65.

Lam R. W. (1989). Light therapy for seasonal bulimia. *American Journal of Psychiatry*, **146**(12), 1640–1.

Lam, R. W., Goldner, E. M. & Grewal, A. K. (1996). Seasonality of symptoms in anorexia and bulimia nervosa. *International Journal of Eating Disorders*, **19**, 35–44.

Lam, R. W., Lee, S. K., Tam, E. M., Grewal, A. & Yatham, L. N. (2001). An open trial of light therapy for women with seasonal affective disorder and comorbid bulimia nervosa. *Journal of Clinical Psychiatry*, **62**(3), 164–8.

Levine, M. D., Marcus, M. D. & Moulton, P. (1996). Exercise in the treatment of binge-eating disorder. *International Journal of Eating Disorders*, **19**, 171–7.

Mehler, P. S. & Weiner, K. L. (1993). Anorexia nervosa and total parenteral nutrition. *International Journal of Eating Disorders*, **14**(3), 297–304.

Morgan, J. F. & Crisp, A. H. (2000). Use of leucotomy for intractable anorexia nervosa: a long-term follow-up study. *International Journal of Eating Disordes*, **27**(3), 249–58.

Morgan, H. G., Purgold, J. & Welbourne, J. (1983). Management and outcome in anorexia nervosa: a standardized prognostic study. *British Journal of Psychiatry*, **143**, 282–7.

National Collaborating Centre for Mental Health (2004). *Other physical interventions in: eating disorders. Core interventions in the treatment and management of anorexia nervosa, bulimia nervosa and related eating disorders.* British Psychological Society and Gaskell, pp. 100–4.

Neiderman, M., Zarody, M., Tattersall, M. & Lask, B.(2000). Enteric feeding in severe adolescent anorexia nervosa: a report of four cases. *International Journal of Eating Disorders*, **28**, 470–5.

Neiderman, M., Farley, A., Richardson, J. & Lask, B. (2001). Nasogastric feeding in children and adolescents with eating disorders: towards good practice. *International Journal of Eating Disorders*, **29**, 441–8.

Pendleton, V. R., Goodrick, G. K., Poston, W. S., Reeves, R. & Foreyt, J. P. (2002). Exercise augments the effects of cognitive-behavioral therapy in the treatment of binge-eating. *International Journal of Eating Disorders*, **31**(2), 172–84.

Pesenti, F., Mavrotheris, S., Serra, C., Lucchio, P. & Pucciarelli, S. (1999). Use of percutaneous endoscopic gastrostomy in anorexia nervosa: case report. *Rivista Italiana di Nutrizione Parenterale ed Enterale*, **17**(1), 24–7.

Pertschuk, M. J., Forster, J., Buzby, G. & Mullen, J. L. (1981). The treatment of anorexia nervosa with total parenteral nutrition. *Biological Psychiatry*, **16**(6), 539–50.

Robb, A. S., Silber, T. J., Orrell-Valente, J. K. *et al.* (2002). Supplemental nocturnal nasogastric refeeding for better short term outcome in hospitalised adolescent girls with anorexia nervosa. *The American Journal of Psychiatry*, **159**(8), 1347–53.

Schwitzer, J., Neudorfer, C. & Fleischhacker, W. W. (1994). Seasonal bulimia treated with fluoxetine and phototherapy. *American Journal of Psychiatry*, **150**(11), 1752.

Serfaty, M. & McCluskey, S. (1998). Compulsory treatment of anorexia nervosa and the moribund patient. *European Eating Disorders Review*, **6**(1), 27–37.

Sundgot-Borgen, J., Rosenvinge, J. H., Bahr, R. & Schneider, L. S. (2002). The effect of exercise, cognitive therapy, and nutritional counselling in treating bulimia nervosa. *Medicine & Science in Sports & Exercise*, **34**(2), 190–5.

Szabo, C. P. & Green, K. (2002). Hospitalized anorexics and resistance training: Impact on body composition and psychological well-being. A preliminary study. *Eating and Weight Disorders*, **7**(4), 293–7.

Sifneos, P. E. (1952). A case of anorexia nervosa treated successfully by leucotomy. *American Journal of Psychiatry*, **109**, 356–60.

Solomon, S. M. & Kirby, D. F. (1990). The refeeding syndrome: a review. *Journal of Parenteral and Enteral Nutrition*, **14**, 90–7.

Thien, V., Thomas, A., Martin, D. & Birmingham, C. L. (2000). Pilot study of a graded exercise program for the treatment of anorexia nervosa. *International Journal of Eating Disorders*, **28**(1), 101–6.

Touyz, S. W., Lennerts, W., Arthur, B. & Beumont, P. J. (1993). Anaerobic exercise as an adjunct to refeeding patients with anorexia nervosa: does it compromise weight gain? *European Eating Disorders Review*, **1**(3), 177–82.

Vandereycken, W., Depreitere, L. & Probst, M. (1987). Body-oriented therapy for anorexia nervosa patients. *American Journal of Psychotherapy*, **41**, 252–9.

Wall, J. H. (1958). Diagnosis, treatment and results in anorexia nervosa. Read at the 114th annual meeting of The American Psychiatric Association, San Francisco, California, May 12–16.

Zamboni, R., Larach, V., Poblete, M. *et al.* (1993). Dorsomedial thalamotomy as a treatment for terminal anorexia: a report of two cases. *Acta Neurochirurgica*, **58**, 34–5.

Zuercher, J. N., Cumella, E. J., Woods, B. K., Eberly, M. & Carr, J. K. (2003). Efficacy of voluntary nasogastric tube feeding in female inpatients with anorexia nervosa. *Journal of Parenteral and Enteral Nutrition*, **27**(4), 268–76.

39

Psychological treatments for eating disorders

Roz Shafran, Pamela K. Keel, Alissa Haedt and Christopher Fairburn

Editor's note

Psychological treatments are now the cornerstone of treatment for eating disorders, with cognitive behaviour therapy having pride of place. This chapter, in conjunction with Chapter 23, shows the importance of setting as a likely determinant of effective treatment, and the relatively limited knowledge we have on the subject. The chapter also illustrates a common problem when the preferred treatment is found to be ineffective; there is often no evidence base for any alternative strategy. The chapter is also a useful reminder not to be too rigid in linking diagnosis to treatment in eating disorders. The frequent changing from one eating diagnosis to another, and the common presentation of EDNOS (eating diorders not otherwise specified) shows the relative lack of utility of the current descriptions when it comes to selecting treatment.

Introduction

It is the task of this chapter to evaluate the evidence on the psychological treatment of eating disorders. The strength of the evidence base for the treatment of anorexia nervosa (AN), bulimia nervosa (BN), binge eating disorder (BED) and remaining eating disorders not otherwise specified (EDNOS; or atypical eating disorders (AEDs)) varies, so each eating disorder will be considered separately. Examination of the evidence base requires the identification and appraisal of the relevant research findings. This has already been done in the UK by the National Institute for Health and Clinical Excellence (NICE) (National Collaborating Centre for Mental Health, 2004), which is the primary source of information on which this chapter is based. In the USA, the *American Psychiatric Association Practice Guidelines for the Treatment of Psychiatric*

Disorders Compendium 2004 provides recommendations for the treatment of eating disorders in a second edition. In common with the other chapters in this book, the confidence in the evidence available is assigned a symbol I–IV. Table 39.1 summarizes the confidence in the data for each of the eating disorders by indicating whether the interventions are first-line, second-line, recommended but not officially endorsed or used despite limited data.

The evidence is considered first for primary care and then for specialist care. Of note, the discussion of psychosocial interventions in primary care settings may have limited relevance for readers in the United States because managed care limits the duration of contact between primary care physicians and patients. In contrast, in the United Kingdom, the first point of contact for patients will be with their general practitioner (primary care physician), regardless of the specific nature of their health complaint. Some patients will be managed entirely in primary care if their eating disorder is relatively straightforward and they appear to be responding well to interventions at this level.

Classification and clinical features of eating disorders

There are three diagnostic categories of eating disorders: anorexia nervosa, bulimia nervosa and atypical eating disorders (referred to in DSM-IV as Eating Disorders Not Otherwise Specified, EDNOS). A further category ('binge eating disorder') has been proposed. Anorexia nervosa is characterized by extreme dietary restriction in order to actively maintain an unduly low body weight (i.e. body mass index ≤ 17.5), amenorrhea in postmenarcheal females not taking an oral contraceptive and the overevaluation of eating, shape, weight or their control. Many patients deny the seriousness of their low weight.

Cambridge Textbook of Effective Treatments in Psychiatry, ed. Peter Tyrer and Kenneth R. Silk. Published by Cambridge University Press.
© Cambridge University Press, 2008.

Table 39.1. Practice Guidelines in the UK and USA

Anorexia nervosa
I   **First-line treatment:**
    None
II **Second-line treatment:**
    None
III **Recommended, but not officially endorsed:**
    Family-based therapy for adolescents
IV **Used with little information available:**
    CBT
    BT
    IPT
    Psychodynamically orientated therapies
Bulimia nervosa
I   **First-line treatment:**
    CBT
II **Second-line treatment:**
    IPT[a]
III **Recommended, but not officially endorsed:**
    IPT[b]
    BT[b]
IV **Used, not endorsed or advised against based on limited data:**
    Psychodynamically informed therapies
    Family-based therapy for adults
Binge eating disorder
I   **First-line treatment:**
    CBT[a]
II **Second line treatment:**
    None
III **Recommended, but not officially endorsed:**
    CBT[b]
    IPT
    BT

[a] In the UK.
[b] In the USA.

Patients with bulimia nervosa share the undue influence of shape and weight on self-evaluation but also experience recurrent episodes of uncontrolled eating ('binges') accompanied by extreme weight control behaviour such as self-induced vomiting, laxative misuse, extreme dietary restriction or excessive exercise. The weight of patients with bulimia nervosa is unremarkable since the extreme weight control behaviour is counteracted by the calorie intake from the binges. In contrast, since binge eating disorder is characterized by binge eating in the absence of extreme weight control behaviour, patients commonly have comorbid obesity. Patients who fall into the EDNOS category have an eating disorder of clinical severity but do not meet criteria for either anorexia nervosa or bulimia

nervosa. For example, patients in this category may consume small amounts of food very frequently and vomit regularly after eating but sustain a normal weight (Keel et al., 2001). The most common eating disorder diagnosis made in clinical practice is EDNOS rather than anorexia nervosa or bulimia nervosa (Fairburn & Bohn, 2005; Fairburn & Harrison, 2003). The common psychopathology among the eating disorders and the migration between them over time has led to the proposition that they share maintaining mechanisms (Fairburn et al., 2003). A factor complicating the interpretation of such findings is the limitations in how the categories have been conceptualized and defined (Keel et al., 2004; Fairburn & Bohn, 2005).

Anorexia nervosa

Primary care

The lack of research in anorexia nervosa in general (see Agras et al., 2004) applies to the investigation of the optimal treatment setting for anorexia nervosa (Fairburn, 2005) (also see Chapter 23). It is not known what proportion of patients are treated in primary care, although clinical guidelines exist on their management (e.g. Kreipe & Yussman, 2003; Powers & Santana, 2002; Waller & Fairburn, 2004). In England and Wales, it is recommended that general practitioners should pay attention to a global clinical assessment that is repeated over time (NICE, 2004, p. 64) that includes BMI, the rate of weight loss in adults or growth rates in children, objective physical signs and relevant laboratory tests. The guidelines state that patients with chronic anorexia nervosa who are not being treated in specialist care should be offered an annual physical and mental health review.

Specialist settings

Anorexia nervosa is usually treated in outpatient, day patient (partial hospitalization) and inpatient settings. There has been just one attempt to randomize patients to different treatment settings (Crisp et al., 1991). Ninety patients with anorexia nervosa were randomized to four treatment conditions: inpatient treatment (followed by post-hospitalization outpatient sessions), two forms of outpatient treatment or a detailed one-off assessment with advice regarding further management. This study was limited by a lack of statistical power and the reluctance of patients to be randomized to the inpatient condition. No differences emerged and it is still the case that there has been little research on either day patient treatment (Zipfel et al.,

2002) or inpatient treatment (Maguire *et al.*, 2003; Vandereycken, 2003). For inpatient settings, open studies suggest that weight regain is aided by focusing on eating and weight (Herzog *et al.*, 1996) and that setting a target rate of weight regain increases the speed of regain (Solanto *et al.*, 1994). There is no evidence suggesting strict behavioural programmes are superior to more flexible ones (Touyz *et al.*, 1984; Vandereycken & Pieters, 1978) and expert opinion suggests that rigid inpatient behaviour modification programmes should not be used in the management of anorexia nervosa (NICE, 2004, p. 65). Instead, a structured symptom-focused intervention with an expectation of weight gain is warranted and wider psychosocial issues should also be addressed.

Outpatient: adolescents

Following inpatient weight restoration, people with anorexia nervosa are likely to be offered some outpatient psychological treatment. Patients are also likely to have received some outpatient intervention prior to being hospitalized and for many, outpatient treatment is their only intervention. Outpatient-based family interventions that directly address the eating disorder are viewed as the treatment of choice for adolescents, although the evidence supporting them is limited (Fairburn, 2005). Only two RCTs comparing family-based treatment with another (non-family) form of treatment have been conducted. In the first study, 21 patients who had just been discharged from inpatient treatment (mean age 16.6 years, mean duration of disorder 1.2 years) were randomized to either 1 year of family-based treatment or 1 year of supportive psychotherapy (Russell *et al.*, 1987). The results showed the family-based treatment was superior to the supportive psychotherapy and this advantage was maintained at 5-year follow-up (Eisler *et al.*, 1997).

A second study of 37 adolescents comparing the family intervention with a psychodynamically orientated treatment found that both interventions were helpful and the only difference was that those in the family intervention had a greater increase in BMI (Robin *et al.*, 1999). However, the relatively greater increase in BMI could be attributable to a period in hospital during their treatment as opposed to differences in the outpatient treatment. As matters stand, family-based treatments are classified as 'III' (see Table 39.1) i.e. recommended as valuable but not officially endorsed as first- or second-line treatment.

Outpatient: adults

Six studies have compared outpatient treatments. Nutritional counselling has been compared with psychotherapy in 30 adolescent and adult outpatients (Hall & Crisp, 1987)

and with cognitive-behavioural therapy in 35 adolescent and adult outpatients (Serfaty *et al.*, 1999). In the latter study, all ten patients randomized to the nutritional counselling dropped out. Differences in treatment completion may be attributable to differences in mean age between treatment groups. The mean age of participants randomized to cognitive-behavioural therapy was 22.1 years, while the mean age of patients randomized to nutritional counselling was 17.9 years (Serfaty *et al.*, 1999). Despite the dramatic differences in treatment completion between conditions, there were no significant outcome differences between groups on BMI, total EDI score, or body dissatisfaction. Behaviour therapy has been compared with cognitive-behaviour therapy and a low-contact control condition in 24 adult patients (Channon *et al.*, 1989) and with cognitive analytic therapy in 30 adult patients (Treasure *et al.*, 1995). No consistent statistically significant findings of note were found in any of these studies.

The largest study comprised 84 patients (mean age 26.3 years; mean duration of the disorder = 6.3 years) (Dare *et al.*, 2001). The patients were randomized to focal psychoanalytic psychotherapy, CAT, family-based treatment, or routine outpatient treatment involving brief sessions with a trainee psychiatrist. Approximately one-third of patients improved significantly, and all three psychotherapies were more effective than the routine treatment for weight, although there were no significant differences in Morgan–Russell scales across the four conditions. In addition, no specific psychotherapy was superior to the others. The superiority of the psychotherapies could either be attributed to the potency of the interventions or to the fact that the routine treatment involved less than half the therapist-patient contact and was delivered by trainees.

The study of Russell and colleagues (1987) described above also included adults and compared treatment conditions in adults with early onset anorexia nervosa ($n = 15$) and late onset anorexia nervosa ($n = 21$). No statistically significant differences emerged between treatments within these adult groups.

In a more recent study, 33 patients whose weight had been restored with inpatient treatment were randomized to receive 12 months of CBT or nutritional counselling (Pike *et al.*, 2003). The CBT was superior to nutritional counselling in terms of the proportion remaining in treatment, relapse rates and meeting criteria for a good outcome. In this study, the superiority of CBT over nutritional counselling could have been partially attributable to antidepressant medication since more patients in the CBT group were receiving antidepressants, and antidepressants have been associated with decreased risk of relapse following weight recovered in patients with anorexia nervosa (Kaye *et al.*, 2001).

Summary

Anorexia nervosa is not usually treated in primary care. There are no officially endorsed first or second lines of treatment for patients diagnosed with anorexia nervosa. For adolescents, family interventions that directly address the eating disorder are recommended as valuable (NICE, 2004, p. 65) or 'with moderate clinical confidence' (APA, 2000, p. 3). The range of therapies to be considered for psychological treatment of anorexia nervosa include cognitive analytic therapy (CAT), behaviour therapy (BT), cognitive-behaviour therapy (CBT), focal dynamic psychotherapy and family interventions focused explicitly on eating disorders (NICE, 2004 p. 64). However, these represent therapies that are often used but not endorsed due to the limited information available to support their efficacy.

Bulimia nervosa

Primary care

Much more is known about the treatment of bulimia nervosa than anorexia nervosa and over 70 RCTs have been conducted (Nakash-Eisikovits *et al.*, 2002; NICE, 2004; Thompson-Brenner *et al.*, 2003; Wilson & Fairburn, 2002). Most studies have been conducted on outpatients in specialist settings and only one has been conducted in primary care. In this recent study, Walsh and colleagues compared the psychological and pharmacological treatment of BN in two primary care clinics in the USA (Walsh *et al.*, 2004). Of the 91 female participants, 15 did not meet full DSM-IV criteria in terms of the frequency or size of the episodes of binge eating. Patients were randomly assigned to receive either 60 mg fluoxetine alone, placebo alone, fluoexetine plus guided self-help or placebo plus guided self-help. The guided self-help was an adaptation of cognitive-behaviour therapy based on previous studies (Carter & Fairburn, 1998; Carter *et al.*, 2003; Loeb *et al.*, 2000; Palmer *et al.*, 2002).

The main finding from this study was that almost 70% of participants dropped out. Some participants reported leaving the study as it was too demanding, whilst others felt that it was not demanding enough. Overall, compared to placebo those who received fluoxetine attended more physician visits, had a greater reduction in binge eating and vomiting, and had a greater improvement in psychological symptoms. There was no evidence of benefit from guided self-help. These findings contrasted with a smaller previous study in primary care using guided self-help. In this case series of 11 patients, 6 did well (Waller *et al.*, 1996).

Specialist settings

There is a large body of scientific research examining the efficacy of a range of psychological interventions for bulimia nervosa (NICE, 2004; Thompson-Brenner *et al.*, 2003; Wilson & Fairburn, 2002). The NICE guidelines endorse cognitive-behavioural therapy as the treatment of choice for BN in adult women, and the APA guidelines stipulate 'cognitive behavioral psychotherapy is the psychosocial treatment for which the most evidence of efficacy currently exists' (APA, 2000, p. 4). These conclusions have been based on multiple randomized controlled trials, for example, 18 RCTs comparing two different forms of psychological treatment (involving 1343 participants) were used as the basis for NICE's recommendations.

The results from these RCTs conducted across the world have been remarkably robust and consistent. Overall, the evidence demonstrates that a specific, eating-disorder focused form of CBT (Fairburn *et al.*, 1993b) is superior to other forms of psychological intervention. This has led to NICE stating that it should be offered to adults with bulimia nervosa as the first-line treatment (NICE, 2004, p. 128). This specific form of CBT is based on a theory of the maintenance of bulimia nervosa (Fairburn, 1981; 1997) and is tailored to changing the mechanisms hypothesized to be responsible for the persistence of the disorder. The duration of treatment is 16 to 20 sessions over 4 to 5 months. Although it is not clear whether adding antidepressants to CBT results in an improved outcome (Wilson & Fairburn, 2002), the APA practice guidelines recommend a combination of antidepressant medication and psychosocial treatment for bulimia nervosa with 'moderate clinical confidence'. On average, the data indicate that a third of patients make a complete and lasting recovery with this specific form of CBT, a substantial proportion are 'much improved' and the great majority of patients maintain their gains (Wilson & Fairburn, 2002). In summary, CBT is not a panacea but it can benefit a substantial proportion of patients and it is clearly superior to the other interventions currently available.

The question of how best to help those patients who fail to respond to CBT or do not want it is a pressing one, since no evidence-based guidelines can be formulated at this time (Fairburn & Harrison, 2003). The leading alternative psychological intervention to CBT is interpersonal psychotherapy (IPT). The results from two treatment trials, one of which was large, suggest that this focal psychotherapy is eventually as effective as CBT but takes 8 to 12 months longer to achieve results comparable to CBT (Fairburn *et al.*, 1993a, b; Agras *et al.*, 2000).

Behaviour therapy (BT) is also an alternative to CBT. Various forms of behaviour therapy have been studied so it is difficult to generalize about them. Almost invariably BT addresses patterns of eating and it may include exposure to food with prevention of response (binge eating or purging). Typically, it does not focus on the overevaluation of shape and weight. Studies of behaviour therapy have demonstrated that it is superior to a waitlist control (Freeman *et al.*, 1988) and it is unlikely that there is any clinically significant difference between BT and CBT at the end of treatment (Cooper & Steere, 1995; Freeman *et al.*, 1988; Thackwray *et al.*, 1993; Wolf & Crowther, 1992). However, there is some evidence to suggest that longer-term (1-year) outcome with this treatment is inferior to outcome with CBT and interpersonal therapy (Fairburn *et al.*, 1993a, b). Furthermore, those forms of BT that involve exposure with response prevention are limited by their aversiveness to patients and the practical difficulties involved in implementing them (Bulik *et al.*, 1998).

There is some evidence that family therapy is inferior to individual therapy in adult BN (Russell *et al.*, 1987). The APA practice guidelines indicate that IPT is 'very useful', behavioural therapy 'may be helpful', and psychodynamically orientated therapies 'may be useful once bingeing and purging are improving'. However, in comparison to the NICE guidelines, the APA guidelines relied more upon clinical opinion than empirical evidence, and the APA guidelines have been criticized as being insufficiently evidence-based (Wilson & Agras, 2001). For adult patients with BN, family therapy and psychodynamically orientated therapies are categorized as 'used, not endorsed or advised against based on limited data' unless CBT, BT, and IPT have been tried and failed.

Format of treatment

The majority of outpatient treatment is conducted on an individual basis. This is consistent with the findings indicating a superior outcome for individual treatment compared to group therapy (Chen *et al.*, 2003), although the reasons for this are debatable (Keel, 2004). Of particular importance is the research addressing the format of cognitive-behavioural therapy (Garvin *et al.*, 1998) and whether it can be delivered effectively in a pure or guided self-help format using a book (e.g. Cooper *et al.*, 1996), the telephone (Palmer *et al.*, 2002), CD-ROM (Bara-Carril *et al.*, 2004) or the internet. The majority of the studies to date show some benefit using the self-help format (e.g. Palmer *et al.*, 2002), although the benefits may be non-specific (Carter *et al.*, 2003). In this latter study, 85 women with bulimia nervosa were randomly assigned to receive one of two self-help manuals or to a waiting list control condition for 8 weeks.

One of the manuals was cognitive behavioural self-help and the other addressed assertiveness. The drop-out rate of 24% was relatively high but comparable to studies with similar sample sizes and an ethnically diverse sample. There was a greater reduction in symptom frequency in both self-help conditions at the end of treatment than for patients who had been on the waiting list but there was no difference between the treatment manuals. As a result of these and other related studies, it is suggested that patients with BN should initially be encouraged to follow a self-help programme that is evidence based. Health care professionals are advised to consider providing direct encouragement and support to patients who are following the programme (NICE, 2004, p. 128). It may be the case that such self-help programmes have an important place in a stepped-care approach to the treatment of BN as they may benefit a subset of patients; however, they are unlikely to be sufficient for the majority of patients. In addition, at present, some self-help studies emphasize 'reduction in frequency' of binge eating as opposed to abstinence from binge eating and purging (e.g. Carter *et al.*, 2003). Results from Mitchell *et al.* (1993) suggest that the combination of low emphasis on abstinence in the context of treatments with lower contact produce worse treatment outcome in bulimia nervosa. In order to truly understand the relative efficacy of self-help and face-to-face interventions, it is vital that the same, and preferably stringent, outcome criteria for recovery (i.e. abstinence of binge eating and purging) are applied across research studies.

Children and adolescents

There has been no research on the treatment of children or adolescents with bulimia nervosa. Expert opinion suggests that the specific form of CBT could be adapted to suit adolescents and the family should also be included where appropriate. Alternatively, a family-based therapy could be adapted to treat adolescents with bulimia nervosa and has been recommended with moderate clinical confidence by APA practice guidelines. However, there is no evidence to support any specific treatment approach in treating children or adolescents at this time.

Summary

Cognitive-behavioural therapy is the universal first-line treatment of choice for bulimia nervosa. In the UK, this was the first time a psychological intervention has been endorsed by the Government as the clear front-runner in treating a clinical disorder. No clear second line of treatment has emerged from the treatment literature. However, both IPT and behaviour therapy are recommended as valuable by

APA guidelines. In contrast, the limited data indicate that psychodynamically orientated therapies and family therapies should be used only if empirically supported treatments have been tried and failed for adults with BN. Self-help may be useful for some patients, although its use in primary care may be limited by high rates of drop-out.

Atypical eating disorders

Atypical eating disorders (or EDNOS) are the most common eating disorder diagnosed in clinical practice (see Fairburn and Bohn, 2005), and epidemiological data support the preponderance of EDNOS among individuals with clinically significant eating disorders (Keel et al., 2006). The absence of research evidence to guide the management of such disorders, other than binge eating disorder, means that clinicians are recommended to treat these patients following the principles advocated for treating the eating disorder that their eating problem most closely resembles. Thus, for conditions resembling anorexia nervosa in adolescent patients, a symptom-focused family-based therapy may be beneficial. For conditions resembling bulimia nervosa in adult patients, cognitive-behaviour therapy, behaviour therapy, and interpersonal therapy may prove useful.

There is a body of evidence, however, about the treatment of binge eating disorder although none that addresses the best service setting. The research on the treatment of binge eating disorder has focused mainly on patients with comorbid obesity. The results show that both CBT and IPT help reduce the frequency of binge eating. In the largest study, 20 weekly sessions of group CBT and group IPT were compared for 162 overweight patients with BED (Wilfley et al., 2002). Binge-eating recovery rates were equivalent for CBT and IPT at posttreatment and at 1-year follow-up, with approximately 60% of patients reporting remission from binge eating at follow-up. The treatments were also equivalent in terms of their reductions in associated eating disorders and psychiatric symptoms. There was only a slight decrease in patients' weight and clinicians are suggested to inform patients that interventions for BED will only have a minimal impact on their weight (NICE, 2004). The conclusion from this and other studies is that there is a range of efficacious interventions for BED, and there is little consistent evidence to favour one treatment over another (NICE, 2004). Reflecting this situation, the APA guidelines remain silent on the issue of treating BED or any other form of EDNOS.

These findings should be considered in light of natural history studies in the USA and UK (Fairburn et al., 2000; Cachelin et al., 1999) and drug trials (for a review see Dingemans et al., 2002) that both suggest that there is a high spontaneous remission rate from BED at least in the short term. There is also a relatively high response to placebo (Dingemans et al., 2002).

Summary

There is little information on the treatment of atypical eating disorders. This is a research priority. The data on BED indicate that a range of interventions may be efficacious but they do not impact greatly on patients' weight. These findings should be considered in light of other studies indicating a high spontaneous remission rate and response to placebo. Moreover, there is no first or second line of treatment for BED. However, CBT and IPT are recommended on the basis of superior outcome to waitlist control.

Conclusions

A large body of research on the treatment of bulimia nervosa means that an evidence-based approach to management is now possible. In particular, CBT is the first-line treatment of choice for bulimia nervosa. Although both IPT and BT have demonstrated efficacy and may be useful if CBT proves unsuccessful, neither has been universally designated as a second line of treatment. Instead, IPT has been endorsed as a second-line treatment in the UK while it remains recommended but not officially endorsed in the US. Both CBT and IPT also appear beneficial for the treatment of binge eating disorder (BED). For adolescents with anorexia nervosa, a symptom-focused family-based intervention is recommended as it appears to be superior to alternative interventions. No evidence-based interventions can be recommended for adults with anorexia nervosa, adolescents with bulimia nervosa, or for patients with atypical eating disorders.

There are many reasons for the lack of research into the treatment of anorexia nervosa (see Agras et al., 2004), primarily the relative rarity of the disorder. In addition, waiting list control conditions have not been utilized within RCTs for anorexia nervosa due to ethical considerations. The same reasons do not apply to atypical eating disorders. Fairburn and Bohn (2005) have suggested new ways of conceptualizing these states that are designed in part to encourage research on their treatment. Generating an evidence-base to guide interventions for these disorders is a research priority.

The level of evidence for each of the interventions discussed in this chapter is summarized in Table 39.2.

Table 39.2. Evidence base for psychological treatments for eating disorder

	Anorexia nervosa	Bulimia nervosa	Binge eating disorder	EDNOS (except binge eating disorder)
Cognitive behaviour therapy	Ib	Ia	Ib	IV
Interpersonal psychotherapy	Ib	Ib	Ib	IV
Family therapy	Ib	Ib	n/a	n/a
Guided self-help	n/a	Ia	Ib	n/a
Behaviour therapy alone	n/a	Not recommended	n/a	n/a
Nutritional counselling alone	Not recommended	Not recommended	n/a	n/a

REFERENCES

Agras, W. S., Walsh, B. T., Fairburn, C. G., Wilson, G. T. & Kraemer, H. C. (2000). A multicenter comparison of cognitive-behavioral therapy and interpersonal psychotherapy for bulimia nervosa. *Archives of General Psychiatry*, **57**, 459–66.

Agras, W. S., Brandt, H. A., Bulik, C. M. *et al.* (2004). Report of the National Institutes of Health workshop on "Overcoming Barriers to Treatment Research in Anorexia Nervosa." *International Journal of Eating Disorders*, **35**, 509–21.

American Psychiatric Association (APA) (2000). Practice guideline for the treatment of patients with eating disorders (revision). *American Journal of Psychiatry*, **157** (suppl. 1), 1–39.

Bara-Carril, N., Williams, C. J., Pombo-Carril, M. G. *et al.* (2004). A preliminary investigation into the feasibility and efficacy of a CD-ROM-based cognitive-behavioral self-help intervention for bulimia nervosa. *International Journal of Eating Disorders*, **35**, 538–48.

Bulik, C. M., Sullivan, P. F., Carter, F. A., McIntosh, V. C. & Joyce, P. R. (1998). The role of exposure with response prevention in the cognitive-behavioural therapy for bulimia nervosa. *Psychological Medicine*, **28**, 611–23.

Cachelin, F. M., Striegel-Moore, R. H., Elder, K. A., Pike, K. M., Wilfley, D. E. & Fairburn, C. G. (1999). Natural course of a community sample of women with binge eating disorder. *International Journal of Eating Disorders*, **25**, 45–54.

Carter, J. C. & Fairburn, C. G. (1998). Cognitive-behavioral self-help for binge eating disorder: a controlled effectiveness study. *Journal of Consulting and Clinical Psychology*, **66**, 616–23.

Carter, J. C., Olmsted, M. P., Kaplan, A. S., McCabe, R. E., Mills, J. S. & Aime, A. (2003). Self-help for bulimia nervosa: a randomized controlled trial. *American Journal of Psychiatry*, **160**, 973–8.

Channon S., de Silva P., Hemsley D. & Perkins R. (1989). A controlled trial of cognitive-behavioural and behavioural treatment of anorexia nervosa. *Behaviour Research and Therapy*, **27**, 529–35.

Chen, E., Touyz, S. W., Beumont, P. *et al.* (2003). Comparison of group and individual cognitive-behavioral therapy for patients with bulimia nervosa. *International Journal of Eating Disorder*, **33**, 241–54.

Cooper, P. J. & Steere, J. (1995). A comparison of two psychological treatments for bulimia nervosa: implications for models of maintenance. *Behaviour Research and Therapy*, **33**, 875–85.

Cooper, P. J., Coker, S. & Fleming, C. (1996). An evaluation of the efficacy of supervised cognitive behavioral self-help bulimia nervosa. *Journal of Psychosomatic Research*, **40**, 281–7.

Crisp, A. H., Norton, K., Gowers, S. *et al.* (1991). A controlled study of the effect of therapies aimed at adolescent and family psychopathology in anorexia nervosa. *British Journal of Psychiatry*, **159**, 325–33.

Dare, C., Eisler, I., Russell, G., Treasure, J. & Dodge, L. (2001). Psychological therapies for adults with anorexia nervosa: randomised controlled trial of out-patient treatments. *British Journal of Psychiatry*, **178**, 216–21.

Dingemans, A. E., Bruna, M. J. & van Furth, E. F. (2002). Binge eating disorder: a review. *International Journal of Obesity*, **26**, 299–307.

Eisler, I., Dare, C., Russell, G. F. M., Szmukler, G., leGrange, D., & Dodge, E. (1997). Family and individual therapy in anorexia nervosa – a 5-year follow-up. *Archives of General Psychiatry*, **54**, 1025–30.

Fairburn, C. G. (1981). A cognitive behavioral approach to the treatment of bulimia. *Psychological Medicine*, **11**, 707–11.

Fairburn, C. G. (1997). Eating disorders. In *Science and Practice of Cognitive Behaviour Therapy*, ed. D. M. Clark & C. G. Fairburn, pp. 209–41. Oxford: Oxford University Press.

Fairburn C. G. & Harrison P. J. (2003). Eating disorders. *Lancet*, **361**, 407–16.

Fairburn, C. G. & Bohn, K. (2005a). Eating Disorder Not Otherwise Specified (EDNOS): an example of the troublesome "Not Otherwise Specified (NOS)" category in DSM IV. *Behaviour Research and Therapy*, **43**(6), 691–701.

Fairburn, C. G. & Bohn, K. (2005b). Evidence-based treatment of anorexia nervosa. *International Journal of Eating Disorders*, **37** Suppl. 526–30.

Fairburn, C. G., Jones, R., Peveler, R. C., Hope, R. A. & O'Connor, M. E. (1993a). Psychotherapy and bulimia nervosa: longer-term effects of interpersonal psychotherapy, behavior therapy, and cognitive-behavior therapy. *Archives of general Psychiatry*, **50**, 419–28.

Fairburn, C. G., Marcus, M. D., & Wilson, G. T. (1993b). Cognitive behavioral therapy for binge eating and bulimia nervosa: a comprehensive treatment manual. In *Binge Eating: Nature, Assessment and Treatment*, ed. C. G. Fairburn, G. T. Wilson, pp. 361–404. New York: Guilford Press.

Fairburn, C. G., Cooper, Z., Doll, H. A., Norman, P. & O'Connor, M. (2000). The natural course of bulimia nervosa and binge eating disorder in young women. *Archives of General Psychiatry*, **57**, 659–65.

Fairburn, C. G., Cooper, Z. & Shafran, R. (2003). Cognitive behaviour therapy for eating disorders: a "transdiagnostic" theory and treatment. *Behaviour Research and Therapy*, **41**, 509–28.

Freeman, C., Barry, F., Dunkeld-Turnbull, J. & Henderson (1988). Controlled trial of psychotherapy for bulmia nervosa. *British Medical Journal*, **296**, 521–5.

Garvin, V., Streigel-Moore, R. H. & Wells, A. M. (1998). Participant reactions to a cognitive-behavioral guided self-help program for binge eating: developing criteria for program evaluation. *Journal of Psychosomatic Research*, **44**, 407–12.

Hall, A. & Crisp, A. H. (1987). Brief psychotherapy in the treatment of anorexia nervosa. Outcome at one year. *British Journal of Psychiatry*, **151**, 185–91.

Herzog, T., Hartmann, A. & Falk, C. (1996). The short-term effects of psychodynamic inpatient treatment of anorexia nervosa with and without an explicit focus on eating pathology – a controlled study. *Psychotherapie Psychosomatik Medizinische Psychologie*, **46**, 11–22.

Kaye, W. H., Nagata, T., Weltzin, T. E. *et al.* (2001). Double-blind placebo-controlled administration of fluoxetine in restricting- and restricting-purging-type anorexia nervosa. *Biological Psychiatry*, **49**(7), 644–52.

Keel, P. K. (2004). Commentary on a multi-dimensional meta-analysis of psychotherapy for bulimia nervosa. *Evidence Based Mental Health*, **7**, 11.

Keel, P. K., Fichter, M., Quadflieg, N. *et al.* (2004). Application of a latent class analysis to empirically define eating disorder phenotypes. *Archives of General Psychiatry*, **61**, 192–200.

Keel, P. K., Mayer, S. A. & Fischer, J. H. (2001). Importance of size in defining binge eating episodes in bulimia nervosa. *International Journal of Eating Disorders*, **29**, 294–301.

Keel, P. K., Heatherton, T. F., Dorer, D. J., Joiner, T. E. & Zalta, A. (2006). Point prevalence of bulimia nervosa in 1982, 1992, and 2002. *Psychological Medicine*, **36**, 119–27.

Kreipe R. E. & Yussman S. M. (2003). The role of the primary care practitioner in the treatment of eating disorders. *Adolescent Medicine*, **14**, 133–47.

Loeb, K. L., Wilson, G. T., Gilbert, J. S. & Labouvie, E. (2000). Guided and unguided self-help for binge eating. *Behaviour Research and Therapy*, **38**, 259–72.

Maguire, S., Surgenor, L. J., Abraham, S. & Beumont, P. (2003). An international collaborative database: its use in predicting length of stay for inpatient treatment of anorexia nervosa. *Australian and New Zealand Journal of Psychiatry*, **37**, 741–7.

Mitchell, J. E., Pyle, R. L., Pomeroy, C. *et al.* (1993). Cognitive-behavioral group psychotherapy of bulimia nervosa: importance of logistical variables. *International Journal of Eating Disorders*, **14**, 277–87.

Nakash-Eisikovits, O., Dierberger, A. & Westen, D. (2002). A multi-dimensional meta-analysis of pharmacotherapy for bulimia nervosa: summarizing the range of outcomes in controlled clinical trials. *Harvard Review of Psychiatry*, **10**, 193–211.

National Collaborating Centre for Mental Health (2004). *Eating Disorders: Core Interventions in the Treatment and Management of Anorexia Nervosa, Bulimia Nervosa and Related Eating Disorders*. London: British Psychological Society and Royal College of Psychiatrists.

National Institute for Clinical Excellence (NICE) (2004). *Eating Disorders Core Interventions in the Treatment and Management of Anorexia Nervosa, Bulimia Nervosa and Related Eating Disorder*. Nice Clinical Guideline No.9. London: National Institute for Clinical Excellence. Available from www.nice.org.uk.

Palmer, R. L., Birchall, H., McGrain, L. & Sullivan, V. (2002). Self-help for bulimic disorders: a randomised controlled trial comparing minimal guidance with face-to-face or telephone guidance. *British Journal of Psychiatry*, **181**, 230–5.

Pike, K. M., Walsh, B. T., Vitousek, K., Wilson, G. T. & Bauer, J. (2003). Cognitive behavior therapy in the posthospitalization treatment of anorexia nervosa. *American Journal of Psychiatry*, **160**, 2046–9.

Powers, P. S. & Santana, C. A. (2002). Eating disorders: a guide for the primary care physician. *Primary Care*, **29**, 81–98.

Robin, A. L., Siegel, P. T., Moye, A. W., Gilroy, M., Dennis, A. B. & Sikand, A. (1999). A controlled comparison of family versus individual therapy for adolescents with anorexia nervosa. *Journal of the American Academy of Child and Adolescent Psychiatry*, **38**, 1482–9.

Russell, G. F. M., Szmukler, G. I., Dare, C. & Eisler, I. (1987). An evaluation of family therapy in anorexia nervosa and bulimia nervosa. *Archives of General Psychiatry*, **44**, 1047–56.

Serfaty, M. A., Turkington, D., Heap, M., Ledsham, L. & Jolley, E. (1999). Cognitive therapy versus dietary counselling in the outpatient treatment of anorexia nervosa: effects of the treatment phase. *European Eating Disorders Review*, **7**, 334–50.

Solanto, M. V., Jacobson, M. S., Heller, L., Golden, N. H. & Hertz, S. (1994). Rate of weight gain in inpatients with anorexia nervosa under two behavioral contracts. *Pediatrics*, **93**, 989–91.

Thackwray, D. E., Smith, M. C., Bodfish, J. W. & Meyers, A. W. (1993). A comparison of behavioral and cognitive-behavioral interventions for bulimia nervosa. *Journal of Consulting and Clinical Psychology*, **61**, 639–45.

Thompson-Brenner, H., Glass, S. & Westen, D. (2003). A multi-dimensional meta-analysis of psychotherapy for bulimia nervosa. *Clinical Psychology Science and Practice*, **10**, 269–87.

Touyz, S. W., Beumont, P. J. V., Glaun, D., Phillips, T. & Cowie, I. (1984). A comparison of lenient and strict operant conditioning programmes in refeeding patients with anorexia nervosa. *British Journal of Psychiatry*, **144**, 517–20.

Treasure, J. L., Todd, G., Brolly, M., Tiller, J., Nehmed, A. & Denman, F. (1995). A pilot study of a randomised trial of cognitive analytical therapy vs educational behaviuoral therapy for adult anorexia nervosa. *Behaviour Research and Therapy*, **33**, 363–7.

Vandereycken, W. (2003). The place of inpatient care in the treatment of anorexia nervosa: questions to be answered. *International Journal of Eating Disorders*, **34**, 409–22.

Vandereycken, W. & Pieters, G. (1978). Short-term weight restoration in anorexia nervosa through operant conditioning. *Scandinavian Journal of Behaviour Therapy*, **7**, 221–36.

Waller, D. & Fairburn, C. G. (2004). Eating disorders. In *Women's Health*, ed. D. Waller & A. McPherson, 5th edn. Chapter 15, pp. 519–51. Oxford: Oxford University Press.

Waller, D., Fairburn, C. G., McPherson, A., Kay, R., Lee, A. & Nowell, T. (1996). Treating bulimia nervosa in primary care: a pilot study. *International Journal of Eating Disorders*, **19**, 99–103.

Walsh B. T., Fairburn C. G., Mickley, D., Sysko, R. & Parides, M. K. (2004). Treatment of bulimia nervosa in a primary care setting. *American Journal of Psychiatry*, **161**, 556–61.

Wilfley, D. E., Welch, R. R., Stein, R. I. *et al.* (2002). A randomized comparison of group cognitive-behavioral therapy and group interpersonal psychotherapy for the treatment of overweight individuals with binge-eating disorder. *Archives of General Psychiatry*, **59**(8), 713–21.

Wilson, G. T. & Agras, W. S. (2001). Practice guidelines for eating disorders. *Behavior Therapy*, **32**, 219–34.

Wilson, G. T. & Fairburn, C. G. (2002). Eating disorders. In *Treatments that Work*, ed. P. E. Nathan & J. M. Gorman, 2nd edn, pp. 559–92. New York: Oxford University Press.

Wolf, E. M. & Crowther, J. H. (1992). An evaluation of behavioral and cognitive-behavioral group interventions for the treatment of bulimia nervosa in women. *International Journal of Eating Disorders*, **11**, 3–15.

Zipfel, S., Reas, D. L., Thornton, C. *et al.* (2002). Day hospitalization programs for eating disorders: a systematic review of the literature. *International Journal of Eating Disorders*, **31**, 105–17.

40

Educational interventions for eating disorders

Mima Simic, Pauline S. Powers and Yvonne Bannon

Editor's note

Despite being relatively small in numbers, specialists in eating disorders have researched their subject more than those in some more established parts of psychiatry and this chapter on educational interventions, including some quite sophisticated studies, illustrates this well. So much of the increasing incidence of eating disorders has been put down to the faulty education of the media and so-called nutrition experts, and whilst the rise is not inexorably upwards as many have suggested, it is more than likely that the slave of fashion combined with the rapid growth of absolutely terrible fast food has promoted fear and wariness in so many people. 'I am afraid to eat', is a statement heard by so many with eating disorders, as though the fact of eating will set free a Pandora's box of conflicting desires and emotions that point towards catastrophe. So there is a clear need for corrective psychoeducation and the beginnings of the evidence base for this are in this chapter.

Educational interventions

Introduction

Educational interventions in medicine involve providing information about risk factors, causes, symptoms, or implications of a disorder, as well as focusing on psychosocial pressures that might influence development or maintenance of a disorder. Target populations may be those at risk of a disorder, people with a disorder or their families/ significant others. Psychoeducation aims to prevent, or improve symptomatology of a mental disorder, engage people in treatment, or improve their adherence to treatment. This involves teaching people about their illness, how to treat it and how to recognize signs of relapse.

Illness-related information and education can be given as general information or as personalized feedback following an evaluation of an individual's specific situation and risks (for a review of the literature on the role of feedback on the process of health behaviour change see DiClemente *et al.*, 2001). The postulated mechanism of action of education or feedback is that these kinds of strategies will facilitate not just a change in knowledge, but critically in attitudes and beliefs and thus motivate the recipient to alter problematic behaviours that lead to the development of a disorder or serve to maintain or worsen it, and promote engagement in and adherence to treatment (Andersen, 1999; Powers & Bannon, 2004) (see also Chapter 6).

Educational interventions are the basis of recently developed Expert Patient and Carer Programmes (Lorig & Holman, 2003) that aim to ensure that people with chronic disorders and their families develop knowledge and essential disease management skills to a point where they are empowered to take responsibilities for the management of their disorder.

Eating disorders tend to be chronic disorders with a wide range of physical and psychological symptoms and sequelae, resulting from starvation or unhelpful weight-loss practices. Those with anorexia nervosa in particular, often underestimate or deny the risks of their disorder and may be reluctant to accept the need for change. Relevant personalized information on risks and consequences may help these people shift the balance between perceived risks and benefits of their disorder towards becoming more accepting of the need for change.

Lack of knowledge or misconceptions about aspects of the disorder abound in people with eating disorder and may maintain symptoms. For example, a person with anorexia nervosa who experiences a sense of fullness after eating only a small amount of food, may believe that she needs to reduce her food intake further. Upon learning that eating little slows gastric emptying and

Cambridge Textbook of Effective Treatments in Psychiatry, ed. Peter Tyrer and Kenneth R. Silk. Published by Cambridge University Press.

'makes food sit in your stomach like a lump of concrete' and that this is reversible with the gradual introduction of larger amounts of food, she may be willing to increase her portions. A person with bulimia nervosa may believe that taking laxatives or inducing vomiting may help her 'get rid of all calories ingested' and may be surprised to find that this is not the case.

The families of people with eating disorders are often very involved in their care, yet lack essential information on how best to support the sufferer. Indeed one of the most common unmet needs identified by families was the lack of appropriate information early on in the stage of the illness (Haigh & Treasure, 2003). Parents may alternate between different extreme and unhelpful beliefs. Beliefs such as that their daughter's disorder may just be a passing phase may lead them to ignore the problem. A view that it is a self-inflicted problem, which she could step out of if she only tried may lead to confrontation about her lack of trying.

Thus in summary, given the chronicity, severity and complexity of eating disorders psychoeducational interventions should play a prominent role in their management, both targeting patients and their families. Indeed, these strategies are recommended as valuable in recent eating disorder guidelines from both sides of the Atlantic (NICE, pg. 7–8, 2004; APA, 2000, pp. 9–13), and such interventions form an integral part of eating disorder treatments of different theoretical orientation, including cognitive-behavioural therapy, family therapy and multi-family group therapy. Yet psychoeducation interventions are rarely used as a stand-alone treatment in eating disorders and evidence for the efficacy of these approaches in eating disorders whether used on their own or in combination with other treatment components is sparse, as is commonplace in complex interventions (Chapter 8). In the following account, the available data on educational interventions targeted towards people with eating disorders and their families or individuals at risk of eating disorders are presented. The possible hazards of educational methods will also be mentioned.

Psychoeducation packages for patients with eating disorders

So far, only five studies have explored the effect of psychoeducational packages on the outcome of eating disorder patients. Most of these were small, non-randomized and used quasi-experimental designs. The only exception is a randomized controlled study by Andrews and colleagues (1996) who compared a computerized health education package with a computer-based placebo programme for patients with bulimia or anorexia nervosa. These

authors found the health education package to be effective in terms of improving knowledge about and attitudes toward eating disordered behaviour. The effect of this intervention on symptoms was not studied.

Ricca and collagues (1997) compared cognitive behavioural therapy (CBT) to a combination of group psychoeducation and fluoxetine in outpatients with bulimia nervosa. Combined group psychoeducation and fluoxetine were as effective as CBT in reducing the number of binge episodes and compensatory behaviours as measured on the Eating Disorder Examination (EDE) 6 months after the beginning of treatment. Both treatments reduced depressive and anxiety symptoms on self-report questionnaires, however, only CBT yielded a significant improvement of overall EDE scores.

In a small cohort of 41 women with bulimia nervosa Davis and colleagues (1990) assessed the clinical significance of change after five sessions of brief group psychoeducation. Between 29% and 56% of subjects showed significant change on instruments measuring bulimic symptoms, drive for thinness, dietary restraint, and body dissatisfaction. By contrast, only a small number of subjects (6%–19%) reported clinically significant change on measures of personality dysfunction and associated psychopathology. In a second study by the same authors (Davis et al., 1997) outcomes of the previous cohort of patients was compared with that of patients who had received seven sessions of group psychotherapy with integrated CBT interventions in addition to the psychoeducation. Both treatments yielded comparable levels of change on measures of specific and non-specific psychopathology. The third study by the same group (Olmsted et al., 1991) compared a cohort of 29 bulimic patients who received the brief group educational programme with a cohort of 30 bulimic patients who received 19 sessions of the CBT. Overall, CBT was superior treatment to the ED, but on several important post treatment outcome measures, both treatments appeared to be equally effective for the subgroup of subjects with less severe symptomatology. In this study educational interventions were found to be significantly more cost-effective than CBT.

Psychoeducation for family members of patients with eating disorders

Psychoeducation is an integral component of family interventions for anorexia nervosa in adolescents and adults, for example in the Behaviour Family System Therapy (Robin et al., 1998) and the Multifamily Group Day Treatment (Eisler et al., 2002; Dare & Eisler, 2000; Treasure et al., 2005). Here, psychoeducational interventions are used as information giving talks explaining the facts about eating disorders, their physical risks and psychological consequences as well as encouragement to families to expand their coping and problem-solving skills in order to manage the illness more effectively.

Two studies have used psychoeducation for parents as stand-alone intervention. In a small randomized controlled trial Geist and colleagues (2000) compared the effects of family therapy to the effects of family group psychoeducation in 25 newly diagnosed adolescents with anorexia nervosa requiring hospitalization. Weight gain following the 4-month period of treatment was equivalent in both groups, however no significant change was reported in psychological functioning by either adolescents or parents. Unfortunately the cost-effectiveness of these interventions was not examined although the authors claim the educational treatment was cheaper.

Uehara and colleagues (2001) explored the effect of the five monthly sessions of multifamily psychoeducation on changes in expressed emotion (EE) in a small cohort of families of people with eating disorders. The rates of high-EE relatives tended to decrease at the end of the intervention, especially for high emotional overinvolment and families' assessment of symptoms. This study provides preliminary evidence to suggest that psychoeducation for the family members of patients with eating disorders may help lower distress and may encourage positive interactions within the family.

Psychoeducation for the prevention of eating disorders

In contrast to the paucity of evidence concerning the efficacy of psychoeducation in full-blown eating disorders, a large number of studies has focused on the use of education for the prevention of eating disorders. Two separate systematic reviews have been conducted. In a Cochrane Database review of interventions for preventing eating disorders in children and adolescents (Pratt & Woolfenden, 2002) only eight randomized controlled studies met criteria for analysis. The meta-analyses showed only one significant effect for two eating disorder programmes based on a media literacy and advocacy approach (Kusel, 1999, Neumark-Sztainer et al., 2000). Both preventions programmes were effective in terms of producing a reduction in the internalization or acceptance of societal ideas relating to appearance at 3 to 6 months follow-up. The reviewers concluded that due to the insufficient evidence of the effectiveness of other programmes, no firm conclusion about the impact of prevention programmes for eating disorders in children and adolescents can currently be drawn.

A second systematic review and meta-analysis by Stice & Shaw (2004) included 38 prevention programmes evaluated in 53 separate controlled trials. These authors distinguished between three generations of prevention programmes. They state:

'The first generation of ED prevention programs delivered didactic psychoeducational material about ED in universal interventions involving all available adolescents. The type of information was implicitly based on the assumption that information about the adverse effects of eating disorders would deter individuals from initiating these maladaptive behaviors. The second generation of prevention programs was also universal in focus and didactic in format but included components focusing on resistance of sociocultural pressures for thinness and healthy weight-control behaviors. These interventions were based on the assumption that sociocultural pressures played a key role in the etiology of eating pathology and that adolescents turned to radical dieting and compensatory behaviors primarily for weight-control purposes. The third generation of interventions has included selective programs that target high-risk individuals with interactive exercises that focus on risk factors that have been shown to predict onset of eating pathology e.g. body dissatisfaction'.

The average effect size for the outcomes of all trials ranged from 0.11 to 0.38 at termination of the programme and from 0.05 to 0.29 at follow-up. Results of the meta-analysis of the effect size moderators have shown that more selective programmes provided to high-risk populations produced significantly larger intervention effects than did (the older) universal programmes. Interactive programmes were more effective than didactic programmes and effects were significantly larger for multi-session programmes offered solely to females over age 15. These factors seemed more important than the actual content of the programmes, although programmes with psychoeducational content were less effective than those without this content for four out of seven outcome measures.

One further prevention study not included in the meta-analysis by Stice and Shaw deserves mentioning. Olmsted and colleagues (2002) studied 85 young women with Type I diabetes mellitus who had disturbed eating attitudes and behaviour. Patients were randomly assigned to either a 6-week psychoeducation programme or treatment as usual. The intervention group had significant reductions on the Restraint and Eating Concern subscales of the Eating Disorder Examination and on the Drive for Thinness and Body Dissatisfaction subscales of the Eating Disorder Inventory, but no improvement in frequency of purging by insulin omission or in haemoglobin A1c levels.

Negative effects of education/information about eating disorders

The equivocal results of some educational efforts to prevent eating disorders has led to speculation that these efforts may actually cause harm. Anecdotal reports suggest that, among some groups, efforts to educate may introduce the recipients to maladaptive eating practices and weight control behaviours. However, both the Cochrane Review (Pratt & Woolfenden, 2002) and the meta-analysis by Stice & Shaw (2004) concluded that there was not sufficient evidence to suggest potentially harmful effects from eating disorder prevention programmes.

In the last few years there has been a proliferation of so-called 'pro-anorexia' sites on the internet (see position statement of the Academy for Eating Disorders; www.aed.org). Although it is widely agreed that these sites promote dangerous and deadly eating practices and efforts have been made to curb access, the sites are still easy to locate. One study (Chesley & Kreipe, 2003) found that these pro-anorexia sites were more organized than traditional sources of information about eating disorders. The danger of the proliferation of these 'pro-anorexia' sites lies in their collusion with the denial that is often a part of clinical presentation of anorexia nervosa. Most probably they also demotivate people with anorexia nervosa from actively seeking treatment that are anyhow not easily available or affordable.

Eating disorder curriculum for primary care providers

Primary care providers have an important role to play in early detection and intervention with eating disorder patients as early intervention fosters good prognosis. A pilot study by Gurney & Halmi (2001) suggests that brief intensive training can increase primary care providers' knowledge resulting in increased rates of screening and detection of eating disorders.

Conclusions

Psychoeducational strategies are recommended as valuable in treatment guidelines from both the UK and the USA but this recommendation is based on clinical consensus, rather than on much evidence of their efficacy. Consequently psychoeducation interventions are not recognized as either first or second line treatment for eating disorders (NICE, pg. 7–8, 2004; APA, 2000, pp. 9–13), although they form an integral part of the eating disorder treatments with proven efficacy like cognitive-behavioural therapy and family therapy. Eating disorder prevention programmes are more extensively researched, and the evidence shows that they are more effective if they are multi-session, interactive, and delivered to high-risk female populations over age 15.

In research terms, the question left to answer is not so much whether to offer eating disorder patients and their families psychoeducation or not, rather future research needs to focus on what kind of education with what aims might be most relevant and effective for whom and at what stage of the illness.

The level of evidence for each of the intervention discussed in this chapter is summarized in Table 40.1.

Table 40.1. Effectiveness of educational treatments for eating disorders

Treatment	Form of treatment	Psychiatric disorder	Level of evidence for efficacy	Comment
Psychoeducation	Computerized education	Anorexia or bulimia nervosa	1b	The package was superior to placebo computer program in terms of improving knowledge about and attitudes toward eating disordered behavior
Psychoeducation	Group psychoeducation	Bulimia nervosa	III	No firm evidence yet
Psychoeducation	Group psychoeducation	Parents of adolescents with anorexia nervosa	Ib	In one small RCT parental group psychoeducation produced similar improvements as family therapy in patients' weight
Psychoeducation	Prevention programmes	Prevention of eating disorders	I	Two systematic reviews reach different conclusions. One, focused on prevention of eating disorders in children and adolescents concludes that the evidence is as yet insufficient to draw firm conclusions. The other SR concludes that interventions targeting high-risk individuals, and which are focused on specific risk factors and use an interactive multi-session format do reduce eating disorder risk

REFERENCES

Andersen, A. E. (1999). Using medical information psychotherapeutically. In *Eating Disorders: A Guide to Medical Care and Complications*, ed. P. S. Mehler & A. E. Andersen. Baltimore: The Johns Hopkins University Press, pp. 192–201.

Andrewes, D. G., O'Connor, P., Mulder, C. *et al.* (1996). Computerised psychoeducation for patients with eating disorders. *Australia and New Zealand Journal of Psychiatry*, **30**, 492–7.

Bell, L. (2003). What can we learn from consumer studies and qualitative research in the treatment of eating disorders? *Eating Weight Disorders*, **8**, 181–7.

Chesley, E. B. & Kreipe, R. E. (2003). Anorexia nervosa and the internet. *Eating Disorder Review*, July/August.

Davis, R., Olmsted, M., Rockert, W., Marques, T. & Dolhanty, J. (1997). Group psychoeducation for bulimia nervosa with and without additional psychotherapy process sessions. *International Journal of Eating Disorders*, **22**(1), 25–34.

Davis, R., Olmsted, M. P. & Rockert, W. (1990). Brief group psychoeducation for bulimia nervosa: assessing the clinical significance of change. *Journal of Consulting and Clinical Psychology*, **58**(6), 882–5.

Di Clemente, C. C., Marinilli, A., Manu Simngh, M. & Bellino, L. (2001). The role of feedback in the process of health Behavior change. *American Journal of Health behavior*, **25**(3), 217–27.

Eisler, I., Dare, C., Hodes, M., Russell, G., Dodge, E. & LeGrange, D. (2000). Family therapy for adolescent anorexia nervosa: the results of a controlled comparison of two family interventions. *Journal of Child Psychology and Psychiatry*, **41**, 727–36.

Eisler, I., LeGrange, D. & Asen, E. (2003). Family interventions. In *Handbook of Eating Disorders*. ed. J. Treasure, U. Schmidt & E. Furth. Chichester, UK: John Wiley & Sons Ltd.

Geist, R., Heinmaa, M., Stephens, D., Davis, R. & Katzman, D. K. (2000). Comparison of family therapy and family group psychoeducation in adolescents with anorexia nervosa. *Canadian Journal of Psychiatry*, **45**, 173–8.

Gurney, V. W. & Halmi, K. A. (2001). An eating disorder curriculum for primary care providers. *International Journal of Eating Disorders*, **30**, 209–12.

Haigh, R. & Treasure, J. L. (2003). Investigating the needs of carers in the area of eating disorders: development of the carers' needs assessment measure (CaNAM). *European Eating Disorder Review*, **11**, 125–41.

Killen, J. D., Taylor, C. B., Hammer, L. D. *et al.* (1993). An attempt to modify unhealthful eating attitudes and weight regulation. *International Journal of Eating Disorders*, **13**, 369–84.

Kusel, A. B. (1999). Primary prevention of eating disorders through media literacy training of girls. *Dissertation Abstracts International B: The Sciences & Engineering*, **60**(4-B), 1859.

Lorig, K. R. & Holman, H. (2003). Self-management education: history, definition, outcomes, and mechanisms. *Annals of Behavior Medicine*, **26**, 1–7.

NICE (2004). *Eating Disorders: Core interventions in the treatment and management of anorexia nervosa, bulimia nervosa and related eating disorders. National Institute for Clinical Excellence*. Clinical Guideline 9, Developed by the National Collaborating Centre for Mental Health, London January.

Neumark-Sztainer, D., Sherwood, N., Coller, T. & Hannan, P. (2000). Primary prevention of disordered eating among preadolescent girls: feasibility and short-term effect of a community-based intervention. *Journal of the American Dietetic Association*, **100**(12).

O'Dea, J. A. & Abraham, S. (2000). Improving the body image, eating attitudes, and behaviors of young male and female adolescents: a new educational approach that focuses on self-esteem. *International Journal of Eating Disorders*, **28**, 43–57.

Olmsted, M. P., Davis, R., Rockert, W., Irvine, M. J., Eagle, M. & Garner, D. M. (1991). Efficacy of a brief group psychoeducational intervention for bulimia nervosa. *Behavior Research Therapy*, **29**(1), 71–83.

Olmsted, M. P., Daneman, D., Rydall, A. C., Lawson, M. L. & Rodin, G. (2002). The effects of psychoeducation on disturbed eating attitudes and behavior in young women with type 1 diabetes mellitus. *International Journal of Eating Disorders*, **32**, 230–9.

Powers, P. S. & Bannon, Y. (2004). Medical co-morbidity of anorexia nervosa, bulimia nervosa, and binge eating disorder. In *Clinical Handbook of Eating Disorders: An Integrated Approach (Medical Psychiatry 26)*, ed. T. Brewerton. New York: Marcel Dekker.

Pratt, B. M. & Woolfenden, S. R. (2002). Interventions for preventing eating disorders in children and adolescents. Cochrane Database of Systematic Reviews, 2, CD002891. Oxford: Update Software Ltd.

Ricca, V., Mannucci, E., Mezzani, B. *et al.* (1997). Cognitive-behavioral therapy versus combined treatment with group psychoeducation and fluoxetine in bulimic outpatients. *Eating Weight Disorders*, **2**(2), 94–9.

Robin, A. L., Gilroy, M. & Dennis, A. B. (1998). Treatment of eating disorders in children and adolescents. *Clinical and Psychological Reviews*, **18**, 421–6.

Stice, E. & Shaw, H. (2004). Eating disorder prevention programs: a meta-analytic review. *Psychology Bulletin*, **130**, 206–7.

Treasure, J. L., Katzman, M., Schmidt, U., Troop, N., Todd, G. & de Silva, P. (1999). Engagement and outcome in the treatment of bulimia nervosa: first phase of a sequential design comparing motivation enhancement therapy and cognitive behavioural therapy. *Behavior Research Therapy*, **37**, 405–18.

Yager, J., Andersen, A., Devlin, M. *et al.* (2000). Practice guideline for the treatment of patients with eating disorders (Revision). *American Journal of Psychiatry*, **157**, 1–39 (Suppl).

Uehara, T., Kawashima, Y., Goto, M., Tasaki, S. I. & Someya, T. (2001). Psychoeducation for the families of patients with eating disorders and changes in expressed emotion: a preliminary study. *Comprehensive Psychiatry*, **42**(2), 132–8.

41

Alternative treatments for eating disorders

Pauline S. Powers, Yvonne Bannon and Adrienne J. Key

Editor's note

This chapter is another illustration for the need for proponents of evidence-based medicine to get over its main message to the wider public. The ability of highly determined and intelligent people to thwart the aims of conventional therapy is very well illustrated in this account. At the same time, there are some useful hints that some of the approaches may be worth investigating further.

Complementary–alternative treatments

Introduction

Both the lay public and identified specialists/practitioners have practised alternative medicine strategies for the treatment of numerous maladies for centuries. Alternative medicinal compounds, a variety of physical treatments, other 'mind' based approaches and spiritual/faith healing are all examples. If we use the definition that an alternative or complementary treatment is one that has not been scientifically validated by randomized controlled trials (RCTs) (but see Chapter 7 to show that this is changing), most treatments in use today for eating disorders would be considered complementary or alternative treatments, including weight restoration programmes and individual psychotherapy for adult anorexia nervosa patients. Another paradox of this definition is that some treatments that have been found to be at least marginally effective in randomized controlled trials, have, nonetheless, not found general acceptance. Examples would include cyproheptadine in hospitalized anorexia nervosa patients (Goldberg *et al.*, 1979) and naltrexone in the outpatient treatment of anorexia or bulimia nervosa (Marrazzi *et al.*, 1995) (see Chapter 37).

A more widely accepted definition for complementary and alternative treatments is the use of treatments outside mainstream medical treatment modalities; that is, treatments not listed as first- or second-line treatments in various guidelines.

NCCAM

In the United States, the National Center for Complementary and Alternative Medicine (NCCAM) is one of 27 institutes and centres that make up the National Institutes of Health (NIH). It was founded in 1998 and funding for that fiscal year was 19.5 million dollars; in 2004 funding had risen to 117.7 million dollars. This federal agency defines complementary and alternative medicine as a group of diverse medical and health care systems, practices and products not presently considered part of conventional medicine. Complementary medicines are defined as those added to conventional treatments and alternative medicines are those used instead of conventional treatments.

The NCCAM (website address: http://www.nccam.nih. gov/health/) sponsors clinical trials in a variety of areas and visitors to the website can locate trials by disease state or by treatment. Table 41.3 is a partial list of complementary and alternative treatments that may be of interest to eating disorder patients. As of the date of this writing, only one clinical trial was listed on this site for eating disorders. It was a study (for which enrollment is now closed) for binge eating disorder comparing meditation-based treatment to psychoeducational techniques and a waiting list control. Also, as of the date of this writing, eating disorders (including anorexia nervosa, bulimia nervosa, and binge eating disorder) were not listed under diseases or conditions. A helpful guide on the NCCAM website is entitled '10 Things to Know About Evaluating Medical Resources on the Web' (see Table 41.1).

Table 41.1. Ten things to know about evaluating medical resources on the web

1. Who runs this site?
2. Who pays for the site?
3. What is the purpose of the site?
4. Where does the information come from?
5. What is the basis of the information?
6. How is the information selected?
7. How current is the information?
8. How does the site choose links to other sites?
9. What information about you does the site collect, and why?
10. How does the site manage interactions with visitors?

From NCCAM website.

Certain celebrity figures have promoted the use of complementary and alternative treatments and have fuelled both their popularity and perhaps the quest to test them by more stringent or acceptable methods. Many patients report the successful use of complementary treatments in a wide spectrum of disorders, usually where conventional medicine has proven limited or ineffective or frequently as an adjunct to accepted treatment. Eating disorders are an example of this, in which, a whole plethora of suggestions have been made. The scientific evidence of clinical effectiveness can, however, remain elusive. In this chapter the nature and extent of various alternative and complementary treatments used by eating disorder patients will be outlined. The results of a literature search will be used to describe the extent of the evidence to support their use. Finally, examples of treatments considered to have promise and in use in some eating disorder treatment facilities but not yet validated will be described.

Complementary and alternative treatments for eating disorders

Conducting a standard database search the following complementary and alternative treatments have been listed as employed/useful in the treatment of eating disorders in descending order of level of scientific evidence: massage, hypnosis, meditation, yoga and herbal remedies. Finally we have commented on anecdotal and patient report on each treatment type based on the authors' knowledge as practitioners in the field of eating disorders.

Massage

The only RCT identified in the search, by Field *et al.* (1998), studied the use of massage therapy in conjunction with standard treatment versus standard treatment alone in 24

adolescents with bulimia nervosa. Patients receiving the massage treatment showed improvement on several behavioural and psychological measures, including reductions in anxiety and depression. The same authors (Hart *et al.*, 2001), also described the use of massage in anorexia nervosa and again found reduced stress levels in the group receiving massage. Taken together, these findings provide preliminary evidence of the utility of massage as an adjunct treatment for eating disorders. A review of the use of massage in many types of conditions including eating disorders offers some hypotheses on potential underlying mechanisms (Field, 2002). Many eating disorder treatment facilities report the use of massage. Anecdotally, patients report beneficial effects including anxiety reduction and a reduction in body dissatisfaction, but there are some negative reports including a heightening in fears of being physically touched, feeling intruded upon and embarrassment.

Mind–body medicine

The field of meditation and hypnosis falls under the heading of mind-body medicine. Barrows & Jacobs (2002) provide a useful introduction and general review of the literature in this field.

Hypnosis

A clinical trial by Griffiths *et al.* (1996) comparing hypnobehavioural therapy with standard CBT for bulimia nervosa found no advantages of either treatment. Two case reports were identified: one reports the use of hypnosis as an adjunct to standard treatment as 'effective' but without definition (Segal, 2000). The second reports the use of 'ego-state' treatment with hypnosis for the treatment of binge eating disorder (Degun-Mather, 2003). The treatment was associated with a reduction in eating related behaviours when other previously attempted therapies had been unsuccessful. The paper reports the patient then successfully returning to CBT. Hypnosis is not commonly practised in eating disorder treatment centres and there is an absence of anecdotal reports from patients.

Meditation

There are many different types of meditation and certain elements are now incorporated into standard treatments; the use of 'mindfulness' is an example of this. A review of Buddhist philosophy and addictive behaviours (Marlatt, 2002), which has included eating disorders in this addictive umbrella, outlines the theoretical underpinning of the philosophy. It examines several concepts in more detail, with mindfulness being one example. Marlatt theorises how these concepts may relate directly to cognitive behavioural therapy.

Table 41.2. Questions to ask to determine characteristics of proposed alternative treatments and practitioners

1. Is the provider credentialed and licensed?
2. Is the provider's experience in treating the patient based on personal clinical experiences with other patients with similar problems? (And, if so, may the patient speak with one of the other patients treated by that provider?)
3. Of what exactly does the therapy consist?
4. How many weeks are likely to pass before the patient and provider decide that the therapy is or is not working?
5. How much will each session cost with or without medications, and what is the anticipated total cost for the specified time period?
6. Are the services covered by third-party payments?
7. What are the potential side effects?
8. With the patient's permission, is the provider willing to communicate diagnostic findings, therapeutic plans, and follow-up information to the patient's conventional providers? Are there any limitations to these communications?

Used with permission from Yager *et al.* (1999).

No RCTs were identified in the search directly related to eating disorders. A cohort study by Kristeller & Hallett (1999) followed 18 obese women with binge eating disorder through a 6-week meditation based group intervention using standard group treatment plus eating specific mindfulness meditation. There were significant reductions in scores on the binge eating scale (BES) and depression and anxiety scores. Time using the eating-related meditations predicted decreases on the BES. A case study (Morishita, 2000) from Japan looked at treatment of a woman with anorexia nervosa with Naikan therapy, an ancient form of psychological treatment involving self-reproach, self-reflection, and meditation. A reduction in eating behaviours and an improvement in mood were reported.

Many eating disorder centres report the use of yoga with or without meditation as part of standard care packages. Only one trial was identified comparing Hatha yoga to aerobics and another unspecified body-orientated exercise group. Hatha proved more beneficial than the comparison treatment and a number of hypotheses about mechanisms are proposed (Daubenmier, 2003). Both yoga and meditation are widely reported by patients as beneficial, helping to improve body and self awareness and achieve relaxation. Some studies focusing on the narratives of individuals who have recovered from eating disorders highlight the spiritual nature of this process as defined by the patients. Their definitions included connection of the many aspects of the self, especially of body and spirit/self/mind; also a connection with others and a connection with nature (Garrett, 1997). It may be that certain core elements of meditation and yoga are useful in CBT/psychological therapies and warrant closer exploration. It may also be that when patients find these practices favourable it enhances alliance with standard treatments which are almost always incorporated into these studies.

Herbalism/homeopathy

Patients and clinicians report multiple uses and abuses of non-prescription drugs. In an interesting case series Yager and colleagues (1999) described a patient with anorexia nervosa who sought conventional treatment at a University eating disorder centre after being referred by her naturopath, general internist and psychologist. She brought with her a large shopping bag of natural remedies that she had been taking and wanted to continue these remedies during her treatment on the inpatient ward. The authors utilize this case to discuss some of the dilemmas around caring for patients who seek both conventional and non-conventional treatments and provide a series of recommendations regarding alternative/complementary treatments. These recommendations include: (1) routinely question patients about alternative and complementary treatments; (2) discuss safety and efficacy; (3) discuss merits of alternative treatments; (4) provide information; (5) learn about alternative therapies; and (6) determine characteristics of proposed alternative treatments and practitioners. Table 41.2 lists specific questions that the patient might ask the potential alternative providers.

Two recent studies have evaluated the use of alternative treatments by patients with eating disorders. In a study of 39 consecutive bulimia nervosa patients seeking treatment, Roerig and colleagues (2003) found that 64% of patients used diet pills and 31% of patients utilized diuretics. In the preceding month, 18% had used diet pills and 21% had used diuretics. These investigators found that a wide range of products had been used and that many which were used had potential toxicities.

In the second study by Trigazis and colleagues (2004), 46 patients with anorexia nervosa, bulimia nervosa, or eating disorder not otherwise specified were given a questionnaire to determine their use of herbal remedies. 37% (17 patients) used herbal remedies. The major reasons for the use of herbal remedies were to decrease appetite and induce vomiting. One-fourth (24%) of patients reported their physicians had asked if they used herbal remedies. Interestingly, the patients were generally satisfied with the traditional health care system and used herbal remedies as complementary rather than alternative treatments.

Ephedra

Ephedra (ephredrine alkaloids) containing products are among the best known herbs used as dietary aids. In April 2004, in the United States, the Food and Drug Administration (FDA) rule banning the sale of dietary supplements containing ephedra became effective. The rule was passed due to concerns over the cardiovascular side effects of ephedra including hypertension and cardiac arrhythmias. Although ephedra may result in short-term weight loss, the hazards, especially when combined with other stimulants such as caffeine, are significant and have resulted in a number of deaths. Despite the rule, however, ephedra-containing products are still available over the internet.

Two case studies were identified of clinicians attempting to treat eating disorders through the use of herbal remedies. One treated a 13-year-old girl with anorexia nervosa with a substance called Juzen-taiho-to, active ingredients were not stated (Wada, 2000). The second case history documents the use of a homeopathic remedy called *Crocus sativa* to treat depression, eating disorder and chilblains in a patient (Geukens, 2001).

Other alternative and complementary treatments reported to be in use by patients but not apparent in the literature review include acupuncture, osteopathy and spiritual or faith healing.

Frequently used treatments not considered mainstream medicine

Although there are many treatments in this category, one example will be given: the use of various non-verbal therapies including art therapy, dance and movement therapy and psychodrama. The use of these treatments rests on the theory that patients with eating disorders, particularly patients with anorexia nervosa, are delayed or regressed in their ability to describe or express emotions (sometimes described as alexithymia, Smith *et al.*, 1997). In addition, patients have been described as delayed in cognitive maturation and are often viewed as being in the concrete operational stage as described by Piaget (1967). Based on these observations, the uses of various non-verbal therapies have been recommended by a number of authors. Although randomized controlled trials have not been done, many of the case reports and case series are poignant and suggest that these methods may help patients access emotions otherwise unavailable to them (Diamond-Raab & Orrell-Valente, 2002).

Conclusions

The definition of complementary and alternative treatments is controversial, but it is clear that many patients utilize various treatments considered outside mainstream

Table 41.3. Effectiveness of treatments listed in NCCAM website possibly related to eating disorders

Treatment	Form of treatment	Psychiatric disorder	Level of evidence for efficacy	Comments
Massage		Bulimia nervosa	Ib	One small study supports the use of massage as an adjunct to inpatient treatment
Hypnosis	Hypnobehavioural therapy	Bulimia nervosa	Ib	One small RCT found no difference between hypnobehavioural therapy and CBT
Psychodrama	Adjunctive to standard treatments	Anorexia and bulimia nervosa	IV	No evidence for effectiveness
Meditation	Includes mindfulness, Naikan therapy, Hatha yoga	Different eating disorders	IV	No evidence of effectiveness
Herbalism/ homeopathy		Different eating disorders	IV	Eating disorder sufferers frequently use herbal remedies to decrease appetite and help them purge
Ephedra		Different eating disorders	IV	The FDA has banned the sale of dietary supplements containing ephedra

Other (ungraded) treatments: Art therapy; Bodywork therapy; Chromium; Dehydroepiandrosterone (DHEA); Guided imagery; Hypnosis; Music therapy; Nutrition; Spirituality; Tai chi; Yoga.

medical practice. Surprisingly, this does not seem to be related to distrust of traditional medicine, but rather these strategies are often used in *addition* to conventional treatments. Since there are actually so few evidence-based treatments for eating disorders that meet the strict criteria of having been demonstrated effective in randomized controlled trials, it is not surprising that alternative and complementary treatments are widely used. Some alternative treatments used by patients with eating disorders are dangerous and/or ineffective, including the herbal dietary aid ephedra. Until more effective treatments are found that are easily accessible, it is likely that use of dangerous alternative treatments will continue.

The level of evidence for each of the interventions discussed in this chapter is summarized in Table 41.3.

REFERENCES

Barrows, K. A. & Jacobs, B. P. (2002). Mind–body medicine, an introduction and review of the literature. *Medical Clinics of North America*, **86**, 11–31.

Daubenmier, J. J. (2003). A comparison of Hatha yoga and aerobic exercise on women's body satisfaction. *Dissertation Abstracts International: Section B: The Sciences and Engineering*, **63**(9-B).

Degun-Mather, M. (2003). Ego-state therapy in the treatment of a complex eating disorder. *Contemporary Hypnosis*, **20**, 165–73.

Diamond-Raab, L. & Orrell-Valente, J. K. (2002). Art therapy, psychodrama, and verbal therapy. An integrative model of group therapy in the treatment of adolescents with anorexia nervosa and bulimia nervosa. *Child and Adolescent Psychiatry Clinics of North America*, **11**, 343–64.

Field, T., Schanberg, S., Kuhn, C. *et al.* (1998). Bulimic adolescents benefit from massage therapy. *Adolescence*, **33**, 554–63.

Field, T. (2002). Massage therapy. *Medical Clinics of North America*, **86**(1), 163–71.

Garrett, C. J. (1997). Recovery from anorexia nervosa: a sociological perspective. *International Journal of Eating Disorders*, **21**, 261–72.

Geukens, A. (2001). Two case histories. *Journal of the American Institute of Homeopathy*, **94**(1), 65–74.

Griffiths, R. A., Hadzi-Pavlovic, D. & Channon-Little, L. (1996). The short-term follow-up effects of hypnobehavioural and cognitive behavioural treatment for bulimia nervosa. *European Eating Disorder Review*, **4**(1), 12–31.

Goldberg, S. C., Halmi, K. A., Eckert, E. D., Casper, R. C. & Davis, J. M. (1979). Cyproheptadine in anorexia nervosa. *British Journal of Psychiatry*, **134**, 67–70.

Hart, S., Field, T., Hernandez-Reif, M. & Nearing, G. (2001). Anorexia nervosa symptoms are reduced by massage therapy. *Eating Disorders*, **9**, 289–99.

Kristeller, J. L. & Hallett, C. B. (1999). An exploratory study of a meditation-based intervention for binge eating disorder. *Journal of Health Psychology*, **4**(3), 357–63.

Marrazzi, M. A., Bacon, J. P., Kinzie, J. & Luby, E. D. (1995). Naltrexone use in the treatment of anorexia nervosa and bulimia nervosa. *International Clinical Psychopharmcology*, **10**, 163–72.

Marlatt, G. A. (2002). Buddhist philosophy and the treatment of addictive behavior. *Cognitive and Behavioral Practice*, **9**(1), 44–50.

Mehler, P. S. & Weiner, K. L. (1993). Anorexia nervosa and total parenteral nutrition. *International Journal of Eating Disorders*, **14**, 297–304.

Morishita, S. (2000). Treatment of anorexia nervosa with Naikan therapy. *International Medical Journal*, **7**(2), 151.

Neiderman, M., Zarody, M., Tattersall, M. & Lask, B. (2000). Enteric feeding in severe adolescent anorexia nervosa: a report of four cases. *International Journal of Eating Disorders*, **28**, 470–5.

NICE: Eating Disorders: Core interventions in the treatment and management of anorexia nervosa, bulimia nervosa and related eating disorders. National Institute for Clinical Excellence. Clinical Guideline 9, Developed by the National Collaborating Centre for Mental Health, London, January 2004.

Piaget, J. (1967). *Six Psychological Studies*. Translated from the French by Anita Tenzer, pp. 3–73. New York: Random House.

Roerig, J. L., Mitchell, J. E., deZwaan, M. *et al.* (2003). The eating disorders medicine cabinet revisited: a clinician's guide to appetite suppressants and diuretics. *International Journal of Eating Disorders*, **33**, 443–57.

Segal, R. (2001). Hypnosis in the treatment of an eating disorder. *Australian Journal of Clinical & Experimental Hypnosis*, **29**(1), 26–36.

Smith, G. J., Amner, G., Johnsson, P. & Franck, A. (1997). Alexithymia in patients with eating disorders: an investigation using a new projective technique. *Perceptual and Motor Skills*, **85**, 247–56.

Trigazis, L., Tennankore, D., Vohra, S. & Katzman, D. K. (2004). The use of herbal remedies by adolescents with eating disorders. *International Journal of Eating Disorders*, **35**, 223–8.

Wada, E. (2000). The successful treatment of a case of anorexia nervosa with Juzen-taiho-to. *Journal of Tokyo Women's Medical College*, **70** (Suppl.), E86–E90.

Yager, J., Siegfreid, S. L. & DiMatteo, T. L. (1999). Use of alternative remedies by psychiatric patients: illustrative vignettes and a discussion of the issues. *American Journal of Psychiatry*, **156**, 1432–8.

Zuercher, J. N., Cumella, E. J., Woods, B. K., Eberly, M. & Carr, J. K. (2003). Efficacy of voluntary tube feeding in female inpatients with anorexia nervosa. *Journal of Parenteral and Enteral Nutrition*, **27**, 268–76.

42

Complex treatments for eating disorders

Scott Crow and Ulrike Schmidt

Editor's note

The decision of where to treat anorexia and bulimia nervosa, and for how long, is a critical part of management. The agonizing that goes into the decision whether to seek treatment at all has been well illustrated in the popular UK radio series *The Archers* in which one of the central characters, Helen Archer, developed excessive dieting and marked loss of weight after the suicide of her partner. (For some reason the script writers insisted her condition was not anorexia nervosa, so they might have been thinking of EDNOS – see Chapter 39.) The difficult task her parents had in getting her to seek treatment – 'there is nothing wrong with me, mum, why do you have to try and control my life?' – and the subtle and delicate way it was finally achieved, shows the importance of matching the treatment of eating disorders to the right setting. This subject, like most complex interventions, is unfortunately not at the stage of giving evidence-based guidelines but at some point the major differences between the type and duration of treatment in different countries will need to be addressed through some formal comparisons.

Introduction

For the greater part of the twentieth century management of anorexia nervosa (AN) was in the hands of non-psychiatrist physicians, and these patients were usually nursed on general medical wards. With the development of psychological models of anorexia nervosa, management of this condition transferred from general medicine to psychiatry or in some European countries to psychosomatic medicine. Specialist eating disorders units emerged within psychiatry. Psychological interventions were developed initially for relapse prevention after weight restoration in hospital and more recently have also been used as a first-line treatment for anorexia nervosa (Treasure & Schmidt, 2004). Day-care programmes have emerged to bridge the gap between in- and outpatient care. The issue of utilizing day care has become increasingly important as health care systems attempt to limit costs and simultaneously provide treatments in the least restrictive settings available.

For bulimia nervosa, which was first described in the late 1970s, psychological models of treatment were available almost instantly (Fairburn, 1981) and outpatient therapy is offered to the majority of cases in Britain and the USA, with day- or inpatient care being reserved for a small group of people with complex and severe comorbidities (Lacey, 1995). The focus of the present chapter will therefore predominantly be on inpatient and day care in the treatment of anorexia nervosa but will adduce evidence on treatment of BN as available.

Inpatient treatment of eating disorders

There is general agreement that inpatient care of anorexia nervosa aimed at stabilizing the patient's physical state is at times medically necessary and may indeed be life-saving in severe cases. Indicators of high medical risk in anorexia nervosa requiring inpatient care have been identified clearly (APA, 2000; Winston & Webster, 2003, NICE, 2004).

However, the need for, and role of, more prolonged inpatient treatments aimed at helping the patient to progress towards full weight recovery by providing a combination of refeeding, physical monitoring and psychosocial interventions is much more controversial (for review, see Vandereycken, 2003). Authors from both sides of the Atlantic have talked about the *'boom in inpatient programmes'* during the 1980s (Vandereycken, 2003) leading

Cambridge Textbook of Effective Treatments in Psychiatry, ed. Peter Tyrer and Kenneth R. Silk. Published by Cambridge University Press.
© Cambridge University Press, 2008.

to an *'abuse of inpatient treatment'* (Garner & Needleman, 1997, p. 53) through *'unnecessary hospitalization of many patients'* (Vandereycken, 2003).

The threshold for initiating inpatient treatment for anorexia nervosa varies widely across different health care systems. In some European countries, such as Germany and Austria, inpatient care is still the norm as a first-line treatment (Rathner & Rainer, 1997; Kächele *et al.*, 1999, 2001), and even a proportion of people with bulimia nervosa are treated as inpatients. In the USA the threshold for inpatient care is relatively low, i.e. a body mass index of less than $16 \, \text{kg/m}^2$ (Garner & Needleman, 1997) or 20% weight loss (American Psychiatric Association, 2000). However, the introduction of managed care has led to tight restrictions on the duration of inpatient care for many. In contrast, in the UK inpatient care is typically reserved for the severely ill with a body mass index of less than $13.5 \, \text{kg/m}^2$ (Winston & Webster, 2003) with little or no restriction on the duration of care.

Where should inpatient care of eating disorder patients take place?

A recent survey of child and adolescent inpatient provision (aged 12 to 18) in England and Wales (O'Herlihy *et al.*, 2003) identified that 20.1% of all beds were occupied by eating disorder patients. About half of these were in general child and adolescent units, the other half in specialist eating disorders units. No comparable figures for adults exist, and it is unknown what proportion of adult eating disorder patients are treated within specialist or generalist inpatient settings. However, general psychiatrists often feel poorly equipped to deal with these patients and the high level of disturbance on many general psychiatric wards makes this an unsuitable environment for what are often extremely vulnerable young females.

There is very little hard evidence on the comparative outcomes produced by specialist or non-specialist inpatient treatment. A study on adult patients with anorexia nervosa who were admitted to a specialist eating disorders unit and who had had previous inpatient care elsewhere in a non-specialist setting, (Council Report, Royal College of Psychiatrists, 1992) showed that weight gain during inpatient treatment was significantly greater during the inpatient episode in a specialist setting. A cohort study by Crisp *et al.* (1992) compared patients from an area without specialist inpatient provision with those admitted to a specialist eating disorder centre. The long-term mortality of patients treated in the specialist centre was significantly lower.

The impact of different types of inpatient programs

From the 1960s onwards, behaviour therapy for anorexia nervosa became increasingly popular, with many articles reporting on the use of operant conditioning techniques (for review, see Schmidt, 1989). The basic operant paradigm consisted of isolating patients from social and material reinforcers that were then re-introduced to them, contingent on weight gain or caloric intake. For a time, this technique became part of many inpatient regimes, because of its efficacy in increasing weight in the short-term. However, operant conditioning approaches have been criticized as coercive and controlling (for review, see Bemis, 1987) and their influence has waned in recent years.

A number of small studies of limited quality have compared different inpatient treatment regimes in randomized controlled trials or clinically controlled studies. Only short-term outcomes are reported (Wullemier, 1975; Eckert, 1979; Touyz *et al.*, 1984; Touyz, 1990; Weizman *et al.*, 1985; Solanto, 1994; Okamoto, 2002; Herzog *et al.*, 1996; Vandereycken, 1985). Nonetheless, some conclusions can be drawn from these studies: There is some evidence that an inpatient programme with an explicit focus on changing eating disorder symptoms and weight is superior to one without such a focus, in terms of producing short term weight gain (Herzog *et al.*, 1996). Importantly also, a strict operant conditioning regime had no advantages over a more lenient regime (Touyz *et al.*, 1984).

Very little is known about the efficacy of different psychological treatments as adjuncts to inpatient treatment and existing studies are of limited quality (Pillay *et al.*, 1987; Goldfarb, 1987).

Duration of inpatient care

A survey of adult inpatients (aged 16 to 64) in NHS facilities in England found that out of all conditions considered eating disorders had the greatest median duration of admissions (36 days) and the highest proportion of patients with a length of stay of greater than 90 days (26.8% of admissions). The comparable figures for schizophrenia and related diagnoses were 28 days and 18.4% respectively (Thompson *et al.*, 2004).

In Germany, Krauth *et al.* (2002) found the mean length of inpatient stay to be 49.8 days for AN and 45.5 days for BN, respectively.

Striegel-Moore *et al.* (2000) reviewed health service use and costs for eating disorders in the USA. 21.5% of women with anorexia nervosa were hospitalized per year with an average length of stay of 26 days, and very much lower hospitalization rates were found for BN and EDNOS. Another US study investigated time trends in hospitalization of eating disorder patients over a 15-year period from 1984 to 1998 examining the records of 1185 eating disorder patients (Wiseman et al., 2001). These authors found a dramatic decrease in mean length of stay from 149.5 days in 1984 to 23.7 days in 1998 due to changes in the economics of health care. Readmission rates increased sharply from 0% during 1984 to 27% of admissions in 1998. Patients with restricting anorexia nervosa were more likely to be readmitted than those with BN. The authors conclude that, for some patients, this change has been deleterious and not cost-effective (Wiseman et al., 2001).

One large prospective naturalistic multi-centre study of inpatients $(n = 1171)$ (anorexia nervosa = 355; anorexia nervosa and bulimia nervosa = 169; bulimia nervosa = 647) conducted in Germany (Kächele et al., 2001) aimed to examine (a) what factors determine the duration of treatment and (b) the relationship between the duration of treatment received and outcome. The duration of inpatient treatment programmes of the 43 participating hospitals varied widely within and between hospitals. The median duration of inpatient treatment was 11.6 weeks for anorexia nervosa and 10.6 weeks for anorexia nervosa – bulimic type. Importantly, patient characteristics explained only 3% of the variance in duration of treatment within hospitals and none of the variance between hospitals. Most of the between-hospital variance in duration of treatment was explained by organizational factors. The same study found an interaction between duration of illness, duration of treatment and outcome. At 2.5 years' follow-up, people with a longer duration of anorexia nervosa or illness had a higher likelihood of good outcome with longer, rather than with briefer, duration of inpatient treatment. In contrast, those with a shorter duration of illness had a higher likelihood of good outcome with briefer inpatient treatment.

In contrast, an Australian multi-centre study of 218 patients with anorexia nervosa (Maguire et al., 2003) found body mass index and having had two to three previous admissions, to make an independent contribution to length of stay, explaining 20% of the variance.

Acceptability and potential harms of inpatient treatment

Patients generally report greater levels of satisfaction with outpatient than with inpatient care (Rosenvinge and Klusmeier, 2000). Adolescents, in particular, have reported finding inpatient treatment difficult, as they feel pressured

and watched, feeling intruded upon and lacking privacy (Brinch et al., 1988; Buston, 2002). Indirect measures of acceptability are treatment uptake and dropout. The lower treatment uptake of inpatient therapy in the study by Crisp et al. (see above) suggests that this was a less acceptable option to a proportion of patients than outpatient psychological treatment. Moreover, dropout from inpatient treatment for anorexia nervosa seems to be higher than that reported for general psychiatric patients (Kahn & Pike, 2001).

It has also been suggested that outpatient programmes may lead to better long-term outcomes than inpatient programmes (Beumont et al., 1993). This may be particularly true for anorexia nervosa in adolescents where outpatient family interventions produce excellent outcomes (e.g. Eisler et al., 2003). One small study by Gowers et al. (2000) followed up adolescents with anorexia nervosa for 2–7 years. Those who had received inpatient treatment had a significantly worse outcome than those never admitted to hospital. Admission was a major predictor of poor outcome and the authors provocatively suggested that inpatient treatment may be harmful for adolescents. However, the findings are confounded by illness severity and the above conclusion therefore seems premature.

Day care treatments for eating disorders

Day care treatments represent an important piece of the continuum of care for individuals with eating disorders. They can either be used as an alternative to admission, or as 'step-down' care from the structure and support of inpatient treatment with the aim to afford patients the chance to continue their recovery in what is increasingly their own environment. Indeed, there is evidence at least in the United States that use of day care following on from inpatient care is increasing, as early discharge from the hospital necessitated by managed care, predicts re-hospitalization (Baran et al., 1995; Wiseman et al., 2001; Gill-Willer et al., in press).

Outcome studies of day care programmes

A number of the existing reports in the literature describe efforts at developing day hospital programmes (Dalle Grave et al., 2001; Thornton et al., 2002; Touyz et al., 2003). However, remarkably little is known at present about the efficacy or effectiveness of day hospital, or about the predictors of success or failure in such treatment (Zipfel et al., 2002). The existing literature on the use of day care programmes in six different centres for eating disorders is reviewed in Table 42.1.

Table 42.1. Outcome studies of day care programmes

Authors	Population	Outcomes
(a) Maddocks et al., 1992 (b) Olmsted et al., 1996 (c) Olmsted et al., 2003	(a) Bulimia (n = 43): comparison of those with and without symptoms at follow-up (b) Bulimia nervosa (n = 166): comparison of rapid and slow responders (c) Anorexia and bulimia nervosa patients: comparison of outcomes from a 5-day programme (n = 468) vs. 4-day programme (n = 288)	(a) Symptomatic patients appeared worse in terms of measures of comorbid psychopathology including depression, self-esteem and social adjustment. (b) Rapid responders were older, had less symptoms at intake and lower preoccupation with binge eating. Rapid responders had a better end of treatment outcome, with less relapse and less frequent use of medication at 2-year follow-up. (c) The 5-day programme led to a higher frequency of abstinence from binge eating and purging and better psychological outcomes. Weight gain was equivalent in the 4-day and 5-day programmes. The 4-day programme was more cost-effective.
Guarda & Heinberg, 2004	Anorexia nervosa (n = 150)	22% left prematurely. Programme completers were admitted to inpatient services at a BMI of 16.1, transitioned to day care at a BMI of 18.3, and discharged from day care at a BMI of 19.6, on average. At discharge, 73% were within 5% of target BMI, and 46% had reached or exceeded target BMI. Average rates of weight gain were 4.3 pounds/week (S.D. 2.0 pounds/week) on the inpatient service and 2.3 pounds/week (S.D. 1.8 pounds/week) in the day care programme. A subanalysis showed that restricting subtype patients had greater weight gain in the day care programme than did purging subtype patients (2.8 pounds/week vs. 1.8 pounds/week). For the first 53 subjects to complete the programme, gains in BMI were maintained at 3 to 6 months follow-up (available for 52%).
Gerlinghoff et al., 1998	65 consecutive patients (65% with BN, 25% with AN)	Average treatment duration 13 weeks. Follow-up assessment on average 17 months after treatment. For people with AN, the average BMI at intake was 15.0 and by the end of treatment it was 18.5. At follow-up, average BMI was 19.1. For people with BN, substantial reductions were seen for binge eating and purging. Additionally, the group as a whole improved on a wide variety of other psychopathology and social/functional measures.
Zeeck et al., 2004	Outcome of day care vs. inpatient care in 18 consecutive BN patients and 18 consecutive non-eating disorder psychiatric patients	50% of those receiving day care treatment met full diagnostic criteria for the last four weeks of treatment, in contrast to only 27.8% of those in inpatient. However, at 18 months follow-up 50% of the day care sample were fully remitted and 26.8% in partial remission.
Dancyger et al., 2003	82 adolescents and young adults mainly with AN	49% of participants met their treatment goals (defined variously as normalization of weight or weight maintenance, or normalization of eating behaviours as specified by the clinical situation). Thirty-eight per cent of subjects left the programme prior to achieving these treatment goals and 13% were transferred to inpatient care.
Williamson et al., 2001	51 patients	Outcomes were similar in terms of length of stay and response rates but day care treatment appeared substantially more cost-effective.

Results for both anorexia nervosa and bulimia nervosa patients are promising and several authors suggest that day care may be a cost-effective alternative to inpatient care (Williamson *et al.*, 2001). However, especially in the context of day treatment of BN, one needs to bear in mind that effective outpatient treatments for BN exist and that, for BN, day care may not be as cost-effective as for AN (Zipfel *et al.*, 2002). No formal examinations of the cost-effectiveness of day care vs. other treatments of eating disorders exist.

Special considerations in day care treatment

In addition to the descriptions of outcome in day care programmes described above, several issues related to the practical utilization of day care treatments as part of the spectrum of care for individuals with eating disorders have also been described. Howard and colleagues (1999) examined the characteristics of individuals who were able to successfully transition from inpatient care to a day hospital programme and found that successful transition was associated with shorter duration of illness, absence of amenorrhoea and a higher BMI, either at the time of admission or transition to day care. Similarly, Franzen *et al.* (2004) studied reasons for dropout from day care treatment. In a sample of 125 patients with bulimia nervosa, 19 (15%) dropped out of treatment. These patients on average had more severe bulimic symptoms, more aggression, more extraversion and more impulsivity.

Tasca and coworkers (2002) examined the nature and role of group climate in eating disorder day hospital groups as compared to non-eating disordered psychiatric day hospital groups. In comparing 61 eating disorder patients with 67 non-eating disordered female psychiatric day hospital patients, these investigators found higher levels of engagement in the eating disorder cohorts but also higher levels of avoidance; they set forth suggestions for how these factors may be useful in facilitating treatment.

Woodside and colleagues described the experience of treating males in the day hospital setting as compared to females (Woodside & Kaplan, 1994). This report described outcome for 334 women and 15 men treated during the same period of time. The authors concluded that, in general, the males and females looked quite similar in terms of characteristics and outcome, and concluded that treating women and men together in mixed gender day hospital programmes was quite feasible.

The issue of adapting family treatment for adolescents with anorexia nervosa has also been addressed by descriptions of the use of multiple family group day treatment (Dare & Eisler, 2000). These investigators describe the adaptation of empirically supported individual family therapy as developed at the Maudsley Hospital (Eisler *et al.*, 1997; Le Grange *et al.*, 1992).

Direct comparison between inpatient, day patient and outpatient care

One systematic review (Meads *et al.*, 1999) compared inpatient treatment with outpatient care. The review identified one randomized controlled trial, addressing this question, which had a 5-year follow-up (Crisp *et al.*, 1991; Gowers *et al.*, 1994). Ninety people with anorexia nervosa were randomized to four treatment groups: inpatient treatment, outpatient treatment (individual and family therapy), outpatient group therapy and assessment interview only. Adherence to allocated treatment differed significantly among groups (adherence rates: inpatient treatment 18/30 (60%), outpatient treatment (individual and family therapy) 18/20 (90%), outpatient group psychotherapy 17/20 (85%), and assessment interview only 20/20 (100%)). Treatment adherence differed significantly between outpatient and inpatient treatment (RR 1.5, 95% CI 1.1 to 2.0). Average acceptance of treatment also varied among groups (20 wks inpatient treatment, 9 outpatient sessions, and 5 group sessions). In the assessment interview-only group, six people had no treatment of any kind in the first year and the others had treatment elsewhere (6 had inpatient treatment, 5 had outpatient hospital treatment, and 3 had at least weekly contact with their general practitioners). Six people in this group spent almost the entire year in treatment. There were no significant differences in mean weight or in the Morgan Russell scale global scores among any of the four groups at 1, 2 and 5 years. The proportion of people with a good outcome with inpatient treatment was 5/29 (17%) at 2 years and 9/27 (33%) at 5 years; with outpatient treatment (individual and family therapy) 4/20 (20%) at 2 years and 8/17 (47%) at 5 years; with outpatient group psychotherapy 5/19 (26%) at 2 years and 10/19 (53%) at 5 years; and with assessment interview only 2/20 (10%) at 2 years and 6/19 (32%) at 5 years. One person died from anorexia nervosa between the assessment and the start of outpatient group treatment, and one of the people allocated to inpatient treatment died from anorexia nervosa by 5 years (Crisp *et al.*, 1991; Gowers *et al.*, 1994).

Since then one further study has appeared, comparing in-patient and outpatient treatment in adolescents with anorexia nervosa (Gowers *et al.*, 2007; Byford *et al.*, 2007). In this study 167 young people with anorexia nervosa (aged 12 to 18) were randomised to one of three treatment conditions: (a) 6 months of a manualised, specialist out-patient treatment, consisting of an initial motivational interview, 12 sessions of individual cognitive-behavioral therapy with parental feedback, parental counselling with the patient (4 to 8 sessions), dietary therapy (4 sessions) and multi-modal feedback monitoring (4 sessions); (b) inpatient treatment within generic Child and Adolescent impatient units with expertise in the treatment of eating disorders; (c) treatment as usual from general child and adolescent mental health services. Adherence to inpatient treatment was poor (i.e. only 50%). At two years there were no differences between groups in clinical outcomes (Gowers et al., 2007). The specialist out-patient group was less costly over the two-year follow-up period (mean total cost £26 738) than the in-patient (£34 531) and general outpatient treatment (£40 794), however this difference was not statistically significant. Nonetheless the out-patient specialist treatment had the highest probability of being cost-effective, supporting the provision of this treatment (Byford et al., 2007).

The systematic review also identified one unpublished study comparing day care with inpatient care (Freeman, 1992) was identified by the systematic review of Meads et al. (1999). The conclusion that can be drawn from this evidence is that for patients with AN which is not so severe as to require emergency intervention, outpatient or day patient treatment may be suitable alternatives (Treasure & Schmidt, 2004; Royal Australian and New Zealand College of Psychiatrists Clinical Practice Guidelines Team for Anorexia Nervosa, 2004).

One study compared inpatient analytic therapy (2 months) with systemic outpatient therapy (15 sessions over 1 year) in patients with bulimia nervosa. Fifty per cent of patients were allocated randomly, the others were allocated according to preference. Both therapies improved symptomatic behaviour as well as other psychosocial outcomes, with no differences between treatments (Jäger et al., 1996).

Differences in UK and US guidance on inpatient and day care treatments for eating disorders

The recent UK NICE (2004) guideline recommends that most adults with anorexia nervosa should be managed on an outpatient basis. Where inpatient treatment is necessary, a structured symptom focused approach with the expectation of weight gain should be provided in order to achieve weight restoration during inpatient treatment. A weekly weight gain of 0.5–1 kg is regarded as optimal. The Guideline specifically cautions against the use of strict behaviour modification programmes. It suggests that psychological treatment should be available during and after inpatient treatment as patients are very vulnerable to post-hospitalization weight loss. No recommendation is made about the kind of psychological treatment to be made available post-hospitalization as there is insufficient evidence to determine the relative effectiveness of different psychotherapies that have been evaluated (such as supportive individual therapy, CBT, nutritional counselling, family therapy) as post-hospitalization treatments. The duration of psychological treatment post-hospitalization should be at least 12 months. The APA Practice Guidelines for treatment of eating disorders acknowledge that selected individuals with AN do well in outpatient treatment but describe a wider variety of

Table 42.2. Effectiveness of treatments for eating disorders

Treatment	Form of treatment	Psychiatric disorder	Level of evidence for efficacy	Comments
Inpatient treatment	Multi-modal treatment involving refeeding; in specialist eating disorders unit	Anorexia nervosa	1b	No difference in outcomes between inpatient, day patient and outpatient treatment in those not so severe as to require emergency treatment
Inpatient treatment	Explicit focus on changing eating disorder symptoms and weight	Anorexia nervosa	IIa	Superior to treatment without focus on eating disorder symptoms, in terms of short-term weight gain
Inpatient treatment	Operant conditioning regimes	Anorexia nervosa	IIa	A strict regime had no advantages over a more lenient one
Inpatient treatment	Inpatient psychoanalytic therapy	Bulimia nervosa	IIa	No difference to outpatient systemic therapy
Day care treatment	Multi-modal treatment in specialist eating disorders unit	Anorexia nervosa	III	Whilst day treatment has shown promise, it is not clear what precisely its status is in the treatment of AN
Day care treatment	Multi-modal treatment in specialist eating disorders unit	Bulimia nervosa	III	Whilst day treatment has shown promise, it is not clear what precisely its status is in the treatment of BN

clinical situations in which hospitalization is recommended. Psychological treatments are strongly advocated, but no specific type of psychotherapy is recommended. The use of medication as a major focus of treatment is discouraged.

Day care is recommended as part of the spectrum of treatment, particularly for anorexia nervosa, in treatment guidelines such as the American Psychiatric Association Practice Guidelines for the Treatment of Patients with Eating Disorders (APA, 2000) and the NICE guidelines (National Collaborating Centre for Mental Health, 2004). Other complex treatment such as home treatment and intensive outreach are in their infancy.

Conclusions

Different health care systems have different thresholds for inpatient admission and the duration of such admissions for anorexia nervosa. These decisions are not usually evidence based and depend mainly on issues such as cost-considerations and how risk-averse a particular health care system is (e.g. what is the potential for being litigated against). Whilst it is difficult at the best of times to mount sufficiently powered treatment trials on anorexia nervosa, future research studies into the relative merits of inpatient, outpatient and day care for this condition are urgently needed and are currently under way.

The level of evidence for each of the interventions discussed in this chapter is summarized in Table 42.2.

REFERENCES

American Psychiatric Association (2000). Practice guideline for the treatment of patients with eating disorders (revision). *American Journal of Psychiatry*, **157** (suppl. 1), 1–39.

Bemis, K. M. (1987). The present status of operant conditioning for the treatment of anorexia nervosa. *Behavior Modification*, **11**, 432–63.

Baran, S., Weltzin, T. & Kaye, W. (1995). Low discharge weight and outcome in anorexia nervosa. *American Journal of Psychiatry*, **152**, 1070–2.

Beumont, P. J. V., Russell, J. D. & Touyz, S. (1993). Treatment of anorexia nervosa. *Lancet*, **341**, 1635–40.

Brinch, M., Isager, T. & Tolstrup, K. (1988). Patients' evaluation of their former treatment for anorexia nervosa (AN). Nordisk psychkatrisk tidsskrift. *Nordic Journal of Psychiatry*, **42**, 445–8.

Buston, K. (2002). Adolescents with mental health problems: what do they say about health services? *Journal of Adolescence*, **25**, 231–42.

Byford, S., Barrett, B., Roberts, C. *et al.* (2007). Economic Evaluation of a randomized controlled trial for adolescent anorexia nervosa – the TOuCAN trial. *British Journal of Psychiatry*, in press.

Crisp, A. H., Norton, K., Gowers, S. *et al.* (1991). A controlled study of the effect of therapies aimed at adolescent and family psychopathology in anorexia nervosa. *British Journal of Psychiatry*, **159**, 325–33.

Crisp, A. H., Callender, J. S., Halek, C. & Hsu, L. K. G. (1992). Long-term mortality in anorexia nervosa: a 20-year follow-up of the St. George's and Aberdeen cohorts. *British Journal of Psychiatry*, **161**, 104–7.

Dalle Grave, R., Ricca, V. & Todesco, T. (2001). The stepped-care approach in anorexia nervosa and bulimia nervosa: progress and problems. *Eating Weight Disorders*, **6**, 81–9.

Dancyger, I., Fornari, V., Schneider, M. *et al.* (2003). Adolescents and eating disorders: an examination of a day treatment program. *Eating and Weight Disorders*, **8**, 242–8.

Dare, C. & Eisler, I. (2000). A multi-family group day treatment programme for adolescent eating disorder. *European Eating Disorders Review*, **8**, 4–18.

Eckert, E. D., Goldberg, S. C., Halmi, K. A., Casper, R. C. & Davis, J. M (1979). Behaviour therapy in anorexia nervosa. *British Journal of Psychiatry*, **134**, 55–9.

Eisler, I., Dare, C., Russell, G. F. M., Szmukler, G. I., Le Grange, D. & Dodge, E. (1997). Family and individual therapy in anorexia nervosa. A 5-year follow-up. *Archives of General Psychiatry*, **54**, 1025–30.

Eisler, I., Le Grange, D. & Asen, E. (2003). Family Interventions. *Handbook of Eating Disorders*. 2nd edn, ed. J., Treasure, U. Schmidt, & E. van Furth, pp. 291–310. Chichester, UK: John Wiley & Sons.

Fairburn C. (1981). A cognitive behavioural approach to the treatment of bulimia. *Psychological Medicine*, **11**, 707–11.

Franzen, U., Backmund, H. & Gerlinghoff, M. (2004). Day treatment group programme for eating disorders: reasons for dropout. *European Eating Disorders Review*, **12**, 153–8.

Freeman, C. (1992). Day patient treatment of anorexia nervosa. *British Review of Bulimia and Anorexia Nervosa*, **6**, 3–8.

Garner, D. M. & Needleman, L. D. (1997). Sequencing and integration of treatments. In *Handbook of Treatment of Eating Disorders*, ed. D. M. Garner and P. E. Garfinkel, pp. 50–66. New York: Guilford Press.

Gerlinghoff, M., Backmund, H. & Franzen, U. (1998). Evaluation of a day treatment programme for eating disorders. *European Eating Disorders Review*, **6**, 96–106.

Goldfarb, L. A., Fuhr, R., Tsujimoto, R. N. & Fischman, S. E. (1987). Systematic desensitisation and relaxation as adjuncts in the treatment of anorexia nervosa: a preliminary study. *Psychological Reports*, **60**, 411–518.

Gowers, S. G., Clark, A., Roberts, C. *et al.* Clinical outcomes of treatments for anorexia nervosa: randomized controlled trial – the TOuCAN trial. *British Journal of Psychiatry*, in press.

Gowers, S., Norton, K., Halek, C. & Crisp, A. H. (1994). Outcome of outpatient psychotherapy in a random allocation treatment study of anorexia nervosa. *International Journal of Eating Disorders*, **15**, 65–77.

Gowers, S. G., Weetman, J., Shore, A., Hossain, F. & Elvins, R. (2000). Impact of hospitalisation on the outcome of adolescent anorexia nervosa. *British Journal of Psychiatry*, **176**, 138–41.

Guarda, A. S. & Heinberg, L. J. (2004). Inpatient and partial hospital approaches to the treatment of eating disorders. In *Handbook of Eating Disorders and Obesity*, ed. J. K. Thompson, pp. 297–320. New Jersey: John Wiley & Sons, Inc.

Herzog, T., Hartmann, A. & Falk, C. (1996). Total symptom-oriented and psychodynamic concept in inpatient treatment of anorexia nervosa. A quasi-experimental comparative study of 40 admission episodes. *Psychotherapie Psychosomatische Medizin und Psychologie*, **46**, 11–22.

Howard, W. T., Evans, K. K., Quintero-Howard, C. V., Bowers, W. A. & Andersen, A. E. (1999). Predictors of success or failure of transition to day hospital treatment for inpatients with anorexia nervosa. *American Journal of Psychiatry*, **156**, 1697–702.

Jäger, B., Liedke, R., Künsebeck, H.-W., Lempa, W., Kersting, A. & Seide, L. (1996). Psychotherapy and bulimia nervosa: evaluation and long-term follow-up of two conflict-orientated treatment conditions. *Acta Psychiatrica Scandinavica*, **93**, 268–78.

Kahn, C. & Pike, K. (2001). In search of predictors of dropout from inpatient treatment for anorexia nervosa. *International Journal of Eating Disorders*, **30**, 237–44.

Kächele, H. for the study group MZ-ESS (1999). Eine multizentrische Studie zu Aufwand und Erfolg bei psychodynamischer Therapie von Eßstörungen. *Psychotherapie und Medizinische Psychologie*, **49**, 100–8.

Kächele, H., Kordy, H., Richard, M. & Research Group TR-EAT. (2001). Therapy amount and outcome of inpatient psychodynamic treatment of eating disorders in Germany: data from a multicenter study. *Psychotherapy Research*, **11**, 239–57.

Krauth, C. (2002). How high are the costs of eating disorders – anorexia nervosa and bulimia nervosa – for German Society? *European Journal of Health Economics*, **3**, 244–50.

Lacey, J. H. (1995). In-patient treatment of multi-impulsive bulimia nervosa. In *Eating Disorders and Obesity*, ed. K. D. Brownell & C. G. Fairburn. New York: Guilford Press.

Le Grange, D., Eisler, I., Dare, C. & Russell, G. F. M. (1992). Evaluation of family therapy in anorexia nervosa: a pilot study. *International Journal of Eating Disorders*, **12**, 347–57.

Maddocks, S. E., Kaplan, A. S., Woodside, D. B., Langdon, L. & Piran, N. (1992). Two year follow-up of bulimia nervosa: the importance of abstinence as the criterion of outcome. *International Journal of Eating Disorders*, **12**, 133–41.

Maguire, S., Surgenor, L. J., Abraham, S. and Beumont, P. (2003). An international collaborative database: its use in predicting length of stay for inpatient treatment of anorexia nervosa. *Australian and New Zealand Journal of Psychiatry*, **37**, 741–7.

Meads, C., Gold, L., Burls, A. & Jobanputra, P. (1999). *In-patient versus out-patient care for eating disorders*. Department of Public Health and Epidemiology. West Midlands Development and Evaluation Service. Report No 17. Birmingham: University of Birmingham.

National Collaborating Centre for Mental Health (2004). *Eating disorders. Core interventions in the treatment and management of anorexia nervosa, bulimia nervosa and related eating disorders*. London: National Institute for Clinical Excellence.

O'Herlihy, A., Worrall, A., Lelliott, P., Jaffa, T., Hill, P. & Banerjee, S. (2003). Distribution and charactiersitics of in-patient child and adolescent mental health services in England and Wales. *British Journal of Psychiatry*, **183**, 847–551.

Okamoto, A., Yamashita, T., Nagoshi, Y. *et al.* (2002). A behavior therapy program combined with liquid nutrition designed for anorexia nervosa. *Psychiatry and Clinical Neuroscience*, **56**, 515–20.

Olmsted, M. P., Kaplan, A. S., Rockert, W. & Jacobsen, M. (1996). Rapid responders to intensive treatment of bulimia nervosa. *International Journal of Eating Disorders*, **19**, 279–85.

Olmsted, M. P., Kaplan, A. S. & Rockert, W. (2003). Relative efficacy of a 4-day versus a 5-day day hospital program. *International Journal of Eating Disorders*, **34**, 441–9.

Pillay, M. & Crisp, A. H. (1981). The impact of social skills training within an established inpatient treatment program for anorexia nervosa. *British Journal of Psychiatry*, **139**, 533–9.

Rathner, G. & Rainer, B. (1997). Annual treatment rates and estimated prevalence of eating disorders in Austria. *Wiener Klinische Wochenschrift*, **109**, 275–80.

Rosenvinge, J. H. & Klusmeier, A. K. (2000). Treatment for eating disorders from a patient satisfaction perspective: a Norwegian replication of a British study. *European Eating Disorders Review*, **8**, 293–300.

Royal Australian and New Zealand College of Psychiatrists Clinical Practice Guidelines Team for Anroexia nervosa. (2004). Australian and New Zealand clinical practice guidelines for the treatment of anorexia nervosa. *Australian and New Zealand Journal of Psychiatry*, **38**, 659–70.

Royal College of Psychiatrists (1992). *Eating disorders (Council Report 14)*. London: Royal College of Psychiatrists.

Schmidt, U. (1989). Behavioural psychotherapy for eating disorders. *International Review Journal of Psychiatry*, **1**, 245–56.

Solanto, M. V., Jacobson, M. S., Heller, L., Golden, N. H. & Hertz, S. (1994). Rate of weight gain of inpatients with anorexia nervosa under two behavioral contracts. *Pediatrics*, **93**, 989–91.

Striegel-Moore, R. H., Leslie, D., Petrill, S. A., Garvin, V. & Rosenheck, R. A. (2000). One-year use and cost of inpatient and outpatient services among female and male patients with an eating disorder: evidence from a national database of health insurance claims. *International Journal of Eating Disorders*, **27**, 381–9.

Tasca, G. A., Flynn, C. & Bissada, H. (2002). Comparison of group climate in an eating disorders partial hospital group and a psychiatric partial hospital group. *International Journal of Group Psychotherapy*, **52**, 409–17.

Thompson, A., Shaw, M., Harrison, G., Verne, J., Ho, D. & Gunnell, D. (2004). Patterns of hospital admission for adult psychiatric illness in England: analysis of Hospital Episode Statistics data. *British Journal of Psychiatry*, **185**, 334–41.

Thornton, C., Beaumont, P. & Touyz, S. (2002). The Australian experience of day programs for patients with eating disorders. *International Journal of Eating Disorders*, **32**, 1–10.

Touyz, S. W., Beumont, P. J., Glaun, D., Phillips, T. & Cowie, I. (1984). A comparison of lenient and strict operant conditioning programs in refeeding patients with anorexia nervosa. *British Journal of Psychiatry*, **144**, 517–20.

Touyz, S. W., Lennerts, W., Freeman, R. J. & Beumont, P. J. (1990). To weigh or not to weigh? Frequency of weighing and rate of weight gain in patients with anorexia nervosa. *British Journal of Psychiatry*, **157**, 752–4.

Touyz, S., Thornton, C., Rieger, E., George, L. & Beaumont, P. (2003). The incorporation of the stage of change model in the day hospital treatment of patients with anorexia nervosa. *European Child and Adolescent Psychiatry*, **12**, 65–71.

Treasure, J. & Schmidt, U. (2004). Anorexia nervosa. *Clinical Evidence*, **12**, 1192–203.

Vandereycken, W. (1985). Inpatient treatment of anorexia nervosa: some research-guided changes. *Journal of Psychiatric Research*, **19**, 2–3, 413–22.

Vandereycken, W. (2003). The place of inpatient care in the treatment of anorexia nervosa: questions to be answered. *International Journal of Eating Disorders*, **34**, 409–22.

Weizman, A., Tyano, S., Wijsenbeek, H. & Ben David, M. (1985). Behavior therapy, pimozide treatment and prolactin secretion in anorexia nervosa. *Psychotherapy and Psychosomatics*, **43**, 136–40.

Williamson, D. A., Thaw, J. M. & Varnado-Sullivan, P. J. (2001). Cost-effectiveness analysis of a hospital-based cognitive-behavioral treatment program for eating disorders. *Behavior Therapy*, **32**, 459–77.

Winston, A. & Webster, P. (2003). Inpatient treatment. In *Handbook of Eating Disorders*. 2nd edn, ed. J. Treasure, U. Schmidt & E. van Furth. Chichester, UK: John Wiley & Sons.

Wiseman, C. V., Sunday, S. R., Klapper, F., Harris, W. A. & Halmi, K. A. (2001). Changing patterns of hospitalization in eating disorder patients. *International Journal of Eating Disorders*, **30**, 69–74.

Woodside, D. B. & Kaplan, A. S. (1994). Day hospital treatment in males with eating disorders – response and comparison to females. *Journal of Psychosomatic Research*, **38**, 471–5.

Wullemier, F., Rossel, F. & Sinclair, K. (1975). La therapie comportementale de l'anorexie nerveuse. *Journal of Psychosomatic Research*, **19**, 267–72.

Zeeck, A., Herzog, T. & Hartmann, A. (2004). Day clinic or inpatient care for severe bulimia nervosa? *European Eating Disorders Review*, **12**, 79–86.

Zipfel, S., Reas, D. L., Thornton C. *et al.* (2002). Day hospitalization programs for eating disorders: a systematic review of the literature. *International Journal of Eating Disorders*, **31**, 105–17.

Personality disorders

Section editors

Anthony Bateman and Mary Zanarini

43

Personality disorder

Anthony Bateman and Mary Zanarini

Editor's note

The literature on effective treatments of the personality disorders is quite large but evidence remains sparse. There are a number of personality disorders for which there is absolutely no evidence and/or no studies examining possible evidence for efficacy, and these disorders, schizoid, histrionic, narcissistic, obsessive-compulsive and dependent are not covered in this chapter (but mentioned in the following one on other less-established treatments for personality disorder). Many descriptions of treatment for these disorders are really combinations of theory with clinical supposition but very little evidence. The evidence for some psychotherapeutic intervention is strongest for borderline personality disorder (BPD) and the evidence for psychopharmacological interventions is strongest for schizotypal personality disorder (STPD). Even well-designed studies are confounded by Axis I and Axis II co-morbidities, and this limits interpretation of the findings. The reader will note the importance given to the structuring and organization of treatment and might also consult the chapter on complex interventions in evaluating the significance of the findings.

Introduction

The definition of personality disorder (PD) remains controversial. Both the DSM-IV and ICD-10 take a categorical approach to the diagnosis of PD defining different types of personality according to descriptive criteria. Tyrer *et al.* (1990), however, found little evidence that categories of personality disorder were helpful in determining response to treatment or indeed that they had any predictive value at all. Research orientated methods rely on structured and semi-structured interviewing or self-report screening measures. Although this improves reliability somewhat, the approach remains unsatisfactory (Pilkonis *et al.*; 1995). Validity is questionable since the underlying construct, which determines diagnosis on Axis II of DSM, relies on self-reported styles of interpersonal function, self-assessment of personal traits, and declared impairment in social roles over a period of time. Interviews utilize direct questions concerning habitual behavioural patterns and self-reported personality descriptions in a manner likely to heighten defensiveness and yield biased data. There is little emphasis on personality functioning in terms of key domains such as work, relationships and self-care (Hill *et al.*, 1989), Developmental history is considered separately from diagnosis and response biases such as a plaintive response set and social desirability response bias have not been taken into consideration.

The clustering of specific trait-related personality disorders into three groupings is an attempt to address this lack of specificity of the diagnostic system. However, the three DSM-IV clusters (the odd-eccentric (Cluster A), the impulsive-erratic (Cluster B), and the anxious-avoidant (Cluster C)) have only face validity, as large cohort studies, which might confirm the stability of such groupings, have not been carried out. There are also indications that the North American and European systems of classification show insufficient levels of agreement (Sara *et al.*, 1996). The usefulness of this approach rests on its intuitive appeal to clinicians, which in its turn may have more to do with the relative ease with which category membership may be identified through the use of prototypes, than with the value of such a system in a scientific description of personality.

Given the problems of diagnosis it will not come as a surprise to the reader to learn that this handicaps evaluation of treatments for personality disorder.

Cambridge Textbook of Effective Treatments in Psychiatry, ed. Peter Tyrer and Kenneth R. Silk. Published by Cambridge University Press.
© Cambridge University Press, 2008.

Assessment of treatment

In order to determine the effectiveness of a treatment for PD it is necessary (a) to define the target population carefully, which in itself can be problematic, as just discussed. In addition co-morbidity has to be considered. Lifetime co-morbidity should not be an exclusion criterion for studies but there is a reasonable argument to exclude individuals with current co-morbidity and to assess subjects, for example, who are not currently depressed or abusing substances; (b) to define treatment adequately and assess its specificity. There is now recognition that personality disorder is a multifaceted condition that can be influenced in many different ways and fully justifies the use of what are now described as 'complex interventions' (Campbell *et al.*, 2000). Complex interventions lead to complex evaluations and consequent greater difficulty in interpreting results; (c) to ensure treatment is superior to no treatment since personality disorders show gradual improvement over time (Zanarini *et al.*, 2003a, 2004a); (d) to demonstrate that treatment impacts on personality rather than merely causing a change in mood or psychiatric symptoms (Clark *et al.*, 2003); (e) to include an adequate follow-up; and (f) to address cost-effectiveness relative to other alternative interventions. Research into effectiveness of treatments for personality disorder has singularly failed to meet most of these requirements.

A further important distinction in determining the value of an intervention is whether its value has been demonstrated in standard practice rather than under strict experimental conditions. This distinction was first highlighted by Schwarz & Lellouch (1967) in discussing differences between randomized trials and is commonly described as the difference between an explanatory trial, i.e. a trial in which treatments are compared under ideal (experimentally manipulated) conditions, and pragmatic trials, in which the study is carried out under the conditions normally pertaining to ordinary practice in which possible confounders to the intervention may be present. Although they can be removed, doing so creates an artificial environment that does not allow the results to be transferred to ordinary practice. Schwarz & Lellouch showed that the results of these trials could be very different even though the treatments under test were the same. As personality disorders are very common in conjunction with other disorders, there is a place for both pragmatic as well as explanatory trials in evaluation of treatment. In evidence-based psychiatry these are sometimes described as trials of efficacy (explanatory) and effectiveness (pragmatic) (Slade & Priebe, 2001). Each has its advantages and disadvantages but, in general, it is common to establish efficacy under controlled conditions first before testing an intervention in conditions of ordinary practice.

Psychotherapy and psychosocial treatments

Meta-analyses

Even though the first meta-analysis of studies of psychotherapeutic treatment for personality disorder was undertaken in 1999, it remains unclear whether the literature is mature enough to withstand the methodology. The relative lack of good quality studies, especially randomized trials, the small number of patients in the trials, the heterogeneity of the personality disorders studied, and the variability of outcome measures across studies means that conclusions can only be tentative. Perry *et al.* (1999) examined the evidence for the effectiveness of psychotherapy for personality disorders in psychotherapy outcome studies. Fifteen studies were located that reported data on pretreatment-to-post-treatment effects and/or recovery at follow-up, including three randomized, controlled treatment trials, three randomized comparisons of active treatments, and nine uncontrolled observational studies. They included psychodynamic/interpersonal, cognitive behaviour, mixed and supportive therapies. All studies reported improvement in personality disorders with psychotherapy. The mean pre–post effect sizes within treatments were large: 1.11 for self-report measures and 1.29 for observational measures. Among the three randomized, controlled treatment trials, active psychotherapy was more effective than no treatment according to self-report measures. In four studies combined, 52% of patients remaining in therapy recovered after a mean of 1.3 years treatment. Recovery was defined as no longer meeting the full criteria for personality disorder. A heuristic model based on these findings estimated that 25.8% of personality disorder patients recovered per year of therapy, a rate sevenfold larger than that in a published model of the natural history of borderline personality disorder (3.7% recovered per year, with recovery of 50% of patients requiring 10.5 years of naturalistic follow-up). It was concluded that psychotherapy is an effective treatment for personality disorders and may be associated with up to a sevenfold faster rate of recovery in comparison with the natural history of disorders.

More recently (Leichsenring & Leibing, 2003) conducted a meta-analysis to address the effectiveness of psychodynamic therapy and cognitive behaviour therapy in the treatment of personality disorders. Studies of psychodynamic therapy and cognitive behaviour therapy that were published between 1974 and 2001 were collected. Only studies that (1) used standardized methods to diagnose personality disorders, (2) applied reliable and valid instruments for the assessment of outcome, and (3) reported data that allowed calculation of within-group effect sizes or assessment of personality disorder recovery rates were included. Fourteen studies of psychodynamic therapy and 11 studies of cognitive-behaviour therapy were included. Psychodynamic studies had a mean follow-up period of 1.5 years compared to only 13 weeks for cognitive-behaviour therapy. Psychodynamic therapy yielded a large overall effect size (1.46), with effect sizes of 1.08 found for self-report measures and 1.79 for observer-rated measures. For cognitive-behaviour therapy, the corresponding values were 1.00, 1.20, and 0.87. For more specific measures of personality disorder pathology, a large overall effect size (1.56) was seen for psychodynamic therapy. Two cognitive-behaviour therapy studies reported significant effects for more specific measures of personality disorder pathology. For psychodynamic therapy, the effect sizes indicate long-term rather than short-term change in personality disorders. They concluded that there is evidence that both psychodynamic therapy and cognitive-behaviour therapy are effective treatments of personality disorders but further studies are necessary that examine specific forms of psychotherapy for specific types of personality disorders and that use measures of core psychopathology. In the last 6 years there have been nearly as many new randomized trials of treatments for personality disorder as were included in Leichenring and Liebing's analysis, so a new systematic review of randomized trials alone is overdue.

We refrain from giving an overview of pharmacotherapy for the group of personality disorders at this time because, outside of the pharmacologic treatment of borderline personality disorder (BPD), there is very little evidence, in fact very few trials at all, for or against the pharmacologic treatment of other personality disorders. The bulk of research on pharmacotherapy (and on psychotherapy as well) has been done with people who have been diagnosed with BPD.

We now turn to the individual personality disorders themselves. The reader will note, however, that not all personality disorders as currently listed in the DSM or ICD are reviewed here. This is because there is little or no data on the effectiveness of treatment for many of the personality disorders, and rather than list them and state that we have no data, we have included a review of treatments for only those personality disorders where there have been some systematic studies of treatment(s) to review.

Paranoid personality disorder

Individuals with paranoid PD are highly suspicious of other people including doctors and often are unable to acknowledge their own negative feelings towards others. This fact alone means that treatment is problematic, but when other characteristics include inappropriate concern that other people have hidden motives, expectation of being exploited by others, inability to collaborate, social isolation, emotional detachment, and overt hostility, treatment becomes nearly impossible. This constellation of characeristics means research on this group of patients is very difficult to conduct because researchers are inevitably seen as having hidden motives. Whatever treatment method is employed, the first step is the development of a moderately trusting relationship.

Psychotherapy

There is no research specifically investigating the outcome of psychotherapeutic treatment for paranoid personality disorder. However, a number of studies have included patients with paranoid PD in assessment of treatment (see mixed personality disorders). In general, the presence of paranoid PD diminishes effectiveness of psychotherapeutic treatment for other co-occurring personality disorders.

Schizotypal personality disorder

Psychological treatment

Most of the interest in schizotypal personality disorder (STPD) has been in its relationship to schizophrenia and hence there is little data on outcome of treatment using psychosocial methods. The Chestnut Lodge follow-up study yielded some data that suggested that patients who had schizophrenia plus STPD and had been treated within the psychotherapeutic milieu did slightly better than patients without STPD (McGlashan, 1986). This unexpected finding has not been explained.

Interestingly, STPD has been one of the few personality disorders to be investigated from a preventive perspective perhaps because of its relationship to schizophrenia (Raine et al., 2003). Eighty-three children were assigned to an experimental enrichment programme from ages 3–5 years and compared with a matched control group at follow-up when the subjects were aged 17 and 23 years. Measures included schizotypal personality and anti-social behaviour. Children who participated in the enrichment programme at ages 3–5 years had lower scores for schizo-typal personality and antisocial behaviour at age 17 years and for criminal behaviour at age 23 years, compared with the control subjects. The beneficial effects of the intervention were greater for children who showed signs of malnutrition at age 3 years, particularly with respect to outcomes for schizotypy at ages 17 and 23 and for antisocial behaviour at age 17. The results are consistent with an increasing body of knowledge that implicates an enriched, stimulating environment in beneficial psychological and behavioural outcomes that could prevent the development of personality disorders.

Pharmacotherapy

Only one paper has been published which has detailed a study of a second-generation agent and STPD (Koenigsberg *et al.*, 2003). Twenty-five (mostly male) patients meeting DSM-IV criteria for STPD (and none with primary BPD) participated in a 9-week, randomized, double-blind, placebo-controlled trial of low-dose risperidone (0.25–1.5 mg/day). Fourteen were randomized to risperidone and 9 to placebo. By week 3, those on active medication showed a significantly greater decline in their negative and general symptoms. By week 7, they showed a significantly greater decline in their positive symptoms. The medication was reasonably well-tolerated in that 57% of the risperi-done-treated subjects completed the trial. There are other studies of pharmacotherapy of STPD, but these studies had subjects who had high co-morbidity rates with BPD, and it is difficult to know how to interpret these studies with respect to STPD. Thiothixene, amoxepine, fluoxetine, and haloperidol were the pharmacologic agents used in these studies.

Borderline personality disorder (BPD)

Psychotherapy and psychosocial treatment

A number of treatments for BPD have emerged over the past decade with psychotherapy being recommended in a US guideline as the primary treatment modality (Oldham *et al.*, 2001). It is not possible to recommend one specific therapy because information from research remains inadequate. It has become clear not only that a number of treatments may be of use but also that any one treatment is only helpful in around 50% of cases. Nevertheless most of research on personality disorder has been with BPD perhaps because these patients differ from most other PDs in frequent help-seeking behaviour and apparent wish to change.

Dynamic psychotherapy

Dynamic psychotherapy has long been recommended for BPD and has now been modified to target the characteristics of the disorder. Initial studies were almost universally of inpatient treatment using prospective one group pretest-posttest designs. Tucker and colleagues (1987) assessed the outcome at 1 and 2 years of 40 of 62 border-line patients treated for between 6 months to 1 year in a specialized unit. Treatment included individual, group and milieu therapies. Improvement in global function, reduction in self-destructive behaviour and suicide attempts, decreased use of hospitalization, and the development of more constructive relationships, all occurred. Copas *et al.* (1984) and McGlashan (1986) retrospectively followed-up 194 psychopathic (3–5 years) and 89 border-line patients (mean 15 years), respectively, with both studies finding symptomatic and behavioural improvement. Stone's (1993) report of up to 20 years follow-up of 550 inpatients, most of whom had received some sort of psychosocial intervention, indicated that 66% of patients were functioning well. Such studies fail to rule out other plausible alternative hypotheses of causality of change such as passage of time or subsequent outpatient treatment. Caution is suggested in ascribing benefits observed to inpatient treatment by a naturalistic five-year follow-up of individuals receiving inpatient treatment at the Cassel Hospital in London (Rosser *et al.*, 1987). Patients with borderline personality disorder (BPD) had a less favourable outcome than those with neurotic pathology, depression, high intelligence, and lack of chronic outpatient history. Whilst longer-term follow-ups are to be applauded, they are hard to interpret because there is a tendency towards regression towards the mean as other therapies are given. This applies to all disorders but as it is conventional to look at long-term improvement before confirming the efficacy of a treatment for personality disorder this complicates evaluation.

The most recent support for a psychoanalytically based approach has come from a randomized study examining the effectiveness of a psychoanalytically oriented partial hospitalization programme using mentalization based treatment (MBT) with standard psychiatric care for patients with borderline personality disorder (Bateman & Fonagy, 1999, 2001). Mentalization entails making sense of the actions of oneself and others on the basis of intentional mental states such as desires, feelings and beliefs. It involves the recognition that what is in the mind is in the mind and reflects knowledge of one's own and others' mental states as mental states. This capacity is enfeebled in borderline patients and so group and individual therapy actively focuses on developing their understanding and recognition of the feelings they evoke in others and the feelings evoked in them by others. Thirty-eight patients with borderline personality disorder, diagnosed according to standardized criteria, were allocated either to MBT or to general psychiatric care (control group) in a randomized control design. Treatment was for 18 months. Outcome measures included frequency of suicide attempts and acts of self-harm, number and duration of inpatient admissions, use of psychotropic medication, and self-report measures of depression, anxiety, general symptom distress, interpersonal function and social adjustment. Data analysis used repeated measures analysis of covariance and non-parametric tests of trend. Patients in the partial hospitalization programme showed a statistically significant decrease on all measures in contrast to the control group which showed limited change or deterioration over the same period. Improvement in depressive symptoms, decrease in suicidal and self-mutilatory acts, reduced inpatient days and better social and interpersonal function began after 6 months and continued to the end of treatment at 18 months (Bateman & Fonagy, 2001). This result suggests that rehabilitative effects were stimulated during the treatment phase, but some treatment continued during the follow-up period. The treatment has also been found to be cost-effective (Bateman & Fonagy, 2003), but as yet the active components of therapy remain unclear, especially because it was not possible to show that mentalization had increased in those patients who showed the most gains. An outpatient version of MBT is currently being evaluated for borderline and antisocial PD in a further randomized controlled trial. The treatment has now been fully manualized (Bateman & Fonagy, 2004, 2006). Treatment interventions are organized to increase the reflective or mentalizing capacity of the patient in the context of group and individual therapy. Although promising, this treatment needs further validation by researchers independent of the originators.

Another manualized dynamic therapy known as transference focused psychotherapy (TFP) is available and gives promising results. In a cohort study (Clarkin et al., 2001), 23 female borderline patients were assessed at baseline and at the end of 12 months of treatment with diagnostic instruments, measures of suicidality, self-injurious behaviour, and measures of medical and psychiatric service utilization. Compared with the year prior to treatment, the number of patients who made suicide attempts significantly decreased, as did the medical risk and severity of medical condition following self-injurious behaviour. In addition, patients during the treatment year had significantly fewer hospitalizations as well as number and days of psychiatric hospitalization compared with the year before. The dropout rate was 19%. Conference reports of a comparison study between patients treated with TFP and a matched untreated control group confirm the benefits of treatment (Clarkin, 2002). Costs have not yet been examined. The outcome of a randomized controlled trial comparing TFP, DBT and supportive psychotherapy is not yet published although its rationale has been described (Clarkin et al., 2004). However, conference reports suggest equivalence in outcome for all treatments. Ninety patients, 92% of whom were female, were randomized. At completion of treatment at 1 year there were no differences between groups on global assessment of functioning, depression scores, social adjustment, anxiety, and measures of self-harm. Interestingly, patients who received TFP showed greatest improvement on reflective function. More careful analysis of the data may show some differences but it appears that non-specific factors of therapy may be as important as specific techniques themselves. This has been suggested by Bateman & Fonagy (2000), who concluded in a review that effective treatments have (a) to be well-structured, (b) to devote considerable effort to enhancing compliance, (c) to have a clear focus whether that focus is a problem behaviour such as self-harm or an aspect of interpersonal relationship patterns, (d) to be theoretically highly coherent to both therapist and patient, sometimes deliberately omitting information incompatible with the theory, (e) to be relatively long-term, (f) to encourage a powerful attachment relationship between therapist and patient, enabling the therapist to adopt a relatively active rather than a passive stance, and (g) to be well integrated with other services available to the patient. All three treatments in this comparative trial meet these criteria.

However, a recently published randomized controlled trial (Giesen-Bloo et al., 2006) throws some doubt on the value of TFP. The treatment, given by personnel fully approved in the treatment methods, in a sample of 88 patients with borderline personality disorder, showed significantly less improvement in TFP than schema-focused cognitive-behaviour therapy over three years and TFP was more expensive. Both groups showed improvement but those in the schema-focused therapy were both greater and more prolonged than TFP. However, the results should be interpreted with caution. First, differences in outcome between the groups can be accounted for almost entirely by the larger dropout early in treatment of patients treated with TFP. Differences in outcome disappear when 'completers' from each group are compared. The larger dropout rate in TFP is of course not a trivial finding. Engaging borderline patients in long-term treatment is important. For furthering our understanding of treatment of borderline patients, first, it would be helpful to know why more dropped out in TFP than SFT. Second, follow-up is required to determine if treatment gains and group differences are maintained. Third, the results of such a long treatment need consideration in the context of follow-on research suggesting that over the same period around 40% of patients would have been expected to have improved (Zanarini *et al.*, 2003). The question might be why gains in treatment were not as large as expected in either or both treatments. Possible negative interaction between therapy and naturalistic outcome have been discussed by Fonagy & Bateman (2006).

Group psychotherapy

Non-controlled studies with day hospital stabilization followed by outpatient dynamic group therapy indicate the utility of the use of groups in BPD (Wilberg *et al.*, 1998). Although not formally psychoanalytic but focusing on relationship management, Marziali & Monroe-Blum have concentrated on group therapy alone without the additional milieu and social components of therapy. In a randomized controlled trial they found equivalent results between group and individual therapy, and they concluded that on cost-effectiveness grounds group therapy is the treatment of choice (Marziali & Monroe-Blum, 1995). But further studies are needed to confirm their findings especially since the treatment offered was less structured than most other treatments and dropout rates were high.

Cognitive analytical therapy

Cognitive analytical therapy (CAT) has been manualized for treatment of borderline personality disorder and many are enthusiastic about its effectiveness. There are some indications that the treatment method may be of help in some patients (Ryle & Golynkina, 2000), and in a small randomized trial (personal communication) patients treated with CAT showed significant improvement over time on a range of clinical measures. But there was no difference between people receiving CAT and those having other psychological treatments and so the effects may be non-specific. However, there was some indication that CAT was judged more helpful than other psychological treatments by borderline patients, which may account for a lower but non-significant attrition rate being found in CAT. A formal randomized trial comparing CAT with 'best available standard care' is currently being carried out with adolescent patients with borderline personality disorder in Victoria, Australia (Ryle, 2004). Preliminary results (Chanen, personal communication to editors) show somewhat similar outcomes.

Cognitive therapy

Cognitive-behavioural formulations of BPD are diverse. In a model derived from 'standard' CBT but modified specifically for personality disorders, Beck and associates (Alford & Beck, 1997) define personality in terms of patterns of social, motivational, and cognitive-affective processes thereby moving away from a primary emphasis on cognitions. However, personality is considered to be determined by 'idiosyncratic structures' known as schemas whose cognitive content gives meaning to the person, and it is these particular schemas that are the cornerstone of cognitive formulations of BPD. Young (1990) has developed a treatment programme for BPD based on early maladaptive schemas (EMS). These are stable and enduring patterns of thinking and perception that begin early in life and are continually elaborated. EMS are unconditional beliefs linked together to form a core of an individual's self-image. Challenge threatens the core identity which is defended with alacrity, guile, and desperation since activation of the schemas may evoke aversive emotions. The EMS gives rise to 'schema coping behaviour' which is the best adaptation to living that the borderline has found. Schema-focused therapy is only just being evaluated but its adherence to the general requirements of an effective treatment enumerated above suggests that it should be reasonably successful. A very recent report has shown its effectiveness and revealed better outcomes than that found with TFP (Giesen-Bloo *et al.*, 2006).

Safran & Segal (1990) have integrated schemas within an interpersonal context arguing that the impact of an individual's beliefs and schemas is not purely cognitive but interacts with interpersonal behaviour which, in turn, has a reciprocal effect on beliefs. This remains theoretical.

Despite all the theoretical developments and the boast that CBT is an evidence-based therapy, it is only fairly recently that there have been randomized controlled trials with treatment outcomes.

Turkat & Maisto (1985) in an uncontrolled trial reported results for 35 patients with a range of personality disorders. Treatment was based on individual formulations. Of 16 cases with outcome data, only 25% showed a positive outcome. Davidson & Tyrer (1996), in an open study, used cognitive therapy for the treatment of two cluster-B personality disorders, antisocial and borderline. They evaluated a brief (ten-session) cognitive therapy approach using single-case methodology, which showed improvement in target problems. Another small ($n = 34$), randomized controlled trial has recently been carried out using brief cognitive therapy, linked to a manual with elements of dialectical behaviour therapy incorporated, in the treatment of recurrent self-harm in those with cluster B personality difficulties and disorders. Self-harm repeaters with a parasuicide attempt in the preceding 12 months were randomly allocated to manual assisted cognitive behaviour therapy (MACT) ($n = 18$), and the rest ($n = 16$) to treatment as usual (TAU). The rate of suicide acts was lower with MACT (median 0.17/month MACT; 0.37/month TAU; $P = 0.11$) and self-rated depressive symptoms also improved ($P = 0.03$) (Evans *et al.*, 1999). The treatment involved a mean of 2.7 sessions and the observed average cost of care was 46% less with MACT ($P = 0.22$). In a more recent large study ($n = 480$), following on from the first, brief manual-assisted cognitive therapy slightly increased the likelihood of self-harm relative to treatment as usual with PD patients and in BPD increased the costs associated with on-going treatment (Tyrer *et al.*, 2004). In a more recent randomized controlled trial of borderline personality disorder with longer treatment (up to 30 sessions), from therapists trained in advance, there was significant benefit on suicidal behaviour ($n = 104$) but a non-significant increase in emergency presentations in those allocated to cognitive-behaviour therapy (Davidson *et al.*, 2006a, 2006b).

The overall evidence in favour of cognitive-behaviour therapy in the treatment of personality disorder is therefore relatively slim with much of it coming from one research group, but it has involved more patients than any other treatment modality. Further studies are currently under way.

Dialectical behaviour therapy (DBT)

DBT is a special adaptation of cognitive-behaviour therapy, which was originally used for the treatment of a group of repeatedly parasuicidal female patients with borderline personality disorder. DBT is a manualized therapy (Linehan, 1993), which includes techniques at the level of behaviour (functional analysis), cognitions (e.g. skills training) and support (empathy, teaching management of trauma) with a judicious mix of ideas derived from Zen Buddhism. The aim of DBT is initially to control self-harm but its main aim is to promote change in the emotional dysregulation that is judged to be at the core of the disorder (Putnam & Silk, 2005; Robins, 2003; Siever *et al.*, 2002). Thus the goal of DBT goes far beyond self-harm reduction. In the initial trial undertaken by its founder, 44 DSM-III-R for borderline personality disorder female patients were admitted to the trial. In addition, they had to have made at least two suicide attempts in the previous five years, with one in the preceding 8 weeks. Twenty-two women patients were assigned to DBT and 22 to the control condition. Assessment was carried out during, and at the end of, therapy, and again after 1-year follow-up

(Linehan *et al.*, 1993). Control patients were significantly more likely to make suicide attempts (mean attempts in control and DBT patients, 33.5 and 6.8, respectively), spent significantly longer as inpatients over the year of treatment (mean 38.8 and 8.5 days, respectively), and were significantly more likely to drop out of those therapies they were assigned to (attrition 50% vs. 16.7%, respectively (Linehan *et al.*, 1991)). Although DBT reduced episodes of self-harm initially, it was less effective in the longer term.

Follow-up was naturalistic and based on the proposition that the morbidity of this group precluded termination of therapy at the end of the experimental period. At 6-month follow-up, DBT patients continued to show less parasuicidal behaviour than controls, though at 1 year there were no between-group differences. At 6 months there were no between-group differences in days in hospital, but at 1 year DBT patients had had fewer days in the hospital. Treatment with DBT for 1 year compared with treatment as usual led to a reduction in the number and severity of suicide attempts and decreased the frequency and length of inpatient admission. However, there were no between-group differences on measures of depression, hopelessness or reasons for living.

The widespread adoption of DBT is both a tribute to the energy and charisma of its founder, Marsha Linehan, and to the attractiveness of the treatment, with its combination of acceptance and change, skills training, excellent manualization, and a climate of opinion that is willing and able to embrace this multifaceted approach (Swenson, 2000). While some have felt that the popularity of DBT is not justified by the strength of the evidence (Tyrer, 2002) and some feel that the conclusions are premature (Levendusky, 2000; Scheel, 2000; Turner, 2000b), currently it is the best validated treatment for BPD. A recent replication of the original study that found, in most respects, findings very similar to the original study, gives further support to its effectiveness (Linehan *et al.*, 2006). In this latest replication, treatment as usual was performed by therapists who were thought to be experts in their practice of non-DBT therapy, and despite these therapists' level of expertise, the results of this study duplicate quite closely the results of the 1991 study. However, the study compared a cohesive group of DBT therapists working as a team with a disparate group of therapists operating a variety of models of therapy, most of whom were working independently. An additional randomized study that supports the findings was performed by Verheul *et al.* (2003). In this study, 58 Dutch women who met DSM-IV criteria for BPD were assigned randomly to either 1 year of DBT or to treatment-as-usual (TAU), i.e. on going treatment in the community. Participants were clinical referrals from both addiction treatment and psychiatric services who were referred because either the therapist or patient or both felt that treatment was not working. Those not randomized to DBT treatment were referred back to their original therapist potentially creating a comparison group of disgruntled patients and therapists. Efficacy was measured in terms of treatment retention and course of high-risk suicidal, self-mutilating and otherwise self-damaging behaviours. The DBT resulted in better retention rates (63% vs. 23%) and significantly greater reductions of self-mutilating behaviours and self-damaging impulsive acts than TAU, especially among those with histories of frequent self-mutilating behaviours. The study suggests DBT is superior to TAU in reducing self-mutilating and otherwise self-damaging impulsive behaviours in patients with BPD; *post-hoc* analyses suggested that those with more severe self-harming behaviour were helped most. Although this study was conducted in the Dutch healthcare system it remains uncertain how well the treatment translates into different healthcare systems. Other studies have either been uncontrolled, too small to add any useful data (Koons *et al.*, 2000; Turner, 2000a) or have shown DBT to be no better than other active treatments such as the 12-step programme for opioid dependence (Linehan *et al.*, 2002).

It is not clear which elements of DBT (individual psychotherapy, skills training, phone consultation, therapist consultation team) make this treatment method effective (Lynch *et al.*, 2006). Two process studies investigated the process of change in DBT by focusing on the possible influence of validation (Linehan *et al.*, 2002; Linehan & Heard, 1993; Shearin & Linehan, 1992) but results are inconclusive. What we know thus far is that adding a DBT skills training group to on going outpatient individual non-DBT psychotherapy does not seem to enhance treatment outcomes. Given that DBT is described as primarily a skills-training approach (Koerner & Linehan, 1992), then, on the one hand, this finding could indicate that the central skills training component of DBT may not be of primary importance. But, on the other hand, individual DBT therapy focuses on the strengthening of skills learned in the skills groups, and trying to combine a skills training group with an individual therapy that ignores or pays minimal attention to skill strengthening may invalidate what the patient has learned in terms of utilizing learned skills in an attempt to cope with everyday functioning. Some disagree with the policy of not admitting patients to hospital, except for a bare minimum period, since some studies show that the time and structure of an inpatient setting can be used to apparently good effect (Bohus *et al.*, 2002). There are also concerns with DBT's focus on treating female-only samples.

Therapeutic community treatments

A therapeutic community (TC) may be defined as an intensive form of treatment in which the environmental setting becomes the core therapy in which behaviour can be challenged and modified, essentially through group interaction and interpersonal understanding. Although they have been in existence in the United Kingdom and Denmark for over 50 years, they have only recently been subjected to direct controlled evaluation. Although the treatments and patient populations treated are so varied that the results are difficult to interpret, the consensus, mainly advanced by proponents of the treatment, is generally favourable. A recent systematic review of the literature (Lees *et al.*, 1999, 2004) concluded that TCs, particularly the so-called 'concept' communities in the United States, were effective but the positive effects were found primarily in substance misusers in secure settings in which there is a considerable degree of coercion and no emphasis is placed on the treatment of personality disorder.

The more common version in Europe is the democratic therapeutic community and no randomized trials have been carried out in this group. However, Dolan and colleagues (Dolan *et al.*, 1997) at the Henderson Hospital, in a creative attempt to find an appropriate control group, used a non-admitted comparison sample to assess the effectiveness of treatment on core symptoms. One hundred and thirty-eight patients were studied of whom 70 were admitted and 67 not admitted either for clinical or for financial reasons. However, this is not a strict comparison group as less than 1 in 7 of those considered for the Henderson Hospital completed treatment (Rutter & Tyrer, 2003). There was significantly greater reduction in core features of personality disorder on the Borderline Syndrome Index (BSI) in the treated group than in the non-admitted group. But using the BSI as a primary outcome measure is inadequate because significant state-dependent fluctuations of core features of personality disorder may occur over time. In a UK study, the BSI has been found to lack validity and to be susceptible to distortion from current symptoms (Marlowe *et al.*, 1996). Further work has suggested that TC treatment may show cost savings over treatment in general psychiatric services primarily because of reducing the need for hospital admission (Davies *et al.*, 1999).

Extended hospital admission is thought to engender pathological dependency and regression (Linehan, 1987), although there is little non-anecdotal evidence for this. In a prospective study of 216 patients with severe personality disorder treated at the Menninger Clinic for variable lengths of time in two psychoanalytically orientated in-patient units. Gabbard *et al.* (2000) found positive change at discharge and 1 year follow-up, with no evidence of deleterious effects due to regression and dependency. Nevertheless Main's (1957) classic paper should act as a reminder that regression and countertransference diffi-culties may pose considerable difficulties for teams treat-ing patients intensively.

As there are now many more treatments available for the treatment of personality disorder, if therapeutic commu-nities are to be considered seriously as a treatment approach, then they need to come into the frame of com-parison studies. Further research should be based upon acceptable experimental designs (Haigh, 2002).

Pharmacotherapy

Numerous cross-sectional studies have documented the high percentage of borderline patients who take psycho-tropic medications (Bender *et al.*, 2001; Zanarini *et al.*, 2001). More recently, a study of the longitudinal course of borderline personality disorder (BPD) (Zanarini *et al.*, 2004b) has documented high rates of intensive polyphar-macy throughout 6 years of prospective follow-up. More specifically, 40% of the borderline patients studied took three or more medications concurrently, 20% took four or more, and 10% took five or more.

Despite this high rate of pharmacotherapy of borderline patients, surprisingly few open-label or controlled medi-cation trials of patients with BPD have been conducted. This is true whether one is referring to first-generation psychotropic medications, such as standard antipsycho-tics or tricyclic antidepressants, or second-generation medications, such as the selective serotonin reuptake inhibitors (SSRIs) or atypical antipsychotics.

We discuss below a careful review of these second gen-eration studies. Only published studies will be described and only studies limited to borderline patients have been included.

Newer antidepressants

Of all the classes of medication, antidepressants have been studied the most frequently. Five open-label trials of SSRIs have been conducted. Three of these have studied the effectiveness of fluoxetine, one has studied the effective-ness of venlafaxine, and one has studied the effectiveness of sertraline.

The open label studies include one by Norden (1989), who studied 12 outpatients in his clinical practice without current major depression meeting DSM-III-R criteria for BPD. Ratings of the effectiveness of 5–40 mg of fluoxetine over 5–26 weeks were made using an overall clinical impression of improvement. All 12 subjects were thought to have improved with 75% rated as substantially improved. Norden states (without reporting supportive data) that symptoms most responsive to fluoxetine appeared to be rejection sensitivity, anger, depressed mood, mood labi-lity, irritability, anxiety, obsessive-compulsive symptoms and impulsivity (including substance abuse and overeat-ing). Cornelius *et al.* (1990) conducted an 8-week, open-label trial of fluoxetine on five patients meeting Diagnostic Interview for Borderlines (DIB) (Gunderson, *et al.*, 1981) and DSM-III criteria for BPD. All five patients had been hospitalized multiple times, had failed other trials of psy-chotropic agents but did not have current major mood disorder or psychosis. There was a significant decrease on 13/20 outcome measures that included diverse areas of psychopathology: depression, impulsivity, hostility, paranoia, psychoticism, somatization and obsessive-compulsive symptoms. Global functioning improved, on average, from the marginal to the good range.

Markovitz *et al.* (1991) conducted a 12-week open-label trial of 80 mg of fluoxetine in 22 'treatment-resistant' subjects who met the DSM-III-R criteria for BPD ($n = 18$) and/or schizotypal personality disorder. Subjects who self-mutilated significantly reduced this behaviour. Additionally, subjects showed significant improvement on those scales of the SCL-90 (Derogatis, 1983) measuring general psychopathology, depression, anxiety, paranoia/psychoticism, obsessive-compulsive symptoms and interpersonal sensitivity. In another open-label study, Markovitz (1995) treated 23 subjects with sertraline (322 mg, SD = 141). After 1 year of treatment, the number of self-injurious patients dropped from 11 to 2 and depression scores on the Beck Depression Inventory (BDI) (Beck *et al.* 1961) were significantly reduced as were the number of episodes of self-injury per week. And Markovitz & Wagner (1995) conducted an open-label trial of venlafaxine (315 mg SD = 96) on 45 DIB and DSM-III-R BPD subjects. Thirty-nine (87%) completed all 12 weeks of the trial. The authors claim that all subscales of the SCL-90 scores decreased significantly over time but only data for the somatization subscale was presented.

Two double-blind, placebo-controlled trials of fluoxe-tine and one of fluvoxamine have also been conducted. Salzman *et al.* (1995) conducted a 13-week study of mildly disturbed symptomatic volunteers with borderline-like traits. Thirteen were randomized to fluoxetine and nine to placebo. Fluoxetine was associated with a significant decrease in anger, independent of improvement in mood. Fluoxetine-treated subjects improved significantly more than placebo-treated subjects on measures of anxiety and depression. Both groups showed significant improvement on the Global Assessment Scale (GAS) over time and both had mean scores in the recovered range (70s) at baseline. Eighty-one percent of the subjects completed the trial.

Markovitz (1995) conducted a 14-week trial involving 17 DIB and DSM-III-R borderline patients (9 on 80 mg of fluoxetine and 8 on placebo). Sixteen met current criteria for a mood disorder (10 for major depression and 6 for bipolar I or II disorder). Many also met criteria for a current anxiety disorder. The subjects taking fluoxetine (78% completion rate) showed a significantly greater response than those in the placebo group (89% completion rate) on all five of the study's outcome measures, (data not shown in original report), including reductions in depression and anxiety. However, it is not clear if fluoxetine was useful for the treatment of BPD or the co-morbid mood/anxiety disorder or some complex admixture of the two.

Rinne *et al.* (2002) conducted a 6-week placebo-controlled, double-blind trial of fluvoxamine in the treatment of 38 (20 to fluvoxamine and 18 to placebo) women with DSM-IV BPD without bipolar or psychotic disorders. About half the subjects were outpatients and the other half were symptomatic volunteers. Current co-morbid diagnoses of unipolar mood disorders and anxiety disorders, including PTSD, were both permitted and common. Those on placebo then crossed over to fluvoxamine treatment while remaining blind to their original treatment status. All subjects then participated in a 12-week open-label trial. Retention through the first six weeks of the trial was high (92%) and was still acceptable even after the full 24 weeks of the study were completed (76%). Subjects treated with fluvoxamine had a significantly greater reduction in their rapid mood shifts that was judged to be independent of a concurrent mood disorder or PTSD than those treated with placebo. However, there were no significant between-group differences on the study's other two outcome measures, anger and impulsivity, after 6 weeks of treatment.

Atypical antipsychotics

Three open-label studies assessed the safety and efficacy of clozapine (253 mg SD = 164). in samples of criteria-defined borderline patients. Frankenburg and Zanarini (1993) studied the efficacy of clozapine in 15 Revised Diagnostic Interview for Borderlines (DIB-R (Zanarini *et al.*, 1989)) and DSM-III-R borderline outpatients. All 15 also met DSM-III-R criteria for psychotic disorder NOS and reported a childhood history of severe abuse but were without concurrent major depression. Subjects

were followed from 2–9 months and re-rated blind to baseline symptom severity and level of psychosocial impairment on the Brief Psychiatric Rating Scale (BPRS [Overall and Gorham, 1962]) and GAS, respectively. There was a significant decrease in positive, negative and general symptoms found and a significant improvement in psychosocial functioning was also found.

Benedetti, Sforzini and Colombo (1998) also studied the efficacy of clozapine (44 mg SD = 19) in 12 DSM-IV BPD inpatients without concurrent major depression or a history of bipolar disorder or a psychotic disorder in an open-label trial. The severity of psychotic symptoms decreased significantly. A wide range of other symptoms, including depression, impulsivity, and affective lability, also improved significantly. In addition, psychosocial functioning improved significantly. Chengappa *et al.* (1999) reported on the use of clozapine in seven BPD women with severe self-mutilation and persistent psychotic symptoms. These subjects were diagnosed with a variety of axis I psychotic disorders and BPD. All subjects had prolonged hospitalizations and five had experienced severe and prolonged childhood abuse. Clozapine treatment was associated with statistically significant reductions in self-mutilation and increase in hospital privileges and four patients were discharged.

Schulz *et al.* (1999a) conducted an eight-week, open-label study of olanzapine (7.7 mg SD = 2.6 at conclusion of the study) in the treatment of 11 symptomatic volunteers meeting DSM-IV criteria for BPD and dysthymic disorder. There were significant reductions in 18 of the 30 outcomes studied including a broad array of symptoms on the SCL-90: obsessive-compulsive, interpersonal sensitivity, depression, anger-hostility, phobic anxiety, paranoia, psychoticism, and overall psychopathology. Significant reductions in symptom severity were found on measures of general psychopathology, schizotypal symptoms and impulsivity but, no significant declines were found on a measure of aggression. There was a significant improvement in Global Assessment of Functioning (GAF) score, with subjects moving, on average, from the fair range to the good range of functioning. Retention was high with 81% of the subjects (9/11) completing all eight weeks of the trial. The average weight gain was 8.9 lbs. (SD = 6.0).

Zanarini & Frankenburg (2001) conducted a 6-month, double-blind, placebo-controlled trial of the efficacy of olanzapine (5.3 mg SD = 3.4 at conclusion of the study) in the treatment of 28 female symptomatic volunteers between the ages of 18–40 meeting both DIB-R and DSM-IV criteria for BPD. Over 75% had a history of individual therapy, over 60% had a history of taking psychotropic medications, and over 10% had been hospitalized for psychiatric reasons. Subjects were not currently depressed and had never met criteria for a bipolar spectrum disorder or a psychotic disorder. Subjects were randomized on a 2:1 schedule with19 patients randomized to olanzapine and 9 to placebo. There were no significant baseline differences found on any of the five scales of the SCL-90 used as outcome measures. Olanzapine was superior to placebo in treating all four core aspects of borderline psychopathology: affect (anxiety), cognition (paranoia), impulsivity (anger/hostility), and interpersonal (interpersonal sensitivity), but no significant difference was found for depression. Retention was good through the first 12 weeks of the study (over 60% of both groups of subjects) but only about 40% of the olanzapine subjects and 11% of the placebo subjects remained in the study all 24 weeks. Olanzapine subjects gained significantly more weight than placebo-treated subjects (2.9 lb (SD = 5.7) vs. a mean loss of 0.8 lb(SD = 2.6)). No tardive dyskinesia or other serious movement disorders were observed.

Bogenschutz and Nurnberg (2004) conducted a 12-week placebo-controlled trial of flexible doses of olanzapine in 40 patients with BPD. Patients with schizophrenia, bipolar disorder or current major depression were excluded. Olanzapine was found to be significantly superior to placebo when considering the total score of the 9 BPD criteria, which were scored on a 1-to-7 Likert scale.

Risperidone has also been studied in an open-label and placebo-controlled manner. Rocca *et al.* (2002) conducted an 8-week, open-label trial of risperidone (3.3 mg SD = 0.5 at conclusion of the study) in 15 DSM-IV BPD patients. While these patients did not currently meet criteria for any axis I disorder, they had spent an average of 12 weeks out of the past 12 months in hospital. There was a significant improvement over time on six of the study's eight outcome measures: general psychopathology, anergia, hostility and suspicion, depression, and aggression and a significant increase in overall functioning as assessed by the GAF (moving from the marginal range to the fair range). Measures of anxiety/depression as well as thought disturbance failed to demonstrate significant change over time. Retention was high with 87% completing all 8 weeks of the trial. Schulz (1999b) also completed a double-blind, placebo-controlled trial of risperidone in borderline patients and found no significant differences between risperidone-treated subjects and placebo-treated subjects.

Nickel *et al.* (2006) performed an 8-week double blind placebo controlled study of 52 patients (26 assigned to aripiprazole, 26 to placebo) with BPD. Intention to treat analysis showed significant improvement in the active medication group for depression, anxiety, anger, and global ratings of psychopathology.

Mood stabilizers

Divalproex sodium

Two open-label studies of DSM-III-R borderline patients being treated with divalproex sodium have been conducted. Stein *et al.* (1995) studied 11 outpatients in an 8-week trial. All were in psychotherapy and none had a current major depression or a history of bipolarity or a psychotic disorder. While 8 of the 11 subjects (73%) completed the trial and half of them were judged to be responders, but significant decreases in psychopathology were found for only two of the study's five main outcomes: subjective irritability as measured by the Modified Overt Aggression Scale (OAS-M) (Coccaro *et al.*, 1991) and general psychopathology as assessed by the SCL-90. Wilcox (1995) conducted a 6-week open-label trial of divalproex sodium. He studied 30 inpatients without co-morbid disorders meeting DSM-III-R criteria for BPD but 6 were on another medication as well. There were significant decreases in both of the study's outcome measures: general psychopathology as measured by the BPRS and number of minutes in seclusion (which was viewed as a measure of agitation). The author concluded that the medication had its greatest effect on anxiety (as rated by the BPRS) and that reduced anxiety led to reduced agitation.

Hollander *et al.* (2001) completed the first placebo-controlled, double-blind study of the efficacy of divalproex sodium in 16 DSM-IV criteria-defined borderline patients. The trail lasted 12 weeks. Twelve subjects were randomized to divalproex sodium and 4 to placebo but 50% of the subjects on active medication dropped out of the study and 100% taking placebo dropped out before completing the study. While no significant between-group differences were found, 42% of subjects taking divalproex sodium were judged to be responders versus none of the subjects being treated with placebo. In addition, substantial reductions in aggression and depression were found for subjects being treated with divalproex sodium.

Frankenburg & Zanarini (2002) conducted a 6-month double-blind, placebo controlled trial of divalproex sodium (850 mg SD = 249) in the treatment of 30 symptomatic volunteers meeting DIB-R and DSM-IV criteria for BPD as well as DSM-IV criteria for co-morbid bipolar II disorder. Twenty were randomized to divalproex sodium and 10 to placebo. Most had histories of outpatient treatment. Those on active treatment experienced significantly greater reductions in three of the study's four outcome measures: interpersonal sensitivity and anger/hostility as measured by the SCL-90 and the total score of the OAS-M. However, depression, as assessed by the SCL-90, did not show a significant between-group difference. Both groups gained, on average, a small but not significantly different amount of weight (2.6 lb (SD = 5.6) vs. 0.3 lb (SD = 4.0)). Retention was quite good through the first eight weeks of the study (70% of those on active compound; 60% of those on placebo). However, only 35% of the subjects treated with divalproex sodium and 40% of the subjects treated with placebo remained in the study all 24 weeks. Given the design of the study, it is not clear whether the mild bipolarity of the subjects was being treated or their borderline lability or both.

Other mood stabilizers

Pinto & Akiskal (1998) studied eight DSM-IV borderline outpatients without a history of a major mood disorder of either a unipolar or bipolar 'nature' in an open-label trial of lamotrigine. Three of these severely ill patients were judged to be responders. The investigators reported in a series of case reports that the impulsive behaviours of these patients were completely eradicated and that they no longer met criteria for BPD.

Other medications Bohus *et al.* (1999) conducted an open-label study of nine female patients meeting DSM-IV and DIB-R criteria for BPD who were treated with naltrexone for dissociative symptoms. Patients reported significant decreases in the duration and intensity of dissociative symptoms and tonic immobility and a substantial but non-significant reduction in analgesia during treatment with this opioid antagonist. In addition, six of nine patients reported a decrease in the mean number of flash-backs per day.

Zanarini and Frankenburg (2003) studied the efficacy of omega-3 fatty acids or more specifically, E-EPA, in an 8-week, double-blind, placebo-controlled trial of 30 female DIB-R and DSM-IV BPD symptomatic volunteers. Most had prior histories of outpatient treatment. Twenty subjects were randomized to the E-EPA group and 10 were to the placebo group. All subjects took 1 gram of 97% pure E-EPA daily and 90% of the subjects in both groups completed the trial. Subjects being treated with E-EPA had significantly greater reductions in both of the study's outcome measures: aggression as measured by the OAS-M and depression as measured by the Montgomery-Asberg Depression Rating Scale (Montgomery & Asberg, 1979). The results of this preliminary study suggest that E-EPA may be a safe and effective form of monotherapy for women with moderately severe borderline personality disorder.

ECT and BPD

Feske *et al.* (2004) studied the response to ECT of three patient groups with current major depression: 20 with BPD, 42 with other personality disorders, and 77 with no axis II disorder. Patients with BPD were found to be less likely to remit from major depression after ECT than those in either comparison group (20% vs. 52% vs. 65%). The authors are unsure of what this finding means other than medication-resistant depressed patients with BPD should be referred for ECT with a lower expectation of success than patients with depression alone or depression plus another axis II disorder. In fact, the response to ECT of these latter two groups was basically the same.

Anti-social personality disorder

People with anti-social personality disorder (ASPD) show a pervasive pattern of disregard for and violation of the rights of others. Their irresponsible and aggressive behaviour begins in childhood and, in adulthood, commonly leads to trouble with the law. They express remorse for their misdemeanors. Some patients within this group represent a high risk to the public and are defined as psychopaths mainly on the basis that they have a high score on the Psychopathy Checklist-Revised (PCL-R), an instrument with demonstrable reliability and some predictive validity (Hare, 1991). In the UK this group will probably make up the bulk of those defined as having Dangerous and Severe Personality Disorder. This new concept has subsequently become a treatment and assessment programme despite the fact that there is little evidence for any effective treatment or good predictability of future violence in personality disordered patients (for discussion, see Maden & Tyrer, 2003).

Not surprisingly, psychopathic and anti-social patients are rarely concordant with the requirements of research trials and so there is limited information about treatment outside the penal system. Most studies examine the impact of treatment on individuals within prison using a pre–post design and are therefore of limited generalizability, although there are a few exceptions. In addition, studies rarely are of ASPD alone because many individuals with this diagnosis show co-morbidity for drug misuse and alcohol problems and seek treatment for these problems rather than the PD itself. A recent review (D'Silva *et al.*, 2004) identified 24 studies specifically related to psychopaths of which only three were of an appropriate design to determine whether treatment was beneficial to this group.

Psychosocial interventions

There are a number of observational studies within secure settings suggestive of some effect of psychosocial interventions on aspects of anti-social function (e.g. Quale & Moore, 1998), but most of these studies use ill-defined treatment, lack information about patient profiles, and criteria for allocation of patients to treatment is vague (Donnelly & Guy, 1998). Hughes & Hogue (1997) studied incarcerated sex offenders considered to have psychopathic disorder and who had a mean score of 21 on the PCL-R. Treatment was not specifically cognitive but from its description it is likely to be within the framework of cognitive-behaviour therapy. Patients received milieu therapy, group therapy designed to change cognitive, emotional and skill functioning and individual therapy as appropriate. On global scores there was significant change for the whole group, although 2 out of a total of 9 patients got worse. Rice et al. (1992) have reported outcomes on patients treated within the Social Therapy Unit at Penetanguishene in Canada. One hundred and seventy-six individuals who had been assessed and treated were matched on a number of variables with a group who had been assessed but not returned to the unit for treatment. Both groups were followed up for 10 years and assessed for general and violent recidivism. There was little difference in outcome between the two groups but the general recidivism rate for non-psychopaths was much lower if they had been treated, whilst that for the psychopaths was reversed; treated psychopaths showed greater recidivism than non-treated psychopaths. Other studies show little effect of treatment on these individuals.

There is very little research into treatment for ASPD within general psychiatric services. Davidson and Tyrer (1996) in their small study discussed above reported detailed clinical data on two of five patients treated with between 9–18 sessions of CBT. Outcomes were broadly positive but interpretation is hampered by the small sample, probable selection bias and lack of information about other patients in the trial. Most other studies outside the penal system investigate patients co-morbid for substance misuse and ASPD (Longabaugh et al., 1994; Project Match Research Group, 1998) or are more concerned with an aspect of behaviour, such as battering, than personality disorder itself (Saunders, 1996). In the latter, study patients with ASPD responded better to CBT treatment in terms of partners' behavioural ratings but there were similar re-offending rates of approximately 50% in 4 years. An early study (Woody et al., 1985) examining the effectiveness of dynamic therapy in opiate dependent men found that co-occurrence of ASPD led to poorer outcomes.

This finding has been confirmed by subsequent studies. A small RCT of substance abusing personality disordered patients (Fisher & Bentley, 1996), some of whom had ASPD, randomized to inpatient or outpatient group treatment using a disease recovery model, suggested that outpatient treatment performed as well as inpatient care and that both were better than a no-treatment comparison.

Avoidant personality disorder

There has been some interest in research on treatment of Avoidant PD (AvPD) but no adequate research on the other Cluster C disorders. Patients with AvPD show a pervasive pattern of social inhibition, feelings of inadequacy and hypersensitivity to negative evaluation. It is one of the more prevalent forms of personality pathology found in clinical and non-clinical populations (Ekselius et al., 2001). Its very nature as a concept also places it on the boundary between Axis 1 and Axis II disorders given its overlap with generalized social phobia (GSP). Clinicians and researchers have differentiated between the two conditions, and some treatment research has looked at the implications for AvPD on the outcome of treatment for GSP. Most studies suggest that patients with GSP with and without AvPD exhibit equivalent levels of change independent of pre-treatment severity (Mersch et al., 1995; van Velzen et al., 1997). One exception is the study by Feske et al. (1996) who found that GSP patients with AvPD showed a lower rate of improvement than those without AvPD.

One recent randomized controlled trial of cognitive behaviour therapy vs. psychodynamic therapy has been carried out in AvPD (Emmelkamp et al., 2006). This study found superior benefit for cognitive-behaviour therapy. Apart from this there are relatively few studies on treatment specific to AvPD, and most studies use an ill-defined group of patients who report social inadequacy. However, many of the trials use randomization to test treatments (Alden, 1989; Marzillier et al., 1976; Stravynski et al., 1982, 1994). These have included behavioural (usually social skills training), cognitive, interpersonal therapy, and supportive-expressive therapy. Patients are often reported to have made substantial gains in all treatment programmes (Barber et al., 1997), but many patients who complete treatment still demonstrate a low level of social function. However, any treatment gains appear to be maintained for up to 1-year after finishing active treatment (Renneberg et al., 1990). Studies that have looked at differential treatment response suggest that CBT may be more effective than IPT but the data is primarily on social and cognitive change rather than relational improvement (Barber & Muenz, 1996). There may be individual differences in how patients respond to different regimens, and patient characteristics may determine how long individuals remain in treatment because obsessional patients showed less attrition (Barber *et al.*, 1997). Alden and Campreol (1993) found that patients who reported problems with interpersonal dependence benefited from a focus on assertiveness and the development of intimate relationships whilst those whose difficulties were avoidance and emotional distance did better with *in vivo* exposure to social situations.

The limited information about treatment of AvPD may be a result of its relegation to the shadow of generalized social phobia (GSP). It is either studied jointly with other personality disorders or from within samples of patients from social phobia clinics where inevitably there is considerable overlap with GSP. Notwithstanding the validity of the diagnosis, purer samples need to be studied and investigated from an interpersonal or relational viewpoint which would fit better with a personality perspective.

Mixed personality disorders

Whilst many of the research protocols discussed in this chapter could be considered as studying mixed personality disorders, there are some studies that recruit a wide-range of personality disordered individuals. In an early randomized trial, Winston *et al.* (1991) showed no difference between short-term dynamic psychotherapy and brief adaptational psychotherapy in a mixed group of personality disorders but both were somewhat superior to a waiting-list control. This study specifically excluded patients with borderline and narcissistic features, although a later study that included some Cluster B disorders produced similar results (Winston *et al.*, 1994).

The relative effectiveness of three psychodynamically orientated treatment models for a mixed group of personality disorders: (a) long-term residential treatment using a therapeutic community approach; (b) briefer inpatient treatment followed by community-based dynamic therapy (step-down programme); and (c) general community psychiatric treatment, has been studied. Initial results suggest that the brief inpatient therapeutic community treatment followed by outpatient dynamic therapy is more effective and more cost-effective than both long-term residential therapeutic community treatment and general psychiatric treatment in the community on most measures including self-harm, attempted suicide and readmission rates to general psychiatric admission wards

(Chiesa *et al.*, 2002, 2004). Follow-up at 36 months has confirmed that patients in the step-down programme continued to show significantly greater improvement than the inpatient group on social adjustment and global assessment of mental health. In addition, they were found to self-mutilate, attempt suicide, and be readmitted significantly less at 24- and 36-month follow-up (Chiesa & Fonagy, 2003). However, the study was not a randomized trial and the groups were not strictly comparable.

Vaglum *et al.* (1990) and Karterud *et al.* (1992) prospectively studied 97 patients, many with personality disorder, (76% had an axis II DSM-III-R diagnosis), treated in a psychodynamically orientated day hospital. The programme was 5 days per week, 7 hours per day and consisted of dynamic, cognitive and expressive therapy. Primary outcome measures were SCL-90 and the Health Sickness Rating Scale. After a mean treatment time of nearly 6 months, symptom outcome was very good for patients with Axis 1 disorders only, good for Cluster C personality disorders, modest for borderline patients, and very modest for schizotypal and other Cluster A patients. They concluded that the containing capacity of a day hospital therapeutic community is substantial and that it may reduce the need for inpatient treatment. Three-year follow-up showed that the gains were maintained but borderline patients, along with schizotypal PD, failed to show improvement in social functioning.

The Norwegian group have also demonstrated that day treatment programmes for PD are generalizable to settings other than University research centres. All patients ($n = 1244$) consecutively admitted to eight different treatment centres in the Norwegian Network of Psychotherapeutic Day Hospitals were screened with the SCID-II. One thousand and ten patients were diagnosed as having PD with avoidant (20%), borderline (22%), and paranoid (12%) being the most frequent. Outcome, as assessed on symptom measures, quality of life, work functioning, and parasuicidal behaviour, was best for BPD, cluster C patients, and PD NOS and poorer for Cluster A patients. Specifically, BPD without a Cluster A co-morbid diagnosis had markedly better outcomes than those with additional paranoid presentations. High dosage of treatment appeared to give no better outcome than low treatment dosage (10 hours per week) and the University unit did no better than units at local hospitals or mental health centres (Karterud *et al.*, 2003).

The MACT study of borderline and anti-social patients described above led to a much larger study but it was not specifically on personality disorder. Seven sessions of MACT were offered to those with recurrent self-harm, 42% of whom had a personality disorder. It differed from other studies in being large ($n = 480$), being multicentred (five centres in Scotland and England), using ordinary therapists (trained in the approach) in the course of their normal work, and offering no special service for those in the trial. The results were, in general, negative in terms of efficacy compared with treatment as usual (which included psychotherapy and problem-solving treatment). Only 60% of patients attended for face-to-face sessions of MACT and for the primary outcome, proportion of patients repeating self-harm, 39% of those allocated to MACT repeated compared with 46% allocated to treatment as usual (TAU) ($P = 0.20$). There were seven suicides, 5 in the TAU group (Tyrer *et al.*, 2003). Frequency of self-harming behaviour was also reduced by 50% in the MACT group compared with TAU, but there was great variation in episodes of self-harm (Tyrer *et al.*, 2004). There was no difference in any of the secondary outcomes. However, important differences between some of these outcomes have been shown between therapists judged as competent after assessment of taped interviews in the study compared with those who were less competent (Davidson *et al.*, 2004). However this simply shows that there are competent and incompetent therapists and presumably the same applies to therapists offering the control treatment. MACT led to a cost-saving of £900 per patient compared with TAU at 6 months but this did not remain significant at 12 months (Byford *et al.*, 2003). Interestingly, in BPD, MACT increased total costs and had less satisfactory results in reducing self-harm in contrast to its effect in other personality disorders (Tyrer *et al.*, 2004).

Limitations of existing studies and directions for future research

In the light of the considerable problems which still exist in conceptualizing and defining personality disorder, separating it from other mental disorders, and designing treatment trials of long term therapy (which have adequate internal as well as external validity), whether psychological or biological, it is perhaps not surprising that our knowledge concerning effective treatments seems still to be somewhat rudimentary. Most studies investigate only small numbers of patients, have inadequate follow-up and have a number of other limitations.

Limitations using BPD as an example

(1) Semi-structured interviews are not always used to identify patients with many subjects recruited through clinical interviews or general knowledge of potential

subjects who were already receiving clinical care by the study's principal investigator or someone working with or for him.

(2) Outcomes measures that were used do not necessarily assess the major psychopathology of the disorder. Thus differences in outcome between groups may be found, but it is often unclear whether the treatment impacted or ameliorated the major psychopathology of the disorder. A clear example of an outcome measure that would assess and score all four major areas of borderline psychopathology is the Zanarini Rating Scale for DSM-IV Borderline Personality Disorder (ZAN-BPD) (Zanarini *et al.*, 2003b). It has good convergent and discriminant validity, high levels of interrater and test–retest reliability, and has been found to be a sensitive measure of change. Thus it can provide a finely grained measure of change, say, from treatment with a particular medication. The overall score provides a change measure for BPD that is equivalent to measures used to assess the efficacy of medications for axis I disorders (e.g. Hamilton Rating Scale for Depression (Hamilton, 1960) and Young Mania Rating Scale (Young *et al.*, 1978))

(3) Often, the sample is made up of Axis II patients, some of whom have a co-morbid Axis I disorder and some of whom do not. While some may argue that a pure Axis II sample is impossible to attain, given the high rates of Axis I co-morbidity (Zanarini *et al.*, 1998), it is important to remember that most of these co-morbid disorders are not chronic in nature. It should be possible to find subjects who, while they have a history of a number of axis I disorders, do not meet criteria for any of them at the time of the Axis II study.

(4) Study samples often consist primarily of treatment-resistant patients. For example, while many patients with BPD might be thought of as treatment resistant, clinical experience suggests that there is a continuum of borderline psychopathology and that many persons with BPD are on the mild, outpatient or non-patient end of the spectrum. Therefore, studying treatment-resistant patients may lead to unnecessarily modest findings or pessimistic conclusions.

(5) There may be major differences in baseline severity levels and these differences in baseline levels of severity are not defined in the study's inclusion (or exclusion) criteria. If a subject is not particularly symptomatic or has mild symptoms at baseline, substantial improvement in these symptoms would be unlikely.

In psychosocial treatments, effective treatment protocols are relatively few in number and, even where they exist, remain largely untested for adherence. Perhaps the manner in which treatment protocols were constructed and delivered may be as important in the success of these treatments as are the interventions that are more specific and theoretically driven. One way of interpreting this observation might be that part of the benefit that severely personality disordered individuals derive from their treatment comes through their experience of being involved in a well-constructed, well-structured and coherent interpersonal endeavour. It seems to us that, from one perspective at least, what may be helpful is the internalization of a thoughtfully constructed structure, the understanding of the inter-relationship of different reliably identifiable components, the causal interdependence of specific ideas and actions, the constructive interactions of professionals, and above all, the experience of being the subject of reliable, coherent and rational thinking. Social experiences such as these are not specific to any treatment modality but rather are correlates of the level of seriousness and the degree of commitment with which teams of professionals approach the problem of caring for this group who may be argued on empirical grounds to have been deprived of exactly such consideration and commitment during their early development and quite frequently throughout their later life (for review see Zanarini & Frankenburg, 1997).

While this suggestion is speculative, it may also be helpful in distinguishing successful from unsuccessful interventions and pointing the way to the creation of even more efficacious protocols in the future. Then the question would arise as to whether treatments meeting such criteria could translate 'well' to a non-research setting, where structure may be less vigorous and treatments become more individually based on the therapist's personality and/or countertransference.

As many psychosocial studies are uncontrolled and as spontaneous remission is a regular feature of patients with personality disorder, especially borderline personality disorder (Zanarini et al., 2003a), we have to be cautious in interpreting the findings. Nonetheless, studies consistently demonstrate modest gains associated with relatively high doses of treatment. Further, there is encouraging evidence that these gains are cost-effective (Gabbard et al., 1997), particularly in terms of savings in healthcare costs.

The review suggests that similar treatments tend to be effective across settings, but the kind of client group for which they are shown to be efficacious varies. Outpatient therapy may be helpful for relatively less severe cases. More severely dysfunctional individuals may gain from treatment in a day hospital or an inpatient setting.

Individuals with avoidant personality disorder appear to respond to social skills training or cognitive therapy, but here generalization beyond the treatment setting remains a problem.

Conclusions

In general, the results of psychotherapeutic treatment of personality disorder are promising to the extent that patients show improvement but disappointing in that no existing treatment helps patients return back to a normal level of function. Although there are now a few randomized controlled trials of treatments there is very little evidence to suggest specificity of any one treatment. Avoidant personality disorder may respond to a limited extent to cognitive behavioural interventions.

Clearly the requirements needed to label a psychotherapeutic treatment as specific and efficacious in the treatment of personality disorder have not been met. Work is urgently needed to identify ways of both better defining and assessing patients. A dimensional approach is most promising. Personality can be formulated from a specific theoretical orientation, a treatment designed accordingly and measures tailored to areas targeted by the treatment. Rather than comparing outcome of different approaches it may be better to ask what are the effective elements of each approach, how may they be combined to make the most efficient and effective treatment, and what is the best time for implementation, in what context and for how long? A match of patient profile and treatment strategy needs to be developed. There may need to be a staged approach of treatment with patients receiving a more supportive therapy as an inpatient or day patient followed by long-term outpatient therapy. Once behavioural stability has been achieved, for example, via DBT, a patient may consolidate the change and add depth through modified psychodynamic or psychoanalytic therapy and that in turn may be further enhanced by involvement in a therapeutic group that targets the interpersonal interactions. More attention should be given to process and dismantling studies as well as to carefully monitored single-case experiments.

Taken together, the results of pharmacological studies suggest several important findings. The first is that most of the medications studied in double-blind, placebo-controlled trials of BPD (and STPD) were found to be efficacious. The second finding is that most of these medications were found to be useful in treating symptoms of both affective dysregulation and impulsive aggression, which have been suggested to be the core dimensions of

Table 43.1. Effectiveness of treatments for personality disorder

Treatment	Form of treatment	Psychiatric Disorder/ Target audience	Level of evidence for efficacy	Comments
Psychotherapeutic	Non-specific	Personality Disorders in general	Ia	All studies (including RCTs) reported improvement with psychotherapy. Improvement was noted whether the therapy was psychodynamic, interpersonal, cognitive behavioural, or supportive. Specific personality disorders or specific treatments were not identified
Psychotherapy	Individual dynamic	Borderline personality disorder	Ib	A number of naturalistic follow-up studies support effectiveness of psychodynamic therapy (III), and there is evidence from RCT of mentalization based treatment (MBT) (1b) Also preliminary reports support effectiveness of Transference Focused Psychotherapy (IIb)
Psychotherapy	Group dynamic	Borderline personality disorder	Ib	Equivalent results when compared with individual psychotherapy but more cost-effective
Psychotherapy	Cognitive analytic	Borderline personality disorder	IIb	Improvement but equal to other psychological treatments. Patients with BPD may show better adherence to this therapy than to others
Psychotherapy	Cognitive and cognitive behavioural	Borderline personality disorder	IIa	Appears to show improvement, but multiple rigorous RCTs have not been performed
Psychotherapy	Dialectic behavioural therapy	Borderline personality disorder	Ia	Better retention rate, decrease in suicidal thoughts, self-destructive and other parasuicidal acts
Psychotherapy	Various cognitive forms	Anti-social personality disorder	III	No effect on outcome though lowered recidivism
Psychotherapy	Various cognitive forms	Avoidant personality disorder	Ia	Behavioural gains are attained but overall impact on social functioning is questionable
Therapeutic community	Milieu and other group therapies	Borderline personality disorder	III	Reduction in borderline symptoms
Day hospital	Psychodynamic orientation	Mixed personality disorders	IIb	Improvement in a number of symptoms with decreased need for inpatient hospitalization, but questionable impact on overall social functioning
Pharmacotherapy	Low-dose risperidone	Schizotypal personality disorder	Ib	Assumption can be made that low doses of other atypical as well as typical antipsychotics would probably be effective depending upon any individual's ability to tolerate side effects
Pharmacotherapy	SSRI – fluoxetine	Borderline personality disorder	Ia	Decrease in anger independent of mood
Pharmacotherapy	SSRI – fluvoxamine	Borderline personality disorder	Ib	Decrease in rapid mood shifts but no change in anger or impulsivity
Pharmacotherapy	SSRIs and other antidepressants (fluoxetine, venlafaxine, sertraline)	Borderline personality disorder	III	Decreases in various symptoms of BPD
Pharmacotherapy	Atypical antipsychotic – clozapine	Borderline personality disorder	III	Most studies confounded by other Axis I or Axis II co-morbid disorders. Improvement shown across a number of symptoms and behaviours
Pharmacotherapy	Atypical antipsychotic – olanzepine	Borderline personality disorder	Ib	Reduced various symptoms of BPD

Table 43.1. (cont.)

Treatment	Form of treatment	Psychiatric Disorder/ Target audience	Level of evidence for efficacy	Comments
Pharmacotherapy	Atypical antipsychotics – risperidone	Borderline personality disorder	III	One study found a reduction in a number of borderline symptoms; another found no difference from placebo
Pharmacotherapy	Atypical antipsychotics – aripiprazole	Borderline personality disorder	Ib	A double blind placebo controlled study found decreased anxiety, depression, anger, and global ratings of psychopathology
Pharmacotherapy	Mood stabilizers – divalproex sodium	Borderline personality disorder	Ib	Decrease in aggression and overall psychopathology. Methodological limitations and diagnostic co-morbidities make results difficult to interpret.
Pharmacotherapy	Mood stabilizers – lamotrigine	Borderline personality disorder	III	Case reports. Improvement in impulsive behaviours
Pharmacotherapy	Omega-3 fatty acids	Borderline personality disorder	Ib	Improvement in aggression and depression

psychopathology underlying BPD (Siever & Davis, 1991). This suggests that the choice of medication can be guided as much by tolerability and safety as by symptom presentation. It also suggests that the common practice of polypharmacy, which has no empirical support, may be unnecessary for most borderline patients. Clearly, more research in this area is needed, both for BPD and other axis II disorders that might be amenable to an adjunctive role for pharmacotherapy.

The level of evidence for each of the intervention discussed in this chapter is summarized in Table 43.1.

REFERENCES

Alden, L. (1989). Short-term structured treatment for avoidant personality disorder. *Journal of Consulting and Clinical Psychology*, **57**, 756–64.

Alden, L. E. & Capreol, M. J. (1993). Avoidant personality disorder: Interpersonal problems as predictors of treatment response. *Behavioural Therapy*, **24**, 357–76.

Alford, B. & Beck, A. (1997). *The Integrative Power of Cognitive Therapy*. New York: Guilford Press.

Barber, J. P. & Muenz, L. R. (1996). The role of avoidance and obsessiveness in matching patients to cognitive and interpersonal psychotherapy: empirical findings from the treatment for depression collaborative research program. *Journal of Consulting and Clinical Psychology*, **64**, 951–58.

Barber, J. P., Morse, J. Q., Krakauer, I. D. *et al.* (1997). Change in obsessive-compulsive and avoidant personality disorders following Time-limited Supportive-expressive therapy. *Psychotherapy*, **34**, 133–43.

Bateman, A. & Fonagy, P. (1999). The effectiveness of partial hospitalization in the treatment of borderline personality disorder – a randomised controlled trial. *American Journal of Psychiatry*, **156**, 1563–9.

Bateman, A. & Fonagy, P. (2000). Effectiveness of psychotherapeutic treatment of personality disorder. *British Journal of Psychiatry*, **177**, 138–43.

Bateman, A. & Fonagy, P. (2001). Treatment of borderline personality disorder with psychoanalytically oriented partial hospitalisation: an 18-month follow-up. *American Journal of Psychiatry*, **158**, 36–42.

Bateman, A. & Fonagy, P. (2003). Health service utilisation costs for borderline personality disorder patients treated with psychoanalytically oriented partial hospitalisation versus general psychiatric care. *American Journal of Psychiatry*, **160**, 169–171.

Bateman, A. & Fonagy, P. (2004). *Psychotherapy for Borderline Personality Disorder: Mentalisation Based Treatment*. Oxford: Oxford University Press.

Bateman, A. & Fonagy, P. (2006). *Mentalization Based Treatment: A Practical Guide*, Oxford: Oxford University Press.

Beck, A. T., Ward, C. H., Mendelson, M. *et al.* (1961). An inventory for measuring depression. *Archives of General Psychiatry*, **4**, 561–71.

Bender, D. S., Dolan, R. T., Skodol, A. E. *et al.* (2001). Treatment utilisation by patients with personality disorders. *American Journal of Psychiatry*, **158**, 295–302.

Benedetti, F., Sforzini, L. & Colombo, C. (1998). Low dose clozapine in acute and continuation treatment of severe borderline personality disorder. *Journal of Clinical Psychiatry*, **59**, 103–7.

Blatt, S. J., Stayner, D. A., Auerbach, J. S. & Behrends, R. S. (1996). Change in object and self-representations in long-term, intensive, inpatient treatment of seriously disturbed adolescents and young adults. *Psychiatry*, **59**, 82–107.

Bogenschutz, M. & Nurnberg, H. (2004). Olanzapine versus placebo in the treatment if borderline personality disorder. *Journal of Clinical Psychiatry*, **65**, 104–9.

Bohus, M., Landwehrmeyer, G., Stiglmayr, C. *et al.* (1999). Naltrexone in the treatment of dissociative symptoms in patients with borderline personality disorder: an open-label trial. *Journal of Clinical Psychiatry*, **60**, 598–603.

Bohus, M., Haaf, B., Simms, T. *et al.* (2002). Effectiveness of inpatient Dialectical Behavioural Therapy for Borderline Personality Disorder: a controlled trial. In *5th ISSPD European Congress on Personality Disorders – Abstracts*, pp. 18. Munich, Germany.

Byford, S., Knapp, M., Greenshields, J. *et al.* (2003). Cost-effectiveness of brief cognitive behaviour therapy versus treatment as usual in recurrent deliberate self-harm: a decision-making approach. *Psychological Medicine*, **33**, 977–86.

Campbell, M., Fitzpatrick, R., Haines, A. *et al.* (2000). A framework for the design and evaluation of complex interventions to improve health. *British Medical Journal*, **321**, 694–6.

Chengappa, K., Ebeling, T., Kang, J. *et al.* (1999). Clozapine reduces severe self-mutilation and aggression in psychotic patients with borderline personality disorder. *Journal of Clinical Psychiatry*, **60**, 477–84.

Chiesa, M. & Fonagy, P. (2003). Psychosocial treatment for severe personality disorder: 36-month follow-up. *British Journal of Psychiatry*, **183**, 356–62.

Chiesa, M., Fonagy, P., Holmes, J. *et al.* (2002). Health Service use costs by personality disorder following specialist and non-specialist treatment: a comparative study. *Journal of Personality Disorders*, **16**, 160–73.

Chiesa, M., Fonagy, P., Holmes, J. *et al.* (2004). Residential versus community treatment of personality disorders: a comparative study of three treatment programmes. *American Journal of Psychiatry*, **161**, 1463–70.

Clark, L. A., Vittengl, J., Kraft, D. *et al.* (2003). Separate personality traits from states to predict depression. *Journal of Personality Disorders*, **17**, 152–72.

Clarkin, J. F. (2002). 5th ISSPD European Congress on Personality Disorders. In *Personality Disorders: Neurobiology and Psychotherapy*. Munich.

Clarkin, J. F., Foelsch, P., Levy, K. *et al.* (2001). The development of a psychodynamic treatment for patients with borderline personality disorder: a preliminary study of behavioural change. *Journal of Personality Disorders*, **15**, 487–95.

Clarkin, J. F., Levy, K. N., Lenzenweger, M. F. *et al.* (2004). The Personality Disorders Institute/Borderline Personality Disorder Research Foundation randomised controlled trial for borderline personality disorder: rationale, methods, and patient characteristics. *Journal of Personality Disorders*, **18**, 52–72.

Coccaro, E., Harvey, P., Kupsaw-Lawrence, E. *et al.* (1991). Development of neuropharmacologically based behavioural assessments of impulsive aggressive behaviour. *Journal of Neuropsychiatry and Clinical Neuroscience*, **3** (Suppl.), 44–51.

Copas, J. B., O'Brien, M., Roberts, J. *et al.* (1984). Treatment outcome in personality disorders: the effect of social, psychological and behavioural variables. *Personality and Individual Differences*, **5**, 565–73.

Cornelius, J., Soloff, P., Perel, J. *et al.* (1990). Fluoxetine trial in borderline personality disorder. *Psychopharmacology Bulletin*, **26**, 151–4.

Davidson, K. & Tyrer, P. (1996). Cognitive therapy for antisocial and borderline personality disorders: single case study series. *British Journal of Clinical Psychology*, **35**, 413–29.

Davidson, K., Norrie, J. & Tyrer, P. (2006a). The effectiveness of cognitive behavior therapy for borderline personality disorder: results from the borderline personality disorder study of cognitive therapy (BOSCOT) trial. *Journal of Personality Disorders*, **20**(5), 450–65.

Davidson, K., Tyrer, P., Gumley, A. *et al.* (2006b). A randomized controlled trial of cognitive behavior therapy for borderline personality disorder: rationale for trial, method, and description of sample. *Journal of Personality Disorders*, **20**, 431–49.

Davidson, K., Scott, J., Schmidt, U. *et al.* (2004). Therapist competence and clinical outcome in the Prevention of Parasuicide by Manual Assisted Cognitive Behaviour Therapy Trial: the POPMACT study. *Psychological Medicine*, **34**, 855–63.

Davies, S., Campling, P. & Ryan, K. (1999). Therapeutic Community provision at regional and district levels. *Psychiatric Bulletin*, **23**, 79–83.

Derogatis, L. R. (1983). *SCL-90R: Administration, Scoring and Procedures – Manual II*. Towson, MD: Clinical Psychometric Research Inc.

Dolan, B., Warren, F. & Norton, K. (1997). Change in borderline symptoms one year after therapeutic community treatment for severe personality disorder. *British Journal of Psychiatry*, **171**, 272–9.

Donnelly, J. & Guy, S. (1998). Evaluation of a first stage pilot project to address offending behaviour in a mentally disordered population in Scotland. *Psychiatric Care*, **5**, 106–8.

D'Silva, K., Duggan, C. & Mccarthy, L. (2004). Does treatment really make psychopaths worse? A review of the evidence. *Journal of Personality Disorders*, **18**, 163–77.

Ekselius, L., Tillfors, M., Furmark, T. *et al.* (2001). Personality Disorder in the general population: DSM-IV and ICD-10 defined prevalence as related to sociodemographic profile. *Personality and Individual Differences*, **30**, 311–20.

Emmelkamp, P. M., Benner, A., Kuipers, A., Feiertag, G. A. Koster, H. C. & van Apeldoorn, F. J. (2006). Comparison of brief dynamic and cognitive-behavioural therapies in avoidant personality disorder. *British Journal of Psychiatry*, **189**, 60–4.

Evans, K., Tyrer, P., Catalan, J. *et al.* (1999). Manual-assisted cognitive-behaviour therapy (MACT): a randomised controlled trial of a brief intervention with bibliotherapy in the treatment of recurrent deliberate self-harm. *Psychological Medicine*, **29**, 19–25.

Feske, U., Mulsant, B., Pilkonis, P. A. *et al.* (2004). Clinical outcome of ECT in patients with major depression and comorbid borderline personality disorder. *American Journal of Psychiatry*, **161**, 2073–80.

Feske, U., Perry, K. J., Chambless, D. L. *et al.* (1996). Avoidant Personality Disorder as a predictor for treatment outcomes among generalised social phobics. *Journal of Personality Disorders*, **10**, 174–84.

Fisher, M. & Bentley, K. (1996). Two group therapy models for clients with a dual diagnosis of substance abuse and personality disorder. *Psychiatric Services*, **11**, 1244–50.

Fonagy, P. & Bateman, A. (2006). Progress in the treatment of borderline personality disorder. *British Journal of Psychiatry*, **188**, 1–3.

Frankenburg, F. R. & Zanarini, M. C. (1993). Clozapine treatment in borderline patients: a preliminary study. *Comprehensive Psychiatry*, **34**, 402–405.

Frankenburg, F. R. & Zanarini, M. C. (2002). Divalproex sodium treatment of women with borderline personality disorder and bipolar II disorder: a double blind placebo controlled pilot study. *Journal of Clinical Psychiatry*, **63**, 442–6.

Gabbard, G. O., Lazar, S. G., Hornberger, J. *et al.* (1997). The economic impact of psychotherapy: a review. *American Journal of Psychiatry*, **154**, 147–55.

Gabbard, G., Coyne, L., Allen, J. *et al.* (2000). Evaluation of intensive in-patient treatment of patients with severe personality disorders. *Psychiatric Services*, **51**, 893–8.

Giesen-Bloo, J., van Dyck, R., Spinhoven, P. *et al.* (2006). Outpatient psychotherapy for borderline personality disorder: randomized trial of schema-focused therapy vs transference-focused psychotherapy. *Archives of General Psychiatry*, **63**, 649–58.

Gunderson, J. G., Kolb, J. E. & Austin, V. (1981). The diagnostic interview for borderline patients. *American Journal of Psychiatry*, **138**, 896–903.

Haigh, R. (2002). Therapeutic community research: past, present and future. *Psychiatric Bulletin*, **26**, 68–70.

Hamilton, M. (1960). A rating scale for depression. *Journal of Neurology, Neurosurgery and Psychiatry*, **23**, 56–62.

Hare, R. (1991). *The Hare Psychopathy Checklist – Revised.* Toronto: Multi-Health Systems.

Hill, J., Harrington, R. C., Fudge, H. *et al.* (1989). Adult personality functioning assessment (APFA): an investigation-based standardised interview. *British Journal of Psychiatry*, **161**, 24–35.

Hollander, E., Allen, A., Lopez, R. *et al.* (2001). A preliminary double blind, placebo controlled trial of divalproex sodium in borderline personality disorder. *Journal of Clinical Psychiatry*, **62**, 199–203.

Hughes, G. & Hogue, T. (1997). First-stage evaluation of a treatment programme for personality disordered offenders. *Journal of Forensic Psychiatry*, **8**, 515–27.

Karterud, S., Vaglum, S., Friis, S. *et al.* (1992). Day hospital therapeutic community treatment for patients with personality disorder: an empirical evaluation of the containment function. *The Journal of Nervous and Mental Disease*, **180**, 238–43.

Karterud, S., Pedersen, G., Bjordal, E. *et al.* (2003). Day treatment of patients with personality disorders: experiences from a Norwegian treatment research network. *Journal of Personality Disorders*, **17**, 243–62.

Koenigsberg, H. W., Reynolds, D. & Goodman, L. (2003). Risperidone in the treatment of schizotypal personality disorder. *Journal of Clinical Psychiatry*, **64**, 628–34.

Koerner, K. & Linehan, M. M. (1992). Integrative therapy for borderline personality disorder: dialectical behaviour therapy. In *Handbook of Psychotherapy Integration*, ed. J. C. G. Norcross, pp. 433–59. New York: Basic Books.

Koons, C., Robins, C. & Tweed, J. (2000). Efficacy of dialectical behavior therapy in women veterans with borderline personality disorder. *Behavior Therapy*, **32**, 371–90.

Lees, J., Manning, N. & Rawlings, B. (1999). *Therapeutic community effectiveness. A systematic international review of therapeutic community treatment for people with personality disorders and mentally disordered offenders.* NHS Centre for Reviews and Dissemination: University of York, CRD Report 17.

Lees, J., Manning, N. & Rawlings, B. (2004). A culture of enquiry: research evidence and the therapeutic community. *Psychiatric Quarterly*, **75**, 279–94.

Leichsenring, F. & Leibing, E. (2003). The effectiveness of psychodynamic therapy and cognitive behavior therapy in the treatment of personality disorders: a meta-analysis. *American Journal of Psychiatry*, **160**, 1223–32.

Levendusky, P. (2000). Dialectical behavior therapy: so far so soon. *Clinical Psychology Science and Practice*, **7**, 99–100.

Linehan, M. M. (1987). Dialectical behavioural therapy: A cognitive behavioural approach to parasuicide. *Journal of Personality Disorders*, **1**, 328–33.

Linehan, M. M. (1993). *The Skills Training Manual for Treating Borderline Personality Disorder.* New York: Guilford Press.

Linehan, M. & Heard, H. (1993). Impact of treatment accessibility on clinical course of parasuicidal patients: reply. *Archives of General Psychiatry*, **50**, 157–8.

Linehan, M. M., Armstrong, H., Suarez, A. *et al.* (1991). Cognitive-behavioural treatment of chronically parasuicidal borderline patients. *Archives of General Psychiatry*, **48**, 1060–64.

Linehan, M. M., Heard, H. L. & Armstrong, H. E. (1993). Naturalistic follow-up of a behavioral treatment for chronically parasuicidal borderline patients. *Archives of General Psychiatry*, **50**, 971–4.

Linehan, M., Dimeff, L., Reynolds, S. *et al.* (2002). Dialectical behavior therapy versus comprehensive validation therapy plus 12-step for the treatment of opioid dependent women meeting criteria for borderline personality disorder. *Drug and Alcohol Dependence*, **67**, 13–26.

Linehan, M. M., Comtois, K. A., Murray, A. M. *et al.* (2006). Two-year randomized controlled trial and follow-up of dialectical behavior therapy vs therapy by experts for suicidal behaviors and borderline personality disorder. *Archives of General Psychiatry*, **63**, 757–66.

Longabaugh, R., Wirtz, P. W., DiClemente, C. C. *et al.* (1994). Issues in the development of client-treatment matching hypotheses. *Journal of Studies on Alcohol.* **12** (Suppl.), 46–59.

Lynch, T. R., Chapman, A. L., Rosenthal, M. Z. *et al.* (2006). Mechanisms of change in dialectical behavior therapy:

theoretical and empirical observations. *Journal of Clinical Psychology*, **62**, 459–80.

Maden, T. & Tyrer, P. (2003). Dangerous and severe personality disorders: a new concept from the United Kingdom. *Journal of Personality Disorders*, **17**, 489–96.

Main, T. (1957). The ailment. *British Journal of Medical Psychology*, **30**, 129–45.

Markovitz, P. J. (1995). Pharmacotherapy of impulsivity, aggression, and related disorders. In *Impulsivity and Aggression*, ed. E. Hollander & D. Stein. Chichester, UK: John Wiley.

Markovitz, P. J. & Wagner, C. (1995). Venlafaxine in the treatment of borderline personality disorder. *Psychopharmacology Bulletin*, **31**, 773–7.

Markovitz, P. J., Calabrese, J., Schulz, S. C. *et al.* (1991). Fluoxetine in treatment of borderline and schizotypal personality disorders. *American Journal of Psychiatry*, **148**, 1064–7.

Marlowe, M. J., O'Neill-Byrne, K., Lowe-Ponsford, F. *et al.* (1996). The borderline syndrome index: a validation study using the personality assessment schedule. *British Journal of Psychiatry*, **168**, 72–5.

Marziali, E. & Monroe-Blum, H. (1995). An interpersonal approach to group psychotherapy with borderline personality disorder. *Journal of Personality Disorders*, **9**, 179–89.

Marzillier, J. S., Lambert, C. & Kelett, J. (1976). A controlled evaluation of systematic desensitisation and social skills training for socially inadequate psychiatric patients. *Behavioural Research and Therapy*, **14**, 225–38.

McGlashan, T. H. (1986). Schizotypal personality disorder. Chestnut Lodge follow-up study: long-term follow-up perspectives. *Archives of General Psychiatry*, **43**, 329–34.

Mersch, P. P., Jansen, M. A. & Arntz, A. (1995). Social phobia and personality disorder: severity of complaint and treatment effectiveness. *Journal of Personality Disorders*, **9**, 143–59.

Montgomery, S. & Asberg, M. (1979). A new depression scale designed to be sensitive to change. *British Journal of Psychiatry*, **135**, 382–9.

Nickel, M. K., Muehlbacher, M, Nickel, C. *et al.* (2006). Aripiprazole in the treatment of patients with borderline personality disorder: a double-blind, placebo-controlled study. *American Journal of Psychiatry*, **163**, 833–8.

Norden, M. J. (1989) Fluoxetine in borderline personality disorder. *Progress in Neuro-Psychopharmacology and Biological Psychiatry*, **13**, 885–93.

Oldham, J., Phillips, K., Gabbard, G. *et al.* (2001). Practice guideline for the treatment of patients with borderline personality disorder. American Psychiatric Association. *American Journal of Psychiatry*, **158**, 1–52.

Overall, J. & Gorham, D. (1962). The brief psychiatric rating scale. *Psychological Reports*, **10**, 799–812.

Perry, J. C., Banon, E. & Ianni, F. (1999). Effectiveness of psychotherapy for personality disorder. *American Journal of Psychiatry*, **156**, 1312–21.

Pilkonis, P. A., Heape, C. L., Proietti, M. S. *et al.* (1995). The reliability and validity of two structured interviews for personality disorders. *Archives of General Psychiatry*, **52**, 1029–33.

Pinto, O. & Akiskal, H. (1998). Lamotrigine as a promising approach to borderline personality: an open case series without concurrent DSM-IV major mood disorder. *Journal of Affective Disorders*, **51**, 333–43.

Project Match Research Group (1998). Therapists effects in three treatments for alcohol problems. *Psychotherapy Research*, **8**, 455–74.

Putnam, K. & Silk, K. R. (2005). Emotion dysregulation and the development of borderline personality disorder. *Development and Psychopathology*, **17**, 899–925.

Quale, M. & Moore, E. (1998). Evaluating the impact of structured group work with men in a high security hospital. *Criminal Behaviour and Mental Health*, **8**, 77–92.

Raine, A., Mellingen, K., Liu, J. *et al.* (2003). Effects of environmental enrichment at ages 3–5 years on schizotypal personality and antisocial behavior at ages 17 and 23. *American Journal of Psychiatry*, **196**, 1627–35.

Renneberg, B., Goldstein, A. J., Phillips, D. *et al.* (1990). Intensive behavioural group treatment of avoidant personality disorder. *Behaviour Therapy*, **21**, 363–77.

Rice, M. E., Harris, G. T. & Cormier, C. A. (1992). An evaluation of a maximum-security therapeutic community for psychopaths and other mentally disordered offenders. *Law and Human Behaviour*, **16**, 399–412.

Rinne, T., van den Brink, W., Wouters, L. *et al.* (2002). SSRI treatment of borderline personality disorder: a randomized, placebo-controlled clinical trial for female patients with borderline personality disorder. *American Journal of Psychiatry*, **159**, 2048–54.

Robins, C. (2003). Dialectical behavior therapy for borderline personality disorder. *Psychiatric Annals*, **32**, 608–16.

Rocca, P., Marchiaro, L., Cocuzza, E. *et al.* (2002). Treatment of borderline personality disorder with risperidone. *Journal of Clinical Psychiatry*, **63**, 241–4.

Rosser, R., Birch, S., Bond, H. *et al.* (1987). Five year follow-up of patients treated with in-patient psychotherapy at the Cassel Hospital for Nervous Diseases. *Journal of the Royal Society of Medicine*, **80**, 549–55.

Rutter, D. & Tyrer, P. (2003). The value of therapeutic communities in the treatment of personality disorder: a suitable place for treatment? *Journal of Psychiatric Practice*, **9**, 291–302.

Ryle, A. (2004). The contribution of cognitive analytic therapy to the treatment of borderline personality disorder. *Journal of Personality* Disorders, **18**, 3–35.

Ryle, A. & Golynkina, K. (2000). Effectiveness of time-limited cognitive analytic therapy of borderline personality disorder: factors associated with outcome. *British Journal of Medical Psychology*, **73**, 197–210.

Safran, J. D. & Segal, Z. V. (1990). *Interpersonal Process in Cognitive Therapy*. New York: Basic Books.

Salzman, C., Wolfson, A., Schatzberg, A. *et al.* (1995). Effect of fluoxetine on anger in symptomatic volunteers with borderline personality disorder. *Journal of Clinical Psychopharmacology*, **15**, 23–9.

Sara, G., Raven, P. & Mann, A. (1996). A comparison of DSM-IIIR and ICD10 personality disorder criteria in an outpatient population. *Psychological Medicine*, **26**, 151–60.

Saunders, D. (1996). Feminist cognitive behavioral and process-psychodynamic treatment for men who batter: interaction of abuser traits and treatment models. *Violence and Victims*, **11**, 393–414.

Scheel, K. (2000) The empirical basis of dialectical behavior therapy: summary, critique, and implications. *Clinical Psychology Science and Practice*, **7**, 68–86.

Schulz, S., Camlin, K., Berry, S. *et al.* (1999a). Olanzapine safety and efficacy in patients with borderline personality disorder and comorbid dysthymia. *Biological Psychiatry*, **46**, 1429–35.

Schulz, S. C., Camlin, K. L., Berry, S. A. *et al.* (1999b). A controlled study of Risperidone for borderline personality disorder. In *7th International Congress on Schizophrenia Research*, pp. 296–297. Santa Fe, New Mexico: Schizophrenia Research.

Schwarz, D. & Lellouch, J. (1967). Explanatory and pragmatic attitudes in therapeutic trials. *Journal of Chronic Diseases*, **20**, 637–48.

Shearin, E. & Linehan, M. M. (1992). Patient–therapist ratings and relationship to progress in dialectical behaviour therapy for borderline personality disorder. *Behaviour Therapy*, **23**, 730–41.

Siever, L. J. & Davis, K. L. (1991). A psychobiological perspective on the personality disorders. *American Journal of Psychiatry*, **148**, 1647–58.

Siever, L. J., Torgersen, S., Gunderson, J. G. *et al.* (2002). The borderline diagnosis III: identifying endophenotypes for genetic studies. *Biological Psychiatry*, **51**, 964–8.

Slade, M. & Priebe, S. (2001). Are randomised controlled trials the only gold that glitters? *British Journal of Psychiatry*, **179**, 286–7.

Stein, D., Simeon, D., Frenkel, M. *et al.* (1995). An open trial of valproate in borderline personality disorder. *Journal of Clinical Psychiatry*, **56**, 506–10.

Stone, M. (1993). Long-term outcome in personality disorders. *British Journal of Psychiatry*, **162**, 299–313.

Stravynski, A., Marks, I. & Yule, W. (1982). Social skills problems in neurotic outpatients: social skills training with and without cognitive modification. *Archives of General Psychiatry*, **39**, 1378–85.

Stravynski, A., Belisle, M., Marcoulier, M. *et al.* (1994). The treatment of avoidant personality disorder by social skills training in the clinic or in real-life settings. *Canadian Journal of Psychiatry*, **39**, 377–83.

Swenson, C. (2000). How can we account for DBT's widespread popularity. *Clinical Psychology: Science and Practice*, **7**, 87–91.

Tucker, L., Bauer, S. F., Wagner *et al.* (1987). Long-term hospital treatment of borderline patients: a descriptive outcome study. *American Journal of Psychiatry*, **144**, 1443–1448.

Turkat, I. D. & Maisto, S. A. (1985). Personality disorders: application of the experimental method to the formulation of personality disorders. In *Clinical Outcome of Psychological Disorders*, ed. D. H. Barlow. New York: Guilford Press.

Turner, R. (2000a). Naturalistic evaluation of dialectical behaviour therapy-orientated treatment for borderline personality disorder. *Cognitive and Behavioural Practice*, **7**, 413–19.

Turner, R. (2000b). Understanding dialectical behaviour therapy. *Clinical Psychology Science and Practice*, **7**, 95–8.

Tyrer, P. (2002). Practice guideline for the treatment of borderline personality disorder: a bridge too far. *Journal of Personality Disorders*, **16**, 113–18.

Tyrer, P., Seivewright, N., Ferguson, B. *et al.* (1990). The Nottingham Study of Neurotic Disorder: relationship between personality status and symptoms. *Psychological Medicine*, **20**, 423–31.

Tyrer, P., Jones, V. & Thompson, S. (2003). Service variation in baseline variables and prediction of risk in a randomised controlled trial of psychological treatment in repeated parasuicide: the POPMACT study. *International Journal of Social Psychiatry*, **49**, 58–69.

Tyrer, P., Tom, B., Byford, S. *et al.* (2004). Differential effects of manual assisted cognitive behaviour therapy in the treatment of recurrent deliberate self-harm and personality disturbance: the POPMACT study. *Journal of Personality Disorders*, **18**, 102–16.

Vaglum, P., Friis, S., Irion, T. *et al.* (1990). Treatment response of severe and nonsevere personality disorders in a therapeutic community day unit. *Journal of Personality Disorders*, **4**, 161–72.

van Velzen, C. J. M., Emmelkamp, P. M. G. & Scholing, A. (1997). The impact of personality disorders on behavioural treatment outcome for social phobia. *Behaviour Research and Therapy*, **35**, 889–900.

Verheul, R., Van Den Bosch, L. M., Koeter, M. W. *et al.* (2003). Dialectical behaviour therapy for women with borderline personality disorder: 12-month, randomised clinical trial in The Netherlands. *British Journal of Psychiatry*, **182**, 135–40.

Wilberg, T., Friis, S., Karterud, S. *et al.* (1998). Outpatient group psychotherapy: a valuable continuation treatment for patients with borderline personality disorder treated in a day hospital? A 3-year follow-up study. *Nordic Journal of Psychiatry*, **52**, 213–22.

Wilcox, J. (1995). Divalproex sodium as a treatment for borderline personality disorder. *Annals of Clinical Psychiatry*, **7**, 33–7.

Winston, A., Pollack, J., McCullough, L. *et al.* (1991). Brief psychotherapy of personality disorders. *Journal of Nervous and Mental Disease*, **179**, 188–93.

Winston, A., Laikin, M., Pollack, J. *et al.* (1994). Short-term dynamic psychotherapy of personality disorders. *American Journal of Psychiatry*, **15**, 190–4.

Woody, G. E., McLellan, T., Luborsky, L. *et al.* (1985). Sociopathy and psychotherapy outcome. *Archives of General Psychiatry*, **179**, 188–93.

Young, J. E. (1990). *Cognitive Therapy for Personality Disorders: A Schema-focused Approach*. Sarasota, Florida: Professional Resource Exchange.

Young, R., Biggs, J., Ziegler, V. *et al.* (1978). A rating scale for mania: reliability, validity, and sensitivity. *British Journal of Psychiatry*, **133**, 429–35.

Zanarini, M. C. & Frankenburg, F. R. (1997). Pathways to the development of borderline personality disorder. *Journal of Personality Disorders*, **11**, 93–104.

Zanarini, M. C. & Frankenburg, F. R. (2001). Olanzapine treatment of borderline patients: a double-blind, placebo-controlled study. *Journal of Clinical Psychiatry*.

Zanarini, M.C. & Frankenburg, F.R. (2003). Omega-3 fatty acid treatment of women with borderline personality disorder. *American Journal of Psychiatry*, **160**, 167–9.

Zanarini, M.C., Gunderson, J., Frankenburg, F.R. *et al.* (1989). The revised Diagnostic Interview for Borderlines: discriminating BPD from other Axis II disorders. *Journal of Personality Disorders*, **3**, 10–18.

Zanarini, M.C., Frankenburg, F.R., Dubo, E. *et al.* (1998). Axis 1 comorbidity of borderline personality disorder. *American Journal of Psychiatry*, **155**, 1733–9.

Zanarini, M.C., Frankenburg, F.R., Khera, G.S. *et al.* (2001). Treatment histories of borderline patients. *Comprehensive Psychiatry*, **42**, 144–50.

Zanarini, M.C., Frankenburg, F.R., Hennen, J. *et al.* (2003a). The Longitudinal Course of Borderline Psychopathology: 6-year prospective follow-up of the phenomenology of borderline personality disorder. *American Journal of Psychiatry*, **160**, 274–83.

Zanarini, M.C., Vujanovic, A.A., Parachini, E.A. *et al.* (2003b). Zanarini rating scale for borderline personality disorder (ZAN-BPD): a continuous measure of DSM-IV borderline psychopathology. *Journal of Personality Disorders*, **17**, 233–42.

Zanarini, M.C., Frankenburg, F.R., Hennen, J. *et al.* (2004a). Axis 1 comorbidity in patients with borderline personality disorder: 6-year follow-up and prediction of time to remission. *American Journal of Psychiatry*, **161**, 2108–14.

Zanarini, M.C., Frankenburg, F.R., Hennen, J. *et al.* (2004b). Mental Health Service utilization by borderline personality disorder patients and Axis II comparison subjects followed prospectively for 6 years. *Journal of Clinical Psychiatry*, **65**, 28–36.

44

Other treatments for persistent disturbances of behaviour

Peter Tyrer and Stephen Tyrer

Editors' note

We were not sure where to place this chapter in this book. Persistent behavioural problems are a feature of many disorders and are discussed at length in the sections on organic disorders, alcohol and substance misuse, schizophrenia and child and adolescent psychiatry. Even when these are all taken into account, there remains a core of behavioural problems that goes beyond the specific diagnostic conditions concerned. These conditions or disorders are probably best considered in the same section as personality disorders as they are behaviours that either are persistent or almost seem to be a part of the person's repertoire. The preceding chapter is admirably comprehensive and covers all personality disorders in the official classification systems but it does not consider a group of interventions that is used frequently in psychiatry but not specifically for a particular diagnostic group, but for behaviour disturbance. A large number of interventions in this management area are for people with intellectual (learning) disability, a discipline which does not appear much elsewhere in this book, partly because, despite its importance, it has a relatively low base for evidence-based interventions.

Introduction

The treatment of persistent behavioural problems is usually lengthy, eventful and frustrating for both therapists and patients. Successful engagement requires commitment and perseverance, and although the therapist often hopes that any abnormal behaviour is a consequence of the disorder being treated by evidence-based therapies and should therefore improve *pari passu* with the other symptoms, all too often the behavioural difficulties persist independently. Sometimes these may be considered to be part of a personality disorder that is almost unrecognized by both therapist and patient. There is a tendency for all therapists to be shy of diagnosing personality disorder in case the label is used pejoratively as a reason for not continuing treatment. Thus, even in populations in which personality difficulties and disorders are highly prevalent, only a minority of staff will consider using this diagnosis (Bowden-Jones *et al.*, 2004). This view is shared by those who appear to have the diagnosis but when confronted with this knowledge choose to do nothing about it. Most people with personality problems have Type R (treatment resisting) rather than Type S (treatment seeking) personalities (Tyrer *et al.*, 2003a), and so it is hardly surprising that, of the 5%–8% of the population whom by epidemiological convention have a personality disorder, only a very small minority, mainly those who are borderline and avoidant, ever present for treatment directly.

When one considers the etiology and development of many persistent disorders this is not surprising. Peter Medawar was awarded the Nobel Prize for Medicine in 1960 for his work with Frank Burnet on the mechanism of acquired immunological tolerance; the young tolerate external antigens because they incorporate them into their own immature immunological systems. Similarly, young people who develop abnormal patterns of behaviour, whether by exposure to environmental insults or through constitutional change, often incorporate them into their still developing psychological systems and accept them as normal. As a consequence, many apparently abnormal features become accepted as intrinsic to normal function (i.e. are egosyntonic). There is also evidence from longitudinal studies that the younger the onset of disturbance, the more likely this is to become egosyntonic and accepted, whereas those with an older onset are more amenable to change (Aarkrog, 1994).

Cambridge Textbook of Effective Treatments in Psychiatry, ed. Peter Tyrer and Kenneth R. Silk. Published by Cambridge University Press.
© Cambridge University Press, 2008.

In this way personality and behavioural disorders differ from most other mental disorders and can be postulated more as diatheses that make a person vulnerable to mental health and behavioural problems rather than being judged as disorders per se (Tyrer, 2006). Treating these conditions requires a subtlety of touch not usually necessary with other conditions. Because of the difficulties, it is more common for researchers to identify populations that might benefit from treatment by identifying their behaviours and the context in which this is displayed rather than making a specific diagnosis.

The main problem in evaluating those with persistent behavioural problems is that treatment is normally not entertained lightly, and this goes some way towards explaining the difficulties in getting adequate studies of treatment that are sufficiently robust to be transferred into ordinary clinical practice. This clearly applies to the complex psychological treatments that require a reasonable level of motivation but may also be equally important in drug treatment, which requires an interpersonal framework in which proper informed discussion of medication can take place (Tasman et al., 2000). This is often lacking in the circumstances of treatment of most of these conditions. This subtlety can either be acknowledged by transferring treatment into indirect approaches to tackle behavioural pathology or by more coercive methods, particularly with dangerous and aggressive behaviour, in which case there is little choice for the patient to take part, or very clear positive reinforcement if and when they do.

Aggressive challenging behaviour

There are a group of disorders within those with learning disability that are not formal diagnoses but are clearly recognized and often present with persistent behavioural problems. People with learning disability may behave in an inappropriate manner for a number of reasons. These include:

(i) poor social awareness
(ii) disinhibited expression of feelings
(iii) boredom or understimulation
(iv) overstimulation
(v) the result of a physical illness, often because of pain or discomfort
(vi) the result of a psychiatric illness.

As there are many causes of this behaviour, it is essential to assess the reasons for this. The classic approach is to use the technique of functional analysis. This impressive epithet means no more than careful observation of the subject concerned over a period of time, ideally 24–48 hours, so that the relationship of antecedent conditions and the consequences of behaviour can be determined (Iwata et al., 1982; O'Neill et al., 1997). This is important as the management of an individual who behaves in an inappropriate way because of overstimulation is very different from that of a bored individual who wishes excitement. It is important also to distinguish episodic behaviours that result from environmental factors from more persistent behaviours that are long-standing and often represent learned behaviours. People in this last group bear some resemblance to those of normal intelligence who have Cluster B personality disorders.

'Challenging behaviour' is the term that is used to describe behaviour of this type. It does not have a simple equivalent in general adult psychiatry but is recognized in the behavioural problems of older people, particularly when cognitive function is impaired (see Chapter 10). Technically, the term refers to behaviours which challenge services, i.e. any behaviour that is socially unacceptable. Thus, it includes behaviours such as belching loudly in a social gathering and picking one's nose in public. For the purposes of this chapter we will confine ourselves to the management of persistent aggressive behaviour.

In learning disability, challenging behaviour is quite different from similar behaviour seen, for example, in anti-social personality disorder. Patients with intellectual impairment are often unaware of social conventions and so may behave inappropriately in social settings. At other times, these behaviours represent uninhibited expression of feelings or as a way of communicating distress or anger. Such behaviour is formally defined as 'any culturally abnormal behaviour(s) of such intensity, frequency or duration that the physical safety of the person or others is likely to be placed in serious jeopardy, or behaviour which is likely to seriously limit use, or result in the person being denied access to, ordinary community facilities' (Emerson et al., 1994). Some 10%–15% of patients with intellectual disability in contact with services exhibit such behaviour (Emerson et al., 2001) with increasing proportions accompanying greater severity of disability (APA, 1994). The scope of challenging behaviour is very wide and in addition to verbal and physical aggression includes temper tantrums, unwanted sexual contact, destruction of property and self-injury. Assessment of personality status is seldom made in this population, and as the prevalence of such disorder varies from less than 1% to 91% in a community setting and 22% to 92% in hospital settings (Alexander & Cooray, 2003), the value of such a diagnosis is dubious.

Treatments for this condition include drug treatments (mainly antipsychotic drugs), general management strategies (of which person-centred planning is the most common), and a range of psychological treatments with wide variation in their degree of evaluation. Most of the conditions described in this section are from the discipline of learning disability. This is not an area where there is a great deal of evidence about the efficacy of interventions, largely because of the difficulties in carrying out randomized controlled trials in those with significant intellectual impairment (Oliver *et al.*, 2002; Willner, 2005). But most of the relevant studies have been carried out in those with behavioural problems as it is these that present the greatest problems in management.

Anger management

The feasibility of conducting RCTs of more conventional psychological interventions has been demonstrated by two recent RCTs of anger management that were conducted amongst people with learning disabilities living in secure settings (Taylor *et al.*, 2002) and in the community (Willner *et al.*, 2002). Both of these studies used randomized allocation either to a waiting list control group or to a group treated over 12 or 9 weeks, respectively, using a package based on the methods introduced by Novaco (1975, 1979) and Black *et al.* (1997), that included both self-management and cognitive techniques. The offenders' study (Taylor *et al.*, 2002) reported significant improvements in anger control in the treated group, as assessed by participants' self-reports. Staff ratings of participants' anger showed similar gains, but the effect was not statistically significant; however, staff rated participants' behaviour on the ward as significantly improved post-treatment and at 1-month follow-up. In the community study (Willner *et al.*, 2002), the treated group improved significantly, relative to the control group and to their own pre-treatment scores, as assessed by participants' self-ratings and by carer ratings. These gains were maintained at 3-month follow-up.

As Willner puts it forcefully 'many people with learning disabilities are capable of engaging with psychological therapies; that there is a wealth of evidence, although largely from methodologically inadequate studies, that such therapies can be beneficial; and that in some contexts, there is no alternative to their use, if people with learning disabilities are to be offered opportunities to relieve their distress' (Willner, p. 84).

Behaviour therapy

Standard behavioural techniques based on operant conditioning were once extremely common in those treated in institutions for those with learning disability, including common behavioural approaches such as 'time out' (removal of the subject to an environment lacking the possibility of social reinforcement), seclusion (Rangecroft *et al.*, 1997), overcorrection and physical restraint. These are often referred to as aversive treatments, sometimes erroneously. Alternative conditioning techniques involving positive reinforcement follow the general principles of contingency management used more commonly now for drug misuse (Petry, 2006). There is also a distinction between, differential reinforcement of other behaviour (DRO) and differential reinforcement of incompatible behaviour (DRI). Most of the evidence for the success of these last two approaches is found with stereotypic behaviour only (LaGrow & Repp, 1984), but the evidence base is very slim and a meta-analysis carried out of all studies between 1976 and 1987 found serious deficiencies with the methodology of most of the investigations (Scotti *et al.*, 1991). These authors concluded that 'the results largely failed to support several widespread assumptions regarding precepts of clinical practice', a message that commonly follows from practice that is based only on supposition and apparent common sense.

A form of DRO has been proposed recently which is termed functional communication (Fisher *et al.*, 2005). This term refers to an approach to help alter inappropriate behaviour by encouraging the individual to communicate his or her wishes in an acceptable way with appropriate reward. This is carried out by reinforcing all efforts by the person undergoing scrutiny to indicate his or her feelings in a non-challenging way. Most studies in this area have been performed on small samples but some studies have shown encouraging effects (Peck Peterson *et al.*, 2005). Furthermore, in a meta-analysis of single-subject research studies (which are particularly prone to publication bias), choice-making as an intervention was shown to be effective in improving behaviour (Shogren *et al.*, 2004).

Cognitive-behavioural therapy

Although cognitive-behaviour therapy has been adapted across the field of learning disability, it has less evidence supporting it than most other areas, largely because of the absence of controlled trials. However, the idea that cognitive-behaviour therapy is not suitable for those with limited intelligence is not an adequate reason for failing to employ this mode of therapy and failure to consider this treatment is said to be misplaced. (Haddock & Jones, 2006). However, only anger management has been evaluated with any degree of rigour in this therapeutic area.

Person-centred planning

Person-centred planning has been introduced to learning disability in an attempt to give greater power to those who have this condition, by a combination of promoting increased choice, listening more to their needs and wishes, building relationships, and promoting better support systems (Browder *et al.*, 1997). It can give voice to those who would otherwise not be heard. Although popular and imbued with common sense, it has not been evaluated using controlled investigations, and there is a lack of studies of this approach in aggressive challenging behaviour.

Nidotherapy

Nidotherapy is a 'collaborative treatment involving the systematic assessment and modification of the environment to minimize the impact of any form of mental disorder on the individual or on society' (Tyrer *et al.*, 2003b). It is based on Charles Darwin's original emphasis in his theory of evolution on the 'survival of the adapted' (subsequently high-jacked by the psychologist, Herbert Spencer, to become 'survival of the fittest'). The notion of improving the adaptation of people to suitable environments rather than trying to change them to be different transfers the emphasis on change in the person to change in the environment. Although environmental changes have always been part of interventions in psychiatry (e.g. going away to the country for a rest cure), these have not been incorporated systematically into a formal treatment strategy until recently.

Nidotherapy can be considered for three forms of mental illness: (a) those in whom no gains in terms of the core features of the disorder can ever be expected (e.g. profound learning disability), (b) people in whom some improvement has been made following direct treatment but this has come to a halt and no further improvement has taken place (e.g. chronic depression, including dysthymia), (c) those for whom treatment may or may not be helpful but this is immaterial as the patient refuses treatment.

The full process of treatment in nidotherapy is described elsewhere (Tyrer & Bajaj, 2005; Tyrer & Kramo, 2006), but generally involves a single therapist (nidotherapist) working closely with the patient to get a full environmental analysis of physical, social and personal environments and then collaboratively constructing a set of planned changes, with time scales, to achieve a better fit between the patient and the environment. This does not involve any direct treatment but often requires considerable skills in acquiring a full understanding of needs and aspirations of the patient, as well as using practical common sense in ensuring that only those environmental goals that are feasible are pursued. When patients are already under the care of a clinical team, the nidotherapist is often placed in the position of advocate in acting on behalf of the patient in negotiating the required environmental changes. These may sometimes run counter to the views of the team.

Evidence base for nidotherapy

Only one randomized controlled trial has been carried out with nidotherapy (Ranger *et al.*, 2007). Fifty-two patients with a severe mental illness and comorbid personality disorder were randomized to nidotherapy plus standard care from an assertive outreach team or standard care alone. The results showed that, after 12 months, the number of days spent in inpatient care in those allocated to nidotherapy was less than half of those randomized to standard treatment, with a corresponding increase in those allocated to (cheaper) supportive placements in the community. Nidotherapy has also been tested in an open trial in those with antisocial personality disturbance leading to a corresponding reduction in aggression, but in the absence of a control group this finding is of limited value (Tyrer & Kramo, 2006). Nidotherapy is currently being evaluated for behaviour disturbance in learning disability, one of its most promising areas of enquiry, but no results are available.

Psychopharmacological treatments

Drug treatment has been used for many years to treat those with learning disability who show behavioural problems and is usually, if not always appropriately, the first choice of management. In the first half of the last century, the choice of treatment included bromides, barbiturates and antihistamines and, more recently, antipsychotic drugs, mood stabilizers and selective serotonin reuptake inhibitors (SSRIs).

Antipsychotic drugs

The extent of use of antipsychotic drugs in learning disability is enormous. In a systematic review Brylewski & Duggan (2004) found over 500 citations to this treatment but only nine randomized controlled trials could be included in the analyses. The authors' conclusion in 1999 that 'these trials provided no evidence as to whether antipsychotic medication does or does not help adults with intellectual disability and challenging behaviour' (Brylewski & Duggan, 1999), might today not be stated quite so negatively, but it is a very unsatisfactory evidence base for a common treatment. What is also alarming is that many clinicians continued to use these medications for years without giving patients a trial without therapy, even though around one in three are able to stop treatment without problems (Ahmed *et al.*, 2000).

Some of these trials, even the less satisfactory ones, are worth looking at more closely, and there is some recent evidence from new randomized trials that could revise this verdict. Van den Borre *et al.* (1993) carried out a complicated cross-over trial involving the administration of risperidone (4–12 mg daily) or placebo to existing medication for 3 weeks followed by placebo wash-out for 1 week and then another 3 weeks treatment using the alternative cross-over medication. Thirty-seven patients were recruited and 30 finished the study. The results suggested a positive effect with risperidone but were completely compromised by differing results in the cross-over arms, a common problem when there are carry-over effects from one treatment to another.

Buitelaar *et al.* (2001) also examined the efficacy of risperidone in a 6-week double-blind, randomized, parallel-group design in the treatment of aggression in 38 hospitalized adolescents with mild, borderline intellectual disability and dull normal intelligence who had a primary diagnosis of DSM-IV disruptive behaviour disorders. Risperidone, at a mean dose of less than 3 mg, was associated with significant improvement in severity of illness and behaviour disturbance. Gagiano *et al.* (2005) compared risperidone (1–4 mg daily, mean 1.45 mg) and placebo in 77 patients with intellectual disability (including 18% with borderline intelligence in the risperidone group) over a 4-week period in a double-blind randomized trial, with outcome determined primarily by the Aberrant Behavior Checklist (ABC). The second author of this chapter (ST) also took part in the recruitment for, and treatment in, this trial (actually begun as two trials which were then amalgamated) but was not informed of, or acknowledged about, its publication, despite repeated attempts to obtain this information. Patients on risperidone improved by 22% more than those allocated to placebo ($P < 0.04$) but those on placebo improved by 31%, showing the extent of non-specific factors in the treatment of aggressive challenging behaviour. Irritability was the first symptom to show differential improvement with risperidone as early as two weeks. Risperidone is now used widely in learning disability units in the United Kingdom, where it is often assumed to be a standard accepted treatment despite not being licensed for this condition. The only independently funded (Department of Health) randomized controlled trial of antipsychotic drug treatment in aggressive challenging behaviour, the NACHBID study, carried out across in 11 centres in the UK

and Australia, compared placebo, risperidone in increasing daily dosage over 12 weeks (1.07–1.78 mg), haloperidol (2.54–2.94 mg) and found placebo to be the most effective drug at the 4 week primary outcome point in reducing aggression (79%), compared with the two active drugs (57%) combined (P = 0.06). The health costs of placebo over periods of treatment of 4 weeks to 6 months was also cheaper and significantly more cost-effective than the two active drugs (Tyrer *et al.*, 2007).

Very recently, a discontinuation study with zuclopenthixol (Haessler *et al.*, 2007) showed possible benefit of the drug, but only in terms of maintaining improvement after treatment. In patients with intellectual disability and challenging behaviour who had improved after treatment, withdrawal of the active drug was followed by a worse outcome in those randomized to placebo compared with zuclopenthixol. However, it would be mistake to assume that a discontinuation study in itself shows evidence of efficacy for reasons which are spelt out more clearly in Chapter 27.

Mood stabilizers

Two randomized trials (Tyrer *et al.*, 1984; Craft *et al.*, 1987) have been carried out with lithium in the treatment of aggressive challenging behaviour in learning disability. Tyrer *et al.* (1984) treated 25 inpatient adults with learning disability and persistent aggressive behaviour in a double-blind cross-over trial lasting 5 months, comparing the effects of lithium with placebo on aspects of aggressive behaviour. All patients were receiving neuroleptic and/or anticonvulsant drugs which were continued during the trial. Seventeen of the patients showed greater improvement with the lithium phase of treatment compared to placebo. Craft *et al.* (1987) in a parallel group trial lasting 4 months involving 42 mentally handicapped patients, compared aggression in patients randomized to lithium and placebo. In the lithium-treated group, 73% of patients showed a reduction in aggression during treatment and somewhat better scores than placebo. Although neither of these studies used an accepted scale, no instrument was available at the time and this was not a major problem in design, the results persuaded the Committee on Safety of Medicines to license lithium for the treatment of aggression in this population. Despite this, the drug is not widely employed in practice.

Topiramate, an anti-epileptic drug, has also shown promise, but only in open trials (Janowsky *et al.*, 2003). Other anticonvulsants, including carbamazepine and sodium valproate, have also been used, but the evidence base for benefit is meagre.

Table 44.1. Effectiveness of treatments for persistent disturbances of behaviour

Treatment	Form of treatment	Psychiatric Disorder	Level of evidence for efficacy	Comments
Functional Communication Training (a form of DRO)	Individual treatment	Behavioural disturbance in moderate or severe intellectual disability	IIb	Evidence from one meta-analysis of single case studies only
Anger management	Group	Challenging behaviour	Ib	Some small evidence of efficacy with maintenance of effects
Cognitive behaviour therapy	Individual	Aggressive challenging behaviour	III	No good comparative studies
Nidotherapy	Individual	Comorbid personality disorder and severe mental illness	Ib	Reduced bed usage with nidotherapy
Person-centred planning	Individual	Learning disability in general	III	No adequate controlled studies
Antipsychotic drugs	Risperidone (1–4 mg)	Aggressive challenging behaviour	Ib	The best evidence to date but still built on very low numbers in company-sponsored trials
Lithium	Standard dosage for correct blood levels	Aggressive challenging behaviour	Ib	Reduction in aggressive behaviour with lithium reasonably well demonstrated
Topiramate	200 mg daily	Aggressive challenging behaviour	III	Case studies only

Selective serotonin reuptake inhibitors

Although selective serotonin reuptake inhibitors (SSRIs) have been used repeatedly for the treatment of aggressive challenging behaviour, there have been no adequate trials of effectiveness and the evidence is circumstantial or based on simple open-label studies (e.g. Janowsky *et al.*, 2005). The positive findings of benefit from these drug company sponsored studies has to be offset against a case-note study of Branford *et al.* (1998) that showed no benefit for these drugs.

Summary and conclusions

In the absence of a good evidence base, it is comfortable to adopt the Hippocratic precept of '*Primum non nocere*' in treating behavioural problems in those with learning disability. However, the recent work on encouraging choice in functional communication training, which is supported by a form of meta-analysis, suggests a way forward in those with less profound intellectual disability. With regard to the use of pharmacological agents a recent systematic review concludes 'If there is an obvious physical or psychological cause for the behaviour, this should be managed in an appropriate way. If no psychiatric disorder can be recognized then non-medication based

management should be considered depending on the formulation. Sometimes, after considering non-medication-based management options, medication may be used either on its own or as an adjunct to no-medication based management.' (Deb *et al.*, 2006, p. 9).

It is hoped that this advice can become less delphic in the future. The findings of the NACHBID study (Tyrer *et al.*, 2007) suggest that the common widespread practice of giving antipsychotic drugs for challenging behaviour needs urgent review and much more research in needed into the effects of psychological interventions to reinforce what is at present a slim evidence base (Table 44.1).

REFERENCES

Aarkrog, T. (1994). *Borderline Adolescents 20 Years Later*. Vojens: PJ Schmidt.

Ahmed, Z., Fraser, W., Kerr, M. P. *et al.* (2000). Reducing antipsychotic medication in people with a learning disability. *British Journal of Psychiatry*, **176**, 42–6.

Alexander, R. & Cooray, S. (2003). Diagnosis of personality disorders in learning disability. *British Journal of Psychiatry*, **182** (Suppl. 44), S28–S31.

American Psychiatric Association (1994). *The Diagnostic and Statistical Manual of Mental Disorders*, 4th edn. Washington: American Psychiatric Association.

Bowden Jones, O., Iqbal, M. Z., Tyrer, P. *et al.* (2004). Prevalence of personality disorder in alcohol and drug services and associated co-morbidity. *Addiction*, **99**, 1306–14.

Branford, D., Bhaumik, S. & Naik (1998). Selective serotonin re-uptake inhibitors for the treatment of perseverative and maladaptive behaviours of people with intellectual disability. *Journal of Intellectual Disability Research*, **42**, 301–6.

Browder, D. M., Bambara, L. M. & Belfiore, P. J. (1997). Using a person-centred approach in community-based institutions for adults with developmental disabilities. *Journal of Behavioral Education*, **7**, 519–28.

Brylewski, J. & Duggan, L. (1999). Antipsychotic medication for challenging behaviour in people with intellectual disability: a systematic review of randomized controlled trials. *Journal of Intellectual Disability Research*, **43**, 360–71.

Brylewski, J. & Duggan, L. (2004). Antipsychotic medication for challenging behaviour in people with learning disability Cochrane Database of Systematic Reviews, **3**, CD000377. Oxford: Update Software Ltd.

Buitelaar, J. K., Van der Gaag, R. J., Cohen-Kettenis, P. & Melman, C. T. M. (2001). A randomized controlled trial of risperidone in the treatment of aggression in hospitalized adolescents with subaverage cognitive abilities. *Journal of Clinical Psychiatry*, **62**, 239–48.

Craft, M., Ismail, I. A., Krisnamurti, D. *et al.* (1987). Lithium in the treatment of aggression in mentally handicapped patients: a double-blind trial. *British Journal of Psychiatry*, **150**, 685–9.

Deb, S., Clarke, D. & Unwin, G. (2006). *Using Medication to Manage Behaviour Problems Among Adults with a Learning Disability: Quick Reference Guide.* Birmingham: University of Birmingham.

Emerson, E., McGill, P. & Mansell, J. (1994). *Severe Learning Disabilities and Challenging Behaviours – Designing High Quality Services.* London: Chapman and Hall.

Emerson, E., Kiernan, C., Alborz, A. *et al.* (2001). The prevalence of challenging behaviors: a total population study. *Research in Developmental Disabilities*, **22**, 77–93.

Fisher, W. W., Adelinis, J. D., Volkert, V. M., Keeney, K. M., Neidert, P. L. & Hovanetz, A. (2005). Assessing preferences for positive and negative reinforcement during treatment of destructive behavior with functional communication training. *Research in Developmental Disabilities*, **26**, 153–68.

Gagiano, C., Read, S., Thorpe, L. *et al.* (2005). Short- and long-term efficacy and safety of risperidone in adults with disruptive behavior disorders. *Psychopharmacology (Berlin)*, **179**, 629–36.

Haddock, K. & Jones, R. S. (2006). Practitioner consensus in the use of cognitive behaviour therapy for individuals with a learning disability. *Journal of Intellectual Disability*, **10**, 221–30.

Haessler, F., Glaser, T. & Beneke, L. J. *et al.* (2007). Zuclopenthixol in aggressive challenging behaviour in learning disability: discontinuation study. *British Journal of Psychiatry*, **190**, 447–8.

Iwata, B. A., Dorsey, M. F., Slifer, K. J. *et al.* (1982). Toward a functional analysis of self injury. *Analysis and Intervention in Developmental Disabilities*, **2**, 1–20.

Janowsky, D. S., Kraus, J. E., Barnhill, L. J. *et al.* (2003). Effects of topiramate on aggressive, self-injurious, and disruptive/destructive behaviors in the intellectually disabled: an open-label retrospective study. *Journal of Clinical Psychopharmacology*, **23**, 500–4.

Janowsky, D. S., Shetty, M., Barnhill, L. J. *et al.* (2005). Serotonergic antidepressant effects on aggressive, self-injurious and destructive/disruptive behaviours in intellectually disabled adults: a retrospective, open-label, naturalistic trial. *International Journal of Neuropsychopharmacology*, **8**, 37–48.

LaGrow, S. J. & Repp, A. C. (1984). Stereotypic responding: a review of intervention research. *American Journal of Mental Deficiency Research*, **88**, 595–609.

O'Neill, R. E., Horner, R. H., Albin, R. W. *et al.* (1997). *Functional Analysis of Problem Behavior: A Practical Assessment Guide*, 2nd edn. Pacific Grove, CA: Brooks/Cole.

Oliver, P. C., Piachaud, J., Done, J. *et al.* (2002). Difficulties in conducting a randomised controlled trial of health service interventions in intellectual disability: implications for evidence-based practice. *Journal of Intellectual Disability Research*, **46**, 340–5.

Peck Peterson, S. M., Caniglia, C., Royster A. J. *et al.* (2005). Blending functional communication training and choice making to improve task engagement and decrease problem behaviour. *Educational Psychology*, **25**, 257–74.

Petry, N. (2006). Contingency management treatments: a uniquely American approach, or perhaps even better suited for European drug abuse treatment? *British Journal of Psychiatry*, **189**, 97–8.

Ranger, M., Barrett, B., Milosevska, K. *et al.* (2007). Nidotherapy in comorbid severe mental illness and personality disorder: a randomised controlled trial. *British Journal of Psychiatry* (submitted).

Rangecroft, M. E. H., Tyrer, S. P. & Berney, T. P. (1997). The use of seclusion and emergency medication in a hospital for people with learning disability. *British Journal of Psychiatry*, **170**, 273–7.

Scotti, J. R., Evans, I. M., Meyer, L. H. *et al.* (1991). A meta-analysis of intervention research with problem behavior: treatment validity and standards of practice. *American Journal on Mental Retardation*, **93**, 233–56.

Shogren, K. A., Faggella-Luby, M., Bae, S. J. & Wehmeyer, M. L. (2004). The effect of choice-making as an intervention for problem behavior: a meta-analysis. *Journal of Positive Behavior Interventions*, **6**, 228–37.

Tasman, A., Riba, M. B. & Silk, K. R. (2000). *The Doctor–Patient Relationship in Pharmacotherapy: Improving Treatment Effectiveness.* New York: Guilford Press.

Taylor, J. L., Novaco, R. W., Gillmer, B. & Thorne, I. (2002). Cognitive-behavioural treatment of anger intensity among offenders with intellectual disabilities. *Journal of Applied Research in Intellectual Disabilities*, **15**, 151–65.

Tyrer, P. (2006). Personality diatheses: a superior explanation than disorder. *Psychological Medicine*, (in press).

Tyrer, P. & Bajaj, P. (2005). Nidotherapy: making the environment do the therapeutic work. *Advances in Psychiatric Treatment*, **11**, 232–8.

Tyrer, P. & Kramo, K. (2006). Nidotherapy in practice. *Journal of Mental Health*, **16**, 117–31.

Tyrer, S. P., Walsh, A., Edwards, D. E. *et al.* (1984). Factors associated with a good response to lithium in aggressive mentally handicapped subjects. *Progress in Neuropsychopharmacology and Biological Psychiatry*, **8**, 751–5.

Tyrer, S. P., Aronson, M. E. & Lauder, J. (1993). The effect of lithium on behavioural factors in aggressive mentally handicapped subjects. In *Lithium in Medicine and Biology*, ed. N. J. Birch, C. Padgham & M. S. Hughes, pp. 119–25. Carnforth: Marius Press.

Tyrer, P., Mitchard, S., Methuen, C. & Ranger, M. (2003a). Treatment-rejecting and treatment-seeking personality disorders: Type R and Type S. *Journal of Personality Disorders*, **17**, 265–70.

Tyrer, P., Sensky, T. & Mitchard, S. (2003b). The principles of nidotherapy in the treatment of persistent mental and personality disorders. *Psychotherapy and Psychosomatics*, **72**, 350–6.

Tyrer, P., Oliver-Africano, P. C., Ahmed, Z. *et al.* (2007). Neuroleptics in the treatment of aggressive challenging behaviour for people with intellectual disabilities (NACHBID trial). *Health Technol Ass* (in press).

Van den Borre, R., Vermote, R., Buttiens, M. *et al.* (1993). Risperidone as add-on therapy in behavioral disturbances in mental-retardation – a double-blind placebo-controlled cross-over study. *Acta Psychiatrica Scandinavica*, **87**, 167–71.

Willner, P. (2005). The effectiveness of psychotherapeutic interventions for people with learning disabilities: a critical overview. *Journal of Intellectual Disabilities Research*, **49**, 73–85.

Willner, P., Jones, J., Tams, R. & Green, G. (2002). A randomised controlled trial of the efficacy of a cognitive-behavioural anger management group for adults with learning disabilities. *Journal of Applied Research in Intellectual Disabilities*, **15**, 224–35.

Sexual and gender identity disorders

Section editors

Michael King and James Barrett

45

Effectiveness of treatments of sexual disorders

Michael King

Editor's note

Treatment for sexual problems is a relatively new venture for psychiatry. If one imagines the evidence base for treatment of all mental disorders in 1906, it has a parallel for sexual therapies today. This granted, a tremendous amount has been achieved in a short time, particularly when one considers that the views of Krafft-Ebing, the author of *Psychopathia sexualis* (Krafft-Ebing, 1886), one of the least evidence-based psychiatric textbooks ever written, were the standard teaching 100 years ago. Krafft-Ebing regarded all sexual problems as indicative of degeneracy, and his book is well summarized by Shorter (1997, p. 96) as 'a classic example of psychiatry run off the rails, of the misuse of scientific authority to demonize cultural preferences'. Now sexual disorders are recognized as problems that people recognize about their own sexual function, not problems from afar decided by censorious public opinion. However, even at this relatively early stage in understanding treatment there is concern that sexual therapy might become a 'life-style issue', with many with normal sexual function wishing to improve their performance for special occasions, and this trivializes what to others are serious difficulties that create much handicap. If we maintain the level of vigilance and common sense shown in this chapter, we should not go too far awry.

Introduction

Claims for a scientific approach to sexual behaviour stem from antiquity (King, 1994). However, the reduction of sexual behaviour into medical terms accelerated in the late nineteenth century with Krafft-Ebing (1886) and Havelock-Ellis (Ellis & Symonds, 1897). Sexual abnormalities were confined to diagnoses that today we would consider paraphilias or sexual deviations and were regarded as either biological disorders or severe psychological pathology amenable to 'working through' in psychoanalysis. Havelock Ellis was more concerned with describing so-called 'normal' sexuality than its pathological expression (Porter & Hall, 1995). Sexual orientation was also a particular obsession of both sexologists and psychoanalysts at least until the 1960s when the behaviourists rose to pre-eminence (King & Bartlett, 1999).

The so-called sexual liberation in Western countries in the 1960s threw off decades of conservative public morality in which it was barely possible to talk about sexual matters. Early seeds of this revolution had appeared immediately after World War II, when Alfred Kinsey and his colleagues shocked America with their pioneering (but methodologically flawed) studies of usual sexual behaviour (Kinsey *et al.*, 1948). In the 1950s and 60s William Masters, a gynaecologist and Virginia Johnson, a psychologist, developed instruments to measure human sexual response and began a project that included direct laboratory observation and measurement of hundreds of men and women while they were having intercourse or masturbating. Based on data collected in this study, they published their book *Human Sexual Response* (Masters & Johnson, 1966). This led inevitably to the conception of sexual dysfunction wherein problems of ordinary sexual behaviour, such as a difficulty initiating or sustaining an erection, became disorders requiring treatment. Sexual therapy expanded rapidly after the publication of Masters and Johnson's subsequent book *Human Sexual Inadequacy* (Masters & Johnson, 1970). This unfortunate title heralded the view that adequacy could be restored in the course of a number of sessions with two skilled therapists. Masters and Johnson advocated a short, intensive therapy in which the dysfunctional couple would book into a hotel and have daily sessions with the therapist

Cambridge Textbook of Effective Treatments in Psychiatry, ed. Peter Tyrer and Kenneth R. Silk. Published by Cambridge University Press.
© Cambridge University Press, 2008.

duo, completing 'homework' later in their room. The treatment combined sexual education with a mainly behavioural intervention aimed at reducing anxiety about sexual performance and increasing the focus on mutually pleasurable sexual arousal. Masters and Johnson claimed that only 20% of couples failed to respond. Helen Kaplan also developed a well-known therapeutic approach in the 1970s, combining a similar behavioural approach with short analytical therapy (Kaplan, 1974). Cognitive theory was introduced into sexual therapy in the 1970s and 1980s (Hawton, 1998) but more recently, therapy for the common sexual dysfunctions has become a post-modern muddle that attempts to integrate education, psychotherapy and medical interventions (Wiederman, 1998), but more is written about this later.

Although the medical view of sex met increasing and well considered criticism (Illich, 1975; Foucault, 1978; Szasz, 1983; Scruton, 1986), it took off at an even greater pace after the British scientist Giles Brindley, who developed intracavernosal drug therapy for erectile dysfunction stepped onto the platform at the American Urological Association meeting in 1983 and displayed his own phentolamine-induced erection (Marks, 2003). A new remedy had arrived that would ensure a man an erection regardless of his sexual or emotional predisposition. The only drawback was the need for an injection into the penis and occasional, unwelcome priapism (prolonged erection). The introduction of oral treatments has been the most recent advance in treatment of erectile dysfunction but it is fast becoming a routine treatment in the hands of primary care physicians (Meuleman, 2003). This increasing substitution of biological for psychological reductionism was largely met with a collective sigh of relief among patients and many in the medical profession for whom the stigma of psychological 'inadequacy' or pathology was unacceptable (Schover & Leiblum, 1994).

Classification of sexual dysfunction

Sexual problems that are not due primarily to physical disorders can be divided into difficulties of desire, arousal, orgasm and pain (Table 45.1). The first three terms arose from the early work of Masters and Johnson (1970) who, as we have seen, were radical in their observational, laboratory-based approach to the study of usual sexual function.

Desire is conceptualized as a wish to engage in sexual activity and the occurrence of sexual fantasies. It is best described as a feeling tone which is common and long lasting. Arousal or excitement is the temporary, immediate feeling of sexual excitement together with the bodily changes that accompany it, such as erection or vaginal lubrication. Orgasm is the peak of sexual pleasure, which is accompanied by genital and perineal muscle contractions, contraction of anal sphincters and (usually) ejaculation in the man. Resolution is the final phase of penile detumnescence, restoration of vaginal volume to normal and physical and mental relaxation. A refractory phase in men then occurs during which it is difficult or impossible to achieve an erection. The phase may last anything between 10 minutes and 48 hours depending on age and physical health.

It is immediately apparent that defining abnormality in any one of these processes is subjective and depends on the values, wishes and sexual knowledge of the potential patient and his or her partner. For example, when is ejaculation considered premature? It seems that Kinsey was unconcerned by the issue concluding on the basis of his extensive interviews with men that 75% reported ejaculating within two minutes of penetration (Kinsey et al., 1948). Definitions that go beyond the DSMIV (Table 45.1) would add that the man has 'little or no voluntary control' over ejaculation (McMahon et al., 2004). DSMIV requires that there be 'clinically significant impairment or distress' for most definitions of disorder. In sexual dysfunction, however, distress may occur exclusively in the partner. For example, in women with hypoactive sexual desire disorder or men with premature ejaculation, it may be only the partner who complains and is responsible for the help-seeking that ensues.

Until the pharmaceutical industry took an interest in the field, the classification of sexual problems in men was relatively uncontroversial beyond the realms of philosophical debate. Now there is widespread concern that epidemiological studies funded by pharmaceutical companies are reporting inflated prevalences of sexual disorders and therefore creating a 'need' for treatment (Akkus et al., 2002; Mirone et al., 2002; Tiefer, 2000). This has in turn led to claims that the pharmaceutical industry is 'building the science of female sexual dysfunction' (Moynihan, 2003). The word *dysfunction* implies a state of *dis-ease* that requires treatment. A woman-centred definition of sexual problems has recently been recommended as an alternative to concepts of sickness and health (Tiefer, 2000; Moynihan, 2003) and the international classifications of sexual dysfunction are currently under review (Vroege et al., 1998; Basson et al., 2000). Some consider that women's sexual function is completely different to men's, in that it is responsive rather than spontaneous and more dependent on emotional closeness with her partner (Basson, 2001). We need further evidence that the common complaints of lack or loss of sexual

Table 45.1. Difficulties of sexual function not explained by medical disorders (based on DSMIV)

Problem Area	Manifested as ...
Desire	• *Hypoactive sexual desire disorder* (persistently or recurrently deficient (or absent) sexual fantasies and desire for sexual activity) • *Sexual Aversion Disorder* (persistent or recurrent extreme aversion to, and avoidance of, all (or almost all) genital sexual contact with a partner)
Arousal	• *Female sexual arousal disorder* (persistent or recurrent inability to attain, or maintain until completion of sexual activity, an adequate lubrication-swelling response of sexual excitement) • *Male erectile disorder* (persistent or recurrent inability to attain, or maintain until completion of sexual activity, an adequate erection)
Orgasm	• *Female orgasmic disorder* (persistent or recurrent delay in, or absence of, orgasm following a normal sexual excitement phase) • *Male orgasmic disorder* (persistent or recurrent delay in, or absence of, orgasm following a normal sexual excitement phase) • *Premature ejaculation (PE)* (persistent or recurrent ejaculation before, on, or shortly after penetration and before the person wishes it)
Pain	• *Dyspareunia (not due to a medical condition)* (recurrent or persistent genital pain associated with sexual intercourse in men or women) • *Vaginismus (not due to a medical condition)* (recurrent or persistent spasm of the musculature of the outer third of the vagina that interferes with sexual intercourse. There may be associated spasm of the internal adductor muscles of the thighs.)

desire in men or women are obstacles to satisfactory sexual relations or that a medical solution is indicated. For many people, reduced sexual interest or response may be a normal adaptation to stress or an unsatisfactory relationship.

This chapter concerns the evidence for effectiveness of treatments of sexual dysfunction. Despite their long history, psychological treatments have accumulated much less evidence of effectiveness than their biomedical counterparts and thus this chapter will inevitably devote much more space to the latter. In fact, research into the efficacy of psychosexual approaches has been gradually declining (Schover & Leiblum, 1994). In addressing the empirical basis for psychosexual therapy, a cynic could be forgiven for describing it as an evidence free zone. A harsher critic might even go so far as to describe it as a theory free zone (Weiderman, 1998). The principal reasons for this gap in the evidence are money and the relative complexity of the undertaking. Not only are there less funds available than for biological research, but also estimating efficacy of a complex psychological intervention for a multifactorial condition that may be the result of complex physical, psychological and cultural factors is a daunting proposition. In particular, we lack evidence for the efficacy of the various components of sex therapy (Weiderman, 1998). As our understanding of sexual dysfunction becomes more

complex, using a similar therapeutic approach to all comers is becoming meaningless (Rosen & Leiblum, 1995).

For the remainder of this chapter I describe the treatment approaches that have been developed to manage the principal sexual dysfunctions and suggest possible avenues for development in the future. In so doing I shall concentrate on the commonest sexual dysfunctions, namely erectile disorder and orgasmic dysfunction in men and hypoactive sexual desire, orgasmic dysfunction and vaginismus in women. I shall finish with a brief review of transsexualism and its management.

Male sexual dysfunction

Sexual disorder in men has been the target of the most extensive and successful expansion of medical treatments. This has meant that we know most about the vascular function and neurophysiology of the male genitals and a brief description of this field is needed for a fuller understanding of current treatments. The penis is composed of two functional compartments, the dorsal, paired corpora cavernosa and the ventral, corpus spongiosum, surrounded by the tunica albuginea. The corpora cavernosa are complex structures composed of smooth muscle fibres, neurones, endothelial lined vascular spaces, coiled arteries and arterioles. The blood supply arises from the paired cavernosal arteries, which are terminal branches of the internal pudendal artery. The helicine arteries, which are branches of the cavernosal artery, open directly into the cavernosal spaces. Blood drains into post-cavernosal venules to reach larger veins that pass through the tunica albuginea and connect with the deep dorsal vein. Blood is retained in the penis during erection by passive compression of the cavernosal venules against the tunica albuginea. Neurological control of erection and ejaculation is complex and incompletely understood. Innervation is by somatic and autonomic nervous systems. The somatic system supplies sensory innervation to the penis and perineal skeletal muscle motor fibres. The sacral parasympathetic neurones are chiefly responsible for initiating and maintaining erection, while sympathetic supply coordinates detumescence and maintains the penis in a flaccid state. Sympathetic activity also predominates in the control of ejaculation. A potential 'ejaculation generator' has been identified in the lumbar spinal cord in rats (Truitt & Coolen, 2002). Several neurotransmitters are involved in erection, but the principal mediator is nitric oxide. Nitric oxide activates the enzyme guanil cyclase, which facilitates the production of guanosine monophosphate (GMP), a potent smooth muscle relaxant. Phosphodiesterases break down GMP and thus blocking their action using phosphodiesterase inhibitors such as *sildenafil* (Viagra) facilitates and prolongs erection. Other active neurotransmitters in the pathway are vasoactive intestinal polypeptide, prostaglandin I_2 and prostaglandin E.

Erectile disorder

As in all diagnoses in this field (and for that matter in psychiatry and medicine as a whole), deciding whether a problem exists requires a degree of subjectivity. The simplest definition is an inability to initiate or sustain a penile erection (hard enough for penetrative sex) until orgasm. The dysfunction may be situational, e.g. with one partner but not with another, or depend on the type of penetration such as oral versus vaginal or anal. It may be primary in that the man has always suffered a degree of difficulty or secondary following a period of normal function. It may occur in all settings including masturbation or only with partners or in particular activities. Figures vary as to its prevalence; in the United Kingdom 8.8% of men of all ages report current erectile disturbance and rates rise with age (Nazareth *et al.*, 2003). Figures for the United States are similar with 7% of 18 to 29-year-olds and 18% of 50 to 59-year-olds

reporting trouble maintaining or achieving and erection (Laumann *et al.*, 1999).

Drug treatments

As already discussed, the earliest successful drug treatments for erectile dysfunction in men were injectables such as *alprostadil* or prostaglandin E. Alprostadil injected into the corpora cavernosa will cause erections that are not mediated by sexual activity. Although running a low risk of priapism, penile pain and fibrosis if used frequently in the longer term, prostaglandin-E remains a useful alternative for men who do not respond to *sildenafil*, particularly after radical prostatectomy. Transurethral preparations of prostaglandin-E are less effective, particularly where there is vascular insufficiency (Porst, 1989; Dinsmore, 2004). Other injectables are *phentolamine*, an alpha-adrenoceptor-blocking drug, and *papaverine*, a non-specific phosphodiesterase inhibitor, neither of which are licensed for use in the United Kingdom. The injectable, intracavernosal drugs are effective but are subject to a high discontinuation rate (Fazio & Brock, 2004). Rates of success in a head-to-head comparison of *alprostadil, papaverine-phentolamine* combination and *papaverine* alone were 72%, 61% and 31%, respectively (Porst, 1989). They are largely reserved for men who fail on oral phospohodiesterase-5 inhibitors and men after radical prostatectomy. Transurethral *alprostadil* is an alternative route of administration to intracavernosal administration but trials have shown mixed response rates of between 30% and 66% of patients noting improvement (Fazio & Brock, 2004). A small open trial has recently suggested that up to 30% of men (including a quarter that had undergone radical prostatectomy) who fail to respond to *sildenafil* may respond to transurethral *alprostadil* (Jaffe *et al.*, 2004).

The first licensed oral drug for erectile dysfunction, the phospohodiesterase-5 inhibitor, *sildenafil*, revolutionized treatment of men with erectile difficulties and has become the first line of treatment (Anon, 2004). By inhibiting breakdown of GMP in penile tissues, it prolongs smooth muscle relaxation and facilitates erection. Adverse effects relate to its action on other phosphodiesterase systems in the body. These include headache, flushing of the skin (particularly of the face and neck), stomach upsets and nasal stuffiness. However, in randomized, controlled studies, only 1% of men stop taking the drug because of adverse effects (Goldstein *et al.*, 1998). The blue visual tinge that is very rarely reported is due to its weak action on phosphodiesterase-6 activity in the retina. Although initial trial reports indicated efficacy rates of 80% to 90%, success in clinical practice is closer to 50% (Morgentaler,

1999). A meta-analysis of trials involving over 2200 men indicated that *sildenafil* led to a higher percentage of successful intercourse attempts (57% to 21%; weighted mean difference 33.7%, CI 29.2, 38.2) than placebo and a greater percentage of men experiencing at least one intercourse success during treatment (83% versus 45%; relative benefit increase 1.8, CI 1.7, 1.9) (Fink *et al.*, 2002). Efficacy in diabetes is about 50% but much lower after radical prostatectomy, particularly if nerve-sparing techniques have not been used. Nitrate drugs are the main contra-indication as, in combination with *sildenafil*, they may lead to profound and life threatening hypotension. *Tadalafil* is a second phosphodiesterase-5 inhibitor with a half-life at least twice that of *sildenafil*, which has recently been approved for prescription in Europe. A review of efficacy trials involving 2102 men had a significant improvement of 6.5 or 8.6 (depending on dose) in erectile function score on the International Index of Erectile Function domain score and a mean success rate of intercourse attempts of 58% and 68%, respectively, compared with 31% in the placebo groups. 71% and 84% reported improved erections at the endpoint vs. 33% on placebo. *Tadalafil* was effective for up to 36 hours after dosing, a much longer window of effect than for *sildenafil*. (Carson *et al.*, 2004). A further drug *vardenafil* appears to have equivalent efficacy and duration of action to *sildenafil* but no meta-analysis of its efficacy has been published to date.

Thus evidence for the phospohodiesterase-5 inhibitors is of the strongest kind. Unfortunately, easy availability of an oral treatment for erectile dysfunction may mean that major psychological factors are overlooked or by-passed. Although *sildenafil* is useful in younger men with primarily psychogenic erectile dysfunction, clinical impression (the lowest form of evidence!) suggests that psychological dependence on using the drug can quickly become established and simply compound the difficulties. Furthermore, there is already evidence that the drug has a street value and can be misused by men with normal sexual function (Tong & Boyer, 2002; Romanelli & Smith, 2004). Where performance anxiety is very high, however, *sildenafil* can reduce tension enough to re-establish a sense of relaxation, help the man to focus on his anxious cognitions and eventually return to normal sexual function (Schover & Leiblum, 1994). It can also be useful in sexual relationships that are unconsummated, particularly where the man loses his erection at the moment of penetration. Possibly its greatest role in men with psychological difficulties is that it gives hope that sexual function can return to normal and gives time for psychological work to proceed. Much more evidence is needed on the efficacy of this approach (Weiderman, 1998).

Apomorphine is a sublingual medication that acts centrally on dopamine systems to promote erection. Two placebo-controlled, randomized trials involving a total of just over 800 men have indicated modest success in terms of proportion of successful attempts at intercourse (von Keitz *et al.*, 2002; Dula *et al.*, 2001). A third trial involved 43 men in a comparison of *apomorphine* with *sildenafil* in which *apomorphine* behaved little differently from placebo in the principal *sildenafil* trials (Perimentis *et al.*, 2004). Its action on dopamine means that it may also increase sexual drive. This latter observation has been under investigation in women and is returned to later in the chapter.

Yohimbine is an indole alkaloid that is found in several plant sources including Rauwolfia root and the bark of the African *Pausinystalia yohimbe* tree. It is a potent, selective alpha$_2$-adrenoceptor antagonist that also has weaker alpha$_1$-adrenoceptor antagonist activity. Its mechanism of action is uncertain but it is thought to affect noradrenergic outflow (sympathetic tone) from the brain. It is sold in several over-the-counter remedies for sexual dysfunction, including low libido. Relatively few randomized trials have been conducted, but it would appear that the drug has a moderate effect on erectile dysfunction at doses of 15 to 30 mg daily. A meta-analysis published in 1998 concluded that *yohimbine* is superior to placebo in the treatment of erectile dysfunction (odds ratio 3.85, 95% confidence interval 6.67 to 2.22) and that serious adverse reactions were infrequent and reversible (Ernst & Pittler, 1998). A further review 2 years later was more conservative in its conclusion suggesting that, since in several trials, the placebo response was also very high conclusions on efficacy were difficult to draw (Tam *et al.*, 2001).

A plethora of complementary (usually herbal) remedies are claimed to have benefit in treating male sexual dysfunction, particularly erectile disorders. Unfortunately there is no evidence of efficacy for any one of them and what is worse some may even have the opposite effect of that intended (Moyad *et al.*, 2004). Given that placebo responses may range up to 30% even in trials of phosphodiesterase inhibitors, it is no surprise that there are many claims of success.

Testosterone replacement in men is beyond the scope of this chapter and is used mainly where hypogonadism is well established (Morgentaler, 1999). There is no good evidence yet for an andropause (male menopause), although there is speculation that androgen insensitivity may occur in later life and respond to testosterone replacement (Gould *et al.*, 2000). A report on modelling the relative costs of the available treatments for erectile dysfunction has suggested that *sildenafil* (and vacuum devices) should be considered as first line management strategies whereas intracavernosal injection, transurethral *alprostadil* and penile implants should be reserved for second or third line treatment (Health Outcomes Research Design Consultants LLC, 2000). This is in accord with clinical opinion and conclusions in the literature on effectiveness.

Psychological treatments

As already discussed, psychological treatment of erectile dysfunction has a long history beginning with psychoanalytical approaches in the early twentieth century (Weiderman, 1998). These treatments gave way to behavioural approaches with Masters and Johnson's recommendations, cognitive and behavioural approaches in the 1980s and systemic and conjoint approaches in the 1980s and 1990s, in which sexual dysfunction was almost always regarded as a problem for the couple rather than the individual (Weiderman, 1998). Unfortunately, we have little in the way of evidence for these treatments. Unresolved Oedipal conflicts or sexual attraction to either parental figure were seen in psychoanalytical theory as the root cause of the erectile difficulty. Oblivious to what must be an almost daily event in low income countries, psychoanalysts thought that a child witnessing sexual behaviour between his or her parents would be traumatized as a result. Working through past experiences and relationships and bringing them into consciousness was considered the aim of therapy. The level of evidence of this approach in any sexual disorder remains at the descriptive and case study level. There have been no well conducted clinical trials of psychoanalytical treatment of sexual dysfunction.

Although there is evidence of positive benefit in cohort studies (Sarwer & Durlak, 1996), traditional sexual therapy using a Masters and Johnson approach has also little controlled trial evidence to back it up. Masters & Johnson regarded anxiety as central to many couple's sexual difficulties. Their 'non-genital sensate focus' advised the couple to abstain from penetrative sex and spend time using massage to 'pleasure' each other without touching each other's genitals. In this way, the man could relax and forget his goal-driven pattern of behaviour. He would notice that erections would return and gain confidence accordingly. The couple would proceed to 'genital sensate focus' when they would fondle each other's genitals and reach orgasm if desired. Penetration would be re-introduced gradually either in a side-to-side or partner-on-top position. Masters & Johnson's early accounts claimed a very high success rate, but this has never been replicated in a high quality clinical trial. Throughout these years, there was little question of the assumption that anxiety was bad for sex. However, the relationship between anxiety

and sexual performance is complex. Although most sex therapists would regard anxiety (and particularly performance anxiety when the man is distracted by sexual 'goals' such as erection and ejaculation rather than allowing himself to be absorbed in the pleasurable experience of sex) as the cause of sexual problems, empirical evidence for this assumption is poor. Anxiety induced by performance demand appears to increase sexual arousal in men and women with no sexual problem and anxiety may only be a problem in people who are *already* dysfunctional (van den Hout & Barlow, 2000) Extreme anxiety, for example in soldiers on the battlefield, may induce erection and even ejaculation in the absence of sexual feelings (Bancroft, 1989).

Just as Helen Kaplan who in the 1970s advocated using brief analytical methods if a behavioural approach failed (Kaplan, 1974), most sex therapists today take a pragmatic approach in which they combine several approaches – psychological and biomedical. Cognitive and behavioural approaches to erectile dysfunction also assume that the man has become distracted by his difficulty, and that this increasing anxiety and despair is acting in a vicious cycle of performance anxiety and preventing recovery. Thus the approach is for the man to be mindful of his thoughts both in fantasized and in actual sexual contact, to explore the evidence for his distorted thoughts and focus his attention on pleasurable sensations in sex, eschewing any notions of goal orientated tasks. Although his partner is encouraged to help him in this venture, it seems that more than one-half of partners of men with erectile dysfunction show very limited interest in accepting help with relationship issues, general sexual issues and lifestyle issues (Lee *et al.*, 1998). The presenting patient is usually a man who wishes to regain a rigid penis with as little (psychological) fuss as possible. Nevertheless, to practitioners in the field this treatment approach appears to bear fruit and has been widely recommended (Hawton, 1998). However, it lacks careful appraisal in large, multicentre trials and brief versions of the approach appear to add no benefit when examined as an adjunct to biological treatments such as intracavernosal *alprostadil* (Van der Windt *et al.*, 2002). Thus the evidence for psychosexual interventions of a cognitive or behavioural type remains at the descriptive level. Given the enthusiasm for assessing the efficacy of similar treatments in other fields such as depression, this is disappointing and probably reflects a further hurdle to good research in this domain, namely the notion that (until the advent of pharmacological treatments and the increased debate about sexual disorders) that erectile dysfunction was a 'lifestyle' problem. It is to be hoped that recent qualitative research revealing the severe psychological impact of such dysfunction will have dispatched that notion once and for all (Tomlinson & Wright, 2004).

Couple sexual therapy, which usually incorporates an eclectic mix of counselling and behavioural techniques, is used for erectile dysfunction. Again, there is little evidence for its efficacy. However, in one small, but interesting trial, couple therapy was combined with a physical treatment. Half of couples receiving therapy were randomized to use a vacuum erectile device and there was limited evidence of efficacy for the combined approach (Wylie *et al.*, 1996).

Despite lack of evidence for effectiveness, pelvic floor muscle (or Kegel) exercises are often recommended as a potential treatment for erectile dysfunction and more particularly premature ejaculation (see below). Such exercises were recently tested in a small randomized trial involving men aged 20 and over with erectile dysfunction of at least 6 months' duration and in whom there were no obvious neurological problems or a history of urological surgery (Dorey *et al.*, 2004). The muscle exercises were combined with manometric biofeedback whereby men could test the degree of their puborectalis muscle contraction using an anal probe connected to a meter. After 3 months men in the intervention group showed significant increases in self-reported erectile function and increased pelvic muscle contraction.

Orgasmic disorders in men

Premature ejaculation

Ejaculation may occur before or after the man (and/or his partner) wants it, or not at all. A common sexual problem in men is ejaculation with minimal stimulation before, on or shortly after penetration, before he wishes it and over which he has little or no voluntary control (McMahon *et al.*, 2004). Prevalence estimates for premature ejaculation vary widely. One estimate in the UK where the problem was regarded as severe was 4% (Nazareth *et al.*, 2003), while in the USA, there are suggestions that a milder form of the problem may occur in up to 30% of men of all ages (Laumann *et al.*, 1999). The etiology of premature ejaculation is unclear. It may be a result of organic causes such as low serum testosterone, major neurological disorders such as multiple sclerosis or even prostatic infection (Jannini *et al.*, 2002). Psychoanalytic theories focused on sadistic or narcissistic tendencies as etiological in premature ejaculation. By ejaculating quickly, the man symbolically prevented his partner reaching orgasm and thus denied her/him sexual satisfaction (Ellis, 1936; Jannini *et al.*, 2002). However, retarded ejaculation was also regarded as an expression of unconscious aggression and anger against

the partner (McMahon *et al.*, 2004). Cultural and evolutionary theories have also been advanced to explain premature ejaculation, in that ejaculation in the mammalian world is usually a very rapid event and speed is likely to be selected for (Metz & Pryor, 2000). Thus our current view of this issue may be cultural as much as medical (Jannini *et al.*, 2002). In fact, causation is likely to be multiple, including a failure to learn to control ejaculation, anxiety and high sexual arousal.

Medical treatments for this problem have been described since *clomipramine* was first reported to retard orgasm in up to 80% of men and women who took it (Monteiro *et al.*, 1987). The drug treatment approaches to premature ejaculation are daily, or as needed, treatment with serotonergic antidepressants. Best randomized trial evidence appears to support the efficacy of most selective serotonin reuptake inhibitors (SSRIs) (except *fluvoxamine*) with little difference between *sertraline, fluoxetine* and *paroxetine* in delaying effect ejaculation (Waldinger *et al.*, 2001; Mendels *et al.*, 1995). Intermittent (i.e. on the day of intercourse) appears to as effective as daily administration for most men (Kolomazník, 2004).

Topical anaesthetics have long been used by men with premature ejaculation. A small randomized trial has recently shown a clear advantage of a *lidocaine-prilocaine* solution over placebo with a five- to six-fold increase in intravaginal ejaculatory latency time (Busato & Galindo, 2004). However, one-third of participants dropped out of the trial. Vaginal hyposensitivity in the partner occurred in only one case. Creams are not particularly popular in clinical practice as they are messy to use, sometimes cause too much anesthesia and occasionally cause allergic dermatitis.

Despite the lack of evidence at the level of a meta-analysis, the American Urological Association has just issued guidelines for the pharmacologic management of premature ejaculation (Montague *et al.*, 2004) in which they recommend *paroxetine, sertraline* and *clomipramine* in continuous or intermittent dosage. Despite lack of evidence of safe, long-term efficacy, they also suggest that a topical anaesthetic applied to the penis combined with use of a condom may be useful.

Retarded ejaculation and anorgasmia

Delayed or retarded ejaculation is a less common, but particularly troubling problem in men with prevalence rates of almost 3% in the UK (Nazareth *et al.*, 2003) and under 2% in the USA (Laumann *et al.*, 1999). The degree of severity ranges from complete absence of orgasm, to experiencing orgasm or emission without orgasm solely during sleep, to orgasm only in masturbation, to men who can be orgasmic with their partner but only during non-penetrative sex. A number of substances including alcohol and antidepressant drugs may inhibit ejaculation.

Evidence for effective pharmacological treatment is poor. Drugs facilitate ejaculation by either a central dopaminergic or anti-serotonergic mechanism of action. Although alpha-adrenergic agonists such a *phenylpropolamide*, *pseudoephedrine* and *ephedrine* have been suggested, their efficacy is doubtful and they have a tendency to cause retrograde ejaculation into the bladder through relaxation of the internal urethral sphincter (Jannini *et al.*, 2002; McMahon *et al.*, 2004). Complete anorgasmia is a rare and usually primary condition that is also unlikely to respond to drug treatment, unless occurring in men with spinal cord injuries (Kamischke & Nieschlag, 2002).

Psychological and behavioural treatments for orgasmic disorders

Like psychological treatments for sexual dysfunction, those for ejaculatory disorders have a long history. They are also of uncertain efficacy, particularly in the longer term (Grenier & Byers, 1995; Kandeel *et al.*, 2001). There is no evidence that psychoanalysis is effective in this condition. Behavioural techniques developed by Masters and Johnson and their colleagues include the squeeze technique, when the penis is pressed lightly just below the glans. This induces a reflex that retards ejaculation. However, it may also lead to loss of erection or ejaculation itself if performed too close to the point of inevitability. Sensate focus can also be used in premature ejaculation to reduce anxiety but as discussed this therapy has not been subjected to a randomized trial. The stop–start technique developed by Semans (1955) and taken up particularly by Kaplan (1974) is one where the man close to orgasm stops moving or actually withdraws his penis. At least one small trial has examined the 'pause–squeeze' technique in combination with antidepressant drugs and reported that it had equal efficacy except in comparison to *paroxetine*. However, this was a very small trial with some methodological difficulties. Cognitive-behavioural therapy with a particular focus on anxiety management is thought to be useful but good evidence for efficacy is lacking. Developing increased tone in the pubococcygeous muscles (so called Kegel exercises after Alfred Kegel who developed them) in which the man clenches his perineal area as if to stop in the middle of micturition, are said to improve ejaculatory control (La Pera & Nicastro, 1996). However, a recent controlled trial found little effect for this treatment.

Delayed ejaculation or anorgasmia that is not secondary to testosterone deficiency or other physical cause may respond to hyperstimulation in masturbation and/or a vibrator applied to the frenulum area of the penis. Once the man has achieved an orgasm on his own, this can be a watershed in that climaxes are reached much more easily thereafter. If he has a partner, he is encouraged to reach orgasm in his or her presence and then begin insertive sexual intercourse just before or at the point of ejaculation. There is only descriptive evidence for this approach. There are many case reports in the literature on psychodynamic, behavioural and cognitive approaches to retarded ejaculation (e.g. Catalan, 1993) but empirical evidence to support any in particular are lacking.

A meta-analysis of bibliotherapy for a range of sexual disorders, most of which concerned orgasmic function, reported a sample size adjusted effect size of 0.5 (van Lankveld, 1998). Bibliotherapy is an intervention in which written material plays a central role and a description of a particular treatment method is typically its focus. This may simply show that simple advice and education is as effective as anything else in these disorders.

Female sexual dysfunction

Female sexual dysfunction has a complex mix of biological, psychological and interpersonal determinants and appears to be age related (Basson *et al.*, 2000). Unfortunately, our knowledge of the physiology of the female sexual response has lagged far behind that of the male. However, there is increasing evidence that the neurological and vascular changes occurring in sexual arousal in men have their counterparts in the clitoral engorgement, vaginal expansion and lubrication seen in women. It is generally accepted that the clitoris is central to sexual arousal in women (Caruso *et al.*, 2004). Neurotransmitter function seen in the male corpora cavernosa appears to be similar in the parallel structure in the clitoris. Women with disorders such as diabetes will commonly have sexual dysfunction just as in men. However, the physical aspects of sexual arousal, lubrication and orgasm are not strongly correlated with sexual distress. Although real interest in female sexual function only took off at the end of the 1990s, some centres now recommend a comprehensive evaluation that includes measurement of serum hormones, vaginal pH, genital vibratory perception thresholds and the use of ultrasonography to measure labial, clitoral vaginal and uterine blood flows (Moynihan, 2003). A detailed psychological assessment is often overlooked in such an approach.

Drugs, such as tricyclic antidepressants and SSRIs that inhibit sexual function in men cause similar dysfunction, such as retarded orgasm, in women (Monteiro *et al.*, 1987).

It also seems likely that androgens are primarily responsible for sexual drive in women (Shifren, 2004; Tuiten *et al.*, 2002). Masters and Johnson stressed that sexual fulfilment is and should be available for all women and that sexual fulfilment through orgasm was the aim for sexual health. This view led to the same reductionist approaches to female sexuality as had occurred earlier for men but has recently been fiercely opposed by writers who are critical of the concept that women's sexual function is defined in terms of men's pleasure and activity. They review evidence going back to Kinsey's early studies that challenge the notion that orgasm through intercourse is necessarily common place in women or even that women regard it as essential to achieving sexual pleasure (Nicolson & Burr, 2003). In a qualitative study of 33 volunteers recruited through advertising in public toilets and notice boards in a teaching hospital and university, they reported that women (1) had a simplistic view of men's sexuality as an uncomplicated drive to satisfy a hunger; (2) regarded their own sexuality as more broadly sensual than men's and not so focused on orgasm; and (3) were in some degree of conflict over 'popular' ideas of female sexuality and their own wishes and desires (Nicholson & Burr, 2003). Unfortunately, the introduction to the paper is so polemical that the reader could be forgiven for assuming the researchers found what they wanted to find. Nevertheless, many of their views are shared by others (Tiefer, 2000; Moynihan, 2003).

Hypoactive sexual desire in women

Lack of sexual desire in women is commonly reported in epidemiological studies and is the commonest problem in women seeking help for sexual dysfunction (Warner *et al.*, 1987). Depending on the narrowness of definition, prevalence rates range between 17% in the UK (Nazareth *et al.*, 2003) and 30% in the USA (Laumann *et al.*, 1999). There are strong associations between low sexual drive and anxiety, depression and discord with spouse or partner (Dunn, 2000). There are also strong associations with use of psychotropic medication (Segraves, 2002). It is also common in the 8 months after childbirth, although less than one-sixth of couples regard the problem as requiring help (Dixon *et al.*, 2000).

When a woman lacks sexual drive, it is well worth asking 'who is complaining?' Thus a recent review of the diagnostic classification in women has suggested that the disorder should be characterized by a persistent lack or deficiency of indicators of sexual desire such as sexual thoughts or fantasies and desire for a partner and that this lack leads to personal distress. Thus this definition does not apply to women who lack desire in certain situations such as marital conflict or at certain times such as menstruation but not in others. Similarly, an imbalance between the woman's desire and that of her partner (given similar age and health) would not necessarily be a sign of disorder (Basson *et al.*, 2000).

Drug treatments

Although sildenafil has been considered as a treatment for low sexual desire in women, research has mainly concentrated on its use in female arousal disorder. If anything, hypoactive sexual desire appears to reduce sildenafil's function in women with arousal disorder (Berman *et al.*, 2003); this is discussed later. Testosterone therapy in women with low sexual drive is currently under investigation and appears to have beneficial effects in women who have undergone oophorectomy and hysterectomy, although placebo response is high (Shifren *et al.*, 2000). However, its use is fraught with the risk of masculinizing side effects (Modelska & Cummings, 2003). Hormone replacement therapy in menopausal women is the main physical treatment that will enhance sexual function through its action on the vaginal epithelium and the vulval and clitoral erectile tissues. Tibolone, a synthetic steroid that has estrogenic, progestogenic and androgenic activity is used to treat menopausal symptoms and may have a place in enhancing sexual function in post-menopausal women (Modelska & Cummings, 2003).

Psychological approaches

Much of the evidence concerning Masters and Johnson's approaches and other individual or couples therapy that were discussed under sexual problems in men are relevant here and do not need to be repeated. Suffice to say that there is little controlled trial evidence for any particular approach. Early trials were small and allocation was not at random (Crowe *et al.*, 1981). However, adopting the Masters and Johnson model of sex therapy for women has received fierce criticism in recent years because it is perceived as equating male and female sexuality, particularly in terms of the response cycle discussed earlier (Nicolson & Burr, 2003). However, advocates of the joint approach contend that such therapy has placed men and women on an equal footing and encourages the view that pleasure in love making is also a female prerogative. They also remind us that female sexual 'emancipation' is a recent historical phenomenon (Bancroft, 2002). Modern sexual therapy for women and their partners concentrates on emotional and sexual communication, dealing with anger and resentment and the identification of insecurity

(Bancroft, 2002). Couple therapy may also take the form of a systemic approach to improve sexual desire in long-term relationships (Clement, 2002). Although widely used as a pragmatic approach, we know little about its overall efficacy or the efficacy of its individual components.

Sexual arousal disorder in women

Lack of arousal in women has been regarded as a disorder in which there is lack of mental excitement or interest and lack of genital engorgement and vaginal lubrication. Depending on what is included in the definition, prevalence rates vary widely from 4% in an English study (Nazareth *et al.*, 2003) to about 25% in a North American report (Laumann *et al.*, 1999). However, the problem is now regarded as wider than that defined in DSMIV which focuses on a lack of genital response (Basson *et al.*, 2000). Some have gone further in suggesting that there are two subtypes of women with arousal dysfunction. In the first, and apparently more common subtype are women who seem unaware that physical arousal is occurring. In the second are women who find arousal unpleasant (Caruso *et al.*, 2004). Evidence for such subtyping, however, is not strong. Main physical etiologies are vascular impairment in disorders such as diabetes and changes associated with reduction of oestrogen at the menopause (Berman *et al.*, 1999). Not surprisingly, sexual dysfunction in diabetic women has received less research attention than that for men. Several studies have suggested that reduced vaginal lubrication makes sexual intercourse unpleasant. Sexual dysfunction is also associated with lower overall quality of marital relationships and more depressive symptoms in diabetic women (Morano, 2003) However, closer scrutiny reveals that objective genital sensory impairment is not well correlated with reported sexual dysfunction, again showing the complexities of sexual dysfunction in women (Erol *et al.*, 2003; Bancroft, 2002; Bancroft *et al.*, 2003).

Drug treatments

If a woman is mentally responsive to her partner, but lacks appropriate increases in genital blood flow, it has been suggested that treatment with phosphodiesterase inhibitors may have a role (Basson, 2001). The success of *sildenafil* in treating erectile disorder in men stimulated the hunt for similar drugs to increase vascular engorgement in the clitoris and labia in women and thus increase sexual arousal and pleasure. Unfortunately, epidemiological evidence also suggested that poor sexual arousal in women in the absence of other issues such as low libido, was much

less commonly found than in men. Making 'objective' assessments of the efficacy of vaso-active drugs such as *sildenafil* and *phentolamine* is also difficult in women. Although measures such as vaginal photoplethysmography (which uses light scattering techniques to measure vasoengorgement) are available, they are invasive and poorly standardized and cannot be easily used in large multicentre trials (Rosen, 2002). However, given that most trials of *sildenafil* and related drugs in men relied on self report meant that similar efforts were perfectly possible in women. Early, uncontrolled studies of *sildenafil* in women with low sexual drive or women on antidepressants had mixed results (Rosen, 2002). Despite one large (Pfizer funded) trial involving menopausal women that suggested some improvements in genital sensation and sexual satisfaction in women with low arousal *without* low libido (Berman *et al.*, 2003), other pharmaceutical industry trials involving about 3000 women produced mixed results and Pfizer has not pursued a licence for *sildenafil* in women (Mayor, 2004). John Bancroft, the former Director of the Kinsey Institute, remarked in that report, 'The recent history of the study of female sexual dysfunction is a classic example of starting with some preconceived and non-evidence-based diagnostic categorisation for women's sexual dysfunction, based on the male model, and then requiring further research to be based on that structure' (Mayor, 2004).

Another drug that has received some attention in women complaining of low arousal is *apomorphine* discussed above in relation to men with sexual dysfunction. *Apomorphine* acts on the noradrenergic–non-cholinergic pathway that modulates nitric oxide. Nitric oxide is thought to be important as a vasodilator in the clitoral corpus cavernosum and vaginal smooth muscle. A daily 2 or 3 mg sustained release dose of *apomorphine* in women with arousal disorders *and* low sexual drive has been shown to improve orgasm, sexual enjoyment and satisfaction in one small placebo, controlled trial (Caruso *et al.*, 2004). Although there was also some increase in sexual desire, it was difficult to know whether this was a secondary phenomenon. In a further example of modelling treatments for low arousal in women on those for men, Padma-Nathan *et al.* (2003) evaluated topical administration of a cream containing the prostaglandin E (*alprostadil*) on arousal in a randomized controlled trial involving 94 women presenting with sexual arousal disorder of at least 6 months' duration. Although not significantly more effective than placebo cream, the authors reported a significant dose response in the alprostadil arm, suggesting that results indicated further evaluation was warranted.

Psychological interventions

Psychological approaches have concentrated on the woman's relationship to her partner or to issues of loss in terms of menopausal or surgical changes in later life. Individual approaches which focus on relaxation and self-focusing to reduce anxiety are also used. For example, use of a vibrator, both alone or with a partner, is frequently recommended and does seem to be effective in bringing about orgasm in some women. Such treatments have run a gauntlet of criticism in their focus on arousal and climax. It is claimed on the basis of detailed, qualitative research that women may be less concerned with achieving orgasm through heterosexual intercourse than with pleasing their partner (Nicolson & Burr, 2003). Wider reviews of the literature do not always concur, however by indicating that there are few major gender differences in attitudes to sexual behaviour, participation in sex and sexual satisfaction (Oliver & Hyde, 1993).

Vaginismus

In this disorder, involuntary vaginal and adductor muscles of the thighs make penetration difficult or impossible. It most commonly presents as primary in young women embarking on their first sexual relationships or secondary following sexual assault or similar trauma. There are no known physical causes and the exact psychological etiology is unknown. However, the condition may be accompanied by a dislike of the body and social anxiety. Sexual arousal and interest are frequently normal. It is not always easy to distinguish from dyspareunia which appears to be a pain syndrome rather than a sexual dysfunction (Meana et al., 1997). Prevalence rates vary between 5% for pure vaginismus according to ICD10 (Nazareth et al., 2003) and 15% for the wider concept of pain during sex (Laumann et al., 1999).

Drug treatments

There are no available drug treatments for vaginismus, although vaginal lubricants may often be used to ease penetration.

Psychological treatments

Over and above non-specific sexual therapy about which little can be added here, behavioural interventions have figured commonly in the management of this condition. This is on the theoretical and intuitive basis that the muscle spasm appears to be a phobic response to a normal stimulus. Desensitization through sensitive physical examination, by encouraging the woman to view her genital area in a mirror or by teaching her to examine herself is attempted. Although encouraging results have been reported from uncontrolled studies, there have been few randomized trials. One example was a trial of desensitization through the use of 'dilators'. This showed that all patients benefited, whether using the dilators or desensitization in imagination (Schnyder et al., 1998). However, use of dilators can also encourage the woman in the common but mistaken belief that there is insufficient room in her vagina for penetration. A recent Cochrane Review has considered all randomized, controlled trials published up to 2002, where treatment for vaginismus was compared to another treatment, either placebo, treatment as usual or a waitlist control (McGuire & Hawton, 2003). Only two trials were identified and neither showed effectiveness for any particular type of intervention.

Transsexualism in men and women

Transsexualism is uncommon. It is included here because it involves assessments by mental health professionals and may entail a complex and invasive process of medical and surgical treatments, but is also described in more detail in Chapter 46. The term transsexualism describes the conviction that despite a normal body, genetic profile and physical development, a person is convinced that their gender has been wrongly 'assigned' and that they should have been born in a body of the opposite sex. Transsexual males outnumber women. It is distinguished from transvestism in which men dress (nearly always) in feminine clothes (or underclothes) to derive sexual arousal and orgasm. Cross-dressing in itself appears not be to be associated with psychopathology (Brown et al., 1996). In fact, dressing and behaving as a woman may have a calming effect for a small proportion of men, no matter what their sexual orientation (Levine, 1993). Although transsexualism is listed as a diagnosis in all international psychiatric diagnostic glossaries, psychiatrists do not regard it as a delusional disorder on the grounds that it is not accompanied by other serious psychopathology (Cohen et al., 1997; Cole et al., 1997). More importantly, the belief is not now considered delusional. Although people with such a belief may be distressed, this is regarded as in keeping with their dilemma. Transsexualism has come to be regarded by some as a mistake of nature that requires correction, rather than variation in the human phenotype. Others view it as a disorder of unknown but probably multifactorial origin.

Awareness of being male or female begins very early in childhood. Infants begin to behave in particular ways in response to biological, social and psychological forces, of which the biological appears to be the most decisive. The sense of being male or female usually develops by age 2 to 4 years. However, the process is not a simple one in nature or degree, nor is it necessarily immutable. The term *gender role* was first used in 1955, while *gender identity* appeared in a press release in 1966 to announce the new clinic for transsexuals at Johns Hopkins Hospital (Money, 1955, 1994). Gender role is defined as the degree to which children respond and behave in ways that are considered characteristic of boys or girls. Girls are encouraged to be conciliatory and co-operative and boys aggressive and competitive (Whiting, 1963; Low, 1989). Family and peers generally discourage gender discordant behaviours, although parents in more recent times have consciously attempted to avoid shaping gender role. Gender role has been regarded as a highly selected characteristic that equips men and women for their respective roles in evolving societies (Stevens & Price, 1996). However, it is readily forgotten how much of it is conceived of in social terms and how concepts of masculinity and femininity differ between cultures (Coleman *et al.*, 1992) and between periods of history in the same culture (Kuchta, 1993).

People uncomfortable with their gender have been described since at least the 1890s (Krafft-Ebing, 1886; Snaith & Hohberger, 1994; Schaefer & Wheeler, 1995). However, by the mid-twentieth century the view arose that transsexuals needed specific psychological and medical management in order to achieve 'gender reassignment' (Money, 1955, 1994). Technological developments in medicine and surgery enabled the establishment of centres for gender reassignment in the United States and Western Europe in the early 1960s. Many people seeking sex reassignment have been convinced since childhood that their gender identity is at variance with their body. For others, the conviction develops in adulthood when sexual excitement arising from cross-dressing declines and a wish to live in the opposite gender role comes to the fore. People seeking reassignment must 'pass' in an opposite sex role in public and private for at least 1 year before being considered for surgery. During this time they almost always take estrogen or testosterone to begin the process of remodelling the body into the desired gender (Blanchard & Steiner, 1990). Men will undergo lengthy treatments of electrolysis or laser treatment to remove body and facial hair. Psychiatrists usually decide over an extended period whether a candidate is convincing in the opposite gender role and can be considered for surgery. We cannot be certain how many people who feel at odds with their biological gender seek gender reassignment. However, epidemiological data from Holland would

suggest that in Western countries, most do so (van Kesteren *et al.*, 1996). Many outcome studies of gender reassignment surgery have also been published. Most claim that candidates achieve satisfactory adaptation to their assigned gender (Blanchard & Steiner 1990; Snaith *et al.*, 1993; Eldh *et al.*, 1997) and that only a small percentage regrets the surgery (Landen *et al.*, 1998). However, outcome is said to be dependent on adequate assessment and preparation and may go wrong (Anon, 1991).

Most biologically female transsexual people in Western countries regard themselves as heterosexual if given the chance to function as the opposite sex. However some, nearly all biologically male, will become technically homosexual in their new role (Blanchard & Sheridan, 1990; Coleman *et al.*, 1992). It also seems that sexual orientation can change following surgical reassignment (Daskalos, 1998). Reports from Eastern cultures, in which most male and female transsexuals are described as homosexual (Tsoi, 1992), indicate that cultural factors are important in the way people in this predicament define their sexuality.

Although transsexualism has become almost an unquestioned status in contemporary psychiatry and medicine, it was not long ago that the requirement (for surgery) that male transsexuals must live as women enraged feminists (Raymond, 1979). The most radical feminist view was that professionals in the field were resolving their 'womb-envy' in trying to create new people. They are believed to fail because transsexuals do not really become women (Daly, 1979). Although the arguments are overstated, they lay bare some of the cultural and temporal assumptions under-pinning the concept of transsexualism.

Concluding remarks

Despite enormous expansion since its origins in the 1960s, sexual therapy is in its infancy in terms of establishing an evidence base for effectiveness. This situation is untenable, given society's much greater openness about sex and sexual problems and the rapid expansion of pharmaceutical and other physical remedies for sexual difficulties. Much greater efforts are needed to understand more about the psychology of the human sexual response as biological treatments are very unlikely to be the complete answer to sexual problems for most people. However, we must constantly recall that we are in a 'minefield' of doubtful self-reporting that Alfred Kinsey first entered when he asked people about their sexual function (Sharp, 2002). People do not always tell us the truth about sex. Furthermore, western culture is steeped in psychoanalytical truths that make us 'people who must not have what they really want, people whose fraught love for their parents has made love a hopeless passion.' (Phillips, 2003). We have a mountain to climb.

The level of evidence for each of the interventious discussed in this chapter is summarized in Table 45.2.

Table 45.2. Effectiveness of treatments for sexual disorders

Treatment	Form of treatment	Psychiatric Disorder	Level of evidence for efficacy	Comments
Phosphodiest-erase-5 inhibitors	Sildefanil (tab)	Erectile dysfunction	Ia	Large effect size, with lower success rates after radical prostatectomy. Contraindicated with nitrates
Phosphodiest-erase-5 inhibitors	Tadalafil (tab)	Erectile dysfunction	la	Longer duration of action (36 hours) and twice half-life of sildefanil
Phosphodiest-erase-5 inhibitors	Vardenafil (tab)	Erectile dysfunction	Ib	Likely to be similar to sildefanil
Dopaminergic drugs	Apomorphine (sublingual)	Erectile dysfunction	Ib	Conflicting results from clinical trials. Probably not as effective as phosphodiesterase-5 inhibitors
Alpha$_2$-adrenoceptor antagonist	Yohimbine (tab)	Erectile dysfunction	Ia	Of some value, but not as effective as other drugs for this condition
Prostaglandins	Alprostadil (intracavernosal injection)	Erectile dysfunction	la	Second-line treatment in view of form of treatment and risk of priapism
Behavioural approaches	Masters & Johnson techniques	Erectile dysfunction	III	Widely used but little tested
Cognitive behaviour therapy	Standard treatment to reduce dysfunctional thinking	Erectile dysfunction	III	Little formal evaluation
Couples sexual therapy	Combined with counselling or physical treatment (e.g. vacuum erectile device)	Erectile dysfunction	IIa	One study supports joint physical/couple counselling approach
Pelvic floor muscle exercises	–	Erectile dysfunction	Ib	One trial showed positive results when biofeedback incorporated
Selective serotonin reuptake inhibitors (SSRIs)	Sertraline, fluoxetine and fluoxetine	Premature ejaculation	Ia	Good evidence
Topical anaesthetics	Lidocaine-prilocaine	Premature ejaculation	Ib	Some evidence of effectiveness
Alpha-adrenergic antagonists	Pseudoephedrine ephedrine	Retarded ejaculation/ anorgasmia	III	No good evidence of efficacy
Pause-squeeze technique	Linked to Masters & Johnson	Retarded ejaculation/ anorgasmia	IIa	Some slight evidence of value
Penile vibrators	–	Retarded ejaculation/ anorgasmia	III	Probably effective to some extent but not tested
Bibliotherapy	Written material only	Disorders of sexual function generally	Ia	Small but consistent level of efficacy
Hormone therapy	Testosterone	Hypoactive sexual drive (women)	III	Possible benefit
Hormone therapy	Estrogen replacement/ tibolone-	Hypoactive sexual drive (women)	III	Little evaluation to date
Phosphodiest-erase-5 inhibitors	Sildefanil (tab)	Poor sexual arousal (women)	Ia	Little evidence of value
Dopaminergic drugs	Apomorphine (sustained release tab)	Poor sexual arousal (women)	Ib	On trial showed benefit
Dilator therapy		Vaginismus	Ia	No evidence of benefit

REFERENCES

Akkus, E., Kadioglu, A., Esen, A. *et al.* (2002). Prevalence and correlates of erectile dysfunction in Turkey: a population based study. *European Urology*, **41**, 298–304.

Anonymous (1991). Transsexualism. *Lancet*, **338**, 603–4.

Anonymous (2004). New oral drugs for erectile dysfunction. *Drugs and Therapeutics Bulletin*, **42**, July.

Bancroft, J. (1989). *Human Sexuality and its Problems.* pp. 128–13. Edinburgh: Churchill Livingston.

Bancroft, J. (2002). The medicalization of female sexual dysfunction: the need for caution. *Archives of Sexual Behavior*, **31**, 451–5.

Bancroft, J., Loftus, J. & Long, J. S. (2003). Distress about sex: a national survey of women in heterosexual relationships. *Archives of Sexual Behavior*, **32**, 193–208.

Basson, R. (2001). Female sexual response: the role of drugs in the management of sexual dysfunction. *American College of Obstetricians and Gynecologists*, **98**, 350–3.

Basson, R., Berman, J., Burnett, A. *et al.* (2000). Report on the international consensus development conference on female sexual dysfunction: definitions and classifications. *Journal of Urology*, **163**, 888–893.

Berman, J. R., Berman, L. A., Werbin, T. J. *et al.* (1999). Clinical evaluation of female sexual dysfunction: effects of age and oestrogen status on subjective and physiologic responses. *International Journal of Impotence Research*, **11** (Suppl.), 31–38.

Berman, J. R., Berman, L. A., Toler, M., Gill, J., Haughie, S. & the Sildenafil Study Group (2003). Safety and efficacy of sildenafil citrate for the treatment of female sexual arousal disorders: a double-blind placebo controlled study. *The Journal of Urology*, **170**, 2333–5.

Blanchard, R. & Sheridan, P. M. (1990). Gender reorientation and psychosocial adjustment. In *Clinical Management of Gender Identity Disorders in Children and Adults*, ed. R. Blanchard & B. Steiner, pp. 159–89. Washington DC: American Psychiatric Press.

Blanchard, R. & Steiner, B. W. (eds) (1990). *Clinical Management of Gender Identity Disorders in Children and Adults.* Washington DC: American Psychiatric Press.

Brown, G. R., Wise, T. N., Costa, P. T., Herbst, J. H., Fagan, P. J. & Schmidt, C. W. (1996). Personality characteristics and sexual functioning of 188 cross-dressing men. *Journal of Nervous and Mental Disease*, **B184**, 265–73.

Busato, W. & Galindo, C. C. (2004). Topical anaesthetic use for treating premature ejaculation: a double-blind, randomized, placebo-controlled study. *BJU International*, **93**, 1081–21.

Carson, C. C., Rajfer, J., Eardley, I. *et al.* (2004). The efficacy and safety of Tadalafil: an update. *BJU International*, **93**, 1276–81.

Caruso, S., Agnello, C., Intelisano, G., Farina, M., Di Mari, L. & Cianci, A. (2004). Placebo-controlled study of the efficacy and safety of daily apomorphine SL intake in premenopausal women affected by hypoactive sexual desire disorder and sexual arousal disorder. *Urology*, **63**, 955–9.

Catalan, J. (1993). Primary male anorgasmia and its treatment: three case reports. *Sexual and Marital Therapy*, **8**(3), 275–82.

Clement, U. (2002). Sex in long-term relationships: a systemic approach to sexual desire problems. *Archives of Sexual Behaviour*, **31**, 241–6.

Cohen, L., de Ruiter, C., Ringelberg, H. & Cohen-Kettenis, P. T. (1997). Psychological functioning of adolescent transsexuals: personality and psychopathology. *Journal of Clinical Psychology*, **53**, 187–96.

Cole, C. M., O'Boyle, M., Emory, L. E. & Mayer, W. J. (1997). Comorbidity of gender dysphoria and other major psychiatric diagnoses. *Archives of Sexual Behaviour*, **26**, 13–26.

Coleman, E., Colgan, P. & Gooren, L. (1992). Male cross-gender behaviour in Myanmar (Burma): a description of the occult. *Archives of Sexual Behaviour*, **21**, 313–21.

Crowe, M. J., Gillan, P. & Golombok, S. (1981). Form and content in the conjoint treatment of sexual dysfunction: a controlled study. *Behavior Research and Therapy*, **19**, 47–54.

Daskalos, C. T. (1998). Changes in the sexual orientation of six heterosexual male-to-female transsexuals. *Archives of Sexual Behaviour*, **27**, 605–14.

Dinsmore, W. (2004). Treatment of erectile dysfunction. *International Journal of STD and AIDS*, **15**, 215–21.

Dixon, M., Booth, N. & Powell, R. (2000). Sex and relationships following childbirth: a first report from general practice of 131 couples. *British Journal of General Practice*, **50**, 223–4.

Dorey, G., Speakman, M., Feneley, R., Swinkels, A., Dunn, C. & Ewings, (2004). Randomised controlled trial of pelvic floor muscle exercises and manometric biofeedback for erectile dysfunction. *British Journal of General Practice*, **54**, 819–25.

Dula, E. S., Bukofzer, R., Perdok, R. J. & George, M. (2001). Apomorphine Study Group. Double-blind, cross-over comparison of 3 mg apomorphine SL with placebo and with 4 mg apomorphine SL in male erectile dysfunction. *European Urology*, **39**, 558–64.

Dunn, K. M. (2000). Satisfaction in the sex life of a general population sample. *Journal of Sexual and Marital Therapy*, **26**, 141–51.

Eldh, H., Berg, A. & Gustafsson, M. (1997). Long-term follow up after sex reassignment surgery. *Scandinavian Journal of Plastic and Reconstructive Surgery and Hand Surgery*, **31**, 39–45.

Ellis, H. (1936). *Studies in the Psychology of Sex.* New York: Random House.

Ellis, H. & Symonds, J. A. (1897). *Sexual Inversion* (Originally Published as Volume 1 – Studies in the Psychology of Sex) reprinted in 1994, USA: Ayer.

Ernst, E. & Pittler, M. H. (1998). Yohimbine for erectile dysfunction: a systematic review and meta-analysis of randomized clinical trials. *Journal of Urology*, **159**(2), 433–6.

Erol, B., Tefekli, A., Sanli, O. *et al.* (2003). Does sexual dysfunction correlate with deterioration of somatic sensory system in diabetic women? *International Journal of Impotence Research*, **15**, 198–202.

Fazio, L. & Brock, G. (2004). Erectile dysfunction: management update. *Canadian Medical Association Journal*, **170**(9), 1429–37.

Fink, H. A., MacDonald, R., Rutks-Indulis, R., Nelson, D. B. & Wilt, T. J. (2002). Sildenafil for male erectile dysfunction: a systematic review and meta-analysis. *Archives of Internal Medicine*, **162**, 1349–60.

Foucault, M. (1978). *The History of Sexuality Volume I An Introduction*. New York: Random House.

Goldstein, I., Lue, T. F., Padma-Nathan, H., Rosen, R. C., Steers, W. D. & Wicker, P. A. (1998). for the sildenafil study group. Oral sildenafil in the treatment of erectile dysfunction. *New England Journal of Medicine*, **338**, 1397–404.

Gould, D. C., Petty, R. & Jacobs, H. S. (2000). The male menopause – does it exist? *British Medical Journal*, **250**, 858–61.

Grenier, G. & Byers, E. S. (1995). Rapid ejaculation: a review of conceptual, etiological and treatment issues. *Archives of Sexual Behaviour*, **24**, 447–72.

Hawton, K. (1998). Sexual dysfunctions. In *Cognitive Behaviour Therapy for Psychiatric Problems. A Practical Guide*, ed. K. Hawton, P. M. Salkovskis, J. Kirk & D. M. Clark. Oxford: Oxford University Press.

Health Outcomes Research Design Consultants LLC (2000). Economic cost of male erectile dysfunction using a decision analytic model: for a hypothetical managed-care plan of 100,000 members. *PharmacoEconomics*, **17**, 77–107.

Illich, I. (1975). *Medical Nemesis. The Expropriation of Health*. London: Marion Boyars.

Jaffe, J. S., Antell, M. R., Greenstein, M., Ginsberg, P. C., Mydlo, J. H. & Harkaway, R. C. (2004). Use of intraurethral alprostadil in patients not responding to sildenafil citrate. *Urology*, **63**, 951–4.

Jannini, E. A., Simonelli, C. & Lenzi, A. (2002). Sexological approach to ejaculatory dysfunction. *International Journal of Andrology*, **25**, 317–23.

Kamischke, A. & Nieschlag, E. (2002). Update on medical treatment of ejaculatory disorders. *International Journal of Andrology*, **25**, 333–44.

Kandeel, F. R., Koussa, V. K. T. & Swerdloff, R. S. (2001). Male sexual function and its disorders: physiology, pathophysiology, clinical investigation and treatment. *Endocrine Reviews*, **22**, 342–88.

Kaplan, H. S. (1974). *The New Sex Therapy: Active Treatment of Sexual Dysfunctions*. Brunner Mazel: New York.

King, H. (1994). Sowing the field: Greek and Roman sexology. In *Sexual Knowledge, Sexual Science*, ed. R. Porter & M. Teich, pp. 29–46. Cambridge: Cambridge University Press.

King, M. B. & Bartlett, A. (1999). British psychiatry and homosexuality. *British Journal of Psychiatry*, **174**, 106–13.

Kinsey, A. C., Pomeroy, W. B. & Martin, C. E. (1948). *Sexual Behaviour in the Human Male*. Philadelphia: Saunders.

Kolomazník, M. (2004). Intermittent administration of sertraline in premature ejaculation. *Psychiatrie*, **8**(2), 100–3.

Krafft-Ebing R. von (1886). *Psychopathia Sexualis Translation C H Chaddock 1894*. Philadephia: F. A. Davis.

Kuchta, D. (1993). The semiotics of masculinity in renaissance England. In *Sexuality and Gender in Early Modern Europe*, ed. J. G. Turner, pp. 233–46. Cambridge: Cambridge University Press.

La Pera, G. & Nicastro, A. (1996). A new treatment for premature ejaculation: the rehabilitation of the pelvis floor. *Journal of Sex and Marital Therapy*, **22**, 22–6.

Landen, M., Walinder, J., Hambert, G. & Lundstrom, B. (1998). Factors predictive of regret in sex reassignment. *Acta Psychiatrica Scandinavica*, **97**, 284–9.

Laumann, E. O., Paik, A. & Rosen, R. C. (1999). Sexual dysfunction in the United States: prevalence and predictors. *Journal of the American Medical Association*, **281**(6), 537–44.

Lee, J. C., Surridge, D. H. C., Morales, A. & Heaton, J. P. W. (1998). Penile rigidity supersedes partner and counselling issues. *Sexual Dysfunction*, **1**, 123–7.

Levine, S. B. (1993). Gender-disturbed males. *Journal of Sexual and Marital Therapy*, **19**, 131–41.

Low, B. S. (1989). Cross-cultural patterns in the training of children: an evolutionary perspective. *Journal of Comparative Psychology*, **103**, 311–19.

Marks, L. S. (2003). Editorial comment 1. *Urology*, **62**, 125–6.

Masters, W. H. & Johnson, V. E. (1966). *Human Sexual Response*. Philadelphia: Williams & Wilkins: Lippincott.

Masters, W. H. & Johnson, V. E. (1970). *Human Sexual Inadequacy*. Boston: Little Brown.

Mayor, S. (2004). Pfizer will not apply for a licence for sildenafil for women. *British Medical Journal*, **328**, 542.

McGuire, H. & Hawton, K. (2003). Interventions for vaginismus. *The Cochrane Database of Systematic Reviews*, **1**, CD001760. Oxford: Update Software Ltd.

McMahon, C. G., Abdo, C., Incrocci, L. *et al.* (2004). Disorders of orgasm and ejaculation in men. *Journal of Sexual Medicine*, **1**(1), 58–65.

Meana, M., Binik, Y. M., Khalifé, S. & Cohen, D. (1997). Dyspareunia: sexual dysfunction or pain syndrome? *Journal for Nervous and Mental Disease*, **185**, 561–9.

Mendels, J., Camera, A. & Sikes, C. (1995). Sertraline treatment for premature ejaculation. *Journal of Clinical Psychopharmacology*, **15**, 341–6.

Meuleman, E. J. H. (2003). Investigations in erectile dysfunction. *Current Opinions in Urology*, **13** 411–16.

Metz, M. E. & Pryor, J. L. (2000). Premature ejaculation; a psychophysiological approach for assessment and management. *Journal of Sex and Marital Therapy*, **26**, 293–320.

Mirone, V., Imbimbo, C., Bortolotti, A. *et al.* (2002). Cigarette smoking as a risk factor for erectile dysfunction: results from an Italian epidemiological study. *European Urology*, **41**, 294–7.

Modelska, K. & Cummings, S. (2003). Tibolone for post menopausal women: a systematic review of randomized trials. *American Journal of Obstetrics and Gynecology*, **188**, 286–93.

Money, J. (1955). An examination of some basic sexual concepts: the evidence of human hermaphroditism. *Bulletin of Johns Hopkins Hospital*, **97**, 301–19.

Money, J. (1994). The concept of gender identity disorder in childhood and adolescence after 39 years. *Journal of Sexual and Marital Therapy*, **20**, 163–77.

Montague, D. K., Jarow, J., Broderick, G. A. *et al.* (2004). AUA guideline on the pharmacologic management of premature ejaculation. *Journal of Urology*, **172**, 290–4.

Monteiro, W. O., Noshirvani, H. F., Marks, I. M. & Lelliott, P. T. (1987). Anorgasmia from clomipramine in obsessive-compulsive disorder. A controlled trial. *British Journal of Psychiatry*, **151**, 107–12.

Morano, S. (2003). Pathophysiology of diabetic sexual dysfunction. *Journal of Endocrinological Investigation*, **26** (Suppl.), 65–9.

Morgentaler, A. (1999). Male impotence. *Lancet*, **354**, 1713–18.

Moyad, M. A., Barada, J. H., Lue, T. F., Mulhall, J. P., Goldstein, I. & Fawzy, A. (2004). Prevention and treatment of erectile dysfunction using lifestyle changes and dietary supplements: what works and what is worthless, part II. *The Urologic clinics of North America*, **31**(2), 259–73.

Moynihan, R. (2003). The making of a disease: female sexual dysfunction. *British Medical Journal*, **236**, 45–7.

Nazareth, I., Boynton, P. & King, M. (2003). Problems with sexual function in people attending London general practitioners: a cross sectional study. *British Medical Journal*, **327**, 423–6.

Nicolson, P. & Burr, J. (2003). What is 'normal' about women's (Hetero)sexual desire and orgasm?: a report of an in-depth interview study. *Social Science and Medicine*, **57**, 1735–45.

Oliver, M. B. & Hyde, J. S. (1993). Gender differences in sexuality: a meta-analysis. *Psychological Bulletin*, **114**, 29–51.

Padma-Nathan, H., Brown, C., Fendl, J., Salem, S., Yeager, J. & Harning, R. (2003). Efficacy and safety of topical alprostadil cream for the treatment of female sexual arousal disorders. (FSAD): a double blind, multicenter, randomized, and placebo-controlled clinical trial. *Journal of Sexual and Marital Therapy*, **29**, 329–44.

Perimenis, P., Gyftopoulos, K., Giannitsas, K. *et al.* (2004). A comparative, crossover study of the efficacy and safety of sildenafil and apomorphine in men with evidence of arteriogenic erectile dysfunction. *International Journal of Importency Research*, **16**, 2–7.

Phillips, A. (2003). Bored with sex? *London Review of Books*, 6 March.

Porst, H. (1989). Prostaglandin E in erectile dysfunction (German language article). *Urologe A*, **28**, 94–8.

Porter, R. & Hall, L. (1995). *The Facts of Life: The Creation of Sexual Knowledge in Britain 1650–1950*. New Haven and London: Yale University Press.

Raymond, J. G. (1979). *The Transsexual Empire*. London: The Womens Press.

Romanelli, F. & Smith, K. M. (2004). Recreational use of sildenafil by HIV-positive and – negative homosexual/bisexual males. *Annals of Pharmacotherapy*, **38**, 1024–30.

Rosen, R. C. (2002). Sexual function assessment and the role of vasoactive drugs in female sexual dysfunction. *Archives of Sexual Behavior*, **31**, 439–43.

Rosen, R. C. & Leiblum, S. R. (1995). Treatment of sexual disorders in the 1990s: an integrated approach. *Journal of Consulting and Clinical Psychology*, **63**, 877–90.

Sarwer, D. B. & Durlak, J. A. (1996). A Field trial of the effectiveness of behavioural treatment for sexual dysfunctions. *Journal of Sexual and Marital Therapy*, **23**, 87–97.

Schaefer, L. C. & Wheeler, C. C. (1995). Harry Benjamin's first ten cases (1938–1953): a clinical historical note. *Archives of Sexual Behaviour*, **24**, 73–93.

Schover, L. R. & Leiblum, S. R. (1994). Commentary: the stagnation of sex therapy. *Journal of Psychology and Human Sexuality*, **6**, 5–30.

Schnyder, U., Schnyder, L. C., Ballinari, P. & Blaser, A. (1998). Therapy for vaginismus: in vivo versus in vitro desensitization. *Canadian Journal of Psychiatry*, **43**, 941–4.

Semans, J. H. (1955). Premature ejaculation: a new approach. *Southern Medical Journal*, **49**, 353–8.

Sharp, D. (2002). Telling the truth about sex. *The Lancet*, **359**, 1084.

Shifren, J. L. (2004). The role of androgens in female sexual dysfunction. *Mayo Clinic Proceedings*, **79** (4 Suppl), S19–24.

Shifren, J. L., Braunstein, G. D., Simon, J. A. *et al.* (2000). Transdermal testosterone treatment in women with impaired sexual function after oophorectomy. *New England Journal of Medicine*, **434**, 682–8.

Shorter, E. (1997). *A History of Psychiatry: From the Era of the Asylum to the Age of Prozac*. Chichester: John Wiley & Sons.

Snaith, P., Tarsh, M. J. & Reid, R. (1993). Sex reassignment surgery. A study of 141 Dutch transsexuals. *British Journal of Psychiatry*, **162**, 681–5.

Snaith, R. P. & Hohberger, A. D. (1994). Transsexualism and gender reassignment. *British Journal of Psychiatry*, **165**, 417–19.

Scruton, R. (1986). *Sexual Desire. A Philosophical Investigation*. London: Weidenfeld & Nicolson.

Segraves, R. T. (2002). Female sexual disorders: psychiatric aspects. *Canadian Journal of Psychiatry*, **47**, 419–25.

Stevens, A. & Price, J. (1996). *Evolutionary Psychiatry*, pp. 162–8. London: Routledge.

Szasz, T. (1983). Speaking about sex: sexual pathology and sexual therapy as a rhetoric. In *Challenges in Sexual Science: Current Theoretical Issues and Research Advances*, ed. C. M. Davis. Lake Mills, IA: The Society for the Scientific Study of Sex.

Tam, S. W., Worcel, M. & Wyllie, M. (2001). Yohimbine: a clinical review. *Pharmacology and Therapeutics*, **91**, 215–43.

Tiefer, L. (2000). Sexology and the pharmaceutical industry: the threat of co-optation. *The Journal of Sex Research*, **37**, 273–83.

Tomlinson, J. M. & Wright, D. (2004). Impact of erectile dysfunction and its subsequent treatment with sildenafil: a qualitative study. *British Medical Journal*, **328**, 1037–40.

Tong, T. & Boyer, E. W. (2002). Club drugs, smart drugs, raves, and circuit parties: an overview of the club scene. *Pediatric Emergency Care*, **18**, 216–18.

Truit, W. A. & Coolen, L. M. (2002). Identification of a potential ejaculation generator in the spinal cord. *Science*, **297**, 1460–1.

Tsoi, W. F. (1992). Male and female transsexuals: a comparison. *Singapore Medical Journal*, **33**, 182–5.

Tuiten, A., van Honk, J., Verbaten, R., Laan, E. & Everaerd, W. (2002). Can sublingual testosterone increase subjective and physiological measures of laboratory-induced sexual arousal? *Archives of General Psychiatry*, **59**, 465.

Van den Hout, M. & Barlow, D. (2000). Attention, arousal and expectancies in anxiety and sexual disorders. *Journal of Affective Disorders*, **61**, 241–56.

Van der Windt, F., Dohle, G. R., van der Tak, J. & Slob, A. K. (2002). Intracavernosal injection therapy with and without sexological counselling in men with erectile dysfunction. *BJU International*, **89**, 901–4.

van Kesteren, P. J., Gooren, L. J. & Megens, J. A. (1996). An epidemiological and demographic study of transsexuals in the Netherlands. *Archives of Sexual Behaviour*, **25**, 589–600.

Van Lankveld, J. J. D. M. (1998). Bibliotherapy in the treatment of sexual dysfunctions: a meta-analysis. *Journal of Consulting and Clinical Psychology*, **66**(4), 702–8.

Von Keitz, A. T., Stroberg, P., Bukofzer, S., Mallard, N. & Hibberd, M. (2002). A European multicentre study to evaluate the tolerability of apomorphine sublingual administered in a forced dose-escalation regimen in patients with erectile dysfunction. *BJU International*, **89**, 409–15.

Vroege, J. A., Gijs, L. & Hengeveld, M. W. (1998). Classification sexual dysfunctions: towards DSM-V and ICD-11. *Comprehensive Psychiatry*, **39**, 333–7.

Waldinger, M. D., Hengeveld, M. W., Zwinderman, A. H. & Olivier, B. (2001). Effect of SSRI antidepressants on ejaculation: a double-blind randomized, placebo-controlled study with fluoxetine, fluvoxamine, paroxetine and sertraline. *Journal of Clinical Psychopharmacology*, **21**(2), 241–2.

Warner, P., Bancroft, J. & Members of the Edinburgh Human Sexuality Group (1987). A regional clinical service for sexual problems: a three year survey. *Sexual and Marital Therapy*, **2**, 115–26.

Weiderman, M. W. (1998). The state of the theory in sex therapy. *The Journal of Sex Research*, **35**, 88–99.

Whiting, B. (ed.) (1963). *Six Cultures: Studies of Child Rearing*. New York: Wiley.

Wylie, K. R., Jones, R. H. & Walters, S. (1996). The potential benefit of vacuum devices augmenting psychosexual therapy for erectile dysfunction: a randomized controlled trial. *Journal of Sexual and Marital Therapy*, **29**, 227–36.

46

Disorders of gender identity

James Barrett

Editor's note

To most psychiatrists the phenomenon of gender identity is a mystery at the edges of their consciousness. This is not surprising, for the conditions subsuming it are rare, and not specifically associated with other psychopathology. The people who have these conditions are now getting increasingly well informed and therefore funnel towards clinics that specialize in the management of these conditions, which often require surgical intervention and close liaison between medical disciplines. This chapter shows a great deal has been learnt in the 40 years since this group first attracted real attention, and the evidence, although limited, indicates the value of intervention.

Note: throughout this chapter the terms 'male' and 'female' refer to sex assigned at birth.

Introduction

Disorders of gender identity have probably always existed, inside and outside Europe (Vietnam, in the case described by Heiman et al., 1975), and as demonstrated in the nineteenth century historical study by Ball et al. (1978). It seems that incidence of transsexualism is very roughly one in 60 000 males and one in every 100 000 females and seems to have remained constant (Landen et al., 1996). These disorders did not come to the attention of psychiatric services, though, until 1966, when Dr Harry Benjamin (then just retired) started to see people with disorders of gender identity in the USA.

From the early 1950s, there were attempts to offer some sort of gender reassignment surgery to people with disorders of gender identity, with some of these cases gaining wider public attention. In the initial years, after the first recognition and description of gender identity problems

by Dr Benjamin, people with gender identity disorders were seen by isolated practitioners, often psychodynamic in orientation and often working in relative isolation. These practitioners, along with surgeons who performed gender reassignment surgery and other interested parties, formed an association named the Harry Benjamin Gender Dysphoria Association.

Initially, problems with gender identity were thought to represent severe mental illness. Beatrice (1985) found the transsexual people studied demonstrated profound psychological dysfunction and concluded that gender reassignment surgery for this group was not the treatment of choice. Levine (1980) reported that, although female patients were significantly healthier than the males, 92% of the males and 58% of the females had psychiatric diagnoses, apart from gender dysphoria. Most of the abnormalities in both groups were character disorders but 8% had schizophrenia.

These sorts of findings have not been seen in larger, recent studies in adults. Haraldsen et al. (2000) found in 86 transsexual people that scores on the Symptom Checklist 90 (SCL-90) were somewhat higher than healthy controls, but that all scores were within the normal range. Cole et al. (1997) studied 318 male and 117 female patients. Less than 10% had problems associated with mental illness, genital mutilation or suicide attempts. Overall, the results supported the view that transsexualism was usually an isolated diagnosis and not part of any general psychopathological disorder. Similar results were found in adolescents (Smith et al., 2001; Cohen et al., 1997), which supported the idea that major psychopathology was not a fundamental underpinning of the development of transsexualism. It seemed that the earlier findings might have represented a sampling bias.

Currently, disorders of gender identity are classified as disorders of adult personality and behaviour in the 10th

Cambridge Textbook of Effective Treatments in Psychiatry, ed. Peter Tyrer and Kenneth R. Silk. Published by Cambridge University Press.
© Cambridge University Press, 2008.

revision of the International Classification of Diseases (ICD-10), and comprise the following: Transsexualism; Dual-role Transvestism; Gender Identity Disorder of Childhood; Other Gender Identity Disorders; Gender Identity Disorder, Unspecified. In the DSM-IV, these disorders would be classified under Sexual and Gender Identity Disorders and would comprise the categories of Gender Identity Disorder; Gender Identity Disorder Not Otherwise Specified; Sexual Disorder Not Otherwise Specified.

Important differential diagnoses include fetishistic transvestism, dysmorphophobia or body dysmorphic disorder, autogynaephilia or transvestic fetishism, and some of the other disorders of personality, including one instance of multiple personality syndrome (Modestin & Ebner, 1995). Occasionally, psychoses may present in such a way as to resemble a gender identity disorder and, increasingly rarely, gay or lesbian people may present as transsexual (Shtasel, 1979).

Whether transvestism is contiguous with transsexualism or distinct from it is a debate that has endured over the decades. It was reported first by Buhrich in 1977. The current diagnostic position includes dual role transvestism but not fetishistic transvestism as a gender identity disorder, and this distinction reflects current uncertainty.

Transsexualism is described in ICD-10 as a desire to live and be accepted as a member of the opposite sex, usually accompanied by a sense of discomfort with one's anatomic sex. There is no formal definition of transsexualism in DSM but most of what is described as transsexualism in ICD is subsumed under Gender Identity Disorder in the DSM. For the diagnosis to be made, transsexual identity should have been present for at least 2 years and must not be a symptom of another mental disorder, such as schizophrenia, or associated with any intersex, genetic, or sex chromosome abnormality. This last stipulation implies that there is never a genetic or hormonal element in transsexualism, and that any such abnormality, if present, would always account for the cross-gender identity. Either or both of these implications may be without foundation.

There is a public and to some extent general psychiatric perception that transsexualism is the only or at least the main disorder of gender identity. That this is probably illusory has been pointed out by Levine (1980) from an analytic perspective, but the illusion persists in part because most dual role transvestites do not come to the attention of psychiatric services. Certainly, transsexualism is the diagnosis for which most treatment evidence is available. There is little research into dual role transvestism, nor much into dysmorphophobia or autogynephilia

per se (Blanchard, 1993a, 1993b, 1993c). Nor into autogynephilia presenting as or relating to a gender identity disorder (Blanchard, 1991, 1993a, 1993b, 1993c), even though these and related areas such as gynandromorphophilia (sexual interest in cross-dressed or anatomically feminized men) (Blanchard & Collins, 1993) are important differential diagnoses and there is the suggestion that non-transsexual disorders of gender identity are more associated with psychopathology (Miach et al., 2000). This is unfortunate, given that it seems an increasing proportion of dual role transvestites are migrating toward full-time living as a woman (Docter et al., 1997). These differential diagnoses may require different management to transsexualism (for example, Blanchard, 1993).

It is now thought possible for transsexualism to be coincidental with another mental illness and yet not caused by it. Successful treatment of a disorder of gender identity in the presence of another psychiatric illness is common and thus paradoxically rarely published but, because teasing the two apart can sometimes be difficult, challenging cases do gain attention. For example, Marks & Mataix-Cols (1988) reported remission of a gender identity disorder with treatment for apparanty coincidental obsessive-compulsive disorder; Puri et al. (1996) reported the successful treatment of an apparently gender dysphoric patient with pimozide; Caldwell and Keshoven (1991) reported a patient whose gender identity problems waxed and waned with his schizophrenic illness and Commander et al. (1990) reported a man whose 'symptomatic transsexualism' responded to the effective treatment of his schizophrenia.

Within this definition, subsets have long been discerned. The most obvious is that of biologically male and female. There is the growing impression that transsexualism may be different in males and females, and this is not reflected in the current classification system (Landen et al., 1988a, 1988b). It seems that female patients display closer ties to their parents and siblings, established stable partnerships more frequently, and usually solely with the same biological sex, and are more satisfied sexually. This is not connected to whether they have undergone surgery (Kockott et al., 1988; Fleming et al., 1985).

Another distinction that is felt by some to be important is that of the sexual orientation of the transsexual person (Clare & Tully, 1989). There is the suggestion that female patients attracted to females differ quite markedly from those attracted to males (Chivers et al., 2000; Dickey & Stephens, 1995), who are said to be more akin to gay men (Coleman et al., 1993). Male patients, especially those sexually attracted to women, tend to present later in life. There is the suggestion that this late presentation may relate to number of earlier marriages and number of children fathered (Blanchard, 1994). Many male patients (almost always sexually attracted to women) would first have been identified as fetishistic transvestites, as noted by Buhrich & McConaghy as early as 1978, and later as dual role transvestites, before meeting the diagnostic criteria for transsexualism (Tsoi, 1992). Those with an early age of onset, low sexual activity, lack of any history of sexual arousal with cross-dressing, same biological sex sexual orientation and some degree of gender identity disorder in childhood have been viewed as 'core' or 'primary' transsexuals and thought to have a better prognosis. This pattern was found by Verschoor & Poortinga (1988) to be more frequent in female patients. A note of caution is sounded by Blanchard & Clemmensen (1985), who noted that it is possible that the differences in the histories produced by transvestites and heterosexual transsexuals are exaggerated to an unknown degree by the motivation of the latter to obtain approval for surgery. Their findings do not diminish the important distinction between these groups, but they do suggest caution in interpreting the self-report data that have frequently been used in comparing them.

Treatment

Most early approaches to the management of transsexualism were purely psychological and involved either an individual patient's case being reported or else publication of a very small series, which could never have amounted to a satisfactory level of evidence. What emerged from these reports was that individual psychotherapy did not act significantly to change the disorder of gender identity although it did help with other aspects of daily living. The failure of psychotherapy alone in these isolated patients led to it never being extensively employed. Instead, surgical approaches to change bodily form closely to resemble that of the opposite sex took the place of psychological treatment. Some psychoanalysts feel that the near abandonment of psychoanalytical approaches was premature, and that such approaches are more possible as psychoanalysis has developed (e.g. Quinodoz, 1988; Chiland, 2001). Others feel that cognitive style and psychological functioning are as yet under-investigated (Midence & Hargreaves, 1997). Lothstein (1981) reports good success with a mixed psychotherapeutic and surgical approach, noting that, of 50 gender dysphoric patients, 70% had adjusted to non-surgical solutions, 20% were receiving treatment

and 10% had received gender reassignment surgery and psychotherapy.

Initially, surgical approaches were also reported individually or in small numbers. This meant that benefit could not be statistically proven, although the case reports were in the main positive, with only occasional negative reports (Van Putten & Fawzy, 1976). The highly charged nature of the topic caused negative results to probably be as likely to be published as positive ones, and the published balance in favour of gender reassignment surgery was thought to be indicative of true (if statistically undemonstrated) benefit. Accordingly, such treatment continued.

The qualification criteria and timing of surgical intervention have always been contentious topics. Often people with disorder of gender identity have pressed for fewer hurdles and earlier intervention, the psychiatrists for more, and later. Before the formation of the Harry Benjamin International Gender Dysphoria Association, it had been possible for individuals with sufficient financial resources to obtain gender reassignment surgery essentially upon request. Outcomes were highly variable, with some said to have been exceedingly poor. The Harry Benjamin International Gender Dysphoria Association set an arbitrary, but not capricious, minimum period for qualification for gender reassignment surgery of at least a year, despite case reports such as that of Levine & Shumaker (1983) suggesting this might be too short a period. This year had to be spent living wholly in the new gender role, with demonstrable psychological and social success. This period was arrived at because it was felt to be the greatest increase from the previous 'surgery on demand' position that surgeons and their patients would be prepared to accept. A greater period was thought probably to be better, but untenable in the political and economic circumstances of the time (Green, personal communication). This period became known as the 'real life test', and was subsequently renamed the 'real life experience'. It became incorporated into a set of 'Minimum Standards of Care' formulated by the Harry Benjamin Gender Dysphoria Association. These standards are periodically revised, the changes at each revision reflecting the ever-changing dynamic between empirical changes in clinical practice, new research evidence, local legal imperatives and patient and political pressures.

Mate-Kole et al. (1988) found that patients who were on a waiting list for surgery showed lower neurotic scores on the Crown-Crisp Experiential Index than those at the assessment stage of clinic attendance, while post-operative transsexuals obtained scores lower than either of the other groups. This suggests that a social change of gender role with hormone treatment is itself helpful, as is subsequent gender reassignment surgery, a finding reiterated by (Blanchard & Clemmensen, 1983), who found a statistically significant negative correlation between depression and social feminization and between tension and social feminization. He also found a significant positive correlation between cohabitation with a male partner and vaginoplasty, reinforcing the findings of Mate-Kole *et al.* (1991).

In general terms, under the Harry Benjamin Gender Dysphoria Association Standards of Care, both male and female patients are required to change gender role prior to a doctor initiating hormone treatment. Such treatment, when it occurs, is with cross-sex hormones. There is debate about any need for antiandrogen or progestrogenic therapy in male patients, but agreement that high dose estrogen therapy is indicated. The treatment seems to be acceptably safe (van Kesteren *et al.*, 1997), with the major risk being that of thromboembolic disease. Female patients require treatment with androgens, either by implant or by intramuscular injection. Oral treatment is anecdotally associated with a raised rate of hepatocellular carcinoma. It is thus ethically and legally challenging to use oral agents.

Children and adolescents with gender identity disorders pose particular problems. Instinctive caution has led to surgery and hormones being delayed, although all the evidence is that with carefully selected patients early surgical intervention carries a good outcome (Cohen-Kettenis & van Goozen, 1997). There is a trend towards postponing puberty by means of GnRH analogues and introducing cross-sex hormone treatment when the child is old enough to give valid consent. There is the suggestion that, for males, an earlier age of onset of transsexualism was associated with better outcome (Tsoi, 1993), which may reflect 'core' transsexualism. The question is rendered more problematic by studies such as that of Davenport (1986), who followed up ten feminine boys, of whom only one became transsexual, and four heterosexual. He concluded that childhood gender dysphoria appears to be a necessary, but not sufficient, factor in a transsexual outcome. The strength, rigidity and persistence of cross-gender behaviour through latency were thought perhaps to predict transsexual outcome.

Those patients who show improved psychological, social, sexual and occupational functioning in their new gender role for a period of at least a year are considered appropriate candidates for gender reassignment surgery. Such surgery has been subject to most investigation, since as treated patient numbers grew, it became possible to assess psychological and social outcomes after gender reassignment surgery more properly and to relate these outcomes to some features of the patients' presenting histories. Regrettably, though many studies show good outcome, most make no greater comment on the selection process for surgery candidature than to delineate what is often little more than a demographic description of the selected group. The process of psychological assessment leading to subsequent selection seemed rarely described in any depth at all, although this has now begun to be addressed (Barrett, 2007).

The timing of surgery was addressed by Mate Cole *et al.* (1991). In a rare, fully controlled study, which established that once patients had been approved for surgery, those fast-tracked showed better psychological function than those who joined a standard waiting list.

The functional results of gender reassignment surgery have been assessed in sexual terms by Green (1998), who noted in passing the lack of rigorous laboratory-based studies. Rehman *et al.* (1999) noted general satisfaction was expressed over the quality of cosmetic (normal appearing genitalia) and functional (ability to perceive orgasm) aspects. Lief & Hubschman (1993) found that orgastic capacity after gender reassignment surgery declined in male patients and increased in female ones. Despite the decrease in orgasm in the males, satisfaction with sex and general satisfaction with the results of surgery were high in both. Blanchard & Legault (1987) separately suggested that, in purely mechanical terms, modest vaginal depth could be compensated for by a change of sexual technique.

There seem to have been good outcomes in settings as disparate as Serbia (Rakic *et al.*, 1996) and Holland (Kuiper & Cohen-Kettenis, 1988) and the strong suggestion from several studies that the technical success of surgery and a subsequent legal recognition of a change of sex relates strongly to good psychological and social outcome (Tsoi & Kok, 1995). Indeed, in one study technical surgical outcome accounted for nearly all the variation in postoperative psychopathology (Ross & Need, 1989). This is reiterated by Stein *et al.* (1990) who reported good outcomes in a group of ten patients, but noted that none reported being discovered as having had a prior operation by their sexual partner, suggesting technically good results in the group. Much worse psychological outcomes were reported by Lindemalm (1986), but in the 13 patients studied, surgical outcome was disappointing. Only one-third of the patients where a vaginal construction was carried out had a functioning vagina, again supporting a connection with surgical outcomes.

It seems increasingly clear that psychological support is needed after surgery (Rehman *et al.*, 1999) to optimize outcomes, since social stressors may persist despite treatment, particularly if the patient has children. In connection with the welfare of children, Green (1978) found there to be no evidence that a change of parental gender role has any effect on the sexual development of children. Despite this, many patients have experienced impaired access to their children on the grounds of their change of gender role.

Suboptimal post-operative outcomes were addressed by Landen et al. (1998), a regression analysis suggesting that regrets about gender reassignment surgery were associated with poor family and friend support, a lack of an earlier history of childhood gender identity disorder and a lack of attraction to the same biological sex. This was reiterated in another study by Blanchard (1989), which found attraction to the opposite biological sex was associated with a poorer outcome. Another study by Bodlund & Kullgren (1996) showed personality disorder and axis II diagnoses to be associated with a worse outcome, and that female patients tend generally to fare better than male. Another study found no pre-operative variables could predict good adjustments for female transsexuals (Tsoi, 1993). Lindemalm et al. (1987) found traumatic loss of both parents in infancy to be associated with poor outcome and an overprotective mother and a distant father with good. Contrary to other reports, high sexual activity and bisexual experience was associated with fair sexual adjustment and with non-repentance after sex change. Completed military service, a history of typically masculine, hard jobs, and a comparatively late (more than 30 years of age) first request for surgery, were found to be negative prognostic factors in sex-reassignment evaluations, and it was thought that both too much and too little ambivalence may suggest a poor prognosis.

Much less studied have been transsexual people who did not have gender reassignment surgery. Kockott & Fahrner (1987) found that those with an unaltered wish for surgery, but who had not had gender reassignment surgery, did not differ substantially from transsexuals who had had surgery. By contrast, the 'hesitating' patients were noticeably older, more often married, more often had children of their own, their partnerships were of long duration, and exclusively with partners of the opposite biological sex. These characteristics had been seen when the diagnosis was first made and were thought to be prognostic for this subgroup. Transsexual people who relinquished their wish for surgery did not differ substantially from transsexuals with an unaltered wish for surgery. Their reasons for relinquishing the wish for surgery could not clearly be established. It was concluded

that it was hesitating patients who required particular scrutiny.

It should not be forgotten that there are a great many surgical procedures apart from gender reassignment surgery that might have the potential to enhance a transsexual person's ability to pass easily in their new gender role. Very few seem evidence based, although rhinoplasty does seem to help, but again this is 'in a selected population' (Hage & Vossen, 1997).

Genital surgery for female patients is a very much more technically challenging procedure and is much less studied and reported. Patients' functional demands are high (Hage et al., 1993) and surgical results often fail to match them. Despite this, one study found that phalloplasty does not appear to be a critical factor in orgasm or in sexual satisfaction, and the authors concluded that it is possible to change one's body image and sexual identity and be sexually satisfied despite inadequate sexual functioning (Lief & Hubschman, 1993). It is strongly suspected that much greater psychological benefit to female patients is conferred by a bilateral mastectomy than by phalloplasty.

Conclusions

Since gender identity disorders were first described, it has so often been said that there is a dearth of evidence to support any treatment approach. This may have become something of a mantra. This is unfortunate because, over the years, this mantra has been repeated much more even as evidence has accumulated that interventions are beneficial. Most of the evidence relates to transsexualism, probably the least common disorder of gender identity, but it is at least now reasonably sound. It suggests that transsexualism is not indicative of serious psychopathology and that in carefully selected patients, with psychological support, a change of social gender role does much to improve the psychological state of the patient and (if the improvement can be sustained for at least a year), gender reassignment surgery will probably further improve it.

In such a difficult subject area as this, it is not surprising that there are, as yet, no controlled trials of different forms of management, but at the rate of current progress, these may not be too far away. Studies of this sort would certainly add a level of credibility not only to the treatment, but to the disorder(s) as well.

The level of evidence for each of the interventions discussed in this chapter is summarized in Table 46.1.

Table 46.1. Effectiveness of treatments for gender identity

Treatment	Form of treatment	Psychiatric disorder/ target audience	Level of evidence for efficacy	Comments
Psychosocial	Psychotherapy	Gender identity disorder/ transsexualism	IV	Did not change the gender identity disorder but perhaps helped with aspects of daily living
Somatic	Gender reassignment surgery	Transsexualism	III	Better psychosocial adjustment (better scores on items of neurosis) than those on a waiting list and those in no treatment, though those on a waiting listed did better than those not in any type of programme. Post-operative psychopathology may be most related to level of satisfaction with the surgery.
Somatic	Hormonal treatment	Transsexxualism	III	Those who were treated with hormones and were living as the opposite gender had better scores on measures of neurosis than those not in treatment but less than those who received actual surgery

REFERENCES

Ball, J. R. & Emmerson, R. (1978). A case of personation. *Medical Journal of Australia*, **2**(5), 198–201.

Barrett, J., ed. (2007). *Transsexualism and Other Disorders of Gender Identity: A Practical Guide to Management*. Radcliffe Medical Publishing.

Beatrice, J. (1985). A psychological comparison of heterosexuals, transvestites, preoperative transsexuals, and postoperative transsexuals. *Journal of Nervous and Mental Disease*, **173**(6), 358–65.

Blanchard, R. (1991). Clinical observations and systematic studies of autogynephilia. *Journal of Sex and Marital Therapy*, **17**(4), 235–51.

Blanchard, R. (1993a). Partial versus complete autogynephilia and gender dysphoria. *Journal of Sex and Marital Therapy*, **19**(4), 301–7.

Blanchard, R. (1993b). Varieties of autogynephilia and their relationship to gender dysphoria. *Archives of Sexual Behavior*, **22**(3), 241–51.

Blanchard, R. (1993c). The she–male phenomenon and the concept of partial autogynephilia. *Journal of Sex and Marital Therapy*, **19**(1), 69–76.

Blanchard, R. (1994). A structural equation model for age at clinical presentation in nonhomosexual male gender dysphorics. *Archives of Sexual Behavior*, **23**(3), 311–20.

Blanchard, R. & Collins, P. I. (1993). Men with sexual interest in transvestites, transsexuals, and she-males. *Journal of Nervous and Mental Disease*, **181**(9), 570–5.

Blanchard, R., Clemmensen, L. H. & Steiner, B. W. (1983). Gender reorientation and psychosocial adjustment in male-to-female transsexuals. *Archives of Sexual behavior*, **12**(6), 503–9.

Blanchard, R., Clemmensen, L. H. & Steiner, B. W. (1985). Social desirability response set and systematic distortion in the self-report of adult male gender patients. *Archives of Sexual behavior*, **14**(6), 505–16.

Blanchard, R., Legault, S. & Lindsay, W. R. (1987). Vaginoplasty outcome in male-to-female transsexuals. *Journal of Sex and Marital Therapy*, **13**(4), 265–75.

Blanchard, R. Steiner, B. W., Clemmensen, L. H. & Dickey, R. (1989). Prediction of regrets in postoperative transsexuals. *Canadian Journal of Psychiatry – Revue Canadienne de Psychiatrie*, **34**(1), 43–5.

Bodlund, O. & Kullgren, G. (1996). Transsexualism – general outcome and prognostic factors: a five-year follow-up study of nineteen transsexuals in the process of changing sex. *Archives of Sexual behavior*, **25**(3), 303–16.

Buhrich, N. & McConaghy, N. (1977a). The discrete syndromes of transvestism and transsexualism. *Archives of Sexual behavior*, **6**(6), 483–95.

Buhrich, N. & McConaghy, N. (1977b). Can fetishism occur in transsexuals? *Archives of Sexual Behavior* 1977, **6**(3): 223–35.

Buhrich, N. & McConaghy, N. (1978). Two clinically discrete syndromes of transsexualism. *British Journal of Psychiatry*, **133**, 73–6.

Caldwell, C. & Keshavan, M. S. (1991). Schizophrenia with secondary transsexualism. *Canadian Journal of Psychiatry – Revue Canadienne de Psychiatrie*, **36**(4), 300–1.

Chiland, C. (2001). The psychoanalyst and the transsexual patient. *International Journal of Psychoanalysis*, **82**(2), 389, author reply 389–92.

Chivers, M. L. & Bailey J. M. (2000). Sexual orientation of female-to-male transsexuals: a comparison of homosexual and non-homosexual types. *Archives of Sexual Behavior*, **29**(3), 259–78.

Clare, D. & Tully, B. (1989). Transhomosexuality, or the dissociation of sexual orientation and sex object choice. *Archives of Sexual Behavior*, **18**(6), 531–6.

Cohen-Kettenis, P. T. & van Goozen, S. H. (1997). Sex reassignment of adolescent transsexuals: a follow-up study. *Journal of the American Academy of Child and Adolescent Psychiatry*, **36**(2), 263–71.

Cole, C. M., O'Boyle, M., Emory, L. E. & Meyer, W. J., 3rd. (1997). Comorbidity of gender dysphoria and other major psychiatric diagnoses. *Archives of Sexual Behavior*, **26**(1), 13–26.

Coleman, E., Bockting, W. O. & Gooren, L. (1993). Homosexual and bisexual identity in sex-reassigned female-to-male transsexuals. *Archives of Sexual Behavior*, **22**(1), 37–50.

Commander, M. & Dean, C. (1990). Symptomatic trans-sexualism. *British Journal of Psychiatry*, **156**, 894–6.

Davenport, C. W. (1986). A follow-up study of 10 feminine boys. *Archives of Sexual Behavior*, **15**(6), 511–17.

Dickey, R. & Stephens, J. (1995). Female-to-male transsexualism, heterosexual type: two cases. *Archives of Sexual Behavior*, **24**(4), 439–45.

Docter, R. F. & Prince, V. (1997). Transvestism: a survey of 1032 cross-dressers. *Archives of Sexual behavior*, **26**(6), 589–605.

Fleming, M., MacGowan, B. & Costos, D. (1985). The dyadic adjustment of female-to-male transsexuals. *Source Archives of Sexual Behavior*, **14**(1), 47–55.

Green, R. (1978). Sexual identity of 37 children raised by homosexual or transsexual parents. *American Journal of Psychiatry*, **135**(6), 692–7.

Green, R. (1998). Sexual functioning in post-operative transsexuals: male-to-female and female-to-male. *International Journal of Impotence Research*, **10** (Suppl. 1), S22–4.

Hage, J. J., Bout, C. A., Bloem, J. J. & Megens, J. A. (1993). Phalloplasty in female-to-male transsexuals: what do our patients ask for? *Annals of Plastic Surgery*, **30**(4): 323–6.

Hage, J. J., Vossen, M. & Becking, A. G. (1997). Rhinoplasty as part of gender-confirming surgery in male transsexuals: basic considerations and clinical experience. *Annals of Plastic Surgery*, **39**(3), 266–71.

Haraldsen, I. R. & Dahl, A. A. (2000). Symptom profiles of gender dysphoric patients of transsexual type compared to patients with personality disorders and healthy adults. *Acta Psychiatrica Scandinavica*, **102**(4), 276–81.

Heiman, E. M. & Cao-Van-Le. (1975). Transsexualism in Vietnam. *Archives of Sexual Behavior*, **4**(1), 89–95.

Kockott, G. & Fahrner, E. M. (1988). Male-to-female and female-to-male transsexuals: a comparison. *Archives of Sexual Behavior*, **17**(6), 539–46.

Kockott, G. & Fahrner, E. M. (1987). Transsexuals who have not undergone surgery: a follow-up study. *Archives of Sexual Behavior*, **16**(6), 511–22.

Kuiper, B. & Cohen-Kettenis, P. (1988). Sex reassignment surgery: a study of 141 Dutch transsexuals. *Archives of Sexual Behavior*, **17**(5), 439–57.

Landen, M., Walinder, J. & Lundstrom, B. (1996). Prevalence, incidence and sex ratio of transsexualism. *Acta Psychiatrica Scandinavica*, **93**(4), 221–3.

Landen, M., Walinder, J., Hambert, G. & Lundstrom, B. (1998a). Factors predictive of regret in sex reassignment. *Acta Psychiatrica Scandinavica*, **97**(4), 284–9.

Landen, M., Walinder, J. & Lundstrom, B. (1998b). Clinical characteristics of a total cohort of female and male applicants for sex reassignment: a descriptive study. *Acta Psychiatrica Scandinavica*, **97**(3), 189–94.

Levine, S. B. (1980). Psychiatric diagnosis of patients requesting sex reassignment surgery. *Journal of Sex and Marital Therapy*, **6**(3), 164–73.

Levine, S. B. & Shumaker, R. E. (1983). Increasingly Ruth: toward understanding sex reassignment. *Archives of Sexual Behavior*, **12**(3), 247–61.

Lief, H. I. & Hubschman, L. (1993). Orgasm in the postoperative transsexual. *Archives of Sexual Behavior*, **22**(2), 145–55.

Lindemalm, G., Korlin, D. & Uddenberg, N. (1986). Long-term follow-up of 'sex change' in 13 male-to-female transsexuals. *Archives of Sexual Behavior*, **15**(3), 187–210.

Lindemalm, G., Korlin, D. & Uddenberg, N. (1987). Prognostic factors vs. outcome in male-to-female transsexualism. A follow-up study of 13 cases. *Acta Psychiatrica Scandinavica*, **75**(3), 268–74.

Lothstein, L. M. & Levine, S. B. (1981). Expressive psychotherapy with gender dysphoric patients. *Archives of General Psychiatry*, **38**(8), 924–9.

Marks, I., Green, R. & Mataix-Cols, D. (2000). Adult gender identity disorder can remit. *Comprehensive Psychiatry*, **41**(4), 273–5.

Marks, I. M. & Mataix-Cols, D. (1988). Four-year remission of transsexualism after comorbid obsessive-compulsive disorder improved with self-exposure therapy. *British Journal of Psychiatry*, **172**, 452–4.

Mate-Kole, C., Freschi, M. & Robin, A. (1988). Aspects of psychiatric symptoms at different stages in the treatment of transsexualism. *British Journal of Psychiatry*, **152**, 550–3.

Mate-Kole, C., Freschi, M. & Robin, A. (1991). A controlled study of psychological and social change after surgical gender reassignment in selected male transsexuals, **158**, 132–3.

Miach, P. P., Berah, E. F., Butcher, J. N. & Rouse S. (2000). Utility of the MMPI-2 in assessing gender dysphoric patients. *Journal of Personality Assessment*, **75**(2), 268–79.

Midence, K. & Hargreaves, I. (1997). Psychosocial adjustment in male-to-female transsexuals: an overview of the research evidence. *Journal of Psychology*, **131**(6), 602–14.

Modestin, J. & Ebner, G. (1995). Multiple personality disorder manifesting itself under the mask of transsexualism. *Psychopathology*, **28**(6), 317–21.

Puri, B. K. Singh, I. (1996). The successful treatment of a gender dysphoric patient with pimozide. *Australian and New Zealand Journal of Psychiatry*, **30**(3), 422–5.

Quinodoz, D. (1998). A fe/male transsexual patient in psychoanalysis. *International Journal of Psycho-Analysis*, **79**(1), 95–111.

Rakic, Z., Starcevic, V., Maric, J. & Kelin, K. (1996). The outcome of sex reassignment surgery in Belgrade: 32 patients of both sexes. *Archives of Sexual Behavior*, **25**(5), 515–25.

Rehman, J., Lazer, S., Benet, A. E., Schaefer, L. C. & Melman, A. (1999). The reported sex and surgery satisfactions of 28 postoperative male-to-female transsexual patients. *Archives of Sexual Behavior*, **28**(1), 71–89.

Ross, M. W. & Need, J. A. (1989). Effects of adequacy of gender reassignment surgery on psychological adjustment: a follow-up of fourteen male-to-female patients. *Archives of Sexual Behavior*, **18**(2), 145–53.

Shtasel, T. F. (1979). Behavioral treatment of transsexualism: a case report. *Journal of Sex and Marital Therapy*, **5**(4), 362–7.

Smith, Y. L., van Goozen, S. H. & Cohen-Kettenis, P. T. (2001). Adolescents with gender identity disorder who were accepted or rejected for sex reassignment surgery: a prospective follow-up study. *Journal of the American Academy of Child and Adolescent Psychiatry*, **40**(4), 472–81.

Stein, M., Tiefer, L. & Melman, A. (1990). Followup observations of operated male-to-female transsexuals. *Journal of Urology*, **143**(6), 1188–92.

Tsoi, W. F. (1992). Male and female transsexuals: a comparison. *Singapore Medical Journal*, **33**(2), 182–5.

Tsoi, W. F. (1993). Follow-up study of transsexuals after sex-reassignment surgery. *Singapore Medical Journal*, **34**(6), 515–17.

Tsoi, W. F., Kok, L. P., Yeo, K. L. & Ratnam, S. S. (1995). Follow-up study of female transsexuals. *Annals of the Academy of Medicine, Singapore*, **24**(5), 664–7.

van Kesteren, P. J., Asscheman, H., Megens, J. A. & Gooren, L. J. (1997). Mortality and morbidity in transsexual subjects treated with cross-sex hormones. *Clinical Endocrinology*, **47**(3), 337–42.

Van Putten, T. & Fawzy, F. I. (1976). Sex conversion surgery in a man with severe gender dysphoria. A tragic outcome. *Archives of General Psychiatry*, **33**(6), 751–3.

Verschoor, A. M. & Poortinga, J. (1988). Psychosocial differences between Dutch male and female transsexuals. *Archives of Sexual Behavior*, **17**(2), 173–8.

Child psychiatry

Section editors

Matthew Hodes and Christopher K. Varley

47

Psychological treatments for children and adolescents

Brian W. Jacobs, Stefanie A. Hlastala and Elizabeth McCauley

Editor's note

This chapter provides an introduction to the various types of psychological treatments currently being provided to children and adolescents. Because the chapter is considered as an overview of psychological interventions, it emphasizes the various types of interventions and reviews some of the techniques of those interventions rather than focusing on the effectiveness of any particular type of intervention. While a table has been provided to review the overall efficacy and effectiveness of psychotherapeutic interventions in this patient age-grouping, more detail will be provided for the effectiveness of these interventions in the sections that discuss specific disorders. Thus the table here probably underestimates the effectiveness of these interventions because they probably are not equally effective across all mental health conditions that impact children. Since the major social context in which children operate is the home (and the school), there is mention made of family therapy as well. The section covers both non-directive and directive individual as well as group therapies. The approaches include dynamic, behavioural and cognitive-behavioural. Family and systemic therapy is reviewed as well as parent and family skills training. Such training and educational interventions also take place in social skills training and problem solving groups.

Psychological treatments

General issues

Children are not small adults. Obvious as it may seem, this fact somehow gets forgotten or becomes an issue that seems overwhelming for those not working in this field. In considering treatments in child and adolescent psychiatry, we must take account of some of the differences so that adaptations of adult treatments can be considered and novel treatments that are more appropriate to children and their situation can be devised and tested. Differences include the complex issue of biological development, an increasingly complex environment as the child grows up and the legal framework designed to protect their welfare.

Family, school and other networks

Much more than adults, children exist in an intricate, dependent context. Disturbance to their environment can result in psychiatric distress and disorder of itself and can add to the difficulties experienced when the root cause of the disorder is predominantly biological.

Initially, children depend for their physical survival on their parents. Failures in early emotional care can lead to biological changes in their brain function which are long-lasting (Heim *et al.*, 2001). The emotional, cognitive and moral environments to which they become exposed are crucial for healthy development. With age, children are exposed to increasingly complex social networks. In Western Society they mix with other children in nursery school and then school. While these networks provide children with opportunities, they also expose them to the complications of peer relationships. Puberty and adolescence present them with increasing finances and exposure to quasi-adult decisions about their lifestyles. Their lack of experience makes them more vulnerable to difficulties. They are still developing emotionally and physically. This ongoing development offers opportunities for greater plasticity to overcome distress and psychiatric disorder in personality development, whilst at the same time making them especially vulnerable. Treatments aimed for children and adolescents have to take these networks and developmental factors into account whatever the particular therapy.

Cambridge Textbook of Effective Treatments in Psychiatry, ed. Peter Tyrer and Kenneth R. Silk. Published by Cambridge University Press.
© Cambridge University Press, 2008.

Confidentiality, consent, legislation and psychological treatments

Confidentiality and consent issues are more complex for children than adults. These issues are pertinent for psychological interventions as well as for other areas of child and adolescent mental health. While parents are usually thought to act in their children's best interests, they probably know less of their children's thoughts and feelings than they think. Parents may know quite a lot about their children's behaviour and actions until adolescence, when the picture becomes increasingly murky as the young person demands independence. Therapists have realized that a child's right of confidentiality, particularly at the lower ends of childhood and adolescence, has to be limited. It is their parents who are most likely to be in a position to protect children from any intention to self-harm. To do so, parents need to be informed.

Confidentiality becomes a pointed matter for adolescents. If it is not respected, they may refuse to see child mental health professionals. Equally, if confidentiality is unthinkingly preserved, their lives may be placed inappropriately at risk at an age when they cannot fully appreciate the consequences of their actions.

In the UK, the picture regarding consent is complex and evolving. Following the case of Gillick (1986), young people are regarded as capable of giving informed consent in their own right if the professional concerned is convinced that they understand the consequences of giving such consent. However, there is currently a higher threshold for a young person being able to refuse consent. Legally, parents or the courts can give consent in the face of a young person's refusal of consent until the age of 18. However, guidance advises against this happening except in extreme circumstances when the young person's life is at risk. This is a controversial situation and it is likely to change too as the treatment of a young person begins to shift into treatment as an adult for these matters from somewhere between the ages of 16 and 18.

In the United Kingdom as elsewhere there is a range of legislation designed to protect the interests of children and young people that does not apply to adults. A principle underlying this legislation requires authorities to consider the needs of the child paramount over those of their carers. This principle shapes the treatments that are designed and implemented for children and young people.

General issues concerning the evidence base for psychological treatments of children and adolescents

More than 1500 empirical studies of psychotherapy for children and adolescents have been conducted (Kazdin, 2000). Studies examining the effects of 'traditional' child psychotherapy (mainly psychodynamic) on functioning indicate that the clinically guided care found in usual practice is not an effective treatment for youth (Weisz et al., 2004). For example, two studies reported overall effect sizes of −0.08 (Weiss et al., 1999) and 0.01 (Weisz et al., 1995) for traditional child psychotherapy applied in clinic settings. Although comprehensive systems of care that provide a case manager and a menu of mental health services increase access to treatment and improve levels of client satisfaction, studies on the effects of these show little evidence of benefit to youth (Bickman et al., 1995; Salzer et al., 1999).

Meta-analyses of research treatments have found effect sizes of 0.71 to 0.79 (Casey & Berman, 1985; Kazdin et al., 1990a, b; Weisz et al., 1987, 1995) for treatment outcomes, indicating that the average child treated with psychotherapy had a better outcome than 76% of control-group children (Weisz et al., 1995). They included treatment outcome studies with children aged 4–18 years old and suggest that the effect size of psychotherapy in youth is similar to the effect size of psychotherapy in adults. The observed loss of treatment effect in an ordinary clinical setting has led to much interest in the question of what constitutes effective vs. efficacious treatment. Until recently, treatment trials have focused on efficacious treatment in carefully controlled research settings rather than in everyday clinics. Currently, there is great interest in what can be effective treatments in the latter (clinical) settings, and funding bodies are increasingly insisting that psychological research is carried out in typical clinical settings rather than teaching hospitals.

Weisz et al. (1995) suggested three plausible explanations for the differential effects found between studies of psychotherapy conducted in research settings vs. those conducted in community clinics: (1) the use of behavioural methods, (2) the use of specific, focused treatment (rather than eclectic approaches), and (3) the use of treatment manuals and therapy adherence monitoring. There is some indication that, in general, behavioural treatments may be more effective than non-behavioural treatments (Casey & Berman 1985; Weisz et al., 1987, 1995). However, there are non-behavioural therapies for specific disorders and/or populations that have been shown to be efficacious (e.g. Interpersonal Therapy for depressed adolescents) (Mufson et al., 1999). It should not be concluded that behavioural therapies are the only effective treatments for children and adolescents.

The existing research literature is dominated by studies examining main effects of treatment without much attention paid to potential moderators of these treatment effects. Some studies of youth with externalizing disorders have found that certain patient variables (e.g. symptom severity, parental psychopathology, family stress and socio-economic disadvantage) moderate treatment outcome (Webster-Stratton & Hammond, 1990; Kazdin, 1995; Kazdin & Wassel, 1999). Other factors are also important when applying psychotherapy for children and adolescents.

Children at higher cognitive developmental levels are able to benefit from more complex interventions (e.g. cognitive interventions aimed to help youth understand the connection between their thinking, emotions and behaviour) than children at lower cognitive developmental levels (Shirk, 2001). Findings from studies specifically examining the relationship between age and psychotherapy outcomes are mixed. Some studies have found no relation between age and treatment effect size (Casey & Berman, 1985), whereas others have found greater effect sizes for adolescents than for younger children (Dush et al., 1989; Durlak et al., 1991; Weisz et al., 1995), while still others found that older youth showed less positive changes in therapy than younger children (Weisz et al., 1987). At this time, there is no consistent pattern found in the research on age and treatment effects. Gender by age interaction were found by Weisz and colleagues (1995) but not in their earlier meta-analysis (Weisz et al., 1987). They suggest that secular trends are responsible or that interventions have become especially sensitive to the treatment needs of adolescent girls.

Not surprisingly, the therapeutic alliance appears to influence the outcome of psychotherapy in youth as well. Children whose parents have a better relationship with the therapist do better in treatment (Kazdin & Wassel, 1999). A bad therapeutic relationship is related to youth and/or their parents prematurely ending treatment (Garcia & Weisz, 2002).

Psychological approaches to treatment for children and adolescents

Behaviour therapy (BT)

Behaviour therapy found early and wide application for child mental health quite widely as it used a problem-solving approach and so was useful across categorical diagnoses. Initially, it was ideologically in opposition to psychodynamic approaches which were much more interested in the psychological meaning of symptoms and in helping children to resolve the conflicts behind these meanings. However, recently there has been an increasing realization among behaviour therapists that the meanings that behaviours carry for the actor and for those around them also require attention to help resolve them.

Behavioural approaches have been widely used with applications for children with learning difficulties and autism spectrum disorders, through children with ADHD and externalizing behaviour disorders to those intensely anxious children and those with obsessional-compulsive disorder. Behaviour therapy has also been applied in the classroom setting to help children stay on task and to promote positive social interactions in the playground (Dolan et al., 1993; Eddy et al., 2000).

The context in which behavioural work is carried out reflects the complexity of development and of family systems and the developmental level of the child. Taking the example of behaviour disorders, delivery of behavioural techniques to parents in recent years has been carried out as direct work with parents (Bank et al., 1991) or to groups of parents (Webster-Stratton, 1996) or in the family setting (Alexander & Parsons, 1982). As children become older, more cognitive elements are introduced (see below).

Cognitive-behaviour therapy (CBT)

Much has been written on the application of cognitive-behavioural therapy to adult disorders. Kendall (2000) and Graham (1998) have collated a growing literature on its application to child and adolescent disorders. Compton and colleagues have recently reviewed the evidence for CBT in the treatment of anxiety and depressive disorders in childhood (Compton et al., 2004). Much of the early work focused on narrow problems such as fears of going out at night (Kanfer et al., 1975) or used particular techniques from the CBT repertoire for adults and adapted them for children, e.g. the use of self-talk (Durlak et al., 1991)). Recently, a more programmatic approach to particular child psychiatric disorders has developed as the range and inter-relationship of cognitive deficits and distortions that are present in particular child mental health disorders is better appreciated (see Hibbs & Jensen, 1996).

Particular adaptations of CBT need to be made for the younger child. The child is seen as working as an equal with the therapist, working empirically with their thoughts and feelings, behaviours and coping style, learning to notice their responses to their own internal and the external cues from important others and the environment and then using this information to alter their responses to responses which are more adaptive and successful. These are complex tasks that have to be simplified by the therapist. As children become more familiar with the techniques the therapists can become more sophisticated in their approach. Often, quite young children are capable of grasping the concepts provided that the language used is modified to be age and developmental stage appropriate. As Ronen (1998) points out, age, gender and cognitive ability will affect the techniques that are used and how they are implemented by the CBT therapist with children and families.

The role of emotions in CBT for children and adolescents has been de-emphasized for two reasons. The first relates to the early theoretical basis of CBT as developed by Beck for adult depression; emotions were seen as outcomes of automatic thoughts and they could be modified through training to have more controlled thoughts. This was a very cognitive model of therapy that may have arisen in reaction to other therapies prominent at the time. More recently, it has been realized that emotions are much more integral to the whole process of thinking. Moreover, cognitions are embedded in feelings by means of differential attention and automatic evaluations (Greenberg et al., 1993).

The second reason connects with normal child development and its distortions, and it is crucial to the application of CBT techniques with children. Essentially, children have a very limited repertoire for the recognition of emotions in infancy. They are helped by sensitive parents to perceive and begin to label their feelings. This ability gradually increases in range and subtlety during childhood and adolescence. Categorizing such emotions tends to lag behind the child's ability to perceive them. Many children who have externalizing disorders come from environments where the naming of emotions is poorly developed (Patterson et al., 1992). For children, the normal process of developing recognition of their own emotions is impaired. This impacts on the child's ability to develop empathy for others and leads to limited and distorted cognitions around social interactions (Dodge, 1985). Additionally, some children may be biologically rather insensitive to emotions. Designing CBT interventions for children and adolescents with particular disorders must take account of these factors and be modified for the particular child's needs.

Certainly a careful multi-axial diagnostic approach is required including an assessment of the child's intellectual level. Adapting the CBT approach for the child's intellectual level is crucial. Similarly, adapting the material so that the child can take an external perspective of his or her own position is essential. This is a conceptual task that younger children can only do with simplified supportive material (Weisz & Weersing, 1999). If an anxious or depressed child has difficulties because of volatile emotions or an inability to evolve solutions or come to a decision, the child will need help with this in its own right as part of the treatment. In general there is a stronger behavioural focus in the CBT programmes designed for children and adolescents with a gradually increasing cognitive

component during adolescence (Brent et al., 1993; Kazdin & Weisz, 1998).

The delivery of CBT to children and adolescents in the context of internalizing disorders is reviewed by Brent et al. (2002). In that account they draw out some general principles of applying CBT to these populations. Children rarely seek treatment by themselves. However, they may resent being brought for help. A working alliance needs to be established and education provided about the methods of CBT so that, particularly for adolescent patients, they can become significantly independent in their treatment and this can improve the chances of treatment success. For younger children involvement of the family in goal setting and in helping the child improve socialization is essential. Though no less important for adolescents, this requires a subtle approach to avoid alienating the young person. These considerations can reduce the dropout rate from therapy (Brent et al., 1993). Often parents are made anxious by their child's difficulties, and a family anxiety management component can improve the outcome of CBT for young, anxious children (Barrett et al., 1996; Brent et al., 1998). Family members can deliver the CBT for their younger children (Barrett et al., 1996; Cohen & Mannarino, 1996). Family discord, poor cohesion and a lack of external support can contribute to treatment being ineffective (Birmaher et al., 2000; Brent et al., 1998; Kolko, 1996)

Family and systemic therapy

Family and systemic therapy has had some successes in empirical research. It is seen as an important approach in child mental health treatments because the child develops in the context of his/her family and is affected by the behaviour and beliefs of other family members.

Interviewing style is very important (Eisler, 2002), both in terms of the type of information that the interviewer is trying to elicit but also because it is so easy to exclude young children by using too adult a style of conversation. The interviewer may need to have drawing materials or play materials (Dare & Lindsey, 1979) and give some time to engaging the child directly and while ensuring that the child understands the conversation as it proceeds.

In general, styles that incorporate behavioural therapy techniques applied in a family context assume greater prominence in intervening with younger children whilst those that are more linked to the family belief systems or discussion of relationship qualities tend to become more useful in later childhood and adolescence. Typically, a behavioural family therapy model will be employed when working with a family with one or more children with oppositional defiant disorder. When working with a family containing a child with anorexia nervosa, a style that combines some elements of a structural family therapy approach with a non-blaming examination of family belief systems is used.

There are exceptions to this generalization. For example, Michael White's approach to externalization provides a method adapted for the young child to begin to grapple with the help of the family with encopresis (White, 1989a, 1989b). It uses a combination of behavioural techniques combined with a simplified approach to the child's belief system that can be acceptable to the close family in enabling the child and family to combat the soiling without blaming the child. Embedded in this method is a simple but important concept, that blame and criticism are very unhelpful for a child's healthy development (Caspi et al., 2004; Seifer et al., 1992). These techniques provide parents with a way of disengaging from strong evoked emotions, while introducing a playful element without losing the basic behavioural techniques that have been shown to work with encopresis.

Not all adolescent problems respond well to an approach based on an improved understanding of family beliefs. Approaches to delinquency in adolescents focusing on these beliefs do not have empirical support. On the other hand, an approach that is largely behavioural but which also involves some negotiation with the adolescent within such a behavioural framework does have an evidence base (see Scott et al., 2001). In addition to this general effect of age and cognitive development on the intervention style with families, Hampson & Beavers (1996) found that under-organized families do better with more structured, directive approaches whilst families that are relatively well-functioning benefit from more narrative/social constructionist approaches .

There is a small research literature developing for family therapy. There is a lack of process research and the outcome research carried out so far is slanted towards behaviourally based interventions. This can lead to a 'truth' that only behavioural family interventions work.

Family therapy is prone to self re-invention. New theoretical frameworks appear with some regularity, and it is sometimes difficult to decide whether or not these are genuine innovations. There is rarely time for the development of manualized treatment approaches, let alone randomized clinical trials before the next development in style of therapy becomes popularized.

Yet family therapy can take pride that many of its ideas have become incorporated into the thinking of child and adolescent mental health practice so that many other professionals take for granted a systemic approach to their work even if they are not practising family therapists. Involving the parents directly in family therapy or in a

parallel cognitive style of therapy that is easily integrated with the child's therapy has been shown to be effective (Kolko, 1996). There are also examples of family therapy techniques being taken up by therapists from other perspectives, such as the use of externalizing in CBT of obsessive-compulsive disorder (March & Mulle, 1998).

There is a recognition among family therapists that there are links between elements of behaviour through increasingly complex ways of assembling these to individual belief systems, family scripts and societal expectations (Campbell et al., 1991). The choice then becomes at what level(s) interventions may usefully be made. With this synthesis it becomes much more possible to integrate thinking about families. It allows the use of elements from behavioural approaches through interpersonal narrative ones and can include psychodynamic thinking to produce a more holistic formulation.

Parent training

Parent and Family Skills training has been developed in the last 30 years and increasing evidence has accrued for its efficacy (Behan & Carr, 2000; Brosnan & Carr, 2000; Kazdin, 1997; Taylor & Biglan, 1998). The programmes have generally concentrated on working with the parents of preschool children and those in middle childhood (Patterson et al., 1975; Webster-Stratton, 1996) but have also been adapted for parents of adolescents (Bank et al., 1991; Dishion & Andrews, 1995).

The goal of these programmes are to improve the relationship between the parents and the target child through age appropriate shared activities, learning to give specific labelled praise to the child and to set up behavioural reward programmes. The methods include a series of non-aggressive techniques for limiting unwanted behaviours in the child. These methods range from the use of withdrawing attention from unwanted behaviours rather than giving them negative attention, to the use of appropriate but limited sanctions and the use of time out. The parents are taught to use these techniques discriminately while trying as far as possible to emphasize and give attention to behaviours that the parents do want rather than those that they wish to extinguish. Characteristic of these programmes is a sophisticated mix of a psycho-educational approach combined with great attention, particularly in the Webster-Stratton suite of programmes, on a collaborative approach to working with the parents (Webster-Stratton & Hammond, 1990, 1997). Programmes often also address difficulties in parents' adult relationships. The goal here is to help parents to teach their children appropriate negotiating and social problem solving skills (e.g. Webster-Stratton, 1996).

Bloomquist & Schnell (2002) review elements of parenting programmes that seem necessary for efficacy. Kazdin (1997) and others have pointed out that a much higher dose (frequency and length of programme) may be necessary in some cases.

Oppositional defiant disorder (ODD) and conduct disorder (CD) are very common in society (Lahey *et al.*, 1999) and form approximately 50%–60% of community child mental health practice and parent skills training is important here. Adaptations of parent training methods have also been used with children who have ADHD (Anastopoulos *et al.*, 1996).

As elsewhere in CAMHS intervention, careful attention needs to be given to the child's developmental stage; they engage with a greater diversity of increasingly complex external systems as they get older. Programmes for disruptive, aggressive adolescents contain the same principles but emphasize age-appropriate negotiation within a clear disciplinary framework and deal with the various temptations and difficulties facing adolescents.

Individual psychodynamic therapy
Psychodynamic approaches to the treatment of children and adolescents have a long history going back to the early development of child mental health services. The theory has changed and evolved since its origins over a century ago. Some aspects of drive theory sometimes still apply with patients but other times it is inadequate. Drive theory, in general, has been replaced by object relations theory. Object relations theory has been seminal to psychodynamic psychotherapists in their thinking about the internal world of the child. Parents and important others are distorted through the child's own defence mechanisms. While defence mechanisms are important in helping the child to obtain some sense of control in phases of his life when he has very limited actual control, unfortunately defences and distorted object relations can become a liability. The development of object relations theory is charted in Greenberg & Mitchell (1990) and its modifications in relation to children can be found in Sandler *et al.* (1980) and Spillius (1988). Much briefer accounts of psychodynamic theory as applied to work with children can be found in Jacobs (1997) and Lanyado & Horn (1999).

With an increasing understanding of early child development through the empirical science of developmental psychology has come a better understanding of how the theoretical models of the child's internal world may have to adapt. Influential in this field for the work of child psychoanalysts and psychotherapists have been the writings of Brazelton & Cramer, 1990; Brazelton & Yogman, 1985.

It is now quite clear that newborn infants are sentient beings with rapidly increasingly complex thought processes and learning soon after birth. This was not realized in earlier psychodynamic writing.

Attachment theory has given rise to the development of a theoretical framework that can more easily be tested empirically with the development of instruments that are thought to measure normal and abnormal activation of the attachment system at various ages in early to middle childhood (Bretherton *et al.*, 1990; Green *et al.*, 2000; Goldwyn *et al.*, 2000). These instruments offer the potential to measure changes in attachment patterns, particularly attachment disorganization.

Working with parents to enable them to support the child's therapy is seen as an essential component of psychodynamic child therapy (Kennedy, 2004). This work with the parents may be intensive in its own right. At other times, group work with parents seems more appropriate particularly when the parent is isolated in reality or through a sense of failure with their child. Meeting others in a similar predicament can be very supportive (Rustin, 1999; Tsiantis, 2000).

Increasingly, child psychotherapists are providing consultation to other professionals working in a variety of settings with distressed children. They are also providing a variety of direct interventions which overlap with other approaches but which retain a psychodynamic approach to their thinking (Hunter, 2001; Rustin, 2003).

Interpersonal therapy (IPT)
Interpersonal therapy for adult depression was adapted for use with adolescents by Mufson and colleagues (Mufson *et al.*, 1993, 1996, 1999). The therapy is designed as a once weekly therapy carried out individually with the adolescent over 12 weeks. The originators describe three phases of treatment. During the first four sessions the aim is to assess the depression, the family and the social context for the adolescent and then negotiate a treatment contact. Parents are used as resources during the assessment. In the second phase, the therapist works with the patient and where necessary conjointly with other family members to address one or two of the problems identified earlier. These may include grief, role disputes or transitions, interpersonal deficits and the particular difficulties of living in a single-parent family. A collaborative approach is made to problem solving. However, there are links to a brief focused psychodynamic approach as well as differences (Fombonne, 1998; Markowitz *et al.*, 1998). The final phase of therapy (sessions 9–12) mainly addresses relinquishing the therapist and establishing a sense of competence to deal with future problems.

The patient is allowed a limited 'sick role' in order to reduce self-blame and criticism from other family members. At the same time the adolescent is encouraged to maintain as many social roles as possible and engage in activities from their previous lifestyle.

Experiential therapies

The evidence base for experiential therapies in child and adolescent mental health is extremely limited. Nonetheless, practitioners use music therapy, art therapy, dance and movement therapies and drama therapy for children and for adolescents in a variety of conditions ranging from autism to severe eating disorders. Practically, it is found that some children are better able to explore their feelings and their interactions through these media than through talking therapies. The interested reader may wish to access the literature through Scott *et al.* (2001).

Group therapy

Group therapies have been surprisingly limited in their application and in research in child and adolescent psychiatry. Despite some lack of enthusiasm for a group approach in the USA (Kazdin *et al.*, 1990a, b; Koocher & Pedulla, 1977) some investigators have shown that these group therapies can be effective interventions (Kolvin *et al.*, 1981). Reid (1999) describes a number of general aspects of group process that may help adolescents.

Some groups have been designed for youngsters trying to come to terms with specific issues such as sexual abuse. Bentovim *et al.* (1988) suggest that group work avoids replication of the secrecy of the abusive experience. The group offers specific support around the conflicts engendered by such abuse and can help these children and adolescents to improve their self-esteem.

The content of groups must be adapted to the appropriate developmental stage of the young people concerned. Groups should probably have a restricted age range because of developmental issues (Kymissis, 1997).

Psychodynamic and other non-directive relationship-based group therapies

Strategies for psychodynamic and other non-directive relationship based group therapies have become more similar over time. Strict psychoanalytical interpretations are less commonly used now, although consideration by the group leader of unconscious processes within the group is common. A clearer focus on current interactions is common.

In thinking about the needs of group members and some aspects of group processes using a psychodynamic developmental framework, certain strategies can be useful. In his active analytic group therapy, Evans (1998) is concerned with both the impact of stressors on the youngster and the youngster's maladaptive (defence driven) responses.

There is a need to balance accessibility with the perfect style of group for the particular child as well as a practical consideration in that adolescents tend to lose their impetus for change unless they get a quick response. Thus, an active analytic group therapy can offer a pragmatic and responsive style. Its aims include:

(a) achievement of age-appropriate tasks
(b) improved style of relating to people
(c) improved coping mechanisms and with a concomitant reduction of anxieties
(d) improved capacity to tolerate frustrations
(e) improved reality testing
(f) improved ability to relinquish patterns of behaviour that have become age inappropriate.

For psychodynamic groups, Kymissis (1997) gives guidance on selection and exclusion criteria for children and adolescents. He suggests that anxiety, poor self esteem, or poor social skills are strong indications for candidacy. Exclusion criteria may include substance abuse, active psychotic symptoms, suicidality or non-compliant continued aggressive behaviour. There is no evidence base for these criteria but they are based on clinical experience.

The techniques used in children's groups include drawing, painting, puppets and group games. Adolescent groups may use fewer accessory materials. The group therapist must attend to group processes that are also seen in adult groups but which may tend to play out at high intensity in a child or adolescent group. Failure to do so can easily result in an ineffective group and a poor outcome.

Client reports and therapist observations suggest that interpretations of patient behaviour and transference in groups in terms of childhood experiences is less useful and much less appreciated than understandings based on current situations (Corder *et al.*, 1981).

Social skills groups and problem-solving skills training

Early attempts in the 1970s at social skills training were divided into those therapists who tried to teach children the micro-skills of social interaction (Argyle, 1969; Spence & Marzillier, 1979) and those who focused more on the macro-patterns of interactions. In general, the latter strategy has been more successful. A third strand has been the development of various social problem-solving programmes (Compas *et al.*, 2002). This has meant that today there are a number of programmes that use elements from both social skills training and also from social problem solving.

Both social skills training and social problem solving training accept that there are deficits in a child's or adolescent's ability to interact with peers. Some claim that the primary deficit is in the child's abilities to analyse the nature of a social interaction and to activate successful prosocial strategies. Others argue that children understand the social situation but lack the skills to take part successfully. A third view gives primacy to a lack of understanding and processing of internal and external emotional cues.

Social skills training has been used in a variety of situations in the treatment of child psychiatric disorders including oppositional defiant disorder (Webster-Stratton &

Hammond, 1997), conduct disorder, anger management (Lochman *et al.*, 1991), attention deficit hyperactivity disorder (Abikoff & Hechtman, 1996; Meichenbaum & Goodman, 1971). Reviews are provided by Baer & Nietzel (1991) and Nolan & Carr (2000). Social skills training has also been applied to child sexual abuse (McGain & McKinzey, 1995; Trowell *et al.*, 2002), drug abuse (Liddle & Dakof, 1995), anxiety disorders (Albano & Barlow, 1996), depression (Clarke & Lewinsohn, 1990; Lewinsohn *et al.*, 1996) and separation and divorce (Alpert-Gillis *et al.*, 1989; Roseby & Deutch 1985). Some of the latter programmes also specifically help children with stress management (Pedro-Carroll *et al.*, 1992). Many of these programmes use social skills training in a group setting but others, particularly those focusing on externalizing disorders in older children, tend to prefer an individual approach.

The level of evidence for each of the interventions discussed in this chapter is summarized in Table 47.1.

Table 47.1. Effectiveness of psychological treatments for children and adolescents

Treatment	Form of treatment	Psychiatric disorder/ target audience	Level of evidence for efficacy	Comments
Clinically guided individual psychotherapy	Psychodynamic and other clinically guided psychotherapies	Child psychiatric disorders in general	Ia, IV	Little evidence for efficacy even when a case management and other comprehensive services added when done in a purely 'clinical' setting (effective) versus effect sizes of approximately 0.75 when carried out in a carefully controlled research setting (efficacious).
Clinically (research) structured individual psychotherapy	Often CBT but other manualized treatments	Child psychiatric disorders in general	IIa	More evidence that behavioural treatments may be more effective than psychodynamic, but definitive studies have yet to be conducted
Family therapy	From psychodynamic and systems through behavioural and cognitive-behavioural	Child psychiatric disorders in general	IIIa	Most empirical research has been done on behavioural therapy which can lead to the (false) impression that this is the only type of family therapy that is effective
Parent and family skills training	Essentially psycho-educational approaches	Child psychiatric disorders in general	IIb	Appears to be particularly useful in externalizing disorders
Group therapy	Psychodynamic and non-directive	Child psychiatric disorders in general	IV	Probably useful in older children and adolescents. Widely used but probably without sufficient empirical support.
Group therapy	Social skills and problem solving (psychoeducational and directive)	Child psychiatric disorders in general	III	Slightly more evidence base than for non-directive groups but still empirical support is quite thin

REFERENCES

(1986). Gillick v. West Norfolk and Wisbech Area Health Authority, AC112.

Abikoff, H. B. & Hechtman, L. (1996). Multimodal therapy and stimulants in the treatment of children with attention deficit hyperactivity disorder. *Psychosocial Treatments for Child and Adolescent Disorders: Empirically based strategies for clinical practice*, ed. E. D. Hibbs & P. S. Jensen, pp. 341–69. Washington DC: American Psychological Association.

Albano, A. M. & Barlow, D. (1996). Breaking the vicious cycle: cognitive-behavioral group treatment for socially anxious youth. *Psychosocial Treatments for Child and Adolescent Disorders: Empirically based strategies for clinical practice*, ed. E. D. Hibbs and P. S. Jensen, pp. 43–62. Washington DC: American Psychological Association.

Alexander, J. F. & Parsons, B. V. (1982). Short term behavioral interventions with delinquent families: Impact on family process and recidivism. *Journal of Abnormal Psychology*, **81**, 219–25.

Alpert-Gillis, L., Pedro-Carroll, J. & Cowen, E. (1989). The children of divorce intervention program: development, implementation and evaluation of a program for young children. *Journal of Consulting and Clinical Psychology*, **57**, 583–9.

Anastopoulos, A. D., Barkley, R. A. & Sheldon, T. L. (1996). Family-based treatment: Psychosocial intervention for children and adolescents with attention deficit hyperactivity disorder. *Psychosocial treatments for child and adolescent disorders empirically based strategies for clinical practice*, ed. E. D. Hibbs & P. S. Jensen. Washington DC: American Psychological Association.

Argyle, M. (1969). *Social Interaction*. London: Methuen.

Baer, R. & Nietzel, M. (1991). Cognitive and behavioural treatments of impulsivity in children: a meta-analytic review of the outcome literature. *Journal of Clinical and Consulting Psychology*, **20**, 400–12.

Bank, L., Marlowe, J. H. Reid, J. B., Patterson, E. R. & Weinrott, M. R. (1991). A comparative evaluation of parent training interventions for families of chronic delinquents. *Journal of Abnormal Child Psychology*, **19**, 15–33.

Barrett, P. M., Dadds, M. R. & Rappee, R. (1996). Family treatment of childhood anxiety: a controlled trial. *Journal of Consulting and Clinical Psychology*, **64**, 333–42.

Behan, J. & Carr, A. (2000). Oppositional defiant disorder. In *What Works with Children and Adolescents? A Critical Review of Psychological Interventions with Children, Adolescents and their Families*, ed. A. Carr. London: Routledge.

Bentovim, A., Elton, A. Hildebrand, J., Tranter, M. & Vizard, E. (1988). *Child Sexual Abuse Within the Family: Assessment and treatment*. London: Wright.

Bickman, L., Guthrie, P. R., Foster, E. M. *et al.* (1995). *Evaluating Managed Mental Health Services: The Fort Bragg Experiment*. New York: Plenum Press.

Birmaher, B., Brent, D. A., Kolko, D. *et al.* (2000). Clinical outcome after short-term psychotherapy for adolescents with major depressive disorder. *Archives of General Psychiatry*, **57**, 29–36.

Bloomquist, M. L. & Schnell, S. V. (2002). *Helping Children with Aggression and Conduct Problems*. New York: Guilford.

Brazelton, T. B. & Cramer, B. G. eds. (1990). *The Eartiest Relationship: Parents, Infants, and the Drama of Early Attachment*. Reading, MA, USA: Addison Wesley/Addison Wesley Longman.

Brazelton, T. B. & Yogman, M. W. eds. (1986). *Affective Development in Infancy*. Westpost, CT, USA: Ablex Publishing.

Brent, D. A., Poling, K., McKain B. & Baughter, M. (1993). A psychoeducational program for families of affectively ill children and adolescents. *Journal of the American Academy of Child and Adolescent Psychiatry*, **32**, 770–4.

Brent, D. A., Roth, C. M., Holder, D. P. *et al.* (1996). Psychosocial interventions for treating adolescent suicidal depression: A comparison of three psychosocial interventions. *Psychosocial Treatments for Child and Adolescent Disorders: Empirically Based Strategies for Clinical Practice*, ed. E. D. Hibbs & P. S. Jensen, pp. 187–206. Washington DC: American Psychological Association.

Brent, D. A., Kolko, D., Birmaher, B. *et al.* (1998). Predictors of treatment efficacy in a clinical trial of three psychosocial treatments for adolescent depression. *Journal of the American Academy of Child and Adolescent Psychiatry*, **37**, 906–14.

Brent, D. A., Gaynor, S. T. & Weersing, V. R. (2002). Cognitive-behavioural approaches to the treatment of depression and anxiety. *Child and Adolescent Psychiatry*, ed. E. Taylor. Oxford: Blackwell Science.

Bretherton, I., Ridgeway, D. & Cassidy, J. (1990). Assessing internal working models of the attachment relationship: an attachment story completion task for 3 year-olds. *Attachment in the Preschool Years: Theory, research and intervention*, ed. M. Greenberg, D. Cicchetti *et al.*, pp. 273–308. Chicago, IL, University of Chicago Press.

Brosnan, R. & Carr, A. (2000). Adolescent conduct problems. In *What Works with Children and Adolescents? A Critical Review of Psychological Interventions with Children, Adolescents and their Families*, ed. A. Carr. London: Routledge.

Campbell, D., Draper, R. & Huffington, C. (1991). *Second Thoughts on the Theory and Practice of the Milan Approach to Family Therapy*. London: Karnac.

Casey, R. J. & Berman, J. S. (1985). The outcome of psychotherapy with children. *Psychological Bulletin*, **98**, 388–400.

Caspi, A., Moffitt, T. E., Morgan, J. *et al.* (2004). Maternal expressed emotion predicts children's antisocial behavior problems: using monozygotic–twin differences to identify environmental effects on behavioral development. *Developmental Psychology*, **40**(2), 149 61.

Clarke, G. N. & Lewinsohn, P. M. (1990). Instructor's manual for the Adolescent Coping with Stress Course for the secondary prevention of depression. *Unpublished Manuscript*.

Cohen, J. A. & Mannarino, A. P. (1996). A treatment outcome study for sexually abused preschool children: Initial findings. *Journal of the American Academy of Child and Adolescent Psychiatry*, **35**(1), 42–50.

Compas, B. E., Benson, M., Benson, M., Boyer, M., Hicks, T. V. & Konik, B. (2002). Problem-solving and problem-solving therapies. In *Child and Adolescent Psychiatry*, ed. M. Rutter & E. Taylor, pp. 938–48. Oxford: Blackwell.

Compton, S. N., March, J. S., Brent, D., Albano, A. M., Weersing, V. & Curry, J. (2004). Cognitive-behavioral psychotherapy for anxiety and depressive disorders in children and adolescents: an evidence-based medicine review. *Journal of the American Academy of Child and Adolescent Psychiatry*, **48**(8), 930–59.

Corder, B. F., Whiteside, L. & Haizlip, T. M. (1981). A study of curative factors in group psychotherapy with adolescents. *International Journal of Group Psychotherapy*, **31**, 345–54.

Dare, C. & Lindsey, C. (1979). Children in family therapy. *Journal of Family Therapy*, **1**, 253–70.

Dishion, T. & Andrews, D. (1995). Preventing escalation in problem behaviours with high-risk adolescents: immediate and one year outcomes. *Journal of Consulting and Clinical Psychology*, **63**, 538–48.

Dodge, K. (1985). Attributional bias in aggressive children. *Advances in Cognitive-Behavioral Research and Therapy*, ed. P. C. Kendall, p. 4. New York: Academic Press.

Dolan, L. J., Kellam, S. G., Brown, C. *et al.* (1993). The short-term impact of two classroom-based preventive interventions on aggressive and shy behaviors and poor achievement. *Journal of Applied Developmental Psychology*, **14**(3), 317–45.

Durlak, J. A., Fuhrman, T. & Lampman, C. (1991). Effectiveness of cognitive behaviour therapy for maladaptive children: a meta-analysis. *Psychological Bulletin*, **110**, 204–14.

Dush, D. M., Hirt, M. L. & Schroeder, H. E. (1989). Self-statement modification in the treatment of child behavior disorders: a meta-analysis. *Psychological Bulletin*, **106**, 97–106.

Eddy, J. M., Reid, J. B. & Fetrow, R. A. (2000). An elementary school-based prevention program targeting modifiable antecedents of youth delinquency and violence: Linking the Interests of Families and Teachers (LIFT). *Journal of Emotional and Behavioral Disorders*, **8**(3), 165–76.

Eisler, I. (2002). Family interviewing: issues of theory and practice. In *Child and Adolescent Psychiatry*, ed. M. Rutter & E. Taylor, pp. 128–40. Oxford: Blackwell Science.

Evans, J. (1998). *Active Analytic Group Therapy for Adolescents*. London and Philadelphia: Jessica Kingsley.

Fombonne, E. (1998). Interpersonal psychotherapy for adolescent depression. *Child Psychology and Psychiatry Review*, **3**(4), 169–75.

Garcia, J. A. & Weisz, J. R. (2002). When youth mental health care stops: Therapeutic relationship problems and other reasons for ending youth outpatient treatment. *Journal of Consulting and Clinical Psychology*, **70**, 439–43.

Goldwyn, R., Stanley, C., Smith, V. & Green, J. M. (2000). The Manchester child attachment story task: Relationship with parental AAI, SAT and child behaviour. *Attachment and Human Development*, **2**(1), 65–78.

Graham, P. (1998). *Cognitive-Behaviour Therapy for Children and Adolescents*. Cambridge: Cambridge University Press.

Green, J. M., Stanley, C., Smith, V. & Goldwyn, R. (2000). A new method of evaluating attachment representations on young school age children: the Manchester child attachment story task. *Attachment and Human Development*, **2**(1), 42–64.

Greenberg, J. R. & Mitchell, S. A. (1990). *Object Relations in Psychoanalytic Theory*. Cambridge, MA and London: Harvard University Press.

Greenberg, L. S., Rice, L. N. & Elliott, R. (1993). *Facilitating Emotional Change: The Moment by Moment Process*. New York: Guilford Press.

Hampson, R. B. & Beavers, R. W. (1996). Family therapy and outcome: Relationships between therapist and family styles. *Contemporary Family Therapy*, **18**(3), 345–70.

Heim, C., Newport, D., Bonsall, R., Miller, A. H. & Nemeroff, C. B. (2001). Altered pituitary–adrenal axis responses to provocative challenge tests in adult survivors of childhood abuse. *American Journal of Psychiatry*, **158**(4), 575–81.

Hibbs, E. D. & Jensen, P. S. (1996). *Psychosocial Treatments for Child and Adolescent Disorders: Empirically Based Strategies for Clinical Practice*. Washington DC: American Psychological Association.

Hunter, M. (2001). *Psychotherapy with Young People in Care: Lost and Found*. London, Routledge.

Jacobs, B. W. (1997). Some aspects of theories of the mind: a psychodynamic perspective. How might they help a judge? In *Rooted Sorrows: Psychoanalytic perspectives on child protection, Assessment, Therapy and Treatment*, ed. N. Wall. Bristol, Family Law, Jordan Publishing.

Kanfer, F. H., Karoly, P. & Newman, A. (1975). Reduction of children's fear of the dark by confidence-related and situational threat related verbal cues. *Journal of Consulting and Clinical Psychology*, **43**, 251–8.

Kazdin, A. E. (1995). Child, parent, and family dysfunction as predictors of outcome in cognitive-behavioral treatment of antisocial children. *Behaviour Research and Therapy*, **33**, 271–81.

Kazdin, A. E. (1997). Practitioner review: psychosocial treatments for conduct disorder in children. *Journal of Child Psychology and Psychiatry*, **38**, 161–78.

Kazdin, A. E. (2000). *Psychotherapy for Children and Adolescents: Directions for Research and Practice*. Oxford and New York: Oxford University Press.

Kazdin, A. E. & Wassel, G. (1999). Barriers to treatment participation and therapeutic change among children referred for conduct disorder. *Journal of Clinical Child Psychology*, **28**, 160–72.

Kazdin, A. E. & Weisz, J. R. (1998). Identifying and developing empirically supported child and adolescent treatments. *Journal of Consulting and Clinical Psychology*, **66**, 19–36.

Kazdin, A. E., Bass, D., Ayres, W. A. & Rodgers, A. (1990a). Empirical and clinical focus of child and adolescent psychotherapy research. *Journal of Consulting and Clinical Psychology*, **58**, 729–40.

Kazdin, A., Siegel, T. & Bass, D. B. (1990b). Drawing on clinical practice to inform research on child and adolescent psychotherapy: survey of practitioners. *Professional Psychology: Research and Practice*, **21**, 189–98.

Kendall, P. C. (ed.) (2000). *Child and Adolescent Therapy: Cognitive-Behavioral Procedures*. New York: Guilford Press.

Kennedy, E. (2004). *Child and Adolescent Psychotherapy: A Systematic Review of Psychoanalytic Approaches*. London: North Central London Strategic Health Authority.

Kolko, D. J. (1996). Individual cognitive behavioral treatment and family therapy for physically abused children and their offending parents: a comparison of clinical outcomes. *Child Maltreatment*, **1**, 322–42.

Kolvin, I., Garside, R. S., Nicol, A. R., MacMillan, A., Wolsterholme, F. & Leitch, I. (1981). *Help Starts Here: The maladjusted child in the ordinary school.* London: Tavistock.

Koocher, G. P. & Pedulla, B. M. (1977). Current practices in child psychotherapy. *Professional Psychology*, **8**, 275–87.

Kymissis, P. (1997). Group therapy. *Child and Adolescent Psychiatric Clinics of North America*, **6**(1), 173–84.

Lahey, B. B., Miller, T. L., Gordon, R. A. & Riley, A. W. (1999). Developmental epidemiology of the disruptive behavior disorders. In *Handbook of Disruptive Behavior Disorders*, ed. H. C. Quay & A. E. Hogan. New York: Kluwer Academic/ Plenum Press.

Lanyado, M. & Horn, A. (eds.) (1999). *Child and Adolescent Psychotherapy: Psychoanalytic Approaches.* London and New York: Routledge.

Lewinsohn, P. M., Clarke, G. N., Rohde, P., Hops, H. & Seeley, J. R. (1996). A course in coping: a cognitive-behavioral approach to the treatment of adolescent depression. *Psychosocial Treatments for Child and Adolescent Disorders: Empirically Based Strategies for Clinical Practice*, ed. E. D. Hibbs & P. S. Jensen, pp. 109–35. Washington DC: American Psychological Association.

Liddle, H. & Dakof, G. (1995). Efficacy of family therapy for drug abuse: Promising but not definitive. *Journal of Marital and Family Therapy*, **21**, 511–43.

Lochman, J. E., White, K. J. & Wayland, K. K. (1991). Cognitive-behavioral assessment and treatment with aggressive children. In *Child and Adolescent Therapy: Cognitive behavioral procedures*, ed. P. C. Kendall. New York: Guilford.

March, J. S. & Mulle, K. (1998). *OCD in Children and Adolescents: A Cognitive Behavioral Treatment Manual.* New York: Guilford Press.

Markowitz, J. C., Svartberg, M. & Swartz, H. A. (1998). Is IPT time-limited psychodynamic psychotherapy? *Journal of Psychotherapy Practice and Research*, **7**(3), 185–95.

McGain, B. & McKinzey, R. (1995). The efficacy of group treatment in sexually abused girls. *Child Abuse and Neglect*, **19**, 1157–69.

Meichenbaum, D. & Goodman, J. (1971). Training impulsive children to talk to themselves: a means of developing self-control. *Journal of Abnormal Psychology*, **77**, 115–26.

Mufson, L., Moreau, D. & Weissman, M. M. (1996). Focus on relationships: interpersonal psychotherapy for adolescent depression. In *Psychosocial Treatments for Child and Adolescent Disorders: Empirically Based Strategies for Clinical Practice*, ed. E. Hibbs & P. S. Jensen. Washington DC: American Psychological Association.

Mufson, L., Moreau, D. & Weissman, M. M. (1999). Efficacy of interpersonal psychotherapy for depressed adolescents. *Archives of General Psychiatry*, **56**, 573–9.

Nolan, M. & Carr, A. (2000). Attention Deficit Hyperactivity Disorder. In *What Works with Children and Adolescents? A Critical Review of Psychological Interventions with Children, Adolescents and their Families*, ed. A. Carr. London: Routledge.

Patterson, G. R. Reid, J. B. (1992). *Antisocial Boys.* Eugene, Oregon: Castalia.

Patterson, G. R., Reid, J. B., Jones, R. R. & Conger, R. E. (1975). *A Social Learning Approach to Family Intervention: Vol 1 Families with Aggressive Children.* Eugene, OR: Castalia.

Pedro-Carroll, J., Alpert-Gillis, L. J. & Cowen, E. L. (1992). An evaluation of the efficacy of a prevention intervention for 4th to 6th grade urban children of divorce. *The Journal of Primary Prevention*, **13**, 115–30.

Reid, S. (1999). The group as a healing whole: group psychotherapies with children and adolescents. In *Child and Adolescent Psychotherapy: Psychoanalytic Approaches*, ed. M. Lanyado & A. Horne. London and New York: Routledge.

Ronen, T. (1998). Linking developmental and emotional elements into child and family cognitive-behavioural therapy. In *Cognitive-Behavioural Therapy for Children and Families*, ed. P. Graham, pp. 1–17. Cambridge: Cambridge University Press.

Roseby, V. & Deutch, R. (1985). Children of separation and divorce: Effects of social role-taking group intervention on fourth and fifth graders. *Journal of Clinical Child Psychology*, **14**, 55–60.

Rustin, M. (1999). Parental consultation and therapy. In *Child and Adolescent Psychotherapy: Psychoanalytic Approaches*, ed. M. Lanyado & A. Horn. London and New York: Routledge.

Rustin, M. J. (2003). Research in the consulting room. *Journal of Child Psychotherapy*, **29**(2), 137–45.

Salzer, M. S., Bickman, L. & Lambert, E. W. (1999). Dose–effect relationship in children's psychotherapy services. *Journal of Consulting and Clinical Psychology*, **67**, 228–38.

Sandler, J., Kennedy, H. & Tyso, R. L. (1980). *The Technique of Child Analysis: Discussions with Anna Freud.* London: Hogarth Press.

Scott, A., Shaw, M. & Joughlin, C. (2001). *Finding the Evidence: A Gateway to the Literature in Child and Adolescent Mental Health.* London, Gaskell: The Royal College of Psychiatrists.

Seifer, R., Sameroff, A. J., Baldwin, C. P. & Baldwin, A. (1992). Child and family factors that ameliorate risk between 4 and 13 years of age. *Journal of the American Academy of Child and Adolescent Psychiatry*, **31**(5), 893–903.

Shirk, S. R. (2001). Development and cognitive therapy. *Journal of Cognitive Psychotherapy*, **15**, 155–63.

Spence, S. & Marzillier, J. S. (1979). Social skills training with adolescent male offenders: 1 Short term effects. *Behaviour Research and Therapy*, **17**, 7–16.

Spillius, E. B. (ed.) (1988). Melanie Klein today. In *New Library of Psychoanalysis*. London and New York: Routledge.

Stern, D. (1985). *The Interpersonal World of the Infant.* New York: Basic Books.

Taylor, T. K. & Biglan, A. (1998). Behavioral interventions for improving child rearing: a review of the literature for clinicians and policy makers. *Clinical Child and Family Psychology Review*, **7**, 41–60.

Trowell, J., Kolvin, I., Weeramanthri, T. *et al.* (2002). Psychotherapy for sexually abused girls: Psychopathological outcome findings and patterns of change. *British Journal of Psychiatry*, **180**, 234–47.

Tsiantis, J. (2000). *Work with Parents: Psychoanalytic Psychotherapy with Child and Adolescents*. London: Karnac Books.

Webster-Stratton, C. (1996). Early intervention with videotape modelling: Programs for families of children with oppositional defiant disorder or conduct disorder. In *Psychosocial Treatments for Child and Adolescent Disorders: Empirically Based Strategies for Clinical Practice*, ed. E. D. Hibbs & P. S. Jensen. Washington DC: American Psychological Association.

Webster-Stratton, C. & Hammond, M. (1990). Predictors of treatment outcome in parent training for families with conduct problem children. *Behaviour Therapy*, **21**, 319–37.

Webster-Stratton, C. & Hammond, M. (1997). Treating children with early onset conduct problems: a comparison of child and parent training interventions. *Journal of Consulting and Clinical Psychology*, **65**, 93–109.

Weiss, B., Catron, T., Harris, V. & Phung, T. M. (1999). The effectiveness of traditional child psychotherapy. *Journal of Consulting and Clinical Psychology*, **67**, 82–94.

Weisz, J. R., Weiss, B., Alicke, M. D. & Klotz, M. L. (1987). Effectiveness of psychotherapy with children and adolescents: a meta-analysis for clinicians. *Journal of Consulting and Clinical Psychology*, **55**, 542–9.

Weisz, J. R., Weiss, B., Han, S. S., Granger, D. A. & Morton, T. (1995). Effects of psychotherapy with children and adolescents revisited: a meta-analysis of treatment outcome studies. *Psychological Bulletin*, **117**, 450–68.

Weisz, J. R. & Weersing, V. R. (1999). Psychotherapy with children and adolescents: efficacy, effectiveness, and developmental concerns. In *Developmental Approaches to Prevention and Intervention*, ed. D. Cicchetti & S. L. Toth, vol. 9, pp. 341–86. Rochester, NY: University of Rochester Press.

Weisz, J.-R., Hawley, K.-M. & Doss, A. J. (2004). Empirically tested psychotherapies for youth internalizing and externalizing problems and disorders. *Child and Adolescent Psychiatric Clinics of North America, Special Issue: Evidence-Based Practice, Part I: Research Update*, **13**(4), 729–815.

White, M. (1989a). The externalising of the problem and the re-authoring of lives and relationships. *Selected Papers*, ed. M. White, pp. 5–28. Adelaide: Dulwich Centre Publications.

White, M. (1989b). Pseudo-encopresis: from avalanche to victory, from vicious to virtuous cycles. *Selected Papers*, ed. M. White, pp. 115–24. Adelaide: Dulwich Centre Publications.

48

Drugs and other physical treatments

Brian W. Jacobs, Jennifer A. Varley and Jon McClellan

Editor's note

This chapter reviews principles and issues that need to be considered in the prescribing of psychotropic medications to children and adolescents. The brain is still developing during this period, and pruning of neurons and synapses goes on during different periods of childhood and adolescence. Fat distribution and protein-binding of medications in this group is different from adults, and issues related to absorption rate and metabolism rate also reveal differences not only between this age grouping and adults but also within different periods of childhood and adolescence. All this suggests that even more caution needs to be taken when prescribing psychotropics to children, even though there are many studies, as revealed by the tables that accompany this chapter, that suggest effectiveness of pharmacologic treatment of psychiatric disorders during childhood and adolescence.

General issues in paediatric psychopharmacology

Currently, an estimated 6% of young people under the age of 20 years in the United States receive prescriptions for psychotropic medication. This number has increased two- to threefold over the past 15 years and now closely approximates rates found in adult populations (Zito *et al.*, 2003). Prescriptions for adolescents and preschoolers have particularly been on the rise in recent years (Martin & Leslie, 2003; Zito *et al.*, 2000). For preschoolers, a threefold increase in stimulant usage in the early 1990s is especially notable (Zito *et al.*, 2000).

In the UK, use of medication is much less and has been less studied. Nonetheless, there has also been a sharp increase in prescribing by child and adolescent psychiatrists over the past decade. Clark (2004) surveying a health region in the North-West of England found 845 incidents of a drug being newly prescribed for a total of 25 different diagnoses using 48 different medications. Seventy-three percent of the medications were accounted for by the eight most commonly prescribed drugs (methylphenidate, methylphenidate/placebo trial, paroxetine, fluoxetine, risperidone, imipramine, dexamphetamine and melatonin). Wong *et al.* (2003) have expressed concerns about this increase in prescribing, especially in reference to the prescribing of psychostimulants such as methylphenidate in some schools.

A tabular review of currently prescribed psychoactive medications is provided in Tables 48.1–48.3.

Ethics and psychotropic drug prescribing

There have been increasing concerns about the lack of evidence for the safety and efficacy of medicines prescribed for children and adolescents. Kennedy (2004, p. 10). summarizes the issue, 'Problems with randomization are compounded in children where the capacity to give informed consent is an issue. Such considerations have inhibited research in many areas including pharmacotherapy where the evidence base for the treatment of child and adolescent psychiatric disturbance is thin (Riddle *et al.*, 2001a; Jureidini *et al.*, 2004).' This has been compounded by the drug industry's reluctance to invest heavily in trials of medication for children.

As evidence increases, the balance of risks and benefits of medications becomes clearer. A recent example of a mix of unpublished and published evidence creating more concern about medication administered to children has been that of the use of SSRI use for depression in children and adolescents. Jureidini *et al.* (2004) chart some of this course. In the USA this has resulted in a black box warning (FDA, October 2004) specifically warning clinicians of

Cambridge Textbook of Effective Treatments in Psychiatry, ed. Peter Tyrer and Kenneth R. Silk. Published by Cambridge University Press.
© Cambridge University Press, 2008.

Table 48.1. Selective serotonin reuptake inhibitors

Medication	Indications	Positive effects	Lacks efficacy	Comments
Fluoxetine	Major depression*	Emslie *et al.*, 1997, 2002 March *et al.*, 2004	Simeon *et al.*, 1990	In moderate – severe persistent depression $n = 439$, fluoxetine superior to both CBT alone and placebo Combined CBT and fluoxetine had highest response rates
	OCD*	Birmaher *et al.*, 2003 Liebowitz *et al.*, 2002 Riddle *et al.*, 1992		
	Elective mutism	Black & Uhde, 1994		$n = 15$ subjects randomized
Paroxetine	Major depression	Braconnier *et al.*, 2003 Keller *et al.*, 2001		Equal efficacy to clomipramine, no placebo controls Superior to placebo and imipramine
Fluvoxamine	Anxiety	RUPP Anxiety Study Group, 2001		Multisite trial, superior to placebo in 8 week trial, included 128 youth with separation anxiety, social phobia or generalized anxiety disorder
	OCD*	Riddle *et al.*, 2001b		Multisite trial, $n = 120$
Sertraline	Major depression	Wagner *et al.*, 2003		Two multisite trials, $n = 376$, pooled analysis, 69% on active drug responded vs. 59% on placebo
	OCD*	March *et al.*, 1998		Multisite trial, $n = 187$
Citalopram	Major depression	Wagner *et al.*, 2004		$n = 174$, 8-week trial, superior to placebo, significant improvement over placebo noted at week 1

*FDA Approved

the increased risk of suicidality in children and adolescents with the use of SSRIs. In the UK, advice from the Committee on the Safety of Medicines resulted in the Department of Health (Department of Health, 2003) dramatically restricting the use of these medications for the treatment of depression in young people under the age of 18. This has affected prescribing practice in the UK (Macey *et al.*, 2005). It remains to be seen whether this will reduce the rate of completed or attempted suicide in depressed adolescents or whether it increases it because of a failure to use medication where it would be beneficial.

Issues in biological development and drug metabolism and distribution

Brain

The rapid development of the brain prenatally and in the early years has major implications for any aspect of the treatment of children and adolescents but perhaps particularly for psychopharmacologic treatment (Carrey *et al.*, 2002). Overdevelopment of neurons and synapses with subsequent pruning occurs in early childhood and then again later in early adolescence (Insel, 1995). Monoamine secreting neurones have been shown in animal models to play an important time-specific role in orientating the arrival of other axons into the cortex (Zecevic & Verney, 1995). These neurotransmitters are detectable by week 5 of human gestation. Serotonin levels in the postnatal cortex of mice are approximately twice those seen in adult mice (Hohman *et al.*, 1988). A similar effect is seen in children aged 3 months to 3 years and the neurotransmitters remain high until a decline after age 5 years (Chugani *et al.*, 1998). These neurotransmitters may be regulating development of neuronal pathways, and in addition there may also be an autoregulation of serotonin pathway development (Lauder *et al.*, 1983) (Whitaker-Azmitia *et al.*, 1996).

We are only beginning to understand the complex development of the brain. This gives good cause to be cautious in the administration of psychotropic medication to children since psychotropic drugs, of course, impact neurotransmitter concentrations.

Table 48.2. Antipsychotic medications

Medication	Indications	Positive effects	Comments
Haloperidol	Autistic disorder	Anderson *et al.*, 1984 Anderson *et al.*, 1989 Campbell *et al.*, 1978 Cohen *et al.*, 1980	Four studies (total $n = 135$), ages 2 to 8 years. Improved stereotypies, withdrawal, irritability, hyperactivity and temper outbursts (dosages 0.25 to 4.0 mg/day)
	Schizophrenia	Spencer *et al.*, 1992	$n = 12$
	Conduct disorder	Campbell *et al.*, 1984	As effective as lithium and superior to placebo
	ADHD	Werry & Aman, 1975 Aman & Werry, 1975	
	Mental retardation	Aman *et al.*, 1989	Slight reduction of stereotypies
Risperidone	Autistic disorder	McCracken *et al.*, 2002	Multisite trial ($n = 101$, mean age 8.8 ± 2.7 years). Improved tantrums, aggression or self-injurious behaviours. Side effects included sedation, increased appetite and drooling.
	Conduct disorder	Findling *et al.*, 2000	Reduced aggression ($n = 20$)
	Mental retardation	Aman *et al.*, 2002	Reduced disruptive problems in 118 youth (ages 5 – 12 years) with subaverage intelligence (IQ range 36 – 84)
		Snyder *et al.*, 2002	Highly significant reduction in disruptive behaviours in 110 children with subaverage intelligence
	Tourette's disorder	Scahill *et al.*, 2003	$n = 26$, significant tic reduction in active drug vs. placebo
Pimozide	Tourette's disorder	Shapiro & Shapiro, 1984	
Chlorpromazine	ADHD	Rapoport *et al.*, 1971 Werry *et al.*, 1966	
Thioridazine	ADHD	Gittelman-Klein *et al.*, 1976	
	Mental retardation	Aman *et al.*, 1991 Aman & White, 1988	Reduction of hyperactivity and conduct problems High dose thioridazine (2.5 mg/kg per day) superior to low dose (1.25 mg/kg per day) in reducing stereotypies and hyperactivity
Ziprasidone	Tourette's disorder	Sallee *et al.*, 2000	$n = 28$, decreased severity and frequency of tics with active drug
Molindone vs. Thioridazine	Conduct disorder	Greenhill *et al.*, 1985	Both drugs reduced aggression, no placebo control
Risperidone vs. Clonidine	Tourette's disorder	Gaffney *et al.*, 2002	Both medications reduced tics
Risperidone vs. pimozide	Tourette's disorder	Gilbert *et al.*, 2004	Risperidone superior to pimozide in decreasing tics, but was associated with greater weight gain
Risperidone/olanzapine vs. haloperidol	Psychotic symptoms	Sikich *et al.*, 2004	$n = 50$, atypicals demonstrated similar, if not better, efficacy as compared to haloperidol.
Haloperidol vs. pimozide	Tourette's disorder	Shapiro *et al.*, 1989	Both drugs superior to placebo, haloperidol was slightly more effective than pimozide
		Sallee *et al.*, 1997	Pimozide was superior to placebo, haloperidol was not
Haloperidol vs. clozapine	Schizophrenia	Kumra *et al.*, 1996	$n = 21$, clozapine superior to haloperidol on clinical measures, but higher rates of adverse effects
Haloperidol vs. loxapine	Schizophrenia	Pool *et al.*, 1976	Both active drugs superior to placebo in 75 adolescents
Molindone vs. Thioridazine	Conduct disorder	Greenhill *et al.*, 1985	Both drugs reduced aggression, no placebo control
Risperidone vs. Clonidine	Tourette's disorder	Gaffney *et al.*, 2002	Both medications reduced tics
Risperidone vs. pimozide	Tourette's disorder	Gilbert *et al.*, 2004	Risperidone superior to pimozide in decreasing tics, but was associated with greater weight gain
Risperidone/olanzapine vs. haloperidol	Psychotic symptoms	Sikich *et al.*, 2004	$n = 50$, atypicals demonstrated similar, if not better, efficacy as compared to haloperidol.
Haloperidol vs. pimozide	Tourette's disorder	Shapiro *et al.*, 1989	Both drugs superior to placebo, haloperidol was slightly more effective than pimozide
		Sallee *et al.*, 1997	Pimozide was superior to placebo, haloperidol was not
Haloperidol vs. clozapine	Schizophrenia	Kumra *et al.*, 1996	$n = 21$, clozapine superior to haloperidol on clinical measures, but higher rates of adverse effects
Haloperidol vs. loxapine	Schizophrenia	Pool *et al.*, 1976	Both active drugs superior to placebo in 75 adolescents

Table 48.3. Mood stabilizers

Medication	Indications	Positive Response	Lacks Efficacy	Comments
Lithium	Mania symptoms*	McKnew et al., 1981		$n=6$
		DeLong & Neiman, 1983		$n=11$
	Bipolar disorder and substance abuse	Geller et al., 1998		Improved both mood and substance abuse disorders
	Disruptive/explosive behaviours	Campbell et al., 1984; 1995	Rifkin et al., 1997	
Carbamazepine	Disruptive/explosive behaviours	Ryan et al., 1999 (review)	Cueva et al., 1996	Sampling and diagnostic issues limit positive findings
	ADHD	Silva et al., 1996		Meta-analysis of published studies supports some efficacy
Valproate	Disruptive/explosive behaviours	Donovan et al., 2000		$n=20$
	Conduct disorder	Steiner et al., 2003		$n=71$, randomized to high or low dose, higher dose had better impulse control

*FDA approved for young people of 12 years and older.

Physical development

Children grow continuously but with a marked growth spurt in early to mid adolescence. This is accompanied by a changing metabolism with some enzyme systems becoming less prominent, whilst others become more so as the child grows up. These changes affect pharmacological handling of medication and potential drug interactions.

Hormones

The hormonal changes of puberty, first evident in children of 6 years or so with changing levels of dehydroepiandrosterone become increasingly relevant. These changes in hormone levels affect young people's psychological development, their self view, and the disorders to which they are vulnerable.

Drug distribution and metabolism

Children's bodies handle drugs differently from adults (Vinks & Walson, 2003). This does not mean that they do not necessarily require smaller doses. Depending on their age, they have lower ratios of adipose tissue to water compared to adults (Kearns & Reed, 1989; Morselli et al., 1980), and pubertal status (Morselli & Pippinger, 1982). These ratios can markedly effect drug distribution as well as the accumulation of fat solvent medicines and their metabolites. The proportion of body fat is greatest during the first year; it then falls until puberty when there is a rise (Milsap & Szefler, 1986). One would therefore expect to see

a higher plasma concentration for the lipophilic neuroleptics and antidepressants in proportion to the dose administered when compared to adults. In fact, the reverse is the case, presumably because of higher rates of drug metabolism and clearance in these younger people.

Drug protein binding also differs between children of different ages and adults (Grandison & Boudinot, 2000). Protein binding can affect the bioavailability of medication differentially between children and adults. Serum albumin concentrations do not change markedly from early childhood so that this will not be a major factor for binding sites for acidic drugs. Alpha-1-acidic glycoprotein, generally more important for basic drugs, does vary with age and also increases with any acute infection; it can increase the binding of drugs such as haloperidol (Schley & Muller-Oerlinghausen, 1983). Protein binding is also affected by diseases that reduce the protein levels. Sodium valproate (used as an anti-epileptic and also as a mood stabilizer) can saturate the protein at therapeutic levels producing sudden toxicity as bioavailability increases.

Relative to their size, children have a greater hepatic metabolic capacity. Their kidneys are more efficient than those of adults in eliminating drugs via that route. Thus given sufficient hydration, children dispose of lithium more rapidly than adults.

There is poor information on the absorption of psychopharmaceuticals by children. However, parents often administer drugs in ways unplanned in their formulation, e.g. crushing tablets, dissolving medications in soft drinks etc. to get children to take them. The effect of these

Table 48.4 Effectiveness of drugs and other physical treatments

Treatment	Form of treatment	Psychiatric disorder/ Target audience	Level of evidence for efficacy	Comments
Psychopharmacology	SSRIs	Depression and anxiety	Ia–IIb	Improvement over placebo in both depressive and anxiety disorders. Greater efficacy in depression. Fluoxetine is the SSRI with the most supporting evidence. OCD is the anxiety disorder most responsive to SSRIs
Psychopharmacology	Antipsychotics	Autism	Ib	Improvement in stereotypies, withdrawal, irritability, temper outburst. Risperidone just approved for autism in USA
Psychopharmacology	Antipsychotics	Schizophrenia	Ib	Superior to placebo. Clozaril may be very effective but side effects even more prominent here
Psychopharmacology	Antipsychotics	Tourette's	Ia	Superior to placebo. Reduces tics and outbursts
Psychopharmacology	Antipsychotics	Conduct disorder	IIb	Studies lack good methodology
Psychopharmacology	Lithium	Bipolar disorder	IIb	Improvement in mood
Psychopharmacology	Mood stabilisers	Disruptive/explosive behaviours	III	Open studies. Other methodological problems
Somatic therapy	ECT	Mood disorders	III	No real comparison studies done. Very small numbers

procedures on the absorption and stability of medicines is largely unknown. Drug concentrations often peak earlier in children than in adults because of a more rapid clearance of the drug by children (Vinks & Walson, 2003). The apparent reduced volume of distribution for drugs in children also reduces the half-life of drugs given to children relative to adults. This can be important in drugs with a narrow therapeutic dose range. For this reason the child may need a more frequent dosing regime than an older adolescent or adult. An example is provided by imipramine which has a half-life of 11–42 hours in children aged 5–12 whilst in adolescents aged 13–16, its half-life increases to 14–89 hours.

Physical therapies

ECT

Child and adolescent psychiatrists have generally been antagonistic to the use of ECT in the UK and elsewhere. Seventy nine per cent surveyed in a UK study said that they had never used ECT in children or adolescents (Parmar, 1993). Similarly, Duffett and colleagues (Duffett et al., 1999), in a survey of members of the Royal College of Psychiatrists, found only 12 young people (of whom only 3 were aged 15 years or less) under age 18 who had been given ECT in 1996. In the USA, there has been some use of ECT in adolescents and guidelines have been provided for its use. In reviewing the existing studies to produce these

guidelines, the authors point out that 'There are few data based indicators regarding when to offer ECT to an adolescent' (Ghaziuddin et al., 2004). More recently there is some evidence from Australia and New Zealand that these countries are becoming more willing to consider its use in adolescents (Walter & Rey, 2003). Taieb and colleagues (Taieb et al., 2000) found that adolescents who had had ECT for a severe mood disorder were generally positive about the treatment. A lack of responsiveness to medication made it easier for the parents to agree to this treatment. Rudnick (2001), in discussing the ethics of ECT for young people, points out the risk of the error of omission, i.e. not giving an effective treatment because of a fear of the risks when there is not much evidence for such risks.

The level of evidence for each of the interventions discussed in this chapter is summarized in Table 48.4.

REFERENCES

Aman, M. G. & Werry, J. S. (1975). The effects of methylphenidate and haloperidol on the heart rate and blood pressure of hyperactive children with special reference to time of action. *Psychopharmacologia*, **43**, 163–8.

Aman, M. G. & White, A. J. (1988). Thioridazine dose effects with reference to stereotypic behavior in mentally retarded residents. *Journal of Autism and Developmental Disorders*, **18**, 355–66.

Aman, M. G., Teehan, C. J., White, A. J., Turbott, S. H. & Vaithianathan, C. (1989). Haloperidol treatment with chronically medicated residents: dose effects on clinical behavior and reinforcement contingencies. *American Journal of Mental Retardation*, **93**, 452–60.

Aman, M. G., Marks, R. E., Turbott, S. H., Wilsher, C. P. & Merry, S. N. (1991). Methylphenidate and thioridazine in the treatment of intellectually subaverage children: effects on cognitive-motor performance. *Journal of the American Academy of Child and Adolescent Psychiatry*, **30**, 816–24.

Aman, M. G., De Smedt, G., Derivan, A., Lyons, B. & Findling, R. L. Risperidone Disruptive Behavior Study Group (2002). Double-blind, placebo-controlled study of risperidone for the treatment of disruptive behaviors in children with sub-average intelligence. *American Journal of Psychiatry*, **159**, 1337–46.

Anderson, L. T., Campbell, M., Grega, D. M., Perry, R., Small, A. M. & Green, W. H. (1984). Haloperidol in the treatment of infantile autism: effects on learning and behavioral symptoms. *American Journal of Psychiatry*, **141**, 1195–202.

Anderson, L. T., Campbell, M., Adams, P., Small, A. M., Perry, R. & Shell, J. (1989). The effects of haloperidol on discrimination learning and behavioral symptoms in autistic children. *Journal of Autism and Developmental Disorders*, **19**, 227–39.

Birmaher, B., Axelson, A. D., Monk, K. *et al.* (2003). Fluoxetine for the treatment of childhood anxiety disorders. *Journal of the American Academy of Child and Adolescent Psychiatry*, **42**, 415–23.

Black, B. & Uhde, T. W. (1994). Treatment of elective mutism with fluoxetine: a double-blind, placebo-controlled study. *Journal of the American Academy of Child and Adolescent Psychiatry*, **33**, 1000–6.

Braconnier, A., Le Coent, R. & Cohen, D; DEROXADO Study Group (2003). Paroxetine versus clomipramine in adolescents with severe major depression: a double-blind, randomized, multicenter trial. *Journal of the American Academy of Child and Adolescent Psychiatry*, **42**, 22–9.

Campbell, D. R. & Kimball, R. R. (1984). Replication of prediction of antidepressant response to lithium: problems in generalizing to a clinical setting. *American Journal of Psychiatry*, **141**, 706–7.

Campbell, M., Anderson, L. T., Meier, M. *et al.* (1978). A comparison of haloperidol and behavior therapy and their interaction in autistic children. *Journal of the American Academy of Child Psychiatry*, **17**, 640–55.

Campbell, M., Small, A. M., Green, W. H. *et al.* (1984). Behavioral efficacy of haloperidol and lithium carbonate. A comparison in hospitalized aggressive children with conduct disorder. *Archives of General Psychiatry*, **41**, 650–6.

Campbell, M., Adams, P. B., Small, A. M. *et al.* (1995). Lithium in hospitalized aggressive children with conduct disorder: a double-blind and placebo-controlled study. *Journal of the American Academy of Child and Adolescent Psychiatry*, **34**, 445–53.

Carrey, N., Mendella, P., McMaster, F. *et al.* (2002). Developmental Psychopharmacology. In *Practical Child and Adolescent Psychopharmacology*, ed. S. Kutcher. Cambridge: Cambridge University Press.

Chugani, D. C., Mizik, O., Chakraborty, P. *et al.* (1998). Human brain serotonin synthesis capacity measured in vivo with alpha-[C11]methyl-L-tryptophan. *Synapse*, **28**, 33–43.

Clark, A. (2004). Incidences of new prescribing by British child and adolescent psychiatrists: a prospective study over 12 months. *Journal of Psychopharmacology*, **18**, 115–20.

Cohen, I. L. Campbell, M., Posner, D. *et al.* (1980). Behavioral effects of haloperidol in young autistic children. An objective analysis using a within-subjects reversal design. *Journal of the American Academy of Child Psychiatry*, **19**, 665–77.

Cueva, J. E., Overall, J. E., Small, A. M. *et al.* (1996). Carbamazepine in aggressive children with conduct disorder: a double-blind and placebo-controlled study. *Journal of the American Academy of Child and Adolescent Psychiatry*, **35**, 480–90.

DeLong, G. R. & Nieman, G. W. (1983). Lithium-induced behavior changes in children with symptoms suggesting manic-depressive illness. *Psychopharmacology Bulletin*, **19**, 258–65.

Department of Health (2003). Selective serotonin reuptake inhibitors – use in children and adolescents with major depressive disorder. http://www.dhsspsni.gov.uk/hssmd49-03.pdf.

Donovan, S. J. Stewart, J. W. Nunes, E. V. *et al.* (2000). Divalproex treatment for youth with explosive temper and mood lability: a double-blind, placebo-controlled crossover design. *American Journal of Psychiatry*, **157**, 818–20.

Duffett, R., Hill, P. & Lelliott, P. (1999). Use of electroconvulsive therapy in young people. *British Journal of Psychiatry*, **175**, 228–30.

Emslie, G. J., Heiligenstein, J. H., Wagner, K. D. *et al.* (2002). Fluoxetine for acute treatment of depression in children and adolescents: a placebo-controlled, randomized clinical trial. *Journal of the American Academy of Child and Adolescent Psychiatry*, **41**, 1205–15.

Emslie, G. J., Rush, A. J., Weinberg, W. A. *et al.* (1997). A double-blind, randomized, placebo-controlled trial of fluoxetine in children and adolescents with depression. *Archives of General Psychiatry*, **54**, 1031–7.

FDA (2004). Suicidality in children and adolescents being treated with antidepressant medications. http://www.fda.gov/cder/drug/antidepressants/SSRIPHA200410.htm.

Findling, R. L., McNamara, N. K., Branicky, L. A. *et al.* (2000). A double-blind pilot study of risperidone in the treatment of conduct disorder. *Journal of the American Academy of Child and Adolescent Psychiatry*, **39**, 509–16.

Gaffney, G. R., Perry, P. J. Lund, B. C. *et al.* (2002). Risperidone versus clonidine in the treatment of children and adolescents with Tourette's syndrome. *Journal of the American Academy of Child and Adolescent Psychiatry*, **41**, 330–6.

Geller, B., Cooper, T. B., Sun, K. *et al.* (1998). Double-blind and placebo-controlled study of lithium for adolescent bipolar disorders with secondary substance dependency. *Journal of the American Academy of Child and Adolescent Psychiatry*, **37**, 171–8.

Ghaziuddin, N., Kutcher, S., Knapp, P. *et al.* (2004). Practice parameter for the use of electroconvulsive therapy with adolescents.

Journal of the American Academy of Child and Adolescent Psychiatry, **43**(12), 1521–39.

Gilbert, D. L., Batterson, J. R., Sethuraman, G. *et al.* (2004). Tic reduction with risperidone versus pimozide in a randomized, double-blind, crossover trial. *Journal of the American Academy of Child & Adolescent Psychiatry*, **43**, 206–14.

Gittelman-Klein, R., Klein, D. F., Katz, S. *et al.* (1976). Comparative effects of methylphenidate and thioridazine in hyperkinetic children. I. Clinical results. *Archives of General Psychiatry*, **33**, 1217–31.

Grandison, M. K. & Boudinot, F. D. (2000). Age related changes in protein binding of drugs: implications for therapy. *Clinical Pharmacokinetics*, **38**, 271–90.

Greenhill, L. L., Solomon, M., Pleak, R. *et al.* (1985). Molindone hydrochloride treatment of hospitalized children with conduct disorder. *Journal of Clinical Psychiatry*, **46**(8Pt 2), 20–5.

Hohman, C., Hamon, R., Batshaw, M. L. *et al.* (1988). Transient postnatal elevation of serotonin levels in mouse neocortex. *Brain Research*, **47**(1), 163–6.

Insel, T. (1995). The development of brain and behavior. In *Psychopharmacology, The Fourth Generation of Progress*, ed. F. Bloom & D. Kupfer. New York: Raven Press.

Jureidini, J. N., Doecke, C. J. & Mansefield, P. R. *et al.* (2004). Efficacy and safety of antidepressants for children and adolescents. *British Medical Journal*, **328**, 879–83.

Kearns, G. L. & Reed, M. D. (1989). Clinical pharmacokinetics in infants and children. A reappraisal. *Clinical Pharmacokinetics*, **17**, 29–67.

Keller, M. B., Ryan, N. D., Strober, M. *et al.* (2001). Efficacy of paroxetine in the treatment of adolescent major depression: a randomized, controlled trial. *Journal of the American Academy of Child and Adolescent Psychiatry*, **40**, 762–72.

Kennedy, E. (2004). *Child and Adolescent Psychotherapy: A Systematic Review of Psychoanalytic Approaches*. London: North Central London Strategic Health Authority.

Kumra, S., Frazier, J. A., Jacobsen, L. K. *et al.* (1996). Childhood-onset schizophrenia. A double-blind clozapine-haloperidol comparison. *Archives of General Psychiatry*, **53**, 1090–7.

Lauder, J. M., Wallace, J. A., Wilkie, M. B. *et al.* (1983). Roles for serotonin in neurogenesis. *Monographs of Neural Sciences*, **9**, 3–10.

Liebowitz, M. R., Turner, S. M., Piacentini, J. *et al.* (2002). Fluoxetine in children and adolescents with OCD: a placebo-controlled trial. *Journal of the American Academy of Child and Adolescent Psychiatry*, **41**, 1431–8.

Macey, M. L., Thompson, M., Santosh, P. J. & Wong, I. C. K.(2005). Effects of The Committee on Safety of Medicines Advice on Antidepressant Prescribing to Children and Adolescents in the UK. *Drug Safety*, **28**, 1151–7.

March, J., Silva, S., Petrycki, S. *et al.* (2004). Treatment for adolescents with depression study (TADS) team. Fluoxetine, cognitive-behavioral therapy, and their combination for adolescents with depression: treatment for Adolescents With Depression Study (TADS) randomized controlled trial. *Journal of the American Medical Association*, **292**, 807–20.

March, J. S., Biederman, J. & Wolkow, R. (1998). Sertraline in children and adolescents with obsessive-compulsive disorder: a multicenter randomized controlled trial. *Journal of the American Medical Association*, **280**, 1752–6.

Martin, A. & Leslie, D. (2003). Trends in psychotropic medication costs for children and adolescents, 1997–2000. *Archives of Paediatric and Adolescent Medicine*, **157**, 997–1004.

McCracken, J. T., McGough, J., Shah, B. *et al.* (2002). Research units on pediatric psychopharmacology autism network. Risperidone in children with autism and serious behavioral problems. *New England Journal of Medicine*, **347**, 314–21.

McKnew, D. H., Cytryn, L., Buchsbaum, M. S. *et al.* (1981). Lithium in children of lithium-responding parents. *Psychiatry Research*, **4**, 171–80.

Milsap, R. L. & Szefler, S. J. (1986). Special pharmacokinetic considerations in children. In *Applied Pharmacokinetic. Principles of Therapeutic Drug Monitoring*, ed. W. E. Evans, J. J. Schentag & W. J. Jusko, pp. 294–330. Spokane WA: Applied Therapeutics Inc.

Morselli, P. L. & Pippinger, C. E. (1982). *Drug Disposition during Development*, pp. 63–70. Washington DC: American Association of Clinical Chemistry.

Morselli, P. L., Franco-Morselli, R., Bossi, L. *et al.* (1980). Clinical pharmacokinetics in newborn and infants. Age related differences and therapeutic implications. *Clinical Pharmacokinetics*, **5**(6), 485–527.

Parmar, R. (1993). Attitudes of child psychiatrists to electroconvulsive therapy. *Psychiatric Bulletin*, **17**, 12–13.

Pool, D., Bloom, W., Mielke, D. H. *et al.* (1976). A controlled evaluation of loxitane in seventy-five adolescent schizophrenic patients. *Current Therapeutic Research, Clinical and Experimental*, **19**, 99–104.

Rapoport, J., Abramson, A., Alexander, D. *et al.* (1971). Playroom observations of hyperactive children on medication. *Journal of the American Academy of Child Psychiatry*, **10**, 524–34.

Research Unit on Paediatric Psychopharmacology Anxiety Study Group (RUPPS) (2001). Fluvoxamine for the treatment of anxiety disorders in children and adolescents. *New England Journal of Medicine*, **344**, 1279–85.

Riddle, M. A., Scahill, L., King, R. A. *et al.* (1992). Double-blind, crossover trial of fluoxetine and placebo in children and adolescents with obsessive-compulsive disorder. *Journal of the American Academy of Child and Adolescent Psychiatry*, **31**(6), 1062–9.

Riddle, M., Kaselic, E. & Frosch, E. (2001a). Paediatric Psychopharmacology. *Journal of Child Psychology and Psychiatry*, **42**(1), 73–90.

Riddle, M. A., Reeve, E. A. Yaryura-Tobias, J. A. *et al.* (2001b). Fluvoxamine for children and adolescents with obsessive-compulsive disorder: a randomized, controlled, multicenter trial. *Journal of the American Academy of Child and Adolescent Psychiatry*, **40**(2), 222–9.

Rifkin, A., Karajgi, B., Dicker, R. *et al.* (1997). Lithium treatment of conduct disorders in adolescents. *American Journal of Psychiatry*, **154**(4), 554–5.

Rudnick, A. (2001). Ethics of ECT for children. *Journal of the American Academy of Child and Adolescence Psychiatry*, **40**, 387.

Ryan, N. D., Bhatara, V. S. & Perel, J. M. (1999). Mood stabilizers in children and adolescents. *Journal of the American Academy of Child and Adolescent Psychiatry*, **38**(5), 529–36.

Sallee, F. R., Nesbitt, L., Jackson, C. *et al.* (1997). Relative efficacy of haloperidol and pimozide in children and adolescents with Tourette's disorder. *American Journal of Psychiatry*, **154**, 1057–62.

Sallee, F. R., Kurlan, R., Goetz, C. G. *et al.* (2000). Ziprasidone treatment of children and adolescents with Tourette's syndrome: a pilot study. *Journal of the American Academy of Child and Adolescent Psychiatry*, **39**, 292–9.

Scahill, L., Leckman, J. F., Schultz, R. T. *et al.* (2003). A placebo-controlled trial of risperidone in Tourette syndrome. *Neurology*, **60**, 1130–5.

Schley, J. & Muller-Oerlinghausen, B. (1983). The binding of chemically different psychotropic drugs to alpha-1-glycoprotein. *Pharmacopsychiatria*, **16**, 82–5.

Shapiro, A. K. & Shapiro, E. (1984). Controlled study of pimozide vs. placebo in Tourette's syndrome. *Journal of the American Academy of Child Psychiatry*, **23**, 161–73.

Shapiro, E., Shapiro, A. K. Fulop, G. *et al.* (1989). Controlled study of haloperidol, pimozide and placebo for the treatment of Gilles de la Tourette's syndrome. *Archives of General Psychiatry*, **46**, 722–30.

Sikich, L., Hamer, R. M., Bashford, R. A. *et al.* (2004). A pilot study of risperidone, olanzapine, and haloperidol in psychotic youth: a double-blind, randomized, 8-week trial. *Neuropsychopharmacology*, **29**, 133–45.

Silva, R. R., Munoz, D. M. & Alpert, M. (1996). Carbamazepine use in children and adolescents with features of attention-deficit hyperactivity disorder: a meta-analysis. *Journal of the American Academy of Child and Adolescent Psychiatry*, **35**, 352–8.

Simeon, J. G., Dinicola, V. F. Ferguson, H. B. *et al.* (1990). Adolescent depression: a placebo-controlled fluoxetine treatment study and follow-up. *Progress in Neuro-Psychopharmacology and Biological Psychiatry*, **14**, 791–5.

Snyder, R., Turgay, A., Aman, M. *et al.* (2002). Risperidone Conduct Study Group. Effects of risperidone on conduct and disruptive behavior disorders in children with subaverage IQs. *Journal of the American Academy of Child and Adolescent Psychiatry*, **41**, 1026–36.

Spencer, E. K., Kafantaris, V., Padron-Gayol, M. V. *et al.* (1992). Haloperidol in schizophrenic children: early findings from a study in progress. *Psychopharmacology Bulletin*, **28**, 183–6.

Steiner, H., Petersen, M. L., Saxena, K. *et al.* (2003). Divalproex sodium for the treatment of conduct disorder: a randomized controlled clinical trial. *Journal of Clinical Psychiatry*, **64**, 1183–91.

Taieb, O., Cohen, D., Mazet P. *et al.* (2000). Adolescents' experience with ECT. *Journal of the American Academy of Child and Adolescence Psychiatry*, **39**(8), 943–4.

Vinks, A. A. & Walson, P. D. (2003). Pharmacokinetics 1: developmental principles. In *Pediatric Psychopharmacology: Principles and Practice* ed. A. Martin, L. Scahill, D. S. Charney & J. F. Leckman. Oxford: Oxford University Press.

Wagner, K. D., Ambrosini, P., Rynn, M. *et al.* (2003). Sertraline Pediatric Depression Study Group. Efficacy of sertraline in the treatment of children and adolescents with major depressive disorder: two randomized controlled trials. *Journal of the American Medical Association*, **290**, 1033–41.

Wagner, K. D., Robb, A. S., Findling, R. L. *et al.* (2004). A randomized, placebo-controlled trial of citalopram for the treatment of major depression in children and adolescents. *American Journal of Psychiatry*, **161**, 1079–83.

Walter, G. & Rey, J. M. (2003). How fixed are child psychiatrists' views about ECT in the young? *The Journal of ECT*, **19**(2), 88–92.

Werry, J. S. & Aman, M. G. (1975). Methylphenidate and haloperidol in children. Effects on attention, memory, and activity. *Archives of General Psychiatry*, **32**, 790–5.

Werry, J. S., Weiss, G., Douglas, V. *et al.* (1966). Studies on the hyperactive child. 3. The effect of chlorpromazine upon behavior and learning ability. *Journal of the American Academy of Child Psychiatry*, **5**, 292–312.

Whitaker-Azmitia, P. M., Druse, M., Walker, P. *et al.* (1996). Serotonin as a developmental signal. *Behaviour Brain Research*, **73**, 19–29.

Wong, I. C., Camilleri-Novak, D., Stephens, P. *et al.* (2003). Rise in psychotropic drug prescribing in children in the UK: an urgent public health issue. *Drug Safety*, **26**(15), 1117–18.

Zecevic, N. & Verney, C. (1995). Development of the catecholamine neurons in human embryos and fetuses, with special emphasis on the innervation of the cerebral cortex. *Journal of Comparative Neurology*, **351**, 509–35.

Zito, J. M., Safer, D. J. & dosReis, S., (2000). Trends in the prescribing of psychotropic medications to preschoolers. *Journal of the American Medical Association*, **283**, 1025–30.

Zito, J. M., Safer, D. J., dosReis, S. *et al.* (2003). Psychotropic practice patterns for youth: a 10-year perspective. *Archives of Pediatric and Adolescent Medicine*, **157**, 17–25.

49

Educational interventions and alternative treatments

Brian W. Jacobs, Michael Storck, Ann Vander Stoep and Wendy Weber

Editor's note

In child and adolescent psychiatry, educational and alternative interventions frequently take place in school, with treatment directed either at the identified individual or with a group of individuals with similar problems, or at the entire class or school or large subsets of the school. There may be educational programmes directed at the teachers who need to be able to handle these troubled children. But interventions can be multi systemic as well and these are in essence directed at the family to help them cope, set limits and deal with the difficult child. But the difficult child may also be removed from the family system and sent to foster care or sent to inpatient hospital. Evidence for any of these interventions is weak but the trend for many of these active and intense interventions suggests a more positive outcome than standard or less intensive treatment.

Interventions in schools

Various interventions are made to help manage young people's psychological difficulties in schools. Examples of these include but are not limited to:

(a) Consultation or training, e.g. to the teacher of a child who has ADHD, may help better manage the child in class
(b) Interventions to deal with school-wide issues such as bullying
(c) Prevention/early intervention programmes designed to inhibit the escalation of difficulties into clinical problems. These programmes may be applied to children in small groups or as a universal programme to classes of children.
(d) Tactics and strategies to help with the psychological difficulties seen in children and staff after traumatic episodes or disasters (Goenjian et al., 1997; March et al., 1998; Yule, 1992).

One advantage of intervening in a school setting is that it is thought to be more certain that one will gain access to the child on a regular basis once appropriate consent has been obtained. Making a whole school or whole class intervention avoids identification of the target child/children. It is hoped that this approach will enhance the understanding and capacity of other children and teachers to help children who have particular types of difficulty, e.g. by improving the social problem solving skills of all class members.

Providing parent skills programmes in the school setting can also be a non-stigmatising way of reaching the parents of vulnerable children. There has been a concern that the parents who are prepared to attend such a programme will only be the anxious parents of those who do not need the help. In practice, this has not been found to be the case (Webster Stratton – personal communication).

Teacher training

Teacher training may be purely educational about particular disorders, e.g. autism, epilepsy ADHD, etc. Alternatively, it may aim to achieve change in classroom management or to intervene specifically in classroom discipline. Often the programmes are based on ones initially developed for the clinic but which have been adapted for the school or other setting.

Small group therapy in school settings

Lochman and others (Lochman et al., 1991; Nelson & Finch, 2000) have developed anger management programmes delivered to small groups of pupils in school settings. Programmes using CBT for youngsters in secondary schools at high risk for depression have also been successfully delivered and results suggest a reduction in the subsequent incidence of affective disorders by almost half (Clarke et al., 1995).

Cambridge Textbook of Effective Treatments in Psychiatry, ed. Peter Tyrer and Kenneth R. Silk. Published by Cambridge University Press.
© Cambridge University Press, 2008.

The history of trying to help selected children improve their social skills through specific programmes in school has not been successful in producing durable changes in the number of friends that the child had (Oden & Asher, 1977), although it was possible to improve the child's social network (Gresham & Nagle, 1980; Oden & Asher, 1977). Using a parent-assisted social skills training for children aged 7–12 delivered to parents who requested access to the social skills programme, Frankel *et al.* (1996) showed promising early results for boys with poor social skills.

Bullying interventions and whole school positive behaviour programmes

Whole school strategies to prevent bullying are reviewed by McCarthy & Carr (2002). School-wide interventions to promote positive behaviour in children with aggressive and conduct problems have been reviewed by Bloomquist & Schnell (2002) in their recent book on interventions for these youngsters. Olweus' work in Norway has been seminal in this field (Olweus *et al.*, 2000).

Successful programmes pay attention to systemic aspects to make sure that there are correct procedures that will be consistently followed throughout the school and to ensure that there is a positive atmosphere in the school (Bloomquist & Schnell, 2002). They create a positive school climate, though sometimes it is thought that creating this positive atmosphere is easier said than achieved. They define behavioural expectations clearly and support positive behaviour. They provide a consistent and effective response to problem behaviours with a clear and predictable hierarchy of responses. There should be strategies that are applied at a whole school level and also strategies that are predictable in classrooms and at the individual level (McCarthy & Carr, 2002). At an individual level, incidents are discussed with the bully, victim and their parents as soon as they are discovered. Sanctions are applied jointly with parents but if an incident cannot be resolved, the bully and not the victim changes class. Victims are given assertiveness training and bully courts may be used in which peers hear both sides of the story.

Whole class interventions as prevention/early intervention

Theoretically, a whole class intervention might enable both change in the high-risk target children but also might produce more highly skilled social behaviour in the children around the target child with the goal of insulating the particular child against his or her particular vulnerability. We know that children quickly decide on the social acceptability of their peers and that these opinions can be difficult to change even if the target child's behaviour has improved in the meantime (Hymel *et al.*, 1990). As many primary schools tend to retain relatively stable classes over several years, a whole class intervention is likely to be beneficial for children vulnerable to developing behavioural difficulties.

Webster-Stratton & Reid (2004) have adapted their clinical social skills and social problem solving skills programme for use as a universal intervention in the classroom. The programme in this setting is intended to protect children vulnerable to developing oppositional defiant disorder and conduct disorder and it is currently being evaluated. The class teacher co-presents this programme, the Dinosaur School, together with a trained Dinosaur School interventionist as a twice weekly lesson during the school. The programme uses puppets about the same size as a 5-year-old child to help the children learn classroom rules, to recognise emotions and to engage in social problem solving scenarios such as how to join games, sharing, paying complements etc that children with behavioural difficulties typically fail in compared with their peers. They take the Dinosaur lessons with their peers. There are many opportunities to practise the skills being learnt during the classes. Between lessons, the teacher uses every opportunity to remind the children about the concepts and helps them to apply them in school. The programme is captivating for children. It has the advantage that the whole cohort of children in the class are given the same language and tools for social negotiation and conflict management. The vulnerable child is, hopefully, in a 'super-skilled' classroom environment during the year and if the class stays together, subsequently.

Reid and colleagues (Eddy *et al.*, 2003; Reid & Eddy, 2004) have delivered a programme with similar principles although with a different style of presentation to grade 2 and grade 5 children. They found that this programme provided some protection against arrest and alcohol use subsequently in middle school.

Multi-systemic therapy

Child mental health services have traditionally engaged families for quite prolonged periods of a year or more. Many of the most vulnerable families would drop out of treatments early after very few sessions. Reviewing their practice Satterfield *et al.* (1981, 1987) found that a variety of different approaches were often required over a prolonged period of 2 years or more for children with ADHD to produce lasting change. This reflected the complexity of these cases.

A high proportion of adolescents who have offended and are involved in the criminal justice system, have psychiatric disorders with estimates as high as 80% (Teplin *et al.*, 2002). Recognizing that psychiatric disorders may reduce the likelihood of successful rehabilitation, the juvenile justice system and government funding have supported the development of evidence-based interventions to reduce criminal recidivism and improve reintegration to home, school, and community.

One therapeutic approach, multi-systemic therapy (MST) (Henggeler *et al.*, 1998) aims to empower parents with the skills and resources needed to successfully deter adolescents from engaging in criminal activities. During the 3–5 months of intervention, MST therapists work with families, schools, and communities to reorganize behavioural contingencies to reinforce protective factors and ameliorate risk factors within all systems in which the adolescent operates. The effectiveness of MST has been supported in controlled clinical trials with impoverished inner-city juvenile offenders and adolescent sexual offenders. Results reveal a decrease in arrests by more than 50% than would be expected with usual service conditions and individual therapy (Borduin *et al.*, 1990, 1995; Henggeler *et al.*, 1986, 1992). MST has been disseminated widely and currently supports licensed sites in 7 countries and 28 states in the USA. Developing similar systems in the UK has been hampered by a chronic lack of resources in CAMHS. Such intensive services have some of the characteristics of inpatient services but are set up to be available in the community and to be highly responsive to family's needs in their own environment.

There have been variable results of intensive home-based treatments. Some programmes have produced reduced symptomatolgy and an improved quality of life (Burns *et al.*, 1996) whilst others have had less encouraging results (Bickman, 1996; Bickman *et al.*, 2000). For effective programmes, the case management has to be of high quality as do the individual components of treatment available within it (Henggeler *et al.*, 1998).

Treatment foster care

Treatment foster care and multi-systemic therapy are described as exemplary service modalities offered to children with psychiatric disorders within the child welfare and juvenile justice systems. At present, more than a half million children in the USA live in foster homes. (Hochman *et al.*, 2004) and the majority of these children are affected by psychiatric illness (Clausen *et al.*, 1998). Children's

mental health conditions can compromise their likelihood of stability in foster care placement. Implemented within child welfare systems since the 1980s, therapeutic (or treatment) foster care (TFC) combines the normalizing influence of family-based foster care with specialized treatment interventions. The goal is to create a structured therapeutic environment within the context of a nurturant family and neighborhood (Chamberlain, 1990; Stroul & Friedman, 1988). TFC is one of the most widely-used forms of out-of-home placement for children with severe emotional and behavioural disorders and it is considered to be the least restrictive form of residential care (Kutash & Rivera, 1996). Core elements of the TFC model include pre-service training and augmented financial support for foster parents. A mental health therapist or case manager is assigned to assist treatment foster parents. Weekly support and training meetings with other TFC parents, 24-hour, 7-day a week on-call access, and respite services are also provided. Studies have shown that youth who participate in TFC experience better post-discharge adjustment and stability compared to youth served in congregate care facilities (Chamberlain & Mihalic, 1998; Chamberlain & Reid, 1991, 1998; Clarke *et al.*, 1995). An innovative variation on TFC called Family-Centered Intensive Case Management (FCICM) has been developed and involves the same kind of specialized training, with intensive professional and peer support, and respite care provided to the child's biological or adoptive family.

There is mixed evidence from trials thus far. The family preservation services (FPS) assessed by the Chamberlain & Rosicky (1995) model keeps the young person at home with parents but includes very intensive home-based and community interventions. The programme takes place over 2 to 4 months, and it requires many hours of professional time each week. It has a mixed outcome as reviewed by Rivera & Kutash (1994). Another randomized controlled trial determined that children who remain at home with their own family while receiving these supports experience the same or better outcomes than children placed in the homes of professional parents (Evans *et al.*, 1994, 1998). Currently, the Department of Health in England is experimenting with a variation of the Chamberlain and Rosicky model of treatment foster-care in the UK.

Inpatient treatment

There is not space in the context of this chapter to review inpatient treatments in detail. There is a radically different model of using inpatient services in the USA and the UK. In recent USA practice, admissions have usually become limited to a few days in length. Martin & Leslie (2003) found that inpatient admissions funded through health insurance in the USA were reduced in length from 14.4 days in 1997 to 11.5 days in 2000. Admissions, that used to treat crisis conditions and situations, have turned their primary focus on to triaging cases for treatment in other services. Admissions are increasingly restricted to cases where there are very high risks of danger, often to others. This state of affairs has raised concern over the past few years (Chang *et al.*, 1996). In the UK, admissions are usually substantially longer with an average of 117 days in a recent study (Jacobs *et al.*, 2004). The admission is used as a treatment in its own right. A recent outcome study in the USA showed some change by discharge but this change was lost by one month later (Dickerson *et al.*, 2001), whilst the UK study of 4 adolescent and 4 children's units with longer admissions produced lasting change at a year post-discharge (Jacobs *et al.*, 2004). Within this study, it was found that longer lengths of stay were associated with a better outcome at 1-year follow-up post-discharge. This differed from the earlier meta-analysis by Pfeiffer & Strzelecki (1990) which found only a modest relationship between length of stay and outcome.

Recent accounts of practice in the UK are given in Green (Green, 2002; Green & Jacobs, 1998). Jacobs and colleagues (Jacobs *et al.*, 2004) suggest that inpatient child and adolescent psychiatry in the UK is an effective treatment for severe complex cases. The treatment reduces the severity from a need for highly specialized services to that of cases more typically seen in community mental health services. The study was not controlled with random allocation because such a design would currently be unethical with these very severe cases but it has a number of internal features that suggest that the improvements seen are not just due to the passage of time.

Complementary and alternative medicine

Complementary medicines are more frequently used in the USA (36%) compared to the UK (10%). (See 'Complementary and Alternative Medicine Use by One Third of US Adults. Media Release: 13 Jan 2005,' 2005 and also see Thomas and Coleman, 2004). An estimated $12.2 billion was spent in out of pocket expenses in 1997. Those with chronic conditions such as depression, anxiety, and attention deficit hyperactivity disorder, are more likely to utilize CAM treatments (Chan, 2002).

One survey of parents in the Washington DC area found that 21% of parents had used CAM treatment for their children (Ottolini *et al.*, 2001). When surveys are conducted in families where the child has a chronic mental health condition such as ADHD, the percent of families utilizing CAM treatments ranges from 12%–64% (Bussing *et al.*, 2002; Chan, 2002). The large variance is most likely due to the definitions of CAM used in each of the surveys. If the survey narrowly defines CAM, fewer individuals report use. However, if the surveys use a broad definition of CAM treatment such as including dietary changes, as many as 64% of children with ADHD have utilized a CAM treatment. While the Internet provides a plethora of testimonials of cures associated with CAM treatments, the scientific research on CAM therapies is limited. As with many pharmaceutical medications, well-controlled trials conducted in paediatric populations are particularly scarce.

It is essential in the clinical exchange for the providers to foster an attitude of openness so that fairlies will be able to ask questions and share information regarding alternative treatments.

The level of evidence for each of the interventions discussed in this chapter is summarized in Table 49.1.

Table 49.1. Effectiveness of educational and educative interventions

Treatment	Form of treatment	Psychiatric disorder/target audience	Level of evidence for efficacy	Comments
Small group therapy in schools	Psychoeducation	School children to prevent depression	Ib	Found reduction in subsequent incidence of affective disorders
Social skills training in schools	Designed course	School children	III	Preliminary evidence of improvement in social skills of boys
Bullying and whole school positive behaviour programmes	Designed programmes	Schools where bullying is a problem	IV	Though practised widely, no real controlled studies found
Whole school prevention programmes	Designed programme	School population	IV	May provide some protection against arrest and alcohol use in middle school

Table 49.1. (cont.)

Treatment	Form of treatment	Psychiatric disorder/target audience	Level of evidence for efficacy	Comments
Multisystemic therapy	Designed programme	General psychiatric disorders of childhood and adolescence	IIa	A decrease in arrest rates
Foster care treatment	Intensive designed treatment	General psychiatric disorders of childhood and adolescence	IIb	Better post-discharge stability
Inpatient treatment	Various programmes	Severe and dangerous behaviour	III	Evidence suggests that longer lengths of stay may be valuable especially in reducing the need for intensive specialty services post-discharge

REFERENCES

Bickman, L. (1996). A continuum of care: more is not always better. *American Psychologist*, **51**, 698–701.

Bickman, L., Lambert, E. W., Andrade, A. R. & Penaloza, R. V. (2000). The Fort Bragg continuum of care for children and adolescents: mental health outcomes over 5 years. *Journal of Consulting and Clinical Psychology*, **68**, 710–16.

Bloomquist, M. L. & Schnell, S. V. (2002). *Helping Children with Aggression and Conduct Problems*. New York: Guilford.

Borduin, C. M., Henggeler, S. W., Blaske, D. M. & Stein, R. J. (1990). Multisystemic treatment of adolescent sexual offenders. *International Journal of Offender Therapy and Comparative Criminology*, **34**, 105–13.

Borduin, C. M., Mann, B. J., Cone, L. T. *et al.* (1995). Multisystemic treatment of serious juvenile offenders: long-term prevention of criminality and violence. *Journal of Consulting and Clinical Psychology*, **63**, 569–78.

Burns, B. J., Farmer, E. M. Z., Angold, A., Costello, E. J. & Behar, L. (1996). A randomized trial of case management for youths with serious emotional disturbance. *Journal of Clinical Child Psychology*, **25**, 476–86.

Bussing, R., Zima, B. T., Gary, F. A. & Garvan, C. W. (2002). Use of complementary and alternative medicine for symptoms of attention-deficit hyperactivity disorder. *Psychiatric Services*, **53**(9), 1096–102.

Chamberlain, P. (1990). Comparative evaluation of specialized foster-care for seriously delinquent youths: a first step. *Community Alternatives: International Journal of Family Care*, **2**, 21–36.

Chamberlain, P. & Mihalic, S. (1998). *Multidimensional Treatment Foster Care*. Boulder: Institute of Behavioral Science, University of Colorado.

Chamberlain, P. & Reid, J. (1991). Using a specialized foster foster-care treatment model for children and adolescents leaving the state mental hospital. *Journal of Community Psychology*, **19**, 266–76.

Chamberlain, P. & Reid, J. B. (1998). Comparison of two community alternatives to incarceration for chronic juvenile offenders. *Journal of Consulting and Clinical Psychology*, **66**, 624–33.

Chamberlain, P. & Rosicky, J. G. (1995). The effectiveness of family therapy in the treatment of adolescents with conduct disorders and delinquency. *Journal of Marital and Family Therapy*, **21**, 441–59.

Chan, E. (2002). The role of complementary and alternative medicine in attention-deficit hyperactivity disorder. *Journal of Developmental Behavioral Pediatrics*, **23**, S37–S45.

Chang, R., Sanacora, G. & Sanchez, R. J. (1996). The need for outcome studies. *Journal of the American Academy of Child and Adolescent Psychiatry*, **35**(5), 557.

Clarke, G. N., Hawkins, W., Murphy, M., Sheeber, L. B., Lewinsohn, P. M. & Seeley, J. R. (1995). Targetted prevention of unipolar depressive disorder in an at risk sample of high school adolescents: a randomized trial of a group cognitive interview. *Journal of the American Academy of Child and Adolescent Psychiatry*, **34**, 312–21.

Clausen, J. M., Landsverk, J., Ganger, W., Chadwick, D. & Litrownik, A. (1998). Mental health problems of children in foster care. *Journal of Child and Family Studies*, **7**(3), 283–96.

Complementary and alternative medicine use by one third of US adults. Media Release: 13 Jan 2005. (2005). *PharmacoEconomics and Outcomes News*, **470**, 8.

Dickerson Mayes, S., Calhoun, S. L., Krecko, V. F., Vesell, H. P. & Hu, J. (2001). Outcome following child psychiatric hospitalization. *Journal of Behavioral Health Services and Research*, **28**, 96–103.

Eddy, J. M., Reid, J. B., Stoolmiller, M. & Fetrow, R. A. (2003). Outcomes during middle school for an elementary school-based preventive intervention for conduct problems: follow-up results from a randomized trial. *Behavior Therapy*, **34**, 535–552.

Evans, M. E., Armstrong, M. I., Thompson, F. & Lee, J.-K. (1994). Assessing the outcomes of parent- and provider-designed systems of care for children with emotional and behavioral disorders. *Psychiatric Quarterly*, **65**, 257–72.

Evans, M. E; Armstrong, M. I, Kuppinger, A. D. Huz, S. & McNulty, T. L.(1998). Preliminary outcomes of an experimental study comparing treatment foster care and family-centered intensive case management. In *Outcomes for Children and Youth with Emotional and Behavioral disorders and their Families: Programs and Evaluation Best Practices*, ed. M.H. Epstein, K. Kutash & A. Duchnowski pp. 543–80. Austin, TX, US: PRO-ED.

Frankel, F., Cantwell, D. P. & Myatt, R. (1996). Helping ostracized children: social skills training and parent support for socially rejected children. In *Psychosocial Treatments for child and Adolescent Disorders: Empirically Based Strategies for Clinical Practice*, ed. E. D. Hibbs & P. S. Jensen.

Goenjian, A. K., Karayan, I., Pynoos, R. S. *et al.* (1997). Outcome of psychotherapy among early adolescents after trauma. *American Journal of Psychiatry*, **154**, 536–42.

Green, J.M. (2002). Provision of intensive treatment: inpatient units, day units and intensive outreach. In *Child and Adolescent Psychiatry*, 4th edn, ed. M. Rutter & E. Taylor Oxford: Blackwell.

Green, J.W. & Jacobs, B.W. (eds.) (1998). *Inpatient Child Psychiatry: Modern Practice Research in the Future*. London: Routledge.

Gresham, F. M. & Nagle, R. J. (1980). Social skills training with children: responsiveness to modelling and coaching as a function of peer orientation. *Journal of Consulting and Clinical Psychology*, **48**, 718–29.

Henggeler, S. W., Rodick, J. D., Borduin, C. M, Hanson, C. L., Watson, S. & Urey, J. R. (1986). Multisystemic treatment of juvenile offenders: effects on adolescent behavior and family interaction. *Developmental Psychology*, **22**, 132–1.

Henggeler, S. W., Melton, G. B. & Smith, L. A. (1992). Family preservation using multisystemic therapy: an effective alternative to incarcerating serious juvenile offenders. *Journal of Consulting and Clinical Psychology*, **60**, 953–61.

Henggeler, S. W., Schoenwald, S. K., Borduin, C.M., Rowland, M. D. & Cunningham, P. B. (1998). *Multisystemic Treatment of Antisocial Behavior in Children and Adolescents*. New York: Guilford.

Hochman, G., Hochman, A. & Miller, J. (2004). Foster Care, voices from the inside. Report Commissioned by The Pew Commission on Children in Foster Care. Washington: Pew Charitable Trusts.

Hymel, S., Wagner, E. & Butler, L. J. (1990) Reputational bias: view from the peer group. In *Peer Rejection in Childhood*, ed. S. R. Asher & J. D. Coie. Cambridge: Cambridge University Press.

Jacobs, B.W., Green, J.M., Kroll, L. *et al.* (2004). *Two and a Half Thousand Hours: The Children and Young Persons Inpatient Evaluation Study (CHYPIE) into Process and Outcome of Inpatient Child and Adolescent Psychiatry*. London: Department of Health. http://kc.nimhe.org.uk/index.cfm?fuseaction=Item.viewResource&intItemID=45078.

Kutash, K. & Rivera, V. R. (1995). Effectiveness of children's mental health services: a review of the literature. *Education and Treatment of Children*, **18**, 443–77.

Kutash, K. & Rivera, V. R. (1996). *What Works in Children's Mental Health Services? Uncovering Answers to Critical Questions*. Baltimore: Brookes.

Lochman, J. E., White, K. J. & Wayland, K. K. (1991). Cognitive-Behavioral assessment and treatment with aggressive children. In *Child and Adolescent Therapy: Cognitive behavioral procedures*, ed. P. C. Kendall. New York: Guilford.

March, J. S., Amaya-Jackson, L., Murray, M. C. & Schulte, A. (1998). Cognitive behavioral psychotherapy for children and adolescents with post-traumatic stress disorder after a single incident stressor. *Journal of the American Academy of Child and Adolescent Psychiatry*, **36**, 554–65.

Martin, A. & Leslie, D. (2003). Psychiatric inpatient, outpatient, and medication utilization and costs among privately insured youths, 1997–2000. *American Journal of Psychiatry*, **160**(4), 757–64.

McCarthy, O. & Carr, A. (2002). Prevention of bullying. In *Prevention: What Works with Children and Adolescents? A Critical Review of Psychological Prevention Programmes for Children, Adolescents and their Families*, ed. A. Carr. Hove, East Sussex: Brunner-Routledge.

Nelson III, W. M. & Finch, A. J. (2000). Managing anger in youth: a cognitive-behavioral intervention approach. In *Child & Adolescent Therapy: Cognitive-Behavioral Procedures*, 2nd edn, ed. P. C. Kendall, pp. 129–170. New York: Guilford Press.

Oden, S. & Asher, S. R. (1977). Coaching children in social skills for friendship making. *Child Development*, **48**, 495–506.

Olweus, D., Limber, S. & Mihalic, S. (2000). *Blueprints for Violence Prevention: Bullying Prevention Program*. Boulder CO: Center for Study and Prevention of Violence.

Ottolini, M. C., Hamburger, E. K., Loprieato, J. O. *et al.* (2001). Complementary and alternative medicine use among children in the Washington, DC area. *Ambulatory Pediatrics*, **1**, 122–5.

Pfeiffer, S. I. & Strzelecki, S. C. (1990). Inpatient psychiatric treatment of children and adolescents: a review of outcome studies. *Journal of the American Academy of Child and Adolescent Psychiatry*, **29**, 847–53.

Reid, J. B. & Eddy, J. M. (2004). Preventive efforts during the elementary school years: the linking the interests of families and teachers project. In *Antisocial Behavior in Children and Adolescents: A Developmental Analysis and Model for Intervention*, ed. J. B. Reid, G. R. Patterson & J. Snyder, pp. 219–33. Washington, DC: American Psychological Association.

Rivera, V. R. & Kutash, K. (1994). *Components of a System of Care. What does the Research Say?* Tampa, FL: University of South Florida Mental Health Institute, Research and Training Center for Children's Mental Health.

Satterfield, J. H., Satterfield, B. & Cantwell, D. P. (1981). Three-year multi-modality study of 100 hyperactive boys. *Journal of Pediatrics*, **98**, 650–5.

Satterfield, J. H., Satterfield, B. & Schell, A. M. (1987). Therapeutic interventions to prevent delinquency in hyperactive boys. *Journal of the American Academy of Child and Adolescent Psychiatry*, **26**, 56–64.

Stroul, B. A. & Friedman, R. M. (1988). Caring for severely emotionally disturbed children and youth. Principles for a system of care. *Children Today*, **17**, 11–15.

Teplin, L. A., Abram, K. M., McClelland, G. M., Dulcan, M. K. & Mericle, A. A. (2002). Psychiatric disorders in youth in juvenile detention. *Archives of General Psychiatry*, **59**(12), 1133–43.

Thomas, K. & Coleman, P. (2004). Use of complementary or alternative medicine in a general population in Great Britain. Results from the National Omnibus survey. *Journal of Public Health*, **26**(2), 152–7.

Webster-Stratton, C. & Reid, M. J. (2004). Strengthening social and emotional competence in young children – the foundation for early school readiness and success incredible years classroom social skills and problem-solving curriculum. *Infants and Young Children*, **17**, 96–113.

Yule, W. (1992). Posttraumatic stress disorder in childhood survivors of shipping disasters: the sinking of the 'Jupiter'. *Psychotherapy Psychosomatics*, **57**, 200–5.

50

Attachment insecurity and attachment disorder

Jonathan Green, Ming Wai Wan and Michelle DeKlyen

Editor's note

Attachment problems can be divided into two broad categories. First, attachment insecurity and disorganization characterize patterns of child/caregiver relationship that represent risk factors for later psychopathology. Second, so-called attachment disorders are categorical disorders of disrupted attachment usually associated with early social deprivation, neglect or maltreatment. These latter include both disinhibited attachment disorder, which reveals itself in indiscriminate sociability, and inhibited attachment disorder. In cases of attachment insecurity, various forms of intervention with parents appear to have effectiveness in increasing parental sensitivity but their impact on attachment per se is less clear cut. These interventions appear to work best when they are relatively brief and specifically target caregiver sensitivity. In more severe cases, especially those involving attachment disorder, interventions may require placement of the children in adoptive homes. 'Holding therapy' lacks empirical support and may pose serious risk to children.

Introduction

Child attachment refers to particular key characteristics of the relationship between child and specific caregiver that are known to be strongly associated with social development and mental health. Research on normative patterns of attachment in infancy find that attachment insecurity (including 'disorganization') is a relative psychosocial risk factor for later development and is best conceptualized as a developmental risk variable on Axis V of a multiaxial classification (Green & Goldwyn, 2002).

Two less common forms of developmental disturbance associated with severe disruption or absence of early attachment relationships are recognized as Axis 1 clinical disorders in both DSM and ICD systems, although neither has yet received robust empirical validation. ICD10 describes two separate syndromes: (1) 'disinhibited attachment disorder', characterized by indiscriminate sociability and associated particularly with the absence of specific early attachment relationships, for instance in institutional care; (2) 'inhibited' or 'reactive' attachment disorder, typically associated with disrupted attachment, neglect or maltreatment. DSM IV defines one 'reactive attachment disorder' with two subtypes which closely parallel the separate disorders in ICD10. To avoid confusion, in this chapter the generic term 'attachment disorder' is used to apply to both syndromes: but the term used in this way thus equates to reactive attachment disorder (RAD) in US usage.

Research into attachment security/insecurity and attachment disorder has been carried out in broadly different contexts, and the relationship between the two concepts is at the early stages of being characterized (Boris *et al.*, 2004; Rutter, 1995). Zeanah & Boris (2000) have suggested they be thought of as occurring on a spectrum. Green (2003) has suggested that attachment disorder in later childhood may be better characterized as an independent social impairment syndrome. Consequently, the treatment evidence relating to the two concepts will be considered separately here.

Interventions for attachment insecurity

Characteristics of the attachment relationship are inferred from either the behaviour of the infant/child within the relationship, particularly on reunion after separation, or

Cambridge Textbook of Effective Treatments in Psychiatry, ed. Peter Tyrer and Kenneth R. Silk. Published by Cambridge University Press.
© Cambridge University Press, 2008.

from the child's 'cognitive representation' of the relationship. Determinants of such child attachments have been found both in caregiver behaviour (responsiveness or sensitivity) and caregiver attachment representation. Intervention strategies have largely addressed one or other of these caregiver aspects in early childhood, either as primary prevention in high risk groups or as intervention in children with attachment insecurity. No interventions have been officially endorsed or widely used.

Behaviourally based interventions focused on increasing caregiver sensitivity

Brief intensive interventions focused on increasing caregiver sensitivity have shown effectiveness. In a randomized clinical trial, three sessions with parents of irritable infants between 6 and 9 months of age from low socioeconomic families (known to be at risk of developing insecure attachment) significantly increased infant security and decreased attachment disorganization at 1 year, compared to controls (Van den Boom, 1994). In another study, three sessions of video feedback on parenting along with written material related to sensitive parenting between 6 and 9 months increased attachment security (Juffer et al., 1997) and reduced attachment disorganization (Juffer et al., 2005). Provision of written material alone was not effective. Similar intervention with mothers of highly reactive at-risk infants found that 67% of infants developed a secure attachment against 56% of controls (Klein Velderman et al., 2006a). More highly reactive infants were more responsive to the intervention. However, these differential effects had washed out at 40 month follow-up (Klein Velderman et al., 2006b) and there was no long-term moderating effect on child behaviour. Sensitivity-focused techniques combined with enhancing motor skills and co-ordination in low birthweight infants was effective in improving attachment security (Sajaniemi et al., 2001). Studies involving other high-risk groups (Bakermans-Kranenburg et al., 1998; Murray et al., 2003) have not found significant intervention effects on attachment, although they have increased parents' sensitivity. Moran et al. (2005) found that treatment was more effective in enhancing parenting responsiveness and attachment security when mothers did not have unresolved attachment states of mind. Little follow-up work has been done.

It appears that carefully tailored behavioural interventions that are brief, use personalized feedback on interaction and sensitivity, and encourage parenting efficacy are effective for the short term. Maternal sensitivity is easier to influence than infant attachment.

Psychodynamic or representation-focused interventions

Two US randomized controlled trials have involved intensive psychodynamic mother–infant psychotherapy work with high risk mothers and their infants. One showed an increase in attachment security and reduced attachment disorganization compared with controls but to a similar degree as a psychoeducational intervention (Cicchetti et al., 2006) and the other observed improved empathy in parenting but no significant alteration in child attachment behaviours (Lieberman et al., 1991). An RCT of toddler–parent psychotherapy with depressed mothers and their toddlers (mean age 20 months) reported a positive effect on toddler security at 36 months (Cicchetti et al., 1999).

Three European studies used representation-focused interventions alone (Murray et al., 2003) or in conjunction with behavioural techniques (Bakermans-Kranenburg et al., 1998; Klein Velderman et al., 2006a). Positive effects were found on maternal mood (Cooper et al., 2003) and sensitivity respectively but no specific effect was found on child attachment status. Bakermans-Kranenburg et al.'s (1998) findings suggest that mothers with a preoccupied attachment representation may benefit differentially from a representation-focused intervention. These studies are based on the premise that changing the mother's underlying cognitions in relation to attachment representation would be most likely to produce long-term benefits for infant attachment security (van IJzendoorn et al., 1995). There is no evidence currently available to either confirm or refute this hypothesis.

Psychosocial support and counselling for caregivers

Psychosocial support and counselling for caregivers is probably the most widely used intervention involving relatively non-specific support over the prenatal period or first 2 years. Three randomized control studies (2 USA, 1 UK) show benefits of such programmes on general maternal functioning and sensitivity in situations of high social adversity but no associated effect on measured infant attachment (Barnard et al., 1988; Beckwith, 1988; Murray et al., 2003). Two US studies in contrast showed no effect on maternal sensitivity but some increase in infant security compared with controls (Jacobson et al., 1991; Lyons-Ruth et al., 1990). Another US study found improvements in maternal mood but little benefit for maternal sensitivity or infant attachment (Gelfand et al., 1996). Thus, while the available evidence is equivocal, it is at best suggestive of some benefit to women who are experiencing social adversity.

Attachment-focused group interventions for parents

There is a preliminary case study of short-term group intervention for insecure parent–child dyads developed by Marvin *et al.* (2002) that combines parent education and psychotherapy to help shift caregivers' views of and interactions with their children. Initial case studies indicate an increase in secure attachments.

Placement with selected foster parents

While this is arguably the most radical intervention involving alternative parenting, it is widely used in high-risk situations. Dozier *et al.* (2001) studied 50 children from very adverse environments typically associated with attachment disorganization who had early alternate care placement (mean 7.7 months). Children were assessed after an average of 9 months in care. Dozier *et al.* found a distribution of attachment patterns similar to low-risk birth families, suggesting that the consequences of the early risk had been avoided by alternative care. Stams *et al.* (2001) studied 146 internationally early-adopted infants at 7 years follow-up compared to birth siblings from the same family. Outcome for adopted children was similar to birth children. Attachment security was related to adoptive mothers' sensitivity and led to better social and cognitive development. Disorganized attachment and temperamental difficulty led to poor later adjustment and cognitive development.

Summary

The above discussion reveals that a variety of programmes have been developed to prevent insecure attachment. A meta-analysis of interventions for enhancing maternal sensitivity and infant attachment (Bakermans-Kranenburg *et al.*, 2003) showed an overall positive but small effect size ($d = 0.20$) on attachment security.

No intervention has been specifically replicated outside its originating centre and comparison is hampered by the diversity of the specifics of the interventions and the heterogeneity of samples and outcome measures used. No interventions are part of recommended treatment in official national guidelines. The most consistent evidence to date supports relatively brief interventions that specifically target caregiver sensitivity and behaviour. There is only little evidence to support psychodynamically oriented approaches. More broadly based, longer-lasting supportive interventions appeared less effective or even counterproductive, although Egeland *et al.* (2000) recommend these longer interventions for high risk samples with multiple problems (e.g. poverty, parent mental illness, abuse history). In more extreme cases

early placement in alternative care may have a positive impact on attachment outcomes. No published studies have developed attachment-based interventions for older children (O'Connor & Zeanah, 2003).

Systematic effectiveness research in this field is at an early stage. Some specific interventions show promise. The choice of a treatment should be guided by its congruence with attachment theory, the clarity of its objectives (e.g. focus on developing caregiver sensitivity or changing internal working models of attachment), and appropriateness to the population (e.g. biological vs. foster parents, multi-risk vs. well-functioning families). The impact of more generic behavioural treatments on attachment as a one-dimensional measure of outcome should be continued with follow-up beyond infancy.

In comparing European with American studies, a number of interesting points surface: (1) European studies have tended to focus on specific high-risk groups (interracial adoptive families, extremely low birthweight infants, infants whose mothers have/had post-natal depression), whereas many American studies involved disadvantaged families whose risk factors are broader, multiple and complex; (2) European interventions have tended to be brief, standardized and behaviourally focused while American studies have often been of relatively open-ended multifaceted psychosocial interventions and psychotherapy; (3) interventions that commenced antenatally have been used by US but not European studies.

Interventions for attachment disorders

No intervention for attachment disorder has been endorsed in national guidelines. There is broad consensus that research has been insufficient to recommend any specific treatment (O'Connor & Zeanah, 2003). Placement in a foster or adoptive home may be the most common intervention. The American Psychiatric Association (2002) specifies that 'holding therapy' is contraindicated for attachment disorder. Nonetheless, its use by practitioners and the related training for foster/adoptive parents is not uncommon in the USA and is gaining popularity in the UK. This has raised concerns among attachment researchers and clinicians (Nilsen, 2003).

Provision of 'normal' caregiving as a non-specific intervention

Smyke *et al.* (2002) compared Romanian children in a 'standard' orphanage with others in a unit designed to provide more consistent caregiving by fewer caregivers and smaller peer groups with a group of never-institutionalized toddlers. Inhibited and indiscriminate behaviours were less evident among children raised in the home-like environments.

While adoption may result in better adjustment for attachment disordered children, indiscriminate social behaviour can be relatively persistent. Nonetheless, 2 or more years after placement, the developmental status of many Romanian orphans had improved (O'Connor et al., 1999; Rutter, 1998). Many had become securely attached (Marvin & O'Connor, 1999) but were still indiscriminately sociable (O'Connor et al., 1999, 2000). Similarly, many adoptees in a Canadian sample became securely attached several months after adoption, but indiscriminate sociability had not diminished (Chisholm et al., 1995, 1998). Further evidence of the relative intransigence of this symptom comes from a longitudinal study of children from residential nurseries in London where indiscriminate sociability was associated with length of time in the institution and lasted longer than most other problems (Hodges & Tizard, 1989).

Psychoeducational intervention with caregivers

Short-term treatment based on the TEACCH programme (Schopler et al., 1995), originally developed for children with autism, resulted in improved social, language and behavioural development in young children with attachment disorder following maternal neglect and depression (Mukaddes et al., 2000, 2004). This intervention focused on supporting parents by teaching them to cope with aggression, to enhance language and to improve self-care skills while practising child-directed play.

'Attachment therapy' or 'holding therapy'

An array of interventions have been promoted under these labels, with the stated goal of providing a 'corrective experience of attunement' (Kelly, 2003), often involving intrusive, coercive and sustained restraint of the child. 'Holding therapy' has been widely criticized for its inconsistency with attachment theory, lack of efficacy research and potentially harmful effects (Steele, 2003). Such interventions have been in use for some years but only one, non-randomized outcome study has been published (Myeroff et al., 1999). This is marred by serious methodological shortcomings, and neither its definition of disorder nor its outcome measures (aggression and delinquency) are specific to RAD.

Summary

Placement of children with attachment disorders in adoptive homes often results in improved functioning, but social and attentional symptoms tend to linger. Much more research is needed to develop and evaluate specific interventions. Effective treatments are likely to include components to: (1) build a nurturant, secure parent–child relationship, (2) address behaviour problems, (3) remediate skill deficits (e.g. language, emotional regulation, and social skills), and (4) support caregivers.

All interventions should utilize what is known about treating the other problems these children may exhibit, such as maltreatment, behaviour problems, language and cognitive delays, attention deficits and poor social skills. Programmes that teach foster parents to manage difficult behaviours are particularly promising (Chamberlain, 1996; Fisher et al., 2000). Studies in the USA and Europe have shown much convergence in this area.

The level of evidence for each of the interventions discussed in this chapter is summarized in Table 50.1.

Table 50.1. Effectiveness of intervention approaches to attachment in security and attachment disorder

Treatment	Form of treatment	Psychiatric Disorder/ Target audience	Level of evidence for efficacy	Comments
Parental sensitivity training	Various short-term interventions	Parents of children at risk of attachment insecurity	Ia	Maternal sensitivity to the infant is increased but the question remains as to whether this actually improves infant attachment.
Psychodynamic or representation-focused interventions	Psychodynamic	Parents of children at risk of attachment insecurity	Ib	Maternal sensitivity to the infant is increased but the question remains as to whether this actually improves infant attachment.
Psychosocial support and counselling for caregivers	Non-specific supportive therapy	Parents of children at risk of attachment insecurity	Ib	Existing data are equivocal but suggest some benefits for the parents

Table 50.1. (cont.)

Treatment	Form of treatment	Psychiatric Disorder/ Target audience	Level of evidence for efficacy	Comments
Attachment focused groups for parents	Short-term group for parents using psychotherapy and parent education	Parents of children at risk of attachment insecurity	IV	Increase in secure attachments
Placement with selected foster parents	Outplacement from family home to foster home	Children at risk of attachment insecurity due to abuse or neglect	III	Outcome appears to be positive and can reduce or eliminate risk of future disturbed attachment patterns
Normal caregiving in alternative situations (i. e. adoption)	Adoption	Children with Attachment Disorder	III	Attachment became more secure, children improved developmental status, but indiscriminate social behaviour persisted.
Psychoeducation for caregivers	TEACCH Programme	Children with Attachment Disorder	III	Improved attachment and behavioural (social and language) adjustment
'Attachment therapy' 'Holding therapy'	Sustained 'holding' of the child	Children with Attachment Disorder	III	Much controversy about the treatment, no substantiated effects on Attachment Disorder, and may pose serious risk to children

REFERENCES

American Psychiatric Association (2002). *Reactive Attachment Disorder: Position Statement*. APA Document No. 200205. Washington, DC: The American Psychiatric Association.

Bakermans-Kranenburg, M. J., Juffer, F. & van IJzendoorn, M. H. (1998). Intervention with video feedback and attachment discussions: does type of maternal insecurity make a difference? *Infant Mental Health Journal*, **19**, 202–19.

Bakermans-Kranenburg, M. J., van IJzendoorn, M. H. & Juffer, F. (2003). Less is more: meta-analysis of sensitivity and attachment interventions in early childhood. *Psychological Bulletin*, **129**, 195–215.

Barnard, K. E., Magyary, D., Sumner, G. *et al.* (1988). Prevention of parenting alterations for women with low social support. *Psychiatry*, **51**, 248–53.

Beckwith, L. (1988). Intervention with disadvantaged parents of sick preterm infants. *Psychiatry*, **51**, 242–7.

Boris, N. W., Hinshaw-Fusilier, S. S., Smyke, A. T., Scheeringa, M. S., Heller, S. S. & Zeanah, C. H. (2004). Comparing criteria for attachment disorders: Establishing reliability and validity in high-risk samples. *Journal of the American Academy of Child and Adolescent Psychiatry*, **43**, 568–77.

Chamberlain, P. (1996). Intensified foster care: Multi-level treatment for adolescents with conduct disorder in out-of-home care. In *Psychosocial Treatments for Child and Adolescent Disorders: Empirically Based Strategies for Clinical Practice*, ed. E. D. Hibbs & P. S. Jensen, pp. 475–95. Washington, DC: American Psychological Association.

Chisholm, K. (1998). A three year follow-up of attachment and indiscriminate friendliness in children adopted from Romanian orphanages. *Child Development*, **69**, 1092–106.

Chisholm, K., Carter, M. C., Ames, E. W. & Morison, S. J. (1995). Attachment security and indiscriminately friendly behavior in children adopted from Romanian orphanages. *Development and Psychopathology*, **7**, 283–94.

Cicchetti, D., Toth, S. L. & Rogosch, F. A. (1999). The efficacy of toddler-parent psychotherapy to increase attachment security in off-spring of depressed mothers. *Attachment and Human Development*, **1**, 34–66.

Cicchetti, D., Rogosch, F. A. & Toth, S. L. (2006). Fostering secure attachment in infants in maltreating families through preventive interventions. *Development and Psychopathology*, **18**, 623–49.

Cooper, P. J., Murray, L., Wilson, A. & Romaniuk, H. (2003). Controlled trial of the short- and long-term effect of psychological treatment of post-partum depression. 1. Impact on maternal mood. *British Journal of Psychiatry*, **182**, 412–19.

Dozier, M., Stovall, K. C., Albus, K. & Bates, B. (2001). Attachment for infants in foster care: the role of caregiver state of mind. *Child Development*, **72**, 1467–77.

Egeland, B., Weinfeld, N. S., Bosquet, M. & Cheng, V. K. (2000), Remembering, repeating, and working through: lessons from attachment-based interventions. In *WAIMH Handbook of Infant Mental Health* (Vol. 4), ed. J. Osofsky, & H. E., Fitzgerald, pp. 35–89. New York: John Wiley & Sons.

Fisher, P. A., Gunnar, M. R., Chamberlain, P. & Reid, J. B. (2000). Preventive intervention for maltreated preschool children: impact on children's behavior, neuroendocrine activity, and foster parent functioning. *Journal of the American Academy of Child and Adolescent Psychiatry*, **39**, 1356–64.

Gelfand, D. M., Teti, D. M., Seiner, S. A. & Jameson, P. B. (1996). Helping mothers fight depression: evaluation of a home-based intervention program for depressed mothers and their infants. *Journal of Clinical Child Psychology*, **25**, 406–22.

Green, J. M. (2003). Are attachment disorders best seen as social impairment syndromes? *Attachment and Human Development*, **5**(3), 259–64.

Green, J. M. & Goldwyn, R. (2002). Annotation: attachment disorganisation and psychopathology: new findings in attachment research and their potential implications for developmental psychopathology in childhood. *Journal of Child Psychology and Psychiatry*, **43**(7), 835–46.

Hodges, J. & Tizard, B. (1989). Social and family relationships of institutional adolescents. *Journal of Child Psychology and Psychiatry*, **30**, 77–97.

Jacobson, S. W. & Frye, K. F. (1991). Effects of maternal social support on attachment: experimental evidence. *Child Development*, **62**, 572–82.

Juffer, F., Hoksbergen, A. C., Riksen-Walraven, J. M. & Kohnstamm, G. A. (1997). Early intervention in adoptive families: supporting maternal sensitive responsiveness, infant–mother attachment, and infant competence. *Journal of Child Psychology and Psychiatry*, **38**, 1039–50.

Juffer, F., Bakermans-Kranenburg, M. J. & van IJzendoorn, M. H. (2005), The importance of parenting in the development of disorganized attachment: evidence from a preventative intervention study in adoptive families. *Journal of Child Psychology and Psychiatry*, **46**, 263–74.

Kelly, V. J. (2003). *Theoretical rationale for the treatment of disorders of attachment. Association for treatment and training in the attachment of children.* (http://bellsouthpwp.net/e/i/eiseles/theoretical_rationale.html).

Klein, Velderman, M., Bakermans-Kranenburg, M. J., Juffer, F. & van IJzendoorn, M. H. (2006a). Effects of attachment-based interventions on maternal sensitivity and infant attachment: differential susceptibility of highly reactive infants. *Journal of Family Psychology*, **20**, 266–74.

Klein Velderman, M., Bakermans-Kranenburg, M. J., Juffer, F. *et al.* (2006b). Preventing preschool externalizing behaviour problems through video-feedback intervention in infancy. *Infant Mental Health Journal*, **27**, 466–93.

Lieberman, A., Weston, D. & Pawl, J. (1991). Preventive intervention and outcome with anxiously attached dyads. *Child Development*, **62**, 199–209.

Lyons-Ruth K, Connell D B, Grunebaum H U, Botein S (1990), Infants at social risk: Maternal depression and family support services. *Child Development*, **61**:85–98.

Marvin, R. & O'Connor, T. G. (1999). The formation of parent–child attachment following privation. Presented at the Biennial Meeting of the Society for Research in Child Development, Albuquerque, NM, April.

Marvin, R., Cooper, G., Hoffman, K. & Powell, B. (2002). The Circle of Security project: attachment-based intervention with caregiver-pre-school child dyads. *Attachment and Human Development*, **4**, 107–24.

Moran, G., Pederson, D. R. & Krupka, A. (2005). Maternal unresolved attachment status impedes the effectiveness of

interventions with adolescent mothers. *Infant Mental Health Journal*, **26**, 231–49.

Mukaddes, N. M., Bilge, S., Alyanak, B. & Kora, M. E. (2000). Clinical characteristics and treatment responses in cases diagnosed as Reactive Attachment Disorder. *Child Psychiatry and Human Development*, **30**, 273–87.

Mukaddes, N. M., Kaynak, F. N., Kinali, G., Besikci, H. & Issever, H. (2004). Psychoeducational treatment of children with autism and reactive attachment disorder. *Autism*, **8**, 101–9.

Murray, L., Cooper, P. J., Wilson, A. & Romaniuk, H. (2003). Controlled trial of the short- and long-term effect of psychological treatment of post-partum depression. 2. Impact on the mother-child relationship and child outcome. *British Journal of Psychiatry*, **182**, 420–7.

Myeroff, R., Mertlich, G. & Gross, J. (1999). Comparative effectiveness of holding therapy with aggressive children. *Child Psychiatry and Human Development*, **29**, 303–13.

Nilsen, W. J. (2003). Perceptions of attachment in academia and the child welfare system: the gap between research and reality. *Attachment and Human Development*, **5**, 303–6.

O'Connor, T. G. & Rutter, M., The English and Romanian Adoptees (ERA) Study Team (2000). Attachment disorder behavior following early severe deprivation: extension and longitudinal follow-up. *Journal of the American Academy of Child and Adolescent Psychiatry*, **39**, 703–12.

O'Connor, T. G. & Zeanah, C. H. (2003). Attachment disorders: assessment strategies and treatment approaches. *Attachment and Human Development*, **5**, 223–44.

O'Connor, T. G., Bredenkamp, D., Rutter, M., The English and Romanian Adoptees (ERA) Study Team (1999). Attachment disturbances and disorders in children exposed to early severe deprivation. *Infant Mental Health Journal*, **20**, 10–29.

Rutter, M. (1995). Clinical implications of attachment concepts: retrospect and prospect. *Journal of Child Psychology and Psychiatry*, **36**, 549–71.

Rutter, M. and the English and Romanian Adoptees (ERA) study team (1998). Developmental catch-up, and deficit, following adoption after severe global early privation. *Journal of Child Psychology and Psychiatry*, **39**, 465–76.

Sajaniemi, N., Mäkelä, J., Salokorpi, T., von Wendt, L., Hämäläinen, T. & Hakamies-Blomqvist, L. (2001). Cognitive performance and attachment patterns at four years of age in extremely low birth weight infants after early intervention. *European Child and Adolescent Psychiatry*, **10**, 122–9.

Schopler, E., Mesibov, G. B. & Hearsey, K. (1995). Structured teaching in the TEACCH system. In *Learning and Cognition in Autism*, ed. E. Schopler, & G. B. Mesibov, pp. 243–68. New York: Plenum.

Smyke, A. T., Dumitrescu, A. & Zeanah, C. H. (2002). Attachment disturbances in young children. I: The continuum of caretaking casualty. *Journal of the American Academy of Child and Adolescent Psychiatry*, **41**, 972–82.

Stams, G. -J. J. M., Juffer, F., van IJzendoorn, M. H. & Hoksbergen, R. A. C. (2001). Attachment-based intervention in adoptive families in infancy and children's development at age 7: two follow-up studies. *British Journal of Developmental Psychology*, **19**, 159–80.

Steele, H. (2003). Holding therapy is not attachment therapy: editor's introduction to this invited Special Issue. *Attachment and Human Development*, **5**, 219.

Van den Boom, D. C. (1994). The influence of temperament and mothering on attachment and exploration: an experimental manipulation of sensitive responsiveness among lower-class mothers with irritable infants. *Child Development*, **65**, 1457–77.

Van IJzendoorn, M. H., Juffer, F. & Duyvesteyn, M. G. C. (1995). Breaking the intergenerational cycle of insecure attachment: a review of the effects of attachment-based interventions on maternal sensitivity and infant security. *Journal of Child Psychology and Psychiatry*, **36**, 225–48.

Zeanah, C. H. & Boris, N. W. (2000). Disturbances and disorders of attachment in early childhood. In *Handbook of Infant Mental Health*, 2nd edn, ed. C. H. Zeanah, pp. 353–68. New York: Guilford Press.

51

Feeding and sleeping disorders in infancy and early childhood

Heather Carmichael Olson, Nancy C. Winters, Sally L. Davidson Ward and Matthew Hodes

Editor's note

This chapter includes separate sections on treatment for feeding and sleeping disorders. These are disorders that truly do apply to the youngest of patients in child psychiatry, though some eating disorders such as rumination as well as some sleep disorders, such as limit setting sleep disorder and perhaps night terrors can extend into late childhood and perhaps, in rare instances, to adolescence. These are disorders for which behavioural treatments, particularly behavioural treatments such as reinforcement, punishment and graduated extinction, often play key roles in intervention. In both of these groups of disorders, parent training and education are important interventions. While medications can be used in both these disorders, they are certainly not the mainstay of treatment, and because of the young age of the patient population, are rarely used except for a very short time. As in much of child psychiatry, there remains a paucity of methodologically sound trials of the various treatments, though there are randomized controlled studies for both of these conditions that support primarily a behavioural approach.

Introduction

This chapter includes separate sections on treatment for feeding and sleeping disorders. These are two common, yet complex topics important in child psychiatry as the field applies to infants and young children (American Psychiatric Association, 2000; Anders & Eiben, 1997; Linscheid, 2004; Manikam & Perman, 2000; Mindell, 1999; World Health Organization, 1993).

Treatment of feeding disorders

Background

Feeding disorders imply a relationship context (Chatoor, 2002) and have both medical and behavioural components that may each receive different emphases in medical or psychiatric literature (Chatoor, 2003; Chatoor et al., 1998; Staiano, 2003). Feeding disorders can be distinguished from failure to thrive (FTT). FTT is generally defined as either: (1) not maintaining expected rate of weight gain over time (e.g. weight <5% on a standardized growth grid); or (2) deviation downward by two major centiles for at least one month duration. FTT is *not* a diagnosis but an *outcome* of any condition that results in growth impairment. The more specific diagnostic term found in the DSM-IV-TR (American Psychiatric Association, 2000) is 'Feeding Disorder of Infancy and Early Childhood'. The diagnosis requires both feeding refusal and growth impairment. However, the ICD-10 definition is broader. Criterion A specifies 'persistent failure to eat adequately, or persistent rumination or regurgitation of food'. Criterion B specifies that 'the child fails to gain weight, loses weight, or exhibits some other significant health problem over at least 1 month' (WHO, 1993). Thus, the broader construct of feeding disturbances or 'Feeding Problems NOS' may include food refusal or disordered eating as a behavioural disturbance that does not necessarily adversely affect growth or physical health (WHO, 1993).

Feeding disturbances are common in children (Reau et al., 1996). Parent concerns about their young children's poor eating are very common and are frequently reported to child health professionals. For example, in one large UK study, parents reported just over 10% of their 3-year-old children had 'faddy eating' and 16% were described as having poor appetite. These symptoms cluster with other behavioural problems and show considerable continuity (Richman *et al.*, 1982). Severe feeding problems that interfere with growth are much less prevalent and occur in 1%–5% of infants (Chatoor, 2002; Linscheid, 1999; Skuse *et al.*, 1992). Yet reported prevalence can reach as high as 80% among children with developmental delays (Burklow *et al.*, 1998; Manikam & Perman, 2000).

Many authors have pointed out the multifactorial etiology of feeding disturbances and have described varied symptom profiles that suggest a variety of classification schema that have changed over time (Chatoor *et al.*, 2001; Iwaniec, 2004; Robb, 2001; Rudolph & Link, 2002; Winters, 2003). The changing nature of what has been classified as a feeding disturbance contributes to the difficulty of generating epidemiological and treatment data when samples and disorders of interest are defined poorly or differently across studies (Drotar, 1990; Fryer, 1988; Rommel *et al.*, 2003; Woolston, 2002).

A primary early target of study and clinical services, 'non-organic failure to thrive' (NOFT), refers to growth failure with no identifiable organic explanation (Reilly *et al.*, 1999). Over the years, considerable research effort centered on establishing different etiologies and their relative contributions to NOFT and other feeding disturbances (Altemeier *et al.*, 1985; Ammaniti *et al.*, 2004; Coolbear & Benoit, 1999; Hawdon *et al.*, 2000; LaGasse *et al.*, 2003, Zangen *et al.*, 2003). Etiologies of feeding disturbances are not well understood but are increasingly seen as multifactorial, and the dichotomy between 'organic' and 'non-organic' failure-to-thrive has fallen out of favour. Recently, authors have proposed feeding disorder subtypes on a continuum from those presumed to have underlying organic etiology, such as oral–motor dysfunction, gastroesophageal reflux or inadequate hunger drive (Hyman, 1994; Tolia, 1995) to those that are primarily behavioural in origin (Chatoor, 2002; Winters, 2003). Given their multifactorial nature and the transactional process of child development, multidisciplinary approaches to treating feeding disturbances have become widespread in both inpatient and outpatient settings (Black *et al.*, 1995). Teams may include a paediatrician, speech or occupational therapist, and nutritionist as well as a social worker, psychologist or other mental health professional. The team provides the skills needed to develop interventions individualized to the child's specific profile of feeding disturbance (Winters, 2003; Zangen *et al.*, 2003). Specific interventions include those that are primarily medical, such as use of a nasogastric or gastrostomy tube feeding to correct malnutrition, as well as those that address behavioural, developmental, or relational

aspects of feeding refusal (Babbit *et al.*, 1994; Benoit, 2000; Chatoor, 2002; Iwaniec, 2004; Maldonado-Duran & Barriguette, 2001; Robb *et al.*, 2001).

Two additional feeding disturbances of interest to the medical and psychiatric community are very briefly discussed here: (1) Pica, which may occur in one-quarter to one-third of young children (Halstead, 1968), is defined as persistent eating of non-nutritive substances for at least 1 month. This non-nutritive ingestion is inappropriate to developmental level, is not part of a culturally sanctioned practice, and is sufficiently severe to receive clinical attention separate from any other mental disorder (American Psychiatric Association, 2000; Woolston, 2002; WHO, 1993). (2) Rumination Disorder is defined as repeated regurgitation and rechewing of food for at least one month. This regurgitation and rechewing is not due to an associated gastrointestinal or other general medical condition, is not part of an eating disorder, and is sufficiently severe to receive attention separate from any other mental disorder (American Psychiatric Association, 2000; Chiall *et al.*, 2003). Within ICD-10, rumination may be subsumed with feeding disorders, but it is not assigned a separate diagnostic category (WHO, 1993).

Treatment approaches by category of feeding disturbance

Feeding disorder of infancy or early childhood (including DSM-IV-TR 307.59 and ICD-10 F98.2: Infant feeding disorder of non-organic origin)

This chapter intentionally omits treatment of children with primarily organic explanations for food refusal such as severe gastroesophageal reflux disease, structurally-based swallowing problems, etc. These problems require appropriate medical interventions. This chapter does discuss treatment of children with a behavioural pattern of food refusal that may emerge from an earlier medical problem. Although many cases of food refusal have no clear etiology, some feeding disturbances appear to be conditioned responses related to prior experiences of irritation or trauma to the oropharynx or oesophagus (Chatoor *et al.*, 2001; Woolston, 2002). These responses have been variously referred to as 'conditioned dysphagia' (Benoit *et al.*, 2000; O'Reilly & Lancioni, 2001), 'oral aversion' (Palmer & Heyman, 1993; Zangen *et al.*, 2003) or, when food refusal follows a known episode of choking, 'post-traumatic feeding disorders' (Benoit & Coolbear, 1998). Other feeding disturbances appear influenced by varied medical factors such as developmental delay associated with neurological impairment such as cerebral palsy or various genetic syndromes, and chronic health conditions such as cystic fibrosis, cardiac disease, etc. (Manikam & Perman, 2000; Rudolph & Link, 2002).

The evidence base for feeding disorder interventions is complicated by several factors. One issue is diversity in study samples that arises from both the heterogeneity of feeding disorders and classification system changes that have occurred over time. Most prior studies defined feeding disturbances as FTT or NOFT, and only recently have researchers used the diagnostic term 'feeding disorder of infancy and early childhood'. Another issue creating complexity is that treatment must be age-specific. Different approaches are required for infants, who are primarily breast- or bottle-fed, versus toddlers or older children who feed themselves and eat a wider variety of foods (Robb, 2001). Finally, there are limited research data upon which to base treatment decisions. Most of the more rigorous controlled trials involve highly structured behavioural interventions for children with primarily organically based disorders or those with a more behavioural etiology.

No national guidelines for treatment of feeding disorders of infancy and early childhood have been established by either the American Academy of Child and Adolescent Psychiatry or the American Academy of Pediatrics. There are no national guidelines for feeding disorders in the UK. In addition, there appear to be no treatments that are widely used. However, this situation could change with an expanded evidence base that addresses efficacy of interventions for subgroups of children with feeding disorders.

Despite this, a variety of treatments that have been recommended as valuable or are commonly used in response to feeding disturbances. Seven major treatment/intervention categories are presented here (with notes about two additional categories).

(1) *Hospitalization*

Hospitalization is warranted in severe cases of malnutrition when the child has not responded to outpatient treatment or in cases where abuse or neglect is suspected (Linscheid and Murphy, 1999; Maggioni and Lifshitz, 1995). Hospitalization offers opportunities for direct observation of feeding, multiple specialty assessments, and introduction of treatment interventions.

(2) *Medical interventions*

Invasive interventions such as enteral feeding (e.g. nasogastric or gastrostomy tube feeding) may be used even in primarily behaviourally based feeding disorders when other interventions are unsuccessful in correcting significant malnutrition (Tolia, 1995).

(3) *Dietary manipulation*

Dietary manipulation is an essential aspect of treatment. Goals are nutritional repletion and achieving 'catch-up' growth. Interventions include structuring mealtimes, instituting a high calorie, high-fat diet, and increasing caloric density by adding a high-calorie formula (Maggioni & Lifschitz, 1995). Dietary manipulation is accompanied by parent education. Often, parent education reveals differences between healthy infant diets vs. the low-fat, low-calorie diets followed by many adults. Dietary strategies can include manipulation of hunger by spacing out meals (Linscheid, 1999).

(4) *Speech or occupational therapy*

Speech or occupational therapy is often used to address the mechanics of eating and/or dealing with sensory problems such as gradual desensitization to advancing textures (Palmer and Heyman, 1993; Winters, 2003).

(5) *Interventions aimed at parent–child interaction*

Interventions aimed at parent–child interaction have been refined over time (e.g. Black & Teti, 1997, Grantham-McGregor et al., 1987). These usually have accompanying parent education that includes establishing regular mealtimes, appropriate seating, age-appropriate food choices and utensils, self-feeding when appropriate, environmental modification to minimize distractions, use of reinforcement, and increasing reciprocal feeding interactions (Black et al., 1999; Linscheid & Murphy, 1999).

(6) *Behaviour modification*

Behaviour modification has been widely used, in both outpatient and intensive (day treatment or hospital) settings (Ahearn et al., 1996; Luiselli, 2000; Reed et al., 2004). Behaviour modification often involves feeding by a behavioural specialist who manipulates reinforcement contingencies and uses extinction strategies (usually negative reinforcement) to eliminate avoidance behaviours. The relative efficacy of positive and negative reinforcement has been examined, and there is some evidence that both are needed (Reed et al., 2004). Accompanying parent training is needed to reintroduce the parent to the feeding situation and teach behaviour modification principles and techniques (Mueller et al., 2003).

(7) *Interventions aimed at parent psychiatric disorder or symptoms*

Abnormal eating attitudes among mothers are significantly associated with childhood feeding problems (McCann et al., 1994; Whelan & Cooper, 2000). Maternal eating disorders may be associated with failure to thrive and feeding disorders in children (Hodes *et al.*, 1997; Russell *et al.*, 1998). Interventions may require treatment for the abnormal eating attitudes and disorder in the parent and, in extreme situations, separation from the mother (Russell *et al.*, 1998). Fathers have not been well studied.

(8) Two additional categories of treatments have been suggested, but are used less commonly without efficacy information available: (a) Medication for the purpose of appetite enhancement has been used with little efficacy data available (Lemons & Dodge, 1998). (b) Developing specialized interventions geared to proposed feeding disorder subtypes or an analysis of the child's individual problems has been suggested but not yet empirically tested (Chatoor, 2003; Linscheid & Murphy, 1999; Maldonado-Duran & Barriguette, 2001; Rommel *et al.*, 2003).

Long-term enteral (nasogastric or gastrostomy) feeding is often used for medically compromised children or those resistant to other interventions. Yet there is some evidence this can result in resistance to oral feeding or food aversion (Benoit *et al.*, 2000), and so recommendations are to use enteral feeding for the shortest period feasible and continue oral feeding throughout (Rudolph & Link, 2002). Not endorsed are two other less common but still utilized practices: (a) Placing children with FTT in foster care should occur only if the home situation is neglectful and/or abusive or caregivers are unable or unwilling to meet children's needs (Sturm & Dawson, 1999) (b) Behaviour modification strategies that are coercive or physically invasive interfere with the child's sense of autonomy and may result in increased food refusal (Birch & Fisher, 1995).

Table 51.1 summarizes selected trials, comparison studies, and open studies. The few large, prospective randomized and quasi-randomized trials show mixed intervention results. This lack of clarity may arise partly because of patient heterogeneity and/or from variation in intensity and specificity of interventions. Community-based studies that involve home health visiting have been less effective. Clinic-based interventions, involving teams, have mostly shown benefit in terms of weight gain and this may reflect the more intensive and targeted intervention that is provided in clinic settings. In well-designed quasi-randomized controlled trials, various interventions show efficacy. In both randomized trials and quasi-randomized trials, effective interventions have included a combination of psychoeducational and behavioural components.

Comparative studies have examined various treatments applied to diverse populations. Multidisciplinary approaches have shown efficacy. Use of speech–language

pathology and/or occupational therapy techniques has resulted in innovative interventions, and careful analysis of sensory or motor-based contributions to feeding problems allows individually tailored treatment. Interventions aimed at parent–child interaction are being refined with increasing information about the nature of specific interactions seen in feeding disorders (Ammaniti *et al.*, 2004; Benoit *et al.*, 2001; Chatoor *et al.*, 2001); these show promise of efficacy and are often applied to younger children. Outpatient and intensive inpatient behaviour modification techniques appear efficacious in the carefully selected situations in which they are applied which are often with very severe feeding disorders. Behavioural research is identifying specific combinations of techniques necessary to produce effective outcomes, with the caveats that retaining focus on underlying behavioural principles is necessary to successfully individualize in clinical settings (Linscheid & Murphy, 1999) and that hunger is an important aspect to consider (Linscheid, 1999). Behavioural components have been catalogued by Kerwin (1999), who also noted that a cost–benefit analysis is important when intrusive procedures are used.

Various open studies have been conducted using different patient samples, various age groups, and different techniques. Interventions generally show efficacy for most, but not all, infants and children with feeding problems when applied to appropriate populations, although outcomes are sometimes limited in success. An important point is that enteral feeding, especially nasogastric tube feeding, can result in resistance to oral feeding or food aversion, and should be used in a limited manner and accompanied by oral feeding throughout.

Some techniques have been recommended based on expert opinion alone, and these techniques seem reasonable candidates for systematic study. These include dietary manipulation (Linscheid, 1999) and interventions logically geared to subtype of the feeding disorder (Chatoor, 2002) or constructed individually to respond to a case analysis of all components contributing to the feeding disorder (Maldonado-Duran & Barriguette, 2001). Only anecdotal evidence is available so far on use of appetite-promoting medications which describes positive effects of cyproheptadine (Lemons & Dodge, 1998). Other appetite-promoting medications such as antidepressants or atypical antipsychotics, have not been studied in young children.

Feeding difficulties and/or mismanagement (feeding problem not otherwise specified) (ICD-10 R63)

This classification refers to feeding difficulties not meeting criteria for 'feeding disorder of infancy and

Table 51.1. Selected studies on feeding disorders

Authors, publication year. US/UK	Population studied / comorbid disorders	Experimental design	Interventions	Results
Prospective randomized controlled trials. *(First two studies listed have relatively large sample size.)*				
Black et al., 1995 US	130 infants >25 months with NOFT	Prospective randomized group comparison	Multidisciplinary clinic + home intervention, weekly for 1 year, vs. clinic only. All children received nutrition intervention at clinic	Growth status improved regardless of intervention group; cognitive status better with home intervention
Casey et al., 1994 US	914 preterm infants (at increased risk for FTT)	Prospective randomized controlled trial	Home visits, weekly while infant 1–3 years, + parent education at child development centre	No difference in multi-element intervention vs. control in incidence of FTT at 3 years
Benoit et al., 2000 US	64 infants with TF and resistance to oral feeding	Prospective randomized controlled trial	At clinic, compared behavioural, 7 sessions, vs. nutritional interventions in discontinuing TF	47% of behavioural group were successes vs. none in nutritional group
Stark, et al., 1996 US	9 children with cystic fibrosis and inadequate intake	Prospective randomized controlled trial	At clinic, behavioural intervention vs. waiting list control	Treatment resulted in weight gain
Turner et al., 1994 US	20 children with feeding problems	Prospective randomized group comparison	Compared behavioural parent training vs. dietary education	Both groups increased appropriate behaviours over time; mothers with behavioural training increased positive attention; weight gain not measured.
Raynor et al., 1999 UK	83 infants mean 26 months, with FTT, presumed non-organic	Prospective randomized controlled trial	Compared clinic attendance vs. clinic attendance + 'intensive' home visiting over 1 year	No differences in growth, but controls had more hospital admissions and missed more clinic appointments.
Wright et al., 1998 UK	206 infants, with FTT (>95% NOFT) identified by community screening (at 9–18 months)	Controlled trial randomized by primary care practice	Intervention: increased advice from health visitor and dietician, 74% paediatric assessment and 16% social work assessment over 2.5 years vs annual weighing	Weight deficit significantly less in intervention group
Comparative or multiple baseline studies not involving randomization. *(First two studies listed have relatively large sample size.)*				
Bithoney et al., 1991	160 children with NOFT	Prospective non-randomized comparison	Multidisciplinary team (53 children) vs. treatment in primary care setting (107)	Children's growth was significantly better with multidisciplinary team care
Drotar et al., 1985	68 infants with NOFT	Group comparison	Two family intervention approaches	No difference in child outcomes between two family intervention strategies (family-centred and parent-centred)
Benoit et al., 2001	28 mother-infant dyads with feeding problems	Group comparison (individually matched dyads)	Compared play-focused parent–infant therapy vs. behavioural feeding-focused intervention	Significant decrease in atypical behaviours and disrupted communication in play-focused intervention; more mothers in play-focused group classified 'non-disrupted' post-intervention
Reed et al., 2004	4 toddlers or children in a day treatment programme for feeding disorders	Case control with crossover design	Non-contingent positive reinforcement (NCR) + escape extinction compared with NCR alone	NCR alone is insufficient to increase intake; escape extinction is needed to increase intake

Table 51.1. (cont.)

Authors, publication year. US/UK	Population studied / comorbid disorders	Experimental design	Interventions	Results
Comparative or multiple baseline studies not involving randomization (cont.)				
Mueller et al., 2003	Parents of 5 children admitted to day treatment programme for feeding disorders	Non-randomized multiple baseline design	Multi-component parent training; examined combinations of components	Two components (verbal instructions and written protocols) achieved parent skills; adding modelling or rehearsal did not improve results
Ahearn et al., 2001	2 children with a history of severe feeding problems	ABAC design with both treatments given and withdrawn	Non-removal of spoon vs. physical guidance	Both treatment packages were effective to create food acceptance; initial exposure facilitate food acceptance in second exposure
Representative open studies				
Babbitt et al., 1994	40 children attending inpatient programme with medically complex, severe feeding disorders	Single site retrospective review	Multidisciplinary approach incorporating behavioural procedures and individualized to child's needs	Among findings: 86% of tube-dependent children at admission took all nutrition and hydration orally by discharge; average weight gain was 0.8 kg
O'Conner & Szekely, 2001	6 infants with frequent breastfeeding, food refusal and FTT	Case series	Multidisciplinary approach including intensive behavioural feeding therapy and intervention with mothers to say no to breastfeeding	Slow catch-up growth; medical problems resulted in 1 death and 1 relapse
Tolia, 1995	7 infants and toddlers with feeding disorders	Case series	Varied treatments including nutritional change, enteral supplements	Continuing supplementation needed in all but 2 cases; in those erratic or tapering supplementation occurred. All showed weight gain, but several still with low weight
Blackman & Nelson, 1984	10 children (<4 years) with developmental disability who have NGTF	Open clinical trial	Behaviour management techniques	Hospital feeding programme more successful in quick return to oral feeding
Chatoor et al., 1997	20 infants with 'infantile anorexia'	Open clinical trial	Psychoeducation and parent training	17/20 infants' parents reported behaviour improvement and weight gain
Benoit & Coolbear, 1998	24 infants with post-traumatic feeding disorder	Open clinical trial	3 component treatment: optimizing hunger, nutritional monitoring, and behavioural therapy (flooding)	Non-responders had more oral resistance to food in their mouths and more related medical problems
Strologo et al., 1996	12 patients with chronic renal failure and NGTF for decreased caloric intake after tube withdrawal	Multisite retrospective review	Examined outcomes following TF withdrawal	8 patients showed persistent eating difficulties after NGTF withdrawal

Key: TF = tube feeding; NGTF = nasogastric tube feeding; FTT = failure to thrive; NOFT = non-organic failure to thrive; NCR = non-contingent reinforcement.
Note: See also Kerwin (1999) & Linscheid (1999) for review of other methodologically sound studies on empirically supported treatments for severe feeding problems.

childhood.' This may include food refusal not significantly impairing growth, refusal of certain food types (e.g. solids or liquids), or very difficult, picky, or slow feeding behaviour (Jacobi et al., 2003; Reau et al., 1996). Early childhood feeding/eating and digestive problems suggest these are correlates of medium predictive power for later eating problems based on retrospective studies (Kotler et al., 2001; Marchi & Cohen, 1990; Rastam, 1992); in contrast, longitudinal prospective studies suggest these are risk factors of unclear predictive power (Jacobi et al., 2004). There are no national guidelines for responding to feeding difficulties and mismanagement in infancy and early childhood that have been established by either the American Academy of Child and Adolescent Psychiatry or the American Academy of Pediatrics. There are no national guidelines for feeding difficulties in the UK. No practices are particularly or widely used.

Most treatment of non-health-impairing feeding difficulties or mismanagement begins by considering child and family distress, and the type of intervention offered depending on distress level. Often parent guidance or education is adequate to change emphasis or decrease pressure during feeding. Medical evaluation of swallowing may be needed and nutritional counselling is also important. If there is no medical abnormality, the mainstay of treatment will be occupational or sensory–motor oriented therapies using systematic desensitization and gradual exposure to increasing textures. Behavioural approaches are also used, with unique treatment packages composed of different components (for review see Kerwin, 1999 and commentary by Linscheid, 1999). Despite evidence to support their general efficacy, there is controversy about using behavioural interventions for less severe feeding problems. There is concern that behavioural interventions may result in control and countercontrol in parent–child interaction and undermine the child's natural motivation to eat (Kerwin, 1999). Invasive medical interventions (such as enteral feeding) are generally not appropriate for children whose feeding problems are not health-impairing, and are seldom used.

Overall there is less literature on non-health-impairing feeding disturbances precisely because they pose less risk to health. Certainly many children have a severely restricted diet or take in enough calories but nonetheless have eating behaviours disturbing to their caregivers. Whether published treatment studies include this population is not always clear, as inclusion criteria may not clarify the extent of growth impairment. Thus conclusions on evidence-based efficacy for this category of feeding problems must be tentative until researchers more clearly define samples under study.

Kerwin (1999) reviewed methodologically adequate studies, not including open studies. He used selection criteria of severe oral feeding problems but not necessarily failure to thrive. While group comparisons were included, studies reviewed primarily used single subject design methodologies (e.g. reversal or multiple baseline), and each study used a unique treatment package composed of different components. Examples of two larger studies of children with less severe feeding problems are given here. Turner et al. (1994) performed a randomized group comparison of behavioural parent training versus dietary education with twenty 18- to 60-month-olds. Findings showed significant increases in appropriate behaviour and decreases in disruptive behaviour over time in both groups, and mothers receiving behaviour training increased positive attention to their children. Madsen et al. (1974) used differential attention and rewards in a reversal design with 46 rural black preschoolers attending Head Start with some success measured as increasing the percentage of children eating meals and the amount consumed at each meal. These examples suggest that conclusions about the efficacy of behavioural interventions can be applied to children with feeding difficulties and/or mismanagement.

Expert opinion supports a phased multiple component treatment approach for these less severe feeding disorders, starting with medical and less invasive interventions. Components can include parent education, medical evaluation with follow-up intervention as needed, nutritional evaluation with follow-up dietary manipulations as needed, such as attention to the pace of eating and calorie/activity balance, sensory–motor oriented therapies, analysis and modification of conditions surrounding the eating situation (such as mealtime conflict), and direct individualized behavioural treatment as needed. Winters (2003) adds that parent therapy may also be important.

Pica (DSM-IV-TR 307.52); pica of infancy and childhood (ICD-10 F98.3)

Pica is defined as the persistent eating of non-nutritive substances for more than one month (American Psychiatric Association, 2000). The behaviour must be developmentally inappropriate and not part of a culturally sanctioned practice. Pica includes eating of a wide variety of substances, can result in many medical risks, including those associated with lead poisoning, and is often considered a self-injurious behaviour (Woolston, 2002). The disorder may occur in association with mental retardation or developmental disabilities, iron deficiency anaemia (Arbiter & Black, 1991; Nchito *et al.*, 2004; Singhi *et al.*, 2003; Vyas & Chandra, 1984) but may also be an isolated pathological behaviour. Understimulation, anxiety and depression may exacerbate pica, but little is known about associated psychopathology (Linscheid & Murphy, 1999). At times, underlying disease that may be related to poverty and malnutrition can cause both pica and nutritional deficiencies (Korman *et al.*, 1990; Linscheid & Murphy, 1999; Nchito *et al.*, 2004; Singhi *et al.*, 2003). Pica is less prevalent in adolescence than in childhood (Marchi & Cohen, 1990), but it may occur in adults during pregnancy or in association with iron deficiency anaemia (Kettaneh *et al.*, 2005). More commonly, however, pica and vitamin deficiencies co-occur in the context of poverty, neglect and poor parental supervision (Linscheid & Murphy, 1999). The most parsimonious causal explanation for pica as a childhood disorder centers around the self-stimulating and self-injurious nature of pica (Fisher *et al.*, 1994), though one must be sure not to overemphasize the improbable assumption that the self-injurious nature of pica is deliberate. Pica has been described as treatment-resistant. Past public policy actions and national public health campaigns have focused on reducing or preventing pica given its role as the major cause of lead poisoning in children (De la Burde & Reames, 1973; Finney *et al.*, 1982).

No national guidelines exist for responding to pica as a disorder in infancy and early childhood. For young children, Linscheid & Murphy (1999) and Woolston (2002) recommend that assessment of pica as a childhood disorder include medical evaluation, assessing home environment and family functioning (for environmental dangers, appropriate developmental stimulation, caregiving practices, and dietary suitability), evaluating the child for cognitive and psychiatric impairments, and careful description and functional analysis of the ingesting behaviour. Recommended treatment for pica has multiple components. Proper supervision of young children and removing access to noxious substances must first be assured. Work with parents focuses on maintaining the child on an adequate and balanced diet, and providing appropriate developmental stimulation. When treatment must go further, behavioural approaches using a combination of techniques are most commonly applied. These interventions are usually paired with parent training with the aim to decrease eating of non-food and/or promote safety. Functional analysis has been used to evaluate and create treatment plans for pica as a self-injurious behaviour (Fisher *et al.*, 1994) and/or an automatically

reinforced behaviour in young children (Piazza *et al.*, 1998). Application of restraints has been used to reduce the risks of pica but may also impact quality of life. Because ethical and quality of life concerns are important in determining treatment for pica, LeBlanc *et al.* (1997) demonstrated development of a multifactorial, data-based decision-making model balancing variables important to treatment and the child's setting. When nutritional difficulties have been identified, supplementation with iron, vitamins and minerals is needed, and such supplementation has been tried as a treatment for pica (Arbiter & Black, 1991; Lofts *et al.*, 1990). A randomized controlled trial was carried out for treatment of pica associated with iron deficiency anemia in 406 African children with geophagy ('eating earth') that was associated with iron deficiency anaemia and gastrointestinal worm infection. Subjects were randomly assigned to iron, multimicronutrient supplementation or placebo groups (Nchito *et al.*, 2004). There was improvement over time but no benefit was found for iron over multimicronutrient supplementation or placebo.

Behavioural treatments in pica are usually studied using carefully controlled, labour-intensive single subject research designs, in which a child's behaviour over time is compared using quantitative data as different treatments are applied or withdrawn. In pica research, typically only a few children are studied who have multiple medical conditions and developmental disabilities, and are at serious risk from pica. Most commonly investigated behavioural treatments have relied on default strategies involving arbitrary reinforcers and punishers, but these treatments have not been consistently found to be effective (Piazza *et al.*, 1998). Behavioural interventions using some combination of differential reinforcement, discrimination training, extinction and punishment have shown only mixed success (Bucher *et al.*, 1976). Duke & Nielen (1993) and Fisher *et al.* (1994) did show significant decreases in pica in controlled settings using treatment packages of response-contingent procedures that included punishment for nonnutritive ingestion. Punishment increases the probability of quickly suppressing self-injurious behaviour (Linscheid & Murphy, 1999). Functional analyses of three patients, including two young children, were conducted to understand the multiple reinforcing functions of pica and to create treatment plans to address socially-motivated components. The analyses found pica reduced for all participants (Piazza *et al.*, 1998). Functional analysis with pica has limits because of variable treatment efficacy and a lack of empirical selection in specific punishers within a treatment package (Fisher *et al.*, 1994). A number of small case series have been published concerning supplementation with chelated zinc (Lofts *et al.*,

1990) and iron supplementation (Arbiter & Black, 1991; Mihailidou *et al.*, 2002). These were effective in treatment for pica associated with deficiencies. Expert opinion supports multiple component assessment and treatment approach with behavioural treatment as needed (Linscheid & Murphy, 1999; Woolston, 2002).

Rumination disorder (DSM-IV-TR 307.53)

Rumination involves voluntarily bringing already-ingested food back into the mouth and then ejecting or rechewing it and swallowing. This process most often is not distressing to the child but enjoyable as though self-stimulating. Rumination often occurs in infants and individuals with mental retardation with prevalence rates estimated from 'rare' (Linscheid & Murphy, 1999) to up to 10% (Fredericks *et al.*, 1998). It may also occur in children and adolescents with or without other disorders (Khan *et al.*, 2000). There is some confusion in the literature between rumination and other conditions, including gastroesophageal reflex, pyloric stenosis, and psychophysiologic vomiting, but these are almost always associated with distress (Chial *et al.*, 2003; Woolston, 2002). Ruling out an organic cause for rumination is important.

While the major concern with rumination is weight loss, social interactions are often also adversely affected and a cause for concern (Linscheid & Murphy, 1999). Rumination is often complicated by comorbid medical or psychiatric conditions that may require additional types of treatment. Recognizing rumination early is essential, as diagnosis is often delayed and then associated with morbidity (Chial *et al.*, 2003). Psychodynamic theories of etiology have been proposed, but behavioural explanations appear more parsimonious and suggest that rumination is a habit maintained by consequences of self-stimulation and/or increased caregiver attention (Linscheid & Murphy, 1999). There are no national guidelines for responding to rumination disorder in infancy and early childhood that have been established by either the American Academy of Child and Adolescent Psychiatry or the American Academy of Pediatrics. There are no national guidelines for rumination disorder in the UK.

Behavioural treatments are the most commonly applied treatments seen as valuable. According to Linscheid & Murphy (1999), treatment begins with environmental and medical assessment to determine the amount of stimulation and seriousness of the child's medical status. Treatments have ranged from nonintrusive counselling directed at the caregiver when rumination is not severe, to very intense, intrusive measures made necessary by life-threatening weight loss and dehydration. Most straightforward is treatment to provide increased attention, interaction, and stimulation. If this is helpful, further intervention is often directed at improving the home environment and caregiver-child interaction. If caregiver psychopathology prevents appropriate stimulation, psychotherapeutic or psychopharmacologic interventions may be needed. In severe cases, behaviourally based aversive conditioning procedures have been applied. For older children who can learn, habit reversal is recommended. This is an empirically supported paradigm where a target problem behaviour can be eliminated by consistent use of an incompatible or competing behaviour, such as diaphragmatic breathing (Chial *et al.*, 2003).

There are only open label studies available to examine effectiveness. In a retrospective case study of 52 patients aged 5 to 20 years treated with behavioural methods including biofeedback, relaxation training, instruction in habit reversal (diaphragmatic breathing) or cognitive therapy improvement was found in 85% of the group (Chial *et al.*, 2003). Other smaller studies also suggest benefit from behavioural methods (Khan *et al.*, 2000), and there are many similar case reports. Mild contingent shock was applied in several studies to treat life-threatening rumination in infants and individuals with mental retardation with very successful outcomes over a brief time period (Linscheid & Cunningham, 1977).

When rumination is not severe, recommended treatment in book chapters is to provide increased attention, interaction, and stimulation, and to maximize home conditions and caregiver-child interaction so this can occur. Behavioural treatments are recommended when health or social interaction consequences become more severe (Table 51.4).

Summary

Critical evaluation and opinion of feeding disorders interventions

Feeding disorders in infants and young children are common but can be serious and potentially life-threatening if untreated. Even when less serious and unlikely to impair health, such disorders can create ongoing family anxiety and stress, require medical attention and other therapies, and raise concern about lasting or future dysfunction. Feeding disturbances may even be correlates or risk factors for later eating disorders in some children. While ideas for best practices and potentially useful classification systems have evolved in the past decade, there are no national guidelines. In fact, there is a surprisingly limited evidence base to guide clinicians, and information about these disorders is not well known clinically in spite of how common feeding problems really are. Programmatic treatment research using clear classification systems and uniform sample definition is needed, and the results must be disseminated to working clinicians. These studies must be explicit in examining various treatments for feeding disorders; careful definition of the samples under study must be emphasized.

Even without a primarily organic explanation for food refusal, medical interventions are typically part of past or current treatment. There is often a medical component to the problem, and medical factors interact with psychosocial factors. However, continuity and comprehensiveness of care are difficult without a multidisciplinary team, and multidisciplinary team approaches appear to be the present standard. Yet most data to support the efficacy of a multidisciplinary approach comes from studies without randomization or with unclear sample definition. Also, a multidisciplinary team approach may be inaccessible or expensive for some families.

Behavioural approaches have a stronger evidence base, yet data do not always clearly guide the full range of clinical treatment because studies have focused primarily on certain types of children (often with significant intellectual disabilities or multiple health problems). Behavioural research needs to be expanded, including attention to controls, populations chosen and defined, how and when to incorporate parents into the process, and how to ensure utilization of techniques once treatment has ended (Kerwin, 1999). In clinical practice, the types of behavioural intervention differ greatly and must be individualized to the configuration of the feeding problem. Behavioural intervention will differ whether a child has associated physical illness, intellectual disabilities, anxiety and/or a feeding disturbance that arises from a past traumatic experience. Further, the child's relationship context plays a role in feeding problem dynamics. Interestingly, well-designed behavioural interventions, which have the strongest empirical support, are not consistently described as part of multidisciplinary team approaches. Approaches geared to subtype or individualized analysis of problem components have not yet been systematically studied, despite strong support for use by experts in the field. Further difficulties arise in developing guidelines and research in view of the heterogeneity of the parents, including mothers, some of whom have abnormal eating attitudes or psychiatric disorders.

Some widely used categories of treatment, such as parent education, sensory–motor approaches, or dietary manipulation, have received little research attention.

Other possible treatments with interesting potential, such as appetite-promoting medications, have not been studied but are subject to all the cautions inherent in using medications with young children.

Programmatic research on pica in children should continue to pursue how functional analysis can be most effective and how to balance risk and quality of life concerns in intervention. Appropriately designed multiple component approaches should be studied with young children whose pica potentially arises from anxiety or associated with other compulsive behaviours. Pica's association with psychopathology in younger children and as a possible risk factor for later bulimia emphasizes the need for research. On a global basis, pica associated with iron and other deficiencies is important and requires further investigation.

The study of rumination appears to be quite limited. While there are very logical rumination treatment techniques that have been described and commonly applied, they have not yet been empirically-supported.

Treatment of sleep disorders

In this section, treatments will be discussed for three common sleep disorders. These include sleep onset association disorder and limit-setting sleep disorder (classified as extrinsic sleep disorders, International Classification of Sleep Disorders (ICSD), Sleep Behaviour Disorder, DC:0–3 diagnostic system, and as a Primary Sleep Disorder, (DSM-IV)), and sleep terrors (classified as a parasomnia (ICSD), Sleep Behaviour Disorder (DC:0–3) and as a Primary Sleep Disorder, (DSM-IV)) (American Academy of Sleep Medicine, 2000; Anders & Eiben, 1997). Sleep disorders that typically occur in middle childhood, adolescence, and adulthood are not covered by this chapter. Comprehensive reviews of empirically supported treatments of limit setting disorder and sleep association disorder and of pharmacotherapy in paediatric insomnia (Mindell, 1999; Owens *et al.*, 2005) are recommended. Because treatment of all sleep disorders requires promoting good sleep hygiene, these principles are described in Table 51.2.

Sleep onset association disorder

Sleep onset association disorder arises when infants and toddlers habitually fall asleep in one environment (usually the parent's arms or bed), and then, after a normal arousal, find themselves in an unfamiliar sleep environment, such as their crib, and are unable to return to sleep until the

Table 51.2. Sleep hygiene in infancy and early childhood

Strictly observe a bedtime routine and time.

Keep the bedtime routine brief, pleasant, predictable, and calming.

Avoid vigorous mental or physical activity in the hour before bedtime.

Avoid hunger at bedtime but schedule mealtime more than an hour before bedtime.

Avoid foods, beverages, and, if possible, medications containing alcohol or caffeine.

Help infants and young children learn to fall asleep alone, without parent intervention.

Keep the sleeping environment cool, dark, and quiet.

Use the bed or crib exclusively for sleeping, not play or feeding.

Television and electronic games should not be in the bedroom.

Avoid excessive fluid intake before bedtime and during the night.

Observe a regular waking up time.

Encourage age-appropriate naps only.

sleep-promoting environment is restored. Considerable parent sleep disruption usually follows, and the typical response by parents unfortunately provides continued reinforcement of the undesirable behaviour.

No national guidelines have been established by either the American Academy of Pediatrics or American Sleep Disorders Association. Graduated extinction, primarily promoted by Ferber (Ferber & Kryger, 1995), is the most commonly applied treatment. Treatment is based on the foundation that the infant, toddler, or preschooler must learn to transition from wakefulness to sleep without parent participation. Parent education about their role in creating and perpetuating sleep disorder comes first. Parents then identify time to devote to changing infant sleep patterns, and they must be committed to success. Ineffective attempts resulting in failure ultimately reinforce the infant's undesirable sleep habits. Treatment involves having the child initiate sleep at night's beginning and return to sleep following spontaneous arousals while remaining in the desired sleeping environment, i.e. the crib. The parent settles the child without removal from the crib. There is a process of progressively longer intervals between interventions throughout the night. Infants gradually learn to initiate sleep on their own, and this usually occurs in less than one week. For older infants or toddlers with long-established patterns, more time may be needed (Ferber & Kryger, 1995). Some parents are not comfortable allowing infants to cry and fuss without intervening, and this parenting style may be predisposed to creating sleep onset association disorder. A

modified Ferber method can include a temporary sleeping area for the parent in the child's room to strengthen parental resolve by allowing more opportunity to sleep. There is a gradual decrease in the amount of time the parent spends in the child's room. This process is slower but very effective (Minde *et al.*, 1993; Minde *et al.*, 1994). Tracking progress by means of a sleep chart may be helpful (Largo & Hunziker, 1984). Scheduled awakenings timed to occur before troublesome awakenings have been suggested, but support for this approach is not widespread (Rickert & Johnson, 1988). Parent education about the importance of sleep onset associations disorders without specific behavioural therapy may be sufficient in some cases. (Eckerberg, 2002)

Some reports suggest that sedating medications are not indicated for sleep onset association disorder in this age group (Owens *et al.*, 2005). Special care should be taken with infants under 6 months in view of the fact that frequent waking may be a normal sleep pattern and the range of risks including sudden infant death syndrome. For these reasons, and in view of the efficacy of behavioural interventions (see below), there is a strong consensus that behavioural approaches should be first line treatments. However antihistamine drugs such as trimeprazine may have a role in the short-term treatment, especially in the context of high parental distress. It is believed that parent choice should influence treatment offered (Anders & Eiben, 1997; Ramchandani *et al.*, 2000). A survey of primary care paediatricians including 671 respondents showed 39% reported using such medications, mainly antihistamines, to treat childhood insomnia (Owens *et al.*, 2003).

In reviewing what evidence might exist for sleep onset disorder, some studies examine treatments for mixed types of infancy sleeping disorders, mostly sleep onset association and limit-setting disorders, so these studies will be included in this section. There are many randomised controlled trials that have been carried out for infants presenting with waking. Psychological interventions evaluated have been based on learning theory, mainly relying on extinction procedures in which parents decrease reinforcement of waking, and the use of strategies to improve sleep hygiene. (See Table 51.2 for sleep hygiene methods). Results of trials evaluating psychological interventions (building on an earlier systematic review by Ramchandani *et al.*, 2000) are shown in Table 51.3. Findings very strongly favour extinction and other behavioural methods to manage sleep problems.

Randomized controlled trials have also been carried out to investigate drug treatments for young children's sleep problems. Five such trials were identified (France

Table 51.3. Randomized controlled trials of behavioural treatments for infancy sleep disorders

Study	Subjects and problems	Interventions	Controls	Outcomes	Results
Rickerts & Johnson, 1988	33 children aged 6–54 months, recruited through newspaper advertisements (waking problems)	Scheduled wakes or extinction	Sleep diary only	Number of night wakes per week	Both interventions better than control ($P < 0.05$)
Pritchard & Appleton, 1988	31 children aged 9–42 months referred for study, with night waking and settling	Extinction programme and support visits	Extinction programme only	Number of night wakes per night	No difference between groups
Seymour et al., 1989	45 children 9–60 months, attendees at family counselling agency with sleep problems (waking and settling)	Sleep programme: Behavioural advice booklet and support, or behavioural advice booklet only	Waiting list	Number of night wakes per week	Both interventions better than control ($P < 0.05$)
Scott & Richards, 1990	90 children aged 1–18 months, referred for study with night waking	Booklet and support visits or booklet only	Sleep diary only	Number of night wakes per night	No difference between treatment groups or control
St James-Roberts et al., 2001	610 children, recruited from postnatal wards	(1) Behavioural programme; leaflet (2) Education group: 10 page guide, dealing with problems + telephone number for advice	Normal services	Sleeping bout > 5 hours at night	At 3 months, behavioural group more likely than other groups to have sleeping bout > 5 hours (OR 2.61 95% CI 1.02–6.69), compared with control group. At 9 months, no group differences in sleeping bouts, but fewer in the behavioural group sought help for sleeping
Hiscock & Wake, 2002	156 children, 6–12 months, mothers reporting sleep problems (waking and settling)	Mothers attended 3 private consultations, learned sleep hygiene, and controlled crying (parents respond to infants crying at increasing time intervals)	Received mailed information sheet on normal sleep patterns	Maternal report of infant sleep problems, and of maternal depression (Edinburgh Postnatal Depression Scale)	More sleep problems resolved in intervention group ($P = 0.005$). Trend to greater improvement in maternal depression after 2 months

et al., 1991, 1999; Montanari *et al.*, 1992; Richman, 1985; Simonoff & Stores, 1987). These were smaller studies, with 20–60 subjects each, with the exception of Montanari *et al.* (1992) that included a placebo group and used trimeprazine (an antihistamine). Of the four studies using trimeprazine, three found drug treatment superior to placebo, although one study found this advantage was not sustained over the long-term (France *et al.*, 1991).

A relatively large prospective non-randomized study (128 historical controls; 164 intervention subjects) compared routine paediatric care to parent education about sleep onset associations and a sleep chart. Intervention infants had 36% fewer night awakenings at age nine months (Adair *et al.*, 1992). A study employing within subject comparison of 208 children using a regular bedtime routine and extinction reported 78% improvement (Seymour *et al.*, 1983). A study of 50 infants assigned to either graduated extinction or its modification (parent sleeping in infant's bedroom) found no treatment differences, with 60% improvement in sleep patterns by parent report for both treatment strategies (Sedeh, 1994).

Two case series showed greater than 80% success using a developmentally-based behavioural approach to sleep disturbance management (Jones & Verduyn, 1983; Largo & Hunziker, 1984). An open trial investigated an individualized approach to increasing maternal sensitivity and settling techniques within a residential setting (Don *et al.*, 2002). Infants were aged less than 20 weeks and had been referred by other services. After 4 days, sleep had improved significantly, and this improvement was maintained one month after discharge (Don *et al.*, 2002). It has also been shown that graded extinction is associated with improved sleep and improved family well-being (Eckerberg, 2004). Book chapters (Ferber & Kryger, 1995; Handford & Vgontzas, 2002; Sheldon *et al.*, 1992), review articles (Minde *et al.*, 1993) and the lay press (Ferber, 1985) also support the intervention of graduated extinction and positive bedtime routines.

Limit-setting sleep disorder

Limit-setting sleep disorder is characterized by inadequate parent enforcement of bedtimes resulting in child refusal to go to bed or stalling techniques ('curtain calls'). This is not a problem until children become ambulatory, able to climb out of a crib and begin to test independence and boundaries. The disorder can persist through adolescence if not addressed. Parenting style related to this disorder may be inconsistent, neglectful, oblivious, or overly permissive (Owens-Stively *et al.*, 1997). In this disorder, once sleep is initiated, there are no abnormalities of sleep architecture or arousal.

No national guidelines have been established by either the American Academy of Pediatrics or American Sleep Disorders Association. Treatment involves parent education emphasizing consistency and supportive firmness without resorting to anger (Ferber & Kryger, 1995; Sheldon *et al.*, 1992). An age-appropriate bedtime ritual with positive routines (pleasant and calming activities) must be implemented and strictly followed. Sleep time may need to temporarily change to coincide with the child's chosen sleep time, but then it is gradually shifted earlier once struggles have resolved (Adams & Richert, 1989). A doorway gate or holding the door closed have been suggested as ways to keep the child physically in the bedroom and emphasize that the parent is in control, but this should be done only under close parental supervision. Any valid fears the child has associated with sleep must be acknowledged and dispelled, and this may require the parent to spend more time in the child's room at sleep onset. Limit-setting sleep disorder may occur in the context of a wider parenting disorder, a chaotic household, or with marital discord. If so, underlying issues should be addressed before determining it is a sleep disorder. Parent education without specific behavioural therapy may sometimes be sufficient treatment (Eckerberg, 2002). Sedating medications are not indicated for limit-setting disorder (Owens *et al.*, 2005). Yet in a survey of 671 primary care paediatricians, 38% reported recommending medications for bedtime struggles and sleep onset delay (Owens *et al.*, 2003).

A small, randomized study of 36 toddlers and preschoolers with bedtime tantrums compared either graduated extinction or a positive bedtime routine with no intervention. The positive routine intervention included scheduling the child's bedtime at the actual sleep time and using pleasant activities before bedtime. Graduated extinction involved putting the child to bed and ignoring undesirable behaviour. Both treatments were more effective than observation alone, and the positive routine group reported improved marital satisfaction (Adams & Rickert, 1989). A comparative study of positive bedtime routines in 45 children (age 5 to 72 months) showed improvement in bedtime behaviour and night awakenings compared to baseline status, based on parent diaries in 70% of subjects (Galbraith *et al.*, 1993). Behavioural therapy was successful in managing six children with bedtime disturbances with concurrent improvement in parent sleep and family satisfaction (Mindell & Duran, 1993).

Sleep terrors

Sleep terrors (previously called 'night terrors') are abrupt events that represent an incomplete arousal from non-rapid eye movement sleep. There is considerable autonomic activation with sweating, tachycardia, screaming, agitation, hyperventilation and tremors. Episodes usually occur during the first half of the night, last several minutes, and are terminated by a sudden return to deep sleep. The child does not remember the event the following morning. The onset is generally between the ages of 2 and 4 years of age and usually resolves spontaneously, though the terrors may peak at 5–7 years with resolution before adolescence (Anders & Eiben, 1997; Chokroverty *et al.*, 2003; Laberge *et al.*, 2000; Sheldon *et al.*, 1992).

No national guidelines have been set forth by either the American Academy of Pediatrics or American Sleep Disorders Association. Therapy begins with reassurance to parents about the benign nature of sleep terrors. Sleep deprivation and sleep schedule disruption should be avoided as these may increase attack frequency. Good sleep hygiene, including age-appropriate naps, should be practised. If episodes include sleep walking, safety measures are needed to prevent injury. Parents should be counselled not to try to arouse the child from sleep, as this can induce confusional arousal and prolong the episode (Adair & Bauchner, 1993; Anders & Eiben, 1997; Chokroverty *et al.*, 2003; Laberge, 2000; Sheldon *et al.*, 1992). Underlying gastroesophageal reflux disease, periodic limb movement disorder, or sleep-disordered breathing may be risk factors for sleep terrors and should be treated if present (Brown, 1996; Goodwin *et al.*, 2004).

A large case series found scheduled awakening just prior to the expected time of night terrors was helpful (Lask, 1988). Hypnosis and relaxation therapy have been recommended for older children (Kohen *et al.*, 1992). Medication is appropriate only when sleep terrors are severe, persistent, and there is safety risk. Other treatable disorders that disrupt sleep or may worsen sleep terrors, such as sleep apnoea, reflux disease, nocturnal seizures, should be ruled out prior to instituting pharmacotherapy. Both benzodiazepines and tricyclic antidepressants have been used (Burstein & Burstein, 1983; Cooper, 1987; Fisher *et al.*, 1973).

A cross-over design found hypnotherapy to be efficacious in subjects with sleep walking (Reid *et al.*, 1981). Four children with dangerous sleep terrors were successfully treated with a short course of imipramine and self-hypnosis, with an additional 7 children successfully treated by self-hypnosis alone (Kohen *et al.*, 1992). Night waking prior to the expected onset of the night terrors was also shown to be effective (Lask, 1988). Book chapters and review articles provide support for parent education and reassurance, coupled with provision of good sleep hygiene and a safe sleep environment for the majority of cases, and brief courses of medication and/or hypnosis for severe cases (Adair & Bauchner, 1993; Ferber & Kryger, 1995; Handford & Vgontzas, 2002; Sheldon *et al.*, 1992).

Summary

Critical evaluation and opinion of sleep disorders treatment

Although effective interventions exist for common sleep disorders among infants and young children, the best approach is preventative (Table 51.5). Two prospective, randomized controlled trials have evaluated the impact of parent education either before or shortly after birth regarding normal infant sleep and infant sleep hygiene. Controls received no specific sleep advice. Both studies demonstrated better initiation and maintenance of sleep in intervention groups with follow up at 6–9 weeks in one study (Wolfson *et al.*, 1992) and 9 months in the other (Kerr *et al.*, 1996). Parent education about the importance of establishing healthy sleep habits early in life should be part of routine health care. National paediatric and sleep medicine associations could sponsor consensus statements outlining appropriate educational content for parents about infant sleep from a behavioural perspective. Incidence of sleep association disorder and limit-setting disorder would likely decrease with this approach. Even though parent education would not prevent development of sleep terrors in susceptible children, parents who understand the benign nature of the disorder would be spared considerable distress, with treatment efforts focused on those rare children with a severe condition.

The level of evidence for each of the interventions discussed in this chapter is summarized in Table 51.4 and 51.5.

Table 51.4. Feeding disorders: level of evidence for efficacy by treatment and form of treatment

Treatment	Form of treatment	Psychiatric disorder/ target audience	Level of evidence for efficacy	Comments
Multidisciplinary approach	Designed programme involving both clinic and home interventions	Feeding disorders	Ia	Growth status improved, and improved cognitive status with home intervention
Multidisciplinary approach	Often individually designed intervention	Pica	IV	Many of the studies come from single case analyses
Multidisciplinary approach	Both home and clinic interventions to increase stimulation and attention	Rumination	IV	Many of the studies come from single case studies
Behavioural intervention	Designed clinic programme	Feeding disorders	Ia	More weight gain with behavioural interventions. Nutritional counselling may or may not add to effectiveness
Behavioural intervention	Reinforcement, discrimination training, extinction, and punishment	Pica	III	Improvement found in pica behaviour but difficult to generalize because many studies are single case studies with specific individualized behavioural intervention
Behavioural (including cognitive) intervention	Biofeedback, relaxation training, habit reversal	Rumination	III	Improvement in 85% of the cases
Parent focused or parent child focused	Designed programmes such as play-focused or psychoeducation	Feeding disorders	III	Improved behaviour and weight gain
Nutritional supplementation	Zinc and/or iron supplementation	Pica	III	Effective for pica associated with deficiencies but not as a general treatment for all situations of pica.

Table 51.5. Sleeping disorders: level of evidence for efficacy by treatment and form of treatment

Treatment	Form of treatment	Psychiatric disorder/ target audience	Level of evidence for efficacy	Comments
Behavioural approaches	Primarily but not limited to graduated extinction	Sleeping onset disorders	Ia	Quite successful and in young infants, results are often obtained within a week
Behavioural approaches	Primarily but not limited to graduated extinction	Limit setting disorders	Ib	Quite successful
Behavioural approaches	Positive bedtime routine	Limit setting disorders	Ib	No more successful than graduated extinction but greater marital satisfaction
Psychopharmacology	Trimeprazine	Sleeping onset disorders	Ia	Effective but some controversy as to whether results can be sustained after medication is stopped
Psychopharmacology	Benzodiazepines Tricyclic antidepressants	Sleep terrors	III	Probably effective but should only be used for short periods of time and medical illnesses need to be ruled out
Parent education	Specific educational programme	Sleeping onset disorders	III	Improvement in sleep and sleep patterns.
Hypnotherapy	Hypnosis	Sleep terrors	III	Useful in older children. Often combined with medications
Night waking	Waking prior to expected onset of sleep terrors	Sleep terrors	III	Reports indicate success

REFERENCES

Adair R. H. & Bauchner, H. (1993). Sleep problems in childhood. *Current Problems in Pediatrics*, **23**, 147–70, 142 (discussion).

Adair R., Zuckerman, B., Bauchner, H., Phillip B. & Levenson, S. (1992). Reducing night waking in infancy: a primary care intervention. *Pediatrics*, **89**, 585–8.

Adams, L. A. & Rickert, V. I. (1989). An approach to infant sleep disorders. *Pediatrics*, **84**(5), 756–61.

Ahearn, W., Kerwin, M., Eigher, P. Shantz, J. & Swearingin, W. (1996). An alternative treatments comparison of two intensive interventions for food refusal. *Journal of Applied Behavior Analysis*, **29**, 321–32.

Ahearn, W. H., Kerwin, M. E., Eicher, P. S. & Lukens, C. J. (2001). An ABAC comparison of two intensive interventions for food refusal. *Behaviour Modification*, **25**(3), 385–405.

Altemeier, W. A., O'Conner, S. M., Sherrod, K. B. & Veitze, P. M. (1985). Prospective study of antecedents for nonorganic failure to thrive. *Journal of Pediatrics*, **106**, 360–5.

American Academy of Sleep Medicine (2000). *The International Classification of Sleep Disorders, Revised*, pp. 159–160. Rochester, MN: Johnson Printing.

American Psychiatric Association (2000). *Diagnostic and Statistical Manual of Mental Disorders*, 4th edn, Text Revision. Washington DC: American Psychiatric Association.

Ammaniti, M., Ambruzzi, A. M., Lucarelli, L., Cimino, S. & D'Olimpio, F. (2004). Malnutrition and dysfunctional mother-child feeding interactions: Clinical assessment and research implications. *Journal of the American College of Nutrition*, **23**(3), 259–71.

Anders, T. F. & Eiben, L. A. (1997). Pediatric sleep disorders: a review of the past 10 years. *Journal of the American Academy of Child and Adolescent Psychiatry*, **36**, 9–20.

Arbiter E. A. & Black, D. (1991). Pica and iron-deficiency anemia. *Child: Care, Health and Development*, **17**(4), 231–4.

Babbit, R. L., Hoch, T. A., Coe, D. A. *et al.* (1994). Behavioral assessment and treatment of pediatric feeding disorders. *Journal of Developmental and Behavioral Pediatrics*, **15**(4), 278–91.

Benoit, D. (2000). Feeding disorders, failure to thrive, and obesity. In *Handbook of Infant Mental Health*, 2nd edn, ed. C. H. Zeanah, pp. 339–352. New York: Guilford Press.

Benoit, D. & Coolbear, J. (1998). Post-traumatic feeding disorders in infancy: Behavioral predicting treatment outcome. *Infant Mental Health Journal*, **19**, 409–91.

Benoit, D., Wang, E. E. L. & Zlotkin, S. H. (2000). Discontinuation of enterostomy tube feeding by behavioral treatment in early childhood: a randomized controlled trial. *Journal of Pediatrics*, **137**, 498–503.

Benoit, D., Madigan, S., Lecce, S., Shea, B. & Goldberg, S. (2001). Atypical maternal behavior toward feeding-disordered infants before and after intervention. *Infant Mental Health Journal*, **22**, 611–26.

Birch, L. L. & Fisher, J. A. (1995). Appetite and eating behavior in children. *Pediatric Clinics of North America*, **4**, 931–55.

Bithoney, W. G., McJunkin, J., Michalek, J., Snyder, J., Egan, H. & Epstein, D. (1991). The effect of a multidisciplinary team approach on weight gain in nonorganic failure-to-thrive children. *Journal of Developmental and Behavioral Pediatrics*, **12**, 254–8.

Black, M. M. & Teti, L. O. (1997). Videotape: a culturally sensitive strategy to promote communication and healthy nutrition among adolescent mothers and their infants. *Pediatrics*, **99**, 432–437.

Black, M. M., Dubowitz, H., Hutcheson, J., Berenson-Howard, J. & Starr, R. H. (1995). A randomized clinical trial of home intervention for children with failure to thrive. *Pediatrics*, **95**(6), 807–14.

Black, M. M., Feigelman, S. & Cureton, P. L. (1999). Evaluation and treatment of children with failure-to-thrive: an interdisciplinary perspective. *Journal of Clinical Outcomes Management*, **6**, 60–73.

Brown, L. W. (1996). Sleep and epilepsy. *Child and Adolescent Psychiatric Clinics of North America*, **5**, 701–14.

Blackman, J. A. & Nelson, C. L. (1984). Reinstituting oral feedings in children fed by gastrosomy tube. *Clinical Pediatrics*, **24**, 434–8.

Bucher, B., Reykdal, B. & Albin, J. (1976). Brief physical restraint to control pica in retarded children. *Journal of Behavior Therapy and Experimental Psychology*, **7**, 141–4.

Burklow, K. A., Phelps, A. N., Schultz, J. R., McConnell, K. & Rudolph, C. (1998). Classifying complex pediatric feeding disorders. *Journal of Pediatric Gastroenterology and Nutrition*, **27**, 143–47.

Burstein, A. & Burstein, A. (1983). Treatment of night terrors with imipramine. *Journal of Clinical Psychiatry*, **44**, 82.

Casey, P. H., Kelleher, K. J., Bradley, R. H., Kellogg, L. W., Kirby, R. S. & Whiteside, L. (1994). A multifaceted intervention for infants with failure to thrive. *Archives of Pediatric and Adolescent Medicine*, **148**, 1071–7.

Chatoor, I. (2002). Feeding disorders in infants and toddlers: diagnosis and treatment. *Child and Adolescent Psychiatric Clinics of North America*, **11**, 163–83.

Chatoor, I. (2003). Food refusal by infants and young children: Diagnosis and treatment. *Cognitive and Behavioral Practice*, **10**, 138–46.

Chatoor, I., Hirsch, R. & Persinger, M., (1997). Facilitating the internal regulation of eating: a treatment model for infantile anorexia. *Infants and young children*, **9**, 12–22.

Chatoor, I., Ganiban, J., Colin, V., Plummer, N. & Harmon, R. (1998). Attachment and feeding problems: a reexamination of nonorganic failure to thrive and attachment insecurity. *Journal of the American Academy of Child and Adolescent Psychiatry*, **37**, 1217–24.

Chatoor, I., Ganiban, J., Harrison, H. & Hirsch, R. (2001). Observation of feeding in the diagnosis of posttraumatic feeding disorder of infancy. *Journal of the American Academy of Child and Adolescent Psychiatry*, **40**(5), 595–602.

Chial, H. J., Camilleri, M., Williams, D. E., Litzinger, K. & Perrault, J. (2003). Rumination syndrome in children and adolescents: Diagnosis, treatment, and prognosis. *Pediatrics*, **111**(1), 158–62.

Chokroverty, S., Hening, W. A. & Walters, A. S. (2003). An approach to the patient with movement disorders during sleep. In *Sleep and Movement Disorders*, ed. S. Chokreverty, W. A. Hening & A. S. Walters, pp. 201–18. Philadelphia, PA: Butterworth Heinemann.

Coolbear, J. & Benoit, D. (1999). Failure to thrive: Risk for clinical disturbance of attachment. *Infant Mental Health Journal*, **20**, 87–104.

Cooper, A. J. (1987). Treatment of coexistent night-terrors and somnambulism in adults with impramine and diazeam. *Journal of Clinical Psychiatry*, **48**, 209–10.

De la Burde, B. & Reames, B. (1973). The prevention of pica, the major cause of lead poisoning in children. *American Journal of Public Health*, **63**(8), 737–43.

Don, N., McMahon, C. & Rossiter, C. (2002). Effectiveness of an individualized multidisciplinary programme for managing unsettled infants. *Journal of Paediatrics and Child Health*, **38**, 563–7.

Drotar, D. (1990). Sampling issues in research with non-organic failure to thrive. *Pediatric Psychology*, **15**, 255–72.

Drotar, D., Nowak, M., Malone, C., Eckerle, D. & Negray, J. (1985). Early psychological outcomes in failure to thrive: predictions from an interactional model. *Journal of Clinical Child Psychology*, **14**, 105–11.

Duke, P. & Nielen, M. (1993). The use of negative practice for control of pica behavior. *Journal of Behavior Therapy and Experimental Psychology*, **24**, 249–53.

Eckerberg, B. (2004). Treatment of sleep problems in families with small children: Is written information enough? *Acta Paediatrica*, **91**, 952–9.

Eckerberg, B. (2002). Treatment of sleep problems in families with young children: effects of treatment on family well-being *Acta Paediatrica*, **93**, 126–34.

Ferber, R. (1985). *Solve Your Child's Sleep Problems*. New York: Simon & Schuster.

Ferber, R. & Kyrger, M. (1995). *Principles and Practice of Sleep Medicine in the Child*, pp. 79–89 & 99–106. Philadelphia: W. B. Saunders Co.

Finney, J. W., Russo, D. C. & Cataldo, M. F. (1982). Reduction of pica in young children with lead poisoning. *Journal of Pediatric Psychology*, **7**(2), 197–207.

Fisher, C., Kahn, E., Edwads, A. & Davis, D. M. (1973). A physiological study of nightmares and night terrors, the suppression of stage 4 night terrors with diazepam, *Archives of General Psychiatry*, **28**, 252–9.

Fisher, W. W., Piazza, C. C., Bowman, L. G., Kurtz, P. F., Sherer, M. R. & Lachman, S. R. (1994). A preliminary evaluation of empirically derived consequences for the treatment of pica. *Journal of Applied Behavior Analysis*, **27**(3), 447–557.

France, K. G., Blampied, N. M. & Wilkinson, P. (1991). Treatment of infant sleep disturbance by trimeprazine in combination with extinction. *Developmental and Behavioral Pediatrics*, **12**, 308–14.

France, K. G., Blampied, N. M., & Wilkinson, P. (1999). A multiple-baseline, double-blind evaluation of the effects of trimeprazine tartrate on infants sleep disturbance. *Experimental and Clinical Psychopharmacology*, **7**, 502–13.

Fredericks, D. W., Carr, J. E. & Williams, W. L. (1998). Overview of the treatment of a rumination disorder for adults in a residential setting. *Journal of Behaviour Therapy and Experimental Psychiatry*, **29**, 31–40.

Fryer, G. E. (1988). The efficacy of hospitalization of nonorganic failure to thrive children: a meta-analysis. *Child Abuse and Neglect*, **12**, 375–81.

Galbraith, L. R., Pritchard, L. & Hewitt, K. E. (1993). Behavioral treatment for sleep disturbance. *Health Visitor*, **66**, 169–71.

Goodivin, J. L., Kaemingk, K. L., Fregosi, R. F. *et al.* (2004). Parasomnias and sleep disordered breathing in Caucasian and Hispanic children – the Tucson children's assessment of sleep apnea study. *BioMed Central Medicine*, **2**, 14 (on line).

Grantham-McGregor, S. M., Schonfield, W. & Powell, C. (1987). The development of severely malnourished children who receive psychosocial stimulation: six year follow-up. *Pediatrics*, **79**, 247–54.

Halstead, J. A. (1968). Geophagia in man: its nature and nutritional effects. *American Journal of Chemical Nutrition*, **21**, 1384–93.

Handford, H. A. & Vgontzas, A. N. (2002). Sleep disturbances and disorders. In *Child and Adolescent Psychiatry: A Comprehensive Textbook*, ed. M. Lewis, pp. 876–888. Philadelphia, PA: Lippincott, Williams & Wilkins.

Hawdon, J. M., Beauregard, N., Slattery, J. & Kennedy, G. (2000). Identification of neonates at risk of developing feeding problems in infancy. *Developmental Medicine and Child Neurology*, **42**, 235–9.

Hiscock, H. & Wake, M. (2002). Randomized controlled trial of behavioural infant sleep intervention to improve infant sleep and maternal mood. *British Medical Journal*, **324**, 1062–8.

Hodes, M., Timimi, S. & Robinson, P. (1997). Children of mothers with eating disorders: a preliminary study. *European Eating Disorders Review*, **5**, 11–24.

Hyman, P. E. (1994). Gastroesophageal reflux: one reason why baby won't eat. *Journal of Pediatrics*, **125**, S103–9.

Iwaniec, D. (2004). *Children who Fail to Thrive*. Chichester, UK: Wiley & Sons Ltd.

Jacobi, C., Agras, W. S., Bryson, S. & Hammer, L. D. (2003). Behavioral validation, precursors, and concomitants of picky eating in childhood. *Journal of the American Academy of Child and Adolescent Psychiatry*, **42**(1), 76–84.

Jacobi, C., Hayward, C., De Zwaan, M., Karemer, H. C. & Agras, W. S. (2004). Coming to terms with risk factors for eating disorders: Application of risk terminology and suggestions for a general taxonomy. *Psychological Bulletin*, **130**(1), 19–65.

Jones, D. P. & Verduyn, C. M. (1983). Behavioral management of sleep problems. *Archives of Diseases of Children*, **58**, 442–4.

Kerr, S. M., Jowett, S. A. & Smith, L. N. (1996). Preventing sleep problems in infants: a randomized controlled trial. *The Journal of Advanced Nursing*, **24**, 938–42.

Kerwin, M. E. (1999). Empirically supported treatments in pediatric psychology: severe feeding problems. *Journal of Pediatric Psychology*, **24**, 193–214.

Kettaneh, A., Eclache, V., Fain, O. *et al.* (2005). Pica and food craving in patients with iron deficiency anemia: a case control study in France. *American Journal of Medicine*, **118**, 185–8.

Khan, S., Hyman, P. E., Cocjin, J. & Di Lorenzo, C. (2000). Rumination syndrome in adolescents. *Journal of Pediatrics*, **136**, 528–31.

Kohen, D. P. Mahowald, M. W. & Rosen, G. M. (1992). Sleep-terror disorder in children: the role of self-hypnosis in management. *American Journal of Clinical Hypnosis*, **34**, 233–44.

Korman, S. H. (1990). Pica as a presenting symptom in childhood celiac disease. *American Journal of Clinical Nutrition*, **51**(2), 139–41.

Kotler, L. A., Cohen, P., Davies, M., Pine, D. S. & Walsh, B. T. (2001). Longitudinal relationships between childhood, adolescent, and adult eating disorders. *Journal of the American Academy of Child and Adolescent Psychiatry*, **40**(12), 1434–40.

Laberge, L. Tremblay, R. E., Vitaro, F. & Montplaisir, J. (2000). Development of parasomnias from childhood to early adolescence. *Pediatrics*, **106**, 67–71.

LaGasse, L. L., Messinger, D., Lester, B. M. *et al.* (2002). Prenatal drug exposure and maternal and infant feeding behavior. *Archives of Diseases in Children: Fetal/Neonatal Education*, **88**, F391–9.

Largo, R. H. & Hunziker, U. A. (1984). A developmental approach to the management of children with sleep disturbances in the first three years of life. *European Journal of Pediatrics*, **142**, 170–173.

Lask, B. (1988). Novel and non-toxic treatment for night terrors. *British Medical Journal*, **297**, 592.

LeBlanc, L. A., Piazza, C. C. & Krug, M. A. (1997). Comparing methods for maintaining the safety of a child with pica. *Research on Developmental Disabilities*, **18**(3), 215–20.

Lemons, P. & Dodge, N. (1998) Persistent failure-to-thrive: a case study. *Journal of Pediatric Health Care*, **12**, 27–32.

Linscheid, T. (1999). Commentary: response to empirically supported treatments for feeding problems. *Journal of Pediatric Psychology*, **24**(3), 215–16.

Linscheid, T. & Cunningham, C. E. (1977). A controlled demonstration of the effectiveness of electric shock in the elimination of chronic infant rumination. *Journal of Applied Behavior Analysis*, **10**, 500.

Linscheid, T. R. & Murphy, L. B. (1999). Feeding disorders of infancy and early childhood. In *Child and Adolescent Psychological Disorders: A Comprehensive Textbook*, ed. S. D. Nether, pp. 139–155. New York: Oxford University Press.

Lofts, R., Schroeder, S. & Maier, R. (1990). Effects of serum zinc supplementation on pica behavior of persons with mental retardation. *American Journal on Mental Retardation*, **95**, 103–9.

Luiselli, J. K. (2000). Cueing, demand fading, and positive reinforcement to establish self-feeding and oral consumption in a child with chronic food refusal. *Behavior Modification*, **24**(3), 348–58.

Madsen, C. H., Madsen, C. K. & Thompson, E. (1974). Increasing rural Head Start children's consumption of middle-class meals. *Journal of Applied Behavior Analysis*, **7**, 257–62.

Maggioni, A. & Lifshitz, F. (1995). Nutritional management of failure to thrive. *Pediatric Clinics of North America*, **42**(4), 791–810.

Maldonado-Duran J. M. & Barriguette, J. A. (2001). Evaluation and treatment of eating and feeding disturbances in infancy. In *Infant and Toddler Mental Health: Models of Clinical Intervention with Infants and Their Families*, ed. J. M. Maldonado-Duran, pp. 309–342. Washington DC: American Psychiatric Publishing, Inc.

Manikam, R. & Perman, J. A. (2000). Pediatric feeding disorders. *Journal of Clinical Gastroenterology*, **30**(1), 3.

Marchi, M. & Cohen, P. (1990). Early childhood eating behaviors and adolescent eating disorders. *Journal of the American Academy of Child Adolescent Psychiatry*, **29**, 112–17.

McCann, J., Stein, A., Fairburn, C. G. & Dunger, D. B. (1994). Eating habits and attitudes of mothers of children with non-organic failure to thrive. *British Medical Journal*, **70**, 234–6.

Mihailidou, H., Galanakis, E., Paspalaki, P., Borgia, P. & Mantzouranis, E. (2002). Pica and the elephant's ear. *Journal of Child Neurology*, **17**, 855–6.

Minde, K., Popiel, K., Leos, N. *et al.* (1993). Evaluation and treatment of sleep disturbances in young children. *Journal of the American Academy of Child Adolescent Psychiatry*, **34**, 521–33.

Minde, K., Faucon, A. & Falkner, S. (1994). Sleep problems in toddlers: Effects of treatment on their daytime behavior. *Journal of the American Academy of Child Adolescent Psychiatry*, **33**, 1114–21.

Mindell, J. A. (1999). Empirically supported treatments in pediatric psychology: bedtime refusal and night waking in young children. *Journal of Pediatric Psychology*, **24**, 465–81.

Mindell, J. A. & Duran, V. M. (1993). Treatment of childhood sleep disorders: generalization across disorders and effects on family members. *Journal of Pediatrics*, **18**, 731–50.

Montanari, G., Schiaulini, P., Covre, A. & Steffan, A., Furlanu, M. (1992). Niaprazine vs chlormethyldiazepam in sleep disturbances in pediatric outpatients. *Pharmacology Research*, **25** (Suppl. 1), 83–4.

Mueller, M. M., Piazza, C. C., Moore, J. W. & Kelley, M. E. (2003). Training parents to implement pediatric feeding protocols. *Journal of Applied Behavior Analysis*, **36** (4), 545–62.

Nchito, M., Geissler, P. W., Mubila, L., Friis H. & Olsen, A. (2004). Effects of iron and multimicronutrient supplementation on geophagy: a two-by-two factorial study among Zambian schoolchildren in Lusaka. *Transactions of the Royal Society of Tropical Medicine and Hygiene*, **98**, 218–27.

O'Conner, M. E. & Szekely, L. J. (2001). Frequent breastfeeding and food refusal associated with failure to thrive: A manifestation of the vulnerable child syndrome. *Clinics in Pediatrics*, **40**(1), 27–33.

O'Reilly, M. F. & Lancioni, G. E. (2001). Treating food refusal in a child with williams syndrome using the parent as therapist in the home setting. *Journal of Intellectual Disabilities Research*, **45**(1), 41–6.

Owens, J. A., Rosen, C. L. & Mindell, J. A. (2003). Medication use in the treatment of pediatric insomnia: results of a survey of community-based pediatricians. *Pediatrics*, **111**, e628–365.

Owens, J. A., Babcock, D., Blumer, J. *et al.* (2005). The use of pharmacotherapy in the treatment of pediatric insomnia in primary care: a consensus meeting summary. *Journal of Clinical Sleep Medicine*, **1**, 49–59.

Owens-Stively, J., Frank, N., Smith, A., Hagino, O., Spirito, A. M. & Al, A. J. (1997). Child temperament, parenting discipline style, and daytime behavior in childhood sleep disorders. *Journal of Developmental and Behavioral Pediatrics*, **18**, 314–21.

Palmer, M. M. & Heyman, M. B. (1993). Assessment and treatment of sensory- versus motor-based feeding problems in very young children. *Infants and Young Children*, **6**, 67–73.

Piazza, C. C., Fisher, W. W., Hanley, G. P. *et al.* (1998). Treatment of pica through multiple analyses of its reinforcing functions. *Journal of Applied Behavioral Analysis*, **31**, 165–89.

Pritchard, A. A. & Appleton, P. (1988). Management of sleep problems in pre-school children. *Early Child Development and Care*, **34**, 227–40.

Ramchandani, P., Wiggs, L., Webb, V. & Stores, G. (2000). A systematic review of treatments for settling problems and night waking in young children. *British Medical Journal*, **320**, 209–13.

Rastam, M. (1992). Anorexia nervosa in 51 Swedish adolescents: premorbid problems and comorbidity. *Journal of the American Academy of Child Adolescent Psychiatry*, **31**, 819–29.

Raynor, P., Rudolf, M. C. J., Cooper, K., Marchant, P. & Cottrell, D. (1999). A randomized controlled trial of specialist health visitor intervention for failure to thrive. *Archives of Disease in Childhood*, **80**, 500–6.

Reau, N. R., Senturia, Y. D., Lebailly, S. A., Christoffel, K. K. (1996). Infant and toddler feeding patterns and problems: Normative data and a new direction. *Developmental and Behavioral Pediatrics*, **17**(3), 149–53.

Reed, G. K., Piazza, C. C., Patel, M. R. *et al.* (2004). On the relative contributions of noncontingent reinforcement and escape extinction in the treatment of food refusal. *Journal of Applied Behavioral Analysis*, **37**, 27–42.

Reid, W. H., Ahmed, I. & Levie, C. A. (1981). Treatment of sleepwalking: a controlled study. *American Journal of Psychology*, **35**, 27–37.

Reilly, S. M., Skuse, D. H., Wolke, D. & Stevenson, J. (1999). Oral-motor dysfunction in children who fail to thrive: organic or non-organic? *Developmental Medicine in Child Neurology*, **41**, 115–22.

Richman, N. (1985). A double-blind drug trial of treatment in young children with waking problems. *Journal of Child Psychology and Psychiatry*, **26**, 591–8.

Richman, N., Stevenson, J. & Graham, P. J. (1982). *Pre-School to School: A Behavioral Study*. London: Academic Press.

Rickert, V. I. & Johnson, C. M. (1988). Reducing nocturnal awakening and crying episodes in infants and young children: a comparison between scheduled awakenings and systematic ignoring. *Pediatrics*, **8**, 203–12.

Robb, A. S. (2001). Eating disorders in children: diagnosis and age-specific treatment. *Psychiatric Clinics of North America*, **24**, 259–70.

Rommel, N., De Meyer, A., Feenstra, L. & Veereman-Wauters, G. (2003). The complexity of feeding problems in 700 infants and young children presenting to a tertiary care institution. *Journal of Pediatric Gastroenterology Nutrition*, **37**, 75–84.

Rudolph, C. D. & Link, D. T. (2002). Feeding disorders in infants and children. *Pediatric Clinics of North America*, **49**(1), 97–112.

Russell, G. F. M., Treasure, J. & Eisler, I. (1998). Mothers with anorexia nervosa who underfeed their children: their recognition and management. *Psychological Medicine*, **28**, 93–108.

Scott, G. & Richards, M. P. M. (1990). Night waking in infants: effect of providing advice and support for parents. *Journal of Child Psychology and Psychiatry*, **31**, 551–67.

Sedeh, A. (1994). Assessment and intervention for infant night waking: parent reports and activity-based home monitoring. *Journal of Consulting and Clinical Psychology*, **62**, 63–8.

Seymour, F. W., Bayfield, G., Brock, P. & During, M. (1983). Management of night-waking in young children. *Australian Journal of Family Therapy*, **4**, 217–22.

Seymour, F. W., Brock, P., During, M. & Poole, G. (1989). Reducing sleep disruptions in young children: evaluation of therapist-guided and written information approaches: a brief report. *Journal of Child Psychology and Psychiatry*, **30**, 913–18.

Sheldon, H. S., Spire, J. P. & Levy, H. B. (1992). *Pediatric Sleep Medicine*, pp. 69–90, 119–135. Philadelphia: W.B. Saunders Company.

Simonoff, E. A. & Stores, G. (1987). Controlled trial of trimeprazine tartrate for night waking. *Archives of Disease in Childhood*, **62**, 253–7.

Singhi, S., Ravishanker, R., Singhi, P. & Nath, R. (2003). Low plasma zinc and iron in pica. *Indian Journal of Pediatrics*, **70**, 139–43.

Skuse, D. Wolke, D. & Reilly, E. (1992). Failure to thrive. Clinical and developmental aspects. In *Developmental Psychopathology*, ed. H. Remschmidt & M. H. Schmidt, pp. 46–71. Lewiston, NK: Hogrefe & Huber.

St James-Roberts, I., Sleep, J., Morris, S., Owen, C. & Gillham, P. (2001). Use of a behavioural programme in the first 3 months to prevent infant crying and sleeping problems. *Journal of Paediatric and Child Health*, **37**, 289–97.

Staiano, A. (2003). Food refusal in toddlers with chronic diseases. *Journal of Pediatric Gastroenterology and Nutrition*, **37**, 225–7.

Stark, L. J., Mulvihill, M. M., Powers, S. W. *et al.* (1996). Behavioral intervention to improve caloric intake of children with cystic fibrosis: treatment versus wait list control. *Journal of Pediatric Gastroenterology and Nutrition*, **22**, 240–53. [Abstract only]

Sturm, L. & Dawson, P. (1999). Working with families: an overview for providers. In *Failure to Thrive and Pediatric Undernutrition: A Transdisciplinary Approach*, ed. D. B. Kessler & P. Dawson pp. 65–76. Baltimore: Brookes Publishing.

Tolia, V. (1995). Very early onset nonorganic failure to thrive in infants. *Journal of Pediatric Gastroenterology and Nutrition*, **20**, 73–80.

Turner, K. M., Sanders, M. R. & Wall, C. R. (1994). Behavioural parent training versus dietary education in the treatment of children with persistent feeding difficulties. *Behavior Change*, **11**, 242–58. [Abstract only]

Vyas, D. & Chandra, R. K. (1984). Functional implications of iron deficiency. In *Iron Nutrition in Infancy and Childhood*, ed. A. Stekel & V. Nestle, pp. 45–49. New York: Raven Press.

Whelan, E. & Cooper, P. J. (2000). The association between childhood feeding problems and maternal eating disorder: A community study. *Psychological Medicine*, **30**, 69–77.

Winters, N. C. (2003). Feeding problems in infancy and early childhood. *Primary Psychiatry*, **10**(6), 30–34.

Wolfson, A., Lacks, P. & Futterman, A. (1992). Effects of parent training on infant sleep patterns, parents' stress, and perceived parental competence. *Journal of Consulting and Clinical Psychology*, **60**, 41–8.

Woolston, J. (2002). Eating and growth disorders in infants and children. In *Child and Adolescent Psychiatry: A Comprehensive Textbook*, ed. M. Lewis, pp. 681–692. Baltimore: Williams & Wilkins.

World Health Organization (1993). *ICD-10: International Classification of Mental and Behavioral Disorders; Diagnostic Criteria for Research, 10th edn*. Geneva, Switzerland: World Health Organization.

Wright, C. M., Callum, J., Birks, E. & Jarvis, S. (1998). Effect of community-based management in failure to thrive: randomized controlled trial. *British Medical Journal*, **317**, 571–4.

Zangen, T., Ciarla, C., Zangem, S. *et al.* (2003). Gastrointestinal motility and sensory abnormalities may contribute to food refusal in medically fragile toddlers. *Journal of Pediatric Gastroenterology and Nutrition*, **37**, 287–293.

52

Evaluating interventions for children with autism and intellectual disabilities

Patricia Howlin and Hower Kwon

Editor's note

Autism and other developmental disorders have led many parents and families to seek alternative or miracle cures because traditional treatment has had, at best, only mild success here. Yet none of these 'miracle treatments' has any evidence of efficacy or effectiveness. Psychopharmacologic interventions that target specific behaviours or symptoms have had some success, and these interventions are more readily used in the USA than in the UK. Educational programmes that provide structure and a predictable schedule and have consistency in the people who deliver the programme do appear to be able to deliver some modest improvement especially if the learning is closely tied to visual cues. Interventions that are behavioural in approach also appear to have some modest success in modifying behaviour especially around communication and social interaction. Again the improvements here are modest and probably have greater success in children who are at the milder end of the developmental disorder or autistic spectrum. A great deal of work needs to be done to empirically test these interventions to identify what elements appear to have the greatest impact on what aspect of these difficult disorders.

Introduction

When the first accounts of autism appeared in the 1940s and 1950s, the condition was considered to be a psychiatric disorder of psychogenic origin. Consequently, the principal treatments were psychoanalysis, medication or interventions such as ECT, as used for patients with psychosis (see Campbell, 1978). Subsequently, autism came to be viewed as a behavioural disorder, and from the mid 1960s onwards there was increasing use of operant approaches. However, these interventions were generally hospital based and focused on the elimination of 'undesirable' behaviours, with frequent use of aversive procedures, including electric shock (Howlin & Rutter, 1987). During the 1970s, recognition of the fundamental cognitive, social and communication deficits underlying the disorder (Rutter, 1972) resulted in a shift to more individually based treatment programmes, with greater recognition of the importance of structured education and of the crucial role of parents in therapy. Over the past three decades there has been increasing integration of home- and school-based programmes, greater involvement of typically developing peers in therapy and a steady movement towards more inclusive education. Furthermore, there is now wide recognition of the need for early intervention and of the role played by communication deficits in causing many of the 'challenging behaviours' frequently associated with autism. Nevertheless, despite such positive trends, the evidence base for treatments for children with autism remains surprisingly weak.

'Miracle cures'

Autism has probably attracted more attention within the field of 'alternative medicine' than almost any other developmental disorder, and claims for miracle treatments and 'cures' abound. On offer are numerous dietary and vitamin treatments, endocrine and other injections, physical therapies (including intensive and systematic exercise, 'facilitated communication', and holding therapy), sensory therapies (including sensory integration, auditory integration, and music therapy), and 'psychoeducational' therapies, such as the Waldon or Son-Rise programmes (see Howlin, 2004).

Despite the dramatic claims made for many of these therapies, evidence for their effectiveness is generally

Cambridge Textbook of Effective Treatments in Psychiatry, ed. Peter Tyrer and Kenneth R. Silk. Published by Cambridge University Press.
© Cambridge University Press, 2008.

lacking. A comprehensive report by the New York State Department of Health Department (1999) of treatments for pre-school children with autism found that, among the several hundred published papers reviewed, only a minority met basic experimental criteria. Moreover, for many of the alternative interventions listed above, no published data exist at all. The review concluded that there was no evidence for the effectiveness of sensory or physically based therapies. Facilitated communication was 'strongly discouraged' and has also been condemned as ineffective and as potentially abusive by the American Psychological Association (1994) and the American Academy of Pediatrics Committee on Children with Disabilities (1998). A Cochrane review of auditory integration training and other auditory therapies (Sinha *et al.*, 2004) concluded that the data in most of these studies were 'unusable', and the three studies that met basic experimental criteria showed no effect of therapy. Of the various quasi-medical or dietary interventions reviewed (secretin, immunoglobulin injections, anti-yeast treatments, vitamin or dietary manipulations), again there is little, if any, evidence of effectiveness. A Cochrane review of previously published studies of vitamin B6 and magnesium treatments for autism (Nye & Brice, 2002) found only one randomized, double-blind trial, and that study showed no benefits compared with placebo. Another Cochrane review of gluten- and casein-free diets for children with autism (Millward *et al.*, 2004) found only one small-scale study that met basic research criteria, and this reported only limited effects. Similarly, recent controlled trials of secretin, a gastro-intestinal peptide hormone claimed to have almost 'miraculous' effects (Horvath *et al.*, 1998; Rimland, 1998), indicate no advantages over placebo (Coniglio *et al.*, 2001; Owley *et al.*, 2001; Sandler *et al.*, 1999). The general conclusion of the New York State Department of Health's review concerning dietary or vitamin therapies was that their use should be discouraged because of significant concerns about side effects. There has been very little consideration, for example, of the consequences of removing basic foodstuffs such as gluten, milk or wheat without ensuring that any resulting dietary deficiencies are adequately compensated for. The possible risks of adding vitamins or other supplements also tend to be almost completely unresearched.

Pharmacological interventions

The use of psychotropic medication for young children with autism varies greatly from country to country. In the UK there is relatively little use of pharmacological treatments for autism per se, although, of course, medication may be necessary for comorbid conditions such as epilepsy (Gringras, 2000). Practitioners in the USA have been far more willing to turn to psychotropic medications for children with autism.

Medications have been largely unsuccessful in treating the core symptoms of autism such as language delay and impaired social functioning. Instead, it is generally accepted that these medications are best used to treat specific problems such as hyperactivity, self-injurious behaviour, depression and irritability, with the hope that improvement in these behaviours will allow individuals with autism to benefit more from educational and other therapeutic approaches. And although the empirical use of psychotropic medications has outpaced the number of studies carefully examining the safety and efficacy of these medications, a growing body of literature supports their use in children and adolescents with autism.

Historically, the antipsychotic agents have been the best-studied class of medications in treating symptoms of autism. Haloperidol (Anderson *et al.*, 1983, 1989; Campbell *et al.*, 1978; Cohen *et al.*, 1980) has been found to reduce stereotypies, withdrawal, hyperactivity, temper tantrums. More recently, in a large multisite, randomized, double-blind trial, risperidone was found to be effective in treating tantrums, aggression, and self-injurious behaviour in children with autism (McCracken *et al.*, 2002). In October 2006, risperidone became the first drug to receive approval by the US FDA for treatment of symptoms related to autism, specifically irritability, aggression, self-injury and tantrums. Several smaller-scale studies support the effectiveness of other atypical antipsychotics such as olanzapine and quetiapine.

Among the classes of antidepressants, selective serotonin reuptake inhibitors (SSRI's) such as fluoxetine, sertraline, and fluvoxamine are being used frequently in efforts to address various problem behaviours in autism. However, only one double-blind placebo-controlled study of an SSRI has been performed, and this study examined the effectiveness of fluvoxamine in adults with autism (McDougle *et al.*, 1996). Fluvoxamine resulted in clinically significant effects on behaviours such as repetitive thoughts and behaviour, aggression, and impaired social relatedness. Numerous smaller-scale studies, case series, and open trials have suggested the usefulness of fluoxetine, sertraline, and paroxetine. Among the older, heterocyclic antidepressants, clomipramine was shown in a double-blind crossover study to be significantly superior to desipramine and placebo in reducing stereotypies and compulsive and ritualized behaviours (Gordon *et al.*, 1993). However, serious side effects were noted, including tachycardia, QT prolongation, seizures, and tremor.

Other psychotropic medications used in treating maladaptive symptoms of autism include alpha-adrenergic agonists such as clonidine and guanfacine, mood stabilizers, and stimulants, but no large controlled trials have been performed. For all of the above-mentioned psychiatric medications, regardless of the presence of carefully controlled studies, additional information about long-term effects is needed, particularly when used with very young children. Again in this population as in many populations of children and adolescents with psychiatric difficulties, psychiatrists in the USA are much more ready and willing to use medications than their counterparts in the UK.

Educational programmes

Rutter & Bartak (1973) confirmed that autistic children exposed to structured, task oriented, 'academic' programmes made significantly better educational and social progress than children in other environments. The TEACCH programme (Teaching and Education of Autistic and Related Communication Handicapped Children (Schopler, 1997)) is among the best known and most widely used, and emphasises individually based teaching, the need for structure, appropriate environmental organization and the use of visual prompts to circumvent communication difficulties. Despite the fact that TEACCH is used in specialist schools for children with autism in countries across the world, empirical validation of its effectiveness is sparse, and the few controlled studies that have been conducted involve very small samples and only short-term follow-ups (Ozonoff & Cathcart, 1998; Panerai et al., 2002). Various other, mostly US based, educational models exist including the Denver programme, the Douglass centre programme, Higashi schools, the Individualized Support Programme, Bright Start, and 'LEAP' (see National Research Council, 2001 for review). There are also some small, short-term studies documenting the potential value of computer-based teaching (Chen & Bernard-Opitz, 1993; Powell & Jordan, 1997; Tjus et al., 2001).

In the UK, the National Autistic Society (1997) promotes the SPELL (Structure, Positive, Empathy, Low Arousal, Links) approach. Other programmes such as the Developmental Intervention Model (Greenspan & Wieder, 1999), the Waldon Program (McGee et al., 1994), the Hanen approach (Sussman, 1999), and the Early Bird Project (Shields, 2001) focus on the encouragement of play and pleasurable interactions between pre-school children with autism and their parents or peers. However, there are very few independent or randomized control trials of these

interventions, but research into this area is beginning to occur (Aldred et al., 2004).

There is also a growing number of programmes specifically designed to overcome social-communication impairments in young children with autism. Two increasingly widely used approaches are the Picture Exchange Communication System (PECS (Bondy & Frost, 1996)) in which children are taught to use symbols and pictures to enhance communication skills, and Social Stories (Grey, 1995), which employs cartoon-type illustrations to help children understand how to respond in social situations. Although there are many anecdotal or single case accounts of the value of these two approaches (many written by the proponents themselves), there are currently no independent, controlled studies of Social Stories. Independent evaluations of PECS (Howlin et al., in press; Yoder & Stone, 2006), whilst reporting positive gains in children's non-verbal communication, found fewer improvements in their verbal skills.

Behavioural programmes for pre-school children

In recent years there has been a steady growth in behaviourally based programmes for toddlers and pre-school children with autism (Rogers, 1998). Among the most widely publicised of these programmes is the Early Intensive Behavioral Intervention (EIBI (Lovaas, 2002)), which employs a highly prescriptive, applied behavioural analysis (ABA) approach. Children are expected to spend at least 40 hours a week in therapy which is supervised (but not conducted) by experienced behavioural consultants. It is recommended that intervention should start at around two years of age and last for 2 years or more. When the programme is followed consistently, major improvements in cognitive ability (30 IQ points or more) are reported. There are also claims that around 47% of participants become 'indistinguishable' from their normally developing peers (Lovaas, 1987; McEachin et al., 1993). However, despite the impressive findings, the number of children involved in the Lovaas studies was only 19 cases. Moreover, criticism has been directed towards proponents of EIBI regarding methodological problems in their studies that shed considerable doubt upon claims of symptomatic improvement in children treated with EIBI (Gresham & MacMillan, 1998).

Generally, the number of participants involved in evaluative studies of early behavioural/educational interventions remains very small. Independent, randomized, controlled trials are virtually non-existent, and many questions remain to be answered concerning the specific effects of these early programmes, since the content is often very eclectic and the relative importance of the different components of treatment is unknown (Lord, 2000). There are many other unanswered questions, for example:

- What are the comparative merits of one-to-one vs. group teaching, or of home-based vs. school-based programmes (Schreibman, 2000)?
- Which children respond best to programmes of this kind? Data here are limited, although there are indications that children with very low IQs are less likely to respond (Smith *et al.*, 1997), and there is some suggestion that those with classic autism may make less progress than those with pervasive developmental disorders (Smith *et al.*, 2000).
- What is the optimal length of time in therapy and at what age should treatment begin? Although Lovaas insists that 40 hours a week of therapy over at least 2 years is essential, positive results have been reported for less intensive programmes (Gabriels *et al.*, 2001; Rogers, 1998).
- What are the longer-term effects on children's social, behavioural and educational outcomes? Is it really valid to claim, as do proponents of EIBI, that the considerable cost in terms of both time and money is justified on the grounds that many children will subsequently no longer require additional or specialist support?

In a study examining EIBI as administered in a non-academic setting, Sheinkopf & Siegel (1998) concluded that early behavioural/educational interventions are a good option for children with autism. They are certainly far better than no intervention or non-specialist school placements. However, they found no evidence in favour of any one approach, any one level of intensity, or any particular degree of structure. Similar conclusions were reached in the New York State Department of Health review (1999). To date, given the current state of research in the field, no one approach has been demonstrated to be generally superior to all others or to be equally effective for all children.

Understanding the research based evidence for effective approaches to intervention

Although research in the field of autism intervention currently lacks large-scale, randomized control designs, conclusions may be drawn from the existing empirical data from well-designed small group and single case studies concerning those components of treatment that are likely to be beneficial and to influence best practice (Koegel *et al.*, 2001).

1. There is evidence of the advantages of individually designed intervention programmes that take into account the individual's cognitive level, severity of autistic symptomatology, and overall developmental level (Anderson & Romanczyk, 1999; Prizant & Rubin, 1999).

2. Many single case and small group studies attest to the importance of structured educational/daily living programmes, with a particular emphasis on visual prompts. By providing children with autism with an environment that is predictable and consistent, confusion and distress can be minimized. Such minimization of variation in the environment can lead to enhanced learning and reductions in stereotyped or disruptive behaviours (Quill, 1995; Schopler, 1997).

3. The more effective treatments take specific account of the core deficits of autism. For example, there are positive advantages of ensuring that the communication used by all those in the child's environment is appropriate for the individual's comprehension level, and that verbal messages are augmented by visual or other means (Howlin, 2004). Beneficial effects are also demonstrated for interventions that focus on the social-communication deficits associated with autism (Rogers, 2000). Specialist training programmes, for example to improve 'Mind-reading' skills (Baron-Cohen, 2000), social understanding (Gray, 1995) and social interactions (Koegel *et al.*, 2001) may also help to enhance social functioning.

4. Stereotyped and ritualistic tendencies are frequently an underlying cause of many behaviour problems and, as these tend to become more unacceptable and/or unmanageable with age, it is important to ensure that parents are helped to develop effective coping strategies in the early years (Howlin, 2004).

5. Many so-called undesirable or challenging behaviours are a reflection of the very limited behavioural repertoires or poor communication skills of autistic children. Again, a focus on skill enhancement and the establishment of effective communication strategies are often the most successful means of reducing difficult or disruptive behaviours (Durand & Merges, 2001; Koegel 2000, Prizant *et al.*, 1997).

6. Family centred treatment approaches appear to ensure more effective generalization and maintenance of skills (Marcus *et al.*, 1997). Although evidence for the relative effectiveness of parent mediated interventions remains limited because of weak experimental design (Diggle *et al.*, 2003), the development of management strategies that can be implemented consistently but in ways that do not demand extensive sacrifice in terms of time, money or other aspects of family life, seems most likely to offer benefits for all involved.

Table 52.1. Effectiveness of treatments for autism and intellectual disabilities in children

Treatment	Form of treatment	Psychiatric disorder/ target audience	Level of evidence for efficacy	Comments
Psychopharmacology	Antipsychotics	Autism and developmentally disabled	Ib	Reduction of temper tantrums, aggression, some stereotypies, and self-injurious behaviour
Psychopharmacology	Antidepressants (SSRIs)	Autism and developmentally disabled	Ib	Improvement of repetitive thoughts and behaviours, aggression, and social relatedness
Psychopharmacology	Antidepressants (TCAs)	Autism and developmentally disabled	IIb	Clomipramine reduced sterotypies and compulsive and ritualized behaviours but substantial side effects
Educational programmes	Multiple models of structured educational interventions	Autism and developmentally disabled	III	Empirical validation remains weak Predictable structure and a heavy emphasis on visual cues appear to be most helpful
Behavioural programmes	Multiple models including Early Intensive Behavioral Intervention (EIBI)	Pre-school children with autism and developmental disorders	III	These are probably effective, but data is needed as to the specificity of the effectiveness and what programmes or what elements of which programmes are effective. It appears that programmes that concentrate on social-communication skills can improve social functioning and interactions

Conclusions

There are no miracle cures for autism, any more than there are for other genetic conditions, such as Down syndrome. The recently published UK 'National Autism Plan for Children' (le Couteur *et al.*, 2003) concluded, on the basis of a detailed literature review, that 'The findings generally support the view that early educational/behavioural programmes are a good option for children with ASD [autistic spectrum disorders], but there is little evidence in support of any one specific methodology or intensity of treatment. Certain pharmacological treatments seem to be effective but further research is required to pinpoint which particular medicines work for which particular children and for which particular types of problem' (p. 87). The report found little or no scientific evidence in support of most other treatments (including diets, vitamins, sensory training, psychoanalysis, or specific programmes such as Son-Rise, Waldon, Daily Life Therapy, or Facilitated Communication), and although a number of parent training programmes, such as Hanen or Early Bird, seemed to offer a good model for intervention, again these had not been adequately assessed. It concludes 'While some of these approaches (with the exception of Facilitated Communication) may be helpful for individual children

with ASD and their families, there is no evidence to support their wider use' (p. 87). Nevertheless, as the present review indicates, there are general approaches to intervention, based on psychological and developmental research that can be used to help children and their families. However, to be effective these must be adapted in order to take account of individual differences and needs.

The level of evidence for each of the interventions discussed in this chapter is summarized in Table 52.1.

REFERENCES

Aldred, C., Green, G. & Adams C. (2004). A new social communication intervention for children with autism: pilot randomised controlled treatment study suggesting effectiveness. *Journal of Child Psychology and Psychiatry*, **45**, 1420–30.

American Academy of Pediatrics Committee on Children with Disabilities (1998). Auditory Integration Training and Facilitated Communication for Autism. *Pediatrics*, **102**, 431–3.

American Psychological Association (1994). *Resolution on Facilitated Communication. August 1994*.

Anderson, S. R. & Romanczyk, R. G. (1999). Continuum-based behavioral models. *Journal of the Association for Persons with Severe Handicaps*, **24**, 162–73.

Anderson, L. T., Campbell, M., Grega, D. M., Perry, R., Small, A. M. & Green, W. H. (1984). Haloperidol in the treatment of infantile autism: effects on learning and behavioral symptoms. *American Journal of Psychiatry*, **141**, 1195–202.

Anderson, L. T., Campbell, M., Adams, P., Small, A. M., Perry, R. & Shell J. (1989). The effects of haloperidol on discrimination learning and behavioral symptoms in autistic children. *Journal of Autism and Developmental Disorders*, **19**, 227–39.

Baron-Cohen, S. (2002). *Mind Reading – The Interactive Guide to Emotions – User Guide and Resource Pack*. Cambridge: University of Cambridge.

Bondy A. & Frost L. (1996). Educational approaches in pre-school: behavior techniques in a public school setting. In *Learning and Cognition in Autism, Current Issues in Autism*, ed. E. Schopler & G. B. Mesibov. New York: Plenum Press.

Campbell, M. (1978). Pharmacotherapy. In *Autism: A Re-Appraisal of Concepts and Treatment*, ed. M. Rutter, & E. Schopler, pp. 337–55. New York: Plenum.

Campbell, M., Anderson, L. T., Meier, M. *et al.* (1978). A comparison of haloperidol and behavior therapy and their interaction in autistic children. *Journal of the American Academy of Child and Adolescent Psychiatry*, **17**, 640–55.

Campbell, M., Schopler, E., Cueva, J. E. & Hallin, A. (1996). Treatment of autistic disorder. *Journal of the American Academy of Child and Adolescent Psychiatry*, **35**, 134–43.

Chen, S. & Bernard-Opitz, V. (1993). Comparison of personal and computer assisted instruction for children with autism. *Mental Retardation*, **31**, 368–76.

Cohen, I. L., Campbell, M., Posner, D., Small, A. M., Triebel, D. & Anderson, L. T. (1980). Behavioral effects of haloperidol in young autistic children. An objective analysis using a within-subjects reversal design. *Journal of the American Academy of Child and Adolescent Psychiatry*, **19**, 665–77.

Coniglio, S. J., Lewis, J. D., Lang, C. *et al.* (2001). A randomized, double-blind, placebo-controlled trial of single-dose intravenous secretin as treatment for children with autism. *Journal of Pediatrics*, **138**, 649–55.

Diggle, T., McConichie, H. R. & Randle, V. R (2003). Parent mediated early intervention for young children with autism spectrum disorder. *Cochrane Database of Systematic Reviews*, **1**, CD 003496. Oxford: Update Software Ltd.

Durand, V. M. & Merges, E. (2001). Functional communication training: a contemporary behavior analytic intervention for problem behavior. *Focus on Autism and Other Developmental Disorders*, **16**, 110–19.

Gabriels, R. L. Hill, D. E., Pierce, R. A. & Rogers, S. J. (2001). Predictors of treatment outcome in young children with autism: a retrospective study. *Autism*, **5**, 399–406.

Gordon, C. T., State, R. C., Nelson, J. E., Hamburger, S. D. & Rapoport, J. L. (1993). A double-blind comparison of clomipramine, desipramine, and placebo in the treatment of autistic disorder. *Archives of General Psychiatry*, **50**, 441–7.

Gray C. A. (1995). Teaching children with autism to 'read' social situations. In *Teaching Children with Autism: Strategies to Enhance Communication and Socialization*, ed. A. Quill, pp. 219–42. New York: Delmar.

Greenspan, S. J. & Wieder, S. (1999). A functional developmental approach to autism spectrum disorders. *Journal of the Association for Persons with Severe Handicap*, **3**, 147–61.

Gresham, F. M. & MacMillan, D. L. (1998). Early Intervention Project: can its claims be substantiated and its effects replicated? *Journal of Autism and Developmental Disorders*, **28**, 5–13.

Gringras, P. (2000). Practical paediatric psychopharmacological prescribing in autism: the potential and the pitfalls. *Autism: International Journal of Research and Practice*, **4**, 229–43.

Horvath, K., Stefanotos, G., Sokolski, K. N., Wachtel, R., Nabors, L. & Tildon, T. (1998) Improved social and language skills after Secretin administration in patients with autistic spectrum disorders. *Journal of the Association of the Academy of Minority Physicians*, **9**, 9–15.

Howlin, P. (2004). *Autism and Asperger syndrome: Preparing for Adulthood*. London: Routledge and Taylor.

Howlin, P. & Rutter, M. (1987). *Treatment of Autistic Children*. Chichester, UK: Wiley.

Howlin, P., Gordon, K, Pasco, G. & Charman, T. (2006). A group randomised, controlled trial of the Picture Exchange Communication System for children with autism. *Journal of Child Psychology and Psychiatry*, **48**, 473–8.

Koegel, L. K. (2000). Interventions to facilitate communication in autism. *Journal of Autism and Developmental Disorders*, **30**, 383–92.

Koegel, R. L., Koegel, L. K. & McNerney, E. K. (2001) Pivotal areas in intervention for autism. *Journal of Clinical Child Psychology*, **30**, 19–32.

Le Couteur, A. (2003). National Autism Plan for Children (NAPC). Produced by NIASA, National Initiative for Autism Screening and Assessment. National Autistic Society, London.

Lord, C. (2000). Commentary: achievements and future directions for intervention research in communication and autism spectrum disorders. *Journal of Autism and Developmental Disorders*, **306**, 393–8.

Lovaas, O. I. (1987). Behavioral treatment and normal education and intellectual functioning in young autistic children. *Journal of Consulting and Clinical Psychology*, **55**, 3–9.

Lovaas, O. I. (2002). *Teaching Individuals with Developmental delays: Basic Intervention Techniques*. Austin, Texas: Pro-Ed.

McCracken, J. T., McGough, J., Shah, B. *et al.*; Research Units on Pediatric Psychopharmacology Autism Network (2002). Risperidone in children with autism and serious behavioral problems. *New England Journal of Medicine*, **347**, 314–21.

McDougle, C. J., Naylor, S. T., Cohen, D. J., Volkmar, F. R., Heninger, G. R. & Price, L. H. (1996). A double-blind, placebo-controlled study of fluvoxamine in adults with autistic disorder. *Archives of General Psychiatry*, **53**, 1001–8.

McGee, G., Daly, T. & Jacobs, A. (1994). Waldon pre-school. In *Preschool Education Programs for Children with Autism*, ed. S. J. Harrris & J. S. Handleman. Austin, Texas: Pro-Ed.

McEachin, J. J., Smith, T. & Lovaas, O. I. (1993). Long-term outcome for children with autism who received early intensive behavioral treatment. *American Journal of Mental Retardation*, **97**, 359–72.

Marcus, L. M., Kunce, L. J. & Schopler, E. (1997). Working with families. In *Handbook of Autism and Pervasive Developmental Disorders*, 2nd edn, D. Cohen & F. Volkmar, pp. 631–49. New York: Wiley.

Millward, C., Ferriter, M., Calver, S. & Connell-Jones, G. (2004). Gluten and casein free diets for autistic spectrum disorders. *Cochrane Database Systematic Reviews*, **2**, cD003498 Oxford: Update Software Ltd.

National Autistic Society (1997). *Approaches to Autism*. London: National Autistic Society.

National Research Council (2001). *Educating Children with Autism*. Committee on Educational Interventions for Children with Autism. Division of Behavioral and Social Sciences and Education. National Research Council. Washington, DC: National Academy Press.

New York State Department of Health (1999). Clinical practice guidelines: report of recommendations. Autism/pervasive developmental disorders. Assessment and intervention for young children (0–6 years). Available at www.health.state.ny.us/ nysdob /eip/menu.htm.

Nye, C. & Brice, A. (2002). Combined vitamin B6-magnesium treatment in autism spectrum disorder. *Cochrane Database of Systematic Reviews*, **4**, CD 003497. Oxford: Update Software Ltd.

Owley, T., McMahon, W., Cook, E. H. *et al.* (2001). Multisite, double-blind, placebo-controlled trial of porcine secretin in autism. *Journal of the American Academy of Child and Adolescent Psychiatry*, **40**, 1293–9.

Ozonoff, S. & Cathcart, K. (1998) Effectiveness of a home program intervention for young children with autism. *Journal of Autism and Developmental Disorders*, **28**, 25–32.

Panerai, S., Ferrante, L. & Zingale, M. (2002). Benefits of the Treatment and Education of Autistic and Communication Handicapped Children (TEACCH) programme as compared with a non-specific approach. *Journal of Intellectual Disability Research*, **46**, 318–27.

Powell, S. & Jordan, R. (eds) (1997). *Autism and Learning: A Guide to Good Practice*. London: David Fulton.

Prizant, B. M. & Rubin, E. (1999). Contemporary issues in interventions for autism spectrum disorders: a commentary. *Journal of the Association for Persons with Severe Handicaps*, **24**, 199–208.

Prizant, B., Schuler A., Wetherby, A. & Rydell, P. (1997). Enhancing language and communication development: language approaches. In *Handbook of Autism and Pervasive Developmental Disorders*, 2nd edn, ed. D. Cohen & F. Volkmar, pp. 572–605. New York: Wiley.

Quill K. A. (ed.) (1995). *Teaching Children with Autism: Strategies to Enhance Communication and Socialization*. New York: Delmar.

Rimland, B. (1998). First secretin efficacy study produces positive results! Editorial comment. *Autism Research Review International*, **15** (2), Insert page 1.

Rogers, S. J. (1998). Empirically supported comprehensive treatments for young children with autism. *Journal of Clinical Child Psychology*, **27**, 168–79.

Rogers, S. J. (2000). Interventions that facilitate socialization in children with autism. *Journal of Autism and Developmental Disorders*, **30**, 399–410.

Rutter, M. (1972). Childhood schizophrenia reconsidered. *Journal of Autism and Childhood Schizophrenia*, **2**, 315–37.

Rutter, M. & Bartak, L. (1973). Special educational treatment of autistic children: a comparative study. II Follow-up findings and implications for services. *Journal of Child Psychology and Psychiatry*, **14**, 241–70.

Sandler, A. D., Sutton, K. A., DeWeese, J., Girardi, M. A., Sheppard, V. & Bodfish, J. W.. (1999). Lack of benefit of a single dose of synthetic human secretin in the treatment of autism and pervasive developmental disorder. *New England Journal of Medicine*, **341**(24), 1801–6.

Schopler, E. (1997). Implementation of TEACCH philosophy. In *Handbook of Autism and Pervasive Developmental Disorders*, 2nd edn, ed. D. J. Cohen & F. R. Volkmar, pp. 767–98. New York: John Wiley.

Schreibman, L. (2000). Intensive behavioral/psychoeducational treatments for autism: research needs and future directions. *Journal of Autism and Developmental Disorders*, **30**, 373–8.

Sheinkopf, S. J. & Siegel, B. (1998). Home-based behavioral treatment for young children with autism. *Journal of Autism and Developmental Disorders*, **28**, 15–23.

Shields, J. (2001). The NAS Early Bird Programme: partnership with parents in early intervention. *Autism: International Journal of Research and Practice*, **5**, 49–56.

Sinha, Y., Silove, N., Wheeler, D. & Willliams, K. (2004). Auditory integration training and other sound therapies for autism spectrum disorders. *Cochrane Database of Systematic Reviews*, **1**, CD 003681. Oxford: Update Software Ltd.

Smith, T., Groen, A. D. & Wynn, J. W. (2000). Randomized trial of intensive early intervention for children with Pervasive Developmental Disorder. *American Journal on Mental Retardation*, **105**, 269–85.

Smith, T., Eikeseth, S., Klevstrand, M. & Lovaas, O. I. (1997). Intensive behavioural treatment for preschoolers with severe mental retardation and pervasive developmental disorder. *American Journal on Mental Retardation*, **102**, 238–49.

Sussman, F. (1999). *More Than Words*. Toronto: The Hanen Program.

Tjus, T., Heimann, M. & Nelson, K. E. (2001). Interaction patterns between children and their teachers when using a specific multi-media and communication strategy. Observations from children with autism and mixed intellectual disabilities. *Autism: International Journal of Research and Practice*, **5**, 175–87.

Yoder, P. J. & Stone, W. L. (2006). A randomized comparison of the effect of two prelinguistic communication interventions on the acquisition of spoken communication in preschoolers with ASD. *Journal of Speech, Language and Hearing Research*, **49**, 698–711.

53

ADHD and hyperkinetic disorder

Paramala J. Santosh, Amy Henry and Christopher K. Varley

Editor's note

Attention deficit and hyperactivity disorder (ADHD) and hyperkinetic disorder (HKD) are not exactly synonymous. ADHD comes from DSM, and there can be some symptoms of inattention and/or impulsivity and hyperactivity, while HKD comes from ICD, and inattention, impulsivity and hyperactivity must all be present for the diagnosis of HKD to be made. Thus ADHD is a broader diagnostic term, and there is clearer evidence for the effectiveness of medications, especially the stimulants, in HKD than in ADHD. Nonetheless, medications, especially first-line treatment with the psychostimulants, has a great deal of data to support its effectiveness. There are less data supporting the use of other non-stimulant drugs such as atomoxetine and bupropion, and the data are less convincing and have smaller effect sizes than the psychostimulants. While psychosocial treatments, particularly behaviour therapy, have evidence for effectiveness, the evidence is not as strong as for the pharmacologic interventions, and the treatments seem more behaviour specific, less generalizable and quite often lose their effectiveness when the treatments end. While combined psychosocial and psychopharmacologic treatments are effective, it appears that most of the effectiveness comes from the pharmacologic intervention, although patients in combined treatment appear to need lower doses of pharmacologic agents.

Introduction

Attention deficit hyperactivity disorder (ADHD) or hyperkinetic disorder (HKD) is a common childhood condition affecting children and youth around the world across various cultures (Biederman et al., 1991; Rohde et al., 2001)). ADHD is characterized by impulsiveness, hyperactivity and/or inattention to a degree that it beyond what is expected in the normal continuum of severity in developmentally similar children. Hyperkinetic disorder is a narrower diagnosis and is a subgroup of ADHD with different implications. There is a genetic component to these disorders.

Hyperkinetic disorder (HKD) is an ICD-10 diagnosis, which requires the presence of inattention, impulsivity and hyperactivity. Symptoms should occur before the age of 6 years and be present in more than one setting. As such, it occurs with a prevalence of about 1.5% in the school-age population. In ICD-10, the presence of another disorder, such as anxiety state, is in itself an exclusion criterion; the expectation is that most cases of HKD will have a single diagnosis. Attention deficit/hyperactivity disorder, on the other hand, is a DSM-IV diagnosis requiring the presence of some symptoms of inattention and/or, impulsivity and hyperactivity. It is a more broadly defined and more common diagnosis. Symptoms should occur before the age of 7 years and cause some impairment in more than one setting. The diagnosis is defined as having subtypes of primarily inattentive, primarily hyperactive–impulsive or combined type. Attention deficit hyperactivity disorder is commonly associated with several co-morbid conditions, such as oppositional defiant disorder, conduct disorder, anxiety disorders, depressive disorders, pervasive developmental disorders, tic disorders and learning disorders (Biederman et al., 1991). ADHD occurs with a prevalence of about 3%–5%. It appears that nearly all cases of HKD should be included within ADHD.

In the UK, traditionally the ICD-10 classification system has been used for diagnosing and treating psychiatric disorders. However, ADHD (DSM-IV based) is increasingly the more familiar diagnosis with both clinicians and families, and is supported by an extensive research literature. European guidelines recommend that assessment

Cambridge Textbook of Effective Treatments in Psychiatry, ed. Peter Tyrer and Kenneth R. Silk. Published by Cambridge University Press.

should consider both diagnostic categories where possible (Taylor *et al.*, 2004). The National Institute of for Health and Clinical Excellence (NICE) guidelines published in 2000 in England and Wales (NICE, 2000) describe 'Severe ADHD' as broadly similar to HKD.

While the typical onset of ADHD is in toddlerhood, preschool or very early school-age years (Barkley 1998), it can continue to affect individuals at least into early adulthood (Weiss & Hechtman, 1993). Attention deficit hyperactivity disorder affects more males than females (roughly 3:1) (Szatmari *et al.*, 1989). It is associated with a variety of functional impairments including problems with academic, family and social functioning (Wells, 2004).

The etiology of ADHD is not known but thought to be multifactorial. There is evidence for genetic vulnerabilities to ADHD, but it is also clear that environmental factors (e.g. toxins, prenatal or perinatal insults, family or environmental adversity) can also contribute to the development and/or expression of this illness (Barkley, 1990).

In recent years, in the United States, the prevalence of ADHD appears to have been rising for unclear reasons (Robinson *et al.*, 1999), and significant controversy has arisen regarding rates of diagnosing ADHD and subsequent prescribing practices. For example, datasets from the early 1990s showed a 2.5-fold increase in prescriptions for ADHD (Safer *et al.*, 1996) and in 1996, epidemiological surveys estimated that between 2% and 7% of American children received a prescription for a stimulant in a 1-year period (Angold *et al.*, 2000). While ADHD is recognized in many cultures, these are remarkable differences between countries in the percentage of youth prescribed medication for this condition.

Co-morbidity is common in ADHD and includes oppositional defiant and conduct disorders, mood and anxiety disorders, specific learning disorders, tics disorders, developmental coordination disorders, and substance abuse. Although some studies from the USA have described high rates of overlap between ADHD and bipolar disorder, consensus is not yet reached on the existence and definition of preadolescent mania.

Children with autism often show hyperactive behaviour and apparent inattention, and autistic symptoms are sometimes seen in those with ADHD (Santosh & Mijovic, 2004). Although both ICD-10 and DSM-IV specifically exclude diagnoses of HKD or ADHD in the presence of pervasive developmental disorders, clinically these children sometimes show a partial response to stimulants, and therefore it is desirable to recognize both disorders when they are present.

This chapter is primarily focused on reviewing the current state of knowledge regarding the treatment of ADHD with a particular emphasis on reviewing controlled intervention trials whenever possible. The difficulty with both psychosocial and pharmacological treatments of ADHD is the lack of maintenance of effects once treatment has been discontinued and the failure of generalization to settings in which treatment has not been active. Situations in which symptoms cause the most impairment should be targeted for treatment.

Pharmacotherapy

Introduction

Medication is usually necessary when treating HKD. It is also to be considered if the disorder meets the DSM-IV criteria for the ADHD syndrome or if psychological treatments have been insufficient alone in managing symptoms.

Greater hyperactivity, inattention and clumsiness in the absence of emotional disorder predict greater positive response to methylphenidate (Taylor *et al.*, 1987). However, it has also been shown that overall symptoms in those with less severe ADHD improve more completely. Medication should be initiated with proper monitoring of target symptoms. Patients without hyperactivity (ADD) may benefit from, and tolerate, lower doses of stimulants.

If hyperactivity is present only in one situation, i.e. at school or at home, then stresses in that situation should be sought and alleviated as the first line of management rather than treatment with medication. With school specific problems, specific learning disabilities should be sought carefully through the assessment of a clinical or educational psychologist. If such problems are present, then adjustment of educational techniques and expectations should be given a try before anti-hyperactivity treatments. If hyperactive behaviour is confined to the home situation, then the possibility of adverse parenting influences should be considered and a parent training approach should be considered. In pervasive and severe cases without autistic or affective co-morbidity, a multimodal treatment approach will be needed.

A very brief overview of the various medications in ADHD follows. In this overview we will include:

- First-line medication: methylphenidate (immediate and extended release), dexamphetamine, (immediate release and extended release)
- Second-line medication: atomoxetine, guanfacine, imipramine, nortriptyline, bupropion, pemoline, clonidine

- <u>Third-line medication</u>: carbamazepine, risperidone, buspirone, venlafaxine
- <u>Experimental medication</u>: moclobamide, nicotine patches, cholinergic agents.

First-line agents – stimulants

Pharmacotherapy with psychostimulants is one of the key elements in the treatment of ADHD. The literature on stimulant medications, methylphenidate, dexamphetamine and pemoline is voluminous. In most cases a stimulant is the first choice medication. More is known about the pharmacologic use of stimulants in children than about any other psychotropic medication in this age population. Its onset of action is rapid, dosage is easy to titrate and positive response often can be predicted from a single dose.

Stimulant medications are the most commonly prescribed psychopharmacologic intervention for children and the most extensively studied treatment for ADHD at this time. Modern formulations of stimulant medications can achieve specialized medication effects (e.g. longer duration of action). To date, there is no compelling evidence of one stimulant preparation being more effective than another (McMaster University Evidence-Based Practice Center, 1998).

The evidence base for the use of methylphenidate (MPH) is based on a substantial evidence base over treatment periods of up to 3 years (Jensen et al., 2004). These studies include many short-term studies, meta-analysis (Jadad et al., 1999), and numerous published clinical guidelines both American and European (American Academy of Child and Adolescent Psychiatry, 1997, 2002; National Institute for Health and Clinical Excellence, 2000; Taylor et al., 1998, 2004). Pemoline has been associated with an increased risk of liver toxicity and liver failure. As a result, it has been removed from the US market. Consequently, recommendations for stimulants in this chapter are in regard to methylphenidate and amphetamine preparations only.

Stimulant medications are effective in treating the core symptoms of ADHD (Schachterr et al., 2001; Spencer et al., 1996). Fonagy (2002) notes that more than 100 trials have documented the efficacy of stimulant medications on the primary symptoms of ADHD. Swanson et al. (1993) estimate the effect size of stimulants on attention and behaviour to be approximately 0.8. These benefits have been observed across settings. Stimulant-treated children with ADHD have fewer disruptive behaviours, more sustained attention and increased task persistence in the classroom, improved on-task behaviours in the home and increased

attentiveness during sporting activities (Abikoff & Gittelman, 1984; Barkley, 1977; Carlson et al., 1992; Elia et al., 1991; Milich et al., 1991; Pelham et al., 1991; Richters et al., 1995).

In addition, positive effects from stimulants have been noted on impairments that are thought to be secondarily associated with ADHD and on some co-morbid symptoms as well. Improvements have been described in terms of academic performance, peer relationships, family interactions, compliance with instructions and self-esteem (Abikoff & Gittelman, 1984; Barkley & Cunningham, 1979; Wells et al., 2000; Whalen et al., 1990). Particularly interesting was Schachar et al's (1987) observation that families with children who have a positive stimulant response are more amenable to psychosocial interventions.

Stimulants appear to be helpful for co-morbid externalizing symptoms, including verbal aggression, physical aggression, covert antisocial behaviour and oppositional behaviour (Hinshaw et al., 1992; Klein et al., 1997; McMahon & Wells, 1998; Schachar et al., 1997). The efficacy of stimulant medications in ADHD with other co-morbid conditions is less clear. Conflicting results have been noted with regard to co-morbid internalizing disorders (American Association of Child and Adolescent Psychiatry, 2002; Fonagy, 2002; March et al., 2000; Spencer et al., 1996) and learning disabilities (Fonagy, 2002; Mayes et al., 1994).

While the majority of studies have assessed the response of school-age children with ADHD to stimulant medication, some researchers have considered the effect of stimulants on children of different ages. The AACAP Official Action Practice Parameter of 2002 identified eight published, double-blind, randomized controlled trials of methylphenidate in 241 preschoolers (American Association of Child and Adolescent Psychiatry, 2002). Six of the eight studies showed methylphenidate to be superior to placebo. All of these were short-term medication trials. A higher rate of side effects was described in this population. In 2000, Smith et al. (2000) identified eight controlled trials of stimulant medications in 214 adolescents with ADHD. All studies found a statistically significant improvement with stimulant medications. Positive effects included improvements in the primary symptoms of the disorder in addition to academic and social behaviour.

Despite the multiple positive findings with regard to short-term stimulant treatment, the long-term effects are less clearly understood. Most stimulant trials have been less than three months in duration. Longer-term studies have examined the effects of stimulant medications from 12 to 24 months. These studies demonstrate continued benefit from stimulants over this time frame (American Association of Child and Adolescent Psychiatry, 2002; Gillberg *et al.*, 1997; MTA Cooperative Group, 1999a). Follow-up studies, however, demonstrate only variable benefits in young adulthood to former ADHD clients who had been treated with stimulants in childhood (Weiss & Hechtman, 1993). Possible benefits are described in areas of self-esteem, social skills, fewer car accidents, less aggression and less need for mental health treatment as adults. In contrast, young adults who were former ADHD children show deficits in comparison to non-ADHD controls across several domains regardless of prior stimulant treatment. These deficits include academic, vocational and financial difficulties. Consequently, there is clearly a need for more study regarding the long-term treatment effects of stimulant medication for ADHD.

Precautions and side effects with stimulants

Stimulants are contraindicated in schizophrenia, hyperthyroidism, cardiac arrhythmias, angina pectoris, glaucoma, or a history of hypersensitivity to drug. Stimulants should be used with caution in youth with hypertension, depression, tics (or family history of Tourette's syndrome), pervasive developmental disorders, severe mental retardation, or a history of substance use disorder.

Even effective treatments have side effects, and a cost–benefit (side effects vs. effectiveness) analysis must always be considered. Aside from the hepatic toxicity associated with pemoline, adverse effects from the other stimulant medications are generally mild. Although the stimulants have an extremely high margin of safety, side effects are similar for all stimulants and increase linearly with dose. Often waiting a few weeks or decreasing the dose eliminates or reduces common side effects such as irritability, headaches, abdominal pain and loss of appetite. Mild appetite suppression is almost universal and may be addressed by giving medication after breakfast and lunch, encouraging a high calorie snack after dinner and reducing the dose on weekends and during the summer. Persistent or severe side effects may require changing drugs. Rebound effects consist of increased excitability, activity, talkativeness, irritability and insomnia beginning 4–15 hours after a dose. Rebound may also be seen as the last dose of the day wears off or may be present for up to several days after sudden withdrawal particularly of high daily doses of stimulants. Sleeplessness is a frequent problem and it is clinically important to distinguish those children whose insomnia is an unwanted effect of the drug from those children whose insomnia may be due to the recurrence (or worsening) of the behavioural difficulties as the medication effect subsides. For the first group of children, the addition of clonidine before bedtime, decreasing the afternoon stimulant dose, or moving it to an earlier time may be sufficient. For the latter group, an evening dose of a stimulant may be helpful. Persistent stimulant related dysphoria may decrease with lowering the dose, but may require switching to a different stimulant or to an antidepressant medication. The use of stimulants for patients with tics has been controversial and is discussed later in this chapter. Growth retardation (decrease in expected weight and height gain) resulting from stimulant use is actually small although it may be statistically significant. Although in general there are no adverse cardiovascular effects of stimulants, black male adolescents may be at a higher risk from mild chronic elevation in blood pressure (Brown & Sexson, 1989). Mixed amphetamine salts were recently withdrawn from the Canadian Market in 2005 by the Canadian Drug Regulatory Agency, following their analysis of reports of several deaths of patients treated with this medication. In the United States, there is currently a warning to clinicians to be aware of possible cardiac side effects particularly in the presence of known cardiovascular illnesses. Whether there is any causal link between use of mixed amphetamine salts and cardiac disease, or mortality is unknown. The reported rates of sudden death on this medication do not exceed reported rates of sudden death on other stimulant medications or the base rate of sudden death in unmedicated youth in this age group.

There is little evidence that stimulants produce a clinically significant decrease in the seizure threshold (Crumrine *et al.*, 1987), and methylphenidate can be used in the presence of well-controlled epilepsy. If seizures worsen or emerge during treatment, then the stimulant treatment plan should be reconsidered. Similarly, while stimulant medications can be misused as substances of abuse, there is little evidence that addiction results from the prescription of stimulants for ADHD. It may be better to use long-acting preparations when there are concerns about diversion or abuse of stimulant medications as these not only are relatively safe but also are difficult to abuse because of the delivery system. Atomoxetine and bupropion may also be useful when abuse of the stimulants is suspected. Additionally, post-marketing surveillance has suggested that on rare occasions stimulants can produce aggression, hypertension and psychotic symptoms.

When children are started on stimulants one needs to monitor pulse, BP at each increase and every 6 months. Weight and height should be charted at least every six months and should be monitored using a growth chart.

Tics, depression, irritability, lack of spontaneity, withdrawal and excessive perseveration should be monitored at each visit. Routine haematological tests are unnecessary.

Second-line agents – non-stimulant medication

The leading drug treatment in ADHD remains the use of central sympathomimetic stimulants. Abundant randomized controlled trials have shown the superiority of this approach over placebo (Santosh & Taylor, 2000) and behaviour therapy (MTA Group Cooperative, 1999a). The stimulants' value has been extended by the introduction of extended release preparations. They have, however, attracted strong public controversy and families are sometimes deterred from the treatment by media publicity. Some families encounter adverse effects of the medication and therefore stop it. Some children do not respond at all.

Effective non-stimulant drugs could have advantages. A different mechanism of action could lead to useful effects on subgroups of children or types of problems that are not helped by current treatments. Drugs without abuse potential might prove more acceptable to prescribers and consumers. Several such drugs are in frequent use, although most are not licensed for the purpose. Atomoxetine is the first non-stimulant drug licensed for use in ADHD.

Atomoxetine

Atomoxetine is a selective norepinephrine reuptake inhibitor that was FDA approved for the treatment of attention deficit hyperactivity disorder in November 2002. The plasma half-life is usually about 4 hours; an active metabolite, 4-hydroxyatomoxetine, is excreted in urine after glucuronidation. In 5% to 10% of people, a polymorphism of the cytochrome enzyme P450 2D6 leads to a longer plasma half-life of up to 19 hours.

Four randomized, double-blind, placebo-controlled trials in children and adolescents demonstrating atomoxetine's effectiveness in treating ADHD are available. One study by Michelson et al. (2001), involved 297 children and adolescents randomly assigned to eight weeks of treatment. Atomoxetine was found to be superior to placebo at doses above 1.2 mg/kg per day in parent ratings of ADHD symptoms. There were no teacher ratings or classroom measures used in this study. Two other controlled trials (Spencer et al., 2002) involved 291 children randomly assigned to 12 weeks of treatment, in which atomoxetine was found to be statistically superior to placebo in parent ratings. There were no teacher ratings or classroom observations reported. A fourth study involved 171 children and adolescents randomly assigned to six weeks of treatment (Michelson et al., 2002). This study also used parent ratings as the primary outcome measure but a teacher rating scale was also used. Atomoxetine was noted to be significantly more effective compared to placebo on both the parent and teacher scales. The primary adverse effects noted with atomoxetine are gastrointestinal upset, decreased appetite, fatigue, dizziness and mild increases in pulse and systolic blood pressure.

Given that atomoxetine is a relatively new medication, there is limited data available about its long-term effects or tolerability. A meta-analysis of information from mixed open-label and controlled trials showed sustained positive effects in subsets of children for at least two years (Kratochvil et al., 2006 and Wilens et al., 2006). There is also little information available comparing atomoxetine directly to established ADHD treatments, although recent unpublished data suggests that atomoxetine is less effective than stimulant medications. Atomoxetine was not available when the 1997 AACAP Practice Parameters were published. At the present time, however, atomoxetine is widely regarded as a promising second-line treatment for ADHD.

Despite its relatively short half life, atomoxetine can be used as either a once daily or twice daily dose and is generally quite safe. It produces minimal increase in BP, heart rate and gastrointestinal symptoms (nausea and vomiting is possible especially during the early part of treatment). It may be useful in those with co-morbid tics, anxiety/depression, or in those who have not responded to stimulants but there are no clear studies to prove this as yet. Symptoms take about 6 weeks to improve with atomoxetine (unlike stimulants), and hence parents have to be informed about this at the start of treatment. Dosage can be initiated at half the required total dose in order to decrease the chances of side effects (especially upper GI effects). There have been reports of rare, but serious, hepatic side effects in patients treated with atomoxetine. The clinical emergence of symptoms of hepatic disorder in patients treated with atomoxetine should result in the withdrawal of this medication and appropriate laboratory assessment.

Tricyclic antidepressants

Antidepressants have been in use for many years. The antidepressants that work in ADHD increase available levels of catecholamines, typically noradrenaline. Although far less studied than stimulants, controlled trials of tricyclic antidepressants in both children and adolescents demonstrate efficacy in the treatment of ADHD (Popper, 1995; Spencer et al., 1996). Tricyclic antidepressants include amitriptyline, desipramine, nortriptyline, imipramine and clomipramine. Historically, they have been the most common second-line pharmacologic treatment for attention deficit hyperactivity disorder following stimulant medications. Desipramine and imipramine have been the most studied among this family of drugs in the treatment of ADHD. It should be noted, however, that tricyclic antidepressants have not been FDA approved for the treatment of attention deficit hyperactivity disorder.

Eighteen controlled trials of tricyclic antidepressants in 310 children and 26 adults with ADHD were identified by Spencer et al. (1996). The majority of trials were short-term (weeks to months). Spencer reports that robust responses were identified in twelve of the controlled trials, moderate responses were identified in five controlled trials and a mixed response was found in one trial. Spencer reports that behavioural symptoms were the most responsive to tricyclic antidepressant treatment based on ratings from clinicians, teachers and parents. Based on data from six of eight controlled trials, Connor et al. (1999) calculated an effect size of 0.44 for tricyclic antidepressants, correlating to moderate improvement. Two controlled trials of tricyclic antidepressants that included ADHD preschoolers showed moderate to robust responses (Spencer et al., 1996). Three controlled trials included adolescents with ADHD and also reported improvement (Spencer et al., 1996).

While tricyclic antidepressants have been noted to demonstrate significant improvement in ADHD symptoms, their use has declined in recent years due to concerns of cardiac arrhythmias and case reports of sudden death in the paediatric population. Drawbacks include potential cardiotoxicity, especially in pre-pubertal children, the danger of accidental or intentional overdose, troublesome sedation, anti-cholinergic side effects, lowering seizure threshold and possibly declining efficacy over time. Parents must be reminded to supervise administration of medication and to keep pills in a safe place. When tricyclic antidepressants are used in the paediatric population, cardiac monitoring at baseline and throughout the course of treatment is essential. This monitoring would include evaluation of vital signs and electrocardiograms. Tricyclic antidepressants are also associated with several side effects that can complicate treatment, including dry mouth, blurred vision, sedation and constipation (Green, 2001). Thus, while tricyclic antidepressants may still have a role in treating ADHD, other agents are often tried first because they offer a more attractive benefit-to-risk profile.

Bupropion

Bupropion is also commonly used as a second-line treatment for ADHD. Adverse effects related to bupropion are generally mild and include sedation, nausea, decreased appetite and dizziness. One serious side effect is that bupropion does lower the seizure threshold and is contra-indicated in patients with a known seizure disorder, eating disorder or at substantial risk for seizures for other reasons. Bupropion has not been FDA approved for any paediatric indication.

Bupropion has been studied in the treatment of paediatric ADHD in two small placebo-controlled trials (Casat et al., 1989; Clay et al., 1988), one larger placebo-controlled four-centre multisite trial (Conners et al., 1996) and one small double-blind crossover study with respect to methylphenidate (Barrickman et al., 1995). For all three placebo controlled trials, bupropion demonstrated significant effects in decreasing ADHD symptoms. Barrickman reported that both bupropion and methylphenidate produced significant improvements in ADHD symptoms and similar effects were described for the two treatments in this small study.

While only these few short-term studies currently document bupropion's effectiveness in treating ADHD, it is a relatively attractive second-line treatment for those who are not at significant risk for seizures given its otherwise relatively benign side effect profile.

Alpha-agonists

Clonidine and guanfacine are central acting alpha-2-adrenergic agonists commonly used in the treatment of paediatric attention deficit hyperactivity disorder. Side effects frequently noted with these medications include sedation, hypotension, tachycardia, dizziness and rash from the transdermal clonidine patch. Neither medication has any FDA approved psychiatric indication. The 1997 AACAP Practice Parameters describe a primarily adjunctive role for alpha agonists in the treatment of ADHD, after more established treatments have been tried (AACAP, 1997).

Connor et al. (1999) did a meta-analysis summarizing the literature with regard to clonidine in the treatment of ADHD (20). Ten studies were identified with some methodologic control involving clonidine in the treatment of ADHD. Several of these studies involved patients with ADHD and a comorbid psychiatric illness (conduct disorder, developmental disorder or tic disorder). Positive effects were reported on ADHD symptoms from all of these studies across parent, teacher and clinician raters. The effect size on ADHD symptoms was 0.58, which correlates to a moderately positive clinical effect.

Pulse and blood pressure should be monitored for bradycardia and hypotension. When discontinuing clonidine, the dose should be tapered rather than stopped suddenly to avoid rebound hypertension. Erratic compliance with medication increases the risk of adverse cardiovascular events. Families should be cautioned about this, and clonidine should not be prescribed if it cannot be administered reliably. Depression and impairment of glucose tolerance can also occur.

Scahill *et al.* (2000) conducted a double-blind, placebo controlled trial of guanfacine in children with ADHD and tic disorders. This study found a significant improvement in teacher ratings of ADHD symptoms and a decrease in tics in the children treated with guanfacine.

Prescribers in clinical practice have commonly combined stimulants and alpha-agonists in the hopes of optimizing ADHD treatment and minimizing side effects. There were case reports of sudden deaths noted in the mid-1990s with regards to this medication combination but no link has been established. Nevertheless, systematic studies of this medication combination are needed. Consequently, while alpha-agonists have become a common pharmacologic intervention for children with ADHD, caution should be used given the limited information available to date regarding their use in this population.

Other pharmacologic interventions

Antipsychotics

Spencer *et al.* (1996) identified 12 controlled trials of antipsychotics in 242 children and adolescents with ADHD. They noted that eight of these studies described moderate or robust improvements, whereas one study found mixed results and three studies reported poor rates of improvement. Gittelman-Klein (1980) reported that no more than 50% of patients with ADHD improve with antipsychotics. Although haloperidol and chlorpromazine do have FDA approval for the treatment of severe behavioural disorders in childhood, traditional antipsychotics can cause serious adverse effects including neuroleptic malignant syndrome and tardive dyskinesias. These medications should be reserved for only the most extreme and treatment-refractory cases.

Other antidepressants

Both fluoxetine and venlafaxine have been tried in open studies with ADHD. Neither medication is FDA approved for this disorder. Since very limited information exists in children with ADHD and because of the recent suggestions of increased suicidal ideation in depressed children treated with these agents, they are not recommended in children.

Carbamazepine

Silva *et al.* (1996) conducted a meta-analysis of carbamazepine use in children with ADHD. They described three double-blind trials involving 53 patients. They report that 71% of those treated with carbamazepine showed a significant improvement compared to 26% of those taking placebo. They calculated an effect size of 1.01 based on these studies.

Carbamazepine is not FDA approved for the treatment of ADHD. Carbamazepine has several significant potential side effects leukopenia, thrombocytopenia, anaemia and hepatic toxicity. Consequently, regular serum monitoring of haematologic and hepatic function is recommended. Due to the potential risks and limited data available, carbamazepine is generally used only in children who have ADHD that has not responded to standard treatments and who have a co-morbid seizure disorder or significant brain damage.

Other medications

Buspirone is a full 5HT1 A agonist at the somatodendritic auto-receptor and a partial agonist at the post-synaptic 5HT1 A receptors. Buspirone acts on the noradrenergic, serotonergic and dopaminergic receptor systems. An open clinical trial has suggested that it can help to improve hyperactivity, impulsivity and oppositionality (Malhotra & Santosh, 1998).

Acetylcholinesterase inhibitors, such as donepezil, have been suggested especially for the treatment of residual cognitive problems in people who have benefited from other drugs on the basis of small-scale open trials (Wilens *et al.*, 2002). Other drugs used in practice include moclobamide and nicotine receptor agonists. A controlled trial of lithium found it to be ineffective in the treatment of ADHD (Greenhill *et al.*, 1973).

Combination of a stimulant and non-stimulant

The problems presented by severe hyperactivity can be very severe and families may become desperate. Clinicians often feel pressed to prescribe unduly high dosages (for which there is no evidence of value) and combinations of drugs, sometimes to target different aspects of the symptom complex. This can be justifiable in extreme cases, but the concurrent use of inadequately evaluated drugs can create hazards and call for specialist advice and careful monitoring. The most common combination currently used for ADHD is a stimulant and clonidine, although there are no published trials of safety or efficacy for this combination. The combination is theoretically appealing due to complementary actions and non-overlapping side effect profiles. Anecdotal clinical experience supports the usefulness of these two drugs especially for children with severe ADHD who cannot be managed satisfactorily with stimulant alone. However, there have been reports of unexplained deaths in three children who at one time had been taking both methylphenidate and clonidine, but the evidence linking the drugs to the deaths is tenuous at best (Fenichel, 1995; Popper, 1995; Swanson *et al.*, 1995). Pending clarification, extra caution is advised when treating children with

cardiac or cardiovascular disease. When combining clonidine with additional medications or if dosing of medication is inconsistent (Swanson *et al.*, 1995), an alternative
strategy might be to substitute dexamphetamine for
methylphenidate or guanfacine for clonidine.

The combination of imipramine and methylphenidate
has been associated with a syndrome of confusion, affective lability, marked aggression and severe agitation (Grob
& Coyle, 1986). The combination of imipramine and
methylphenidate can increase plasma levels of imipramine. As blood levels of desipramine can increase unpre-
dictably with methylphenidate, blood levels may be
necessary for monitoring, if this combination is used.

Developmental trajectory and medication response

- **ADHD in preschoolers**: Behavioural interventions such
  as parent training approaches are useful. Stimulants are
  probably less effective than in school-going children
  and produce greater side effects (Kratochvil *et al.*, 2004).
- **ADHD in school-going children**: Medication is superior
  to behavioural interventions in this age group. Behavioural
  interventions are essential when treating co-morbidity in
  ADHD.
- **ADHD in adolescence**: Non-compliance with medication is a greater problem in treatment of adolescents
  due to their desire to avoid taking medication during
  school hours and the increased prevalence of stimulant
  related dysphoria. The risk of misuse of stimulants is
  increased in adolescents. Giving or selling medication
  to peers is more common than abuse by the patient
  themselves. The drug interactions that could result
  from undisclosed substance misuse should always be
  bourne in mind. Extended release stimulant preparations or atomoxetine are good options in this group.
  Adolescents with ADHD demonstrated significantly
  less variability and better driving performance in one
  study when receiving an extended release preparation
  compared to dosing a short-acting stimulant three
  times daily (Cox *et al.*, 2004).
- **ADHD in adults**: It is difficult to develop clinical skills in
  the management of residual adult manifestations of
  developmental disorders without clinical experience
  with their presentation in childhood. Adult patients
  are increasingly seeking treatment for the symptoms of
  ADHD, and physicians need practice guidelines. Adult
  ADHD often presents differently from childhood ADHD.
  Because adult ADHD can be co-morbid with other disorders and has symptoms similar to those of other
  disorders, it is important to consider the differential
  diagnoses. Physicians should work with patients to provide feedback about their symptoms, to educate them

about ADHD, and to set treatment goals. Treatment for
ADHD in adults should include a medication trial,
restructuring of the patient's environment to make it
more compatible with the symptoms of ADHD, and
ongoing supportive management to address any residual
impairment and to facilitate functional and developmental improvements (Weiss & Weiss, 2004). Atomoxetine is
licensed to be used in adults. Both stimulants and atomoxetine are effective in adults but the effect size is
marginally lower than in children.

Pharmacological management of HKD in Europe
The importance of treating hyperactivity is established. A
variety of different clinical traditions have evolved within
Europe. In some countries, notably Britain and France,
there has been widespread public hostility to the use of
psychotropic medication for this purpose. European
guidelines exist for managing hyperkinetic disorder
(Taylor *et al.*, 1998, 2004). Indeed, much of the persisting
controversy seems to arise over one question: the extent to
which a narrower definition of hyperkinetic disorder or a
broader definition of attention deficit/hyperactivity disorder (AD/HD) should guide clinical practice. There is little
doubt that children with the severe form of disorder
termed 'hyperkinetic disorder' in ICD-10 (see below)
should receive specific treatment. The recent re-analyses
of the Multimodal Treatment Study of Children with
ADHD (MTA study) shows that HKD is more stimulant
responsive than ADHD, and less responsive to behavioural
interventions alone (Santosh *et al.*, 2005). Co-morbid conditions such as conduct disorder, anxiety and depressive
disorders appear to benefit from combined treatment with
stimulants and behavioural treatment (Santosh *et al.*, 2005).

Psychosocial interventions

Despite medication remaining the mainstay of treatment,
other adjunctive treatments may be necessary to optimise
outcomes. Training of social competence may be important especially in those who have poor social skills.
Individual psychotherapy may be helpful in managing
low self-esteem and family support. Psychoeducation,
and respite care may also be useful. Remedial education
may also help some patients. Appropriate psychosocial
interventions for co-morbid conditions are essential.

Behaviour therapy and cognitive-behavioural therapy

Behaviour therapy is commonly used to address both the
primary symptoms of ADHD and the associated functional

impairments in daily life. The overall goal is to prevent and discourage maladaptive behaviours while rewarding and eliciting positive behaviours. In children, behaviour therapy typically involves the assessment of an individual child's particular deficits and the typical contexts and outcomes of the problematic behaviour. The behaviour therapy then, to promote alternative behaviours in the child, develops alternative contexts and outcomes. Behaviour therapy frequently applies the principles of learning theory, including the use of contingency management to influence child behaviour. Cognitive-behavioural therapy (CBT) combines these elements of behaviour therapy with cognitive therapy techniques such as self-monitoring and problem-solving. Behaviour therapy and CBT can be applied in various settings including home and/or school. Behaviour therapy has been shown to improve the classroom behaviour of ADHD children in the short-term relative to control settings without behaviour modification interventions (Carlson et al., 1992).

The 1997 AACAP Practice Parameters note, however, that while behaviour therapy does appear to be effective, the effects do not appear to be sustained after the treatment is discontinued, and the effects do not appear to generalize beyond the situation where the treatment is implemented (American Academy of Child and Adolescent Psychiatry, 1997). Studies that have directly compared behaviour therapy alone to stimulant medication alone show that behaviour therapy is generally not as effective as stimulant medication (Carlson et al., 1992). Cognitive-behavioural therapy has had mixed results in studies with ADHD children. Hinshaw et al. (1984), for example, found that children who participated in CBT as part of a summer programme demonstrated more successful coping with provocative social situations compared to peers who did not receive the CBT intervention. Subsequent studies, however, have raised concerns that CBT does not appear to offer benefits beyond the behavioural component alone. CBT appears to share the same disadvantages as behaviour therapy with regard to generalization to new settings and with regard to efficacy relative to stimulant medication.

Social skills training

Social skills training has been utilized in various formats trying to address the social skill deficits commonly associated with ADHD. This form of treatment typically uses cognitive and behavioural strategies to address these skill deficits. Social learning theory is also frequently used through modelling. Social skills training has been offered both individually and in groups to children with ADHD.

While limited information exists about the efficacy of social skills training, it appears that social skills training is typically most effective in group settings where peer interactions allow skill building most naturally.

Parent training

Parent training typically offers psychoeducation and training in the principles of learning theory to the parents of children with ADHD in order to promote positive behaviour and minimize negative behaviour in their children. Social learning theory may also be incorporated into the treatment by modelling from the therapist. Controlled studies of parent training interventions show improved functioning in both ADHD children and their parents, including improved compliance and more rapid task completion in ADHD children, decreased symptom ratings by parents and decreased parent stress with improved parental self-esteem (Anastopoulos et al., 1993; Pisterman et al., 1989). Similar interventions can be offered to teachers in order to expand the benefits into the school setting.

Family therapy

Structural family therapy focuses on altering common maladaptive patterns of communication and functioning within families. While family therapy is often provided to ADHD families, there is limited efficacy data available. Barkley et al. (1992) compared structural family therapy to behaviour therapy and to problem-solving and communication training in a randomized trial with 61 adolescents with ADHD. All three interventions demonstrated significant decreases in negative communications, decreases in family conflicts and improvements in school adjustment. No significant differences in outcome were noted between the three treatment groups. In all treatment groups, less than 30% of the group showed significant improvement and less than 20% recovered.

Combined treatments

Multimodal treatment is very common with ADHD. Medications are commonly combined with behaviour therapy and/or parent training interventions. Several randomized studies have attempted to evaluate the benefits of combining these treatment interventions.

Klein et al. (1997) studied 89 children with ADHD randomized to either methylphenidate alone, behaviour therapy with parent training, teacher consultation and a placebo or a combination treatment that included both methylphenidate and psychotherapeutic interventions. Klein's data showed that while some teacher ratings were improved with combination treatment, no significant benefit was noted on clinician or parent ratings with combination treatment compared to medication alone. Horn *et al.* (1991) studied 117 children with ADHD randomized to low-dose stimulant medication alone, high-dose stimulant medication alone and each stimulant medication dose combined with parent training and child self-control training. While adding the psychotherapy did not offer additional benefit compared to the stimulant medication alone, it appeared that the combination of low-dose stimulant medication with the psychotherapeutic interventions resulted in the same outcome as high-dose stimulant medication alone.

The MTA Cooperative Group, funded by the National Institute of Mental Health, conducted a study of 539 children with ADHD comparing medication interventions alone, intensive psychotherapeutic interventions alone (parent training, behaviour therapy, teacher consultation and school-based interventions), the combination of medication and intensive psychotherapeutic interventions and a control group receiving treatment-as-usual in the community (MTA, 1999a). While the combined intervention was significantly better compared to the psychotherapeutic interventions alone at addressing parent and teacher ratings of core symptoms, parent ratings of oppositional behaviour, internalizing symptoms and reading achievement, the combined treatment did not demonstrate significant benefits compared to medication intervention alone. However, the children in the combined treatment group required 20% less medication than the medication treatment only group. Subsequent data analysis also

suggested a trend for children with co-morbid anxiety disorders to respond better to combined treatment compared to medication-only treatment (MTA, 1999b).

Duration of treatment

Treatment trial evidence shows continued benefits of treatment for periods up to 36 months. Discontinuation trial evidence shows that many children can ultimately discontinue their medications without symptom recurrence. Adult trial evidence shows continued efficacy of treatment into adulthood. It is recommended that a trial of treatment discontinuation be undertaken every 12 months. Nevertheless, long-term treatment may be necessary in a subgroup of subjects.

Conclusions

Attention-deficit hyperactivity disorder is a common condition affecting children and adolescents that causes significant morbidity. It is a treatable condition with an extensive body of research available regarding treatment interventions. There are clear limitations, however in the current state of knowledge. Currently, more research is needed in long-term treatment outcomes, non-stimulant pharmacologic interventions, non-pharmacologic interventions, combined pharmacologic interventions and multimodal interventions.

The level of evidence for each of the interventions discussed in this chapter is summarized in Table 53.1.

Table 53.1. Effectiveness of treatments for ADHD and hyperkinetic disorder

Treatment	Form of treatment	Psychiatric disorder/ target audience	Level of evidence for efficacy	Comments
Psychopharmacology	Stimulants: Methyphenidate, amphetamine salts	ADHD, HKD	Ia	Multiple trials support their use as effective in not only core symptoms of ADHD (increased attention, decreased disruptive behaviours across many settings) and some secondary symptoms as well (academic performance, peer and family interactions). They appear to work across age groups and not only with children. Most studies have been short term
Psychopharmacology	Non-stimulant: Atomoxetine	ADHD, HKD	Ia	Found to be significantly more effective in parent and teacher ratings for core symptoms of ADHD than placebo
Psychopharmacology	Non-stimulant: tricyclic antidepresaants	ADHD, HKD	Ia	Moderate effectiveness especially with respect to behavioural symptoms. Stimulants overall are more effective

Table 53.1. (cont.)

Treatment	Form of treatment	Psychiatric disorder/ target audience	Level of evidence for efficacy	Comments
Psychopharmacology	Non-stimulant: Bupropion	ADHD, HKD	Ib	Appears to be an effective second-line treatment
Psychopharmacology	Non-stimulant: Clonidine	ADHD, HKD	Ib	Effect size of 0.58 (moderately effective treatment)
Psychopharmacology	Non-stimulant: guanfacine	ADHD, HKD	IIa	Studied with children with ADHD and tics. Improvement in both
Psychopharmacology	Non-stimulant: antipsychotics	ADHD, HKD	IIa	Are effective in about 50% of the cases but because of side effects, should only be used in the most treatment resistant cases
Psychopharmacology	Non-stimulant: carbamazepine	ADHD, HKD	IIa	Are effective in about 3/4s of the cases but because of side effects, should only be used in the most treatment resistant cases
Psychosocial intervention	Behaviour therapy	ADHD, HKD	IIa	Appears effective but not as effective as psychopharmacological interventions. Results do not appear to be generalizable from the specific studied behaviour. Results do not sustain themselves after termination of treatment
Psychosocial intervention	Behaviour therapy	ADHD, HKD	IIb	Questions raised as to whether adding a cognitive component add anything to the effectiveness of the behavioural approach alone
Psychosocial intervention	Social skills training	ADHD, HKD	IV	If it works, works best in a group setting
Psychosocial intervention	Parent training	ADHD, HKD	IIa	Improved functioning in both parents and children
Psychosocial intervention	Family therapy	ADHD, HKD	IIb	Appears to decrease negative communication and family conflicts and improves school performance. Effective in about 30%

REFERENCES

AACAP Official Action (1997). Practice Parameters for the Assessment and Treatment of Children, Adolescents, and Adults with Attention-Deficit/Hyperactivity Disorder. *Journal of the American Academy of Child and Adolescent Psychiatry*, **36** (10) Suppl., 85S–121S.

AACAP Official Action (2002). Practice Parameter for the Use of Stimulant Medications in the Treatment of Children, Adolescents and Adults. *Journal of the American Academy of Child and Adolescent Psychiatry*, **41**(2) Suppl., 26S–49S.

Abikoff, H. & Gittelman, R. (1984). Does behaviour therapy normalize the classrrom behaviour of hyperactive children? *Archives of General Psychiatry*, **41**, 449–54.

Anastopoulos, A. D., Shelton, T. L., DuPaul, G. J. & Guevremont, D. C. (1993). Parent training for attention-deficit hyperactivity disorder: Its impact on parent functioning. *Journal of Abnormal Child Psychology*, **21**, 581–95.

Angold, A., Erkanli, A., Egger, H. L. & Costello, E. J. (2000). Stimulant treatment for children: a community perspective. *Journal of the American Academy of Child and Adolescent Psychiatry*, **39**, 975–94.

Barkley, R. A. (1977). A review of stimulant drug research with hyperactive children. *Journal of Child Psychology and Psychiatry*, **18**, 137–65.

Barkley, R. A. (1990). *Attention-deficit Hyperactivity Disorder: A Handbook for Diagnosis and Treatment.* New York: Guilford Press.

Barkley, R. A. (1998). *Attention Deficit Hyperactivity Disorder: A Handbook for Diagnosis and Treatment*, 2nd edn. New York: Guilford Press.

Barkley, R. A. & Cunningham, C. E. (1979). The effects of methylphenidate on the mother–child interactions of hyperactive children. *Archives of General Psychiatry*, **36**, 201–8.

Barkley, R. A., Guevremont, D. C., Anastopoulos, A. D. & Fletcher, K. E. (1992). A comparison of three family therapy programs for treating family conflicts in adolescents with attention-deficit hyperactivity disorder. *Journal of Consulting and Clinical Psychology*, **60**(3), 450–62.

Barrickman, L. L., Perry, P. J., Allen, A. J. *et al.* (1995). Bupropion versus methylphenidate in the treatment of attention deficit/hyperactivity disorder. *Journal of the American Academy of Child and Adolescent Psychiatry*, **34**, 649–57.

Biederman, J., Newcorn, J. & Sprich, S. (1991). Comorbidity of attention deficit hyperactivity disorder with conduct, depressive, anxiety and other disorders. *American Journal of Psychiatry*, **148**, 564–77.

Brown, R. T. & Sexson, S. B. (1989). Effects of methylphenidate on cardiovascular responses in attention deficit hyperactivity disordered adolescents. *Journal of Adolescent Health Care*, **10**, 179–83.

Carlson, C. L., Pelham, W. E., Milich, R. & Dixon, J. (1992). Single and combined effects of methylphenidate and behaviour therapy on the classroom performance of children with attention-deficit hyperactivity disorder. *Journal of Abnormal Child Psychology*, **20**, 213–32.

Casat, C. D., Pleasants, D. Z., Schroeder, D. H. & Parler, D. W. (1989). Bupropion in children with attention deficit disorder. *Psychopharmacology Bulletin*, **25**, 198–201.

Clay, T. H., Gualtieri, C. T., Evans, R. W. & Guillion, C. M. (1988). Clinical and neuropsychological effects of the novel antidepressant bupropion. *Psychopharmacology Bulletin*, **24**, 143–8.

Conners, K., Casat, C. D., Gualtieri, C. *et al.* (1996). Bupropion hydrochloride in attention deficit disorder with hyperactivity. *Journal of the American Academy of Child and Adolescent Psychiatry*, **35**, 1314.

Connor, D. F., Fletcher, K. E. & Swanson, J. M. (1999). A meta-analysis of Clonidine for symptoms of attention-deficit hyperactivity disorder. *Journal of the American Academy of Child and Adolescent Psychiatry*, **38**, 151–9.

Cox, D. J., Merkel, R. L., Penberthy, J. K., Kovatchev, B. & Hankin, C. S. (2004). Impact of methylphenidate delivery profiles on driving performance of adolescents with attention-deficit/hyperactivity disorder: a pilot study. *Journal of the American Academy of and Child Adolescent Psychiatry*, **43**(3), 269–75.

Crumrine, P. K., Feldman, H. M., Teodori, J., Handen, B. L. & Alvin, R. M. (1987). The use of methylphenidate in children with seizures and attention deficit disorder. *Annals of Neurology*, **22**, 441–2.

Elia, J., Borcherding, B. G., Rapoport, J. L. & Keysor, C. S. (1991). Methylphenidate and dextroamphetamine treatments of hyperactivity: are there true nonresponders? *Psychiatry Research*, **36**, 141–55.

Fenichel, R. R. (1995). Combining methylphenidate and clonidine: the role of post-marketing surveillance. *Journal of Child and Adolescent Psychopharmacology*, **5**, 155–6.

Fonagy, P. (2002). Attention-deficit/hyperactivity disorder. In *What Works for Whom? A Critical Review of Treatments for Children and Adolescents*, ed. P. Fonagy, M. Target, D. Cottrell, J. Phillips & Z. Kurtz.

Gillberg, C., Melander, II., con Knorring, A. L. *et al.* (1997). Long term stimulant treatment of children with attention-deficit hyperactivity disorder symptoms. *Archives of General Psychiatry*, **54**, 857–64.

Gittelman-Klein, R. (1980). Diagnosis and drug treatment of childhood disorders: attention deficit disorder with hyperactivity. In *Diagnosis and Drug Treatment of Psychiatric Disorders: Adults and Children*, ed. D. F. Klein, R. Gittelman-Klein, F. Quitkin & A. Rifkin. Baltimore: Williams & Wilkins.

Green, W. H. (2001). *Child and Adolescent Clinical Psychopharmacology*, 3rd edn. Philiadelphia: Lippincott Williams and Wilkins.

Greenhill, L. L., Rieder, R. O., Wender, P. H., Bushsbaum, M. & Zahn, T. P. (1973). Lithium carbonate in the treatment of hyperactive children. *Archives of General Psychiatry*, **28**, 636–40.

Grob, C. S. & Coyle, J. T. (1986). Suspected adverse methylphenidate-imipramine interactions in children. *Journal of Developmental and behavioural Pediatrics*, **7**(4), 265–7.

Hinshaw, S. P., Henker, B. & Whalen, C. K. (1984). Cognitive-behavioural and pharmacologic interventions for hyperactive boys: comparative and combined effects. *Journal of Consulting and Clinical Psychology*, **52**, 739–49.

Hinshaw, S. P., Heller, T. & McHale, J. P. (1992). Covert antisocial behaviour in boys with attention-deficit hyperactivity disorder: External validation and effects of methylphenidate. *Journal of Consulting and Clinical Psychology*, **60**, 274–81.

Horn, W. F., Ialongo, N. S., Pascoe, J. M. *et al.* (1991). Additive effects of psychostimulants, parent training, and self-control therapy with ADHD children. *Journal of the American Academy of Child and Adolescent Psychiatry*, **30**, 233–40.

Jadad, A. R., Booker, L., Gauld, M. *et al.* (1999). The treatment of attention-deficit hyperactivity disorder: an annotated bibliography and critical appraisal of published systematic reviews and metaanalyses. *Canadian Journal of Psychiatry*, **44**(10), 1025–35.

Jensen, P. S., Eaton Hoagwood, K., Roper, M. *et al.* (2004). The services for children and adolescents–parent interview: development and performance characteristics. *Journal of the American Academy of Child and Adolescent Psychiatry*, **43**(11), 1334–44.

Klein, R. G., Abikoff, H., Klass, E., Ganeles, D., Seese, L. M. & Pollack, S. (1997). Clinical efficacy of methylphenidate in conduct disorder with and without attention deficit hyperactivity disorder. *Archives of General Psychiatry*, **54**, 1073–9.

Kratochvil, C. J., Wilens, T. E., Greenhill, L. L. *et al.* (2006). Effects of long-term atomoxetine treatment for young children with attention-deficit/hyperactivity disorder. *Journal of the American Academy of Child and Adolescent Psychiatry*, **45**(8), 919–27.

Kratochvil, C. J., Greenhill, L. L., March, J. S., Burke, W. J. & Vaughan, B. S. (2004). The role of stimulants in the treatment of preschool children with attention-deficit hyperactivity disorder. *CNS Drugs*, **18**(14), 957–66.

Malhotra, S. & Santosh, P. J. (1998). An open clinical trial of buspirone in children with attention-deficit/hyperactivity disorder. *Journal of the American Academy of Child and Adolescent Psychiatry*, **37**(1), 61 71.

March, J. S., Swanson, J. M., Arnold, L. E. *et al.* (2000). Anxiety as a predictor and outcome variable in the multimodal treatment study of children with ADHD (MTA). *Journal of Abnormal Child Psychology*, **28**, 527–41.

Mayes, S., Crites, D., Bixler, E., Humphrey, F. & Mattison, R. (1994). Methylphenidate and ADHD: Influence of age, IQ, neurodevelopmental stutus. *Developmental Medicine and Child Neurology*, **36**, 1099–107.

McMahon, R. J. & Wells, K. C. (1998). Conduct problems. In *Treatment of Childhood Disorders*, 2nd edn, ed. E. J. Mash & R. A. Barkley. New York: Guilford Press.

McMaster University Evidence-Based Practice Center (1998). *The Treatment of Attention-Deficit/Hyperactivity Disorder: An Evidence Report* (Contract 290-97-0017). Washington, DC: Agency for Health Care Policy and Research.

Michelson, D., Faries, D., Wernicke, J. *et al.* (2001). Atomoxetine in the treatment of children and adolescents with attention-deficit/hyperactivity disorder: a randomized, placebo-controlled, dose-response study. *Pediatrics*, **108**(5), e83.

Michelson, D., Allen, A. J., Busner, J. *et al.* (2002). Once-daily atomoxetine treatment for children and adolescents with attention deficit hyperacivity disorder: a randomized, placebo-controlled study. *American Journal of Psychiatry*, **159**, 1896–901.

Milich, R., Carlson, C. L., Pelham, W. E. & Licht, B. G. (1991). Effects of methylphenidate on the persistence of ADHD boys following failure experiences. *Journal of Abnormal Child Psychology*, **19**, 519–36.

MTA Cooperative Group (1999a). Moderators and mediators of treatment response for children with attention-deficit/hyperactivity disorder. *Archives of General Psychiatry*, **56**, 1088–96.

MTA Cooperative Group (1999b). A 14-month randomized clinical trial of treatment strategies for attention deficit hyperactivity disorder. *Archives of General Psychiatry*, **56**, 1073–85.

National Institute for Health and Clinical Excellence (2000). Guidance on the use of methylphenidate for ADHD. http://www.nice.org.uk/pdf/Methylph-guidance13.pdf.

Pelham, W. E., Vodde-Hamilton, M., Murphy, D. A., Greenstein, J. & Vallano, G. (1991). The effects of methylphenidate on ADHD adolescents in recreational, peer group and classroom settings. *Journal of Clinical Child Psychologist*, **20**, 293–300.

Pisterman, S., McGrath, P., Firestone, P., Goodman, J. T., Webster, I. & Mallory, R. (1989). Outcome of parent-mediated treatment of preschoolers with attention deficit disorder with hyperactivity. *Journal of Consulting and Clinical Psychology*, **57**, 628–35.

Popper, C. W. (1995). Combining methylphenidate and clonidine: pharmacologic questions and news reports about sudden death. *Journal of Child and Adolescent Psychopharmacology*, **5**, 157–66.

Richters, J. E., Arnold, L. E., Jensen, P. S. *et al.* (1995). NIMH Collaborative Multisite Multimodal Treatment Study of Children with ADHD: Background and rationale. *Journal of the American Academy of Child and Adolescent Psychiatry*, **34**, 987–1000.

Robinson, L. M., Sclar, D. A., Skaer, T. L. & Galin, R. S. (1999). National trends in the prevalence of attention-deficit/hyperactivity disorder and the prescribing of methylphenidate among school-age children: 1990–1995. *Clinical Pediatrics*, **38**, 209–17.

Rohde, L. A., Barbosa, G., Polanczyk, G. *et al.* (2001). Factor and latent class analysis of DSM-IV ADHD symptoms in a school sample of Brazilian adolescents. *Journal of the American Academy of Child and Adolescent Psychiatry*, **40**(6), 711–18.

Safer, D. J., Zito, J. M. & Fine, E. M. (1996). Increased methylphenidate usage for attention deficit disorder in the 1990s. *Pediatrics*, **98**, 184.

Santosh, P. J. & Mijovic, A. (2004). Social impairment in Hyperkinetic Disorder – relationship to psychopathology and environmental stressors. *European Child and Adolescent Psychiatry*, **13**(3), 141–50.

Santosh, P. J. & Taylor, E. (2000). Stimulant drugs. *European Child and Adolescent Psychiatry*, **9** (Suppl. 1), 127–43.

Scahill, L., Chappell, P. B., Kim, Y. S. *et al.* (2000). Guanfacine in the treatment of children with tic disorders and ADHD: a placebo-controlled study. (Abstract, 40th Annual NCCDEU meeting.) *Journal of Child and Adolescent Psychopharmacology*, **10**, 250.

Schachar, R. J., Taylor, E., Wieselberg, M., Thorley, G. & Rutter, M. (1987). Changes in family function and relationships in children who respond to methylphenidate. *Journal of the American Academy of Child and Adolescent Psychiatry*, **26**, 728–32.

Schachar, R., Tannock, R., Cunningham, C. & Corkum, P. (1997). Behavioural, situational, and temporal effects of treatment of ADHD with methylphenidate. *Journal of the American Academy of Child and Adolescent Psychiatry*, **36**, 754–63.

Schachter, H. M., Pham, B., King, J., Langford, S. & Moher, D. (2001). How efficacious and safe is short-acting methylphenidate for the treatment of attention-deficit disorder in children and adolescents? A meta-analysis. *Canadian Medical Association Journal*, **165**(11), 1475–88.

Silva, R. R., Dinohra, M. D., Munoz, M. D. & Alpert, M. (1996). Carbamazepine use in children and adolescents with features of attention-deficit hyperactivity disorder: a meta-analysis. *Journal of the American Academy of Child and Adolescent Psychiatry*, **35**, 352–8.

Smith, B. H., Waschbusch, D. A., Willoughby, M. T. & Evans, S. (2000). The efficacy, safety, and practicality of treatments for adolescents with attention-deficit/hyperactivity disorder (ADHD). *Clinical Child and Family Psychology Review*, **3**(4), 243–67.

Spencer, T., Biederman, J., Wilens, T., Harding, M., O'Donnell, D. & Griffin, S. (1996). Pharmacotherapy of attention deficit hyperactivity disorder across the life cycle. *Journal of the American Academy of Child and Adolescent Psychiatry*, **35**, 409–32.

Spencer, T., Heiligenstein, J. H., Biederman, J. *et al.* (2002). Results from 2 proof-of-concept, placebo-controlled studies of atomoxetine in children with attention-deficit/hyperactivity disorder. *Journal of Clinical Psychiatry*, **63**(12), 1140–7.

Swanson, J. M., McBurnett, K. & Wiwal, T. (1993). Effect of stimulant medication on children with attention deficit disorder: A 'review of reviews'. *Exceptional Children*, **60**, 154–62.

Swanson, J. M., Flockhart, D., Udrea, D., Cantwell, D., Connor, D. & Williams, L. (1995). Clonidine in the treatment of ADHD: questions about safety and efficacy (letter to the editor). *Journal of Child and Adolescent Psychopharmacology*, **5**, 301–4.

Szatmari, P., Offord, D. R. & Boyle, M. H. (1989). Ontario Child Health Study: prevalence of attention deficit disorder with hyperactivity. *Journal of Child Psychology and Psychiatry and Allied Disciplines*, **30**, 219–30.

Taylor, E., Schachar, R., Thorley, G., Wieselberg, H. M., Everitt, B. & Rutter, M. (1987). Which boys respond to stimulant medication?

A controlled trial of methylphenidate in boys with disruptive behaviour. *Psychological Medicine*, **17**, 121–43.

Taylor, E., Sergeant, J., Doepfner, M. *et al.* (1998). Clinical guidelines for hyperkinetic disorder. European Society for Child and Adolescent Psychiatry. *European Child and Adolescent Psychiatry*, **7**(4), 184–200.

Taylor, E., Dopfner, M., Sergeant, J. *et al.* (2004): European clinical guidelines for hyperkinetic disorder – first upgrade. *European Child and Adolescent Psychiatry*, **13** (Suppl. 1), I7–30.

Weiss, M. D. & Weiss, J. R. (2004). A guide to the treatment of adults with ADHD. *Journal of Clinical Psychiatry*, **65** (Suppl. 3), 27–37.

Weiss, G. & Hechtman, L. T. (1993). *Hyperactive Children Grown Up. 2nd edn. ADHD in Children, Adolescents, and Adults*. New York: Guildford Press.

Wells, K. C., Pelham, W. E., Kotkin, R. A. *et al.* (2000b). Psychosocial treatment strategies in the MTA study: Rationale, methods, and critical issues in design and implementation. *Journal of Abnormal Child Psychology*, **28**, 483–505.

Wells, K. C. (2004). Treatment of ADHD in children and adolescents. In *Handbook of Interventions that Work with Children and Adolescents: Prevention and Treatment*, ed. P. M. Barrett & T. H. Ollendick. Chicherter, UK: John Wiley & Sons, Ltd.

Wells, K. C., Epstein, J. N., Hinshaw, S. P. *et al.* (2000a). Parenting and family stress treatment outcomes in attention-deficit/hyperactivity disorder (ADHD): an empirical analysis in the MTA Study. *Journal of Abnormal Child Psychology*, **28**, 543–53.

Whalen, C. K, Henker, B. & Granger, D. A. (1990). Social judgment processes in hyperactive boys: effects of methylphenidate and comparisons with normal peers. *Journal of Abnormal Child Psychology*, **18**, 297–316.

Wilens, T. E., Biederman, J., Wong, J., Spencer, T. J. & Prince, J. B. (2002). Adjunctive donepezil in attention deficit hyperactivity disorder youth: case series. *Journal of Child and Adolescent Psychopharmacology*, **10**(3), 217–22.

Wilens, T. E., Newcorn, J. H., Kratochvil, C. J. *et al.* (2006). Long-term atomoxetine treatment in adolescents with attention-deficit/hyperactivity disorder. *Journal of Pediatrics*, **149** (1), 112–19.

54

Oppositional defiant disorder and conduct disorder

Brent Collett, Stephen Scott, Carol Rockhill, Matthew Speltz and Jon McClellan

Editor's note

This chapter refers to both oppositional defiant disorder and conduct disorder under the broader term of Conduct Problems. The chapter reveals that many interventions have been shown to be effective in this group of patients, and even in some instances for the effectiveness to last long after the intervention has ended. Interventions that focus on parent training or on family interventions have been shown to have positive impact. These interventions are effective if delivered to the individual parents or families or to groups of parents or families. Psychopharmacology for this group of patients is used much more readily in the USA than in the UK, and effectiveness has been shown for the psychostimulants, clonidine and risperidone. As always, the care needs to be individualized. The authors lament the fact that, while there is a very great need for interventions among this diagnostic population, the availability of the psychosocial interventions is quite limited in both the UK and USA.

Introduction

Conduct disorder (CD) is characterized by persisting, inappropriate and severe antisocial behaviour. In ICD 10, CD is an overarching term that includes oppositional defiant disorder (ODD) as a milder subtype typically found in younger children and CD as more severe form found in older youths. In DSM IV, they are classified as separate disorders. ODD and CD are the most common reasons for referral for psychiatric care for boys (Meltzer *et al.*, 2003). Because of the overlap between these diagnoses and other forms of antisocial behaviour, much of the treatment literature uses the broad term 'conduct problems' (CP) rather than focusing on a single diagnostic construct.

Many influences contribute to the causation of CP. Child factors include genetic and biological vulnerability (Scourfield *et al.*, 2004); difficult temperament (Rothbart & Bates, 1998); a neuropsychological profile characterized by deficient verbal skills and executive functioning, inattentiveness, overactivity and impulsiveness (Pennington & Ozonoff, 1996); insecure attachment (Speltz *et al.*, 1999); and a propensity to interpret ambiguous social situations as hostile, and to generate aggressive rather than prosocial responses to conflict (Dodge *et al.*, 1986). Parent factors include irritability and explosiveness; inconsistent, overly rigid and inflexible discipline; inadequate supervision; low warmth and involvement; and limited use of strategies to increase prosocial behaviour (Chamberlain & Patterson, 1995; DeKlyen *et al.*, 1998). As children enter school, interactions with teachers are often challenging since the CP is often complicated by poor academic achievement (Hinshaw, 1992). Within the peer group, children with CP are more likely to be rejected by normal peers and may associate with deviant peers who provide encouragement of increasingly serious antisocial behaviour (Dishion *et al.*, 1991). Following assessment, these causal and risk factors can be used directly as targets for treatments.

Most evidence-based treatments for CP are intended for delivery by specialty care providers (e.g. child/adolescent psychiatrists, clinical child psychologists), and many treatments require specialized training and ongoing treatment fidelity monitoring. However, due to the limited availability of mental health resources in many areas, primary care physicians often play a key role in initial triage and ongoing treatment such as medication management. Most of these interventions are intended for outpatient or community settings. In fact, though psychiatric hospitalization may be necessary, there is little or no evidence that inpatient admissions lead to gains that are maintained after the child is returned to their family. In the USA, the American

Cambridge Textbook of Effective Treatments in Psychiatry, ed. Peter Tyrer and Kenneth R. Silk. Published by Cambridge University Press.
© Cambridge University Press, 2008.

Academy of Child and Adolescent Psychiatry (AACAP, 1997) has published practice parameters for the treatment of CD, and several excellent reviews of the evidence based CP treatments have been published (Brestan & Eyberg, 1998; Farmer *et al.*, 2002; Woolfenden *et al.*, 2002).

Psychological interventions

Several psychological interventions for CP are considered 'well-established' or 'probably efficacious' by evidence-based standards (Chambless & Hollon, 1998), and these are referenced in the American Association of Child and Adolescent Psychiatry parameters (AACAP, 1997). The appropriateness of these interventions varies with the patient's developmental level, the unique risk factors contributing to the evolution of CP, and co-morbidities. For example, parenting skills interventions are very effective with young children though somewhat less so with older children and adolescents (Dishion & Patterson, 1992; Ruma *et al.*, 1996). More advanced cognitive development may facilitate participation in the individual or group therapies described below (Forehand & Wierson, 1993). Engagement in therapy tends to be difficult with this population with dropout rates of up to 60% (for a review, see Kazdin, 1996a). Practical measures, such as assisting with transportation, providing childcare, and holding sessions in the evening or at other times to suit the family, are all likely to facilitate retention.

Parenting skills

Parenting programmes are designed to improve parents' behaviour management skills and the quality of the parent–child relationship. Though there is variability among programmes, most target skills such as promoting play and developing a positive parent–child relationship, using praise and rewards to increase desirable social behaviour, giving clear directions and rules, using consistent and calm consequences for unwanted behaviour, and reorganizing the child's day to prevent problems. Parenting interventions may also address distal factors likely to inhibit change (e.g. parental drug/alcohol abuse, maternal depression and relational violence between parents). Treatment can be delivered in individual parent–child appointments or in a parenting group. Individual approaches offer the advantages of in vivo observation of the parent–child dyad and therapist coaching and feedback regarding progress. *Living with Children* (Patterson & Gullion, 1968) and *Parent Child Interaction Therapy* (PCIT [Eyberg, 1988]) are two examples of well-validated individual programmes. Group treatment has been shown to be equally effective and offers opportunities for parents to share their

experience with others who are struggling with a disruptive child. Group treatments emphasize discussion among group leaders and parents and may use videotaped vignettes of parent–child interactions that illustrate the 'right' and 'wrong' ways to handle situations. Two well-known group treatments are the *Incredible Years Program* (IY (Webster-Stratton, 1981)) and the *Positive Parenting Program* (Triple-P (Sanders & Markie-Dadds, 1996; Sanders *et al.*, 2000b)). See Table 54.1 for detailed descriptions.

Behavioural parent training is the most extensively studied treatment for CP, and there is considerable empirical support for its effectiveness (Weisz *et al.*, 2004). The *Living with Children* and *IY* programmes are both considered 'well established' with multiple randomized trials (Patterson *et al.*, 1982; Webster-Stratton *et al.*, 2001a) and replications by independent research groups (Brotman *et al.*, 2005; Fleishman, 1981; Fleishman & Szykula, 1981; Scott *et al.*, 2001). There have also been randomized trials showing the effectiveness of *PCIT* and *Triple P* (Bor *et al.*, 2002; Sanders *et al.*, 2000a), and there is at least one independent replication of the PCIT model (Nixon *et al.*, 2003). Studies suggest that behavioural parent training leads to short-term reductions in antisocial behaviour, with moderate to large effect sizes of $d = 0.5$ to 0.8. Though 'normalization' of children's behaviour following treatment (i.e. post-treatment scores within the average range on rating scale or behavioural observation measures) is sometimes achieved (Reid *et al.*, 2003), this is not consistently observed. In other words, although children in treatment may show statistically significant and robust decreases in behaviour problems relative to controls, many continue to have more problems than typically developing peers. Follow-up studies suggest enduring effects at up to 6-years post-treatment (Hood & Eyberg, 2003; Reid *et al.*, 2003).

Family interventions

Various forms of family therapy have been applied to the treatment of CP, particularly for adolescents and their families. As with the parenting skills training approaches, these treatments often include elements to teach parents behavioural strategies for managing child behaviour. Recognizing the developmental transitions in this age group, treatments may also include focus on increased monitoring and supervision, parent–child communication and negotiation, and helping parents advocate for their child in the community (e.g. with school personnel, juvenile justice). Other community systems with an emphasis on helping families to utilize available supports may be included. For particularly acute cases, treatment may include out of home placement. A few family treatment

Table 54.1. Behavioural parent training interventions

Intervention	Target population	Treatment duration	Description	Availability/resources
Living with Children	Children ages 3–12 yrs and caregivers	Parents are asked to read one of the companion books, and attend 6–8 sessions	Individual parent training model. Treatment focuses on teaching parents to use behavioural principles such as: behaviour tracking, establishing a positive reinforcement system (token economy, praise, privileges) to increase desired behaviours, and using time-out and/or response cost (e.g. removal of privileges) for problem behaviours. Other issues (e.g. marital conflict, family crises) are addressed as needed.	Treatment manual by Patterson. (1975b). Resources for parents include Patterson (1976) *Living with Children* and Patterson (1975a) *Families*
Parent–child interaction therapy	Children ages 3–6 yrs and caregivers. Modified versions have been used with younger/older children	8–12 1-hour sessions, plus 'boosters' as needed	Clinic-based individual parent training model. Treatment includes 2-stages. During the first stage ('child's game'), parents receive coaching in child-directed play. During the second stage, parents receive coaching in giving effective directions, setting limits, and using time-out effectively. During in-session coaching sessions, parents wear an ear piece (i.e. 'bug-in-the-ear') and the therapist coaches them to use target skills while watching through a one-way mirror.	Treatment manual by Hembree-Kigin & McNeil (1995). More information, including downloadable forms, available at www.pcit.org
Incredible years	Children ages 2–6 yrs and caregivers	8–12 2-hour sessions	Group parent training model, applicable for clinic or community settings (e.g. preschool). Groups of 12–14 parents meet regularly with a group facilitator/therapist to discuss child behaviour management strategies. Videotaped vignettes are used to illustrate key principles and strategies. Additional treatment components are available for teacher training and child group social skills training.	Materials and training resources at www.incredibleyears.com
Positive parenting program (Triple-P)	Children ages 1–14 yrs and caregivers. Most studies have been with children approx. 2–6 yrs	Up to 12 1-hour sessions	Group/individual parent training model, applicable for clinic or community settings. Programme includes multiple levels of intervention, including: (1) universal/community wide efforts (media promotions); (2) seminars and/or individual consultation for parents with a specific concern; (3) time-limited, focused behavioural parent training for parents with specific concerns about their child's development; (4) standard behavioural parent training for the parents of children with more severe behavioural problems, delivered in group, individual, or self-directed formats; and (5) individualized intervention, including standard behavioural parent training, home visits, mood/stress management for parents, and partner support skills	Treatment and theoretical rationale described by Sanders *et al.* (2000b). Materials and training resources at www.triplep.net

approaches have been systematically investigated and validated. Though these programmes are potentially costly to the community and healthcare system, Aos *et al.* (2004) have reported that these programmes may result in a net savings, when the costs associated with recidivism are considered. Examples reviewed here include *Functional Family Therapy* (FFT (Alexander & Parsons, 1982; Barton & Alexander, 1981)), *Multisystemic Therapy* (MST (Henggeler *et al.*, 1998, 2002), and *Multidimensional Treatment Foster Care* (MTFC (Chamberlain, 1994; 2003)) (see Table 54.2).

As a group, these interventions have been well studied by their originators, with a few independent replications. Studies of *FFT* have demonstrated improved family communication and reduced recidivism compared to controls (Alexander & Parsons, 1973; Barton *et al.*, 1985; Gordon *et al.*, 1995). In families who have received *FFT*, youth continue to show lower rates of criminal offence well into early adulthood than controls (Gordon *et al.*, 1995). These positive findings have been replicated in a Swedish sample (Hansson *et al.*, 2004). The effectiveness of *MST* has been studied in multiple trials including samples of chronic, often violent juvenile offenders. Relative to control youth receiving 'treatment as usual', those who have received *MST* evidence improved family interactions in direct behavioural observations (Borduin *et al.*, 1995; Henggeler *et al.*, 1986, 1992), are less likely to be placed out of the home (Henggeler *et al.*, 1999; Schoenwald *et al.*, 2000), and have a lower rate of re-arrests (Borduin *et al.*, 1990; Henggeler *et al.*, 1997). Depending on the functional domain assessed, effect sizes range from $d = 0.11$ (peer relations) to 0.76 (observed family interactions) (Curtis *et al.*, 2004). Many of these benefits are maintained at follow-up evaluations up to 15-years post-treatment (Schaeffer & Borduin, 2005). Studies of effectiveness are under way by other research groups (Henggeler & Lee, 2003). Chamberlain and colleagues have shown that, compared to other out-of-home placements, *MTFC* results in decreased youth behaviour problems and self-reported delinquency, lower runaway and arrest rates, and fewer days of incarceration (Chamberlain & Moore, 1998; Chamberlain & Reid, 1998; Eddy *et al.*, 2004). For foster parents and the foster care system, *MTFC* results in better behaviour management strategies, retention of foster parents, and fewer disruptions in child placements (Fisher *et al.*, 2000). We are not aware of replications by researchers not affiliated with *MTFC*'s developers.

Youth interpersonal skills

Cognitive-behavioural therapy (CBT) targets the social-cognitive errors and limited prosocial behavioural repertoires observed in CP children who are mainly of school-age and older, though elements of CBT have been included in treatments for preschoolers. These interventions may be delivered in individual or group therapy formats. Though groups offer several advantages (e.g. opportunities to practice peer interactions), it is worth noting that there is some research documenting iatrogenic effects in adolescents with CP (Dishion *et al.*, 1999). This appears to be particularly problematic in larger groups and those with inadequate therapist supervision, where youth may learn deviant behaviour from their peers. A lower patient–therapist ratio is therefore recommended for group work. Two of the more popular treatment models for school-age youth and adolescents are Kazdin's *Problem Solving Skills Training with in vivo Practice* (PSST-P (Kazdin, 1996b)) and Lochman & Wells's (1996) *Coping Power Program*. Recently, Webster-Stratton *et al.* (2001b, 2004) have added a group child social skills training component to their *IY* programme. This programme, *Dinosaur School*, is intended for preschoolers and early school-age children. The programmes are described in greater detail in Table 54.3.

In two randomized controlled studies, Kazdin *et al.* (1987, 1989) found that *PSST* results in significant decreases in deviant behaviour and increases in prosocial behaviour. Outcomes were superior to a client-centred, relationship-based treatment and were maintained at 1-year follow-up. The addition of in vivo practice and a parent training component have both been found to enhance outcomes (Kazdin & Wassell, 2000; Kazdin *et al.*, 1989). Evaluations of the *Coping Power* programme demonstrate reductions in aggression and substance use, and improved social competence (Lochman & Wells, 2002a, 2002b). Treatment effects were maintained at 1-year follow-up, particularly for those who also received a parent training components (Lochman & Wells, 2004). Both of these programmes are considered 'probably efficacious', though replications by independent research groups are needed. In studies by Webster-Stratton *et al.* (2001b, 2004), *Dinosaur School* has been found to result in significant decreases in behaviour problems and increased prosocial behaviour; treatment gains appeared to be maintained after 1 year. There is at least one independent replication of the *IY* programme, including the *Dinosaur School* component (Hutchings *et al.*, 2004).

Psychopharmacology

At present, there are no pharmacological interventions approved specifically for CP. Nonetheless, medications

Table 54.2. Family interventions

Intervention	Target population	Treatment duration	Description	Availability/Resources
Functional family therapy	Children/adolescents ages 10–18 yrs and families	8–12 1-hour sessions	Combination of family systems and behavioural interventions. Treatment focuses on parent–child communication, inter-parental consistency, parental supervision and monitoring of child behaviour, and negotiating rules and consequences for rule violations. Treatment progresses through three phases: (1) engagement/motivation, (2) behaviour change, and (3) generalization.	Treatment and theoretical foundations are described in Alexander and Parsons (1982). Further information and resources at www.fftinc.com
Multisystemic therapy	Children/adolescents ages 10–17 yrs and families	3–5 months	Broad-based family/community treatment emphasizing the context in which a young person and their family functions. Treatment takes place in the youth's home/community, and includes efforts to help the family draw upon available support systems (e.g. peer group, extended family, community agencies). Therapists carry a low caseload (i.e. 4–6 families), but are expected to be available to families 24-hours per day, 7 days per week. Treatment is guided by nine core principles that include, for example: treatment should be positive and strength-focused; interventions should be present focused, action orientated, and well-defined; intervention effectiveness should be monitored continuously, with the treatment team taking ultimate responsibility for overcoming barriers to care.	Treatment manuals by Henggeler *et al.* (1998) and Henggeler *et al.* (2002). Treatment description, supporting research articles, and contact information provided at www.mstservices.com
Multidimensional treatment foster care	Children/adolescents ages 3–18 years in foster care, foster caregivers, and families of origin Most studies have been with children approx. ages 12–17	NA (ongoing services throughout foster care placement)	In the context of out-of-home/foster care placement, care is provided by a treatment team consisting of: trained foster parents, a programme supervisor, a family therapist, an individual therapist, a youth skills trainer, a daily telephone contact person, and (as needed) a consulting psychiatrist. Considerable training and support is provided to foster parents to facilitate management of the youth's behaviour and retention in the foster family. Given that many youth will return to their families of origin, training and family therapy are also provided for biological families. Youth receive individual skills training and supportive therapy, as well as psychiatric medication consultation when needed. The treatment team also collaborates with school personnel and other community agencies as needed.	Description provided in Chamberlain (1994, 2003). Treatment description, supporting research articles, and contact information are provided at www.mtfc.com

Table 54.3. Youth interpersonal skills interventions

Intervention	Target population	Treatment duration	Description	Availability/resources
Problem solving skills training with in vivo practice	Children/ adolescents ages 7–13 years	12–20 1-hour sessions	Individual training in interpersonal cognitive problem solving techniques. Focus is on identifying problem situations, learning a series of problem-solving steps, and applying the steps to hypothetical situations, in role plays, and in real-life situations. Therapeutic strategies include games, therapist modelling, and role-play with therapist feedback. A token system is used in session to reinforce youths' efforts to practise target skills. Parents are involved periodically for conjoint sessions, and may receive behavioural parent training as an adjunctive treatment.	Treatment described in Kazdin (2003). A treatment manual is in development for dissemination
Coping power programme	Children ages 8–12 years	33 one-to-one-and-a half-hour group sessions, with periodic (at least monthly) individual meetings	Group training focusing on interpretation of social cues, generating prosocial solutions to problems, and anger management/arousal reduction strategies. Treatment is delivered in groups of 5–7 youth by a therapist and co-therapist. Sessions include imagined scenarios, therapist modelling, role plays with corrective feedback, and assignments to practise outside of sessions. Parent and teacher training components have also been developed as adjunctive treatments.	Treatment described in Lochman & Wells (1996)
Dinosaur School	Children ages 4–8 years	20–22 2-hour group sessions.	Group training (roughly 6 children/group) in interpersonal problem solving for young children. Sessions include discussion of hypothetical situations and possible solutions, therapist modelling of prosocial responses, and practise role playing with therapist feedback. Videotaped vignettes are used to present situations for discussion. Puppets are used for interactive role plays, as well as child-friendly cue cards, colouring books, and cartoons. The Dinosaur School programme dovetails with other interventions in the Incredible Years programme, including parent and teacher training. There is also an accompanying classroom curriculum.	Materials and training information available at www.incredibleyears.com

are used relatively frequently and increasingly in this population in the USA (Zito et al., 2000; Steiner et al., 2003; Turgay, 2004). Primary care physicians are often placed in the position of managing such medications. Concerns have been raised about this practice because primary care clinicians often lack adequate training in developmental psychopathology and because primary practice often does not allow adequate time for thorough

assessment and monitoring (Vitiello, 2001). In the UK medication would not generally be supported as good practice because, as discussed below, well-replicated trials of effectiveness are limited, particularly for children with CP without ADHD.

The best-studied pharmacological interventions for youth with CP are psychostimulants (e.g. methylpheni-date), as used with children with co-morbid ADHD and CP. There is evidence that reduction in hyperactivity/impulsivity will also result in reduced CP (Connor *et al.*, 2002; Gerardin *et al.*, 2002). Other approaches have tended to target reactive aggression/over-arousal, primarily in highly aggressive and psychiatrically hospitalized youth. These include medications targeting affect dysregulation (e.g. buspirone, clonidine), mood stabilizers (e.g. lithium, carbamazepine), and neuroleptics (e.g. risperidone).

There is at least some evidence supporting psychopharmacological intervention for CP, though in many cases samples have been small and/or treatment design limited. It is also important to note that, in contrast to most of the psychological approaches reviewed, these treatments have greater risk for side effects and their effectiveness does not endure after therapy is discontinued. Further, research on the use of medication in disruptive preschoolers is lacking. Connor *et al.* (2002) published a meta-analytic review of placebo-controlled studies examining the effects of stimulants on aggression. The authors identified two studies of patients with a primary diagnosis of CD (with and without co-morbid ADHD; Kaplan *et al.*, 1990; Klein *et al.*, 1997). Both studies showed robust decreases in aggression following treatment (effect sizes of roughly $d = 0.75$ to 1.5). Klein *et al.* (1997) found that improvements in CD symptoms were independent of ADHD symptom reduction. Comparable effects were observed in studies examining the effects of stimulants on children with primary ADHD and co-morbid CP (average effect size $d = 0.84$ on measures of overt aggression, and $d = 0.69$ on measures of covert aggression).

Clonidine has also been examined, both as a single treatment approach and in combination with psychostimulants. In a small (i.e. $n = 8$ per treatment group), placebo-controlled study, Connor *et al.* (2000) showed that clonidine alone led to reduced oppositional defiant symptoms, and the combination of stimulants plus clonidine resulted in greater improvement than stimulants or clonidine alone. Comparable findings were reported by Hazell & Stuart (2003) in a larger placebo-controlled, randomized trial (stimulants plus placebo vs. stimulants plus clonidine). However, it should be noted that the use of polypharmacy treatment also carries the risk of increased side effect risks (Impicciatore *et al.*, 2001).

In other studies, risperidone has been shown to be efficacious for the treatment of aggressive youth with CD. Findling *et al.* (2000), in a small ($n = 10$ per group),

double blind, placebo-controlled study, found significant short-term reductions in aggression. Recently, the Risperidone Disruptive Behaviour Study Group has published the results of larger trials (e.g. $n = 110$) using a placebo-controlled, double blind design to study the effects of risperidone in children with subaverage IQ and CP. Results have been encouraging, suggesting that risperidone results in significant improvements in behaviour versus placebo (Aman *et al.*, 2002; Research Units on Pediatric Psychopharmacology Autism Network, 2005; Snyder *et al.*, 2002). While Malone *et al.* (2000) found that lithium reduced aggression and hostility in psychiatrically hospitalized youth, others have failed to show effectiveness in outpatient samples (Klein., 1991) and in studies of shorter treatment intervals (12-weeks or less (Rifkin *et al.*, 1997)).

Finally, uncontrolled (open trials) studies have suggested that carbamazepine reduces aggression and explosive behaviour (Kafantaris *et al.*, 1992; Mattes, 1990). However, carbamazepine failed to outperform placebo in a more recent, double-blind placebo-controlled study (Cueva *et al.*, 1996).

Conclusions

As the above review demonstrates, psychological therapies are the mainstay of treatment for CP (see Table 54.4 for a summary of the evidence base for psychological and psychiatric interventions). However, despite this strong evidence base, in both the USA and the UK, only a small percentage of youth receive any treatment and even fewer receive empirically supported interventions. Further, the 'effectiveness' of these interventions as practiced in community settings tends to lag behind documented 'efficacy' in controlled trials (Curtis *et al.*, 2004). As can already be seen in recent efforts with many of the interventions described above, the next generation of evidence-based treatments for CP will likely include much greater attention to dissemination, including strategies for ongoing training and supervision of practitioners to ensure treatment fidelity. The ultimate goal, of course, being to ensure that children with these disorders have access to high quality, empirically based care.

The level of evidence for each of the interventions discussed in this chapter is summarized in Table 54.4.

Table 54.4. Effectiveness of treatments for oppositional defiant disorder and conduct disorder

Treatment	Form of treatment	Psychiatric disorder/ target audience	Level of evidence for efficacy	Comments
Parenting skills	Living with children	Individual parent training model	Ia	Among the oldest parent-training programmes, used as a model for many of the newer interventions
Parenting skills	Parent–child interaction therapy	Individual parent training model	Ib	Currently being disseminated for use with high risk groups (e.g. parents with a history of abusing their child)
Parenting skills	Incredible years	Group parent training model	Ia	Evidence-based teacher training and child social skills groups are also available, making this a desirable choice for multi-modal intervention
Parenting skills	Positive Parenting Program (Triple-P)	Group and individual parent training model	Ib	Unique given inclusion of multiple levels of intervention (i.e. ranging from public service announcements to targeted interventions for higher-risk children/families)
Family interventions	Functional family therapy	Combined family systems and behavioural interventions	Ib	Data from delinquent juveniles showing long-term reductions in recidivism. Cost-effectiveness data indicate net savings to the community
Family interventions	Multisystemic therapy	Community treatment of family. Intensive with support always available	Ia	Adequate implementation requires considerable staff involvement and commitment. Cost-effectiveness data indicate net savings to the community
Family interventions	Multidimensional treatment foster care	Intensive multidimensional care in foster home	Ib	Enduring effects at up to 4-years post-intervention. Cost-effectiveness data indicate net savings to the community relative to regular foster care
Youth interpersonal skills	Problem solving skills training with in vivo practice	Individual cognitive behavioural training	Ib	Decreases in deviant and increases in prosocial behaviour. Improvements in family and parent functioning have been observed in addition to child behaviour improvements
Youth interpersonal skills	Coping power programme	Group training especially on interpersonal cues and skills. Can have a parent training component	Ib	Reduced aggression and substance misuse and increased social competence
Youth interpersonal skills	Dinosaur School	Group training in interpersonal skills for young children	Ib	Decrease in behavioural problems and improved social behaviour. Can be integrated along with other components from the IY programme
Psychopharmacology	Psychostimulants	Patients with CP	Ia	Decreased in aggression that appears to be independent of/in addition to reduced ADHD symptoms
Psychopharmacology	Clonidine	Patients with CP	Ib	Reduced oppositional defiant symptoms
Psychopharmacology	Psychostimulants + Clonidine	Patients with CP	Ib	Improvement may be better than with either agent alone
Psychopharmacology	Risperidone	Patients with CP	Ib	Significant improvement in behaviour, including those with CP as well as developmental delay

REFERENCES

Alexander, J.F. & Parsons, B.V. (1973). Short-term behavioral intervention with delinquent families: impact on family process and recidivism. *Journal of Abnormal Psychology*, **81**, 219–25.

Alexander, J.F. & Parsons, B.V. (1982). *Functional Family Therapy*. Monterey, CA: Brooks/Cole.

Aman, M.G., De Smedt, G., Derivan, A., Lyons, B. & Findling, R.L.; Risperidone Disruptive Behavior Study Group. (2002). Double-blind, placebo-controlled study of risperidone for the treatment of disruptive behaviors in children with subaverage intelligence. *American Journal of Psychiatry*, **159**, 1337–46.

American Academy of Child and Adolescent Psychiatry (1997). Practice parameters for the assessment and treatment of children and adolescents with conduct disorder. *Journal of the American Academy of Child and Adolescent Psychiatry*, **36**, 122S–39S.

Aos, S., Lieb, R., Mayfield, J., Miller, M. & Pennucci, A. (2004). *Benefits and costs of prevention and early intervention programs for youth*. Retrieved from www.wsipp.wa.gov/rptfiles/04-07-3901.pdf

Barton, C. & Alexander, J.F. (1981). Functional family therapy. In *Handbook of Family Therapy*, ed. A.S. Gurman & D.P. Kniskern, pp. 403–43. New York: Brunner/Mazel.

Barton, C., Alexander, J.F., Waldron, H., Turner, C.W. & Warburton, J. (1985). Generalizing treatment effects of Functional Family Therapy: three replications. *American Journal of Family Therapy*, **13**, 16–26.

Bor, W., Sanders, M.R. & Markie-Dadds, C. (2002). The effects of the Triple P-positive Parenting Program on preschool children with co-occurring disruptive behavior and attentional/hyperactive difficulties. *Journal of Abnormal Child Psychology*, **30**, 571–87.

Borduin, C.M., Henggeler, S.W., Blaske, D.M. & Stein, R.J. (1990). Multisystemic treatment of adolescent sexual offenders. *International Journal of Offender Therapy and Comparative Criminology*, **34**, 105–13.

Borduin, C.M., Mann, B.J., Cone, L.T. (1995). Multisystemic treatment of serious juvenile offenders: long-term prevention of criminality and violence. *Journal of Consulting and Clinical Psychology*, **63**, 569–78.

Brestan, E.V. & Eyberg, S.M. (1998). Effective psychosocial treatments of conduct-disordered children and adolescents: 29 years, 82 studies, and 5,272 kids. *Journal of Clinical Child Psychology*, **27**, 180–9.

Brotman, L.M., Gouley, K.K., Chesir-Teran, D., Dennis, T., Klein, R.G. & Shrout, P. (2005). Prevention for preschoolers at high risk for conduct problems: immediate outcomes on parenting practices and child social competence. *Journal of Clinical Child & Adolescent Psychology*, **34**, 724–34.

Chamberlain, P. (1994). *Family connections: Treatment Foster Care for adolescents*. Eugene, OR: Northwest Media.

Chamberlain, P. (2003). *Treating chronic juvenile offenders: Advances made through the Oregon Multidimensional Treatment Foster Care model*. Washington, DC: American Psychological Association.

Chamberlain, P. & Moore, K.J. (1998). A clinical model of parenting juvenile offenders: a comparison of group versus family care. *Clinical Child Psychology and Psychiatry*, **3**, 375–86.

Chamberlain, P. & Patterson, G.R. (1995). Discipline and child compliance in parenting. In *Handbook of Parenting, Vol. 4: Applied and Practical Parenting*, ed. M.H. Bornstein pp. 205–25. Hillsdale, NJ: Lawrence Erlbaum Associates.

Chamberlain, P. & Reid, J. (1998). Comparison of two community alternatives to incarceration for chronic juvenile offenders. *Journal of Consulting and Clinical Psychology*, **6**, 624–33.

Chambless, D.L. & Hollon, S.D. (1998). Defining empirically supported therapies. *Journal of Consulting and Clinical Psychology*, **66**, 7–18.

Connor, D.F., Barkley, R.A. & Davis, H.T. (2000). A pilot study of methylphenidate, clonidine, or the combination in ADHD comorbid with aggressive oppositional defiant or conduct disorder. *Clinical Pediatrics*, **39**, 15–25.

Connor, D.F., Glatt, S.J., Lopez, I.D., Jackson, D. & Melloni, R.H. (2002). Psychopharmacology and aggression. I: A meta-analysis of stimulant effects on overt/covert aggression-related behaviors in ADHD. *Journal of the American Academy of Child and Adolescent Psychiatry*, **41**, 253–61.

Cueva, J.E., Overall, J.E. Small, A.M., Armenteros, J.L., Perry, R. & Campbell, M. (1996). Carbamazepine in aggressive children with conduct disorder: a double-blind and placebo-controlled study. *Journal of the American Academy of Child & Adolescent Psychiatry*, **35**, 480–490.

Curtis, N.M., Ronan, K.R. & Borduin, C.M. (2004). Multisystemic therapy: a meta-analysis of outcome studies. *Journal of Family Psychology*, **18**, 411–19.

DeKlyen, M., Biernbaum, M.A., Speltz, M.L. & Greenberg, M.T. (1998). Fathers and preschool behavior problems. *Developmental Psychology*, **34**, 264–75.

Dishion, T.J. & Patterson, G.R. (1992). Age effects in parent training outcome. *Behavior Therapy*, **23**, 719–29.

Dishion, T.J., Patterson, G.R., Stoolmiller, M. & Skinner, M.L. (1991). Family, school, and behavioral antecedents to early adolescent involvement with antisocial peers. *Developmental Psychology*, **27**, 172–80.

Dishion, T.J., McCord, J. & Poulin, F. (1999). When interventions harm: peer groups and problem behavior. *American Psychologist*, **54**, 755–64.

Dodge, K.A., Pettit, G.S., McClaskey, C.L. & Brown, M.M. (1986). Social competence in children. *Monographs of the Society for Research in Child Development*, **51**, 1–85.

Eddy, M.J., Bridges, R. & Chamberlain, P. (2004). The prevention of violent behavior by chronic and serious male juvenile offenders: a 2-year follow-up of a randomized clinical trial. *Journal of Family Psychology*, **12**, 2–8.

Eyberg, S.M. (1988). Parent–child interaction therapy: integration of traditional and behavioral concerns. *Child and Family Behavior Therapy*, **10**, 33–48.

Farmer, E.M., Compton, S.N., Bums, B.J. & Robertson, E. (2002). Review of the evidence base for treatment of childhood psychopathology: externalizing disorders. *Journal of Consulting and Clinical Psychology*, **70**, 1267–302.

Findling, R. L., McNamara, N. K., Branicky, L. A., Schluchter, M. D., Lemon, E. & Blumer, J. L. (2000). A double-blind pilot study of risperidone in the treatment of conduct disorder. *Journal of the American Academy of Child and Adolescent Psychiatry*, **39**, 509–16.

Fisher, P. A., Gunnar, M. R., Chamberlain, P. & Reid, J. B. (2000). Preventive intervention for maltreated preschool children: impact on children's behavior, neuroendocrine activity, and foster parent functioning. *Journal of the American Academy of Child and Adolescent Psychiatry*, **39**, 1356–64.

Fleishman, M. J. (1981). A replication of Patterson's 'Intervention for boys with conduct problems.' *Journal of Consulting and Clinical Psychology*, **49**, 342–51.

Fleishman, M. J. & Szykula, S. A. (1981). A community setting replication of a social learning treatment for aggressive children. *Behavior Therapy*, **12**, 115–22.

Forehand, R. & Wierson, M. (1993). The role of developmental factors in planning behavioral interventions for children: disruptive behavior as an example. *Behavior Therapy*, **24**, 117–41.

Gerardin, P., Cohen, D., Mazet, P. & Flament, M. F. (2002). Drug treatment of conduct disorder in young people. *European Neuropsychopharmacology*, **12**, 361–70.

Gordon, D. A., Graves, K. & Arbuthnot, J. (1995). The effect of functional family therapy for delinquents on adult criminal behavior. *Criminal Justice and Behavior*, **22**, 60–73.

Hansson, K., Johansson, P., Drott-Englen, G. & Benderix, Y. (2004). Functional Family Therapy in child psychiatric practice. *Nordisk Psykologi*, **56**, 304–20.

Hazell, P. L. & Stuart, J. E. (2003). A randomized controlled trial of clonidine added to psychostimulant medication for hyperactive and aggressive children. *Journal of the American Academy of Child and Adolescent Psychiatry*, **42**, 886–94.

Hembree-Kigin, T. L. & McNeil, C. B. (1995). *Parent–child Interaction Therapy*. New York: Plenum.

Henggeler, S. W. & Lee, T. (2003). Multisystemic treatment of serious clinical problems. In *Evidence-based Psychotherapies for Children and Adolescents*, ed. A. E. Kazdin & J. R. Weisz, pp. 301–22. New York: Guilford.

Henggeler, S. W., Rodick, J. D., Borduin, C. M., Hanson, C. L., Watson, S. M. & Urey, J. R. (1986). Multisystemic treatment of juvenile offenders: effects on adolescent behavior and family interactions. *Developmental Psychology*, **22**, 132–41.

Henggeler, S. W., Melton, G. B. & Smith, L. A. (1992). Family preservation using multisystemic therapy: an effective alternative to incarcerating serious juvenile offenders. *Journal of Consulting and Clinical Psychology*, **60**, 953–61.

Henggeler, S. W., Melton, G. B., Brondino, M. J., Scherer, D. G. & Hanley, J. H. (1997). Multisystemic therapy with violent and chronic juvenile offenders and their families: the role of treatment fidelity in successful dissemination. *Journal of Consulting and Clinical Psychology*, **65**, 821–33.

Henggeler, S. W., Schoenwald, S. K., Borduin, C. M., Rowland, M. D. & Cunningham, P. B. (1998). *Multisystemic treatment of antisocial behavior in children and adolescents*. New York: Guilford.

Henggeler, S. W., Pickrel, S. G. & Brondino, M. J. (1999). Multisystemic treatment of substance abusing and dependent delinquents: outcomes, treatment fidelity, and transportability. *Mental Health Services Research*, **1**, 171–84.

Henggeler, S. W., Schoenwald, S. K., Rowland, M. D. & Cunningham, P. B. (2002). *Serious emotional disturbance in children and adolescents: Multisystemic therapy*. New York: Guilford Press.

Hinshaw, S. P. (1992). Externalizing behavior problems and academic underachievement in childhood and adolescence: causal relationships and underlying mechanisms. *Psychological Bulletin*, **111**, 127–55.

Hood, K. & Eyberg, S. M. (2003). Outcomes of parent–child interaction therapy: mothers' reports on maintenance three to six years after treatment. *Journal of Clinical Child and Adolescent Psychology*, **32**, 419–29.

Hutchings, J., Lane, E., Owen, R. E. & Gwyn, R. (2004). The introduction of the Webster-Stratton Incredible Years Classroom Dinosaur School Programme in Gwynedd, North Wales: a pilot study. *Educational and Child Psychology*, **21**, 4–15.

Impicciatore, P., Choonara, I., Clarkson, A., Provasi, D., Pandolfini, C. & Bonati, M. (2001). Incidence of adverse drug reactions in paediatric in/out-patients: a systematic review and meta-analysis of prospective studies. *British Journal of Clinical Pharmacology*, **52**(1), 77–83.

Kafantaris, V., Campbell, M., Padron-Gayol, M. V., Small, A. M., Locascio, J. J. & Rosenberg, C. R. (1992). Carbamazepine in hospitalized aggressive conduct disorder children: an open pilot study. *Psychopharmacology Bulletin*, **28**, 193–9.

Kaplan, S. L., Busner, J., Kupietz, S., Wassermann, E. & Segal, B. (1990). Effects of methylphenidate on adolescents with aggressive conduct disorder and ADDH: a preliminary report. *Journal of the American Academy of Child and Adolescent Psychiatry*, **29**, 719–23.

Kazdin, A. E. (1996a). Dropping out of child therapy: Issues for research and implications for practice. *Clinical Child Psychology and Psychiatry*, **1**, 133–56.

Kazdin, A. E. (1996b). Problem solving and parent management in treating aggressive and antisocial behavior. In *Psychosocial Treatments for Child and Adolescent Disorders: Empirically-based Strategies for Clinical Practice* ed. E. S. Hibbs & P. S. Jensen, pp. 377–408. Washington, DC: American Psychological Association.

Kazdin, A. E. (2003). Problem-solving skills training and parent management training for conduct disorder. In *Evidence-based Psychotherapies for Children and Adolescents*, ed. A. E. Kazdin & J. R. Weisz. New York: Guilford.

Kazdin, A. E. & Wassell, G. (2000). Therapeutic changes in children, parents, and families resulting from treatment of children with conduct problems. *Journal of the American Academy of Child and Adolescent Psychiatry*, **39**, 414–20.

Kazdin, A. E., Esveldt-Dawson, K., French, N. H. & Unis, A. S. (1987). Problem-solving skills training and relationship therapy in the treatment of antisocial child behavior. *Journal of Consulting and Clinical Psychology*, **55**, 76–85.

Kazdin, A. E., Bass, D., Siegel, T. & Thomas, C. (1989). Cognitive-behavioural treatment and relationship therapy in the treatment of children referred for antisocial behaviour. *Journal of Consulting and Clinical Psychology*, **57**, 522–35.

Klein, R. (1991). *Preliminary results: lithium effects in conduct disorders.* In CME Syllabus and Proceedings Summary, 144th Annual Meeting of the American Psychiatric Association, New Orleans, pp. 119–120.

Klein, R. G., Abikoff, H., Klass, E., Ganeles, D., Seese, L. M. & Pollack, S. (1997). Clinical efficacy of methylphenidate in conduct disorder with and without attention deficit hyperactivity disorder. *Archives of General Psychiatry*, **54**, 1073–80.

Lochman, J. E. & Wells, K. C. (1996). A social-cognitive intervention with aggressive children: prevention effects and contextual implementation issues. In *Prevention and Early Intervention: Childhood Disorders, Substance Use and Delinquency*, ed. R. Peters & R. J. McMahon, pp. 111–43. Thousand Oaks, CA: Sage.

Lochman, J. E. & Wells, K. C. (2002a). Contextual social cognitive mediators and child outcome: a test of the theoretical model in the Coping Power Program. *Development and Psychopathology*, **14**, 945–67.

Lochman, J. E. & Wells, K. C. (2002b). The Coping Power Program at the middle school transition: universal and indicated prevention effects. *Psychology of Addictive Behaviors*, **16**, 540–54.

Lochman, J. E. & Wells, K. C. (2004). The coping power program for preadolescent aggressive boys and their parents: outcome effects at the 1-year follow-up. *Journal of Consulting and Clinical Psychology*, **72**, 571–8.

Malone, R. P., Delaney, M. A., Luebbert, J. F., Cater, J. & Campbell M. (2000). A double-blind placebo-controlled study of lithium in hospitalized aggressive children and adolescents with conduct disorder. *Archives of General Psychiatry*, **57**, 649–54.

Mattes, J. A. (1990). Comparative effectiveness of carbamazepine and propranolol for rage outbursts. *Journal of Neuropsychiatry and Clinical Neurosciences*, **2**, 159–64.

Meltzer, H., Gatward, R., Goodman, R. & Ford T. (2003). Mental health of children and adolescents in Great Britain. *International Review of Psychiatry*, **15**, 185–7.

Nixon, R. D., Sweeney, L., Erickson, D. B. & Touyz, S. W. (2003). Parent-child interaction therapy: a comparison of standard and abbreviated treatments for oppositional defiant preschoolers. *Journal of Consulting and Clinical Psychology*, **71**, 251–60.

Patterson, G. R. (1975a). *Families: Applications of Social Learning to Family Life* (revised edn). Champaign, IL: Research Press.

Patterson, G. R. (1975b). *A Guide for the Professional for Use with Living with Children and Families.* Champaign, IL: Research Press.

Patterson, G. R. (1976). *Living with Children: New Methods for Parents and Teachers* (revised edn). Champaign, IL: Research Press.

Patterson, G. R. & Gullion, M. E. (1968). *Living with Children: New Methods for Parents and Teachers.* Champaign, IL: Research Press.

Patterson, G. R., Chamberlain, P. & Reid, J. B. (1982). A comparative evaluation of a parent training program. *Behavior Therapy*, **13**, 638–50.

Pennington, B. F. & Ozonoff, S. (1996). Executive functions and developmental psychopathology. *Journal of Child Psychology and Psychiatry*, **37**, 51–87.

Reid, M. J., Webster-Stratton, C. & Hammond, M. (2003). Follow-up of children who received the incredible years intervention for oppositional-defiant disorder: maintenance and prediction of 2-year outcome. *Behavior Therapy*, **34**, 471–91.

Research Units on Pediatric Psychopharmacology Autism Network (2005). Risperidone treatment of autistic disorder: longer-term benefits and blinded discontinuation after 6 months. *American Journal of Psychiatry*, **162**, 1361–9.

Rifkin, A., Karajgi, B., Dicker, R. *et al.* (1997). Lithium treatment of conduct disorders in adolescents. *American Journal of Psychiatry*, **154**, 554–5.

Rothbart, M. K. & Bates, J. E. (1998). Temperament. In *Handbook of Child Psychology, 5th edn., Vol 3. Social, Emotional, and Personality Development*, ed. W. Damon & N. Eisenberg, pp. 105–76. Hoboken, NJ: John Wiley & Sons.

Ruma, P. R., Burke, R. V. & Thompson, R. W. (1996). Group parent training: Is it effective for children of all ages? *Behavior Therapy*, **27**, 159–69.

Sanders, M. R. & Markie-Dadds, C. (1996). Triple P: a multi-level family intervention program for children with disruptive behavior disorders. In *Early Intervention and Prevention in Mental Health*, ed. P. Cotton & H. Jackson, pp. 59–85. Melbourne: Australian Psychological Society.

Sanders, M. R., Markie-Dadds, C., Tully, L. A. & Bor, W. (2000a). The Triple P-Positive Parenting Program: a comparison of enhanced, standard, and self-directed behavioral family intervention for parents of children with early onset conduct problems. *Journal of Consulting and Clinical Psychology*, **68**, 624–40.

Sanders, M. R., Markie-Dadds, C. & Turner, K. M. T. (2000b). Theoretical, scientific, and clinical foundations of the Triple P-Positive Parenting Program: a population approach to the promotion of parenting competence. *Parenting Research and Practice Monograph*, **1**, 1–21.

Schaeffer, C. M. & Borduin, C. M. (2005). Long-term follow-up to a randomized clinical trial of multisystemic therapy with serious and violent juvenile offenders. *Journal of Consulting and Clinical Psychology*, **73**, 445–53.

Schoenwald, S. K., Ward, D. M., Henggeler, S. W. & Rowland, M. D. (2000). MST vs. hospitalization for crisis stabilization of youth: placement outcomes 4 months post-referral. *Mental Health Services Research*, **2**, 3–12.

Scott, S., Spender, Q., Doolan, M., Jacobs, B. & Aspland, H. (2001). Multicentre controlled trial of parenting groups for childhood antisocial behaviour in clinical practice. *British Medical Journal*, **323**, 1–7.

Scourfield, J., Van den Bree, M., Martin, N. & McGuffin, P. (2004). Conduct problems in children and adolescents: a twin study. *Archives of General Psychiatry*, **61**, 489–96.

Snyder, R., Turgay, A., Aman, M. & Risperidone Conduct Study Group (2002). Effects of risperidone on conduct and disruptive behavior disorders in children with subaverage IQs. *Journal of the American Academy of Child and Adolescent Psychiatry*, **41**, 1026–36.

Speltz, M. L., DeKlyen, M. & Greenberg, M. T. (1999). Attachment in boys with early onset conduct problems. *Development and Psychopathology*, **11**, 269–285.

Steiner, H., Saxena, K. & Chang, K. (2003). Psychopharmacologic strategies for the treatment of aggression in juveniles. *CNS Spectrums*, **8**, 298–308.

Turgay, A. (2004). Aggression and disruptive behavior disorders in children and adolescents. *Expert Review of Neurotherapeutics*, **4**, 623–32.

Vitiello, B. (2001). Psychopharmacology for young children: clinical needs and research opportunities. *Pediatrics*, **108**, 983–9.

Webster-Stratton, C. (1981). Modification of mothers' behaviors and attitudes through a videotape modeling group discussion program. *Behavior Therapy*, **12**, 634–42.

Webster-Stratton,C., Reid, J. & Hammond, M. (2001a). Preventing conduct problems, promoting social competence: a parent and teacher training partnership in head start. *Journal of Clinical Child Psychology*, **30**, 283–302.

Webster-Stratton, C., Reid, J. & Hammond, M. (2001b). Social skills and problem-solving training for children with early-onset conduct problems: who benefits? *Journal of Child Psychology and Psychiatry*, **42**, 943–52.

Webster-Stratton, C., Reid, M. J. & Hammond, M. (2004). Treating children with early-onset conduct problems: inter vention outcomes for parent, child, and teacher training. *Journal of Clinical Child and Adolescent Psychology*, **33**, 105–24.

Weisz, J. R., Hawley, K. M. & Doss, A. J. (2004). Empirically tested psychotherapies for youth internalizing and externalizing problems and disorders. *Child and Adolescent Psychiatric Clinics of North America*, **13**, 729–815.

Woolfenden, S. R., Williams, K. & Peat, J. K. (2002). Family and parenting interventions for conduct disorder and delinquency: a meta-analysis of randomised controlled trials. *Archives of Disease in Childhood*, **86**, 251–6.

Zito, J. M., Safer, D. J., dosReis, S., Gardner, J. F., Boles, M. & Lynch, F. (2000). Trends in the prescribing of psychotropic medications to preschoolers. *Journal of the American Medical Association*, **283**, 1025–30.

55

Treatment of depressive disorders in children and adolescents

Kelly Schloredt, Rachel Gershenson, Christopher K. Varley, Paul Wilkinson and Ian Goodyer

Editor's note

The treatment of depression in children and adolescents has commanded much attention in the news in both the USA and the UK. In the UK, there are very strong guidelines against the use of any SSRI antidepressants except fluoxetine, and the guidelines urge that, if fluoxetine is used, it should be used only in moderate to severe cases and should always be accompanied by some psychotherapeutic efforts. In the USA, the advice is somewhat less strict in that SSRIs other than fluoxetine are not advised against, but there is a 'block box' issued that reminds clinicians to weigh the costs vs. the benefits of SSRI usage. One of the costs of using SSRIs may be an increase in suicidal ideation if not actual suicide among users of these medications, though the evidence here is not as strong as critics of SSRI usage would like it to be. Psychotherapeutic treatments, especially cognitive-behavioural treatment (CBT) and interpersonal therapy (IPT) have been shown to be effective interventions for depression in youth. Yet there are also questions not to its effectiveness per se, but as to the duration of the effectiveness. The current thinking in the treatment of depression in both children and adolescents suggests that in milder depression one should try non-pharmacologic treatments at first, and if they do not prove to be effective, then pharmacologic treatment can be added. In moderate to severe depression, a combined psychopharmacologic-psychotherapeutic approach is called for, perhaps with some family therapy or family or parental educational interventions added.

Introduction

In the United States, the prevalence rates of dysthymic disorder (DD) and major depressive disorders (MDD) in children and adolescents range from 0.6% to 8.2% (Fleming & Offord, 1990; Garrison et al., 1992, Kashani et al., 1987a, 1987b; Lewinsohn et al., 1993, 1994). While these rates tend to be lower during the childhood years, they increase dramatically during adolescence. For example, it is reported that 1 in 20 adolescents suffer from MDD at any point in time, 20% of adolescents have at least one episode of clinical depression by age 18, and 65% of adolescents report transient or less severe depressive symptoms (Lewinsohn et al., 1993). In a national survey in the UK (Meltzer et al., 2003), 10% of children aged 5–15 had a mental disorder, with 4% having anxiety or depression and about 1% having depression. Childhood depression is persistent, compromises the process of development by interfering with academic and social functioning, and represents a primary risk factor for substance use and suicide (Baer et al., 1998; Birmaher et al., 1996a; Gjerde & Westenberg, 1998; Hammen, 1997). As such, the need for effective treatments is crucial.

Most recently, the UK National Institute for Health and Clinical Excellence (2005) has published guidelines for the treatment of depression in this population. Psychological treatment is the treatment of choice, and antidepressant medication is shunned for mild depression. In moderate to severe depression, the use of fluoxetine is approved but the guideline suggests that it should be used cautiously and only in conjunction with ongoing psychological treatment. The United States practice parameters for the treatment of children and adolescents with depressive disorders suggest the utilization of a multi-method approach that takes into consideration the severity of the illness, the motivation of the patient and patient's family, the severity of other psychiatric and/or medical conditions, and the provision of treatment in the least restrictive safe environment (Birmaher et al., 1998). In line with these recommendations, empirical studies completed within the USA support both psychopharmacological and psychosocial interventions for MDD in children and adolescents with some limitations. As there have been very few controlled studies examining treatment options for children and adolescents with DD, the studies reviewed center largely on MDD.

Pharmacotherapy

The psychopharmacologic treatment of depression in children and adolescents has become increasingly common in the USA (Delate *et al.*, 2004; Zito *et al.*, 2002), though in the UK, as stated above, there is more hesitation and controversy regarding the treatment of depression in children with antidepressants. Recent guidance by the UK Medicines and Healthcare products Regulatory Agency (MHRA, 2003) state that for children under 18, the only SSRI for which the evidence suggested that the benefits outweighed the risks was fluoxetine. Published (Emslie *et al.*, 1997, 2002; Keller *et al.*, 2001; Wagner *et al.*, 2003) and unpublished RCT data were presented.

SSRIs

Until 1997, no double-blind, placebo-controlled trials of antidepressant medication had demonstrated efficacy in the treatment of youth with MDD. Although there had been prior trials with a number of different medications, including both tricyclic antidepressants and monoamine oxidase inhibitors, all had negative results (Emslie *et al.*, 1997). The first double-blind, placebo-controlled trial of antidepressant medication to demonstrate efficacy was conducted with the selective serotonin reuptake inhibitor (SSRI), fluoxetine. In this first study, 96 children and adolescents were randomized to either fluoxetine (20 mg) or placebo; and they were seen weekly over 8 weeks. Those in the fluoxetine condition showed a 56% response rate compared to 33% in the placebo condition (Emslie *et al.*, 1997). A second fluoxetine study of 219 youth found that 41% of youth being treated with fluoxetine achieved remission, whereas only 20% of youth remitted on the placebo (Emslie *et al.*, 2002). Based on these results, the Food and Drug Administration (FDA) in the USA authorized fluoxetine for treatment of major depression in children and adolescents.

A number of other SSRIs have been studied in children and adolescents including paroxetine (Keller *et al.*, 2001), sertraline (Wagner *et al.*, 2003), citalopram (Wagner *et al.*, 2004), and venlafaxine (Mandoki *et al.*, 1997). Data from these studies, however, have been difficult to decipher.

Although there are findings to suggest that these medications are well tolerated, the evidence for the efficacy of these agents in depressed youth is limited, and the MHRA concluded that there were no or minimal benefits and increased side effects (possibly including increased suicidality) for paroxetine, sertraline, citalopram and venlafaxine. Thus on one hand, there is some evidence in favour of SSRI medication with response rates as high as 70% (Emslie *et al.*, 1997; Wagner *et al.*, 2003). On the other hand, clinical significance for some SSRI agents is lacking in that the overall effect of the medication is low (Wagner *et al.*, 2004), and/or the effect over and above what is observed in the placebo condition is minimal (Emslie *et al.*, 1997, 2002; Wagner *et al.*, 2003, 2004). For example, a study involving citalopram showed a 36% response rate for the drug condition compared to a 24% response rate for the placebo (Wagner *et al.*, 2004). To complicate matters further, still other studies have shown no evidence of benefit from SSRI treatment at all (Mandoki *et al.*, 1997; Milin *et al.*, 1999).

Thus while SSRIs have emerged as the psychopharmacologic treatment of choice in the USA with some caution and only fluoxetine has emerged as the treatment of choice in the UK with depressed youth, such treatment has grown controversial. A debate has arisen, accompanied by formal regulatory action in Great Britain and the USA, concerning the use of some SSRIs with children and adolescents. At the center of the debate lie concerns regarding the extent of benefit in trials reported as positive, the number of unpublished trials showing negative results, and possible mood related side effects associated with SSRI use, particularly suicidal thinking and suicide attempts. In June 2003, the MHRA declared paroxetine contraindicated for the treatment of major depression in individuals under age 18 (Duff, 2003b). Approximately one week later, the FDA in the USA followed suit (US Food and Drug Administration, 2003). Since that time, a number of other SSRI medications have been declared contraindicated for use in depressed youth by the MHRA in Great Britain including, venlafaxine, citalopram, escitalopram, sertraline, nefazodone and mirtazapine, with the notion that the risks of treatment with these agents outweigh the benefits (Duff, 2003a). The only SSRI felt to have a favourable risk–benefit ratio is that of fluoxetine (Whittington *et al.*, 2004).

Many UK child and adolescent psychiatrists disagreed with this advice to restrict SSRI usage to fluoxetine because they felt that the data was really incomplete for the following reasons: most of the studies excluded patients with co-morbid conditions, more severe depression and pre-existing suicidality. Therefore, it is very difficult to extrapolate the findings to patients with more severe depression seen in clinics. In particular, there may be a greater medication–placebo difference in more severe depression; the studies to date may underestimate the efficacy of medication for the most at-risk from recurrent disorder and suicide attempts.

Yet to fuel the controversy further, some other psychiatrists have suggested that the evidence for the efficacy of fluoxetine is not reliable enough, in particular that there was no statistically significant difference on the primary endpoints (proportion of subjects meeting pre-defined remission criteria) in the first two studies which are generally seen as showing the efficacy of fluoxetine (Jureidini *et al.*, 2004). Despite their criticisms of the use of SSRIs in this population, a meta-analysis (Jureidini *et al.*, 2004) of the five published RCTs of SSRIs (not including Treatment for Adolescents with Depression Study (TADS)) showed a small, but statistically significant, effect size of 0.26 (95% confidence interval 0.13 to 0.40).

The FDA in the USA undertook a review process parallel to the MHRA. US academicians responding to the issue have taken exception to the cautionary recommendations, arguing, among other issues, that the interpretation of the data is flawed in that there are no statistically significant differences in rates of suicidality between drug and placebo conditions in the individual studies examined by the MHRA and FDA (Brent & Birmaher, 2004, American College of Neuropsychopharmacology, 2004; Simon *et al.*, 2006). However, meta-analysis of all the paediatric SSRI studies has demonstrated significantly increased suicidality and self-harm events in those given SSRI compared with placebo (Dubicka *et al.*, 2006, Hammad *et al.*, 2006, Kaizar *et al.*, 2006). However, absolute differences are small: for example, Dubicka and colleagues demonstrated self-harm or suicidality in 4.8% of children and adolescents given SSRI, and 3.0% in those given placebo. Despite the response from the academic community, the FDA issued a 'black box' regarding an increased risk of suicidal behavior in children and adolescents treated with antidepressant medication (US Food and Drug Administration, 2004). Following the issuance of the black box warning there has been a significant decrease in the annual number of prescriptions written for antidepressants in the USA, following several years of increasing numbers of prescriptions. Perhaps the only issue that is clear in this debate is that when antidepressants are used currently, practitioners must fully inform their patients and families of possible side effects and devote increased attention during follow-up to signs of suicidality, agitation, and clinical worsening of symptoms.

Subsequent to these debates, the results of the TADS were published (March *et al.*, 2004). Data from the TADS study has reinforced that fluoxetine is more effective than placebo (effect size: 0.68; positive response rates: fluoxetine 61%, placebo 35%) and more effective than CBT alone (positive response rate: 43%). Treatment reduced suicidality in all groups. Although participants receiving an SSRI had more suicide-related adverse events than the non-SSRI participants, the difference between the groups was not significant.

In summary, while some depressed children and adolescents appear to benefit from antidepressant medication, studies show that up to 40% are 'non-responders' (Keller *et al.*, 2001; Reinecke *et al.*, 1998). This fact, coupled with the controversy over potential negative side effects of antidepressant use, highlights the need for effective psychosocial treatment options for depressed youth. Nonetheless, the debate as to the appropriateness of the use of SSRIs in children and adolescents continues. In view of the lack of evidence for other treatments (particularly psychological treatments) in severe depression, and the fact that subjects in treatment studies tended to have less severe depression, it is generally accepted that SSRIs are still an important treatment for severe depression. Certainly in the UK at the present time, fluoxetine should be used first-line.

Tricyclic antidepressants (TCAs)

A Cochrane meta-analysis (Hazell *et al.*, 2004) found 13 RCTs comparing oral TCAs with placebo in 506 children and adolescents aged 6 to 18. Results suggested marginal effectiveness in reducing depressive symptoms for depressed adolescents (effect size = −0.47, 95% confidence interval −0.92 to −0.02) but not children (effect size = 0.15, 95% confidence interval −0.34 to 0.64). There was no significant difference in improvement rates in either age group. There were significantly higher rates of side effects in the TCA groups.

Birmaher *et al.* (1998) investigated amitriptyline in 27 adolescents with 'treatment resistant' depression. Most had already had a course of antidepressants (including SSRIs). There was no significant difference between amitriptyline and placebo. However, small studies such as this are unable to pick up that a small number of adolescents may respond to a TCA when nothing else has been successful, and, under specialist supervision and with careful monitoring, TCAs may be an appropriate treatment.

Other antidepressants

A review of unpublished RCT data (MHRA, 2004) concluded that there was no evidence for the efficacy of mirtazepine and that mirtazepine caused side-effects, but that mirtazepine did not cause an increase in suicidality. Small uncontrolled case series have shown improvements in clinical condition in depressed adolescents with bupropion (Daviss *et al.*, 2001; Glod *et al.*, 2003), nefazodone (Goodnick *et al.*, 2000) and phenelzine (Strober *et al.*, 1998). There have been no published controlled trials with these, or other, psychotropic agents with putative antidepressant effects.

Somatic treatments

Electroconvulsive therapy (ECT)

The use of ECT in children and adolescents is a controversial topic in the USA and UK alike. Although a review of the recent literature completed by the American Academy of Child and Adolescent Psychiatry (2004) for the purposes of developing US practice parameters suggests that ECT may be an effective treatment for adolescents with unipolar and bipolar disorders, data remains insufficient in assessing the utility of ECT in children with unipolar and bipolar disorders (Rudnick, 2001). Electroconvulsive therapy is very rarely used in the UK for depressed adolescents. A comprehensive survey (Duffett *et al.*, 1999) suggested that in 1996, ECT was used for eight adolescents aged less than 18 years in the whole UK. This is due to concerns about side effects (particularly cognitive) and the ethical issues of using such a treatment in young people unable to give consent. Its use in affective disorders tends to be restricted to cases where a very urgent response is needed due to risk of death (4 out of 8 cases in the above survey) and/or in severe and treatment-resistant depression (6 out of 8 cases). It is considered best practice to obtain a second opinion before proceeding with ECT.

There have been no randomized trials of ECT in adolescents. A systematic review (Walter *et al.*, 1999b) of published case reports and case series showed that 33/52 (64%) adolescents with major depression and 25/35 (71%) adolescents with psychotic depression showed remission or marked improvements after ECT. As this is based on published cases, publication bias is likely, but these results show that a large number of cases of severe and treatment-resistant cases of depression do improve with ECT. Side effects tended to be mild and transient, including headache, muscle ache, nausea and memory problems. Modern ECT techniques are likely to cause less side effects (Walter *et al.*, 1999b). While short-term memory problems are common, small studies (Cohen *et al.*, 2000) have suggested that there are no long-term

effects on memory. Despite these side effects, an Australian study (Walter *et al.*, 1999a) of people who had had ECT during adolescence showed that the majority (69%) would have it again if indicated and would recommend it to others (77%). Ninety-two per cent of subjects said that the illness or the medication were worse experiences than the ECT.

Current US practice parameters for the use of ECT with adolescents suggests that ECT can be considered as an appropriate treatment option when adolescents have had two or more trials of pharmacotherapy with poor response, or the severity of the adolescent's symptoms preclude the amount of time that would be needed to show a psychopharmacological treatment response (AACAP, 2004). In addition, these practice parameters highlight the absolute need for consent from the adolescent's legal guardian, with a preference to also obtain consent/assent from the adolescent, the need to follow state and institutional guidelines, the need to use techniques that have been shown to have the greatest efficacy and the fewest side effects, and the need for systematic pre- and post-treatment evaluations that include the assessment of both symptoms and cognitive functioning (AACAP, 2004).

Psychotherapy

While the body of research on psychosocial interventions is growing rapidly, there exist only a small number of controlled studies. Although the treatment literature covers a variety of psychotherapeutic schools of thought, such as psychodynamic therapy (Bemporad, 1988) and supportive group treatment (Fine *et al.*, 1991), cognitive-behavioral therapy (CBT) and interpersonal therapy (IPT) have been more widely studied in controlled trials, and as a result, will be the focus of this review.

Cognitive-behavioural therapy (CBT)

The most thoroughly researched psychosocial intervention in depressed youth is that of CBT, which aims to alter depressogenic behaviours and cognitions through a variety of techniques including mood monitoring, pleasant events scheduling, and challenging automatic thoughts/beliefs. It has been delivered to adolescents in both individual and group formats with remarkably consistent results. Initial studies were conducted primarily in school settings with children identified as depressed via elevated scores on self-report questionnaires. These studies have shown short-term superiority for CBT over no-treatment or waitlist conditions (Curry, 2001). In a meta-analysis by Lewinsohn & Clarke (1999), CBT was found to have an estimated overall effect size of 1.27 (large effect). As 63% of the patients across the studies analyzed made clinically significant improvements by the end of treatment, CBT was deemed an effective treatment for adolescent depression. Similar conclusions were drawn from the meta-analyses of Marcotte (1997) and Reinecke *et al.* (1998), where the magnitude of reported effect sizes ranged from 0.41 (small) to 1.70 (large). There are a number of individual studies where improvement rates for children and adolescents with depressive disorders ranged from 54.0% to 66.7% (Brent *et al.*, 1997; Clarke *et al.*, 1999; Wood *et al.*, 1996).

A meta-analysis (Harrington *et al.*, 1998) of six randomized controlled trials compared CBT with control interventions in the acute stage treatment of 400 8–19 year olds with depressive disorders. Remission rates were 59% and 41% in the CBT and control conditions, respectively. The authors concluded that methodological quality of the primary studies was only moderate and subjects tended to less severe impairment than subjects in tricyclic antidepressant studies. Jayson *et al.* (1998) showed that more severe social impairment reduced the efficacy of CBT.

The recent Treatment for Adolescents with Depression Study (TADS, March *et al.*, 2004), a single large RCT (around 110 subjects per group) with more rigorous methodology, compared CBT with fluoxetine, placebo and combined fluoxetine and CBT. It showed no difference in effectiveness between CBT and placebo, and that fluoxetine alone was more effective than CBT alone. Interestingly, CBT plus fluoxetine was more effective than fluoxetine alone. The authors suggested that these results may have shown CBT alone to be ineffective as patients were more severely depressed than in earlier studies.

The above studies used experienced mental health professionals to provide CBT. One RCT (Kerfoot *et al.*, 2004) trained and supervised social workers in CBT for their clients with depressive symptoms (as defined by self-rated Mood and Feelings Questionnaire score of at least 23). Half of the sample had major depressive disorder. There were no differences between the CBT and non-CBT groups.

Clinic based studies of youth presenting with MDD report mixed results. Brent *et al.* (1997, 1998), enrolled and randomly assigned 107 adolescents with MDD into 12–16 weeks of treatment with CBT, systemic behavioural family therapy (SBFT), and non-directive supportive therapy (NST). Short-term outcomes revealed decreased depressive cognitions among those in the CBT group

(Brent *et al.*, 1997), but there is some evidence that the CBT was only more effective when there was a co-morbid anxiety disorder (Brent *et al.*, 1998). Despite the initial advantage of CBT in the acute treatment of adolescent MDD, however, no long-term advantage was realized with reference to rates of remission, recovery, recurrence, and level of functioning (Birmaher *et al.*, 2000). A study by Wood, Harrington & Moore (1996) similarly revealed a clear advantage of CBT over relaxation training in the acute treatment of childhood and adolescent depressive disorders. In this study, the initial advantage of CBT, however, was significantly diminished 6 months post-treatment.

These findings have led some investigators to examine ways in which treatment gains from CBT might be maintained. For example, one study examined whether booster sessions following acute treatment with group CBT would reduce the rate of recurrence of MDD in adolescents. The study found that while boosters did not reduce recurrence rate at follow-up, they did appear to speed the recovery of those still depressed after acute treatment (Clarke *et al.*, 1999).

Interpersonal therapy (IPT)

In contrast to CBT, interpersonal therapy (IPT) aims to reduce depressive symptoms and increase interpersonal functioning by connecting symptoms to problem areas such as grief, role disputes, role transitions, and interpersonal sensitivities (Mufson *et al.*, 1999). Originally developed for depressed adult outpatients, IPT has been manualized for adolescents (IPT-A) by Mufson and colleagues (Mufson *et al.*, 1999) and applied in both clinic and school settings (Mufson *et al.*, 1994, 1999, 2004). Initial evaluation of the 12-week treatment course suggested positive gains, with the majority of adolescents reporting few depressive symptoms and maintaining improvements in social functioning at 1-year follow-up (Mufson & Fairbanks, 1996; Mufson *et al.*, 1994). These findings were replicated in a larger, control study utilizing a sample of 48 clinic-referred adolescents who met criteria for MDD (Mufson *et al.*, 1999). In this study, the authors found that IPT-A was efficacious in reducing depressive symptoms and improving social functioning and interpersonal problem solving in acutely depressed adolescents. Significantly more IPT-A treated adolescents met recovery criteria and were rated by their treating clinicians to be less depressed than their control group peers at the end of treatment. In a randomized effectiveness study of IPT-A delivered within a school based health clinic, it was found that adolescents meeting criteria for a depressive disorder (e.g. MDD, dysthymia, adjustment disorder with depressed mood) and treated with IPT-A experienced greater symptom reduction and improved overall functioning compared to their peers receiving 'treatment at usual' (Mufson *et al.*, 2004).

Rosselló & Bernal (1999) compared IPT and CBT to each other, as well as to a waiting-list control. The study was limited by the sole use of (unblinded) self-report questionnaires and small numbers. The study suggested that both treatments were significantly better than control, but that there was no significant difference in efficacy between them.

Family therapy

Although CBT and IPT-A have received the most empirical support in the literature on the treatment of child and adolescent depression, some investigators have begun to highlight the importance of family work in depression treatment (Cotrell, 2003; Dujovne *et al.*, 1995), and others have begun to develop specific family based interventions, e.g. family therapy for the treatment of depressed adolescents (FTDA (Diamond & Siqueland, 1995)) and stress busters (Asarnow *et al.*, 2002). Family interventions will likely be an area of increased investigation in years to come and at least from a clinical perspective would appear promising in the treatment of depressed youth. While family discord can be an important aetiological factor in paediatric depression, randomized controlled trials have shown family therapy for the whole family (Brent *et al.*, 1997; Harrington *et al.*, 1998) and for parents alone (Lewinsohn *et al.*, 1990) to be no more effective than control treatments.

Issues to consider in treatment of youth depression

In examining psychopharmacologic and psychotherapeutic interventions as a whole, the results are quite similar. Regardless of the type of intervention, approximately 40% of depressed youth are 'non-responders' to treatment (Keller *et al.*, 2001; Reinecke *et al.*, 1998), and of those who 'respond' to acute treatment, relapse rates within 1 year following treatment are significant (Birmaher *et al.*, 2000). The true test in discerning which forms of intervention are most efficacious in treating depressed children and adolescents involve studies which pit such interventions, whether psychopharmacological or psychotherapeutic, directly against each other in randomized controlled trials. Three types of this kind of study are beginning to emerge, studies which pit medication against medication, therapy against therapy, or medication against therapy.

Birmaher *et al.* (1996b) identify the need for controlled studies in large samples of depressed youth comparing specific classes of antidepressants, but to date, no such studies exist. Several studies, some noted above, have compared psychosocial treatments to each other. As briefly stated above, a study comparing CBT, IPT, and waiting-list control conditions in depressed Puerto Rican adolescents, for example, found both CBT and IPT to be efficacious in significantly reducing depressive symptoms when compared to waiting-list controls (Rosselló & Bernal, 1999). In this trial, however, IPT outperformed CBT in that 82% of adolescents receiving IPT were deemed 'functional' after treatment, compared to 59% of adolescents receiving CBT. Nevertheless, these data should be interpreted cautiously, as the waitlist control participants were not evaluated at follow-up, only self-report measures of depression were utilized, and co-morbidity was not assessed. Furthermore, cultural modifications were made to the treatment that could limit generalizability.

Although the above study favored IPT over CBT, Brent *et al.* (1997) report an initial advantage of CBT over SBFT and NST, however, this effect does not hold long-term (Birmaher *et al.*, 2000). As briefly stated above, in the only randomized controlled trial comparing medication with psychotherapy in the treatment of depressed youth, investigators in the Treatments for Adolescents with Depression Study (TADS) compared groups of depressed adolescents receiving medication alone (fluoxetine), psychotherapy alone (CBT), combined treatment (fluoxetine + CBT), or placebo (March *et al.*, 2004). In this landmark trial sponsored by the National Institute of Mental Health, fluoxetine combined with CBT had a response rate of 71% and was found to be superior to fluoxetine alone (63% response rate), CBT alone (43% response rate), and placebo (31% response rate) in the acute treatment of depression in adolescents. More recent studies in the USA (Clarke *et al.*, 2005) and UK (I.M. Goodyer *et al.*, unpublished data) showed no significant differences in depressive symptoms nor recovery rates between SSRI plus treatment as usual and SSRI, treatment as usual plus CBT. Melvin *et al.* (2006) compared sertraline, CBT and combined sertraline and CBT, and demonstrated that CBT was more effective than sertraline and there was no difference between combined and single treatments.

Summary

Although there is evidence concerning the effectiveness of both pharmacotherapy and psychotherapy in the treatment of childhood and adolescent depressive disorders, limited response rates for both pharmacotherapy and psychotherapy have led to the recommendation in US practice parameters for the use of 'combined' treatment (Birmaher *et al.*, 1998), a conclusion supported by the NICE guidelines which emphasize that psychopharmacologic treatment should not be undertaken without some concurrent psychotherapy (National Institute for Health and Clinical Excellence, 2005). This approach develops further credence given the severity of the costs of depression, both psychosocial and academic, as well as the psychosocial and developmental context in which depressive disorders emerge. Although the best science to date would suggest that this is perhaps the most promising route for practitioners to take in terms of offering the most efficacious treatment, much further research is needed to clarify this position. In particular, there is a need for studies that employ:

- Randomized controlled trials comparing single and combined therapies of both a pharmacologic and psychological nature within the same design;
- Diagnostic algorithms, which employ the use of multiple methods and scientifically valid and reliable measures of psychopathology, allowing for the systematic and careful definition and delineation of categories of depressed children and adolescents (e.g. MDD versus dysthymia);
- Psychotherapeutic interventions that are not only manualized but have built in checks for treatment integrity such that results are generalizable;
- Longitudinal designs that evaluate efficacy longer than 6–12 months after treatment; and
- Designs that examine the impact of development, age, gender, ethnicity, culture, and co-morbidity on the efficacy of treatment interventions.

Conclusions

There is some evidence to support the use of some of the physical and psychological treatments used for paediatric depression, particularly fluoxetine, IPT and CBT. However, this evidence is rather limited, particularly by the fact that most of the studies have been carried out on young people with non-severe depression and/or no suicidality. It is difficult to extrapolate this evidence to guide us in the treatment of the most unwell patients that we see in our clinical practice. In particular, we may find that more severely depressed patients find it more difficult to use psychological treatments; conversely more severely depressed young people may show a much greater response to antidepressants than to placebo.

In addition to trying to apply this limited evidence, it is important to take into account the views of our patients and their carers. They may be very reluctant to use medication, particularly in view of the recent concerns about side effects and suicidality. Conversely, they may not want or be able to come to a clinic for regular psychological treatment, a process that may involve hard work and the changing of ideas and behaviours. In addition, we are constrained by our resources. Significant numbers of child and adolescent psychiatry clinics do not have trained CBT therapists and very few have IPT therapists though that appears to be changing in both the UK and the USA.

Thus while it is incumbent upon us to consider evidence-based treatments, we must also consider the natural history of an episode of depression. Current evidence has shown that the median time to full remission is between 28 and 39 weeks with around 70% of patients recovered by 72 weeks (Goodyer *et al.*, 2003). Many treatments may be operating to accelerate time to recovery.

Finally there is evidence that is beginning to accumulate that dysfunctional family and friendship patterns of behaviour may prevent remission by maintaining non-depressive co-morbid disorders (Goodyer *et al.*, 1997). These deserve management in their own right, despite the fact that they have no direct effect on the cessation of depressive symptoms. This emphasizes the importance of treating the whole child in his or her social context and not just as an operational diagnosis.

With all of the above in mind, investigators should continue to develop and examine innovative treatments, for it would appear that the most efficacious treatments currently available only work for a subset of depressed youth, and some are associated with great controversy. Ultimately, the 'best' and 'most efficacious' treatment for depressive disorders in children and adolescents will likely vary with the individual child or adolescent based on age, gender, family history and presenting symptomatology, such as sleep disturbance, cognitive symptoms, school, peer and self-esteem difficulties.

The level of evidence for each of the interventions discussed in this chapter is summarized in Table 55.1.

Table 55.1. Effectiveness of treatments for depressive disorders in children and adolescents

Treatment	Form of treatment	Psychiatric disorder/ target audience	Level of evidence for efficacy	Comments
Pharmacotherapy	SSRIs	Childhood and adolescent depression	Ia	Only SSRI showing significant improvement in symptoms is fluoxetine. Much controversy about the use of SSRIs in this age group. Other SSRIs and other newer antidepressants have little or negative evidence for effectiveness
Electroconvulsive therapy	(ECT)	Childhood and adolescent depression	III	Recommendation only when depression is so severe that safety or welfare of the patient is at immediate risk
Psychotherapy	Cognitive behavioural	Childhood and adolescent depression	Ia	Meta-analyses reveal effect size from 0.41 to 1.70. Improvement in the range of somewhere between 50% and 70%
Psychotherapy	Interpersonal therapy	Childhood and adolescent depression	Ia	There are RCTs here, but caution should be used because the RCTs have all been conducted by the same group. One study showed both CBT and IPT to be better than waiting list, but CBT and IPT were equally effective
Psychotherapy	Family therapy	Families with and parents with children with childhood and adolescent depression	IV	While it is thought that the family system impacts the depression in childhood and adolescence, little empirical evidence exists to support this viewpoint

REFERENCES

American Academy of Child and Adolescent Psychiatry (2004). Practice parameter for use of electroconvulsive therapy with adolescents. *Journal of the American Academy of Child and Adolescent Psychiatry*, **43**(12), 1521–39.

American College of Neuropsychopharmacology (2004). Executive Summary: Preliminary report of the Task Force on SSRIs and suicidal behavior in youth. http://www.acnp.org/exec_summary.pdf.

Asarnow, J.R., Scott, C.V. & Mintz, J. (2002). A combined cognitive-behavioral family education intervention for depression in children: a treatment development study. *Cognitive Therapy & Research*, **26**(2), 221–9.

Baer, J.S., MacLean, M.G. & Marlatt, G.A. (1998). Linking etiology and treatment for adolescent substance abuse: toward a better match. In *New Perspectives on Adolescent Risk Behavior*, ed. R. Jessor, pp. 182–211. New York: Cambridge University Press.

Bemporad, J.R. (1988). Psychodynamic treatment of depressed adolescents. *Journal of Clinical Psychiatry*, **49** (Suppl). 26–31.

Birmaher, B., Ryan N.D., Brent, D., Dahl, R.E., Kaufman, J. & Williamson, D.E. (1996a). Child and adolescent depression: a review of the past ten years. Part I. *Journal of the American Academy of Child and Adolescent Psychiatry*, **35**, 1427–39.

Birmaher, B., Ryan, N.D., Williamson, D.E., Brent, D.A. & Kaufman, J. (1996b). Childhood and adolescent depression: a review of the past 10 years. Part II. *Journal of the American Academy of Child and Adolescent Psychiatry*, **35**, 1575–83.

Birmaher, B., Brent, D.A. & Benson, R.S. (1998). Summary of the practice parameters for the assessment and treatment of children and adolescents with depressive disorders. *Journal of American Academy of Child and Adolescent Psychiatry*, **37**, 1234–8.

Birmaher, B., Brent, D.A., Kolko, D. *et al.* (2000). Clinical outcome after short-term psychotherapy for adolescents with major depressive disorder. *Archives of General Psychiatry*, **57**, 29–36.

Brent, D.A., Holder, D., Kolko, D. *et al.* (1997). A clinical psychotherapy trial for adolescent depression comparing cognitive, family, and supportive therapy. *Archives of General Psychiatry*, **54**, 877–85.

Brent, D.A., Kolko, D., Birmaher, B., Baugher, M., Bridge, J., Roth, C. & Holder, D. (1998). Predictors of treatment efficacy in a clinical trial of three psychosocial treatments for adolescent depression. *Journal of American Academy of Child and Adolescent Psychiatry*, **37**, 906–14.

Brent, D.A. & Birmaher, B. (2004). British warnings on SSRI's questioned. *Journal of the American Academy of Child and Adolescent Psychiatry*, **43**(4), 379–80.

Clarke, G.N., Rohde, P., Lewinsohn, P.M., Hops, H. & Seeley, J.R. (1999). Cognitive-behavioral treatment of adolescent depression: Efficacy of acute group treatment and booster sessions. *Journal of American Academy of Child and Adolescent Psychiatry*, **38**, 272–9.

Clarke, G., Debar, L., Lynch, F. *et al.* (2005). A randomized effectiveness trial of brief cognitive-behavioral therapy for depressed adolescents receiving antidepressant medication. *Journal of the American Academy of Child and Adolescent Psychiatry*, **44**, 888–98.

Cohen D., Taieb O., Flament M. *et al.* (2000). Absence of cognitive impairment at long-term follow-up in adolescents treated with

ECT for severe mood disorder. *American Journal of Psychiatry*, **157**, 460–2.

Cottrell, D. (2003). Outcome studies of family therapy in child and adolescent depression. *Journal of Family Therapy*, **25**(4), 406–16.

Curry, J. F. (2001). Specific psychotherapies for childhood and adolescent depression. *Biological Psychiatry*, **49**(12), 1091–100.

Daviss, W. B., Bentivoglio, P., Racusin, R., Brown, K. M., Bostic, J. Q. & Wiley, L. (2001). Bupropion sustained release in adolescents with comorbid attention-deficit/hyperactivity disorder and depression. *Journal of the American Academy of Child and Adolescent Psychiatry*, **40**, 307–14.

Delate, T., Gelenberg, A. J., Simmons, V. A. & Motheral, B. R. (2004). Trends in the use of antidepressants in a national sample of commercially insured pediatric patients, 1998 to 2002. *Psychiatric Services*, **55**(4), 387–91.

Diamond, G. & Siqueland, L. (1995). Family therapy for the treatment of depressed adolescents. *Psychotherapy: Theory, Research, Practice, Training*, **32**, 77–90.

Dubicka, B., Hadley, S. & Roberts, C. (2006). Suicidal behaviour in youths with depression treated with new-generation antidepressants: meta-analysis. *British Journal of Psychiatry*, **189**, 393–8.

Duff, G. (2003a). Safety and efficacy of the SSRI class in the treatment of paediatric major depressive disorder. Expert Working Group on Safety of Medicines. Available at: http://www.mhra.gov.uk/news/2003.htm#ssri.

Duff, G. (2003b). Safety of Seroxat (paroxetine) in children and adolescents under 18 years – contraindication in the treatment of depressive illness. United Kingdom's Department of Health's Chairman of Committee of Safety of Medicine's message on paroxetine. Available at: http://www.mhra.gov.uk/news/2003.htm#june.

Duffett, R., Hill, P. & Lelliott, P. (1999). Use of electroconvulsive therapy in young people. *British Journal of Psychiatry*, **175**, 228–30.

Dujovne, V. F., Barnard, M. U. & Rapoff, M. A. (1995). Pharmacological and cognitive behavioral approaches in the treatment of childhood depression: a review and critique. *Clinical Psychology Review*, **15**(7), 589–611.

Emslie, G. J., Rush, A. J., Weinberg, W. A. *et al.* (1997). A double blind, randomized, placebo-controlled trial of fluoxetine in children and adolescents with depression. *Archives of General Psychiatry*, **54**, 1031–7.

Emslie, G. J., Heiligenstein, J. H. & Wagner, K. D. (2002). Fluoxetine for acute treatment of depression in children and adolescents: a placebo-controlled, randomized clinical trial. *Journal of the American Academy of Child and Adolescent Psychiatry*, **41**, 1205–15.

Fine, S., Forth, A., Gilbert, M. & Haley, G. (1991). Group therapy for adolescent depressive disorder: a comparison of social skills and therapeutic support. *Journal of American Academy of Child and Adolescent Psychiatry*, **30**, 79–85.

Fleming, J. E. & Offord, D. R. (1990). Epidemiology of childhood depressive disorders: A critical review. *Journal of American Academy of Child and Adolescent Psychiatry*, **29**, 571–80.

Garrison, C. Z., Addy, C. L. K., Jackson, K. L., McKeown, R. E. & Waller, J. L. (1992). Major depressive disorder and dysthymia in young adolescents. *American Journal of Epidemiology*, **135**, 792–802.

Gjerde, P. F. & Westenberg, P. M. (1998). Dysphoric adolescents as young adults: A prospective study of the psychological sequelae of depressed mood in adolescence. *Journal of Research on Adolescence*, **8**(3), 377–402.

Glod, C. A., Lynch, A., Flynn, E., Berkowitz, C. & Baldessarini, R. J. (2003). Open trial of bupropion SR in adolescent major depression. *Journal of Child and Adolescent Psychiatry Nursing*, **16**, 123–30.

Goodnick, P. J., Jorge, C. A., Hunter, T. & Kumar, A. M. (2000). Nefazodone treatment of adolescent depression: an open-label study of response and biochemistry. *Annals of Clinical Psychiatry*, **12**, 97–100.

Goodyer, I. M., Herbert, J., Tamplin, A., Secher, S. M. & Pearson, J. (1997). Short-term outcome of major depression: II. Life events, family dysfunction, and friendship difficulties as predictors of persistent disorder. *Journal of the American Academy of Child and Adolescent Psychiatry*, **36**, 474–80.

Goodyer, I. M., Herbert, J. & Tamplin, A. (2003). Psychoendocrine antecedents of persistent first-episode major depression in adolescents: a community-based longitudinal enquiry. *Psychological Medicine*, **33**, 601–10.

Hammad, T. A., Laughren, T. & Racoosin, J. (2006). Suicidality in pediatric patients treated with antidepressant drugs. *Archives of General Psychiatry*, **63**, 332–9.

Hammen, C. (1997). *Depression*. Hove, England: Psychology Press/Erlbaum.

Harrington, R., Kerfoot, M., Dyer, E. *et al.* (1998). Randomized trial of a home-based family intervention for children who have deliberately poisoned themselves. *Journal of the American Academy of Child and Adolescent Psychiatry*, **37**, 512–18.

Jayson, D., Wood, A., Kroll, L., Fraser, J. & Harrington, R. (1998). Which depressed patients respond to cognitive-behavioral treatment? *Journal of the American Academy of Child and Adolescent Psychiatry*, **37**, 35–9.

Jureidini, J. N., Doecke, C. J., Mansfield, P. R., Haby, M. M., Menkes, D. B. & Tonkin, A. L. (2004). Efficacy and safety of antidepressants for children and adolescents. *British Medical Journal*, **328**, 879–83.

Kaizar, E. E., Greenhouse, J. B., Seltman, H. & Kelleher, K. (2006). Do antidepressants cause suicidality in children? A Bayesian meta-analysis. *Clinical Trials*, **3**, 73–90.

Kashani, J. H., Beck, N. C., Hoeper, E. W. *et al.* (1987a). Psychiatric disorders in a community sample of adolescents. *American Journal of Psychiatry*, **144**, 584–9.

Kashani, J. H., Carlson, G. A., Beck, N. C. *et al.* (1987b). Depression, depressive symptoms, and depressed mood among a community sample of adolescents. *American Journal of Psychiatry*, **144**, 931–4.

Keller, M. B., Ryan, N. D., Strober, M. *et al.* (2001). Efficacy of paroxetine in the treatment of adolescent major depressive disorder: A randomized, controlled trial. *Journal of American Academy of Child and Adolescent Psychiatry*, **40**, 762–72.

Kerfoot, M., Harrington, R., Harrington, V., Rogers, J. & Verduyn, C. (2004). A step too far? Randomized trial of cognitive-behaviour therapy delivered by social workers to depressed adolescents. *European Child and Adolescent Psychiatry*, **13**, 92–9.

Kroll, L., Harrington, R., Jayson, D., Fraser, J. & Gowers, S. (1996). Pilot study of continuation cognitive-behavioral therapy for major depression in adolescent psychiatric patients. *Journal of the American Academy of Child and Adolescent Psychiatry*, **35**, 1156–61.

Lewinsohn, P. M., Clarke, G. N., Hops, H. *et al.* (1990). Cognitive-behavioral treatment for depressed adolescents. *Behavior Therapy*, **21**, 385–401.

Lewinsohn, P. M., Hops, H., Roberts, R. E., Seeley, J. R. & Andrew, J. A. (1993). Adolescent psychopathology, I: Prevalence and incidence of depression and other DSM-III-R disorders in high school students. *Journal of Abnormal Psychology*, **103**, 133–44.

Lewinsohn, P. M., Clarke, G. N., Seeley, J. R. & Rohde, P. (1994). Major depression in community adolescents: age at onset, episode duration, and time to recurrence. *Journal of American Academy of Child and Adolescent Psychiatry*, **33**, 809–18.

Lewinsohn, P. M. & Clarke, G. N. (1999). Psychosocial treatments for adolescent depression. *Clinical Psychology Review*, **19**(3), 329–42.

Mandoki, M. W., Tapia, M. R., Tapia, M. A., Summer, G. S. & Parker, J. L. (1997). Venlafaxine in the treatment of children and adolescents with major depression. *Psychopharmacology Bulletin*, **33**, 149–54.

March, J., Silva, S., Petrycki, S. *et al.* (2004). Fluoxetine, cognitive-behavioral therapy, and their combination for adolescents with depression: Treatment for Adolescents With Depression Study (TADS) randomized controlled trial. *Journal of the American Medical Association*, **292**, 807–20.

Marcotte, D. (1997). Treating depression in adolescence: A review of the effectiveness of cognitive-behavioral treatments. *Journal of Youth and Adolescence*, **26**(3), 273–83.

Meltzer, H., Gatward, R., Goodman, R. & Ford, T. (2003). Mental health of children and adolescents in Great Britain. *International Review of Psychiatry*, **15**, 185–7.

Melvin, G. A., Tonge, B. J., King, N. J., Heyne, D., Gordon, M. S. & Klimkeit, E. D. (2006). A comparison of cognitive-behavioural therapy, sertraline, and their combination for adolescent depression. *Journal of the American Academy of Child and Adolescent Psychiatry*, **45**, 1151–61.

MHRA (2003). http://www.mhra.gov.uk/news/2003.htm#ssri, Vol. 2004, Medicines and Healthcare products Regulatory Agency.

MHRA (2004). http://medicines.mhra.gov.uk/ourwork/monitor safequalmed/safetymessages/ssrioverview_101203.htm, Vol. 2004, Medicines and Healthcare products Regulatory Agency.

Milin, R. P., Simeon, J. & Spenst, W. P. (1999). Poster presented at the 46th Annual American Academy of Child and Adolescent Psychiatry Meeting, Chicago, IL. October 19–21. [abstract] NR67: 104–5.

Mufson, L. & Fairbanks, J. (1996). Interpersonal psychotherapy for depressed adolescents: a one year naturalistic follow-up study.

Journal of the American Academy of Child and Adolescent Psychiatry, **35**, 1145–55.

Mufson, L., Moreau, D., Weissman, M. M., Wickmaranted, P., Martin, J. & Samoilov, A. (1994). Modification of interpersonal psychotherapy with depressed adolescents (IPT-A): Phase I and II studies. *Journal of the American Academy of Child and Adolescent Psychiatry*, **33**, 695–705.

Mufson, L., Weissman, M. M., Moreau, D. & Garfinkel, R. (1999). Efficacy of interpersonal psychotherapy for depressed adolescents. *Archives of General Psychiatry*, **56**, 573–9.

Mufson, L., Dorta, K. P., Wickramarante, P., Nomura, Y., Olfson, M. & Weissman, M. (2004). A randomized effectiveness trial of interpersonal psychotherapy for depressed adolescents. *Archives of General Psychiatry*, **61**, 577–84.

National Institute for Health and Clinical Excellence. (2005). CG28 Depression in children and young people: Full guideline. http://www.nice.org.uk/pdf/cg028fullguideline.pdf.

Reinecke, M. A., Ryan, N. E. & DuBois, D. L. (1998). Cognitive-behavioral therapy of depression and depressive symptoms during adolescence: A review and meta-analysis. *Journal of the American Academy of Child and Adolescent Psychiatry*, **37**, 26–34.

Rosselló, J. & Bernal, G. (1999). The efficacy of cognitive-behavioral and interpersonal treatments for depression in Puerto Rican adolescents. *Journal of Consulting & Clinical Psychology*, **67**(5), 734–45.

Rudnick, A. (2001). Ethics of ECT for children (Letters to the Editor). *Journal of the American Academy of Child and Adolescent Psychiatry*, **40**(4), 387.

Simon, G. E., Savarino, J., Opereskalski, B. & Wang, P. S. (2006). Suicide risk during antidepressant treatment. *American Journal of Psychiatry*, **163**, 41–7.

Strober, M., Pataki, C. & DeAntonio, M. (1998). Complete remission of 'treatment resistant' severe melancholia in adolescents with phenelzine: two case reports. *Journal of Affective Disorders*, **50**, 55–8.

US Food and Drug Administration (2003). FDA statement regarding the anti-depressant Paxil for pediatric population. FDA Talking Paper, June 19. Available at: http://www.fda.gov/bbs/topics/ANSWERS/2003/ANS01230.html.

US Food and Drug Administration (2004). Suicidality in children and adolescents being treated with antidepressant medications. FDA Public Health Advisory, October 15. Available at: www.fda.gov/cder/drug/antidepressants/SSRIPHA200410.htm.

Wagner, K. D., Ambrosini, P., Rynn, M. *et al.* (2003). Efficacy of sertraline in the treatment of children and adolescents with major depressive disorder: two randomized controlled trials. *Journal of the American Medical Association*, **290**, 1033–41.

Wagner, K. D., Robb, A. S., Findling, R. L., Jin, J., Gutierrez, M. M. & Heydorn, W. E. (2004). A randomized, placebo-controlled trial of citalopram for the treatment of major depression in children and adolescents. *American Journal of Psychiatry*, **161**(6), 1079–83.

Walter, G., Koster, K. & Rey, J. M. (1999a). Electroconvulsive therapy in adolescents: experience, knowledge, and attitudes of recipients. *Journal of the American Academy of Child and Adolescent Psychiatry*, **38**, 594–9.

Walter, G., Rey, J. M. & Mitchell, P. B. (1999b). Practitioner review: electroconvulsive therapy in adolescents. *Journal of Child Psychology and Psychiatry*, **40**, 325–34.

Whittington, C. J., Kendall, T., Fonagy, P., Cottrell, D., Cotgrove, A. & Boddington, E. (2004). Selective serotonin reuptake inhibitors in childhood depression: systematic review of published versus unpublished data. *The Lancet*, **363**, 1341–5.

Wood, A., Harrington, R. & Moore, A. (1996). Controlled trial of a brief cognitive-behavioral intervention in adolescent patients with depressive disorders. *Journal of Child Psychology and Psychiatry and Allied Disciplines*, **37**, 737–46.

Zito, J. M., Safer, D. J., DosReis, S. *et al.* (2002). Rising prevalence of antidepressant treatment for US children and adolescents. *Pediatrics*, **109**, 721–7.

56

Treatment of psychoses in children and adolescents

Anthony James and Jon McClellan

Editor's note

This section discusses treatment of psychoses in children and adolescents. The psychoses here are caused by schizophrenia or bipolar disorders, and the treatment of other psychoses that occur in youth, such as in developmental disorders, is discussed elsewhere. The most effective treatments for psychoses appear to be with the antipsychotic medications, and the atypical antipsychotics are used here. The chapter on child and adolescent psychopharmacology covers in much more detail the issues that need to be considered when prescribing psychotropic medication to children. Overall, children and adolescents may be more sensitive to the extrapyramidal and the weight gain side effects when compared to their adult counterparts, and this is so even when the choice of antipsychotic medication is an atypical. Atypicals appear effective in both schizophrenia and bipolar disorder, and in bipolar disorder appear to work better when combined with mood stabilisers. Evidence for family therapy and cognitive-behavioural therapy is scant, and even the scant evidence does not provide a solid basis for effectiveness of these interventions in families or patients with either bipolar disorder or schizophrenia. ECT may be used in the most severe of the patients in this population, but ECT is much more effective in mood disorders, especially depression, than in schizophrenia or other psychotic states or disorders.

Introduction

There is a lack of researched-based evidence, particularly randomized controlled trials (RCTs), to guide the clinician in making decisions on the treatment of psychosis in children and adolescents. Although there are evidence-based treatments for the use of antipsychotic medications in other disorders (McClellan & Werry, 2003), as well as reviews and texts addressing the use of atypical medications in paediatric psychopharmacology (Findling & McNamara, 2004; Kucher, 2002; Wagner, 2004), at this time treatment decisions must be based on data extrapolated from adults, plus open trials, cases studies or clinical anecdote. Since current evidence suggests that early onset schizophrenia (EOS) is continuous with the later-onset form, adapting the adult literature is reasonable. However, developmental considerations must be taken into account given there are important differences from adults. For example early onset schizophrenia generally has a more severe course, is less treatment responsive, has more severe initial and progressive brain abnormalities (Jacobsen et al., 1998), and may have a higher genetic loading (Nicolson et al., 2000).

Pharmacological treatment

Schizophrenia

Both the NICE (National Institute for Clinical Excellence, 2002) guidelines for adults developed in the UK, and Practice Guidelines for the Treatment of Patients with Schizophrenia developed by the American Psychiatric Association (APA, 2004) advocate the use of second generation antipsychotics as first line treatment for first-episode schizophrenia. Clozapine was recommended for treatment resistant cases (inadequate response or unacceptable side effects with two antipsychotics, one being atypical, each used for a minimum of 6–8 weeks). Atypicals are thought to have less extrapyramidal side effects, and to be more effective against negative symptoms, and in general are better tolerated than the traditional antipsychotics. There are conflicting views on whether the newer atypicals are, however, more effective in equivalent doses.

Cambridge Textbook of Effective Treatments in Psychiatry, ed. Peter Tyrer and Kenneth R. Silk. Published by Cambridge University Press.

Table 56.1. Randomized controlled–trials (RCTs) of antispychotic medication in the treatment of schizophrenia in children and adolescents

Study	Age (years)	Numbers	Drug dose mean (SD) mg/day	Trial	Outcome P value
Paillere-Martinot et al., 1995	$20^* \pm 4$	10 amisulpride 10 placebo	50	Double-blind 6 weeks	↓BPRS $P = 0.04$ ↓SANS $P = 0.02$ ↓SAPS $P = 0.02$ Ami > Placebo
Kumra et al., 1996	14.0 ± 2.3	10 Clozapine 11 Haloperidol	Cloz 176 ± 149 Hal 16 ± 8	Double-blind 6 weeks	↓BPRS $P = 0.04$ ↓SANS $P = 0.02$ ↓SAPS $P = 0.02$ Cloz > Hal
Sikich et al., 2004	14.8 ± 2.8	19 Risperidone 16 Olanzapine 7 Haloperidol	Ris 3.3 ± 1.5 Olan 12.3 ± 4.5 Hal 5.3 ± 1.7	Double-blind 8 weeks plus extension	↓BPRS $P = 0.001$ Ris ↓BPRS $P = 0.001$ Olan ↓PBRS $P = 0.01$ Hal
Shaw et al., 2006	11.7 ± 2.3 Cloz vs. 12.8 ± 2.4 Olan	12 Clozaril 12 Olanzapine		Double-blind 8 weeks with 2-year open follow-up	↓SANS $P = 0.04$ Cloz > Olan; both Cloz and Oln ↓SAPS ↓SANS;↓ GGI-S ↓ BPRS-24
Mozes et al., 2006	11.1 ± 1.5	12 Risperidone 12 Olanzapine	Ris 1.6 ± 1.0 Olan 8.8 ± 4.4	Open trial 12 weeks	↓ PANSS $P < 0.001$ similar efficacy but completion, rates Ris 69% Olan 91%

There has been a largely negative Cochrane review (Geddes *et al.*, 2000) as well as a more recent positive meta-analysis (Davis *et al.*, 2003). A recent systematic review and meta-analysis of 15 studies of antipsychotics in children an adolescents (up to the year 2003) (Armenteros *et al.*, 2006) showed an average response in 8 studies employing atypicals of 55.7% compared to 72.3% in the 13 studies using typicals. The difference was significant at a trend level ($z = 1.65$ $P < 0.10$) with an effect size d 0.36 in favour of the typicals. The review was, however, limited by the methodological quality of the studies, which included only two RCTs of typical medications – loxapine (Pool *et al.*, 1978) and haloperidol (Spencer *et al.*, 1992). The more recent RCTs for the atypicals were not included. The consensus appears to be that atypicals or second generation antipsychotics may be as effective, except for clozapine which is superior but which is reserved for resistant cases because of the risk of agranulocystosis.

In this youth age group, there are only two RCTs involving antipsychotics for the treatment of schizophrenia. One trial demonstrated a superiority of clozapine over haloperidol (Kumra *et al.*, 1996), while Shaw *et al.* (2006) demonstrated a superiority of clozapine over olanzapine for negative symptoms, but with more adverse side effects (Table 56.1). In addition, Sikich *et al.* (2004), found risperidone, olanzapine and haloperidol to be similarly effective for youth with an array of early onset psychotic disorders,

but the group across all the medications had greater weight gain and extrapyramidal side effects than typically seen with adults (McConville & Sorter, 2004). An RCT of low dose amisulpiride versus placebo involving young adults (mean age 20 years (SD 4)) demonstrated a beneficial effect on negative symptoms with the active medication (Paillere-Martinot *et al.*, 1995).

There is a large publicly funded multi-site RCT under way, 'Treatment of Early Onset Schizophrenia Spectrum Disorders' (TEOSS). TEOSS was designed to compare the effectiveness and safety of molindone, risperidone and olanzapine in youth with schizophrenia spectrum disorders, and will be completed in 2007. However, although the blind is not yet broken, it is important to note that the olanzapine arm was prematurely discontinued due to excessive weight gain (Sikich *et al.*, 2006).

At the time that this chapter was originally written, there were ten open trials for clozapine ($n = 216$), 13 open trials for risperidone ($n = 152$), seven open trials for olanzapine ($n = 158$), and five open trials for quetiapine ($n = 55$) (Table 56.2). There are no open trials for ziprasidone or aripiprazole. All of the open trials described positive responses. A preliminary study of 24 adolescents with first episode schizophrenia did not demonstrate an association with treatment response in those with repeat alleles (>7) polymorphism on the dopamine receptor DRD4 gene (Zalsman *et al.*, 2003b), although the small sample size limits the findings. Psychopharmacogenetics may become an important aspect of planned treatments in the future.

Bipolar disorder

For bipolar disorder, an RCT comparing adjunctive treatment (DelBello *et al.*, 2002) showed that quetiapine 450 mg/day and divalproate (20 mg/kg) were more effective than divalproate and placebo (F 1.27 = 5.0, P = 0.03). Quetiapine (400–600 mg/day) and divalproex (serum level 80–120 μg/l) are equally effective, although quetiapine had a quicker onset of action (DelBello *et al.*, 2006). The evidence base for the use of lithium in youths is, however, limited, with only two RCTs – of lithium use adolescent mania and comorbid substance abuse (Geller *et al.*, 1998), and lithium discontinuation (Kafantaris *et al.*, 2004). A large open trial of lithium (Kafantaris *et al.*, 2003) showed that lithium was efficacious in treating psychotic mania in combination with antipsychotic drugs. The antipsychotic drugs, quetiapine (DelBello *et al.*, 2002, 2006) olanzapine (Frazier *et al.*, 2001), risperidone (Frazier *et al.*, 1999) and aripiprazole (Biederman *et al.*, 2005) appear effective in treating juvenile mania, although combination therapy, of an antipsychotic agent and a mood stabilizer, is likely to be necessary, especially in those with psychosis. In an open trial of 29 patients, a combination of lithium and an antipsychotic (haloperidol) produced a 64% response rate after 4 weeks of treatment; however, relapse was common on discontinuation of the antipsychotic with only 29% (8/29) remaining stable (Kafantaris *et al.*, 2001). The effect of psychotic symptoms in a manic presentation is not clear with the finding from an RCT study of lithium discontinuation, which showed no difference in relapse rates between those with and without psychotic features (Kafantaris *et al.*, 2004).

Early intervention

There has been a tremendous expansion of interest in the area of intervening early in disorders which psychotic features (both bipolar disorder as well as schizophrenia) despite reservations over false positives and unnecessary stigmatization. Prodromal detection and intervention remains controversial particularly in view of the lack of clear evidence of biological and possibly cognitive deterioration being linked to duration of untreated psychosis. Nevertheless, prevention of psychosocial deterioration seems a worthwhile goal (McConville & Sorter, 2004).

A Cochrane review in 2004 (Marshall & Lockwood, 2004) suggested benefit for early intervention studies although results from ongoing trials are needed to allow more definitive analyses. The greater acceptability and lower risk profile of atypicals has encouraged their use in prodromal studies involving young subjects less than 35 years old. An early intervention study in high risk cases of 59 young persons who were randomly allocated to CBT (n = 29) or combination of CBT and low dose risperidone (mean 1.3 mg/day) (n = 31), showed that at six months fewer in the group receiving active interventions progressed to psychosis ((3/31) 9.7% vs. (10/28) 36%; P = 0.03) (McGorry *et al.*, 2002). The effect wore off after discontinuation, and this suggested that the intervention may delay, but not prevent, the development of psychosis. A further small prodromal study of four high risk and six first episode adolescents with schizophrenia (Cannon *et al.*, 2002) using 1.0 mg – 1.8 mg/day of risperidone in a 8–12 week open trial showed a significant 30% reduction in thought disorder and a 100% improvement in verbal learning. The benefits of active intervention in the treatment of psychosis were shown in a Dutch study of 76 adolescents and young adults who had a 15.5% relapse rate during the trial period followed by a 52% relapse rate over the next 60 months (Linszen *et al.*, 2001). A naturalistic study of 50 adolescents with prodromal symptoms or in the prepsychotic stage treated with olanzapine or risperidone for a 1 year showed considerable improvement on a number of measures (Cornblatt *et al.*, 2000). The PRIME study, a multi-centre study involving a double-blind clinical trial of olanzapine versus placebo for prodromal symptomatic patients (n = 60, mean age 17.8, SD.4.8) found 16.1% of subjects treated with olanzapine converted to psychosis vs. 37.9% of those receiving placebo. Although the hazard ratio for conversion was 2.5 greater in the placebo group, the result was not statistically significant due to the low power of the study. Those treated with olanzapine gained on average 8.79 kg (SD 9.0) vs. 0.3 kg (SD. 4.2) in the placebo group (McGlashan *et al.*, 2006).

It has been suggested that atypical antipsychotics may be neuroprotective, possibly by releasing neuroprotective proteins, i.e. brain-derived neurotroptic factor (BDNF), or by altering gene expression enhancing cholinergic transmission, or inducing neurogenesis (McConville & Sorter, 2004). Longitudinal neuroimaging studies, notably in subjects with treatment-resistant childhood-onset schizophrenia (Rapoport, 2004b), show a loss of grey matter in adolescence, which did not appear to be affected by the use of atypical drugs. These changes may represent the neurodevelopmental progression of the disorder against the backdrop of normal brain development. Thus, although medication status was not correlated with MRI findings, treatment may still be protective at the neuronal level. There is some evidence in adults that suggests a protective effect for antipsychotics (Lieberman

Table 56.2. Open-trials of antipsychotic medication in the treatment of schizophrenia in children and adolescents

(a) Clozapine

Study	Age (years)	Numbers	Drug dose mean (SD) mg/day	Trial	Outcome P value
Clozapine					
Siefen & Remschmidt, 1986	18.1(57% <18)	21	Clozapine 352 mg/day (75–800)	133 days	80% improved
Schmidt et al., 1989	10–21(16.8)	57 (53 scz, 2 = mood, 2 = PDD)	Clozapine 285 mg (75–800)	311 days	88% improved, 7% no change, 5% worse
Piscitelli et al., 1994	6–18(14.1)	11	Clozapine 350 mg	6 weeks	↓ BPRS, BHS
Reimschmidt et al., 1994	11–18	36	Clozapine Mean dose 330 mg/day (range 50–800 mg/day)	Open trial 154 days	3 patients no response 6 patients discontinued treatment 27 patients notable symptomatic improvement
Frazier et al., 1994	12–18	11	Clozapine 330 mg (125–900)	6 weeks	> 50% improved BPRS, CGAS, BHS, SAPS, SANS, AIMS
Levkovitch et al., 1994	14–17(16.6)	13	Clozapine 240 mg	154 days	BPRS 77% improved
Abczynska et al., 1995	NA	31	Clozapine 240 mg	NA	Improved
Schulz et al., 1996	14–22	20	Clozapine 307 mg (75–600)	30 weeks	↑
Turetz et al., 1997	9–13	11	Clozapine 227.3 mg/day (s.d. 34.4)	Open trial 16 weeks	Symptoms ↓ in BPRS and PANSS especially positive symptoms
Kumra et al., 1998	13.6 ± 1.5	15	Clozapine 317 ± 147 mg/day	Open label 8 weeks	8/15 53% responders

(b) Olanzapine and quetiapine

Study	Age (years)	Numbers	Drug dose mean (SD) mg/day	Trial	Outcome P value
Olanzapine					
Kumra et al.,1998	15.3 mean range 6–18	8	Olanzapine 17.5 ± 2.3 mg (12.5–20)	Open label 8 weeks	17%↓ BPRS total score 27% ↓Negative symptoms 1% ↓ Positive symptoms
Sholevar et al., 2000	6–13	15	Olanzapine 2.5 –5 mg/day	12 days	67% moderate or greater improvement
Bardenstien et al., 2000	17.3 mean 16–18	16	Olanzapine 5–15 mg/day	6 weeks open trial	37% ↓ PANSS ↓CGI
Frazier et al., 2001	5–14	23 bipolar	Olanzapine 2.5- 20 mg/day	Open label trial 8 weeks	Response rate 61% (> 30% ↓ in Y-MRS) $P < 0.001$
Mozes et al., 2003	12.5 ± 1.1 11–14.	9	Olanzapine 5 mg on day 5 10 mg in week 3 Six patients – 20 mg in week 5. Average dose 15.6 mg ± 4.6	Open Label 12 weeks	↓ BPRS 32% p = 0.05 ↓ PANSS 21% ns. Improvement maintained at 1 year in 8 patients. Side effects were mild
Findling et al., 2003a	13.8 ± 1.5 12–17	16	Olanzapine 2.5 mg increased to 20 mg	Open Label 8 weeks	↓ PANSS,CGI and CGAS ↓ in both positive and negative symptoms $P < 0.0005$
Ross et al., 2003	6–15	20	Olanzapine Treating clinician was free to vary or discontinue dosing and use additional medication	Open label 1 year	BPRS-C Positive symptoms ↓ by 6 weeks BPRS-C Negative symptoms ↓ after 1 year 74% of subjects treatment responders with greater than 20% reduction in total BPRS-C and impairment mild or better $P < 0.004$
Dittmann et al., 2003	12–21	96	Olanzapine 14.2 ± 4.7 mg/day	Open label 6 weeks	↓ BPRS $P < 0.01$ CGI $P < 0.01$

Table 56.2. (cont.)

Study	Age (years)	Numbers	Drug dose mean (SD) mg/day	Trial	Outcome P value
Quetiapine					
McConville et al., 2000	12.3–15.9	10	Quetiapine 50 mg increasing to 800 mg /day	23 days	↓ BPRS, SANS, CGI $P < 0.001$
Shaw et al., 2001	15.1 ± 2.2 13–15	15	Quetiapine mean dose 467 mg/day (300–800 mg)	Open trial 8 weeks	↓ BPRS, CGI, PANSS, Y-MRS $P < 0.001$

(c) Risperidone

Study	Age (years)	Numbers	Drug dose mean (SD) mg/day	Trial	Outcome P value
Risperidone					
Armenteros et al., 1997	11–18	10	Risperidone: 2.0 mg/day followed by 1.0 mg increments. Doses ranged from 4–10 mg/day (mean 6.6 mg)	Open pilot study 6 weeks	↓ PANSS, BPRS and CGI $P < 0.007$
Hrdlicka et al., 1998	14–18 mean 15.8	11	Mean 3.5 mg/day		CGI good response in 63%
Drtilkova, 1999	13–17	16	Children 2.6 mg/day, adolescents 3.8 mg/day	Open trial 5–8 weeks	↓ PANSS, and CGI 75% improvement
Kaleda et al., 2000	16–20	56	Risperidone 4–11 mg b.i.d (mean 5.6 mg) Haloperidol 4.5–20 mg b.i.d (mean 11.5 mg)	Open comparative 3 months	Ris: (GCI) 40% very much improvement, 53.3% much improvement, 6.6% minimal improvement. Hal: 19.3% very much improvement, 30.7% much, 26.9% minimal. PANSS positive ↓ 57.7% Ris ↓ 42.1% Hal PANSS negative ↓ 45.2% Ris ↓19.7% Hal 30% improvement in thought and behaviour disturbance
Cannon et al., 2002	10	10	Risperidone 1.0 –1.8 mg/day	8–12 week open trial	PANSS ↓28% $P < 0.01$ BPRS ↓30.11% $P < 0.01$ CGI↓31.36% $P < 0.01$
Zalsman et al., 2003	15.5–20 mean 17.3 ± 1.3	11	Risperidone 3.1 ± 1.6 mg/day	Open label 6 weeks	Ineffective in treatment of negative signs on PANSS

PANSS Positive and Negative Syndrome Scale for Schizophrenia.
BHS Bunney–Hamburg Scale.
BPRS Brief Psychiatric Rating Scale.
CGI Clinical Global Impression.
Y-MRS Young Mania Rating Scale.

et al., 2001). Clinically, atypical agents are associated with cognitive improvement in adults (Harvey et al., 2003), with some similar findings in adolescents (Martsenkovsky et al., 2002; Sikich et al., 2001).

Side effects of psychopharmacologic intervention

The pharmacokinetics of olanzapine, quetiapine and risperidone are not substantially different in youths from adults, but the side effect profile does differ with higher rates of extrapyramidal side effects for risperidone and greater weight gain for risperidone and particularly olanzapine. Haloperidol, olanzapine, and risperidone appear equally effective, but haloperidol produces more extrapyramidal side effects (Gothelf et al., 2003). A retrospective study of 97 children and adolescents treated with atypicals showed 4% of patients treated with quetiapine developed extrapyramidal side effects (EPS), compared to 7% for olanzapine and 19% for risperidone (Grcevich et al., 2001). The sensitivity to extrapyramidal side effects is age related, probably due to the greater number of D_1 and D_2 receptors in the striatum in infancy; the number of these receptors reduces over time (Lewis, 1998). There are reports of weight gains of over 40 kg in adolescents taking clozapine (Theisen et al., 2001). A systematic review of antipsychotic medications in youths (Armenteros et al., 2006) found weight gain was greater with atypicals −4.5 kg vs. 1.2 kg for the older typicals. There are also reports of hyperglycemia and hypercholesterolemia (Bloch et al., 2003) in juveniles taking atypicals and cases of induced diabetes as well (Koller et al., 2004). However, an epidemiological case-controlled study (involving only 20 out of 3147 subjects less than 20 years) found an increased risk of developing diabetes for olanzapine but not risperidone (Koro et al., 2002). Hyperprolactinaemia is seen with risperidone, less so with olanzapine, and was not found in the one report examining quetiapine (Shaw et al., 2001). Longer-term studies with children with various diagnoses show that the initial hyperprolactinaemia seen with risperidone decreases over time, eventually returning to near normal levels (Findling et al., 2003b).

The side effects of clozapine include hyper-salivation, sedation, cardiac abnormalities and seizures (Kumra et al., 1996; Wehmeier et al., 2004) and potentially fatal agranulocystosis. Thus there is the need for regular blood level monitoring. The pharmacokinetics of clozapine is somewhat different in children and adolescents with higher levels of the active metabolite, norclozapine, than clozapine (Frazier et al., 2003). This is the reverse of the situation in adults where norclozapine levels are 10%–25% less than clozapine levels. Measurement of drug levels may be helpful, as clinical response correlates with clozapine levels, while adverse effects vary with norclozapine levels. There

are reports of myocarditis, pericarditis and cardiomyopathy associated with clozapine use, however, systematic review of its use with 36 youths showed one case of pericarditis (Wehmeier et al., 2004). Cardiac monitoring including routine use of an ECG is necessary.

Family therapy

In adults, numerous trials support the effectiveness of psychoeducational family interventions for reducing relapse and reducing symptom severity (APA, 2004). The length of therapy may be as important as the approach (Pilling et al., 2002a). Although family therapy is often used with families of adolescents with psychotic disorders, there is very limited research evidence, with only one trial of family therapy. In a small Norwegian trial (Rund et al., 1994), 12 patients (9 with schizophrenia, 1 with schizophreniform psychosis, 1 schizotypal personality disorder and 1 with schizoaffective disorder) were compared with 12 patients (all 12 with schizophrenia) who had received treatment as usual from the same hospital previously. All had been hospitalized at the time of entry into the study and followed up after 2 years. The intervention group received family meetings, at first weekly then reduced to monthly, as well as parent and patient problem-solving therapies, welfare support, housing, and home visits. There were no significant differences between groups in terms of change in GAS score or time spent in hospital (53 weeks (experimental) versus 69 weeks (control)) but the overall cost was $30 000 (US) less per patient in the experimental group, despite the extra input. Youth with poor premorbid psychosocial functioning benefited the most from the psychoeducational interventions. Clinical improvement was associated with the families expressed emotion ratings changing from high to low.

A 9-year longitudinal study of family therapy for young persons with schizophrenia (15–26 years), following an initial inpatient treatment, showed no effect on relapse rates or on levels of expressed emotion, and it seemed that the family therapy was less effective in the younger group (Lenior et al., 2002). A pilot study of adolescent patients with schizophrenia and bipolar disorder (S. Browning, unpublished data) that compared family therapy (10 patients), CBT (9 patients) and inpatient treatment as usual (9 patients), showed a trend for greater improvement in both active intervention groups.

Miklowitz and colleagues (2004) describe an open treatment trial of adjunctive family-focused psychoeducational treatment for bipolar adolescents (FFT-A) The family focused psychoeducation treatment (FFT-A) is administered in 21 outpatient sessions and consists of psychoeducation, communication enhancement training, and problem solving skills training. A trial with 20 bipolar adolescents (11 boys, 9 girls; mean age 14.8 +/−1.6) found that the combination of FFT-A and mood stabilizing medications was associated with improvements in depression symptoms, mania symptoms, and behavior problems over 1 year. The results of an ongoing larger RCT are awaited.

CBT

For adults, there is accumulating evidence for the effectiveness of CBT in schizophrenia in the acute and chronic stages (Pilling *et al.*, 2002b). A sub-analysis of a large CBT trial in schizophrenia (SoCRATES) (Tarrier *et al.*, 2004) showed a benefit of supportive counselling over CBT for those under 21 years of age (Haddock *et al.*, 2006). Indeed, younger subjects fared worse and were more difficult to engage in psychological therapies. There are no reported RCTs of CBT in this age group, although a pilot study of HIT (hallucination focused integrative treatment) applied cognitive techniques and coping skills, reduced voices and anxiety in 65% of 14 adolescents with schizophrenia (Jenner *et al.*, 2001).

Cognitive remediation (Ueland *et al.*, 2004) does not appear effective in this age range or even more generally (Pilling *et al.*, 2002b), nor is there any evidence of efficacy of social skills training (Pilling *et al.*, 2002b).

ECT

ECT is rarely used in adolescents. There are no RCTs, but case series and reports support its use in severe life-threatening psychotic depression or treatment resistant mania. The response rate for psychotic disorders is 50%–60% (Ghaziuddin *et al.*, 2004). The Practice Parameter of the American Academy of Child and Adolescent Psychiatry recommends ECT for adolescents when there is lack of response to at least two trials of pharmacological treatment or severe symptoms preclude waiting for a response to pharmacological treatment (Ghaziuddin *et al.*, 2004). In general in adults, ECT is found to be more effective in mood than in schizophrenic disorders.

Conclusions

As in adults, the mainstay of the treatment of psychosis in this age group is pharmacological. There is, however, a paucity of evidence and further RCTs are needed, particularly in view of the differing patient characteristics and experience of adverse effects in younger patients, A promising area is the development and evaluation of the combination of drug treatments with other therapeutic modalities such as CBT.

The level of evidence for each of the interventions discussed is summarized in Table 56.3.

Table 56.3. Effectiveness of treatments for psychoses in children and adolescents

Treatment	Form of treatment	Psychiatric disorder/ target audience	Level of evidence for efficacy	Comments
Psychopharmacology	Atypical antipsychotics	Youth with schizophrenia	Ia	As effective as typical antipsychotics. May cause more weight gain in youth than adults. Improvement in BPRS< SANS, SAPS
Psychopharmacology	Combined antipsychotic and mood stabiliser	Youth with bipolar illness	Ib	Youth appear to do better on a combination of an antipsychotic and a mood stabilizer, especially if psychotic features present
Psychopharmacology	Early pharmacologic intervention	Psychoses	IIb	Intervention appears to be effective but little evidence if early intervention impacts long-term course and/or ability to remain well after intervention is stopped
Family therapy	Family therapy and other psychoeducational programmes to families	Families of patients with schizophrenia	IIa	Some but not consistent evidence of family therapy being better than TAU though not necessarily better than CBT
Psychotherapy	Cognitive-behavioural therapy	Schizophrenia	III	No real methodologically sound studies and evidence for or against not very strong though some evidence that younger children may do worse in psychological therapies

REFERENCES

Abczynska, M., Kazmirek, Z., Syguda, J. & Terminska, T. (1995). Own experience (1989–1994) in the treatment of adolescent schizophrenic paranoid syndromes with Leponex produced by Sandoz Company. *Psychiatric Policy*, **29**, 79–85.

American Psychiatric Association (APA) (2004). Practice guideline for the treatment of patients with schizophrenia., Second Edition. *American Journal of Psychiatry*, **161**(Suppl. 2), 1–56.

Armenteros, J. L., Whitaker, A. H., Welikson, M., Stedge, D. J. & Gorman J. (1997). Risperidone in Adolescents with Schizophrenia: an Open Pilot Study. *Journal of American Academy Child Adolescent Psychiatry*, **36**, 694–700.

Armenteros, J. & Davies, M. (2006). Antipsychotics in early-onset schizophrenia. Systematic review and meta-analysis. *European Journal of Child and Adolescent Psychiatry*, **15**, 141–8.

Bardenstein, L., Kurashov, A. & Mozhginski Y. (2000). Olanzapine in the treatment of first-episode schizophrenia in adolescents. *International Journal of Neuropsychopharmacology*, **3**(Suppl. 1).

Biederman, J., McDonnell, M., Wozniack, J. *et al.* (2005). Aripiprazole in the treatment of pediatric bipolar disorder: a systematic chart review. *CNS Spectrum*, **10**, 141–8.

Bloch, Y., Vardi, O., Mendlovic, S., Levkovitz, Y., Gothelf, D. & Ratzoni, G. (2003). Hyperglycaemia from olanzapine treatment in adolescents. *Journal of Child and Adolescent Psychopharmacology*, **13**, 97–102.

Cannon, T. D., Huttunen, M. O., Dahlstorm, M., Larmo, I., Rasanen, P. & Juriloo, A. (2002). Antipsychotic drug treatment in the prodromal phase of schizophrenia. *American Journal of Psychiatry*, **159**(7), 1230–2.

Cornblatt, B., Ditkowsky, K., Becker, J., Pappadopulos, E., Coscia, D. & Obuchowski, M. (2000). The Hillside RAPP clinic: why the sudden interesting the schizophrenia prodrome? *Biological Psychiatry*, **47**, 29S.

Davis, J., Chen, N. & Glick, I. D. (2003). A meta-analysis of the efficacy of second generation antipsychotics: *Archives of General Psychiatry*, **60**, 553–64.

DelBello, M., Schwiers, M. L., Rosenberg, H. L. & Strakowski, S. M. (2002). A double-blind, randomized, placebo-controlled study of quetiapine as adjunctive treatment for adolescent mania. *Journal of the American Academy of Child and Adolescent Psychiatry*, **41**, 1216–23.

DelBello, M., Kowatch, R., Adler, C. *et al.* (2006). A double-blind randomized pilot study comparing quetiapine and divalproex for adolescent mania. *Journal of the American Academy of Child and Adolescent Psychiatry*, **45**, 305–13.

Dittmann, R. W., Hagenah, U., Junghanss, J. *et al.* (2003). Efficacy and safety of olanzapine in adolescents with schizophrenia. Presented at the 50th Congress of the American Academy of Child and Adolescent Psychiatry, Oct 14–19 2003, Florida, US, p. 165.

Drtilkova, I. (1999). Risperidone in children and adolescents with schizophrenic disorders. *Ceska: A Slovenska Psychiatrie*, **95** (Suppl.), 22–9.

Findling, R. L. & McNamara, N. K. (2004). Atypical antipsychotics in the treatment of children and adolescents: clinical applications. *Journal of Clinical Psychiatry*, **65** (Suppl. 6), 30–44.

Findling, R. L., Kusumakar, V., Danemen, D., Moshang, T., De Smedt, G. & Binder, C. (2003a). Prolactin levels during long-term risperidone treatment in children and adolescents. *Journal of Clinical Psychiatry*, **64**(11), 1362–9.

Findling, R. L., McNamara, N. K., Youngstorm, E. A., Branicky, L. A., Demeter, C. A. & Schulz, C. (2003b). A prospective, open-label trail of olanzapine in adolescents with schizophrenia. *Journal of American Academy Child Adolescent Psychiatry*, **42**(2), 170–5.

Frazier, J. A., Gordon, C. T., McKenna, K., Lenane, M. C., Jih, D. & Rapoport J. L. (1994). An open trail of clozapine in 11 adolescents with childhood-onset schizophrenia. *Journal of the American Academy of Child and Adolescent Psychiatry*, **33**(5), 658–63.

Frazier, J. A., Meyer, M. C., Biederman, J. *et al.* (1999). Risperidone treatment for juvenile bipolar disorder: a retrospective chart review. *Journal of American Academy Child Adolescent Psychiatry*, **38**(8), 960–5.

Frazier, J. A., Biederman, J., Tohen, M. *et al.* (2001). A prospective open-label treatment trial of olanzapine monotherapy in children and adolescents with bipolar disorder. *Journal of Child and Adolescent Psychopharmacology*, **11**(3), 239–50.

Frazier, J. A., Cohen, L. G., Jacobsen, L. *et al.* (2003). Clozapine pharmacokinetics in children and adolescents with childhood-onset schizophrenia. *Journal of Clinical Psychopharmacology*, **23**(1), 87–91.

Geddes, J., Freemantle, N., Harrison, P. & Bebbington, P. (2000). Atypical antipsychotics in the treatment of schizophrenia: systematic overview and meta-regression analysis. *British Medical Journal*, **321**, 1371–6.

Geller, B., Cooper, T., Sun, K. *et al.* (1998). Double-blind and placebo-controlled study of lithium for adolescent bipolar disorder with secondary substance dependency. *Journal of the American Academy of Child and Adolescent Psychiatry*, **37**, 171–8.

Ghaziuddin, N., Kutcher, S. P. & Knapp P. and American Academy of Child and Adolescent Psychiatry Work Group on Quality Issues (2004). Summary of the practice parameter for the use of electroconvulsive therapy with adolescents. *Journal of American Academy Child Adolescent Psychiatry*, **43**(1), 119–22.

Gothelf, D., Apter, A., Reidman, J. *et al.* (2003). Olanzapine, risperidone and haloperidol in treatment of adolescent patients with schizophrenia. *Journal of Neutral Transmission*, **110**(5), 545–60.

Grcevich, S., Melamed, L. & Richards, R. (2001). Comparative side effects of atypical antipsychotics in children and adolescents. Presented at the 8th biennial meeting of the International Congress on Schizophrenia Research: April 28-May. Whistler, Canada.

Haddock, G., Lewis, S., Bentall, R., Dunn, G., Drake, R. & Tarrier, N. (2006). Influence of age on outcome of psychological treatments in first-episode psychosis. *Britsih Journal of Psychiatry*, **188**, 250–6.

Harvey, P. D., Green, M. F., McGurk, S. R. & Meltzer, H. Y. (2003). Changes in cognitive functioning with risperidone and olanzapine treatment: a large-scale, double-blind, randomized study. *Psychopharmacology*, **169**, 404–11.

Hrdlicka, M., Propper, L., Vinar, O., *et al*. (1998). Risperidone in the acute treatment of schizophrenia in adolescents. *Ceska: A Slovenska Psychiatrie*, **94**, 131–6.

Jacobsen, L. K. & Rapoport, J. L. (1998). Research update: childhood-onset schizophrenia: implications, of clinical and neurobiological research. *Journal of Child Psychology and Psychiatry*, **39**, 202–10.

Jenner, J A. & van de Willage, G. (2001). HIT, hallucination focused integrative treatment as early intervention in psychotic adolescents with auditory hallucinations: a pilot study. *Acta Psychiatrica Scandinavica*, **101**, 148–52.

Kafantaris, V., Coletti, D., Dicker, R., Padula, G. & Kane, J M. (2001). Adjunctive antipsychotic treatment of acute mania in adolescents with bipolar psychosis. *Journal of the American Academy of Child and Adolescent Psychiatry*, **40**, 1448–56.

Kafantaris, V., Coletti, D., Dicker, R., Padula, G. & Kane, J. M. (2003). Lithium treatment of acut mania in adolescent: a large open trial. *Journal of the American Academy of Child and Adolescent Psychiatry*, **432**, 1038–45.

Kafantaris, V., Coletti, D., Dicker, R. *et al*. (2004). Lithium treatment of acute mania in adolescents: a placebo-controlled discontinuation study. *Journal of the American Academy of Child and Adolescent Psychiatry*, **43**, 984–93.

Kaleda, V. G., Oleichik, I. V., Artioukh, V. V. & Naddour, S. A. (2000). Risperidone vs Haloperidol in the therapy of adolescent schizophrenia and schizoaffective disorders: an open comparative medium-term efficacy and tolerability study: *The International Journal of Neuropsychopharmacology*, **3** (Suppl.1), S99–S100.

Koller, E. A., Cross, J. T. & Schneider. B. (2004). Risperidone-associated diabetes mellitus in children: *Pediatrics*, **113**(2), 421.

Koro, C. F., Fedder, D. O., L'Italien, G. J. *et al*. (2002). Assessment of independent effect of olanzapine and risperidone on risk of diabetes among patients with schizophrenia: population based nested case-control study. *British Medical Journal*, **325**, 243–7.

Kucher, S. P. (2002). *Practical Child and Adolescent Psychopharamcology*. Cambridge: Cambridge University Press.

Kumra, S., Frazier, J. A., Jacobsen, L. K. *et al*. (1996). Childhood-onset schizophrenia: a double-blind clozapine-haloperidol comparison. *Archives of General Psychiatry*, **53**, 1090–7.

Kumra, S., Jacobsen, L. K., Lenane, M. *et al*. (1998). Childhood onset schizophrenia: an open label study of olanzapine in adolescents. *Journal of American Academy Child Adolescent Psychiatry*, **37**(4), 377–85.

Lenior, M. E., Dingemans, P. M., Schene, A. H., Hart, A. A. & Linszen, D. H. (2002). The course of parental expressed emotion and psychotic episode after family intervention in recent-onset schizophrenia: A longitudinal study. *Schizophrenic Research*, **57**(2–3), 183–90.

Lieberman, J. A., Perkins, D., Belger, A. *et al*. (2001). The early stages of schizophrenia: speculations on pathogenesis, pathophysiology, and therapeutic approaches. *Biological Psychiatry*, **50**, 884–97.

Levkovitch, Y., Kaysar, N., Kronnenberg, Y. Hagai, H. & Gaoni, B. (1994). Clozapine for schizophrenia (letter). *Journal of Academy of Child and Adolescent Psychiatry*, **20**, 697–712.

Lewis, R. (1998). Typical and atypical antipsychotics in adolescent schizophrenia: efficacy, tolerability, and differential sensitivity to extrapyramidal symptoms. *Canadian Journal of Psychiatry*, **43**, 596–604.

Linszen, D. Dingemans. P. & Lenior, M.(2001). Early intervention and a five year follow up in young adults with a short duration of untreated psychosis: ethical implications. *Schizophrenia Research*, **51**(1), 55–61.

Marshall, M. & Lockwood, A. (2004). Early intervention for psychosis (Cochrane Review). In *The Cochrane Library*, **2**. Chichester, UK: Wiley.

Martsenkovsky, I., Bikshaeva, Y., Martsenskovska, I., Drughinska, O., Rudzinska, M. & Prokopenko, N. (2002). Risperidone improves cognitive function in adolescents with first episode of schizophrenia. Abstract 3rd International Conference on Early Psychosis, Denmark, pp. 25–8.

McClellan, J. M. & Werry, J. S. (2003). Evidence-based treatments in child and adolescent psychiatry: an inventory. *Journal of the American Academy of Child and Adolescent Psychiatry*, **42**(12), 1388–400.

McConville, B. J. Arvanitis, L. A., Thyrum, P. T. *et al*. (2000). Pharmacokinetics, tolerability, and clinical effectiveness of quetiapine fumarate: an open-label trial in adolescents with psychotic disorders. *Journal of Clinical Psychiatry*, **61**(4), 252–60.

McConville, B. J. & Sorter, M. T. (2004). Treatment challenges and safety considerations for antipsychotic use in children and adolescents with psychoses. *Journal of Clinical Psychiatry*, **65** (Suppl. 6), 20–9.

McGlashan, T. H., Zipursky, R. B., Perkins, D. *et al*. (2006). Randomized, double-blind trial of olanzapine versus placebo in patients prodromally symptomatic for psychosis. *American Journal of Psychiatry*, **163**, 790–9.

McGorry, P. D., Yung, A. R., Phillips, L. J. *et al*. (2002). Randomized controlled trial of interventions designed to reduce the risk of progression to first-episode psychosis in a clinical sample with subthreshold symptoms: *Archives General Psychiatry*, **59**, 921–8.

Miklowitz, D., George, E., Axelson, D. *et al*. (2004). Family-focused treatment for adolescents with bipolar disorder. *Journal of Affective Disorder*, **Suppl. 1**, S113–128.

Mozes, T., Greenberg, Y., Spivak, B., Tyano, S., Weizman, A. & Mester, R. (2003). Olanzapine treatment in chronic drug-resistant childhood-onset schizophrenia: an Open-Label study. *Journal of Child and Adolescent Psychopharmacology*, **13**(3), 311–17.

Mozes, T., Ebert, T., Michal, Spivak, B. & Weizman, A. (2006). An open-trial randomized comparison of olanzapine versus risperidone of childhood-onset schizophrenia. *Journal of Child and Adolescent Psychopharmacology*, **16**, 393–403.

National Institute for Clinical Excellence. (2002). Guidance for the Use of Newer (Atypical) Antispychotic Drugs for the Treatment of Schizophrenia. Technology Appraisal Guidance. No 43. London: NICE, 2002.

Nicolson, R., Lenane, M., Singaracharlu, S. *et al.* (2000). Premorbid speech and language impairments in childhood-onset schizophrenia: association with risk factors. *American Journal of Psychiatry*, **157**, 794–800.

Paillere-Martinot, M., Lecrubier, Y., Martinot, J. & Martinot, J. (1995). Improvement of some schizophrenia deficit symptoms with low doses of amisulpiride: *American Journal of Psychiatry*, **152**, 130–3.

Pilling, S., Bebbington, P., Kuipers, E. *et al.* (2002a). Psychological treatments in schizophrenia: I Meta-analyses of family intervention and cognitive behavioural therapy: *Psychology Medicine* **32**(5), 763–82.

Pilling, S., Bebbington, P., Kuipers, E. *et al.* (2002b). Psychological treatments in schizophrenia: II Meta-analyses of randomized controlled trials of social skills training and cognitive remediation: *Psychology Medicine* **32**(5), 783–91.

Piscitelli, S. C., Frazier, J. A., McKenna, K. *et al.* (1994). Plasma clozapine and haloperidol concentrations in adolescents with childhood-onset schizophrenia. *Journal of Clinical Psychiatry*, **55**(9, Suppl. B), 94–7.

Pool, D., Bloom, W., Mieke, D., Reniger, I. & Gallant, D. (1978). A controlled evaluation of loxatine in seventy-five adolescent schizophrenic patients. *Current Therapy Research*, **24**, 559–66.

Rapoport, J. L. (2004). Childhood schizophrenia: a progressive neurodevelopmental disorder. *International Journal of Neuropsychopharmacolgy*, **7**(Suppl. 1), S22.

Reimschmidt, H., Schulz, E. & Martin, P. D. M. (1994). An open trial of clozapine in thirty-six adolescents with schizophrenia. *Journal of Child and Adolescent Psychopharmacology*, **4**(1), 31–41.

Reimschmidt, H., Hennighausen, K., Clement, H. W., Heiser, P. & Schulz, E. (2000). The use of atypical neuroleptics drugs in child and adolescent psychiatry. *European Child and Adolescent Psychiatry*, **9**, I/9–I/19.

Ross, R. G., Novins, D., Farley, G. K. & Adler, L. E. (2003). A 1-year open-label trial of olanzapine in school-age children with schizophrenia. *Journal of Child and Adolescent Psychopharmacology*, **13**, 301–9.

Rund, B. R. (1994). The relationship between psychosocial and cognitive functioning in schizophrenic patients and expressed emotion and communication deviance in their parents. *Acta Psychiatrica Scandinavica*, **90**(2), 133–40.

Schmidt, M. H., Trott, G. F., Blanz, B. & Nissen, G. (1989). Clozapine medication in adolescents. In *Psychiatry: A World Perspective, vol 1. Proceedings of the 8th World Congress of Psychiatry*, ed. C. N. Stefanis, A. D. Rabavilas, & C. R. Soldatos, Athens, Greece; October 12–19. Amsterdam, the Netherlands: Excerta Medica, 1100–04.

Schulz, B., Fleischhaker, C. & Remschmidt, H. E. (1996). Correlated changes in symptoms and neurotransmitter indices during maintenance treatment with Clozapine or conventional neuroleptics in adolescents and young adults with schizophrenia. *Journal of Child and Adolescent Psychopharmacology*, **6**, 119–31.

Shaw, J. A., Lewis, J. E., Pascal, S. *et al.* (2001). A study of the quetiapine: efficacy and tolerability in psychotic adolescent. *Journal of Child and Adolescent Psychopharmacology*, **11**, 415–25.

Shaw, P., Sporn, A., Gogtay, N. *et al.* (2006). Childhood-onset schizophrenia. *Archives of General Psychiatry*, **63**, 721–30.

Sholevar, E. H., Baron, D. A. & Hardie, T. L. (2000). Treatment of childhood-onset schizophrenia with olanzapine. *Journal of Child and Adolescent Psychopharmacology*, **10**, 69–78.

Siefen, G. & Remschmidt, H. (1986). Results of treatment with clozapine in schizophrenic adolescents. *Zeitschrift Kinder Jugenpsychiatrie*, **14**, 245–7.

Sikich, L., Hooper, S. R., Malekpour, A. H., Sheitman, B. B. & Lieberman, J. A. (2001). A double blind comparison of typical versus atypical agents on selected neurocognitive functions in children and adolescents with psychotic disorders. *Schizophrenia Research*, **49**(Suppl. 1–2), 245.

Sikich, L., Hamer, R. M., Bashford, R. A, Sheitman, B. B. & Lieberman, J. A. (2004). A pilot study of risperidone, olanzapine, and haloperidol in psychotic youth: a double-blind, randomized, 8-week trial. *Neuropsychopharmacology*, **29**(1), 133–45.

Sikich, L., Findling, R., McClellan, J., Frazier, J. & Vitiello, B. (2006). Initial findings from early-onset schizophrenia spectrum research group. Symposium 53rd Annual meeting of the American Academy of Child and Adolescent Psychiatry, San Diego, California, USA, October 24–29.

Spencer, E., Kafantaris, V., Padron-Gayol, M., Rosenberg, C. & Campbell, M. (1992). Haloperidol in schizophrenic children: early findings from a a study in progress. *Psychopharmacology Bulletin*, **28**, 183–6.

Tarrier, N., Lewis, S., Haddock, G. *et al.* (2004). Cognitive-behavioural therapy in first-episode and early-onset schizophrenia. 18-month follow-up of a randomised controlled trial. *British Journal of Psychiatry*, **184**, 231–9.

Theisen, F M., Cichon, S., Linden, A., Martin, M., Remschmidt, H. & Hebebrand, J. (2001). Clozapine and weight gain. *American Journal of Psychiatry*, **158**, 816.

Turetz, M., Mozes, T., Tohen, P. *et al.* (1997). An open trial of clozapine in neuroleptic-resistant childhood-onset schizophrenia. *British Journal Psychiatry*, **170**, 507–10.

Ueland, T. & Rund, B. R. (2004). A controlled randomized treatment study: the effects of a cognitive remediation program on adolescents with early onset psychosis. *Acta Psychiatrica Scandinavica*, **109**(1), 70–4.

Wagner, K D. (2004). Treatment of childhood and adolescent disorders. In *Textbook of Psychopharamacolgy*, 3rd edn, ed. A. F. Schatberg & C. B. Nemeroff, Chapter 57, pp. 949–1007. Washington, DC: American Psychiatric Publishing Inc.

Wehmeier, P., Schuler-Springorum, M., Heiser, P. & Remschmidt, H. (2004). Chart review for potential features of myocarditis, pericarditis, and cardiomyopathy in children and adolescents treated with clozapine. *Journal of Child and Adolescent Psychopharmacology*, **14**, 267–71.

Zalsman, G., Carmon, E., Martin, A., Bensason, D., Weizman, A. & Tyano, S. (2003a). Effectiveness, safety and tolerability of risperidone in adolescents with schizophrenia. An open-label study.

Journal of Child and Adolescent Psychopharmacology, **13**(3), 319–27.

Zalsman, G., Frisch, A., Lev-Ran, S. *et al.* (2003b). DRD4 Exon III polymorphism and responder response to risperidone in Israeli adolescents with schizophrenia: a pilot pharmacogenetic study. *European Neuropsychopharmacology*, **13**, 1853–5.

57

Anxiety disorders

Christopher K. Varley, Angeles Diaz-Caneja and Elena Garralda

Editor's note

Treatment of anxiety disorders in children and adolescence is dominated by treatment with cognitive-behavioural therapy or with techniques from cognitive-behavioral therapy. These types of therapies are the first-line treatments among youth with a variety of anxiety disorders including school phobia, elective mutism, PTSD, social phobia, generalized anxiety disorder, panic disorder and obsessive-compulsive disorder. As the disorders become more severe, then medications are recommended, but psychopharmacologic treatment in children is not as widely encouraged as in adults. Also, given that the SSRIs are, in general, the major class used in the treatment of anxiety disorders, and given that there are concerns with respect to suicidal ideation and acts among young people on SSRIs, these pharmacologic interventions are not viewed as first-line treatments. And yet there is much more methodologically sound evidence for pharmacologic treatment than for CBT. The best data we have, for both behavioural/cognitive behavioural as well as psychopharmacological intervention is, with obsessive-compulsive disorder.

Introduction

Anxiety disorders are common in childhood occurring in 3%–13% of all children and adolescents (Anderson *et al.*, 1987; Costello & Angold, 1995; Kashani & Orvashel, 1990). Children typically present with more than one anxiety disorder. Co-morbidity, primarily with depression, is common. Anxiety disorders are associated with significant impairments in multiple functional domains (Costello *et al.*, 1999; Klein & Pine, 2002). Since anxiety disorders may persist into adulthood (Pine *et al.*, 1998), effective treatment is important.

Treatments of anxiety disorders in children and adolescents have often been drawn from the adult literature as few controlled studies have been carried out with children and adolescents. Recently, randomized controlled trials have been published, but, because of limitations, e.g. small number of participants, inclusion criteria and co-morbidity among participants such as other anxiety disorders or depression, the results need to be taken cautiously. Pharmacotherapy for anxiety disorders in children and adolescents is not generally approved in the UK (except sertraline and fluvoxamine for OCD) and in the USA (except for sertraline, fluvoxamine, fluoxetine and clomipramine for OCD). Clinicians may use medications based on their clinical expertise or experience (off-licence/off label).

The American Academy of Child and Adolescent Psychiatry (AACAP) has published practice parameters to guide the clinician in the management of anxiety disorders, post-traumatic stress disorders and obsessive-compulsive disorders (AACAP, 1997, 1998a, 1998b). In Europe, the European Society of Child and Adolescent Psychiatry has published guidelines only for OCD (Thomsen, 1998). The Royal College of Psychiatrists (Scott *et al.*, 2001) and recent books have summarized the evidence of treatment for mental disorders, including anxiety disorders (Carr, 2000; Target & Fonagy, 1996). These guidelines suggest that psychoeducation about the diagnosis (symptoms, treatment, prognosis) is important before any formal treatment. Family is considered an important part of the treatment and should be included in any management plan (AACAP, 1997, 1998a, 1998b).

In this review, we consider management of anxiety disorders in children and adolescents and try to assess the effectiveness of treatments. First, we will consider mixed or non-specified anxiety disorders. Secondly, we will focus on treatment for specific anxiety disorders. Some studies are mentioned in more than one section.

Cambridge Textbook of Effective Treatments in Psychiatry, ed. Peter Tyrer and Kenneth R. Silk. Published by Cambridge University Press.
© Cambridge University Press, 2008.

Anxiety disorders in general (includes social anxiety disorder)

Psychotherapy – cognitive-behavioural therapy

Studies in this area either did not have defined inclusion criteria regarding diagnosis or included youth with mixed anxiety disorders. Psychological interventions such as cognitive-behavioural therapy (CBT) have proved effective in a number of studies (randomized controlled trials or quasi-experimental studies) with participants having generalized anxiety disorder (GAD), SAD, and social phobia. Two RCTs (Kendall, 1994; Kendall et al., 1997) found that individual CBT group showed clinically significant reduction in anxiety compared with a wait list control group. Barret et al. (1996) compared CBT or CBT and family anxiety management programme to a control group. Both intervention groups had clinically significant reductions in anxiety compared with a control group. The improvements were sustained at 1-year follow-up. The group receiving the combined treatment fared better in the long term.

Effectiveness of group CBT with and without parental involvement has been studied (Flannery-Schroeder & Kendall, 2000; Manassis et al., 2002). Results showed that treated children improved with either individual or group treatment. However, children with higher social anxiety may respond preferentially to individual treatment (Manassis et al., 2002).

Psychopharmacology

Pharmacological treatment, mainly tricyclic antidepressants (TCAs), selective serotonergic reuptake inhibitors (SSRIs), and benzodiazepines have been extensively researched in adults with anxiety disorder (Roy-Byrne & Cowley, 2002). In children, there are few studies. Bernstein et al. (2000) carried out a small RCT comparing imipramine and placebo in adolescents with school refusal and anxiety disorders. Imipramine was superior to placebo.

SSRIs have been studied among children and adolescents with mixed anxiety disorders in two randomized controlled trials (Birmaher et al., 2003; Research Unit of Paediatric Psychopharmacology Anxiety Study Group (RUPPS), 2001). In the 8 weeks RUPPS study of fluvoxamine, 76% of children with social phobia, SAD and/or GAD on medication improved compared to 28% on placebo. In the Birmaher 12-week study of fluoxetine, 61% responded on medication vs. 35% on placebo. Fluoxetine was generally well tolerated.

In a follow-up open study (RUPPS, 2002), participants were divided in three groups and followed for 6 months: (a) continuing with fluvoxamine; (b) placebo non-responders switched to fluvoxamine; (c) fluvoxamine non-responders switched to fluoxetine. Results were that 94% in the continue on fluvoxamine group continued with low anxiety, 56% of the placebo switched to fluvoxamine improved, and 71% of fluvoxamine non-responders improved when switched to fluoxetine.

Other antidepressants may be considered although data is limited for use in children and adolescents (Emslie et al., 1999). Benzodiazepines can be considered in acute anxiety situations, but no effectiveness has been proved (Graee et al., 1994)

Generalized anxiety disorder (GAD)

Psychotherapy – cognitive-behavioural therapy

Behavioural techniques and CBT are recommended as first-line treatment. If symptoms are severe, pharmacological measures can be considered. Other therapies should be considered depending on the symptoms (AACAP, 1997). Cognitive therapy includes systematic desensitization, exposure and response prevention (ERP), extinction, counter-conditioning, modelling and operant techniques (Barret et al., 1996; Kendall, 1994; Kendall et al., 1997).

Pharmacotherapy

There is some, but limited, controlled evidence of the efficacy of medications in GAD. Venlafaxine XR was examined in an 8-week multi-centre RCT (Rynn et al., 2002). There was a highly significant reduction in the ratings on anxiety scales. Dosing was titrated from 37.5 to 225 mg/day. Side effects included weakness, decreased appetite, pain and somnolence. There was a discontinuation rate of 2% on both venlafaxine and placebo.

Sertraline was studied in a 9-week RCT in 22 children and adolescents with GAD (Rynn et al., 2001). Hamilton Anxiety Scale and CGI showed significant differences in favour of sertraline over placebo beginning at week 4. The RUPPS study of fluvoxamine included children with GAD and demonstrated efficacy (Rynn et al., 2001).

The TCAs have been used in adults (Klein et al., 1992), but their evidence has not been proved in children. Other medication used in adults such as benzodiazepines or beta-blockers do not have evidence of efficacy in controlled trials in children and adolescents. However, benzodiazepines may be used with caution in anticipatory anxiety and panic disorder (Simeon et al.,1992).

Specific phobia (including school phobia)

Psychotherapy – cognitive-behavioural therapy

Specific phobias should first be approached with behavioural and cognitive-behavioural treatment. Systematic desensitization and exposure and response prevention (ERP) have proved to be efficacious. When there are associated complications, individual and/or family psychotherapy should be considered (AACAP, 1997). Clinically, behavioural treatments have been used extensively.

School phobia has been managed within a CBT or behavioural approach. Uncontrolled studies have possible efficacy of behavioural management. Blagg & Yule (1984) compared three interventions for school phobia: family-based behaviour therapy with in vivo flooding and the child returning to school immediately; hospital-based inpatient programme including milieu therapy, educational and occupational therapy, pharmacological treatment, and liaison with parents and school; and home tuition with a psychotherapy programme for the child and parents. In vivo exposure was superior to the other two interventions, with return to school. Improvement was maintained a year after the study. Limitations were that subjects were not randomly allocated to treatment interventions.

In a RCT of CBT, educational support therapy, and waiting list control, CBT was effective compared to the control (King et al., 1998). However, CBT was not superior to educational-support therapy. Both treatments were effective in reducing anxiety and depression. There was evidence for efficacy of group CBT for children with anxiety disorders in a study by Flannery-Schroeder & Kendall (2000). Children were randomly assigned to individual CBT, group CBT, or a waiting list control with improvement in the two intervention groups.

Psychopharmacology

Results of pharmacological treatment of school phobia have been inconsistent. One study showed that imipramine was significantly better than placebo in facilitating school attendance and reducing anxiety symptoms (Gittelman-Klein & Klein, 1971). Other studies showed no differences (Berney et al., 1981; Bernstein et al., 1990; Klein et al., 1992). Differences in the findings may be explained in terms of sample size, administered dosage, presence of co-morbid disorders (depression, separation anxiety), and type and control of concurrent therapies (behavioural therapy). No studies have compared psychological and pharmacological interventions.

Psychotherapy and psychopharmacology

Medication adjuvant of behavioural or CBT treatment can be considered. In an 8-week study comparing CBT plus imipramine to CBT and placebo in the treatment of school refusal, medication and CBT were significantly more efficacious in improving school attendance and decreasing depression (Bernstein et al., 2000). The children had co-morbid anxiety and depression. At 1 year follow-up, no differences were found between both groups in severity of depression or in prevalence of anxiety or depressive disorders. Thus, benefit of maintenance treatment in children with school refusal and co-morbid disorder remains unclear (Bernstein et al., 2001).

Liaison between school, family and services with emphasis on gradual reintegration in school of the child is essential. CBT or supportive counselling during the integration can be helpful.

Social phobia (including selective mutism)

The AACAP (1997) recommends CBT (individual or group) and behavioural therapy to promote successful experience in social interactions as first-line treatment. Family interventions should be considered.

Psychotherapy – cognitive-behavioural therapy

Several clinic-based treatments have been published. Social effectiveness therapy for children (Beidel & Turner, 1998) combines group sessions of social skills and individual exposure sessions to address social anxiety. It was superior to study-skills and test-taking skills (Testbusters) at 6 months follow-up (Beidel et al., 2000). Social Skills Training, with or without parental involvement, was superior to a wait list control (Spence et al., 2000). Cognitive-behavioural group therapy for adolescents was beneficial in a preliminary study (Albano et al., 1995). A RCT of 3 weeks of CBT vs. a waiting list for children with social phobia found CBT demonstrated significant improvement on the majority of child, parent and interviewer reports of social anxiety symptoms (Gallagher-Heather et al., 2004).

Psychopharmacology

Paroxetine was studied in social phobia (Wetherhold et al., 2002). There was a highly significant difference in 319 youths (mean age 9 years) treated with paroxetine (78%) vs. placebo (38%) having a positive response. The mean dose was 25 mg/day. The side effect profile was typical for the SSRIs with headache, nausea, sedation and activation, with a 5% dropout due to adverse events. Other serotonergic agents (paroxetine, sertraline and nefazodone) were tried in a case series to treat children with social phobia with a positive clinical response and were well tolerated (Mancini *et al.*, 1999).

Fluoxetine has been studied in children with selective mutism in case reports (Black *et al.*, 1992). In a 9-week open trial of 21 children, 76% showed benefit with fluoxetine with decreased anxiety and increased speech in social settings (Dummit *et al.*, 1996), and in a 12-week RCT of 15 children there was significantly greater improvement in parent-rated outcome measures on fluoxetine (Black & Uhde, 1994).

The small number of participants and mixed results make it difficult to interpret the role of medication in elective mutism. However, the RUPPS (2001) study of fluvoxamine included some children with social phobia. However, medications used in adults with social phobia are not recommended in children (Labellarte *et al.*, 1999).

Panic disorder

Few studies about treatment of this condition in youth have been published. Because of limited research, treatment of panic disorder should be a combination of psychoeducation for the child and family with subsequent CBT. Addition of small doses of benzodiazepines if symptoms are very severe can be used for a limited time while psychological treatment is organized. SSRIs can be considered.

In adults, TCAs, monoamine oxidase inhibitors and benzodiazepines are used, but they are not recommended in children (AACAP, 1997). An open study of SSRIs in children with panic disorders showed that the symptoms improved (Renaud *et al.*, 1999). However, the children also had depressive symptoms.

Post-traumatic stress disorder (includes adjustment disorders)

Exposure to life-threatening stressors can lead to PTSD in all ages (March *et al.*, 1998a). Treatment should be comprehensive and include both the parent and the child, trauma focused therapy, psychoeducation about PTSD, and address non-PTSD behavioural and emotional difficulties. Medication (SSRIs) can be used adjuvant with psychological interventions if depressive or panic symptoms are present (AACAP, 1998a).

Controlled treatment intervention studies have not been done with adjustment disorders. Treatment guidelines generally follow recommendations for PTSD.

Psychotherapy – cognitive-behavioural therapy

Seven randomized trials comparing a trauma-specific CBT to no treatment or credible alternative have demonstrated the superiority of CBT on at least some outcomes for sexually abused, multiply traumatized, disaster and community violence exposed children (Cohen *et al.*, 2000, 2003). Deblinger *et al.* (1996, 1999), Cohen & Mannarino (1996); Cohen *et al.* (2004), Cohen & Mannarino (1997) and Trowell *et al.* (2002) have studied trauma-focused CBT (TF-CBT) in sexual abuse of children and adolescents and have showed improvement with this intervention. Involvement of family did not affect outcome (King *et al.*, 2000). One study comparing TF-CBT and supportive therapy found no differences (Celano *et al.*, 1996). This type of intervention includes teaching anxiety management skills, correcting maladaptive cognitions, and gradual exposure/desensitization. Most have a parental component.

If focused on other situations such as exposure to a single stressor (March *et al.*, 1998a) or exposure to violence (Stein *et al.*, 2003), group CBT intervention may be more efficacious. March *et al.*'s study (1998a) consisted of group CBT for children exposed to a single stressor. Fifty-seven per cent of the participants who met the criteria for PTSD did not meet criteria for PTSD after treatment. At 6-month follow up 12/14 subjects were free of PTSD. However, there was no control group. Stein *et al.* (2003) conducted a RCT of CBT for children with PTSD and depression resulting from exposure to violence. After 3 months, the intervention group had lower scores on symptoms for PTSD, depression and psychosocial dysfunction.

There is little data to support other psychological interventions. Early reports suggested that PTSD could be prevented by early intervention using debriefing, but no studies support this. Psychodynamic psychotherapy does not have any supporting evidence.

Psychopharmacology

Psychopharmacologic treatments are widely used to treat childhood PTSD, but no rigorous, empirical research has evaluated effectiveness. A survey of child and adolescent psychiatrists indicated that 95% had used SSRIs and other medications (Cohen *et al.*, 2003). A group of 25 paediatric burn patients, aged 2–19, with acute stress disorder aged 2 to 19 received imipramine or chloral hydrate for 7 days in a randomized double-blind design (Robert *et al.*, 1999).

Imipramine was more effective than chloral hydrate. In all cases, the combined serum levels were less than 40 nanograms/ml. The initial dose of imipramine was 1 mg/kg per day, with a maximum dose of 100 mg.

In a recent review of pharmacotherapy for PTSD in adults, SSRIs (sertraline and paroxetine) were the treatment of choice following successful controlled trials (Schoenfeld et al., 2004). Medication (SSRIs) should be used adjuvant with psychological interventions, if depressive or panic symptoms are present (AACAP, 1997).

Eye movement desensitization and reprocessing (EMDR)

No controlled studies have evaluated the benefits and risks of EMDR in children and adolescents. Chemtob et al. (2002) showed an improvement in PTSD symptoms after three sessions of EMDR in children presenting with PTSD symptoms a year after a disaster in an uncontrolled field study. Improvement was maintained after 6 months.

The final word with PTSD would be that trauma focused-CBT should be used as first line, with subsequent pharmacotherapy.

Obsessive-compulsive disorder

Obsessive-compulsive behaviour in children and adolescents appears to be the condition with best evidence for efficacy of treatment. In the USA, AACAP guidelines (1998a) recommend behavioural therapy or medication as initial treatment. In Europe, the recommendations are similar (Thomsen, 1998). However, the clinical impression is that a combination of behavioural therapy and medication with SSRIs is the preferred treatment in severe cases.

Psychotherapy – behaviour therapy and cognitive-behavioural therapy

Open trials showed that CBT involving ERP (exposure and response prevention) was efficacious (Benazon et al., 2002; Franklin et al., 1998; Piacentini et al., 2002). However, no protocol manual, use of medication in some participants, small sample size and open administration of the treatment are the limitations of these studies. In some studies, manualized group CBT has showed efficacy in the treatment of OCD (Cordioli et al., 2003; Thienemann et al., 2001).

Participation of the family is crucial in the treatment to help the child overcome obsessive thoughts and compulsions. Other studies have investigated integrating CBT and family treatment (CBFT) with improvement not only in the child's symptoms but also in the family's anxiety (Waters et al., 2001). Barret et al. (2004) showed that CBFT was as effective in reducing OCD symptoms for children and adolescents as individual treatment.

Drug treatment should be first line if children are overwhelmed by the symptoms or family is unable to engage in treatment. Where possible it should be used in combination with ERP (AACAP, 1998b).

Psychopharmacology

Antidepressants are the first pharmacological option. The SSRIs and clomipramine have showed effectiveness in several randomized control trials. In more detail, antidepressant medications that been found to be effective include fluoxetine (Liebowitz et al., 2002; Riddle et al., 1992), fluvoxamine (Riddle et al., 1996), sertraline (March et al., 1998b; The Paediatric OCD Treatment Study (POTS) Team, 2004), paroxetine (Geller et al., 2004), and clomipramine (Flament et al., 1985; Leonard et al., 1989). A small open-label study tried citalopram (Thomsen 1997).

Fluvoxamine was studied in a 10-week, multi-centre group parallel study of paediatric outpatients (Riddle et al., 1996). Patients were titrated to a total daily dose of approximately 100 mg/day over the first 2 weeks with subsequent dosage adjustment within a range of 50 to 200 mg/day on a b.i.d. schedule, with the following results vs. placebo: very much improved (21% vs. 11%); much improved (18% vs. 17%); minimally improved (37% vs. 22%).

Sertraline was studied in youth to the age of 6, with benefit as well as safety in a RCT of 187 children and 80 adolescents with a dose range of 25–200 mg/day (March et al., 1998b). The dosages were titrated up to a dose of 200 mg/day. On sertraline, 42% were rated as very much improved vs. 26% on placebo. Of this group, 132 were examined for long-term efficacy (Wagner et al., 2003). Forty-seven per cent completed the 52-week trial, and 70% of all subjects who entered this phase of the study experienced at least partial remission, with 47% achieving full remission. The mean daily dosage at the end of treatment was 151 ± 54 mg.

Fluoxetine demonstrated statistically significant efficacy in a RCT in children and adolescents (Riddle et al., 1992). However, in another RCT that examined the efficacy of fluoxetine, Liebowitz et al. (2002) found that the response rates of those receiving active drug ($n = 21$) vs. those on placebo ($n = 22$) did not differ significantly at the end of the initial 8-week acute phase of treatment. However, the fluoxetine group ($n = 12$) who continued treatment through the subsequent 8-week maintenance

Table 57.1. Psychopharmacological interventions

| Disorder | Evidenced-based psychopharmacological interventions (based on double-blind placebo-controlled studies of adequate statistical power) | |
	Youth	Adults (Roy-Byrne & Cowley, 2002; Lydiard, 1996)
Separation anxiety disorder	Fluvoxamine (RUPPS, 2001)	N/A
	Fluoxetine (Birmaher *et al.*, 2003)	
Selective mutism	None to date	N/A
Panic disorder, with or without agoraphobia	None to date	Imipramine
		Clonazepam
		Alprazolam
		Lorazepam
		Diazepam
		Venlafaxine
		Sertraline
		Paroxetine
		Citalopram
		Fluoxetine
		Fluvoxamine
Specific phobia	None to date	None to date
Social phobia	Fluvoxamine (RUPPS, 2001)	Selective serotonergic reuptake inhibitors
	Paroxetine (Wetherhold *et al.*, 2002)	
	Fluoxetine (Birmaher *et al.*, 2003)	Benzodiazepines
Obsessive-compulsive disorder	Clomipramine (Flament *et al.*, 1985; Leonard *et al.*, 1989)	Clomipramine
	Fluoxetine (Liebowitz *et al.*, 2002)	Fluoxetine
	Paroxetine (Geller, 2002)	Paroxetine
	Fluvoxamine (Riddle *et al.*, 1996)	Fluvoxamine
	Sertraline (March, 1998a, b; POTS, 2004)	Sertraline
		Citalopram
Acute stress disorder	None to date	None to date
Post-traumatic stress disorder	None to date	Sertraline
		Paroxetine
Generalized anxiety disorder	Fluvoxamine (RUPPS, 2001)	Buspirone
	Venlafaxine (Rynn *et al.*, 2002)	Alprazolam
	Fluoxetine (Birmaher *et al.*, 2003)	Clonazepam
Anxiety secondary to medical condition or substance induced	None to date	None to date
Adjustment disorder with anxiety	None to date	None to date

phase showed a statistically significant reduction in symptoms as compared to the placebo group ($n = 7$). Fluoxetine was generally well tolerated.

Paroxetine was studied in a multi-centre, 10-week RCT in 203 children and adolescents (Geller *et al.*, 2004). The dose range of paroxetine was from 10–50 mg. There was significant reduction of OCD symptoms on paroxetine versus placebo, though 10.2% of patients discontinued treatment on paroxetine vs. 2.9% on placebo due to adverse events.

In the most comprehensive study of OCD, CBT and sertraline and their combination were studied in a population of 112 patients, ages 7 through 17. CBT alone ($P = 0.003$), sertraline alone ($P = 0.007$) and combined treatment ($P = 0.001$) were superior to placebo (The Pediatric OCD Treatment Study (POTS) Team, 2004). Combined treatment also proved superior to CBT alone ($P = 0.008$) and to sertraline alone ($P = 0.006$), which did not differ from each other. The rate for clinical remission for combined treatment was 53.6%, CBT alone 39.3%, sertraline alone 21.4% and placebo 3.6%. The three active treatments proved acceptable and well tolerated with no evidence of treatment emergent harm to self or others.

Augmentation of medication has been considered, but no effectiveness has been proved and likely increases risk of side effects. In a meta-analysis of pharmacotherapy trials in paediatric obsessive-compulsive disorder, clomipramine was superior to SSRIs, but it should not be first line because of side effects and risk of cardiac arrhythmias (Geller *et al.*, 2003)

Conclusions

The evidence supports the initial use of CBT, followed by psychopharmacology if CBT is not successful. Severely anxious patients may initially require psychopharmacologic treatment as well as CBT. An algorithm following these guidelines has been developed (Labellarte *et al.*, 1999). While there are published guidelines for the psychopharmacologic treatment of children with PTSD, these should be considered as tentative in the absence of controlled data. SSRIs are first-line interventions, and tricyclic antidepressants and venlafaxine are second-line agents. Benzodiazepines are considered second- or third-line agents (Table 57.1).

The best evidence for psychopharmacologic treatment is for OCD, for both SSRIs and clomipramine. There are important safety issues to consider regarding side effects of pharmacological treatment of anxiety in youth. In Great Britain, SSRIs are contraindicated in the treatment of major depression in youth, with the exception of fluoxetine and fluvoxamine (MHRA, 2004). In the United States, a 'Black Box warning' has been issued by the FDA regarding suicidality, including suicidal ideation and attempts,

for antidepressants in children and adolescents for treatment of both depression and anxiety disorders (US Federal Drug Administration, 2004). The pooled analysis of all controlled trials of antidepressants in children and adolescents identifies a heightened risk in the treatment of major depression (4% of suicide related behaviour vs. 2% on placebo) and also in the treatment of anxiety. Anxiety disorders are often co-morbid with depressive disorders, so awareness of possible mood related side effects is essential, as is the provision of informed consent, and careful monitoring of treatment response. There are also potential cardiovascular concerns regarding TCAs in youth, which also require careful cardiac monitoring (Varley, 2001).

While much research remains to be done there is evidence of efficacy of a number of interventions for anxiety disorders in children and teens. Non-specific measures of parent education and illness education to parents and patients may be helpful. There is a need for holistic, comprehensive treatment with attention to specific psychopharmacologic and psychotherapy needs, attention to family matters, dealing with abuse issues, freedom from substance abuse, promotion of healthier life style choices such as exercise, and use of peer support groups. There is a need for teamwork and effective communication between team members. A rising number of well-done, large, placebo-controlled studies provide increased support for both medication and for psychotherapy to inform evidence-based treatment.

The level of evidence for each of the interventions discussed in their chapter is summarized in Table 57.2.

Table 57.2. Effectiveness of treatments for anxiety disorder

Treatment	Form of treatment	Psychiatric disorder/ target audience	Level of evidence for efficacy	Comments
Psychotherapy	Cognitive-behavioural therapy	Anxiety disorder in general in children and adolescents	Ia	Reduction in anxiety that was maintained at one year follow-up. Those receiving CBT plus a family management programme fared even better
Psychotherapy	Cognitive-behavioural therapy and techniques	GAD	IV	Recommended as first-line treatment but no real controlled studies
Psychotherapy	Cognitive-behavioural therapy and techniques	Specific phobias	IIb	Recommended as first-line treatment and efficacy has been established
Psychotherapy	Cognitive-behavioural therapy and techniques	School phobia	III	Behavioural treatment with in vivo flooding better that hospitalization or home schooling plus psychotherapy
Psychotherapy	CBT (Individual or group)	Social phobia	IIa	A number of clinic-based studies supports its effectiveness

Table 57.2. (cont.)

Treatment	Form of treatment	Psychiatric disorder/ target audience	Level of evidence for efficacy	Comments
Psychotherapy	CBT	Panic Disorder	IV	Little research but recommended as first-line treatment
Psychotherapy	Trauma focused-CBT	Post-traumatic stress disorder	Ib	Multiple controlled studies plus RCTs to support this intervention
Psychotherapy	CBT with exposure response prevention (ERP)	Obsessive-compulsive disorder	Ib	Found to be effective. CBT with ERP recommended as first-line treatment
Psychopharmacology	Tricyclic antidepressants (TCAs)	Anxiety disorder in general in children and adolescents	Ib	Imipramine improved school refusal and anxiety
Psychopharmacology	SSRIs	Anxiety disorder in general in children and adolescents	Ia	Particularly evidence for fluvoxamine and fluoxetine with somewhere between 50% and 75% responding
Psychopharmacology	SSRIs SNRIs	GAD	Ib	RCTs with venlafaxine, fluoxetine, and fluvoxamine
Psychopharmacology	Tricyclic antidepressants	School phobia	III	Some studies show significant improvement; other studies do not show improvement (Imipramine)
Psychopharmacology	SSRIs	Social phobia Selective mutism	Ia	RCTs with fluoxetine primarily but other SSRIs are effective. Paroxetine also found effective but its use in children and adolescents is currently not encouraged
Psychopharmacology	SSRIs	Panic disorder	III	Medications used for panic disorder in adults are not recommended though open studies have revealed that panic disorder symptoms improved with SSRIs in this age grouping
Psychopharmacology	SSRIs	PTSD	IIa	Controlled trials have been conducted with sertraline and paroxetine. 95% of adolescent psychiatrists have used SSRIs to treat PTSD symptoms in their patients
Psychopharmacology	SSRIs Clomipramine	Obsessive-compulsive disorder	Ia	Repeatedly found to be effective. SSRIs recommended over clomipramine due to side effect differences
Psychopharmacology plus Psychotherapy	TCAs plus CBT	School phobias	IIa	Combination was better that CBT alone. But no difference between groups at one year
Psychopharmacology plus Psychotherapy	SSRI plus CBT	Obsessive-compulsive disorder	Ib	Combined treatment more effective (54%) than the SSRI (sertraline) alone (21%) or CBT alone (395) or placebo alone (4%)

REFERENCES

Albano, A. M., Marten, P. A., Holt, C. S., Heimberg, R. G. & Barlow, D. H. (1995). Cognitive behavioural group treatment for social phobia in adolescents. A preliminary study. *Journal of Nervous and Mental Disease*, **183**(10), 649–56.

American Academy of Child and Adolescent Psychiatry (AACAP) (1997). Practice parameters for the assessment and treatment of children with anxiety disorders. *Journal of the American Academy of Child and Adolescent Psychiatry*, **36** (Suppl.), S4–26.

American Academy of Child and Adolescent Psychiatry (1998a). Practice parameters for the assessment and treatment of children and adolescents with posttraumatic stress disorders.

Journal of the American Academy of Child and Adolescent Psychiatry, **37** (Suppl.), S27–45.

American Academy of Child and Adolescent Psychiatry (1998b). Practice parameters for the assessment and treatment of children and adolescents with obsessive-compulsive disorders. *Journal of the American Academy of Child and Adolescent Psychiatry*, **37** (Suppl.), S4–26.

Anderson, D. J., Williams, S., McGee, R. & Silva, P. A. (1987). DSM-III disorders in preadolescent children: prevalence in large sample from the general population. *Archives of General Psychiatry*, **44**, 69–76.

Barret, P. M., Dadds, M. R. & Rapee, R. M. (1996). Family management of childhood anxiety: a controlled trial. *Journal of Consulting and Clinical Psychology*, **65**, 366–80.

Barret, P., Healy-Farrell, L. & March, J. (2004). Cognitive-behavioural family treatment of childhood obsessive-compulsive disorder: a controlled trial. *Journal of the American Academy of Child and Adolescent Psychiatry*, **43**, 46–62.

Beidel, D. C. & Turner, S. M. (1998). *Shy Children, Phobic Adults: Nature and Treatment of Social Phobia*. Washington, DC: American Psychological Association.

Beidel, D. C., Turner, S. M. & Morris, T. L. (2000). Behavioural treatment of childhood social phobia. *Journal of Consulting Clinical Psychology*, **68**, 1072–80.

Benazon, N. R., Ager, J. & Rosenberg, D. R. (2002). Cognitive behaviour therapy in treatment-naïve children and adolescents with obsessive-compulsive disorder: an open trial. *Behaviour Research and Therapy*, **40**(5), 529–539.

Berney, T., Kolvin, I., Bhate, S. R. *et al.* (1981). School phobia: a therapeutic trial with clomipramine and short term outcome. *British Journal of Psychiatry*, **138**, 110–18.

Bernstein, G. A., Garfinkel, B. D. & Borchardt, C. M. (1990). Comparative studies of pharmacotherapy for school refusal. *Journal of the American Academy of Child and Adolescent Psychiatry*, **29**, 773–81.

Bernstein, G. A., Borchardt, C. M., Perwien, A. R. *et al.* (2000). Imipramine plus cognitive-behavioural therapy in the treatment of school refusal. *Journal of Child and Adolescent Psychiatry*, **39**(3), 276–83.

Bernstein, G. A., Hektner, J. M., Borchardt, C. M. & McMillan, M. H. (2001). Treatment of school refusal: one-year follow-up. *Journal of Child and Adolescent Psychiatry*, **40**(2), 206–13.

Birmaher, B., Axelson, D. A., Monk, K. *et al.* (2003). Fluoxetine for treatment of childhood anxiety disorders. *Journal of the American Academy of Child and Adolescent Psychiatry*, **42**, 415–23.

Black, B. & Uhde, T W. (1994). Treatment of elective mutism with Fluoxetine: A double-blind placebo-controlled study. *Journal of the American Academy of Child and Adolescent Psychiatry*, **33**, 1000–6.

Black, B., Uhde, T. W. & Tancer, M. E. (1992). Fluoxetine for the treatment of social phobia. *Journal of the American Academy of Child and Adolescent Psychiatry*, **29**, 36–44.

Blagg, N. R. & Yule, W. (1984). The behavioural treatment of school refusal. *Behavioural Research Therapy*, **22**, 119–27.

Carr, A. (ed) (2000). *What Works with Children and Adolescents? A Critical Review of Psychological Interventions with Children, Adolescents and Their Families*. London: Routledge.

Celano, M., Hazzard, A., Webb, C. & McCall, C. (1996). Treatment of traumagenic beliefs among sexually abused girls and their mothers: an evaluation study. *Journal of Abnormal Child Psychology*, **24**, 1–17.

Chemtob, C, M., Nakashima, J. & Carlson, J. G. (2002). Brief treatment for elementary school children with disaster-related post-traumatic stress disorder: a field study. *Journal of Clinical Psychology*, **58**, 99–112.

Cohen, J. A. & Mannarino, A. P. (1996). A treatment study for sexually abused preschool children: initial findings. *Journal of the American Academy Child and Adolescent Psychiatry*, **35**, 42–50.

Cohen, J. A. & Mannarino, A. P. (1997). A treatment study of sexually abused preschool children: outcome during 1-year follow-up. *Journal of the American Academy Child and Adolescent Psychiatry*, **36**, 1228–35.

Cohen, J. A., Berliner, L. & March, J. S. (2000). Treatment of children and adolescents. In *Effective Treatments for PTSD*, ed. E. B. Foa, T. M. Keane & M. J. Friedman, pp. 106–39. New York: Guilford Press.

Cohen, J. A., Berliner, L. & Mannarino, A. P. (2003). Psychosocial and pharmacological interventions for child crime victims. *Journal of Traumatic Stress*, **16**(2), 175–86.

Cohen, J., Deblinger., E, Mannarino, A. P. & Steer, R. A. (2004). A multisite, randomised controlled trial for children with sexual abuse-related PTSD symptoms. *Journal of the American Academy of Child and Adolescent Psychiatry*, **43**(4), 393–402.

Cordioli, A., Heldt, E., Bochi, D. B. *et al.* (2003). Cognitive-behavioural group therapy in obsessive-compulsive disorder: a randomised clinical trial. *Psychotherapy and Psychosomatics*, **72**, 211.

Costello E. & Angold A. (1995). Epidemiology. In *Anxiety Disorders in Children and Adolescents*, ed. J. March, pp. 109–24. New York: Guilford Press.

Costello, E. J., Angold, A. & Keeler, G. P. (1999). Adolescent outcomes of childhood disorders: the consequences of severity and impairment. *Journal of the American Academy of Child and Adolescent Psychiatry*, **38**, 121–8.

Deblinger, E., Lippman, J. & Steer, R. (1996). Sexually abused children suffering post-traumatic stress symptoms: initial treatment outcome findings. *Child Maltreatment*, **1**, 310–21.

Deblinger, E., Steer R. & Lippmann, J. (1999). Two-year follow-up study of cognitive behavioural therapy for sexually abused children suffering post-traumatic stress symptoms. *Child Abuse and Neglect*, **23**, 1371–8.

Dummit, E. S., Klein, R. G., Asche, B., Martin, J. & Tancer, N. K. (1996). Fluoxetine treatment of children with selective mutism: an open trial. *Journal of the American Academy of Child and Adolescent Psychiatry*, **35**, 615–21.

Emslie, G., Walkup, J., Pliszka, S. & Ernst, M. (1999). Nontricyclic antidepressants: current trends in children and adolescents. *Journal of the American Academy of Child and Adolescent Psychiatry*, **38**(5), 517–28.

Flament, M., Rapoport, J. L., Beg, C. *et al.* (1985). Clomipramine treatment of childhood obsessive-compulsive disorder, *Archives of General Psychiatry*, **42**, 977–88.

Flannery-Schroeder, E. & Kendall, P. C. (2000). Group versus individual cognitive-behavioural treatment for youth with anxiety disorders: a randomised clinical trial. *Cognitive Therapy and Research*, **3**, 251–78.

Franklin, M., Kozak, M., Cashman, L., Coles, M., Rheingold, A. & Foa, E. (1998). Cognitive-behavioural treatment of paediatric obsessive-compulsive disorder: an open clinical trial. *Journal of American Academy of Child and Adolescent Psychiatry*, **37**(4), 412–19.

Gallagher-Heather, M., Rabbin, B. A. & McCloskey, M. S. (2004). A brief group cognitive-behavioural intervention for social phobia in childhood. *Journal of Anxiety Disorders*, **18**(4), 459–79.

Geller, D., Biederman, J., Stewart, E. *et al.* (2003). Which SSRI? A meta-analysis of pharmacotherapy trials in paediatric obsessive compulsive disorder. *American Journal of Psychiatry*, **160**, 1919–28.

Geller, D. A., Wagner, K. D. & Emslie, G. (2004). Paroxetine treatment in children and adolescents with obsessive-compulsive disorder: a randomised, multicenter, double-blind, placebo-controlled trial. *Journal of the American Academy of Child and Adolescent Psychiatry*, **43**, 1387–96.

Gittelman-Klein, R. & Klein, D. F. (1971). Controlled imipramine treatment of school phobia. *Archives of General Psychiatry*, **25**, 199–215.

Graee, F., Milner, J., Rizzotto, L. & Klein, R. (1994). Clonazepam in childhood anxiety disorders. *Journal of the American Academy of Child and Adolescent Psychiatry*, **33**, 372–6.

Kashani, H. & Orvashel, H. (1990). A community study of anxiety in children and adolescents. *American Journal of Psychiatry*, **147**, 313–18.

Kendall, P. (1994). Treating anxiety disorders in children: results of a randomised clinical trial. *Journal of Consulting and Clinical Psychology*, **62** (1), 100–10.

Kendall, P. C., Flannery-Schroeder, E. & Panichelli-Mindel, S. M. *et al.* (1997). Therapy for youths with anxiety disorders: a second randomised clinical trial. *Journal of Consulting and Clinical Psychology*, **65**(3), 366–80.

King, N., Tonge, B., Heyne, D. *et al.* (1998). Cognitive behavioural treatment of school-refusing children: a controlled evaluation. *Journal of the American Academy of Child and Adolescent Psychiatry*, **37**(4), 395–403.

King, N, J., Tange, B. J., Mullen, P. *et al.* (2000). Treating sexually abused children with posttraumatic stress symptoms: a randomized clinical trial. *Journal of the American Academy of Child and Adolescent Psychiatry*, **39**, 1347–55.

Klein, R. G. & Pine, D. S. (2002). Anxiety disorders. In *Child and Adolescent Psychiatry: Modern Approaches*, ed. M. Rutter & E. Taylor, 4th edn. London: Blackwell Science Ltd.

Klein, R. G., Kopelwicz, H. S. & Kanner, A. (1992). Imipramine treatment in children with separation anxiety. *Journal of the American Academy of Child and Adolescent Psychiatry*, **31**, 21–8.

Labellarte, M. J., Ginsburg, G. S., Walkup, J. T. & Riddle, M. A. (1999). The treatment of anxiety disorders in children and adolescents. *Society of Biological Psychiatry*, **46**, 1567–78.

Leonard, H. L., Swedo, S. E., Rapaport, J. L. *et al.* (1989). Treatment of obsessive-compulsive disorder with clomipramine and Desipramine in children and adolescents: a double-blind crossover comparison. *Archives of General Psychiatry*, **46**, 1088–92.

Liebowitz, M. R., Turner, S. M., Piacentini, J. (2002). Fluoxetine in children and adolescents with OCD: a placebo-controlled trial. *Journal of the American Academy of Child and Adolescent Psychiatry*, **41**, 1431–8.

Manassis, K., Mendlowitz, S. L., Scapillato, D. *et al.* (2002). Group and individual cognitive-behavioural therapy for childhood anxiety disorders: a randomised trial. *Journal of the American Academy of Child and Adolescent Psychiatry*, **41**, 1423–30.

Mancini, C., Van-Ameringen, M., Oakman, R. & Farvolden, P. (1999). Serotonergic agents in the treatment of social phobia in children and adolescents: a case series. *Depression and Anxiety*, **10**(1), 33–9.

March, J. S., Amaya-Jackson, L., Murray, M. D., Cathryn, M. & Schulte, A. (1998a). Cognitive behavioural psychotherapy for children and adolescents with posttraumatic stress disorder after a single incident stressor. *Journal of the American Academy of Child and Adolescent Psychiatry*, **37**, 585–93.

March, J. S., Biederman, J., Wolkow, R. *et al.* (1998b). Sertraline in children and adolescents with obsessive-compulsive disorder: a multi-center randomized controlled trial. *Journal of the American Medical Association*, **280**(20), 1752–6.

MHRA (2004). Advice on SSRIs in Children from the Committee on Safety in Medicine. February 12, 2004. Available at: http://medicines.mhra.gov.uk/aboutagency/regframework/csm/csmhome.htm.

Piacentini, J., Bergman, R. L., Jacobs, C., McCracken, J. T. & Kretchman, J. (2002). Open trial of cognitive behaviour therapy for childhood obsessive-compulsive disorder. *Journal of Anxiety Disorders*, **16**(2), 207–19.

Pine, D. S., Cohen, P., Gurley, D., Brook, J. & Ma, Y. (1998). The risk for early adulthood anxiety and depressive disorders in anxiety and depressive disorders. *Archives of General Psychiatry*, **55**, 56–64.

Renaud, J., Birmaher, B., Wassick, S. C. & Bridge, J. (1999). Use of selective serotonin reuptake inhibitors for the treatment of childhood panic disorder: a pilot study. *Journal of Child and Adolescent Psychopharmacology*, **9**(2), 73–83.

Research Unit on Paediatric Psychopharmacology Anxiety Study Group (RUPPS) (2001). Fluvoxamine for the treatment of anxiety disorders in children and adolescents. *New England Journal of Medicine*, **344**(17), 1279–85.

Research Unit of Paediatric Psychopharmacology Anxiety Study Group (RUPPS) (2002). Treatment of paediatric anxiety disorders: an open label extension of the research units on paediatric psychopharmacology anxiety study. *Journal of Child and Adolescent Psychopharmacology*, **12**(3), 175–88.

Riddle, M. A., Scahill, L., King, R. A. *et al.* (1992). Double-blind crossover trial of fluoxetine and placebo in children and adolescents with obsessive-compulsive disorder. *Journal of American Academy of Child and Adolescent Psychiatry*, **31**, 1062–9.

Riddle, M. A., Claghorn J. & Gaffney, G. (1996). Fluvoxamine for children and adolescents with OCD: a controlled multi-center trial. Presented at the 43rd Annual Meeting of the American Academy of Child and Adolescent Psychiatry, Philadelphia, October.

Robert, R., Blakeney, P. E., Villarreal, C., Rosenberg, L. & Meyer, W. J. (1999). Imipramine treatment in pediatric burn patients with symptoms of acute stress disorder: a pilot study. *Journal of the American Academy Child and Adolescent Psychiatry*, **38**(7), 873–82.

Roy-Byrne, P. P. & Cowley, D. S. (2002). Pharmacological treatments for panic disorder, generalized anxiety disorder, specific phobia and social anxiety disorder. In *A Guide to Treatments that Work*, ed. P. E. Nathan & J. M. Groman, 2nd edn, pp. 337–65. New York: Oxford University Press.

Rynn, M. A., Siqueland, L. & Rickels, K. (2001). Placebo-controlled trial of sertraline in the treatment of children with generalized anxiety disorder. *The American Journal of Psychiatry*, **158**(12), 2008–14.

Rynn, M. A., Kunz, N. R. & Lamm, L. W. (2002). Venlafaxine XR for treatment of GAD in children and adolescents. Presented at the American Academy Child Adolescent Psychiatry Annual meeting, October 24, 2002 San Francisco, California.

Schoenfeld, F., Marmar, C. & Neylan, T. (2004). Current concepts in pharmacotherapy for Posttraumatic Stress Disorder. *Psychiatric Services*, **55**, 519–31.

Scott, A., Shaw, M. & Joughin, C. (2001). *Finding the Evidence: A Gateway to the Literature in Child and Adolescent Mental Health*. London: Gaskell.

Simeon, J. G., Ferguson, H. B., Knott, V. *et al.* (1992). Clinical, cognitive, and neurophysiological effects of alprazolam in children and adolescents with overanxious and avoidant disorders. *Journal of American Academy of Child and Adolescent Psychiatry*, **31**, 29–33.

Spence, S. H., Donovan, C. & Brechman-Toussaint, M. (2000). The treatment of childhood social phobia: the effectiveness of a social skills training-based cognitive-behavioural intervention, with and without parental involvement. *Journal of Child Psychology and Psychiatry, and Allied Disciplines*, **41**(6), 713–26.

Stein, B. D., Jaycox, L. & Kataoka, S. *et al.* (2003). A mental health intervention for schoolchildren exposed to violence: a randomised controlled trial. *Journal of the American Medical Association*, **290**, 603–11.

Target, M. & Fonagy, P. (1996). The psychological treatment of child and adolescent psychiatric disorders. In *What Works for Whom*, ed. A. Roth & P. Fonagy. London: Guilford Press.

The Pediatric OCD Treatment Study (POTS) Team. (2004). Cognitive-behavior therapy, sertraline, and their combination for children and adolescents with obsessive-compulsive disorder: the pediatric OCD treatment study (POTS) randomised controlled trial. *Journal of the American Medical Association*, **292**(16), 1969–76.

Thienemann, M., Martin, J., Cregger, B., Thompson, H. B. & Dyer-Friedman, J. (2001). Manual-driven group cognitive-behavioural therapy for adolescents with obsessive-compulsive disorder: a pilot study. *Journal of American Academy of Child and Adolescent Psychiatry*, 1254–60.

Thomsen, P. H. (1997). Child and adolescent obsessive-compulsive disorder treated with citalopram: Findings from an open trial of 23 cases. *Journal of Child and Adolescent Psychopharmacology*, **7**, 156–66.

Thomsen, P. H. (1998). Obsessive-compulsive disorder in children and adolescents. Clinical guidelines. *European Child and Adolescent Psychiatry*, **7**, 1–11.

Trowell, J., Kolvin, I., Weeramanthri, T. *et al.* (2002). Psychotherapy for sexually abused girls: psychopathological outcome findings and patterns of change. *British Journal of Psychiatry*, **180**, 234–47.

US Food and Drug Administration (2004). Antidepressant use in children, adolescents, and adults. October 15. Available at: http://www.fda.gov/cdept/drug/antidepressant/default.htm.

Varley, C. K. (2001). Sudden death related to selected tricyclic antidepressants in children: epidemiology, mechanisms and clinical implications. *Paediatric Drugs*, **3**(8), 613–27.

Wagner, K. D., Cook, E. H., Chung, H. & Messig, M. (2003). Remission status after long-term sertraline treatment of pediatric obsessive-compulsive disorder. *Journal of Child and Adolescent Psychopharmacology*, **13**(Suppl. 1), S53–60.

Waters, T. L., Barret, P. M. & March, J. S. (2001). Cognitive-behavioural family treatment of childhood obsessive-compulsive disorder: preliminary findings. *American Journal of Psychotherapy*, **55**, 372.

Wetherhold, E. A., Carpenter, D. J. & Bailey, A. J. (2002). Efficacy of paroxetine in childhood and adolescent social anxiety disorder. Presented at the American Academy of Child and Adolescent Psych Annual meeting, October 24, 2002 San Francisco, California.

58

Treatment of eating disorders in children and adolescents

Matthew Hodes, Rose Calderon, Cora Collette Breuner and Christopher K. Varley

Editor's note

As is the situation in many disorders of childhood and adolescence, there is very little good data to support any particular type of intervention in eating disorders that occur during this time period. While all would agree on multi-modal treatment, there are no RCTs to examine that particular type of intervention. What little evidence there is to support any type of intervention leads us to primarily family therapy interventions in this patient population. While there may be a need for psychopharmacology, cognitive-behavioral therapy and nutrition counseling, there is little evidence that can point us to better outcomes when these other interventions are employed. There is probably a role for hospitalization here, but hospitalizations keep people alive but do not necessarily alter the long-term outcome. Both the USA and the UK have practice guidelines, but these guidelines are not rooted in interventions that have withstood methodological rigor.

Introduction

There are now abundant data showing that eating disorders, including anorexia and bulimia nervosa, originate in late childhood and early adolescence (American Academy of Pediatrics, Committee on Adolescence, 2003). The vast majority of patients with eating disorders are diagnosed prior to age 25 years, with the age of onset for anorexia nervosa peaking between ages 13 and 15 years and onset of bulimia nervosa peaking between 17 and 25. Evidence for an increased incidence exists for bulimia nervosa (for example) from cohort studies (Bushnell *et al.*, 1990; Kendler *et al.*, 1991). While there is not good evidence for an increased incidence of anorexia nervosa (Fombonne, 1995), in recent years there may be help seeking at an earlier stage for this

disorder (Lucas *et al.*, 1991). Current prevalence rates for anorexia range from 0.5%–1.0% in females and 0.1% in males (Hsu, 1996). Bulimia nervosa is less prevalent in those under 18 years of age. Bulimic behaviors are more prevalent in females with estimates of 1%–3% in females (Bulik, 2002) and less than 0.2% in males (Carlat & Camargo, 1991; Hsu, 1996; Robb & Dadson, 2002).

Eating disorders are associated with functional impairment and extensive psychiatric co-morbidity (Casper, 1998; Cooper, 1995; Hsu *et al.*, 1993; Striegel-Moore *et al.*, 2003; Wonderlich & Mitchell, 1997). Over the course of their eating disorder, these patients often withdraw from activities and social interaction and suffer impairment in their ability to function in academic and work settings (Bulik, 2002). Depression and anxiety are particularly common co-morbidities for anorexia nervosa and bulimia nervosa. It has been reported that 50%–70% of patients with anorexia and bulimia also have a depressive disorder (Geist *et al.*, 1998; Halmi *et al.*, 1991; Zaider *et al.*, 2000), and co-morbid anxiety disorders, particularly social phobia, are common among patients with anorexia nervosa or bulimia nervosa (Braun *et al.*, 1994; Halmi *et al.*, 1991; Herzog *et al.*, 1992). It should be noted that these symptoms may precede and place youth at risk for developing anorexia or may follow from the physiological effects of malnutrition (Golden, 2003). Patients with bulimia also frequently suffer from mood and anxiety disorders (Bulik *et al.*, 1997; Godart *et al.*, 2000), as well as substance abuse (Wells & Sadowski, 2001). Bulimia is often associated with affective dysregulation as evidenced by high rates of self-injurious behavior (Schmidt *et al.*, 1992) and Cluster B personality disorder diagnoses (Casper, 1998; Holderness *et al.*, 1994; Mitchell *et al.*, 1991; Skodol *et al.*, 1993; Wonderlich & Mitchell, 1997). For both anorexia and bulimia nervosa, obsessive-compulsive disorder (OCD) is a common co-morbid diagnosis (Bellodi *et al.*, 2001).

Cambridge Textbook of Effective Treatments in Psychiatry, ed. Peter Tyrer and Kenneth R. Silk. Published by Cambridge University Press.
© Cambridge University Press, 2008.

Despite this relatively broad literature base, our understanding of the treatment of eating disorders in children and adolescence is limited as few controlled treatment studies have been carried out. Managing the growing population of youngsters with eating disorders seeking treatment requires a judicious integration of the available evidence-based treatments obtained with this age group, use of treatments derived from an understanding of mechanisms of the disorder, and inferences from research with adults with eating disorders (Gowers & Bryant-Waugh, 2004).

Because of the complexity of anorexia and overlap of symptoms with other common co-morbid psychiatric conditions, it is unclear if treatment is to be successful whether multiple aspects of the illness must be addressed simultaneously or in sequence or, whether by solely addressing the anorexia, the other co-morbid concerns will also resolve. A primary example is the extent to which children and adolescents with eating disorders need to be medically stable and cognitively intact before psychotherapy interventions can be utilized. Therefore, therapists often employ an eclectic approach to treatment and work closely with medical and nutrition providers. Treatment provision may be influenced by the apparent suitability of the individual taking into account their understanding, intellectual ability and the appropriateness of language based or more abstract therapies. Working with an interdisciplinary model of treatment which includes pediatrics or general medicine, nutrition and mental health provides the most comprehensive treatment approach when all providers are in regular contact with one another and share a similar philosophy in the understanding and treatment of the disorder.

With the exception of family based interventions, there is little research to support the efficacy of the more commonly used treatment approaches described below for anorexia nervosa. Despite the lack of a well-informed research literature, these interventions are reported to be useful by both clinicians and clients (Lask & Bryant-Waugh, 2000; McDermott *et al.*, 2002).

Psychotherapies and other psychosocial interventions

Psychoeducation

Psychoeducation is based on the assumption that eating disorder adolescents possess misconceptions about the factors that lead to and maintain the illness. The goal of psychoeducation is to reduce the resistance to treatment by increasing the adolescent's and parent's awareness of the scientific evidence regarding factors that perpetuate eating disorders and to secure the engagement and partnership of the teen for changing their behaviors (Lask, 2000). Psychoeducation is a preliminary step for enhancing the understanding of eating disorders and is considered an integral component of cognitive-behavioral therapy. Information is offered on the multiple causes of eating disorders, cultural influences, physiology of body weight, effects of starvation, the importance of restoring normal eating patterns, the ill effects of vomiting, laxatives, and other weight controlling substances or practices, medical and physical complications, determining a healthy body weight and muscle to fat body composition, and relapse prevention (Garner, 1997).

Cognitive-behavioral therapy

Specific techniques of cognitive-behavioral therapy include the use of cognitive restructuring which addresses characteristic eating disordered attitudes about weight and shape and provides extensive psychoeducation as described above. The challenge of using CBT with patients with anorexia nervosa is they often lack motivation for weight gain and this must be addressed first in the initial phase of treatment in order to cultivate and sustain motivation for change. Clients with bulimia nervosa do not necessarily require weight gain as a sign of successful outcome but rather ending the binge/purge behaviors. Thus motivation and subsequent engagement in a CBT approach may be easier for them. Garner *et al.* (1997) present a detailed model for the use of CBT in the treatment of anorexia, and Wilson *et al.* (1997) present CBT approaches to the treatment of bulimia nervosa.

Systematic reviews have demonstrated the benefits of CBT compared with placebo or waiting list controls for adults with bulimia nervosa (Hay *et al.*, 2004; Jacobi *et al.*, 1997; Whittal *et al.*, 1999). The first randomised trial of cognitive behaviour therapy for adolescents with bulimia nervosa showed this was associated with more rapid improvement than family therapy (Schmidt *et al.*, 2007). One study of anorexia nervosa that included many adolescents found that CBT was superior to nutritional counselling alone (Serfaty, 1999). Another small study of anorexia nervosa that had some adolescent patients provided data on 18 who completed treatments and did not find a difference between CBT and behavioural family therapy (Ball & Mitchell, 2004).

Psychodynamic psychotherapy

There is a long tradition of using psychodynamic psychotherapy for the treatment of children and adolescents with eating disorders (Magagna, 2000). Some authorities advocate that it should be included in the range of therapies in a comprehensive approach to management (Lask, 2000). However, there is no evidence that it is effective. In the only relevant study identified, comparison was made with behavioral systems family therapy (see Table 58.1, Robin *et al.*, 1994, 1999). Adolescents with anorexia nervosa provided with the psychodynamic psychotherapy achieved less weight gain than those who had the family therapy, and against expectation, they did not achieve greater gains in ego functioning than those receiving the family treatment.

Narrative therapy

Narrative therapy focuses on the problem being the problem itself, rather than considering the problem to be a surface manifestation of a central core or self issue. The problem influences the person, and the person can take responsibility for his or her relationship with the problem. Narrative therapy promotes the use of externalizing language to objectify and scrutinize the problem, not the person. It allows for personification of the problem and reverses the vocabulary of self-blame, allows for alliances to form against the problem, pathologizes the culture not the individual, and promotes identification and acts of resistance against the problem while cultivating authority in the individual over the problem. The therapist listens for differences, exceptions, and 'unique outcomes', and the therapist stories them to encourage personal agency and change so as to construct a life apart from the problem (White & Epston, 1990). This approach is helpful in allowing objectification of the eating disorder illness rather than the identified person with an eating disorder as being one and the same with the eating disorder and being further defined as a person unwilling to change his or her behavior. Narrative therapy provides a framework by which to allow strong alliances to be drawn between the therapist/spouse/parent/caring others and the client to work together against the illness. This approach promotes useful language and construction of small steps to reclaim one's own 'story' or life rather than the destruction of life that is orchestrated by the illness. Maisel *et al.* (2004) provide detailed applications of this approach in the treatment of anorexia and bulimia. Yet there is little data to support or refute it.

Interpersonal therapy (IPT)

This was originally developed for use with depressed patients but has been shown to be an effective treatment for bulimia (Fairburn, 1997). Although there have not been any studies of its use with adolescent eating disorders, its effectiveness with adult bulimia nervosa (Fairburn *et al.*, 1995) and benefit in adolescent depression (Mufson *et al.*, 1999) suggest this may be a useful treatment.

Body image therapy

Body image distortion and over-emphasis of self-worth being dependent on body image are hallmark diagnostic criteria of eating disorders. Body image therapy is a systematic approach to transforming the teen's relationship with his or her body from a self-defeating struggle to an experience of self-acceptance and enjoyment. Body image therapy is best utilized as an adjunct intervention to treatments that directly address the primary symptoms of the eating disorder (Cash, 1997).

Motivation interviewing and enhancement

Motivation interviewing and enhancement can be a helpful intervention tool for those teens with chronic, entrenched patterns of eating disordered behaviors, especially those who are being brought to treatment by parents or under court order rather than arriving at treatment with their own desire for change. A key ingredient in the initial phase of treatment for anorexia is cultivating and sustaining motivation for change. Assessment of the stage of change (e.g. precontemplation, contemplation, preparation, action, maintenance) is useful to determine where treatment should begin (Prochaska & DiClemente, 1992). Because most clients start at the precontemplation stage, the initial aim is to heighten awareness of the dangers of the eating disorder in order to move the teen to the contemplation stage. Once at the contemplation stage, then awareness of the problem with maintaining the eating disorder must be further fortified such that a commitment to change is established with agreed upon goals for outcome. This may then allow for movement into the more advanced stages of preparation and action. Clients with anorexia may have setbacks in their motivation stage as the reality of weight gain occurs and fearfulness, ambivalence and dissonance obstruct their thinking patterns. They may need to be taken through the stages of motivation multiple times by revisiting and building on previous conversations and successes. Again, this intervention has not been evaluated with the younger age group, but evidence from treatment discontinuation and the attitudes and behaviors of adolescents in treatment suggest this is an important area for further development (Gowers & Bryant-Waugh, 2004).

Table 58.1. Controlled studies of family treatment for adolescent anorexia nervosa

Research centre authors	Sample	Age years (range) at entry to trial	Measures of change	Treatment	End of treatment outcome and FU
St George's, London Hall & Crisp, 1987	30 All <85% MPMW All amenorrhoea	19.5 13–27	weight MR scales CCEI	All OP (1) 12 sessions PFT (2) 12 sessions dietary	Weight: no difference groups. Only dietary group > baseline MR changes only reported at 1 year FU, PFT > dietary on social and sexual adjustment
Crisp *et al.*, 1991 Gowers *et al.*, 1994	90 AN DSM IIIR	22	weight MR scales	(1) IP (2) 12 sessions PFT + 4 sessions dietary (3) 10 sessions group + 4 sessions dietary (4) Assessment only	All treatment groups > 4. Similar changes 1,2,3. Poor compliance all groups. 2 year FU, group 3 > group 4 on weight and socioeconomic functioning
Maudsley, London Russell *et al.*, 1987 Eisler *et al.*, 1997	DSM III: 21 EOSH	16.6 (1.7) CCEI	weight MR scales	All IP for weight restoration. Then RA to 1 year of: (1) family therapy (2) individual	According to groups: (1) For weight and all MR subscales (except mental state) family therapy (2) individual. FT at 5 year FU.
Le Grange *et al.*, 1992a, b	18 DSM IIIR 12–17	15.3 (1.8)	weight MR scales EE, FACES	All OP, RA to 32 weeks of: (1) conjoint family therapy (2) separated family therapy	Significant improvement all measures, Good outcome associated with better family function No differences between treatments.
Dare *et al.*, 2000 Eisler *et al.*, 2000 Eüler *et al.*, 2007	40 ICD 10 11–17	15.5 (1.6)	weight MR scales EE, FACES EAT, EDI MFQ	All OP, RA to 52 weeks of: (1) conjoint family therapy (2) separated family therapy	Significant improvement in all measures of adolescent and family function. Conjoint therapy greater improvement depression, interpersonal mistrust. Separated therapy greater improvement weight gain for high EE families. Benefit maintained at 5-year FU.
Detroit, USA Robin *et al.*, 1994 1999	37 DSM IIIR	12–20	weight EAT, BSQ, EDI, BDI, PARQ	IP for weight restoration if <75% healthy weight RA to (1) BFST (2) EOIT	Weight: BFST > EOIT. Eat attitudes, mood, family relationships, improved, no treatment differences.
Toronto, Canada Geist *et al.*, 2000,	25 DSM-IV weight <90% IBW	12–17.4 years 14.9 (1.7)	weight EDI, BSI CDI, FAM-III,	in-patient weight to 90% IBW RA: (1) 8 sessions family therapy (2) 8 sessions family group psychoeducation	No significant differences between family interventions

Abbreviations: AN : anorexia nervosa; OP: outpatient; FU: follow up; MPMW: matched population mean weight; MR: Morgan Russell scales; CCEI Crown Crisp Experiential Index; PFT: psychodynamic and family therapy; Dietary: dietary counselling. PFT: psychodynamic and family therapy; EOSH: early onset short history; MR: Morgan Russell scales; CCEI Crown Crisp Experiential Index; EE: expressed emotion; FACES: Family Adaptability and Cohesion Evaluation Scale; EAT: Eating Attitudes Test; EDI: Eating Disorders inventory; MFQ: Mood and Feelings Questionnaire; IP: inpatient; OP: outpatient; RA: random allocation; BSQ: Body Shape Questionnaire; BDI: Beck Depression Inventory; PARQ: Parent Adolescent Relationship Questionnaire; BFST: behavioral family systems therapy; EOIT: ego-oriented individual therapy; IBW: ideal body weight; BSI: brief symptom inventory; CDI: children's depression inventory; FAM-III: family assessment measure.

Meal support therapy (MST)

This can be defined as a combination of social modeling, psychoeducation, and cognitive-behavioral techniques that are aimed at stabilizing and normalizing eating behaviors in individuals with eating disorders. Additionally, MST is a present orientated intervention to be used 'in the moment' with adolescents struggling to eat during a meal. Hall *et al.* (2004) regard the supervision, emotional support, reassurance and education offered in order to help the teen complete each meal or snack as the key therapeutic elements of MST. The rationale of MST is to provide this structure and encouragement through modeling, CBT techniques and family therapy approaches to stabilize and normalize eating behaviors in order to facilitate further treatment and recovery.

Family therapy interventions

Considerable work has been carried out on the family therapy of adolescent anorexia nervosa (for reviews, see Eisler, 2005; Le Grange & Lock, 2005). The rather different models of Bruch (1973, 1978, 1982), Minuchin *et al.* (1975, 1978), and Selvini-Palazzoli (1974; Selvini-Palazzoli *et al.* 1978) have converged. They agree that the families with an adolescent with anorexia nervosa have (a) a high level of closeness that typically involves the sufferer and one of her parents, usually mother, (b) hidden but ongoing conflict between the parents, and (c) a lack of expressed warmth and emotion recognition in the families. These formulations have produced specific approaches to intervention that include directive elements (especially in the Minuchin's model of structural family therapy) and the reframing and avoidance of blame, a point emphasized in Selvini–Palazolli's model.

During the 1970s and 1980s a number of open trials were reported by these groups and others whom they influenced (Eisler, 2005; Le Grange & Lock, 2005). Clearer evidence for their effectiveness came from randomized controlled trails (see Table 58.1).

Details of the adequate reports are given in the table but a number of caveats need to be mentioned in relation to these studies. First, only the study by Crisp *et al.* (1991) compares an active psychological intervention with assessment only or 'inactive treatment'. The mean age of the patients was 22 years, although some were adolescents. In addition, the psychological therapy offered was a composite that included family sessions. Secondly, amongst the studies that focus only on adolescents (Table 58.1), the family intervention was offered at different stages in the management of the anorexia nervosa.

Thus the Russell *et al.* (1987) study provided family intervention following hospital admission for weight restoration, all those in the Le Grange study (1992b) were outpatients, and in the Eisler *et al.* (2000) study, 4 out of 40 (10%) were hospitalized during the course of outpatient family therapy, mainly because of low weight. In the Robin *et al.* (1999) study, 16 out of 34 (43%) had been hospitalized initially. Only the Robin *et al.* (1994, 1999) studies compared family intervention with individual psychodynamic therapy.

Some tentative conclusions can be drawn from these studies. Firstly, family interventions that have a directive element and which focus on the parents guiding their adolescent offspring to eat more are associated with more rapid improvement than individual psychological treatments, and/or no intervention. Secondly, by the end of treatment over 12–15 months, most will make good progress. For example, combining the results of the Le Grange *et al.* (1992b) and Eisler *et al.* (2000) studies, carried out in the same centre with the same kinds of family intervention, 70% (of the 58) achieved good or intermediate outcome (defined as achieving healthy weight). Thirdly, in the studies by Le Grange *et al.* (1992b), Eisler *et al.* (2000), and Robin *et al.* (1999), the improvement occurs not only in weight but also in eating attitudes and mood, even in the absence of specific therapies targeting these areas. Fourthly, during the course of improvement, there is significant improvement in family relationships, involving both parents and the adolescent sufferer, as well as improvement in the relationship between the parents (Eisler *et al.*, 2000; Hodes, 2003). Fifthly, it has been found that in families with high conflict, separated family therapy, in which parents and the sufferer are seen separately, shows advantages over conjoint family therapy (Eisler *et al.*, 2000; Euler *et al.*, 2007).

A more recent development in family intervention for anorexia nervosa has been the provision of multi-family groups (Dare & Eisler, 2000; Scholz & Asen, 2001). The only randomized controlled trial of multi-family groups is a small study that did not show this intervention was superior to conjoint family therapy (Geist *et al.*, 2000). There has also been an awareness of the need to manualize the treatments, and this manualization in some instances has now been carried out (Le Grange *et al.*, 2005; Lock *et al.*, 2001).

Only two systematic investigations have been reported of family intervention one with bulimia nervosa in young people. One open trial with eight adolescents (mean age 16.5, SD 1.21 years) provided conjoint family therapy similar to that used in Le Grange *et al.* (1992b) and Eisler *et al.* (2000). It was found that, during the course of the intervention, there was significant reduction in binge eating, vomiting and laxative use and improvement in general outcome (Dodge *et al.*, 1995). The first randomized trial for treatment of adolescents with bulimia nervosa showed that family therapy was associated with less rapid improvement than cognitive behaviour therapy guided self-care (Schmidt *et al.*, 2007). However this study included older adolescents some of whom were not living at home with parents (in family therapy group mean age was 17.9 years, SD 1.6, 17% were not living with at least one parent). Other single case studies suggest that family therapy for adolescent bulimia nervosa may be useful (Le Grange & Lock, 2003).

Nutrition counseling

The goal of nutrition counseling is to provide individualized assessment and treatment regarding the physiological aspects of an eating disorder. These aspects include metabolic needs, energy needs for growth and development, activity needs, food and nutrition needs, effects of semi-starvation, body composition and body image. The nutritionist facilitates the teen's understanding of what he or she needs from a physiological standpoint and to learn how to apply it to their own body. The goal is to normalize food intake to help individuals achieve normal hunger and satiety signals so they can fuel themselves adequately to support health and allow them to achieve their life goals (Dixon Docter, personal communication, 2004). Nutritional counseling has not promoted itself to be a primary treatment but rather an important component to a comprehensive treatment plan. In one RCT (Serfaty, 1999), CBT was compared with nutritional counseling for 35 patients with anorexia nervosa (mean age 21 years, youngest 16 years). All patients who received nutritional counseling had dropped out by 3 months, resulting in a lack of follow up data for this group. At follow up, 16/23 of the CBT group no longer met criteria for anorexia nervosa. While these data should not be taken to mean that nutritional counseling could not be helpful as part of an overall intervention, they do suggest that CBT may have some active ingredients, and may have a useful place in the repertoire of psychological treatments.

Psychopharmacology

If significant psychiatric symptoms are persistent, then consideration of psychotropic medications may be warranted as part of a comprehensive treatment plan, although the primary treatment for anorexia nervosa is

eating (Gowers & Bryant-Waugh, 2004). That said, there are no controlled trials with children and adolescents with eating disorders that can inform treatment. Evidence is from clinical impressions and multiple single case studies.

Most commonly prescribed medications for youngsters with anorexia nervosa are antidepressant medications which target both symptoms of depression and anxiety (Mitchell *et al.*, 2003). There is evidence of benefit in the treatment of major depression in children and adolescents with the selective serotonergic uptake inhibitor fluoxetine (SSRIs), but controlled trials have not specifically been done in the co-existing conditions of major depression and anorexia nervosa. Depression associated with anorexia nervosa improves with family treatment directed at weight gain and family relationships (Eisler *et al.*, 2000). Furthermore, some patients with anorexia nervosa, investigated in open trials of SSRI's (e.g. citalopram) deteriorate (Bergh *et al.*, 1996). On the other hand, for some youngsters the depression persists despite some weight gain, and for this group a case may be made for the use of fluoxetine (Gowers & Bryant-Waugh, 2004). By way of contrast, there is substantial evidence for the benefit of antidepressants, mostly SSRIs, in adult bulimia nervosa (Bacaltchuk & Hay, 2003). Adolescents with bulimia nervosa may also be offered this treatment if there is reluctance to use psychological treatments or failure to progress with them

In the presence of very high levels of anxiety, particularly at mealtimes, other medications to reduce anxiety have been tried on a case-by-case basis. Benzodiazepines, particularly the long acting agent clonazepam, are at times prescribed, with uneven clinical success (Mitchell *et al.*, 2003).

Atypical antipsychotics are used increasingly in the United States and some European centres for children and adolescents with anorexia nervosa. Multiple single case studies of children and adolescents with severe anorexia treated with olanzapine resulted in significant clinical improvement (Boachie *et al.*, 2003; Dennis *et al.*, 2006; Mehler *et al.*, 2001). The underlying rationale for antipsychotic medication is the need to change the fixed distorted belief systems of eating disorder psychopathology. Another rationale is the well-known propensity of some of the atypical antipsychotic medications such as olanzapine to cause weight gain. They may also reduce anxiety and agitation which may be associated with increased compliance with other aspects of therapy.

Medical concerns and management

The medical management of the adolescent with an eating disorder requires knowledge of the physical presentations and quick attention to the medical complications that may occur (American Academy of Pediatrics, Committee on Adolescence, 2003; Golden *et al.*, 2003; Rome & Ammerman, 2003; Misra *et al.*, 2004). Physical symptoms include dry skin, cold intolerance, acrocyanosis, constipation, bloating, lanugo hair, scalp hair loss, early satiety with delayed gastric emptying, weakness, fatigue or low energy, short stature, delayed puberty, primary or secondary amenorrhea, nerve compression, breast atrophy, atrophic vaginitis and pitting edema of extremities. There is a potential for irreversible growth retardation if bone maturation and closure of epiphyseal plates has not occurred (Kreipe *et al.*, 1995). In bulimia nervosa there may be mouth sores, pharyngeal trauma, dental caries, heartburn, chest pain, muscle cramps, weakness, bloody diarrhea (in laxative abusers), bleeding or easy bruising, irregular periods or amenorrhea, fainting and swollen parotid glands. It is imperative to recognize signs of worsening physical status in these young patients as the mortality for those with eating disorders is the highest among psychiatric conditions including deaths from physiologic causes and suicides.

Vitals signs should include height, weight, orthostatic blood pressure and pulse and temperature. Laboratory assessment for girls with eating disorders include: blood urea, potassium, sodium, chloride, bicarbonate, calcium, magnesium, phosphate, creatinine, full blood picture, erythrocyte sedimentation rate, electrocardiogram, urinalysis, urine pregnancy test and dual-energy radiograph absorptiometry (DEXA) scan of spine or hip.

Myocardial impairment

Myocardial abnormalities noted in adolescents with eating disorders may be categorized into physiologic adaptations, such as sinus bradycardia, sinus arrhythmia, low blood pressure or myocardial abnormalities (Kreipe & Harris, 1992). The bradycardia noted in girls with anorexia nervosa might be due to increased cardiac vagal activity (Kolial *et al.*, 1994). In anorexia nervosa, a pulse differential of greater than 30 beats/min, especially if there is resting bradycardia, suggests excess vagal tone that is counterbalanced by excess standing sympathetic tone. In normal-weight patients with bulimia, hypovolemia is reflected in this pulse differential (Kriepe *et al.*, 1994). Prolonged QT interval, fatal ventricular dysrhythmias, and abnormal contractility have been noted in both adults and adolescents (Isner *et al.*, 1985; Cooke *et al.*, 1994; Swenne & Larsson, 1999; Swenne, 2000). These abnormalities can be reversed after weight has been regained (Mont *et al.*, 2003). Patients with prolonged QT interval should be monitored for hypokalemia or hypomagnesemia, especially if they vomit or take laxatives. Caffeine and exercise

should be avoided to prevent a fatal arrhythmia in those with a diurnal heart rate less than 50 and a nocturnal heart rate less than 46 (Rome & Ammerman, 2003).

Electrolyte abnormalities

Refeeding the adolescent may cause hypophosphatemia which can be corrected with supplemental phosphorus orally twice per day (Rome & Ammerman, 2003). Hypokalemia, noted predominantly in bulimic patients, should be treated with oral potassium until potassium equilibrates or patient stops vomiting (Palla & Litt, 1988; Greenfeld *et al.*, 1995).

Osteoporosis

Peak bone mass is acquired during the teenage years (Gordon & Nelson, 2003). Hypoestrogenemic osteopenia may be seen in as many as 50% of adolescents with eating disorders (Soyka *et al.*, 1999, 2002). This may be due to an acquired growth hormone resistance, low DHEAS, low IGF-1 and elevated cytokines such as osteoprotegerin (Gordon *et al.*, 2002a; Misra *et al.*, 2003a, 2003b). The impact that this may have on the developing bone mass in young woman can have significant deleterious effects in the adult. The treatment of an abnormal DEXA scan in the patient with an eating disorder has been controversial. It is known that weight-recovered patients had improved BMD (bone mineral density (Treasure *et al.*, 1987)). Estrogen replacement has not been shown to be an effective treatment for decreased bone mineral densities in adolescents except in those with exceedingly low weight (Golden, 2003; Kreipe *et al.*, 1993; Klibanski *et al.*, 1995). There have been two trials using DHEA, one for three months and the other for a year. Neither study showed a significant change in BMD (Gordon *et al.*, 1999, 2002b). Dexamethasone has not been shown to affect BMD in patients with anorexia (Gorson *et al.*, 2000). Two studies have shown a positive effect on BMD in those with anorexia using bisphosphonates, one of which was performed with adolescents (Golden *et al.*, 2005; Miller *et al.*, 2004).

Amenorrhea

The absence of menses in the adolescent with an eating disorder is caused by starvation and weight loss associated hypothalamic dysfunction (Laughlin *et al.*, 1998). This may be due to a decrease in leptin levels and thyroid dysfunction (Warren *et al.*, 1999). Amenorrhea may occur in one-third of normal weight bulimics (Levine, 2002). Hypothalamic amenorrhea may have significant longterm effects on fertility. Weight recovery is clearly required for a patient to conceive (Kreipe & Mou, 2000; Perkins *et al.*, 2001).

Growth retardation

There is growing concern that growth is affected in children and adolescents with eating disorders. In one study, girls who presented before menarche trended down in their height and weight curves at least one-year before weight loss occurred (Swenne & Thurfjell, 2003). A separate study showed that girls with a premenarchal presentation of their anorexia nervosa did not achieve their genetic height potential (Lantzouni *et al.*, 2002). In adolescent males with anorexia nervosa followed for 4 years, growth retardation was noted during their illness. Weight restoration was associated with 'catch up' growth but targeted height was not achieved (Modan-Moses *et al.*, 2003).

Hospitalization in the adolescent

If greater than 30% of ideal body weight has been lost, hospitalization should be considered (Lask, 2000; Rome, 2003). Criteria for hospitalization are noted in Table 58.2.

Touyz *et al.* (1995) report weight gain and improvements in eating attitudes and behaviors and mood during the course of hospitalization. Only one randomized controlled trial has compared the benefits of admission with no treatment or outpatient psychological therapies (Crisp *et al.*, 1991). As can be seen from Table 58.1, the group of young women, which included some in the teenage years, achieved greater improvement if they were assigned to one of the active treatment groups. A further study has questioned the medium to long-term benefits of admission for adolescent anorexia nervosa (Gowers *et al.*, 2000). This cohort study of adolescents (mean age at presentation 15.2 years) found that presenting weight as well as initial global functioning (indicated by Morgan Russell scales) was strongly associated with outcome 2–7 years later. More striking, 3/21 treated as inpatients had good outcome at 4 years compared with 31/51 of those who had never been admitted. A cohort study cannot definitively address the question of benefits from admission (as the two groups those admitted and those not admitted were not the same at entry into the study). However, the results are a reminder that there is still no evidence that admission of adolescents is associated with improved medium to long-term outcome.

Within the context of the inpatient unit, a number of studies have been carried out that have bearing on the management approach. First, the strict behavioral approaches that were widely used resulted in dissatisfaction from the patients and criticism by those who argued that they would prevent psychological development (Bruch, 1974). This resulted in investigation of a more

Table 58.2. Criteria for hospitalization in anorexia

Sinus bradycardia, rate less than 45 beats per minute
Other arrhythmia, including prolonged corrected
  QT interval
Hypothermia (temperature < 97.5 °F)
Orthostatic hypotension by pulse or by blood pressure
Precipitous weight loss in a short time period
Severe electrolyte imbalances (potassium < 3.0,
  phosphorus < 2.0)
Unable to eat or drink, acute food refusal
Intractable vomiting
Marked depression, with suicidal ideation and intent
Failure to progress in outpatient treatment, especially when risk
  of growth delay

lenient approach which was no less successful in achieving weight restoration than the strict operant techniques (Touyz *et al.*, 1984). This led to the widespread use of the more flexible approach that is more in keeping with current practice which seeks to achieve a greater partnership with patients and their parents (Touyz *et al.*, 1995). Weight gain of 1.5 kg per week is expected but if less is achieved there may be some reduction of freedom but no restriction of access to personal possessions. The second line of investigation concerns supplemental nocturnal nasogastric refeeding. It has been shown that in a randomized controlled trial amongst adolescent girls, weight gain was more rapid with nasogastric feeding (Robb *et al.*, 2002). While this intervention might only be used in extreme circumstances, it is important to keep this evidence in mind for effectiveness in relation to weight gain. Finally, it has been shown that the frequency of weighing (daily compared with three times weekly) does not affect weight restoration in the inpatient setting (Touyz *et al.*, 1990).

Practice guidelines for treatment

In 2000, the American Psychiatric Association published a revision of their 1993 Practice Guidelines for the Treatment of Patients with Eating Disorders (American Psychiatric Association Practice Guidelines, 2000). These practice guidelines are not specific to adolescents nor are they considered national guidelines as are those promoted by NICE in the UK. Despite these limitations, the APA Treatment Guidelines offer a comprehensive overview for treatment and is helpful in orienting practitioners new to the treatment of eating disorders. It also outlines an historical overview of the illness, diagnostic criteria, epidemiology and

Table 58.3. Core concepts of therapies used in the treatment of child and adolescent eating disorders

- Interdisciplinary and coordinated care provider approach: medicine, nutrition, and psychotherapy (individual, family, and/or group)
- Psychoeducation to promote understanding to both the client and family members regarding the medical, nutritional, and psychosocial aspects of the eating disorder and recovery process
- Provide an objective conceptualization of the eating disorder as being separate from the individual in order for the patient, family, and treatment providers to form an alliance against the illness
- Cultivate parents as healthy role models for their son or daughter re: eating, exercise, stress management and communication skills, this may extend to parents taking charge of the teen's eating until the teen can assume this responsibility
- Promote healthy and realistic interpersonal relationships in order to supplant the relationship the adolescent has with the eating disorder
- Establish or re-establish new measures of success or basis for self-esteem versus perfectionism or unrealistic media images
- Challenge body image distortions and cultivate acceptance of the uniqueness of one's own body
- Provide alternate internal 'dialogues' to challenge the voice of the eating disorder and promote rational, conscious decision making and behavior change
- Implement clear recovery goals and steps toward behavior change related to specific ED behaviors (e.g. decrease purging, increase normal eating patterns and diversity of foods, exercise management, decrease restricting, tolerate weight gain and resumption of menses)
- Improve interpersonal communication skills, self-advocacy skills, affective awareness and tolerance for negative affect
- Develop a balanced lifestyle of work/school, recreation, social relationships and community involvement
- Treat co-morbid psychiatric disorders (e.g. depression, anxiety, OCD, self-harming behaviors)
- Develop distress tolerance and relaxation skills
- Provide an accepting and nurturing therapeutic model balanced with continuous challenging of maladaptive beliefs and behaviors

demographic data, treatment principles and alternatives, basic medical and nutrition guidelines, medication efficacy, psychosocial treatments, treatment planning strategies, common co-morbid psychiatric disorders, concurrent medical conditions, and ideas for future research. Many of the points are listed in Table 58.3.

Within the UK, the National Institute of Clinical Excellence has published guidelines on the management of eating disorders (NCCMH, 2004). With regard to children and adolescents with anorexia nervosa, the only guideline that is graded as B (based on adequately designed studies without randomization) concerns the recommendation that 'family intervention that directly addresses the eating disorder should be offered' (NCCMH, 2004). With regards to bulimia nervosa, there is only one paragraph regarding psychological treatments in this younger group. This states that they may be 'treated with CBT-BN adapted as needed to suit their age, circumstances and level of development and including the family as appropriate'. The many other treatment and service recommendations for anorexia nervosa that are made are assigned category C (i.e. based on expert committee reports, or based on extrapolation from studies with control or comparison groups), are similar to the numerous practice points made in this review. This rather sanguine interpretation of the evidence arises because of the rigorous nature of the standards used,

including the need for adequately powered studies, use of manualized treatments and random allocation.

There is little knowledge about the treatments that are provided for children and adolescents with eating disorders. Some services provide 'a comprehensive treatment approach', with availability of a range of interventions including psychodynamic therapy (Lask, 2000). Management in this model would involve youngsters receiving many treatments concurrently which would place a high level of demand on them, their parents, and service providers. Alternative approaches would be more parsimonious; and if outpatient management is appropriate, start with psychoeducation, nutritional counseling and family intervention, and then add treatments in relation to the progress that is made and continuing psychopathology.

One survey has been carried out into the treatments that are provided across Europe (Gowers et al., 2002). There were considerable variations with respect to the availability of inpatient and day services, and the range of psychological treatments (Gowers et al., 2002). Psychotropic drugs including SSRIs, antipsychotics and minor tranquilizers appear to be quite widely used.

A final note concerns the treatment of children and adolescent with eating disorders that do not reach the criteria for anorexia nervosa or bulimia. They may have occasional binge eating or dietary restriction with some degree of

Table 58.4. Effectiveness of treatments for eating disorders in children and adolescents

Treatment	Form of treatment	Psychiatric disorder/ target audience	Level of evidence for efficacy	Comments
Psychotherapy	Cognitive behavioral therapy	Eating disorders	Ib	CBT results in more rapid response than family therapy for bulimia nervosa. For anorexia nervosa some adult studies included adolescents, with some evidence that CBT > nutritional counselling alone
Psychotherapy	Interpersonal therapy	Bulimia	III	No trials on children or adolescents but evidence from adult studies suggest it may be useful in this younger age group as well
Psychotherapy	Motivation interviewing and enhancement	Eating disorders	IV	May work with adolescents and increase treatment uptake; inadequately investigated in adolescents
Family therapy	Various forms of structured and systemic family therapy	Anorexia	Ia	Weight gain. Better relationships among identified patients and parents. Better relationships between parents
Psychopharmacology	SSRIs (especially fluoxetine)	Eating disorders	III	Evidence from studies with adults might apply to adolescents as well. Some studies show worsening with citalopram. A greater body of evidence for treatment success with SSRIs for bulimia than for anorexia
Psychopharmacology	Atypical antipsychotics (especially olanzapine)	Anorexia	III	May help change fixed ideas about body and weight and may also, because of weight gain side effect, directly contribute to weight gain
Hospitalization	Multidisciplinary intervention	Primarily for anorexia	III	May be necessary especially in life-threatening situations. Little data as to the long effect of hospitalization

weight loss and often a high level of eating and weight preoccupation with characteristic fear of fatness. Such individuals may make up half of those referred to services (Nicholls *et al.*, 2000). They may reach the criteria for Eating Disorders Not Otherwise Specified, with regard to DSM-IV (American Psychiatric Association, 1994), or partial syndromes of anorexia nervosa or bulimia nervosa ICD-10 (WHO, 1992), and in these people there may be a high level of distress and social impairment. The evidence base does not give explicit guidance on how to manage this group, but it would seem clinically appropriate to follow the general treatment principles outlined in Table 58.3. Clinical impressions are that specific treatments should be chosen that will target the most impairing and dangerous behavior, i.e. follow the guidelines for anorexia nervosa for those who have low weight and the treatment of bulimia nervosa for those who are binge eating.

The level of evidence for each of the interventions discussed in this chapter is summarized in Table 58.4.

REFERENCES

American Academy of Pediatrics, Committee on Adolescence (2003). Identifying and treating eating disorders. *Pediatrics*, **111**(1), 204–11.

American Psychiatric Association (1994). *Diagnostic and Statistical Manual of Mental Disorders*, 4th edn. Washington, DC: American Psychiatric Association.

American Psychiatric Association Practice Guidelines (2000). Practice guidelines for the treatment of patients with eating disorders (Revision). *Supplement to The American Journal of Psychiatry*, **151**(1), 1–39.

Bacaltchuk, J. & Hay, P. (2003). Antidepressants versus placebo for people with bulimia nervosa. *Cochrane Database Systematic Review*, CD003391. Oxford: Update Software Ltd.

Ball, J. & Mitchell, P. (2004). A randomized controlled study of cognitive behavior therapy and behavioral family therapy for anorexia nervosa patients. *Eating Disorders*, **12**, 303–14.

Bellodi, L., Cavallini, M. C., Bertelli, S., Chiapparino, D., Riboldi, C. & Smeraldi, E. (2001). Morbidity risk of obsessive-compulsive spectrum disorders in first-degree relatives of patients with eating disorders. *American Journal of Psychiatry*, **158**, 563–9.

Bergh, C., Eriksson, M., Lindberg, G. & Sodersten, P. (1996). Selective serotonin reuptake inhibitors in anorexia. *Lancet*, **348**, 1459–60.

Boachie, A., Goldfield, G. S. & Spettigue, W. (2003). Olanzapine use as an adjunctive treatment for hospitalized children with anorexia nervosa: case reports. *International Journal of Eating Disorders*, **33**, 98–103.

Braun, D. L., Sunday, S. R. & Halmi K. A. (1994). Psychiatric comorbidity in patients with eating disorders. *Psychological Medicine*, **2**, 859–67.

Bruch H. (1973). *Eating Disorders: Obesity, Anorexia Nervosa and the Person Within*. New York: Basic Books

Bruch, H. (1974). Perils of behaviour modification in the treatment of anorexia nervosa. *Journal of the American Medical Association*, **230**, 1419–22.

Bruch, H. (1978). *The Golden Cage. The Enigma of Anorexia Nervosa*. Cambridge, MA: Harvard University Press.

Bruch, H. (1982) Anorexia nervosa: therapy and theory. *American Journal of Psychiatry*, **139**, 1531–8.

Bulik, C. M. (2002). Eating disorders in adolescents and young adults. *Child and Adolescent Psychiatric Clinics of North America*, **11**(2), 201–18.

Bulik, C. M., Sullivan, P. F., Fear, J. & Joyce, P. R. (1997). Eating disorders and antecedent anxiety disorders: a controlled study. *Acta Psychiatrica Scandinavica*, **92**, 101–7.

Bushnell, J. A., Wells, J. E., Hornblow, A. R., Oakley-Brown, M. A. & Joyce, P. (1990). Prevalence of three bulimia syndromes in the general population. *Psychological Medicine*, **20**, 671–80.

Carlat, D.J. & Camargo, C.A. (1991). Review of bulimia nervosa in males. *American Journal of Psychiatry*, **148**, 831–43.

Cash, T. (1997). *The Body Image Workbook: An 8-Step Program for Learning to Like Your Looks*. Oakland: New Harbinger Publications.

Casper, R.C. (1998). Depression and eating disorders. *Depression and Anxiety*, **8**(Suppl. 1), 96–104.

Cooke, R., Chambers, J., Singh, R. *et al.* (1994). QT interval in anorexia nervosa. *British Heart Journal*, **1**(72), 69–73.

Cooper, P. J. (1995). Eating disorders and their relationship to mood and anxiety disorders. In *Eating Disorders and Obesity: A Comprehensive Handbook*, ed. K. D. Brownell & C. G. Fairburn, pp. 159–64. New York: Guilford Press.

Crisp, A. H., Norton, K. W. R., Gowers, S. G. *et al.* (1991). A controlled study of the effect of therapies aimed at adolescent and family psychopathology in anorexia nervosa. *British Journal of Psychiatry*, **159**, 325–33.

Dare, C., Chania, E., Eisler, I., Hodes, M. & Dodge, E. (2000). The eating disorder inventory as an instrument to explore change in adolescents in family therapy for anorexia nervosa. *European Eating Disorders Review*, **8**, 369–83.

Dare, C. & Eisler, I. (2000). A multi-family group day treatment programme for adolescent eating disorder. *European Eating Disorders Review*, **8**, 4–18.

Dennis, K., Le Grange, D. & Bremer, J. (2006). Olanzapine use in adolescent anorexia nervosa. *Eating and Weight Disorders*, **11**, e53–56.

Dodge, E., Hodes, M., Eisler, I. & Dare, C. (1995) Family therapy for bulimia nervosa in adolescents: An exploratory study. *Journal of Family Therapy*, **17**, 59–77.

Eisler, I. (2005). The empirical and theoretical base of family therapy and multiple family day therapy for adolescent anorexia nervosa. *Journal of Family Therapy*, **27**, 104–31.

Eisler, I., Dare, C., Russell, G. F. M., Szmukler, G. I., Le Grange, D. & Dodge, E. (1997). Family and individual therapy in anorexia nervosa. A 5-year follow-up. *Archives of General Psychiatry*, **54**, 1025–30.

Eisler, I., Dare, C., Hodes, M., Russell, G. F. M., Dodge, E. & Le Grange, D. (2000). Family therapy for adolescent anorexia nervosa: the results of a controlled comparison of two family interventions. *Journal of Child Psychology and Psychiatry*, **41**, 727–36.

Eisler, I., Simic, M., Russell, G. F. M. & Dare, C. (2007). A randomised controlled treatment trial of two forms of family therapy in anorexia nervosa in adolescent anorexia nervosa: a five-year follow-up. *Journal of Child Psychology and Psychiatry*, **48**, 552–60.

Fairburn, C. (1997). Interpersonal psychotherapy for bulimia nervosa. In *The Handbook of Treatment for Eating Disorders*, 2nd edn, ed. D. M. Garner & P. E. Garfinkel, pp. 278–94. New York: Guilford Press.

Fairburn, C. G., Norman, P. A., Welch, S. L., O'Connor, M. E., Doll, H. A. & Peveler, R. C. (1995). A prospective study of outcome in bulimia nervosa and the longterm effects of three psychological treatments. *Archives of General Pyshciatry*, **52**, 304–12.

Fombonne, E. (1995) Anorexia nervosa: no evidence of an increase. *British Journal of Psychiatry*, **166**, 462–71.

Garner, D. M. (1997). Psychoeducational principles in treatment. In *The Handbook of Treatment for Eating Disorders*, 2nd edn, ed. D. M. Garner & P. E. Garfinkel, pp. 145–77. New York: Guilford Press.

Garner, D. M., Vitousek, P. K. M. (1997). Cognitive-behavioral therapy for anorexia nervosa. In *The Handbook of Treatment for Eating Disorders*, 2nd edn, ed. D. M. Garner & P. E. Garfinkel, pp. 94–144. New York: Guilford Press.

Geist R., Davis, R. & Heinman, M. (1998). Binge/purge symptoms and comorbidity in adolescents with eating disorders. *Canadian Journal of Psychiatry*, **43**, 507–12.

Geist, R., Heinmaa, M., Stephens, D., Davis, R. & Katzman, D. K. (2000). Comparison of family therapy and family group psychoeducation in adolescents with anorexia nervosa. *Canadian Journal of Psychiatry*, **45**, 173–8.

Godart, N. T., Flamant, M. F., Lecrubier, Y. & Jeammet, P. (2000). Anxiety disorders in anorexia nervosa and bulimia nervosa: co-morbidity and chronology of appearance. *European Psychiatry*, **15**, 38–45.

Golden, N.H. (2003). Eating disorders in adolescence and their sequelae. *Best Practice and Research in Clinical Ostetrics and Gynaecology*, **17**(1), 57–73.

Golden, N.H., Katzman, D.K., Kreipe, R.E. *et al.* (2003). Eating disorders in adolescents: position paper of the Society for Adolescent Medicine. *Journal of Adolescent Health*, **33**(6), 496–503.

Golden, N.H., Jacobson, M.S., Igelsia, E. (2005). Alendrolate for the treatment of osteopenia in anorexia nervosa: a randomized double blind placebo-controlled trial. *Journal of Adolescent Health*, **36**(2), 103.

Gordon, C.M. & Nelson, L.M. (2003). Amenorrhea and bone health in adolescents and young women. *Current Opinion in Obstetrics and Gynecology*, **15**, 377–84.

Gordon, C.M., Grace, E., Emans, S.J., Goodman, E., Crawford, M. & Leboff, M. (1999). Changes in bone turnover markers and menstrual function after short term oral HDHEA in young women with anorexia nervosa. *Journal of Bone and Mineral Research*, **14**, 136–45.

Gordon, C.M. Emans, S.J. Durant, R.H. *et al.* (2000). Endocrinologic and physiologic effects of short term dexamethasone in anorexia nervosa. *Eating and Weight Disorders*, **5**(3), 175–82.

Gordon, C.M., Goodman, E., Emans, S.J. *et al.* (2002a). Physiologic regulators of bone turnover in young women with anorexia nervosa. *Journal of Pediatrics*, **14**(1), 64–70.

Gordon, C.M., Grace, E., Emans, S.J. *et al.* (2002b). Effects of oral dehydroepiandrosterone on bone density in young women with anorexia nervosa: a randomized trial. *Journal of Clinical Endocrinology and Metabolism*, **87**, 4935–41.

Gowers, S. & Bryant-Waugh, R. (2004). Management of child and adolescent eating disorders: The current evidence base and future directions. *Journal of Child Psychology and Psychiatry*, **45**, 63–83.

Gowers, S., Norton, K., Halek, C. & Crisp, A.H. (1994). Outcome of outpatient psychotherapy in a random allocation treatment study of anorexia nervosa. *International Journal of Eating Disorders*, **15**, 165–77.

Gowers, S.G., Weetman, J., Shore, A., Hossain, F. & Elvins, R. (2000). Impact of hospitalization on the outcome of adolescent anorexia nervosa. *British Journal of Psychiatry*, **176**, 138–41.

Gowers, S.G., Edwards, V.J., Fleminger, S. *et al.* (2002). Treatment aims and philosophy in the treatment of adolescent anorexia nervosa in Europe. *European Eating Disorders Review*, **10**, 271–80.

Greenfeld, D., Mickley, D., Quinlan, D.M. & Roloff, P. (1995). Hypokalemia in outpatients with eating disorders. *American Journal of Psychiatry*, **152**, 60–3.

Hall, A. & Crisp, A.H. (1987) Brief psychotherapy in the treatment of anorexia nervosa. Outcome at one year. *British Journal of Psychiatry*, **151**, 185–91.

Hall, D., Leichner, P., Calderon, R. & Caufield, S. (2004). *Meal Support Manual: Introduction for Parents, Friends and Caregivers*. Published and distributed by the BC Children's Hospital, Vancouver, BC, Canada.

Halmi, K.A., Eckert, E., Marchi, P., Sampugnaro, V., Apple, R. & Cohen, J. (1991). Comorbidity of psychiatric diagnoses in anorexia nervosa. *Archives of General Psychiatry*, **48**, 712–18.

Hay, P.J., Bacalchuk, J. & Stefano, S. (2004). Psychotherapy for bulimia nervosa and binge eating. *Cochrane Review. The Cochrane Library*, **3**, CD000562. Oxford: Update Software Ltd.

Herzog, D.B., Keller, M.B., Lavori, P.W., Kenny, G.M. & Sacks NR. (1992). The prevalence of personality disorders in 210 women with eating disorders. *Journal of Clinical Psychiatry*, **53**, 147–52.

Hodes, M. (2003) *The Family Treatment of Adolescent Anorexia Nervosa: Changes in the Adolescent and Parental Expressed Emotion*. Unpublished PhD thesis, Kings College, University of London.

Holderness, C., Brooks-Gunn, J. & Warren, M. (1994). Comorbidity of eating disorders and substance abuse: Review of the literature. *International Journal of Eating Disorders*, **16**, 1–35.

Hsu, L.K.G. (1996). Epidemiology of the eating disorders. *Psychiatric Clinics of North America*, **19**, 681–700.

Hsu, L.K.G., Kaye, W. & Weltzin, T. (1993). Are the eating disorders related to obsessive-compulsive disorder? *International Journal of Eating Disorders*, **14**, 305–18.

Isner, J., Roberts, W., Heymsfield, S. & Yager, J. (1985). Anorexia nervosa and sudden death. *Annals of Internal Medicine*, **102**, 49–52.

Jacobi, C., Dahme, B. & Rustenbach, S. (1997). Comparison of controlled psycho and pharmacotherapy studies in bulimia anorexia nervosa [in German]. *Psychotherapy Psychpsomatik Midizinische Psychologie*, **47**, 346–64.

Kendler, K.S., Maclean, C., Neale, M., Kessler, R., Heath, A. & Eaves, L. (1991). The genetic epidemiology of bulimia nervosa. *American Journal of Psychiatry*, **148**, 1627–37.

Klibanski, A., Biller, B.M.K., Schoenfeld, D.A., Herzog, D.B. & Saxe, V.C. (1995). The effects of estrogen administration on trabecular bone loss in young women with anorexia nervosa. *Journal of Clinical Endocrinology and Metabolism*, **80**, 898–904.

Kolial, M., Bonyhay, I., Jokkel, G. & Szonyi, L. (1994). Cardiac hyperactivity in adolescent anorexia nervosa. *European Heat Journal*, **15**, 1113–18.

Kreipe, R.E. & Harris, J.P. (1992). Myocardial impairment in eating disorders. *Pediatric Annals*, **21**, 760–8.

Kreipe, R.E. & Mou, S.M. (2000). Eating disorders in adolescents and young adults. *Obstetric and Gynecology Clinics of North America*, **27**(1), 101–24.

Kreipe, R.E., Hicks, D., Rosier, R. & Puzas, J. (1993). Preliminary findings on the effects of sex hormones on bone metabolism in anorexia nervosa. *Journal of Adolescent Health*, **14**, 319.

Kreipe, R.E., Goldstein, B., DeKing, D.E., Tipton, R. & Kempski, M.H. (1994). Heart rate power spectrum analysis of autonomic dysfunction in adolescents with anorexia nervosa. *International Journal of Eating Disorders*, **16**, 159–65.

Kreipe, R.E., Golden, N.H., Katzman, D.K. *et al.* (1995). Eating disorders in adolescents: a position paper for the Society of Adolescent Medicine. *Journal of Adolescent Health*, **16**, 476–9.

Lantzouni, E., Frank, G.R., Golden, N.H. & Shenker, R.I.. (2002). Reversibility of growth stunting in early onset anorexia nervosa: a prospective study. *Journal of Adolescent Health*, **31**(2), 162–5.

Lask, B. (2000). Overview of management. In *Anorexia Nervosa and Related Eating Disorders in Childhood and Adolescence*, 2nd edn, ed. B. Lask & R. Bryant-Waugh, pp. 167–85. Hove, East Sussex: Psychology Press, Taylor and Francis Group.

Lask, B. & Bryant-Waugh, R. (2000). *Anorexia Nervosa and Related Eating Disorders in Childhood and Adolescence*, 2nd edn. Hove, East Sussex: Psychology Press, Taylor and Francis Group.

Laughlin, G. A., Dominguez, C. E. & Yen, S. S. (1998). Nutritional and endocrine–metabolic aberrations in women with functional hypothalamic amenorrhea. *Journal of Clinical Endocrinology and Metabolism*, **83**, 25–32.

Le Grange, D. & Lock, J. (2003). Family-based therapy for adolescents with bulimia nervosa. *American Journal of Psychotherapy*, **57**, 237–51.

Le Grange, D. & Lock, J. (2005). The dearth of psychological treatment studies for anorexia nervosa. *International Journal of Eating Disorders*, **37**, 79–91.

Le Grange, D., Eisler, I., Dare, C. & Hodes, M. (1992a). Family criticism and self-starvation: a study of expressed emotion. *Journal of Family Therapy*, **14**, 177–92.

Le Grange, D., Eisler, I., Dare, C. & Russell, G. F. M. (1992b). Evaluation of family therapy in anorexia nervosa: a pilot study. *International Journal of Eating Disorders*, **12**, 347–57.

Le Grange, D., Binford, R. & Loeb, K. L. (2005). Manualized family–based treatment for anorexia nervosa. *Journal of the American Academy of Child and Adolescent Psychiatry*, **44**, 41–6.

Levine, R. L. (2002). Endocrine aspects of eating disorders in adolescent. *Adolescent Medicine State of the Art Reviews*, **13**(1), 129–43.

Lock, J., Le Grange, D., Agras, W. S. & Dare, C. (2001). *Treatment Manual for Anorexia Nervosa. A Family-Based Approach*. New York: Guilford Press.

Lucas, A.R., Beard, C.M., O'Fallon, W.M. *et al.* (1991). 50-year treands in the incidence of anorexia nervosa in Rochester, MN: a population-based study. *American Journal of Psychiatry*, **148**, 917–22.

Magagna, J. (2000). Individual psychotherapy. In *Anorexia Nervosa and Related Eating Disorders in Childhood and Adolescence*, 2nd edn, ed. B. Lask & R. Bryant-Waugh, pp. 227–63. Hove, East Sussex: Psychology Press, Taylor and Francis Group.

Maisel, R., Epston, D. & Borden, A. (2004). *Biting the Hand That Starves You: Inspiring Resistance to Anorexia/Bulimia*. New York: Norton Press.

McDermott, B.M., Harris, C. & Gibbon, P. (2002). Individual psychotherapy for children and adolescents with an eating disorder: from historical precedent toward evidence-based practice. *Child and Adolescent Psychiatric Clinics of North America*, **11**(2), 311–30.

Mehler, C., Wewetzer, C., Sculze, U., Warnke, A., Theisen, F. & Dittmann R.W. (2001). Olanzapine in children and adolescents with chronic anorexia nervosa: a study of five cases. *European Child and Adolescent Psychiatry*, **10**, 151–7.

Miller, K. K., Greico, K. A., Mulder, J. (2004). Effects of risedronate on bone density in anorexia nervosa. *Journal of Clinical Endocrinology and Metabolism*, **89**(8), 3903–6.

Minuchin, S., Baker, L., Rosman, B. T., Liebman, R., Milman, L. & Todd, T. I. (1975). A conceptual model of psychosomatic illness in childhood. *Archives of General Psychiatry*, **32**, 1031–8.

Minuchin, S., Rosman, B.l. & Baker, T. (1978). *Psychosomatic Families: Anorexia Nervosa in Context*. Cambridge, MA: Harvard University Press.

Misra, M., Miller, K.K., Bjornson, J. *et al.* (2003a). Alterations in growth hormone secretory dynamics in adolescent girls with anorexia nervosa and effects on bone metabolism. *Journal of Clinical Endocrinology and Metabolism*, **88**, 5615–23.

Misra, M., Soyka, L. A., Miller, K. K. *et al.* (2003b). Serum osteoprotegerin in adolescent girls with anorexia nervosa. *Journal of Clinical Endocrinology and Metabolism*, **88**(8), 3816–22.

Misra, M., Aggarwal, A., Miller, K. K. *et al.* (2004). Effects of anorexia nervosa on clinical, hematologic, biochemical, and bone density parameters in community-dwelling adolescent girls. *Pediatrics*, **114**, 1574–83.

Mitchell, J.E., Specker, S.M. & de Zwaan, M. (1991). Comorbidity and medical complications of bulimia nervosa. *Journal of Clinical Psychiatry*, **52**(Suppl. 10), 13–20.

Mitchell, J.E., de Zwaan, M. & Roerig, J.L. (2003). Drug therapy for eating disorders. *Current Drug Targets – CNS and Neurological Disorders*, **2**(1), 17–29.

Modan-Moses, D., Yaroslavsky, A., Novikov, I. *et al.* (2003). Stunting of growth as a major feature of anorexia nervosa in male adolescents. *Pediatrics*, **111**(2), 270–6.

Mont, L. Castro, J. Herreros, B. *et al.* (2003). Reversibility of cardiac abnormalities in adolescents with anorexia nervosa after weight recovery. *Journal of the American Academy of Child and Adolescent Psychiatry*, **42**(7), 808–13.

Mufson, L., Weissman, M.M., Moreau, D. & Garfinkel, P. (1999). Efficacy of interpersonal psychotherapy for depressed adolescents. *Archives of General Psychiatry*, **56**, 573–9.

National Collaborating Centre for Mental Health (NCCMH) (2004) *Eating Disorders: Core Interventions in the Treatment and Management of Anorexia Nervosa, Bulimia Nervosa and Related eating Disorders*. London: National Institute for Clinical Excellence.

Nicholls, D., Chater, R. & Lask, B. (2000). Children into DSM don't go: a comparison of classification systems for eating disorders in childhood and early adolescence. *International Journal of Eating Disorders*, **28**, 317–24.

Palla, B. & Litt, I. (1988). Medical complications of eating disorders in adolescents. *Pediatrics*, **81**, 613–23.

Perkins, R. B., Hall, J. E. & Martin, K. A. (2001). Aetiology, previous menstrual function and patterns of neuroendocrine disturbance as prognostic indicators in hypothalamic amenorrhoea. *Human Reproduction*, **16**(10), 2198–205.

Prochaska, J. O. & DiClemente, C. C. (1992). Stages of change in the modification of problem behaviors. In *Progress in Behavior Modification*, ed. M. Hersen, R.M. Eisler & P.M. Miller, pp. 184–214. Sycamore, IL: Sycamore Press.

Robb, A. S. & Dadson, M. J. (2002). Eating disorders in males. *Child and Adolescent Psychiatric Clinics of North America*, **11**(2), 399–418.

Robb, A. S., Silber, T. J., Orrell-Valente, J. K. *et al.* (2002). Supplemental nocturnal nasogastric refeeding for better short-term outcome in hospitalized adolescent girls with anorexia nervosa. *American Journal of Psychiatry*, **159**, 1347–53.

Robin, A. L., Siegel, P. T., Koepke, T., Moye, A. W. & Tice, S. (1994). Family therapy versus individual therapy for adolescent females with anorexia nervosa. *Developmental and Behavioral Pediatrics*, **15**, 111–16.

Robin, A. L., Siegel, P. T., Moye, A. W., Gilroy, M., Dennis, A. B. & Sikand, A. (1999). A controlled comparison of family versus individual therapy for adolescents with anorexia nervosa. *Journal of the American Academy of Child and Adolescent Psychiatry*, **38**, 1482–9.

Rome, E. S. (2003). Eating disorders. *Obstetrics and Gynecology Clinics of North America*, **30**(2), 353–77.

Rome, E. S. & Ammerman, S. (2003). Medical complications of eating disorders: an update. *Journal of Adolescent Health*, **33**(6), 418–26.

Russell, G. F. M., Szmukler, G. I., Dare, C. & Eisler, I. (1987). An evaluation of family therapy in anorexia nervosa and bulimia nervosa. *Archives of General Psychiatry*, **44**, 1047–56.

Schmidt, U., Hodes, M. & Treasure, J. (1992). Early onset bulimia nervosa: who is at risk? Retrospective case-control study. *Psychological Medicine*, **22**, 623–8.

Schmidt, U., Lee, S., Beecham, J. *et al.* (2007). A randomised controlled trial of family therapy and cognitive behaviour therapy guided self-care for adolescents with bulimia nervosa and related disorders. *American Journal of Psychiatry*, **164**, 591–8.

Scholz, M. & Asen, E. (2001). Multiple family therapy with eating disordered adolescents: concepts and preliminary results. *European Eating Disorders Review*, **9**, 33–42.

Selvini-Palazzoli, M. (1974). *Self Starvation: From the Intrapsychic to the Transpersonal Approach to Anorexia Nervosa.* London: Chaucer Publishing.

Selvini-Palazzoli, M., Boscolo, L., Cechin, G. & Prata, G. (1978). *Paradox and Counterparadox.* New York: Jason Aronson.

Serfaty, M. A. (1999). Cognitive therapy versus dietary counseling in the outpatient treatment of anorexia nervosa: effects of the treatment phase. *European Eating Disorders Review*, **7**, 334–50.

Skodol, A. E., Oldham, J. M., Hyler, S. E., Kellman, H. D., Doidge, N. & Davies, M. (1993). Comorbidity of DSM-III-R eating disorders and personality disorders. *International Journal of Eating Disorders*, **14**, 403–16.

Soyka, L., Grinspoon, S., Levitsky, L., Herzog, D. & Klibanski, A. (1999). The effects of anorexia nervosa on bone metabolism in female adolescents. *Journal of Clinical Endocrinology and Metabolism*, **84**, 4489–96.

Soyka, L., Misra, M., Frenchman, A. *et al.* (2002). Abnormal bone mineral accrual in adolescent girls with anorexia nervosa. *Journal of Clinical Endocrinology and Metabolism*, **87**, 4177–85.

Striegel-Moore, R. H., Seeley, J. R. & Lewinsohn, P. M. (2003). Psychosocial adjustment in young adulthood of women who experienced an eating disorder during adolescence. *Journal of the American Academy of Child and Adolescent Psychiatry*, **42**(5), 587–93.

Swenne, I. (2000). Heart risk associated with weight loss in anorexia nervosa and eating disorders: electrocardiographic changes during the early phase of refeeding. *Acta Paediatrica*, **89**(4), 447–552.

Swenne, I. & Larsson, P. T. (1999). Heart risk associated with weight loss in anorexia nervosa and eating disorders: risk factors for QTc interval prolongation and dispersion. *Acta Pediatrica*, **88**(3), 304–9.

Swenne, I. & Thurfjell, B. (2003). Clinical onset and diagnosis of eating disorders in premenarcheal girls is preceded by inadequate weight gain and growth retardation. *Acta Paediatrica*, **92**(10), 1133–7.

Touyz, S. W., Beumont, P. J. V., Glaun, D., Phillips, T. & Cowie, I. (1984). A comparison of lenient and strict operant conditioning programmes in refeeding patients with anorexia nervosa. *British Journal of Psychiatry*, **144**, 517–20.

Touyz, S. W., Lennerts, W., Freeman, R.J. & Beumont, P. J. V. (1990). To weigh or not to weigh? Frequency of weighing and rate of weight gain in patients with anorexia nervosa. *British Journal of Psychiatry*, **157**, 752–4.

Touyz, S. W., Garner, D. M. & Beumont, P. J. V. (1995). The inpatient management of the adolescent patient with anorexia nervosa. In *Anorexia and Bulimia Nervosa: Eating Disorders in Adolescence*, ed. H-Ch. Steinhausen, pp. 247–70. Berlin, New York: Walter de Gruyter.

Treasure, J. L., Russell, G. F., Fogelman, I. & Murby, B. (1987). Reversible bone loss in anorexia nervosa. *British Medical Journal Clinical Research Education*, **295**(6596), 474–5.

Warren, M. P., Voussoughian, F., Geer, E. B., Hyle, E. P., Adberg, C. L. & Ramos, R. H. (1999). Functional hypothalamic amenorrhea: hypoleptinemia and disordered eating. *Journal of Clinical Endocrinology and Metabolism*, **84**(3), 873–7.

Wells, L. A. & Sadowski, C. A. (2001). Bulima nervosa: an update and treatment recommendations. *Current Opinion in Pediatrics*, **13**, 591–7.

White, M. & Epston, D. (1990). *Narrative Means to Therapeutic Ends.* New York: Norton Press.

Whittal, M. L., Agras, W. S. & Gould, R. A. (1999). Bulimia nervosa: a meta analysis of psychosocial and pharmacological treatments. *Behavioral Therapy*, **30**, 117–35.

Wilson, G. T., Fairburn, C. G. & Agras, W. S. (1997). Cognitive-behavioral therapy for bulimia nervosa. In *The Handbook of Treatment for Eating Disorders*, 2nd edn, ed. D. M. Garner & P. E. Garfinkel, pp. 67–93. New York: Guilford Press.

Wonderlich, S. A. & Mitchell, J. E. (1997). Eating disorders and comorbidity: empirical, conceptual and clinical implications. *Psychopharmacology Bulletin*, **33**, 381–90.

World Health Organization (1992). *The ICD-10 Classification of Mental and Behavioural Disorders.* Geneva: World Health Organization.

Zaider, T. L., Johnson, J. G. & Cockell, S. J. (2000). Psychiatric comorbidity associated with eating disorder symptomatology among adolescents in the community. *International Journal of Eating Disorders*, **28**, 58–67.

Appendix I: Summary of specific drugs having evidence of effectiveness in mental disorders

Michele Sie and Sally Guthrie

Because the individual drugs are too many to deserve separate description in the text of the rest of the book we have listed all those that are considered to be effective and indicated the conditions for which they are licensed to treat (in UK and USA) and any special properties that distinguish them from others in the same group. This allows cross-referencing and easy identification of the uses of a particular treatment. To help the reader, these are given in alphabetical order. (Please note that all drugs have an *approved* name that is universal and a *proprietary* name that varies by company and country; our order is that of the approved name; '*NA*' indicates the drug is 'not available'.)

Appendix I. Psychiatric medications marketed in the United Kingdom and the United States

Drug	Proprietary names	Drug class	Form of drug (and licensed indication)	Adult daily dosage range (mg unless otherwise indicated)	Special features
Acamprosate	Campral EC® – UK and US	Modulates glutamate and GABA neurotransmission	Tablet (alcohol dependence)	1332–1998	Best given immediately after abstinence has been achieved
Acebutalol	Sectral® – UK and US	Beta-adrenoceptor blocking drugs	Tablet (hypertension, angina, arrhythmias)	100–200	See propranolol Off-label indication
Alprazolam	Xanax® – UK and US	Benzodiazepine	Tablet (anxiety short term)	1–3	First used extensively in panic disorder Off-label indication
Alprostadil	Caverject® – US Viridal Duo® – UK	Prostaglandin E₁	Injection (Intracavernosal)	1.25–40 (60) 2–3 micrograms times per week (depends on product)	Dose adjusted according to duration of erection If erection lasts more than 4 hours must seek medical advice
	MUSE® – UK	Urethral application (Erectile Dysfunction)	0.25–1 7 doses per week		
Amantadine	Symmetrel® – UK and US	Dopamine agonist	Capsule Syrup (Parkinson's disease NOT drug induced EPSE)	100–400	Off-label use for antipsychotic induced hyperprolactinaemia – risk of worsening psychosis
Amisulpride	generic Solian® – UK – US NA	Dopamine antagonist Atypical Antipsychotic	Tablet Syrup (Schizophrenia)	50–300 (negative symptoms) 400–1200 (positive symptoms)	Specific D2/D3 antagonist
Amitriptyline hydrochloride	generic Triptafen® – UK generic Elavil® – US	Serotonin and Noradrenaline reuptake inhibition Tricyclic Antidepressant	Tablet Solution (depression)	75–200	For moderate to severe depression Sedative Arrhythmias and heartblock dangerous in O/D Withdrawal effects reported
Apomorphine	Uprima® – UK Apokyn* – US	Centrally acting dopamine agonist	Sublingual Tablet (erectile dysfunction)	2–3 20 minutes before sexual activity 8 hours between doses	Limited absorption from sublingual site May increase sexual drive
Aripiprazole	Abilify® – UK and US	Dopamine partial agonist Atypical Antipsychotic	Tablet (schizophrenia)	Titrated by 5 mg per week to 15–30 Optimum dose 15	Dose titration to reduce nausea and vomiting, insomnia and restlessness
Barbiturates	Amytal® – Amobarbital – UK and US Sodium Amytal®–amobarbital sodium – UK and US Soneryl® – butobarbital – UK – US NA	Potentiate inhibition through the GABA receptors	Tablets (Severe intractable insomnia in those already taking barbiturates)	100–200	No longer recommended for use in insomnia due to level of tolerance, dependence and withdrawal. Should never be stopped suddenly
				60–200	
				100–200	
	Secanal Sodium® – Secobarbital sodium – UK – US NA			100	

Drug	Brand / Country	Class / Mechanism	Formulation (indication)	Dose range	Notes
Benperidol	Anquil® – UK – US *NA*	Dopamine antagonist Butyrophenone Typical Antipsychotic	Tablet (control of deviant antisocial sexual behaviour)	0.25–1.5	Evidence of effect value lacking High incidence EPSE
Benzatropine	Cogentin® – UK generic Cogentin® – US	Antimuscarinic	Injection (IM or IV)	1–2	Tablets no longer available in UK
Bromocriptine	generic Parlodel® – UK and US	Dopamine agonist	Tablet (Parkinson's disease NOT drug induced EPSE)	Titrated to 10–40	Off-label use for antipsychotic induced hyperprolactinaemia – risk of worsening psychosis
Buspirone	generic Buspar® – UK and US	Serotonin 5HT1A agonist	Tablet (Anxiolytic)	10–45	Short term use
Carbamazepine	generic Tegretol® – UK and US	anti-epileptic blockade of voltage-sensitive sodium channels reducing membrane excitability	Tablets; Syrup (prophylaxis of bipolar unresponsive to lithium, tonic clonic seizures, trigeminal neuralgia)	100–1600	Induces liver enzymes and may reduce levels of other medications Carbamazepine level may be useful and recommended level is higher than in epilepsy 7–12 mg/l
Chloral Hydrate	generic – UK and US	Hypnotic	Solution (Insomnia short term)	500–2000	Limited role dependence and tolerance
Chlordiazepoxide	generic – UK generic Librium® – US	Benzodiazepine	Capsule (anxiety short term, alcohol withdrawal)	30–100 40–200	Used mainly in alcohol withdrawal, seen as low abuse potential
Chlorpromazine	generic Largactil® – UK generic Thorazine® – US	Dopamine antagonist Phenothiazine Antipsychotic typical	Tablet; Solution; Injection	75–1000	Marked sedation Moderate antimuscarinic and EPSE Injection not recommended as causes pain and severe postural hypotension
Citalopram	generic Cipralex® – UK generic Celexa® – US	Selective serotonin reuptake inhibitor (SSRI) antidepressant	Tablet; Oral Drops (depression, panic disorder)	20–60 10–60	For moderate to severe depression 8 mg Oral drops = 10 mg tablet
Clomethiazole	Heminevrin® – UK – US *NA*	Hypnotic	Capsules; Syrup (in elderly only, severe insomnia short term use, restlessness and agitation)	1–2 caps 3 caps	Dependence and tolerance occur. Respiratory depression
Clomipramine	generic Anafranil® – UK and US	Serotonin and Noradrenaline reuptake inhibitor Tricyclic Antidepressant	Capsule (depression, phobia and obsessional states)	10–250 25–250	For moderate to severe depression Sedative Arrhythmias and heart block dangerous in O/D Withdrawal effects reported Off-label use for premature ejaculation
Clonazepam	Rivotril® – UK Klonopin® – US	Benzodiazepine	Tablet (epilepsy, myoclonus, status epilepticus)	0.5–8	Off-label use anti-epileptic – being used as an anxiolytic
Cloral Betaine	Welldorm® – UK – US *NA*	Hypnotic	Tablets; Elixir (Insomnia short term)	707–3535	Limited role dependence and tolerance

Appendix I. (cont.)

Drug	Proprietary names	Drug class	Form of drug (and licensed indication)	Adult daily dosage range (mg unless otherwise indicated)	Special features
Clozapine	Clozaril® Zaponex® Denzapine® – UK Clozaril® generic – US	Dopamine antagonist Antipsychotic Atypical	Tablet (schizophrenia in patients unresponsive or intolerant to conventional antipsychotics)	Slowly titrated to 200–450 mg Max 900 mg	Mandatory FBC monitoring for agranulocytosis. Patient and physician must be registered with monitoring service. High affinity for D4 receptor
Diazepam	generic Valium® – UK and US	Benzodiazepine	Tablet Syrup (short term use anxiety and insomnia)	5–30	Long-acting dependence and tolerance
Dosulepin	generic Prothiaden® – UK – US NA	Serotonin and Noradrenaline Reuptake inhibition Tricyclic Antidepressant	Capsule, tablet (Depression)	75–225	For moderate to severe depression Sedative Arrhythmias and heart block dangerous in O/D linked to high fatality Withdrawal effects reported
Fluoxetine	generic Prozac® – UK and US	Selective serotonin reuptake inhibitor (SSRI) Antidepressant	Capsule (major depression, Bulimia nervosa, OCD)	20–80 60–80 20–80	For moderate to severe depression Long half life
Flupenthixol	Depixol® – UK – US NA	Dopamine antagonist Thioxanthene Antipsychotic typical	Tablet	6–18	Less sedating than chlorpromazine
Flupenthixol	Fluanxol® – UK – US NA	Dopamine antagonist	Tablet (depression)	1–3	Mode of action in depression unclear
Flupenthixol Decanoate	Depixol® – UK – US NA	Dopamine antagonist Thioxanthene Antipsychotic typical	Depot injection	12.5–400/week Maintenance dose every 2–4 weeks	IM Test dose (20 mg) required
Fluphenazine	Moditen® – UK generic Prolixin® – US	Dopamine antagonist Phenothiazine Antipsychotic typical	Tablet (schizophrenia and other psychosis, mania, management of severe anxiety, agitation, excitement, violent or dangerous impulsive behaviour)	4–20 2–4	Marked EPSE Mild Sedation and antimuscarinic
Fluphenazine Decanoate	generic Modecate® – UK Prolixin Dec® – US	Dopamine antagonist Antipsychotic typical	Depot injection (maintenance in schizophrenia and other psychoses)	12.5–50/week Maintenance dose every 2–5 weeks	IM Test dose required

Drug	Brand names	Class	Form (indication)	Dose	Notes
Fluvoxamine	generic Faverin® – UK Luvox® – US	Selective serotonin reuptake inhibitor (SSRI) Antidepressants	Tablet (Depression, OCD)	50–300	Due to liver enzyme inhibition interacts with numerous medication
Haloperidol	generic Serenace® – UK generic Haldol® – US	Dopamine antagonist Butyrophenone Antipsychotic typical	Tablet / Liquid / Injection (IM or IV) (schizophrenia and other psychosis, mania, management of severe anxiety, agitation, excitement, violent or dangerous impulsive behaviour)	50–300 / 3–30 / 2–18	Marked EPSE Mild Sedation and antimuscarinic / Administer antimuscarinic with injection / Close physical observations with IM administration BP, pulse, temp, hydration, level of consciousness every 5–10 minutes for 1 hour then every 30 mins until active
Haloperidol Decanoate	Haldol® – UK Haldol Dec® – US	Dopamine antagonist Antipsychotic Typical	Depot injection (maintenance in schizophrenia and other psychoses)	12.5–75/week Maintenance dose every 4 weeks	IM Test Dose required
Hyoscine Hydrobromide	Kwells® – UK – US *NA*	Antimuscarinic	Tablet (motion sickness)	0.3–0.9	Off-label indication used for clozapine induced hypersalivation should be sucked for effect
Imipramine	generic – UK generic Tofranil® – US	Serotonin and Noradrenaline reuptake inhibition Tricyclic Antidepressant	Tablet (depression)	75–300	For moderate to severe depression Less sedative Antimuscarinic effects Arrhythmias and heart block dangerous in O/D
Isocarboxazid	generic – UK – US *NA*	Monoamine-oxidase inhibitors (MAOI) Antidepressant	Tablet (depression)	Initially 30–60 Maintenance 10–40	Withdrawal effects reported Useful in refractory and atypical depression as well as phobic states. Tyramine containing foods must be avoided as well as some sympathomimetic medications
Lithium Carbonate	Pradel® Camcolit® Liskonium® – UK generic Lithobid® Eskalith® – US	Anti-manic	Tablet (treatment and prophylaxis of mania, bipolar disorder, and recurrent depression; aggressive or self mutilating behaviour)	According to trough blood level (0.5–1.0 mmol/l) taken after at least 4 days on same dose Slow release once daily, immediate release twice daily	Prescribe by brand as differences in bioavailability and release profile Should not be stopped suddenly
Lithium Citrate	Li Liquid® Priadel® – UK generic – US	Anti-manic	Syrup (treatment and prophylaxis of mania, bipolar disorder, and recurrent depression; aggressive or self mutilating behaviour)	According to trough blood level (0.5–1.0 mmol/l) taken after at least 4 days on same dose twice daily dosing	Prescribe by brand as slight differences in concentration 5 ml (520 mg or 509 mg depending on brand) Lithium Citrate syrup = 200 mg Lithium Carbonate Should not be stopped suddenly

Appendix I. (cont.)

Drug	Proprietary names	Drug class	Form of drug (and licensed indication)	Adult daily dosage range (mg unless otherwise indicated)	Special features
Lofepramine	generic Gamanil® – UK – US *NA*	Serotonin and Noradrenaline reuptake inhibition Tricyclic Antidepressant	Tablet (depression)	140–210	For moderate to severe depression Less sedative Appears less dangerous in overdose Withdrawal effects reported
Lorazepam	generic Ativan® – UK and US	Benzodiazepine	Tablet Injection (IM/IV) (short term use in anxiety or insomnia)	1–4 25–30 micrograms/kg	Short Acting Dependence and Tolerance
Lormetazepam	generic – UK – US *NA*	Benzodiazepine	Tablet (Insomnia short term)	0.5–1.5	Shorter acting, little or no hangover, Dependence and Tolerance
Mirtazapine	generic Zispin® – UK generic Remeron® – US	NASSA Noradrenergic and Serotonergic Specific Antidepressant	Tablet (major depression)	15–30	Sedative Weight gain
Moclobemide	generic Manerix® – UK – US *NA*	Reversible MAOI Antidepressant	Tablet (depression; social phobia)	300–600	Prolonged action, cumulative
Nitrazepam	generic Mogadon® – UK – US *NA*	Benzodiazepine	Tablets Syrup (Insomnia short term)	5–10	
Nortriptyline	Allegron® – UK generic Pamelor® – US	Serotonin and Noradrenaline reuptake inhibition Tricyclic Antidepressant	Tablet (depression)	75–150	For moderate to severe depression Less sedative Antimuscarinic effects Arrhythmias and heart block dangerous in O/D Withdrawal effects reported
Olanzapine	Zyprexa® – UK & US	Dopamine antagonist Antipsychotic Atypical	Tablet Velotab® Injection IM (schizophrenia, mania, preventing recurrence in bipolar)	10–20	May cause weight gain which could be associated with increased risk of diabetes and dyslipidaemias
Orphenadrine	generic Disipal® – UK – US *NA*	Antimuscarinic	Tablet Solution (drug induced EPSE but not TD)	150–400	May cause insomnia – no later than 6 pm Possibility of abuse
Oxazepam	generic – UK generic Serax® – US	Benzodiazepine	Tablet (anxiety short term)	15–120	Shorter acting, withdrawal syndrome dependence and tolerance
Oxprenolol	generic – UK – US *NA*	Beta-adrenoceptor blocking drugs	Tablet (anxiety symptoms short term)	40–80	See propranolol
Papaverine	UK *NA* Para-Time SR* US	Non-specific phosphodiesterase inhibitor Smooth muscle relaxant	Injection (Intracavernosal) Not licensed in UK	30–60	maximum once a day, two days in a row or three times a week

Drug	Brand	Class	Formulation (indication)	Dose (mg)	Comments
Paroxetine	generic Seroxat® – UK generic Paxil® – US	Selective serotonin reuptake inhibitor (SSRI) antidepressant	Tablet Liquid (major depression, OCD, panic disorder, social phobia, PTSD, GAD)	20–50 or 60 dependant on indication	Recommended dose for depression, social anxiety disorder, GAD and PTSD is 20 mg/d. For OCD and Panic Disorder is 40 mg/d. There is no evidence to support benefits with the use of higher doses. Short half life, can cause withdrawal effects if missed doses. Off-label use for premature ejaculation
Pericyazine	Neulactil® – UK – US *NA*	Dopamine antagonist Phenothiazine Antipsychotic typical	Tablet (schizophrenia)	25–1000	Moderate Sedation Marked antimuscarinic Mild EPSE CATIE 2
Perphenazine	Fentazin® – UK generic Trilafon® – US	Dopamine antagonist Phenothiazine Antipsychotic typical	Tablet (schizophrenia and other psychosis, mania, management of severe anxiety, agitation, excitement, violent or dangerous impulsive behaviour)	12–24	Marked EPSE Mild Sedation and antimuscarinic
Phenelzine	Nardil® – UK and US	Monoamine-oxidase inhibitors (MAOI) Antidepressant	Tablet (depression)	Initially 45–90 Maintenance – lowest possible dose 15 mg on alternate days may be sufficient	Useful in refractory and atypical depression as well as phobic states. Tyramine containing foods must be avoided as well as some sympathomimetic medications
Phentolamine	Rogitine® – US	Alpha adrenoceptor blocking drugs	Injection (hypertensive episodes due to phaeochromocytoma)	0.5–1 Intracavernosaly maximum once a day, two days in a row or three times a week	Off-label indication added to papaverine if inadequate response
Pimozide	Orap® – UK and US	Dopamine antagonist diphenylbutylpiperidone Antipsychotic typical	Tablet (schizophrenia, paranoid psychosis)	2–20	ECG prior to initiation and annually. Not to be given with other antipsychotics, medications that are known to prolong QT interval or cause electrolyte imbalance
Pipotiazine Palmitate	Piportil® – UK – US *NA*	Dopamine antagonist Phenothiazine Antipsychotic typical	Depot injection	12.5–50/week Maintenance dose every 4 weeks	IM Test Dose required
Pirenzapine	– UK *NA* – US *NA*	Selective M1/M4 muscarinic antagonist	Tablets Not licensed in UK	50–150	Off label indication used for clozapine induced hypersalivation M-4 receptors are prominent in salivary glands should be sucked for effect

Appendix I. (cont.)

Drug	Proprietary names	Drug class	Form of drug (and licensed indication)	Adult daily dosage range (mg unless otherwise indicated)	Special features
Procyclidine	generic Kemadrin® Arpicolin® – UK Kemadrin® – US	Antimuscarinic	Tablet Syrup Injection (drug induced EPSE but not TD)	7.5–30	May cause insomnia – no later than 6 pm Possibility of abuse
Promethazine	Phenergan® – UK and US	Antihistamine	Tablet (night sedation and insomnia short term)	25–50	May be of use if benzodiazepine tolerant.
Propranolol	generic – UK generic Inderal® – US	Beta adrenoceptor blocking drugs	Tablet Solution (anxiety with palpitations, sweating, tremor)	40–120	Reduce autonomic symptoms, e.g. palpitations, tremor but not muscle tension or psychological symptoms. Avoid in Asthma
Quetiapine	Seroquel® – UK and US	Dopamine antagonist Antipsychotic atypical	Tablet (schizophrenia; mania)	50–750 100–800	Recommended treatment dose at least 600 mg/d
Reboxetine	Edronax® – UK – US *NA*	Selective noradrenaline reuptake inhibitor (NARI) Antidepressant	Tablet (depression)	8–12	May have a role in increasing energy
Risperidone	Risperdal® – UK and US	Dopamine antagonist Antipsychotic atypical	Tablet Liquid Orodispersible (acute and chronic psychoses, mania)	2–16 normal dose range 4–6	Doses above 6 mg/day increase the risk of EPSE doses above 10 mg/day should only be used if benefit outweigh risks Hyperprolactinaemia
Risperidone	Risperdal Consta® – UK & US	Dopamine antagonist Antipsychotic atypical	Long Acting Injection (schizophrenia and other psychoses in patients tolerant to oral risperidone)	Following trial of oral risperidone to test tolerability and response 25–50 every two weeks, dose adjusted at least every 4 weeks	Oral Cover must be maintained for at least 4–6 weeks to allow for release of risperidone and steady state plasma levels to be achieved. The oral should then be slowly tapered off
Sertraline	generic Lustral® – UK Zoloft® – US	Selective serotonin reuptake inhibitor (SSRI) antidepressant	Tablet Liquid (depression, OCD, PTSD in women)	50–200 50–200 25–200	For moderate to severe depression Off label use for premature ejaculation
Sildefanil	Viagra® – US	Phosphodiest-erase-5 inhibitors	Tablet (erectile dysfunction)	25–100 mg one hour before sexual activity	Effective in 50% of cases, contraindicated with nitrates
Sodium Valproate	generic Epilim® – UK generic Depakene® – US	anti-epileptic? enhances GABA activity	Tablets Syrup (all forms of epilepsy)	600–2500	Off label use as a mood stabilizer or treatment of Clozapine induced seizures. Trough plasma level after at least 5 days at steady dose may be of benefit Range 50–125 mg/l

Drug	Brand/generic	Class/action	Formulation (indication)	Dose	Comments
Sulpiride	generic Dolmatil® – UK – US *NA*	Dopamine antagonist Substituted benzamide Antipsychotic typical	Tablets Solution (schizophrenia)	400–2400 (Max 800 in negative symptoms)	Although classed as typical has effect on negative symptoms at low doses and less EPSE's than other typicals Hyperprolactinaemia occurs
Tadalafil	Cialis® – US	Phosphodiesterase-5 inhibitors	Tablet (erectile dysfunction)	10–20 mg 30 minutes before sexual activity	Effective for up to 36 hours after dosing, contraindicated with nitrates
Temazepam	generic – UK generic Restoril® – US	Benzodiazepine	Tablets Solution (Insomnia short term)	10–40	Shorter acting, little or no hangover, withdrawal syndrome
Tibolone	Liv-al® – US	Synthetic steroid with oestrogenic, progestogenic and androgenic activity	Tablets (short term symptoms of oestrogen deficiency)	2.5	May enhance sexual function in post-menopausal women
Tranylcypromine	generic – UK Parnate® – US	Monoamine-oxidase inhibitors (MAOI) Antidepressant	Tablet (depression)	Initially 10bd increased after 1 week to 10 om 20 at lunch second dose must be given before 3 pm Maintenance – usually 10 od	Useful in refractory and atypical depression as well as phobic states. Tyramine containing foods must be avoided as well as some sympathomimetic medications Considered most hazardous of MAOI's due to stimulant action
Trazadone	generic Molipaxin® – UK generic Desyrel® – US	Serotonin reuptake inhibitor and serotonin 2 antagonist Antidepressant	Capsules Tablets Liquid (depression, anxiety)	150–600 75–300	Sedative effects Reduced anxiety, no sexual dysfunction dangerous in O/D
Trifluoperazine	generic Stelazine® – UK and US	Dopamine antagonist Phenothiazine Antipsychotic typical	Tablet (schizophrenia and other psychosis, agitation, excitement, violent or dangerous impulsive behaviour, Management of severe anxiety)	10 – (No max stated in BNF) but 50 is suggested 2–6	Marked EPSE Mild Sedation and antimuscarinic Release profile of tablets similar to slow release capsules
Trihexyphenidyl	generic Broflex® – UK generic Artane® – US	Antimuscarinic	Tablet Syrup (drug induced EPSE but not TD)	1–20	May cause insomnia – no later than 6 pm Possibility of abuse
Trimipramine	Surmontil® – UK and US	Serotonin and Noradrenaline reuptake inhibition Tricyclic Antidepressant	Capsule Tablet (Depression)	50–300	For moderate to severe depression Sedative Arrhythmias and heart block dangerous in O/D Withdrawal effects reported

Appendix I. (cont.)

Drug	Proprietary names	Drug class	Form of drug (and licensed indication)	Adult daily dosage range (mg unless otherwise indicated)	Special features
Valproic Acid (semisodium valproate)	Depakote® – UK and US	Antimanic ? enhances GABA activity	Tablet (Mania associated with BAD)	750–2000 patients receiving doses above 45 mg/kg/day should be closely monitored	May have a better bioavailability than sodium valproate. Trough levels after at least 7 days on same dose that are in the range of 80 mg/l–120 mg/l have been associated with more rapid resolution of symptoms
Vardenafil	Levitra® – US	Phosphodiesterase-5 inhibitors	Tablet (erectile dysfunction)	10–20 mg 25–60 minutes before sexual activity	Contraindicated with nitrates
Venlafaxine	Efexor® – UK and US	Serotonin and Noradrenaline reuptake inhibition (SNRI) Antidepressant	Tablet Capsule XL (depression, GAD)	75–375 75–225 75	Causes insomnia Nausea and vomiting associated with dose titration Contraindicated in uncontrolled hypertension, and in patients with a very high risk of a serious cardiac ventricular arrhythmia Withdrawal effects reported
Zolpidem	Stilnoct® – UK Ambien® – US	Hypnotic	Tablets (Insomnia short term up to 4 weeks)	10	Short-acting tolerance and dependence have been reported
Zopiclone	Zimovane® – UK – US *NA*	Hypnotic	Tablets (Insomnia short term up to 4 weeks)	7.5	Short-acting tolerance and dependence have been reported
Zuclopenthixol Acetate (acuphase)	Clopixol Acuphase® – UK – US *NA*	Dopamine antagonist Thioxanthene Antipsychotic typical	Injection IM (short term management of acute psychosis, mania, or exacerbation of chronic psychosis)	50–150 repeated IF NECESSARY after 2–3 days Max duration of treatment 2 weeks Max number of injections = 4 Max cumulative dose = 400 mg	Onset of action 2–8 hours. Close physical observations see Haloperidol IM
Zuclopenthixol Decanoate	Clopixol® – UK – US *NA*	Dopamine antagonist Thioxanthene Antipsychotic typical	Depot injection	100–600/week Maintenance dose every 1–4 weeks	IM test dose (100 mg) required
Zuclopenthixol Dihydrochloride	Clopixol® – UK – US *NA*	Dopamine antagonist Thioxanthene Antipsychotic typical	Tablet (schizophrenia and other psychosis)	30–150	

FURTHER READING

BNF 51 March 2006. *British Medical Association*, ed. D. Mehta, London: Pharmaceutical Press.

Stahl, S.M. (1999). *Psychopharmacology of Antidepressants*. London: Martin Dunitz.

Hirschfeld, R.M.A., Baker, J.D., Wozniak, P., Tracy, K. & Sommerville, K.W. (2003). The safety and early efficacy of oral-loaded Divalproex versus standard-titration divalproex, lithium, olanzapine, and placebo in the treatment of acute mania associated with bipolar disorder. *Journal of Clinical Psychiatry*, **64** (7), 841–6.

Taylor, D.M., Paton, C. & Kerwin, R. (2005–6). *The Maudsley 2005–2006 Prescribing Guidelines 8th edn*. London: Taylor and Francis.

Appendix II: Key to effectiveness tables

Ia   Evidence from meta-analysis of randomized controlled trials
Ib   Evidence from at least one randomized controlled trial
IIa Evidence from at least one controlled study without randomization
IIb Evidence from at least one other type of quasi-experimental study
III Evidence from non-experimental descriptive studies, such as comparative studies, correlation studies and case-control studies
IV   Evidence from expert committee reports or opinion and/or clinical experience of respected authorities

US Agency for Health Care Policy and Research Classification (AHCPR) (US Department of Health and Human Services, Public Health Service, Agency for Health Care Policy and Research. Acute pain management: operative or medical procedures and trauma. Rockville, MD: Agency for Health Care Policy and Research Publications 1992).

Index